Primary Cardiology

SECOND EDITION

Eugene Braunwald, MD, MD(hon), ScD(hon)

Chief Academic Officer
Partners HealthCare System
Hersey Distinguished Professor of Medicine
Faculty Dean for Academic Programs at Brigham and Women's Hospital
and Massachusetts General Hospital
Harvard Medical School
Boston, Massachusetts

Lee Goldman, MD, MPH

Julius R. Krevans Distinguished Professor and Chair
Department of Medicine
Associate Dean for Clinical Affairs
School of Medicine
University of California, San Francisco
San Francisco, California

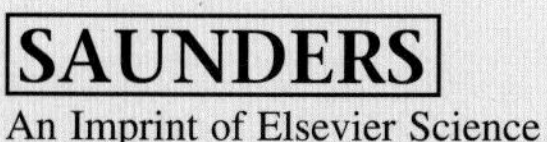

An Imprint of Elsevier Science

SAUNDERS
An Imprint of Elsevier Science

The Curtis Center
Independence Square West
Philadelphia, Pennsylvania 19106

PRIMARY CARDIOLOGY ISBN 0–7216–9444–6

Notice

Medicine is an ever-changing field. Standard safety precautions must be followed, but as new research and clinical experience broaden our knowledge, changes in treatment and drug therapy may become necessary or appropriate. Readers are advised to check the most current product information provided by the manufacturer of each drug to be administered to verify the recommended dose, the method and duration of administration, and the contraindications. It is the responsibility of the treating physician, relying on experience and knowledge of the patient, to determine dosages and the best treatment for each individual patient. Neither the Publisher nor the author assumes any liability for any injury and/or damage to persons or property arising from this publication.

The Publisher

First Edition 1998. Second Edition 2003.

Library of Congress Cataloging-in-Publication Data
Primary cardiology / [edited by] Eugene Braunwald, Lee Goldman.–2nd ed.
p. ; cm.
Rev. ed. of: Primary cardiology / [edited by] Lee Goldman, Eugene Braunwald. ©1998.
Includes bibliographical references and index.
ISBN 0–7216–9444–6
1. Heart–Diseases. 2. Cardiology. I. Braunwald, Eugene. II. Goldman, Lee. III. Primary cardiology.
[DNLM: 1. Cardiovascular Diseases–diagnosis. 2. Cardiovascular Diseases–therapy. 3. Primary Health Care–methods. WG 120 P952 2003]
RC681 .P72 2003
616.1′2–dc21 2002030219

Acquisitions Editor: Thomas Moore
Developmental Editor: Lynne Gery
Project Manager: Jennifer Ehlers
Book Designer: Steven Stave
Indexer: Angela Holt

BS/PAR

Printed in China.

Last digit is the print number: 9 8 7 6 5 4 3 2 1

Dedicated to
Elaine, Karen, Allison, Jill, Dana, Alex, Mara, Elise, Cari,
Benjamin, and Rachel
and to
Jill, Jeff, Daniel, and Robyn

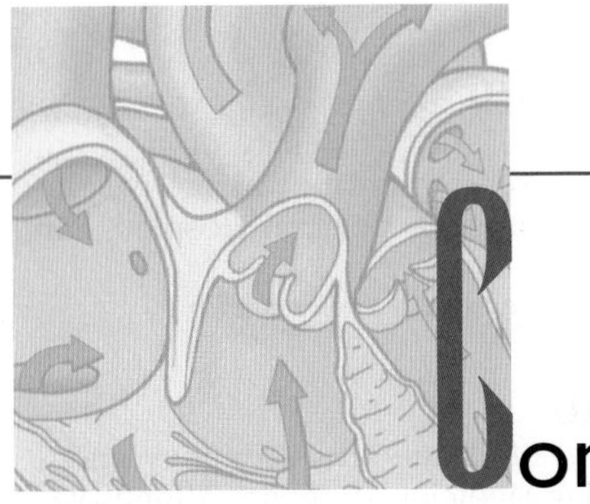

Contributors

Joshua S. Adler, MD
Assistant Clinical Professor of Medicine, and Director of Ambulatory Services, Department of Medicine, University of California–San Francisco; San Francisco, California
Approach to the Patient Undergoing Noncardiac Surgery

Karen P. Alexander, MD
Assistant Professor of Medicine, Division of Cardiology, Duke University Medical Center, Durham, North Carolina
Approach to the Elderly Patient with Heart Disease

Robert A. Barish, MBA, MD
Professor of Surgery and Medicine and Associate Dean for Clinical Affairs, University of Maryland School of Medicine, Baltimore, Maryland
Approach to Cardiovascular Emergencies

Neal L. Benowitz, MD
Professor of Medicine, Psychiatry, and Biopharmaceutical Sciences, University of California–San Francisco, San Francisco, California
Smoking and Smoking Cessation

Henry R. Black, MD
Charles J. and Margaret Roberts Professor of Preventive Medicine and Professor of Internal Medicine and Pharmacology, RUSH Medical College of RUSH University; Associate Vice President for Research, RUSH-Presbyterian-St. Luke's Medical Center, Chicago, Illinois
Diagnosis and Management of Patients with Hypertension

Eugene Braunwald, MD, MD(hon), ScD(hon)
Chief Academic Officer, Partners HealthCare System; Hersey Distinguished Professor of Medicine and Faculty Dean for Academic Programs, Brigham and Women's Hospital and Massachusetts General Hospital, Harvard Medical School, Boston, Massachusetts
The Clinical Examination; Recognition and Management of Patients with Unstable Angina and Non–ST Elevation Myocardial Infarction; Recognition and Management of Patients with Acute Myocardial Infarction

Blase A. Carabello, MD
The WA "Tex" and Deborah Moncrief, Jr. Professor of Medicine and Vice Chairman, Department of Medicine, Baylor College of Medicine; Medical Care Line Executive, Houston Veterans Affairs Medical Center, Houston, Texas
Recognition and Management of Patients with Valvular Heart Disease

Pamela Charney, MD
Clinical Professor of Medicine, Albert Einstein College of Medicine, Bronx, New York; Program Director, Internal Medicine Residency, Norwalk Hospital, Norwalk, Connecticut
Approach to the Woman with Heart Disease, Including During Pregnancy

Kanu Chatterjee, MB
Professor of Medicine and Lucie Stern Professor of Cardiology and Director, Gallo-Chatterjee Center for Cardiac Research, Division of Cardiology, Department of Medicine, University of California–San Francisco, San Francisco, California
Recognition and Management of Patients with Stable Angina Pectoris

Melvin D. Cheitlin, MD
Professor of Medicine Emeritus and Former Chief of Cardiology, San Francisco General Hospital, University of California–San Francisco, San Francisco, California
Recognition and Management of Adults with Congenital Heart Disease

Glenn M. Chertow, MD, MPH
Associate Professor of Medicine, and Director of Clinical Services, Division of Nephrology, University of California–San Francisco Medical Center, San Francisco, California
Approach to the Patient with Edema

G. William Dec, MD
Associate Professor of Medicine, Harvard Medical School; Director of Clinical Cardiology, Masachusetts General Hospital, Boston, Massachusetts
Recognition and Management of Patients with Cardiomyopathies

William J. Elliott, MD, PhD
Professor of Preventive Medicine, Internal Medicine, and Pharmacology, RUSH Medical College of RUSH University; Attending Physician, RUSH-Presbyterian-St. Luke's Medical Center, Chicago, Illinois
Diagnosis and Management of Patients with Hypertension

David Feller-Kopman, MD
Instructor in Medicine, Harvard Medical School; Physician, Beth Israel Deaconess Medical Center, Boston, Massachusetts
Approach to the Patient with Dyspnea

Elyse Foster, MD
Professor of Clinical Medicine and Anesthesia and Director of the Adult Echocardiography Laboratory and Adult Congenital Heart Disease Service, University of California–San Francisco, San Francisco, California
Recognition and Management of Adults with Congenital Heart Disease

Leonard I. Ganz, MD
Associate Professor of Medicine, University of Pittsburgh School of Medicine; Director of Cardiac Electrophysiology, Cardiovascular Institute, University of Pittsburgh Medical Center, Pittsburgh, Pennsylvania
Approach to the Patient with Asymptomatic Electrocardiographic Abnormalities

J. Michael Gaziano, MD, MPH
Associate Professor of Medicine, Harvard Medical School; Physician, Brigham and Women's Hospital and VA Boston Healthcare System, Boston, Massachusetts
Screening for Coronary Heart Disease and Its Risk Factors

C. Michael Gibson, MD
Associate Professor of Medicine, Harvard Medical School; Associate Chief of Cardiology, Beth Israel–Deaconess Medical Center, Boston, Massachusetts
Recognition and Management of Patients with Stable Angina Pectoris

Samuel Z. Goldhaber, MD
Associate Professor of Medicine, Harvard Medical School; Director of Venous Thromboembolism Research Group and Anticoagulation Service, Brigham and Women's Hospital, Boston, Massachusetts
Pulmonary Embolism, Deep Venous Thrombosis, and Cor Pulmonale

Lee Goldman, MD, MPH
Julius R. Krevans Distinguished Professor and Chair, Department of Medicine, and Associate Dean for Clinical Affairs, School of Medicine; University of California–San Francisco, San Francisco, California
Evidence-Based Medicine; Clinical Decision Making; Approach to the Patient with Chest Pain; Approach to the Patient Undergoing Noncardiac Surgery; Recognition and Management of Patients with Stable Angina Pectoris

Nora Goldschlager, MD
Professor of Clinical Medicine, University of California–San Francisco; Associate Chief, Division of Cardiology, San Francisco General Hospital, San Francisco, California
Recognition and Management of Patients with Bradyarrhythmias

Alan T. Hirsch, MD
Associate Professor of Medicine and Radiology and Director of Vascular Medicine Program, Minnesota Vascular Diseases Center, University of Minnesota Medical School, Minneapolis, Minnesota
Recognition and Management of Peripheral Arterial Disease

Mark A. Hlatky, MD
Professor of Health Research and Policy and of Medicine; Chair of Department of Health Research and Policy, Stanford University School of Medicine, Stanford, California
Approach to the Patient with Palpitations

Frank B. Hu, MD, PhD
Associate Professor, Department of Nutrition and Epidemiology, Harvard School of Public Health, Boston, Massachusetts
Other Risk Factors for Coronary Heart Disease: Diet, Lifestyle, Psychological Disorders, and Estrogen Deficiency/Hormone Replacement Therapy

Wishwa N. Kapoor, MD, MPH
Professor of Medicine, University of Pittsburgh School of Medicine; Chief, Division of General Internal Medicine, University of Pittsburgh Medical Center, Pittsburgh, Pennsylvania
Approach to the Patient with Syncope

Adolf W. Karchmer, MD
Professor of Medicine, Harvard Medical School; Chief, Division of Infectious Diseases, Beth Israel Deaconess Medical Center, Boston, Massachusetts
Recognition and Management of Patients with Infective Endocarditis

Vineet Kaushik, MD*
Cardiac Electrophysiology Fellow, Division of Cardiology, University of California–San Francisco, San Francisco, California
Recognition and Management of Patients with Tachyarrhythmias

Kenneth R. Kidd, MD
Consultant, Whitewater Family Practice, Whitewater, Wisconsin
Recognition and Management of Patients with Pericardial Disease

Robert H. Knopp, MD
Professor of Medicine, University of Washington School of Medicine; Chief, Section of Metabolism, Endocrinology, and Nutrition, Harborview Medical Center, Seattle, Washington
Dietary Fat and Lipid Disorders

*Deceased

Thomas H. Lee, MD
Associate Professor of Medicine, Harvard Medical School; Chief Medical Officer, Partners Community Healthcare, Boston, Massachusetts
Cardiac Noninvasive Testing

JoAnn E. Manson, MD, DrPH
Professor of Medicine, Harvard Medical School; Chief of Division of Preventive Medicine, Brigham and Women's Hospital, Boston, Massachusetts
Other Risk Factors for Coronary Heart Disease: Diet, Lifestyle, Psychological Disorders, and Estrogen Deficiency/Hormone Replacement Therapy

Jacob M. Mishell, MD
Fellow in Cardiology, University of California–San Francisco, San Francisco, California
Recognition and Management of Patients with Bradyarrhythmias

Jerome F.X. Naradzay, MD
Adjunct Clinical Assistant Professor of Emergency Medicine, New York College of Osteopathic Medicine, Old Westbury, New York
Approach to Cardiovascular Emergencies

Rick A. Nishimura, MD
Professor of Medicine, Mayo Clinic and Mayo Foundation; Consultant in Cardiovascular Diseases, Mayo Foundation, Rochester, New York
Recognition and Management of Patients with Pericardial Disease

Peter J. Norton, MD
Instructor in Cardiology, University of Southern California School of Medicine, Los Angeles, California
Approach to the Patient with a Heart Murmur

Patrick T. O'Gara, MD
Associate Professor of Medicine, Harvard Medical School; Director of Clinical Cardiology and Vice Chair of Medicine, Brigham and Women's Hospital, Boston, Massachusetts
Approach to the Patient with Cardiac Enlargement; Recognition and Management of Patients with Diseases of the Aorta: Aneurysms and Dissection

Robert A. O'Rourke, MD
Professor of Medicine, Division of Cardiology, University of Texas Health Science Center, San Antonio, Texas
Approach to the Patient with a Heart Murmur

Steven Z. Pantilat, MD
Assistant Clinical Professor of Medicine, University of California–San Francisco; Director of Comfort Care Suites, Moffitt-Long Hospital, University of California–San Francisco Medical Center, San Francisco, California
Approach to End-of-Life Care for the Patient with End-Stage Heart Disease

Eric D. Peterson, MD, MPH
Associate Professor of Medicine, Division of Cardiology, Duke University School of Medicine; Director of Cardiovascular Outcomes Research, Duke Clinical Research Insitute, Durham, North Carolina
Approach to the Elderly Patient with Heart Disease

Melvin M. Scheinman, MD
Professor of Medicine, University of California–San Francisco; Chief, Cardiac Electrophysiology Section, Moffit-Long Hospital, University of California San Francisco Medical Center, San Francisco, California
Recognition and Management of Patients with Tachyarrhythmias

Richard M. Schwartzstein, MD
Associate Professor of Medicine, Harvard Medical School; Clinical Director, Division of Pulmonary and Critical Care Medicine, Beth Israel Deaconess Medical Center, Boston, Massachusetts
Approach to the Patient with Dyspnea

Scott D. Solomon, MD
Assistant Professor of Medicine, Harvard Medical School; Director of Noninvasive Cardiology, Brigham and Women's Hospital, Boston, Massachusetts
Principles of Echocardiography

Lynne Warner Stevenson, MD
Associate Professor of Medicine, Harvard Medical School; Codirector of Cardiomyopathy/Heart Failure, Brigham and Women's Hospital, Boston, Massachusetts
Recognition and Management of Patients with Heart Failure

Paul D. Thompson, MD
Professor of Medicine, University of Connecticut, Farmington, Connecticut; Director of Preventive Cardiology and Cardiovascular Research, Hartford Hospital, Hartford, Connecticut
Exercise and Heart Disease

Sandra Wainwright, MD
Senior Resident, Internal Medicine, Norwalk Hospital, Norwalk, Connecticut
Approach to the Woman with Heart Disease, Including During Pregnancy

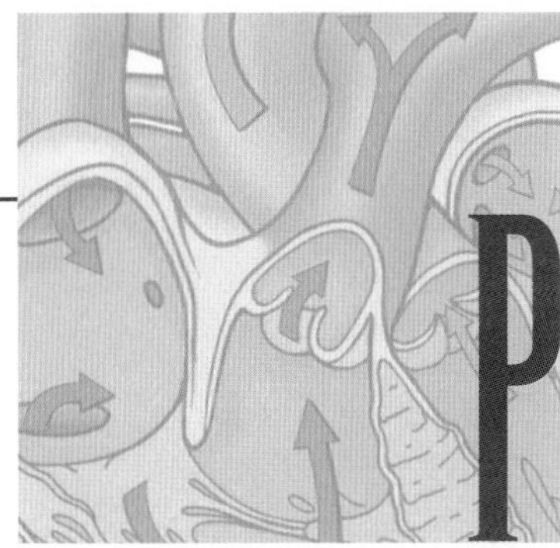

Preface

Despite a more than 50% reduction in the age-adjusted coronary heart disease death rates since the early 1960s, heart disease remains the leading cause of death in the United States. Cardiovascular symptoms, signs, and diseases continue to be a major determinant of office visits and hospital admissions. In the current era of managed care, the primary care physician is assuming increasing responsibility for the care of the patient with known or suspected cardiovascular disease, as well as for the prevention of such disease.

Although numerous texts address issues related to heart disease, *Primary Cardiology* has been conceived and designed to fill what we believe to be a critical gap: it is intended to be an authoritative, yet user-friendly, text for primary care physicians, internists, and family physicians—and other physicians who have not specialized in cardiovascular diseases. We believe that primary care physicians need and deserve a text that is more sophisticated than a manual, yet more succinct and focused than an encyclopedic text written for the cardiovascular specialist. *Primary Cardiology* is designed to provide more clinically applicable information than is available in standard medical textbooks and to go beyond the texts in primary care and ambulatory care, which usually focus on conditions seen in outpatients.

Primary Cardiology is divided into four parts. Part I (Chapters 1 through 5) covers fundamental principles that underlie evidence-based medicine and the translation of advances in science to the practice of medicine. Part 2 (Chapters 6 through 17) emphasizes rational approaches to common presenting cardiovascular symptoms, signs, and situations frequently faced by the primary care physician. Part 3 (Chapters 18 through 23) describes key approaches to screening for asymptomatic coronary disease and its prevention. Part 4 (Chapters 24 through 38) focuses on the evaluation and management of a variety of cardiovascular disorders that the primary care physician encounters commonly.

This second edition has been thoroughly revised and includes new chapters on the approach to the patient with ECG abnormalities; echocardiography; screening for coronary artery disease; dietary fats; exercise; hormone replacement therapy; smoking cessation; and peripheral arterial diseases.

It is our hope that *Primary Cardiology*, written by nationally recognized experts, will capture the essence of the ideal consultative interaction, which quickly summarizes the most important evidence-based literature and provides a targeted approach to solving the problem at hand. The algorithms, flow diagrams, and guidelines in this book are the natural extension of the background and evidence on which they are based.

We are grateful to our authors who worked so well with us in creating a new and different type of textbook. In our offices, Kathryn Saxon (Boston) and Vida Lynum (San Francisco) were critical to the preparation of this book. At W.B. Saunders, we are grateful to our publisher and to Thomas Moore (editor), Lynne Gery (senior developmental editor), Jennifer Ehlers (project manager), and Frank Polizzano (publishing services manager).

We hope that the readers, especially primary care physicians and internists who now render most cardiac care, as well as trainees who aspire to these important responsibilities, will find that *Primary Cardiology* fills an important niche, helps them to be better informed, and, most importantly, aids them in the care of their patients on a daily basis.

Eugene Braunwald, MD   Lee Goldman, MD

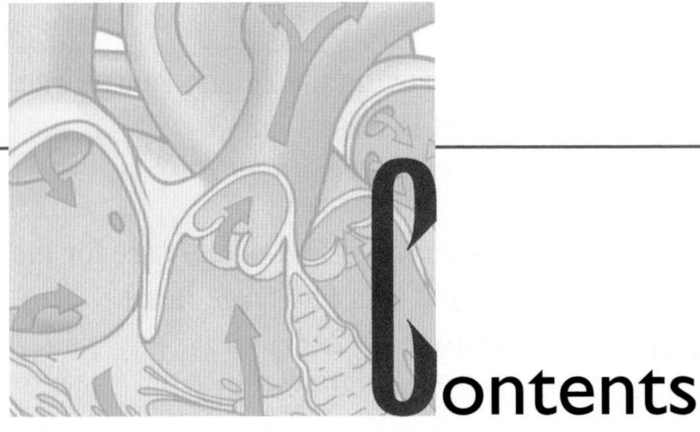

Contents

PART 1

Cardiologic Principles for the Primary Care Physician 1

PART 2

Approach to Common Cardiac Problems 81

PART 1

Cardiologic Principles for the Primary Care Physician

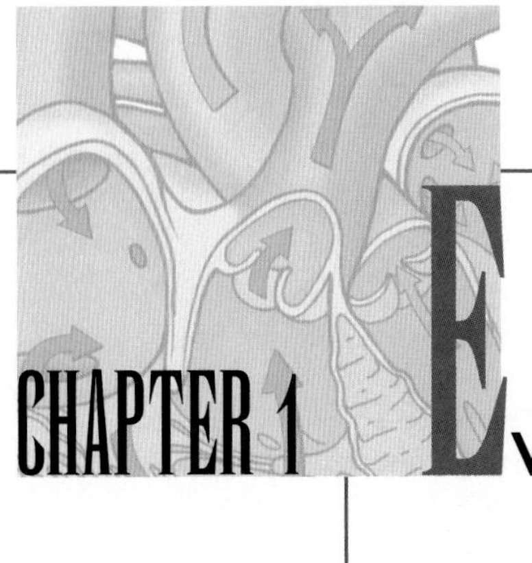

CHAPTER 1 Evidence-Based Medicine

Lee Goldman

Decisions in cardiology and, for that matter, all of medicine are increasingly being driven by objective evidence from well-designed randomized trials rather than by uncontrolled observations or the experiential teachings of senior professors.[1–3] This evidence-based approach has led to the examination or reexamination of virtually every cardiologic practice of the past several decades. Before this new use of evidence, digitalis, which is now known to have no significant effect on mortality in patients with heart failure, was thought to be *the* cornerstone of therapy for such patients, whereas beta-blockers, which are now known to prolong survival in many patients with heart failure, were thought to be absolutely contraindicated in this setting (see Chapter 28).

To understand evidence-based medicine, it is critical to appreciate key issues related to study design and the analysis of clinical data. These methods can be applied to questions of diagnosis, prognosis, cause, and therapy.

OVERVIEW OF STUDY DESIGN

(Box 1–1)

Prospective cohort studies identify subjects *before* the outcome of interest has developed—whether it is a diagnosis such as coronary artery disease in the Framingham Heart Study or whether an *endpoint such as death* occurs in a cohort of patients with known congestive heart failure—and then systematically observe these patients to determine those in whom *the outcome develops.* Traditional *cohort* studies monitor subjects without imposing any specific management interventions so that the *natural history* can be determined and, if possible, explained in part by whatever baseline characteristics are influencing the prognosis.

Prospective cohort studies are sometimes subdivided into *prolective* studies, which specifically gather baseline data as part of a planned clinical research study, and *retrolective* studies, which rely on medical and administrative data that were routinely gathered as part of clinical care before the specific study was conceived. Prospective studies that directly assess therapeutic decisions are best designed as *randomized controlled trials* in which the randomization process is used to distribute both known and unknown confounding factors (which might influence outcome) evenly among patients receiving different randomized therapies. Although sophisticated, multivariate analytic techniques can theoretically adjust for measurable differences between patients who receive different nonrandomized treatments, the major benefit of randomization is that it should result in an unbiased distribution of the full range of unmeasured or poorly measured factors that may influence both treatment decisions and outcome.

Retrospective studies begin by selecting subjects in whom the outcome has already occurred and then look backward to assess potential predisposing risk factors. These studies are subject to a wide variety of biases

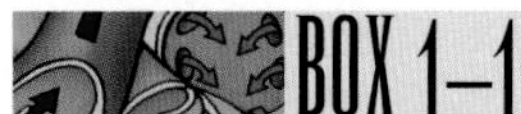

BOX 1–1

Overview of Study Design

I. Cohort study (prospective)

A. To determine causes of a disease

Population free of disease	→	Sample followed	→	Incident cases of new disease

B. To determine natural history in patients with a disease

Population of patients with a known disease	→	Sample followed	→	Cases with pre-specified outcomes (e.g., death or decline in functional status)

II. Case-control study (retrospective)

Patients with the disease or already with a pre-specified outcome	→	Look back to determine exposure to possible risk factors or causes

III. Cross-sectional study

Patients with characteristic of interest	↔	Look at same time to see other characteristics

related to recall or recording of exposure and risk factors in the past and are therefore weaker in study design than prospective cohort studies or randomized clinical trials are. The most common type of retrospective study in the medical literature is a case-control study in which *cases* with the disease or outcome of interest are compared with *controls* who do not have the outcome in terms of their *relative exposure* to potential risk factors. This approach has also been used more recently to raise questions about the potential hazards of antihypertensive medications as risk factors for sudden death.

Cross-sectional studies compare characteristics and outcomes at the same point in time. For example, a study might report on the percentage of patients with heart failure who have normal left ventricular systolic function.

BOX 1–2

Incidence and Prevalence

$$\text{Incidence (any given time period)} = \frac{\text{New cases}}{\text{Population at risk}} \Big/ \text{Time period}$$

$$\text{Prevalence} = \frac{\text{Total cases}}{\text{Population at risk}}$$

$$\text{Prevalence} = \text{Incidence} \times \text{Average life expectancy}$$

Cohort Studies

Incidence

Cohort studies are ideal for determining the *incidence* of disease, which is the number of subjects with new onset of disease divided by all those at risk (Box 1–2). For example, the incidence of major bleeding in patients treated with oral anticoagulants may be 5% at 1 year and 3% in each subsequent year, for a cumulative incidence of 11% at 3 years. By comparison, *prevalence* refers to the total number of individuals with the disease at any given time. For example, there may be 6 million prevalent cases of coronary heart disease in the United States. By simple arithmetic, the prevalence of a given chronic disease is approximately equal to its annual incidence multiplied by the average life expectancy of patients with the disease.

In calculating the incidence rate, individuals in whom an endpoint develops are the numerator, and the population or group of patients at risk is the denominator. The generalizability of a study depends on whether the denominator is clinically relevant and represents the types of patients that a physician may see. For example, early studies of the natural history of mitral valve prolapse were based on patients referred to tertiary centers, presumably because of their higher risk characteristics. It is not surprising that this denominator was associated with a higher rate of outcome events than when subsequent studies evaluated the natural history of unselected consecutive patients with mitral valve prolapse in the general population.

Outcomes/Endpoints

In cohort studies, the outcome of interest may be death, a morbid event such as myocardial infarction, functional status, quality of life, satisfaction, cost, or any other clinically cogent endpoint. For a study to be relevant for clinical practice, the endpoints must be clinically important and reproducible. To minimize bias, the investigators who determine whether an endpoint has occurred should be blinded regarding the presence or absence of the putative risk factors for that endpoint.

Risk Factors

Although some texts distinguish risk factors for the development of a disease from prognostic factors that influence the subsequent course after onset of the disease, this definition is somewhat artificial and should not obscure the fact that both types of studies use similar designs. Risk factors or prognostic factors may include the full spectrum of clinical data gathered by physicians, from historical factors to physical examination and laboratory data. The ability of these various clinical characteristics to predict risk or prognosis can be measured by their univariate association with the endpoint of interest or by their independent *multivariate* association. The impact of such factors may be measured in terms of their *absolute risk*, *relative risk*, and *attributable risk* (Box 1–3). Relative risk is calculated by dividing the incidence in subjects with the risk factor by the incidence in subjects without the risk factor. Many of the strongest risk factors for the development of coronary artery disease, such as smoking and hypercholesterolemia, have a relative risk of about 3 or less. Another approach is to assess attributable risk, which is the incidence of the endpoint in patients with the risk factor minus the incidence in those without the risk factor. When multiplied by the potential population at risk, the attributable risk provides an assessment of the magnitude of disease or disability that may be attributed to the risk factor in the entire population of interest.

Studies of Prognosis

In studies of prognosis, it is important that an *inception cohort* be assembled so that patients are enrolled at a well-defined point along the course of their disease. For example, an inception cohort of patients with acute myocardial infarction would enroll patients either at the time of the infarction or at some pre-specified point such as immediately after hospital discharge or 30 days later. Construction of an inception cohort is especially important to avoid *lead-time bias*, whereby patients in whom the disease is diagnosed sooner will live longer and may be mistakenly thought to do better simply because their follow-up began at an earlier stage of the disease.

Case Fatality and Survival Curves

The *case fatality* rate is defined as the number of patients who die of an event or a disease divided by the total number with it. For some diseases such as acute myocardial infarction, the case fatality rate has a relatively short time horizon, such as during the initial hospitalization. However, one might also determine that among patients with unoperated critical aortic stenosis, nearly all patients ultimately die of the aortic stenosis or its complications, thus yielding a disease-specific case fatality rate of nearly 100% over the lifetime of the patient.

The survival of a cohort is commonly measured by calculating a *survival curve*, in which the probability of survival is plotted against the time of follow-up.[4] Alternatively, sometimes the Y-axis will instead plot the number of events or the mortality rate. In either situation, *survival analysis* considers not only the number of events that occur but also their timing, and it recognizes that individual subjects in a study may be monitored for various periods, either because they were enrolled at different times or because some are lost to

BOX 1–3

Calculating Absolute Risk, Relative Risk, and Attributable Risk

Example 1:

Absolute incidence (risk) of death (death rate) per year in patients with a risk factor	15/1000 = 1.5%
Absolute incidence (risk) of death (death rate) per year in patients without a risk factor	5/1000 = 0.5%
Relative risk in patients with a risk factor vs. those without it	3.0
Risk attributable to a risk factor	10/1000 = 1.0%

Example 2: Effect of a Relative Risk of 2.0 in a Population of 1 Million Depending on the Baseline Absolute Risk

	SUBJECTS WITHOUT A RISK FACTOR	SUBJECTS WITH A RISK FACTOR
Absolute risk	0.5%	1%
Relative risk		2.0
Attributable risk		0.5%
Population attributable risk		5000
Absolute risk	5%	10%
Relative risk		2.0
Attributable risk		5%
Population attributable risk		50,000

follow-up. Thus, a survival curve will calculate a time-specific *hazard rate* and use the hazard rate to draw each subsequent portion of the curve (Fig. 1–1). It is critical to recognize that the decline in the survival curve during any time interval is reflected by the percentage of endpoints in patients who are at risk during the interval. Patients who are censored, either because their eligible follow-up time has not extended into this time period or because they were lost to follow-up, do not appear in either the numerator or the denominator. A comparison of prognosis between two groups requires that their entire survival curves be compared; comparison at just one point in time somewhere along the curve is subject to substantial bias by those who might retrospectively pick that time because of what the data show.

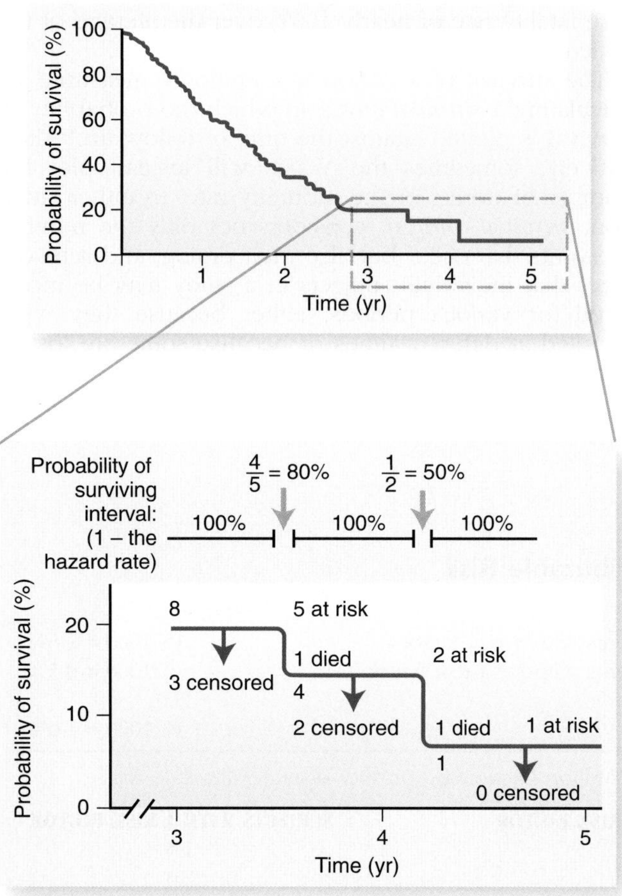

FIGURE 1–1. A typical Kaplan-Meier survival curve with detail for one part of the curve. The curve considers the hazard rate (deaths in patients at risk) in each time period. (Adapted from Fletcher RH, Fletcher SW, Wagner EH: Clinical Epidemiology: The Essentials, 2nd ed. Baltimore, Williams & Wilkins, 1988.)

Bias in Cohort Studies

One major potential bias in cohort studies relates to the ways in which cohorts are selected. Theoretically, a cohort study *samples* a larger population of patients for whom the study subjects are supposed to be representative. If the cohort specifically selects sicker patients, those who have been referred to a certain medical center, those who have survived some particular stress or event, or those who just happen to be available, the cohort will not be *generalizable* to the broader sample from which it was theoretically drawn.

A second major bias in cohort studies relates to loss to follow-up. It can never be assumed that those who are lost to follow-up are completely represented by those for whom follow-up information is available. Although there is no magic rate of loss to follow-up that must be achieved in every study, the acceptable lost-to-follow-up rate depends on the rate of the endpoint of interest. For example, if 50% of patients with heart failure die by the end of 2 years, a 3% or 4% lost-to-follow-up rate will have little effect on assessment of risk or prognostic factors. By comparison, if an event is very uncommon and occurs in only 2% or so of patients, the same 3% or 4% lost-to-follow-up rate may introduce major biases if it is assumed that even 25% or 30% of patients who are lost to follow-up had truly died.

A third major source of bias in cohort studies is the unblinding of investigators, in which those who are familiar with the potential risk factors or treatments are also identifying the outcome. In such circumstances, the risk factors may become self-fulfilling prophecies when potentially biased investigators are assessing them. This bias can be minimized by having different individuals assess risk factors and outcomes and by having strict definitions for both risk factors and outcomes.

Advantages of cohort studies include their ability to measure incidence, their ability to assess risk factors and prognostic factors before the outcome is known, and their potential ability to study multiple outcomes in the same patients. Disadvantages are the need to enroll many subjects if the outcome is uncommon or delayed, the need to monitor patients for a protracted period, and the inability to control for differences in medical treatments or to assess the true impact of various therapeutic interventions.

RANDOMIZED CONTROLLED TRIALS

Randomized trials represent a subgroup of cohort studies in which a treatment option is randomly allocated.[5] Although careful observational cohort studies can detect large effects of treatments on morbidity or mortality[6] and oftentimes predict what will be found in subsequent randomized trials, major discrepancies have occurred for treatments such as postmenopausal estrogen for the prevention of heart disease in women[7] (see Chapter 15). Most studies randomly distribute half the patients into two groups—one that receives the new, experimental treatment and another that receives placebo or standard treatment. Placebo controls are always preferable to a "no treatment" group because it is via the placebo that the patient is blinded regarding the treatment group. By blinding patients, it is possible to include outcomes that might be biased by knowledge of the treatment being received, such as functional status and quality of life, as well as outcomes such as the use of medical resources. Ideally, physicians who are caring for the patients are also blinded, and when both the patient and the caring physician have been blinded, the study is called *double blind.* In many situations in cardiology, especially when comparing interventions such as angioplasty and coronary artery bypass grafting, it is impossible to blind either the patient or the caring physician. In such circumstances, assessment of "hard" endpoints such as death and myocardial infarction is unlikely to be biased, but measurement of "soft" endpoints such as the severity of angina or quality of life may be influenced by the fact that both the patient and the physician know which treatment the patient received. For intermediate endpoints such as hospitalization and performance on a treadmill test, it is important to be sure that the definitions are sufficiently stringent and reproducible to reduce bias. The core laboratories that interpret test results and the data and safety monitoring boards that decide whether to continue or terminate the trial should also be blinded regarding group assignment so that their judgments will not be biased.

Study Design

Although most clinical trials randomize patients evenly between two alternative strategies, some trials may randomize patients to more than two groups, especially if low-dose and high-dose interventions are to be compared with standard care. Articles should explicitly detail the randomization process, which is usually via sealed envelopes or telephone relay of a centralized process generated by a random number sequence.[5]

Compliance

In randomized trials, one of the key issues is whether patients comply with the intervention. For a one-time intervention such as angioplasty or coronary artery bypass grafting, the issue of compliance seems straightforward. However, it is critical to remember that patients are enrolled in a randomized trial at the time that they are randomized and that some interval always elapses between randomization and receipt of the assigned treatment. Even if patients do not receive the assigned treatment, be it a medication or surgical intervention, they must remain in the group to which they were randomized under the *intention-to-treat principle* (Fig. 1–2). Patients who do not receive the assigned treatment are, by definition, fundamentally different from those who do, and it is critical that *all* patients be included in the final results of the study regardless of whether they received the assigned treatment or

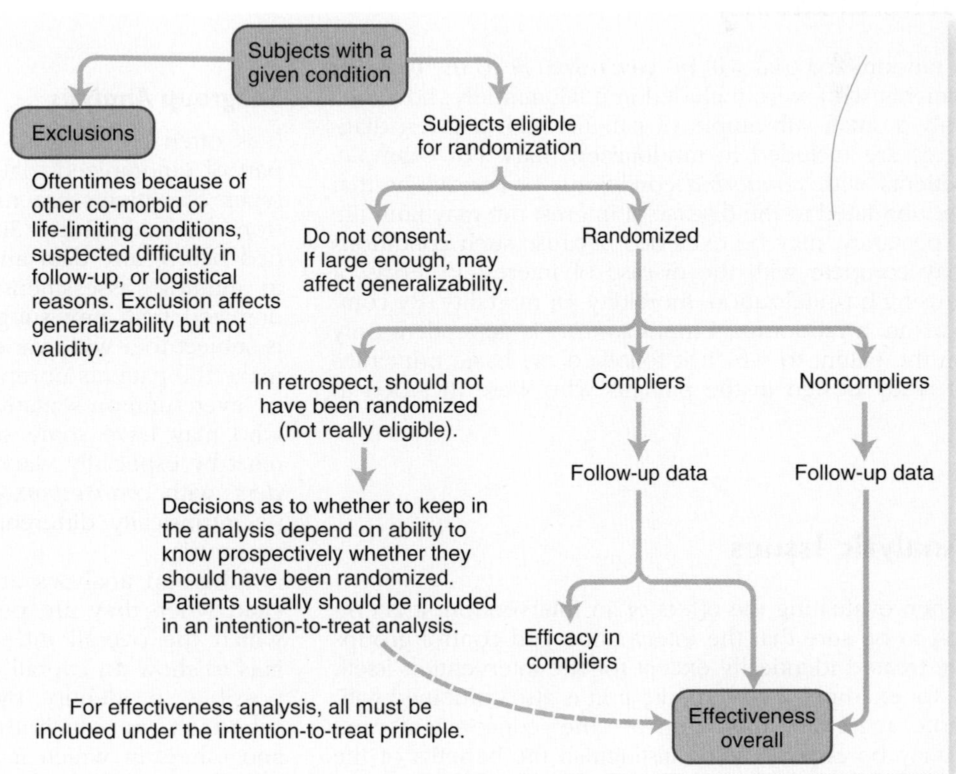

FIGURE 1–2. Randomized trials: enrollment, exclusions, and the intention-to-treat principle.

complied with it. It is only by such an intention-to-treat analysis that investigators can determine whether the treatment is *effective*, that is, does more good than harm in those who are assigned to receive it at the time that a physician must make a clinical decision. For example, in the original Veterans Administration study of coronary artery bypass graft surgery versus medical therapy for patients with stable angina, some argued that those who were randomized to receive bypass graft surgery but died before receiving it should not be counted as "surgical deaths." At that time, however, it was common for patients awaiting elective surgery to wait many weeks, and therefore the *strategy* of choosing coronary artery bypass grafting versus medical therapy had to include the waiting period for the invasive alternative. Otherwise, the sickest patients randomized to surgery, who of course were those most likely to die while awaiting it, would have been excluded from the surgical arm, thereby including only the less sick surgical patients and hence making surgery look better than it should have. Of course, if delay or noncompliance leads to a marked diminution in the effectiveness of the therapeutic alternative, one should try to find a new strategy that will minimize delay and maximize compliance. Sometimes the term *efficacious* is used to assess whether an intervention improves outcome in those who actually receive and comply with it. Studies of *efficacy* normally serve as a prelude to improved strategies that ultimately show whether the intervention is more *effective* as well.

Generalizability

A randomized trial will be *generalizable* to the types of patients who were included in it. Commonly, however, only a small subsample of patients with a given diagnosis are included in randomized trials. For example, patients with *co-morbid* conditions, or conditions that are unrelated to the disease of interest but may limit life expectancy, may be excluded because such conditions may compete with the disease of interest in terms of causing hospitalization, morbidity, or mortality. By comparison, a randomized trial's *validity* is dependent only on the extent to which it followed the basic principles of study design in the patients who were included in it.

Analytic Issues

When evaluating the effect of an intervention, it is critical to be sure that the intervention and control groups are treated identically except for the intervention itself. If, for example, a new medication is also combined with more aggressive follow-up or other concomitant care, it may be impossible to distinguish the benefits of the medication itself from the benefits of the other accompanying treatments.

Although randomization should create groups with equal baseline risk at the beginning of a trial, the randomization process itself is imperfect. One of the key tables in a randomized trial must compare the baseline characteristics of the intervention and control groups. Even if none of the factors differ significantly between the two groups, it is common to adjust for any baseline differences when reporting the effects of the study to be sure that the impact of the intervention is distinguished from any potential differences in baseline prognosis.

Magnitude of Effect

In assessing whether the results of a randomized trial may be useful for an individual physician, it is critical to understand the magnitude of the treatment effect. Although randomized trials often report the percent reduction in the occurrence of an endpoint (similar to a decline in relative risk), for the individual patient and physician, the absolute magnitude of the treatment effect (the change in absolute risk) may be critical in weighing the value of the intervention against other options. Another way to quantify the impact of an intervention is to estimate the number of patients who must be treated to achieve a particular benefit, such as the number of patients who must be treated to save a life or a year of life. For example, if an intervention reduces mortality from 6% to 4% in 1 year, absolute risk is reduced 2%, relative risk is reduced 33%, and 50 patients need to be treated for 1 year to save a life.

Subgroup Analysis

It is often tempting to perform *subgroup analyses* as part of randomized trials to determine whether certain types of patients are more likely to benefit or suffer from the intervention. Such subgroups should be specified before any data analysis to avoid biases inherent in multiple assessments of the data. Within a randomized trial, any subgroup that is not pre-specified is subject to a wide variety of selection biases that may make the patients unrepresentative of others in the trial or even unrepresentative of nonrandomized patients who may have some similar characteristics. A reader must be especially wary of trials that compare *responders* with *nonresponders* because responders may be intrinsically different in terms of their underlying prognosis.

Subgroup analyses are generally more likely to be valid when they are performed as part of a study in which the overall difference is large. When a study fails to show an overall difference, it is virtually always possible to identify by retrospective analysis some subgroups in which the intervention was beneficial and others in which it appeared to be harmful; such findings may generate hypotheses for future testing but should not be considered definitive.

Other Biases

The *Hawthorne effect* describes the fact that decisions and care may improve simply because people realize that they are being observed while participating in a trial rather than because of the specific intervention itself. *Regression to the mean* describes the tendency for measurements that are the most extreme initially to move more toward the mean on remeasurement, even if no intervention has occurred. For example, if subjects are chosen because of elevated blood pressure on one measurement, many will be selected because of a reading that is unusually high for them. On repeat measurement, the apparent improvement in blood pressure in many individuals will be a function of nothing more than the intrinsic fluctuation back toward their own mean blood pressure.

The major advantage of randomized trials is that they provide the least biased way to assess the benefit or harm of interventions. However, by definition, *randomized trials* are undertaken only to test something that is thought to be better than no treatment or the current standard of care. Hence, randomized trials are not performed with the intent of identifying interventions that are thought to be harmful, such as smoking. Randomized trials are also disadvantaged by their expense and logistic difficulties.

Quasi-experimental Studies

In some situations, *quasi-experimental* approaches may be required because randomization is impractical or unreasonably expensive. Quasi-experimental designs are most appropriate in situations in which a program is being evaluated rather than when the treatment of individual patients is being studied. For example, if care at an institution is re-engineered in such a way that standard care can no longer be delivered or its delivery would be hopelessly *contaminated*, or influenced, by the intervention, it may be appropriate to have a control group from another institution or time period. Quasi-experimental designs are subject to a variety of biases, including an inability to be sure that patients in the intervention group are similar to those in the control group. In addition, temporal or secular changes unrelated to the intervention itself may be more important than the intervention. In interpreting quasi-experimental studies, it is critical to be sure that adequate concurrent controls have been enrolled and that secular influences have been excluded or adjustments have been made for them. One approach is to perform a *time series* study in which the program is implemented in some time periods and not in others, with time periods alternated to provide an adequate control for secular and other influences.

CASE-CONTROL STUDIES

Because it is not ethical to randomize patients to receive interventions that are thought to be harmful, other study designs must be found to assess the cause of many diseases. In situations in which the risk factor is common and the outcome of interest occurs with a reasonably high frequency and in a reasonably short time frame, cohort studies can assess causative factors. However, in circumstances in which the outcome is unusual, an alternative design is the case-control study. In this approach, *cases* are patients with the disease and *controls* are subjects without it. These two groups are compared in terms of their *exposure* to various potential risk factors.

Commonly, a case-control study will be *retrospective* such that patients are identified after they already have the outcome (i.e., they are a *case*) and are then asked or surveyed to determine previous exposure. Alternatively, cases may be the relatively few individuals in whom an endpoint developed as part of a cohort study, and to maximize both efficiency and power, they may be compared with randomly selected or matched control patients from that same cohort. In general, case-control studies become more powerful as the ratio of controls to cases increases to about 3:1 to 4:1, but little incremental power is gained from further increasing the number of nondiseased controls in either a case-control or a cohort study. For example, in a large cohort study of 10,000 people, intracranial bleeding may develop in only 100, and it might be interesting to gather additional data on aspirin exposure or a family history of polycystic kidney disease. Rather than gathering the data on 9900 controls, the study might select 3 or 4 nonbleeding controls per case of bleeding and gather the additional data on this smaller sample. This *nested case-control* study within a larger cohort study is more efficient than including all the cohort patients in whom the endpoint did not develop—especially if additional measurements must be made on patients who are included in the case-control study.

Case-control studies are subject to a number of biases, including how the cases and controls are defined and how the exposure is measured. Because cases and controls may differ in a variety of factors other than the exposure being studied, it is common to adjust for these factors by using multivariate methods or by *matching* patients based on key characteristics such as age and sex.

In choosing cases and controls, it is important that the two groups be as similar as possible other than that the case has the outcome of interest. Potential exposure must be measured in similar ways in both groups, and it is critical to be sure that the exposure truly preceded the outcome. Furthermore, the conclusions of case-control studies are more likely to be valid if a clear dose-response gradient can be established such that greater degrees of exposure result in a higher likelihood of disease or more severe disease. For example, if smoking is associated with coronary disease, more smoking should carry an even larger risk. When a case-control study identifies a potentially harmful exposure, consideration should be given to trying to confirm the harmful effect in a cohort study.

Because case-control studies arbitrarily select the number of patients with and without the disease, they cannot measure incidence or relative risk. Instead, they calculate an odds ratio (Box 1–4). Case-control studies are usually able to identify risk factors that have odds ratios of 2 or more, but they are not generally very useful for identifying exposures that increase the odds of an endpoint by less than that magnitude.

Case-control studies suffer from the fact that the population at risk is generally undefined, cases are selected on the basis of their availability rather than by being sampled from a defined population, and controls are selected by the investigator in the hope that they will somehow be appropriate for comparison with the cases. Exposure must commonly be recalled rather than being observed, and incidence rates and relative risk cannot be calculated. Nevertheless, case-control studies represent an efficient way to assess possible risk factors and were, for example, the method by which the increased cardiovascular risk associated with homocysteine was first noted.

DATA ANALYSIS

Statistics provide a mechanism for analyzing observations and determining whether clinically important differences exist.[4] Some clinical variables can be measured on a continuous scale, such as systolic blood pressure, and a mean value and standard deviation can be assessed. Others, such as the intensity of a systolic murmur, may be graded on an ordinal scale in which most individuals have a normal value (no murmur) and the number of patients with an abnormality declines as its severity increases.

Reproducibility or *reliability* refers to whether the same result would be obtained if the measurement were repeated. This property should be contrasted with *validity*, which determines whether the measurement is an accurate reflection of reality. Ordinal measurements are oftentimes "soft" data that require clinical judgment rather than an automated machine. Nevertheless, assessment of functional status, quality of life, satisfaction, and the like can be "hardened" by standardized techniques that make them more reproducible. For example, standardized, validated questionnaires have been developed to measure functional capacity, health status, and quality of life and have reproducibility and validity that compare favorably with that of a typical radiographic test.

Because humans vary from time to time, it is not surprising that any measurement, be it blood pressure or functional status, may also vary. By statistical convention, a measurement may be considered abnormal if the chance is less than 1 in 20 that it would be observed in a normal individual. However, for many laboratory tests, this statistical criterion is far too lenient because just by chance each person would be abnormal on something if enough factors were measured. This principle of *multiple testing* demonstrates that statistical definitions of normal must be tempered by clinical judgment.

Specific types of statistical approaches are most appropriate for specific types of data (Table 1–1). Most of these tests can be performed easily by a variety of statistical packages on a personal computer.

Multivariate analysis can consider many potential factors and assess their importance independent of other factors. The various methods (Box 1–5) generally proceed by selecting the most important factor associated with the endpoint and then sequentially selecting the second most important factor, the third most important factor, and so on. Multivariate analysis can be used to assess the independent importance of risk factors or to adjust for a variety of known risk factors in determining whether an additional factor adds incremental importance.[2, 4]

When multiple factors are being tested, it may be more appropriate to define statistical significance as less

BOX 1–4

Calculation of the Odds Ratio in Case-Control Studies and Comparison with a Relative Risk Calculation from a Cohort Study

		CASES WITH THE OUTCOME		CONTROLS WITHOUT THE OUTCOME		TOTAL
Exposure present		A		B		A + B
Exposure absent		C		D		C + D
Total		A + C		B + D		
Odds ratio in a case-control study	=	$\frac{\frac{A/(A+C)}{C/(A+C)}}{\frac{B/(B+D)}{D/(B+D)}}$	=	$\frac{A/C}{B/D}$	=	$\frac{AD}{BC}$
Relative risk in a cohort study	=	$\frac{A/(A+B)}{C/(C+D)}$				

TABLE 1–1

Overview of How to Choose Statistical Tests

Type of Measure	Comparison of Two Groups of Different Individuals to Each Other	Comparison of Same Individuals to Themselves—Two Measurements on Each	Comparison of Three or More Groups of Different Individuals	Comparison of Same Individuals to Themselves—Three or More Measurements on Each	Association of Two Different Variables with Each Other—Each Measured in the Same Individual
Continuous and either normally distributed or measured in many subjects (e.g., blood pressure)	Unpaired t test	Paired t test	Analysis of variance	Repeated measures analysis of variance	Pearson correlation coefficient or linear regression
Ordered but in few categories or not normally distributed	Mann-Whitney rank sum test	Wilcoxon signed-rank test	Kruskal-Wallis statistic	Friedman statistic	Spearman rank correlation coefficient
Categorical—often dichotomous (two categories) and usually five or fewer categories	Chi-square test or Fisher exact test	McNemar's test	Chi-square test	Cochrane Q	Contingency coefficient

Adapted from Glantz SA: Primer of Biostatistics, 3rd ed. New York, McGraw-Hill, 1992. Copyright © by McGraw-Hill, Inc. Used by permission of McGraw-Hill Book Company.

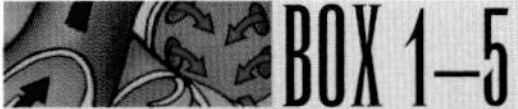

BOX 1–5

Statistical Approaches

PARAMETRIC MULTIVARIATE ANALYSES

Create an equation that weights the various predictive factors and adds them up to give a score

$$ax_1 + bx_2 + cx_3 \ldots + \text{constant}$$

where a, b, and c are the respective weights for variables x_1, x_2, x_3

Linear regression analysis: Preferred when the predictive variables are continuous (e.g., blood pressure) and the outcome is also continuous (e.g., left ventricular mass)

Logistic regression analysis: Preferred when the predictive variables are both continuous and dichotomous (e.g., blood pressure, family history of stroke) and the outcome is continuous (e.g., risk of stroke)

Discriminant analysis: Preferred when the outcome variable is in more than two ordered categories (e.g., no complications, major complications without death, death)

RECURSIVE PARTITIONING ANALYSIS

Sequentially splits subjects into subgroups based on factors that discriminate between those with and those without the outcome of interest

Most useful when predictive factors are dichotomous and the outcome is dichotomous (e.g., live or die), especially if predictive factors have strong interrelationships

than 1 chance in 100 ($P < .01$) rather than less than 1 chance in 20 ($P < .05$). Regardless of the definition of statistical significance, the question of clinical importance must also be addressed. In these situations, relative risk and attributable risk (Fig. 1–3) may be as important as the P value. For randomized trials, it may be appropriate to calculate the *number needed to treat,* that is, the number of patients who must receive an intervention to save one life or to avoid one endpoint.[4, 5]

By convention, statistical tests may be considered *one tailed* or *two tailed.* A two-tailed test considers whether either of two options being compared may be better or worse than the other (see Fig. 1–3). A one-tailed test estimates the probability of whether option A is better than option B, but not the converse (the possibility that B may be better than A). Although clinical investigators are often tempted to use one-tailed tests under the assumption that a new option may be better than a previous option but it could not possibly be worse, statistical convention and most journals require that two-tailed tests be used. Simply put, the P value reported for a two-tailed test will be twice as large as the P value reported for a one-tailed test and, hence, less likely to demonstrate conventional statistical significance.

It is common in the medical literature to calculate *confidence intervals* around a point estimate. The 95% confidence interval indicates the range in which 95% of individuals are estimated to fall or the range in which the results are estimated to occur 95% of the time if the experiment were repeated multiple times.

Whereas the P value estimates the likelihood that an observed difference may be due to chance, the *power*

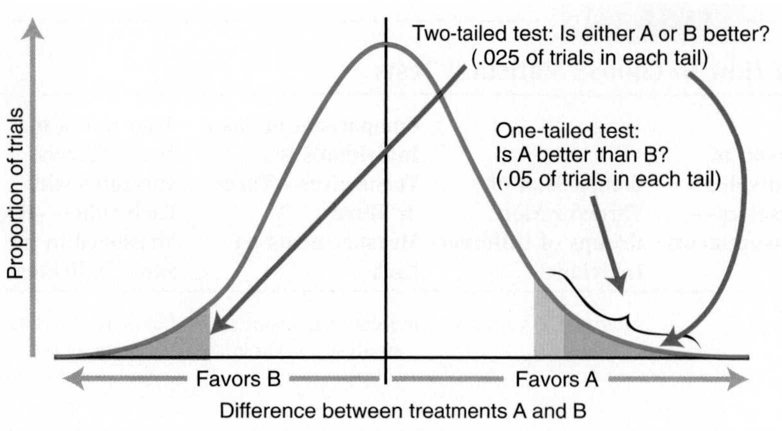

FIGURE 1–3. One- and two-tailed tests of statistical significance where $P_x = .05$. A larger observed difference in favor of treatment is required for statistical significance if during analysis it is assumed that either A or B might be better. (Adapted from Fletcher RH, Fletcher SW, Wagner EH: Clinical Epidemiology: The Essentials, 2nd ed. Baltimore, Williams & Wilkins, 1988.)

TABLE 1–2

Alpha and Beta Error: *P* Values and the Definition of Power

		Truth in the Population from Which the Study Sample Was Chosen	
		Association	***No Association***
Findings in the study	Significant association (e.g., $P < .05$)	Correct	Type I (alpha) error* (association found by a 1 in 20 chance even though it does not truly exist)
	Not a significant association (e.g., $P > .05$)	Type II (beta) error† (association not found, often because the study was too small to have sufficient power to detect a statistically significant relationship)	Correct

*The acceptable alpha error is usually .05 (1 in 20), but it may be .01 or lower.

†The acceptable beta error is usually about .20 (1 in 5; power of 80%), but it may be .10 (power of 90%) or even .05 (power of 95%) if it is very important not to miss an association.

of a study estimates the likelihood that it will be able to find a true difference if one exists (Table 1–2). Commonly, randomized trials are designed to have a power of at least 80% for finding a relevant difference if one does indeed exist, but sometimes the power might be increased if it is extremely important to be sure that such a difference does not exist. A study's power is calculated before the study is conducted; when the final data are presented, they should be reported in terms of the confidence intervals around any observed differences.

META-ANALYSIS

Because even the largest studies oftentimes do not have power sufficient to exclude a small difference, *meta-analysis* is a method for combining the results of randomized trials to increase aggregate sample size and see whether differences truly exist. Meta-analyses are more likely to be useful if the studies being combined are similar, if the studies represent current medical treatments, and if it is unlikely that any *publication bias* has occurred such that positive studies have been reported but negative studies have not.[8, 9]

In formal meta-analyses, standardized methods are used to be sure that all potentially relevant studies have been identified, that they meet the criteria for methodologic rigor, and that the results are combined in statistically appropriate ways. The results of meta-analyses are commonly presented in a summary figure that shows the relative harm or benefit found in individual studies (with their 95% confidence intervals), as well as the pooled estimate of the effect of the intervention overall (Fig. 1–4).

In general, meta-analyses are more useful for summarizing the results of multiple large trials than the results of very small studies, which may be more subject to bias. Thus, meta-analyses appear to supplement rather than substitute for large clinical trials, and they are more useful when the preceding trials are generally consistent than when they are used to resolve major differences among studies. For example, meta-analyses

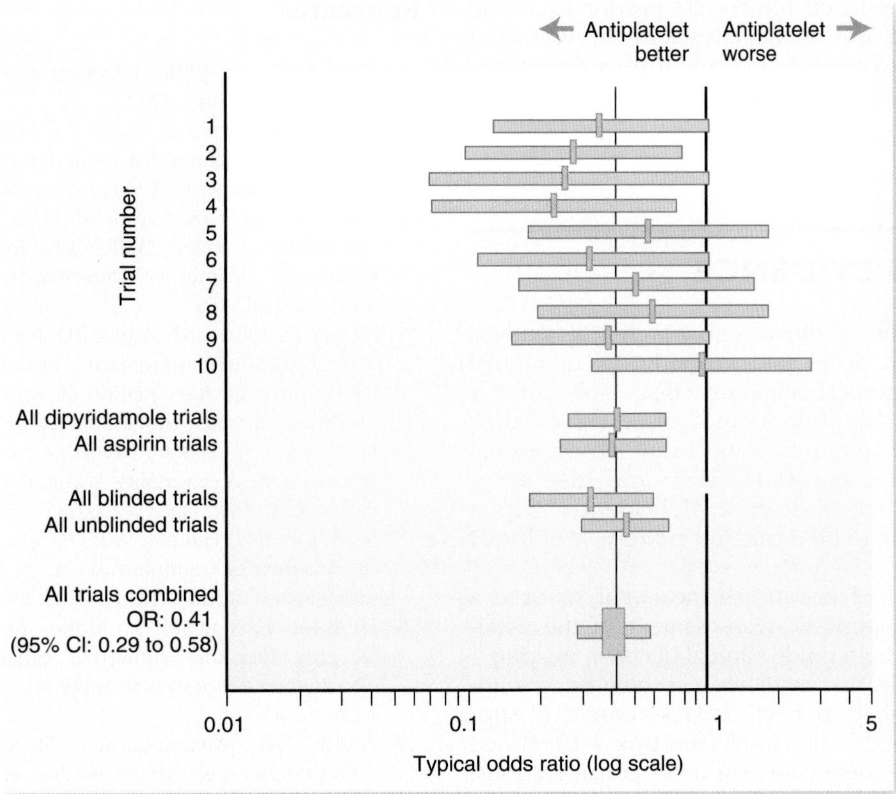

FIGURE 1–4. Odds ratio (OR) plots (logarithmic scale) for randomized trials of antiplatelet therapy or control in addition to warfarin to prevent thromboembolism in patients with prosthetic heart valves. The center of each horizontal line represents the OR for the individual trial, and the ends of the horizontal line represent the 95% confidence intervals (CIs). Trials are also subdivided by the type of antiplatelet therapy (dipyridamole or aspirin) to demonstrate that the type of antiplatelet therapy makes no difference, as well as by blinded versus unblinded trials to demonstrate that the benefit of antiplatelet agents is even greater in studies with the preferred (blinded) study design (also see Chapter 32). The solid vertical line represents an OR of 1; to the left of the line (OR < 1) favors antiplatelet therapy, and to the right of the line (OR > 1) favors control or placebo. The bottom line and the center of the box represent the pooled OR, and the ends of the horizontal line represent the pooled 95% CI. (Adapted from Massel D, Little SH: Risks and benefits of adding antiplatelet therapy to warfarin among patients with prosthetic heart valves: A meta-analysis. J Am Coll Cardiol 2001;37:569–578.)

BOX 1–6

Grading of Levels of Evidence

Level 1

1a	Evidence from large randomized clinical trials (RCTs) or systematic reviews (including meta-analyses) of multiple randomized trials that collectively have at least as much data as one single well-defined trial
1b	Evidence from at least one "all or none" high-quality cohort study in which *all* patients died/failed with conventional therapy and some survived/succeeded with the new therapy (e.g., chemotherapy for tuberculosis or meningitis or defibrillation for ventricular fibrillation) or in which many died/failed with conventional therapy and *none* died/failed with the new therapy (e.g., penicillin for pneumococcal infections)
1c	Evidence from at least one moderate-sized RCT or a meta-analysis of small trials that collectively has only a moderate number of patients
1d	Evidence from at least one RCT
Level 2	Evidence from at least one high-quality study of nonrandomized cohorts that did and did not receive the new therapy
Level 3	Evidence from at least one high-quality case-control study
Level 4	Evidence from at least one high-quality case series
Level 5	Opinions from experts without reference or access to any of the foregoing (e.g., argument from physiology, bench research, or first principles)

Adapted from Yusuf S, Cairns JA, Camm AJ, et al (eds): Evidence-Based Cardiology. London, BMJ Publishing Group, 1998, p xxvi.

of thrombolysis predicted the results eventually found in large megatrials, but meta-analyses of the effects of magnesium and nitroglycerin in acute myocardial infarction have been discrepant with the results of subsequent megatrials.

GRADING EVIDENCE

Based on the rigor of the design of clinical studies, systems have been developed to grade the quality of evidence in the medical literature (Box 1–6). Level 1 evidence requires data from a randomized clinical trial. Level 2 evidence requires data from observational studies. Case-control studies (level 3) and case series (level 4) provide lesser degrees of evidence. Expert opinion, though not to be dismissed entirely, is of lower quality (level 5).

Whether performed as a formal meta-analysis or as a systematic review, periodic reassessment of the available evidence can help guide clinical decision making.[10] For treatment decisions, evidence can also be categorized by how well its benefit or lack thereof is supported by the available literature (see Box 1–6). Based on the quality of evidence and on other considerations, numerous practice guidelines have been developed by the American Heart Association and the American College of Cardiology (see Chapter 2).

References

1. Barton S (ed): Clinical Evidence, Issue 7. London, BMJ Publishing Group, 2002.
2. Guyatt G, Rennie D (eds): Users' Guide to the Medical Literature: A Manual for Evidence-Based Clinical Practice. Chicago, American Medical Association, 2002.
3. Yusuf S, Cairns JA, Camm AJ, et al (eds): Evidence-Based Cardiology. London, BMJ Publishing Group, 1998.
4. Glantz SA. Primer of Biostatistics, 4th ed. New York, McGraw-Hill, 1997.
5. Moher D, Schulz KF, Altman D, for the CONSORT Group: The CONSORT statement: Revised recommendations for improving the quality of reports of parallel-group randomized trials. JAMA 2001;285:1987–1991.
6. MacMahon S, Collins R: Reliable assessment of the effects of treatment on mortality and major morbidity, II: Observational studies. Lancet 2001;357:455–462.
7. Ioannidis JPA, Haidich A-B, Pappa M, et al: Comparison of evidence of treatment effects in randomized and nonrandomized studies. JAMA 2001;286:821–830.
8. McAuley L, Tugwell P, Moher D: Does the inclusion of grey literature influence estimates of intervention effectiveness reported in meta-analyses? Lancet 2001;356: 1228–1231.
9. Petitti DB: Meta-analysis, Decision Analyses, and Cost-Effectiveness Analyses, 2nd ed. New York, Oxford University Press, 2000.
10. The Cochrane Library. Available at www.update_software.com.

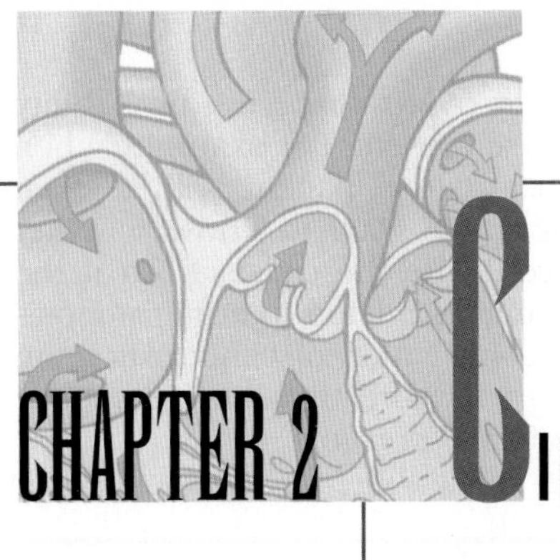

CHAPTER 2 Clinical Decision Making

Lee Goldman

Clinical decision making is a complicated process based on experience, judgment, and reasoning that should simultaneously integrate information from the medical literature and a variety of other sources. Although *decision making* should not be confused with *decision analysis*, which is a quantitative method for analyzing medical information, it should incorporate the quantitative results of randomized clinical trials and other studies that form the substance of what is often called *evidence-based medicine* (see Chapter 1).

Medical decision making generally proceeds through a five-step process that *first* begins with elicitation of pertinent historical information related to the chief complaint and history of the present illness. The past medical history and physical examination may be specially targeted to pursue possibilities uncovered by the original questioning, in addition to providing a standard body of background information. *Second*, the physician may choose from a variety of diagnostic tests, which in cardiology oftentimes includes different options for obtaining the same type of information. For example, the left ventricular ejection fraction may be measured by echocardiography (transthoracic or transesophageal), by a radionuclide ventriculogram, or by a contrast ventriculogram. In the *third* step, the results of diagnostic tests are used to modify or adjust the probabilities or hypotheses that were generated from the original history and physical examination. In the *fourth* phase, the potential risks and benefits of additional diagnostic tests and therapeutic interventions are compared so that the physician may develop a set of recommendations for the patient. *Fifth*, a plan or alternative plans are discussed with the patient, the patient's comparative preferences for various options are considered, and a plan is implemented.

HISTORY AND PHYSICAL EXAMINATION

During the initial medical history, the physician should pursue complaints that may be cardiac in origin with the understanding that the importance of the cardiac abnormality may be far greater than the severity of the patient's initial complaint. For example, even very mild anginal pain may be the first key symptom of coronary artery disease. The same complaint would be far less important if it could be proved to be related to a musculoskeletal abnormality. Because even minor complaints that may be consistent with cardiac disease could be the first symptom of severe pathoanatomic abnormalities with dire and sudden clinical consequences, it is critical that complaints of chest discomfort, shortness of breath, dizziness, or edema be investigated in sufficient detail to determine whether they are early warning signs for important cardiac disease.

When investigating complaints potentially consistent with cardiac disease, an experienced physician will generate a list of important diseases that could cause the complaint and then ask additional questions in an order that helps determine whether more serious potential causes of the symptom are present. In a process termed *iterative hypothesis testing*, the clinician will sequentially investigate the likelihood of various causes of the symptom or sign rather than asking all imaginable questions in a standardized order. For example, in a patient who complains of chest discomfort, the physician should focus on the location and quality of the discomfort and how it may be provoked or relieved. The physician should determine whether the pain is precipitated by exercise, emotion, eating, deep breathing, or changes in position (see Chapter 7). Depending on the patient's response, a series of questions would be asked to try to reinforce or discard the diagnostic suspicion. For example, if the pain is pleuritic in nature, the physician would ask about previous viral symptoms and risk factors for venous thromboembolic disease. It must be emphasized that this focused approach does not obviate the need for a complete history and physical examination, and the history and physical examination should reinforce and influence each other.

Both the history and physical examination will be more helpful if the physician is precise in the way that questions are asked and how the physical examination is performed. Patients' responses to questions may vary from time to time, and it is often helpful to ask the same question in different ways to be sure that the responses are consistent. On physical examination, many of the key findings that are used for diagnostic decision making, such as the presence and intensity of a murmur, may be poorly reproducible from time to time and from observer to observer.

Because of the poor reproducibility of many physical findings, it is important for the clinician to listen or observe carefully and to also look for corroborating information. For example, if the jugular veins appear to be distended, the finding of hepatomegaly, hepatojugular reflux, or peripheral edema would tend to confirm the abnormality. A precordial systolic murmur suggestive of aortic outflow obstruction may be confirmed by auscultation over the carotid arteries. In addition, by using a variety of bedside maneuvers, careful cardiac auscultation can often accurately predict the cause of a systolic murmur (see Chapter 11).

Diagnostic tests may be especially important to confirm suspicions raised by the history or physical examination. For example, the findings of bibasilar rales and a clearly enlarged heart on physical examination in a patient with dyspnea on exertion may be readily ascribed to heart failure. However, the same apparent physical findings in the absence of symptoms of heart failure would not be nearly as definitive and should prompt additional evaluation, such as a chest radiograph, to assess whether heart failure is present. Even when all the data support the diagnosis of heart failure, a chest radiograph may be useful to assess the severity of the heart failure, and an echocardiogram may be critical for evaluating the cause and severity of any underlying left ventricular dysfunction or valvular abnormalities (see Chapter 4).

In weighing clinical information, physicians tend to have great difficulty in estimating accurate probabilities. Part of the problem is related to reliance on vague and ill-defined terms such as *often* or *unlikely*. Physicians also tend systematically to overestimate the probability that unusual conditions are present. For example, when a systolic murmur is heard in a patient with angina, heart failure, or syncope, it is vital to know whether critical aortic stenosis could be the cause. Even if the probability that the murmur is related to aortic stenosis is very small, a cardiac consultation or echocardiogram may still be important to be sure that this potentially fatal but curable cause is not present.

DIAGNOSTIC TESTING

No diagnostic test is perfect. Even a test such as coronary arteriography, which may be considered the gold standard for the diagnosis of coronary disease, has an imperfect correlation with autopsy findings. Similarly, a pulmonary angiogram, which is generally considered the gold standard for the diagnosis of pulmonary embolism, is also imperfect.

Because diagnostic tests provide useful but not perfect information, it is critical that their results be integrated with findings from the history and physical examination. The history and physical examination provide a *prior probability* that a condition in question, such as critical aortic stenosis, is present. This probability can then be modified by the results of a diagnostic test such as an echocardiogram. Although an echocardiogram should be an accurate way to determine the gradient across an aortic valve (see Chapter 32), this gradient may decline as severe left ventricular dysfunction develops. Hence, a gradient of 50 or 60 mm Hg may represent only moderate stenosis in a patient with normal left ventricular function, whereas a gradient of 30 mm Hg may represent severe stenosis in a patient with markedly compromised left ventricular function. Therefore, cardiac catheterization with simultaneous measurement of both the aortic valve gradient and cardiac output may be required to achieve the best possible in vivo estimate of the severity of aortic valve stenosis, with the recognition that even this estimate may not be perfect.

Because diagnostic tests do not provide perfect information, it is critical to understand the terminology commonly used to assess the accuracy of a diagnostic test (Table 2–1). Whereas the clinician tends to think about the patient in terms of the probability of a disease, such as critical aortic stenosis, after a test such as an echocardiogram, the postechocardiogram probability is dependent not only on the result of the echocardiogram but also on the pretest likelihood of aortic stenosis. This pretest likelihood in an individual patient is the equivalent of the *prevalence* of the disease in a population of patients with the same characteristics. Using this general approach, a single test with known sensitivity and specificity will yield different probabilities of disease, depending on the pretest probability of the condition in question (Fig. 2–1).

The same phenomenon can be understood by considering it from a population perspective. For example,

TABLE 2–1

Definitions of Commonly Used Terms in Epidemiology and Decision Making

Test Result	Disease State: *Present*	Disease State: *Absent*
Positive	*a* (true positive)	*b* (false positive)
Negative	*c* (false negative)	*d* (true negative)
Prevalence (prior probability)	$= (a + c)/(a + b + c + d)$	= All patients with the disease/All patients tested
Sensitivity (true-positive rate)	$= a/(a + c)$	= True-positive test results/All patients with the disease
Specificity (true-negative rate)	$= d/(b + d)$	= True-negative test results/All patients without the disease
False-negative rate	$= c/(a + c)$	= False-negative test results/All patients with the disease
False-positive rate	$= b/(b + d)$	= False-positive test results/All patients without the disease
Positive predictive value	$= a/(a + b)$	= True-positive test results/All positive test results
Negative predictive value	$= d/(c + d)$	= True-negative test results/All patients with negative results
Overall accuracy	$= (a + d)/(a + b + c + d)$	= True-positive + true-negative test results/All tests
Likelihood ratio for a positive test	$= \dfrac{a/(a+c)}{b/(b+d)}$	= True-positive rate/False-positive rate
Likelihood ratio for a negative test	$= \dfrac{d/(b+d)}{c/(a+c)}$	= True-negative rate/False-negative rate

Adapted from Fauci AS, Braunwald E, Isselbacher KJ, et al (eds): Harrison's Principles of Internal Medicine, 14th ed. New York, McGraw-Hill, 1998, p. 10.

the likelihood of different exercise test results in patients with differing severity of coronary artery disease is reasonably known from the medical literature. The prevalence of this varying severity of coronary disease in the population can also be estimated. Based on these two estimates, the expected results of exercise testing can be projected, and the likelihood of varying levels of disease severity, given a particular exercise test result, can be calculated (Fig. 2–2).

Sensitivity and Specificity

The sensitivity and specificity of a test do not depend on the prevalence of the disease in the population being studied or the probability of the disease in an individual. However, both sensitivity and specificity are dependent on the *spectrum* of patients being studied. For example, if a new enzyme assay for the diagnosis of acute myocardial infarction is evaluated in 50 patients with obvious acute myocardial infarction based on electrocardiographic criteria and in 50 normal college students, it will appear to have near-perfect sensitivity and specificity. If, however, the same test is applied to 100 patients with suspicious symptoms who are being evaluated as part of a protocol to rule out myocardial infarction, both the sensitivity and the specificity will be far lower; in fact, given the absence of a true gold standard, the precise sensitivity and specificity may be difficult, if not impossible, to determine.

For many diagnostic tests the result is not dichotomous (i.e., normal vs. abnormal) but, instead, may be interpreted on a continuum. Whether this continuum is the level of a cardiac enzyme, the number of millimeters of ST segment depression on exercise testing, or the measured gradient across a valve during Doppler echocardiography, judgment must be used to determine what value or values should guide medical decision making. One way to assess this inherent tradeoff between defining normal so as to provide high sensitivity (such as diagnosing postangioplasty myocardial infarction in a patient with minimal cardiac enzyme elevation) versus emphasizing high specificity (such as requiring a threefold or fourfold increase in cardiac enzyme values as a criterion for a postprocedure infarction) is to evaluate various definitions of an abnormal test result. This principle can be depicted by a *receiver operating characteristic curve,* which graphically displays the sensitivity and specificity associated with various test results (Fig. 2–3).

In many situations, tests may be valued because of their high sensitivity or high specificity, but not both. For example, when an electrocardiogram shows 1 mm or more of ST segment elevation in two or more contiguous leads in a patient with acute chest pain, the likelihood of acute myocardial infarction is very high. In the absence of evidence for conditions such as acute pericarditis or aortic dissection, where the risk of thrombolysis is very high, these patients are considered appropriate for immediate thrombolysis or catheterization with probable primary angioplasty because the electrocardiographic result is unlikely to be a false positive (i.e., it is highly specific); even if it is, however, the risk of aggressive therapy in the few false-positive cases is far outweighed by the benefit for the vast majority of true-positive cases. In other settings, a

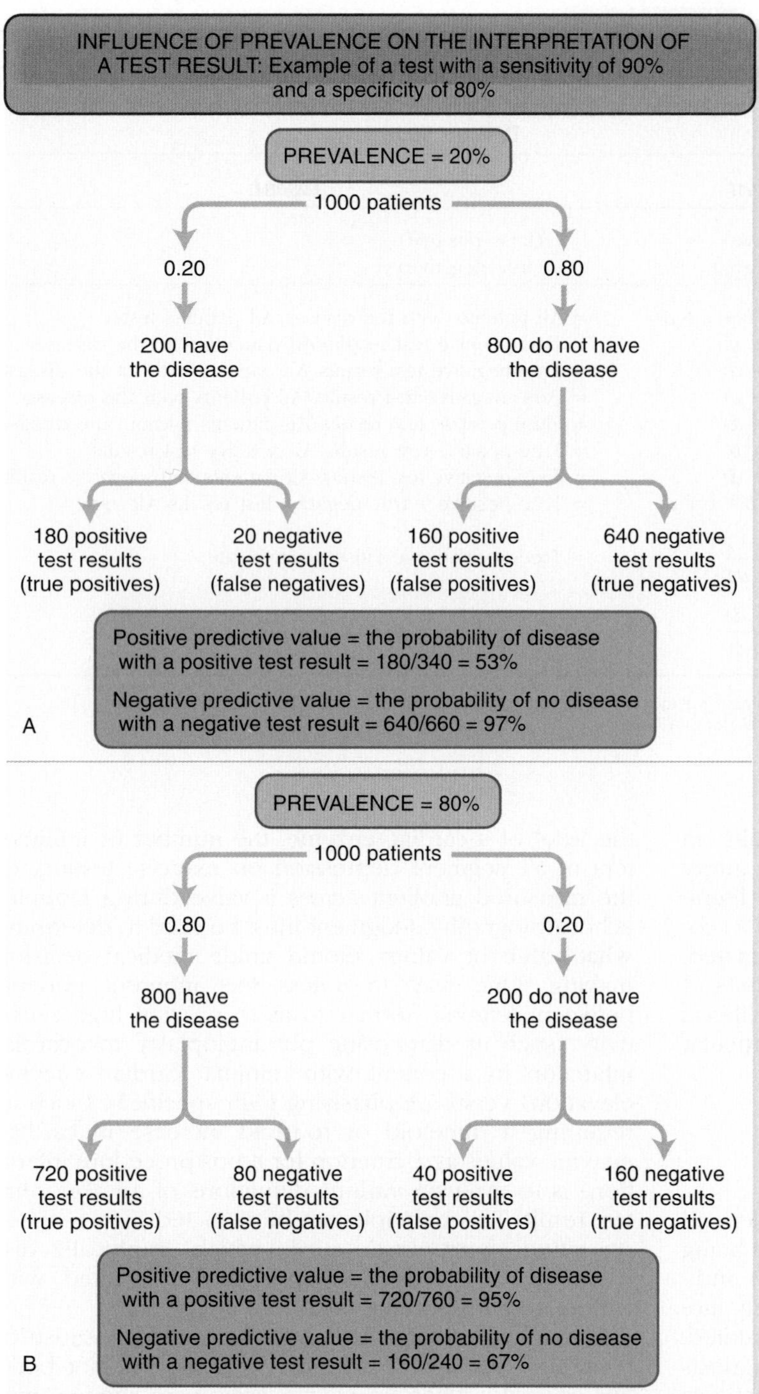

FIGURE 2–1. The influence of prevalence on the interpretation of a test result.

test may be valued because of its very high sensitivity. For example, cardiac enzyme abnormalities may represent false-positive elevations in patients with skeletal muscle trauma, alcohol ingestion, or a variety of other conditions, but unlike the electrocardiographic criteria of ST segment elevation, such abnormalities are virtually always found in patients with acute myocardial infarction. By combining a sensitive test with a specific test, such as the combination of cardiac enzymes with an electrocardiogram, a physician may be able to integrate information and avoid both false-positive and false-negative diagnoses. Alternatively, sometimes a single test, such as a pulmonary angiogram for the diagnosis of pulmonary embolism, has sufficiently high sensitivity and specificity to serve as the ultimate arbiter of a clinical diagnosis, even though it is not a perfect predictor of the pathoanatomy.

A set of principles for evaluating and applying the results of studies of diagnostic tests can be used as a general approach to interpreting the medical literature (Box 2–1). It is critical that a test be compared with the results of an independent gold standard performed and

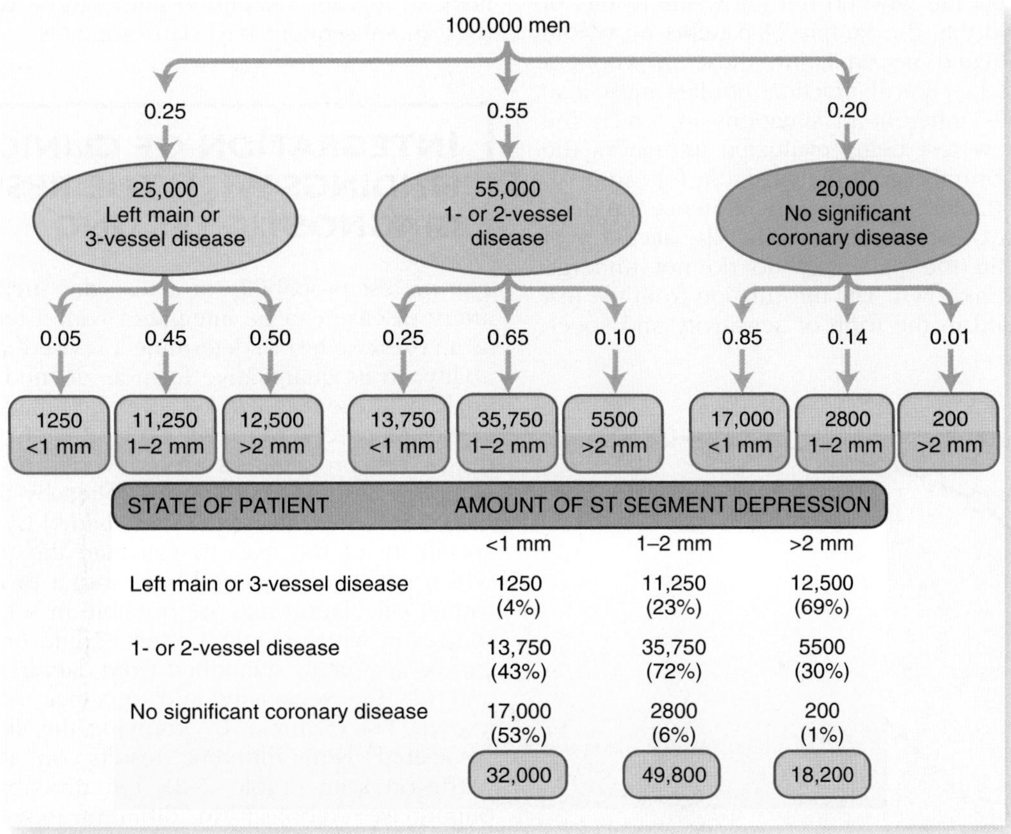

FIGURE 2–2. Cohort flow model of Bayes' rule for interpretation of an exercise tolerance test in a 50-year-old man with typical angina. Consider a cohort of 100,000 such men: 25% have left main or three-vessel disease, 55% have one- or two-vessel disease, and 20% are free of significant coronary disease. If the conditional probabilities of less than 1 mm, 1 to 2 mm, and greater than 2 mm of ST segment depression are as shown and determine how many men from each diagnostic subgroup will have each finding, of the 1250 + 13,750 + 17,000 (or 32,000) men with less than 1 mm of ST segment depression, 17,000, or 53%, will have no significant coronary disease, 43% will have one- or two-vessel disease, and 4% will have left main or three-vessel disease. (Data from Diamond GA, Forrester JS: Analysis of probability as an aid in the clinical diagnosis of coronary artery disease. N Engl J Med 1979;300:1350.)

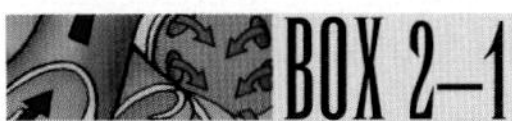

Evaluating and Applying the Results of Studies of Diagnostic Tests

ARE THE RESULTS OF THE STUDY VALID?

Primary guides

Did the study include an independent, blind comparison with a reference standard?

Did the patient sample include an appropriate spectrum of patients to whom the diagnostic test will be applied in clinical practice?

Secondary guides

Did the results of the test being evaluated influence the decision to perform the reference standard?

Were the methods for performing the test described in sufficient detail to permit replication?

WHAT ARE THE RESULTS?

Are likelihood ratios for the test results presented or are the data necessary for their calculation provided?

WILL THE RESULTS HELP ME IN CARING FOR MY PATIENTS?

Will the reproducibility of the test result and its interpretation be satisfactory in my setting?

Are the results applicable to my patient?

Will the results change my management?

Will patients be better off as a result of the test?

From Jaeschke R, Guyatt GH, Sackett DL, for the Evidence-Based Medicine Working Group: Users' guides to the medical literature. III. How to use an article about a diagnostic test. B. What are the results and will they help me in caring for my patients? JAMA 1994;271:703–707.

interpreted by people who do not know the results of the new test and that the sample of patients on whom the test is evaluated be similar to those in whom it would be used in clinical practice. Studies must also avoid the biases inherent in situations in which the result of the new test being evaluated influences the decision to perform the gold standard test; for example, if the results of thallium scintigraphy influence the decision to perform coronary angiography, the accuracy of the scintigram in the patients who do not undergo angiography is unknown. The information from the test must be provided in the form of sensitivity and specificity so that the likelihood ratio can be calculated and used in subsequent bayesian estimates.

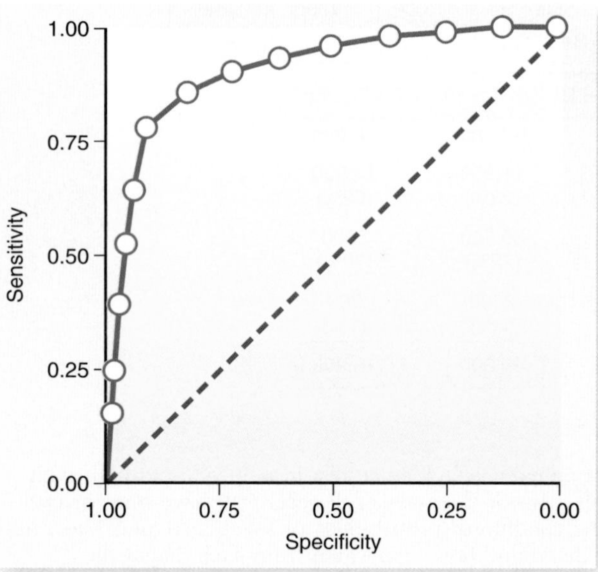

FIGURE 2–3. For any diagnostic test, an increase in sensitivity will be associated with an inherent tradeoff that lowers specificity. Better tests are associated with curves closer to the upper left corner, whereas tests near the 45-degree angle are of little value. The curve can be used to help decide the definition of a normal as compared with an abnormal test result.

INTEGRATION OF CLINICAL FINDINGS WITH THE RESULTS OF DIAGNOSTIC TESTING

The pretest probability of a disorder such as coronary artery disease can be integrated with a test result such as an exercise test to determine a revised, posttest probability. In its quantitative form as defined by *bayesian* analysis, these data can be combined mathematically to arrive at a precise probability (Fig. 2–4). In this example, the pretest probabilities are converted to odds as in a gambling wager and then multiplied by the likelihood ratio (the sensitivity of the test divided by 1, minus the specificity of the test) to calculate the posttest odds, which are then converted back into a probability. This formal calculation may be possible in selected circumstances in which (1) the pretest diagnostic probabilities can be accurately quantified from data in the literature, and (2) the sensitivity and specificity of a test are known. For example, by knowing the likelihood ratio associated with different results on a ventilation-perfusion scan (Table 2–2), the probability of acute pulmonary embolism in different types of patients with these scan findings can be estimated (Table 2–3). A similar, simple approach can help estimate the probability of coronary disease given varying results on exercise testing and thallium scintigraphy in patients with typical anginal pain, patients with atypical pain potentially consistent with coronary disease, or asymptomatic patients in the age range in which coronary disease is often found (Figs. 2–5 through 2–7). Similar information can also be generated via graphs that help integrate prior probabilities with diagnostic test results (Fig. 2–8). In other circumstances, such formal calculations may be impossible or inappropriate because of inadequate information on the pretest probability or on the

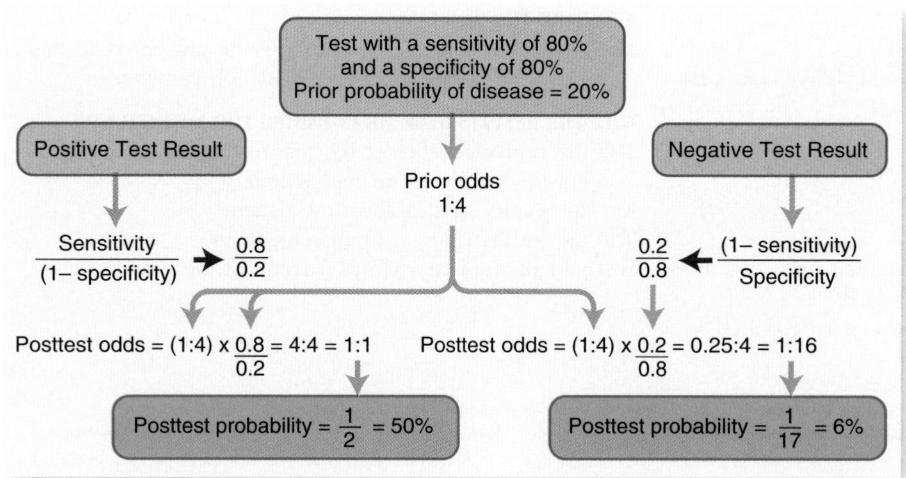

FIGURE 2–4. Bayesian analysis using odds and likelihood ratios to calculate a posttest probability.

TABLE 2–2

Test Properties of Ventilation-Perfusion ($\dot{V}/\dot{Q}$) Scanning

	Pulmonary Embolism				
	Present		*Absent*		
$\dot{V}/\dot{Q}$ Scan Result	***No.***	***Proportion***	***No.***	***Proportion***	**Likelihood Ratio**
High probability	102	102/251 = 0.406	14	14/630 = 0.022	18.3
Intermediate probability	105	105/251 = 0.418	217	217/630 = 0.344	1.2
Low probability	39	39/251 = 0.155	273	273/630 = 0.433	0.36
Normal/near normal	5	5/251 = 0.020	126	126/630 = 0.200	0.10
Total	251	—	630	—	—

From Jaeschke R, Guyatt GH, Sackett DL, for the Evidence-Based Medicine Working Group: Users' guides to the medical literature. III. How to use an article about a diagnostic test. B. What are the results and will they help me in caring for my patients? JAMA 1994;271:703–707. Copyright 1994, American Medical Association.

TABLE 2–3

Pretest Probabilities, Likelihood Ratios of Ventilation-Perfusion Scan Results, and Posttest Probabilities in Two Patients with Pulmonary Embolus

Pretest Probability, % (Range)*	Scan Result (LR)	Posttest Probability, % (Range)*
78-Year-Old Woman with Sudden Onset of Dyspnea after Abdominal Surgery		
70 (60–80)	High probability (18.3)	97 (96–99)
70 (60–80)	Intermediate probability (1.2)	74 (64–83)
70 (60–80)	Low probability (0.36)	46 (35–59)
70 (60–80)	Normal/near normal (0.1)	19 (13–29)
28-Year-Old Man with Dyspnea and Atypical Chest Pain		
20 (10–30)	High probability (18.3)	82 (67–89)
20 (10–30)	Intermediate probability (1.2)	23 (12–34)
20 (10–30)	Low probability (0.36)	8 (4–16)
20 (10–30)	Normal/near normal (0.1)	2 (1–4)

*The values in parentheses represent a plausible range of pretest probabilities. That is, although the best guess regarding the pretest probability is 70%, values of 60% to 80% would also be reasonable estimates.

LR, likelihood ratio.

From Jaeschke R, Guyatt GH, Sackett DL, for the Evidence-Based Medicine Working Group: Users' guides to the medical literature. III. How to use an article about a diagnostic test. B. What are the results and will they help me in caring for my patients? JAMA 1994;271:703–707. Copyright 1994, American Medical Association.

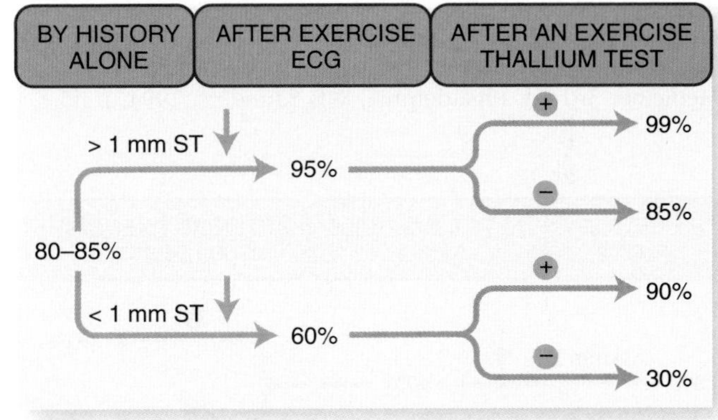

FIGURE 2–5. Approximate probability of coronary artery disease before and after noninvasive testing in a patient with typical angina pectoris. These percentages demonstrate how the sequential use of an electrocardiogram (ECG) and an exercise thallium test may affect the probability of coronary artery disease in a patient with typical angina pectoris. (Redrawn from Branch WB Jr [ed]: Office Practice of Medicine, 3rd ed. Philadelphia, WB Saunders, 1994, p 45.)

sensitivity or specificity of the diagnostic test, but the general bayesian approach may still be helpful.

A key assumption in bayesian analysis is that a test adds new, incremental information above and beyond what is already previously known. If a test simply duplicates previous information, it is not helpful. For example, an estimation of ejection fraction by a radionuclide ventriculogram does not add new, independent information to a similar estimation by echocardiography. In contrast, the information obtained by thallium or sestamibi scintigraphy appears to add incrementally to information that can be obtained from the history, physical examination, and standard exercise electrocardiogram.

The Threshold Approach

Diagnostic tests are most helpful when they change a probability across a decision-making threshold. Oftentimes, this threshold is not 50% and may well be far lower. For example, a test that lowers the probability of aortic dissection to 49% would not be considered reassuring because the decision-making threshold for proceeding in the evaluation and potential treatment of this life-threatening condition should be lower. In such

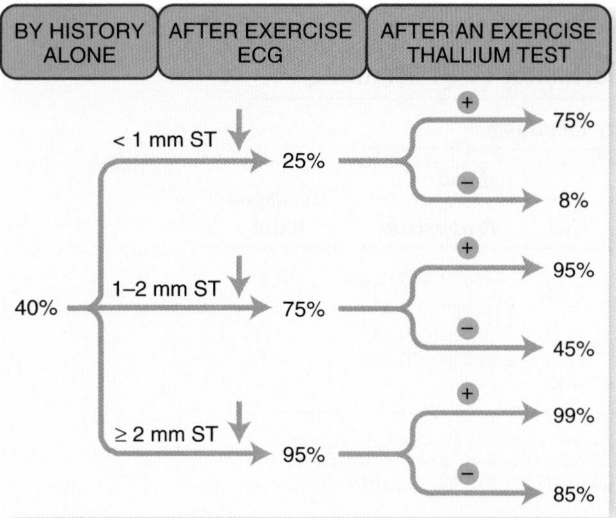

FIGURE 2–6. Approximate probability of coronary artery disease before and after noninvasive testing in a patient with atypical angina symptoms. ECG, electrocardiogram. (Redrawn from Branch WB Jr [ed]: Office Practice of Medicine, 3rd ed. Philadelphia, WB Saunders, 1994, p 45.)

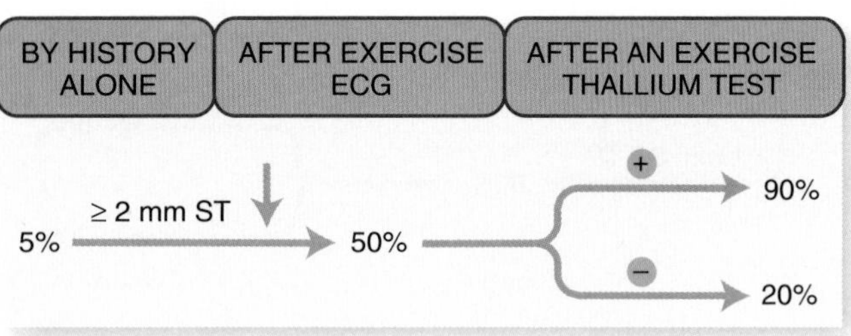

Figure 2–7. Approximate probability of coronary artery disease before and after noninvasive testing in an asymptomatic subject in the coronary artery disease age range. ECG, electrocardiogram. (Redrawn from Branch WB Jr [ed]: Office Practice of Medicine, 3rd ed. Philadelphia, WB Saunders, 1994, p 45.)

a situation, a test must be sensitive enough for detecting aortic dissection so that a negative test result reduces the probability to a sufficiently low level. In other situations, it may be useful to divide patients into three different probability groups: one appropriate for immediate treatment, one appropriate for further testing, and one in which no further evaluation is indicated. Unfortunately, for many conditions the precise threshold that should guide clinical decision making has not been determined.

Diagnostic tests may be useful for confirming a finding on physical examination, reassuring a patient, or reassuring the physician. However, they are most likely to be useful when they may lead to a sufficient change in the diagnostic probability that the management of a patient will be altered.

In deciding whether to order a test, the physician must decide not only whether the test is sufficiently

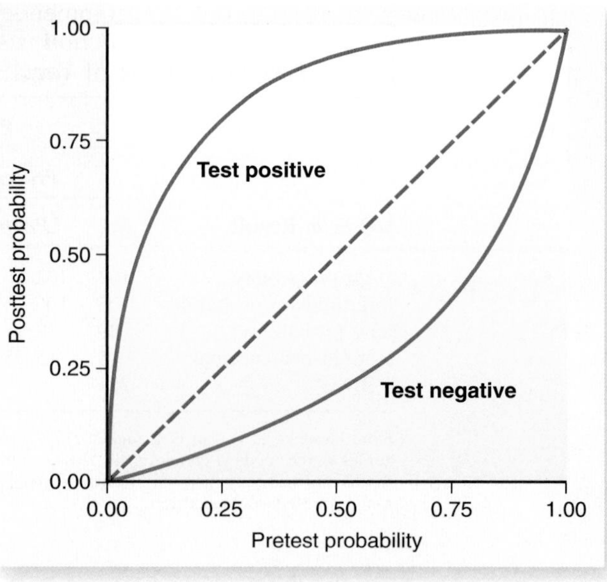

FIGURE 2–8. How the pretest probability affects the posttest probability of disease. The same test result has far different implications depending on the pretest probability.

accurate (high sensitivity and specificity) for the condition in question but also how likely it is that the patient has the condition under consideration, what the adverse consequences would be if the condition were missed or the patient were inappropriately treated for a condition that is not present, and how likely it is that the test will have a sufficient impact on the probability of disease to influence the diagnosis or treatment. In making these decisions, the physician must consider the benefits, risks, and cost of the test, as well as other alternatives such as continued observation or proceeding immediately to another test or empiric treatment.

Various studies on the ordering patterns and impact of cardiac nuclear medicine procedures and echocardiograms have found that such tests lead to an appropriate change in diagnosis in about 20% to 25% of cases and to an appropriate change in therapy in about 10% of cases in which they are ordered. These findings do not imply that all tests that do not lead to a change in diagnosis or management were inappropriate to order, unless they did not meet the criteria enumerated previously.

Prediction Rules

Aggregated information from large numbers of patients in data banks or prospective cohort studies can be used to assess the pretest probability for various diagnoses or outcomes.[1] When appropriately validated in prospective testing, these probabilities can be used to guide clinical decision making. For example, data on many thousands of patients with chest pain have been used to derive estimates of the likelihood that such patients are having an acute myocardial infarction and to then validate these estimates prospectively (see Fig. 6–1).

When probabilities are used to derive recommended decisions, they may be used to create a *prediction rule.* For prediction rules to be useful, they must be derived and tested in patient populations that are relevant to the clinician and must use clinical findings or diagnostic tests that are both readily available and reproducible.

WEIGHING RISKS AND BENEFITS

All clinicians intuitively compare the risks of tests and treatments with their probable benefits. In some situations, definitive data from large randomized trials may be available so that this process is simple and straightforward, such as the value of reperfusion therapy for acute myocardial infarction. In other situations, however, an individual patient may not be similar to those who have been included in randomized trials, or the precise question may not have been subjected to an appropriate trial. In these circumstances, decision analysis provides a quantitative method for comparing risks with benefits.[2] It should be emphasized that formal decision analysis is oftentimes much too cumbersome to be used by individual physicians, but published decision analyses may help guide decisions in the absence of definitive data from randomized trials. However, decision analyses can be no more accurate than the data on which they are based, and sometimes the uncertainties are sufficiently large that the analyses cannot be considered conclusive.

Decision Analysis

A typical decision analysis (Fig. 2–9) considers the choices (decisions) that the physician must make (the square box or node labeled *A*), as well as the probabilities of the various events that may depend on each decision (circular nodes *B* to *S*). For each of these probabilities, an estimate is commonly derived from the literature or based on the best possible expert opinion. Each of the possible ultimate outcomes is then assigned a *utility* or relative value. An outcome of perfect health may be assigned a utility of 1.0, whereas death may be assigned an outcome of zero. Outcomes that are associated with survival in less than perfect health may be assigned utilities based on the cumulative quality of life associated with the outcome, such as life with angina or after a cerebrovascular accident. After a utility corresponding with the outcome has been assigned to each terminal branch of the decision tree, all the terminal branches related to a choice (decision) node can be summed and averaged to determine the *expected value* of the choices emanating from that node. The preferred decision would be the one that yields the highest average expected value after all its potential outcomes have been considered.

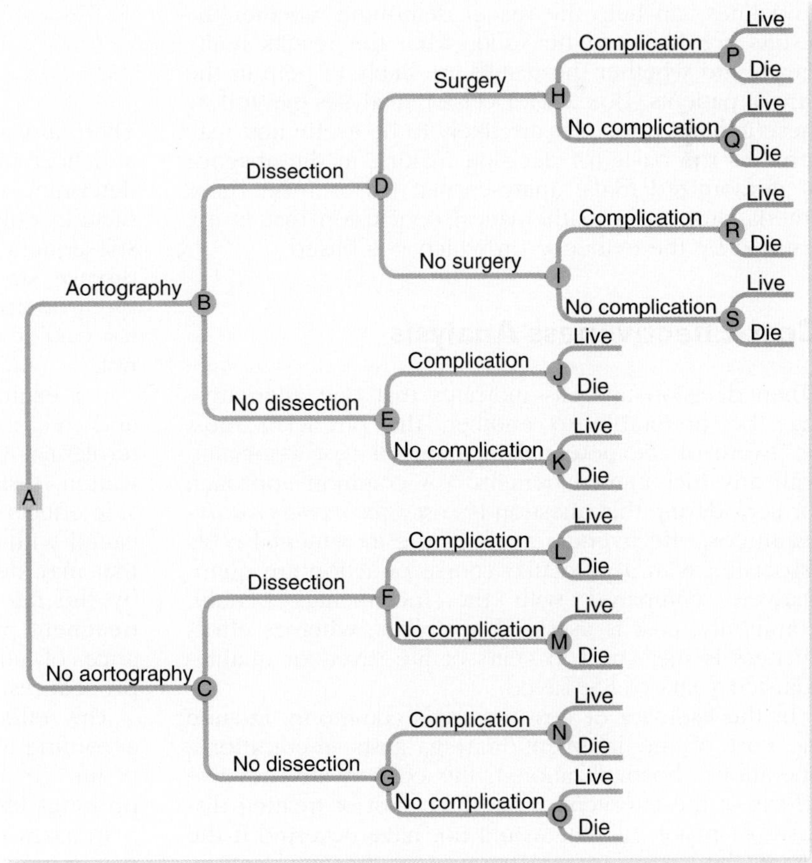

FIGURE 2–9. Simplified decision tree for deciding whether to perform aortography in a patient who has a suspected aortic dissection, assuming that surgery is performed only if the results of aortography are positive. The *square* node represents the decision point, and the *round* nodes denote the chance events for which probabilities can be estimated.

Decision analyses often require estimates and sometimes even guesswork to assign the necessary probabilities and utilities. For example, although it is critical to adjust future years of life for their quality, especially in patients in whom a complication such as intracranial hemorrhage may develop or in those who derive an advantage such as a smaller infarction with less heart failure, these adjustments often cannot be determined accurately.

Because decision analysis is so inherently dependent on a variety of estimates, it is critical that *sensitivity analyses* be performed to demonstrate how conceivable differences in each of these estimates or assumptions will alter the ultimate conclusions. Many decision analyses intentionally use conservative estimates to demonstrate that an intervention is still valuable despite such conservatism, or they may include more radical assumptions to prove that the intervention is safe despite the most hazardous of assumptions.

Sometimes, decision analyses will demonstrate a dramatic difference between two options and definitively influence decision making even in the absence of a randomized trial. In other situations, the analysis may reveal that the decision is such a close call that either alternative is reasonable, or it may suggest that unmeasured or unmeasurable factors should be the ultimate arbiter of decision making, such as a patient's preferences or local experience or expertise. Even when the analysis seems to be definitive, care must be taken to be sure that other, unconsidered factors would not alter the conclusion.

In evaluating decision analyses, several general guidelines can help the reader determine whether the results are likely to be valid, what the results really mean, and whether the results are likely to help in the care of patients (Box 2–2). Decision analyses that follow these general principles are likely to be useful and may serve as the basis for decision making in the absence of randomized trials; analyses that fail to meet these criteria propose a mathematical conclusion that is not justified by the evidence on which it is based.

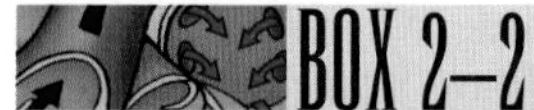

Users' Guides for Clinical Decision Analysis

ARE THE RESULTS VALID?

Were all the important strategies and outcomes included?

Was an explicit and sensible process used to identify, select, and combine the evidence into probabilities?

Were the utilities obtained in an explicit and sensible way from credible sources?

Was the potential impact of any uncertainty in the evidence determined?

WHAT ARE THE RESULTS?

In the baseline analysis, does one strategy result in a clinically important gain for patients? If not, is the result a toss-up?

How strong is the evidence used in the analysis?

Could the uncertainty in the evidence change the result?

WILL THE RESULTS HELP ME IN CARING FOR MY PATIENTS?

Do the probability estimates fit my patients' clinical features?

Do the utilities reflect how my patients would value the outcomes of the decision?

From Richardson WS, Detsky AS, for the Evidence-Based Medicine Working Group: Users' guides to the medical literature. VII. How to use a clinical decision analysis? A. Are the results of the study valid? JAMA 1995;273:1292–1295.

Cost-Effectiveness Analysis

When decision analysis indicates that one alternative may be preferable to another, the physician must be aware of the potential incremental cost associated with any incremental benefit.[3, 4] A common approach for considering this question is *cost-effectiveness analysis.* In cost-effectiveness analysis, the incremental costs associated with a particular course of action are quantitatively compared with the incremental benefit. Commonly, cost is assessed in dollars, whereas effectiveness is measured in years of life saved or quality-adjusted years of life saved.

In the estimate of cost, analyses commonly include the cost of the intervention (e.g., tests, medications, operations, hospitalizations), the cost of any adverse effects of the intervention, and the cost of treating diseases or problems that would not have occurred if the patient had not survived because of the intervention. Then, any savings from medications, tests, procedures, and hospitalizations that are avoided are deducted to determine the net cost. For simplicity, most analyses include only disease-specific subsequent costs, so the subsequent cost of cardiovascular disease (e.g., heart disease, stroke) is considered in a patient who is saved by thrombolysis, but the potential eventual cost of care for cancer or Alzheimer's disease among survivors is not.

For example, consider a comparison of medication and no medication in patients with hypercholesterolemia. The cost would include the cost of the medication, tests needed to monitor the medication, and side effects of the medication, as well as any cost associated with the potential treatment of coronary disease that may develop in the additional days of life gained by the intervention. The savings associated with the treatment program include those related to the avoidance of subsequent myocardial infarction, coronary procedures, or other medications.

The effectiveness of an intervention is estimated according to how it changes life expectancy or quality of life. An intervention may be worthwhile because it prolongs life, improves quality, or does both.

In assessing both cost and benefit, it is important to determine when each will be realized. For many health care programs, cost is incurred immediately in the form of medications or procedures, whereas the benefit may be delayed until well into the future. Because other events or unexpected developments may occur in the interim, the expectation or even promise of future benefit is not generally valued as highly as the realization of immediate benefit. This principle, commonly called *discounting*, is independent of monetary inflation and recognizes the common aphorism that a bird in the hand is worth two in the bush. In simple terms, if one had $10 to spend, one would rather see an immediate benefit than a promise of a similar benefit 5 years from now.

The Cost-Effectiveness Ratio

Very few health interventions both reduce cost and increase quality-adjusted life expectancy. In the calculation of a *cost-effectiveness ratio*, the relative benefit to be gained from an investment in different health programs can be assessed and compared. In such an approach, it is critical that the *incremental cost* and *incremental benefit* of the program be assessed. For example, because streptokinase is already known to be beneficial at a reasonable cost in comparison to conservative treatment of patients with acute myocardial infarction and ST segment elevation, any assessment of tissue plasminogen activator or primary angioplasty should be compared with streptokinase, unless the patient has a contraindication to it, rather than with conservative treatment.

Just as the interpretation of a diagnostic test depends not only on its own intrinsic sensitivity and specificity but also on the previous probability or prevalence in patients on whom it is being used, cost-effectiveness analysis depends not only on the cost and effectiveness of the intervention but also on the risk status of patients in whom the intervention is being considered. The same intervention may be associated with a very favorable cost-effectiveness ratio in high-risk patients but a much less favorable ratio in low-risk patients (Box 2–3). A common metric for a favorable cost-effectiveness ratio is the $35,000 to $50,000 per year of life saved by chronic renal dialysis, a cost that American society has indicated it is willing to pay.

It is oftentimes difficult to compare cost-effectiveness ratios from one study with those of another because of their varying assumptions. As noted previously, some analyses may have used particularly conservative or generous assumptions to prove a point, and it is difficult to update both the clinical and the cost assumptions of studies that were performed in the past.

CLINICAL GUIDELINES

Based on the state of clinical evidence (see Chapter 1) and on a consideration of the risks, costs, and benefits of various tests or treatments, physicians and organizations have increasingly tried to develop guidelines for

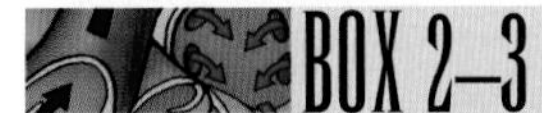

BOX 2–3

Example of Cost, Effectiveness, and Cost-Effectiveness for a Hypothetic Intervention in 10,000 Patients for 5 Years* (High-Risk Patients versus Low-Risk Patients)

	HIGH RISK		LOW RISK	
	Untreated	*Treated*	*Untreated*	*Treated*
Annual death rate	10%	5%	1%	0.5%
Years of life saved†	0	5209	0	614
Cost of treatment ($ millions) at $2000/yr	0	90.5	0	99.0
Annual CABG rate	6%	3%	0.6%	0.3%
Cost/CABG	$20,000	$20,000	$20,000	$20,000
Annual MI rate	4%	2%	0.4%	0.2%
Cost/MI	$10,000	$10,000	$10,000	$10,000
Annual rate of other events	4%	2%	0.4%	0.2%
Cost/other event	$5000	$5000	$5000	$5000
Medical costs ($ millions)	70.0	39.7	8.8	4.4
Total cost ($ millions)	70.0	130.2	8.8	103.4
Total cost difference ($ millions)		60.2		94.8
Approximate cost/yr of life saved		$11,500		$155,000

*Simplified so that the intervention reduces all risks by 50%, neither costs nor health effects are discounted, all patients are assumed to die at midyear, and the analysis considers only the first 5 years.

†By life-table analysis.

CABG, coronary artery bypass graft surgery; MI, myocardial infarction.

From Goldman L, Garber AM, Grover SA, Hlatky MA: Task Force 6. Cost effectiveness of assessment and management of risk factors. J Am Coll Cardiol 1996;27:1020–1030. Reprinted with permission from the American College of Cardiology.

medical practice. Guidelines, which are usually voluntary, provide consensus approaches to reducing the use of unnecessary tests and treatments and increasing the use of tests and treatments that have been shown to be beneficial at a reasonable cost. Guidelines have the potential to reduce inappropriate variations[5] in practice patterns and to make major improvements in the outcomes of individual patients and entire populations.[6] Although some physicians have been reluctant to embrace guidelines for a variety of reasons ranging from disagreement with individual guidelines to fear about the loss of autonomy,[7] the American Heart Association and American College of Cardiology have increasingly developed and promulgated a wide range of clinical guidelines, many of which serve as the basis for the evidence-based recommendations in this text (Box 2–4).

DISCUSSIONS WITH PATIENTS AND DERIVATION OF THE FINAL PLAN

In conjunction with quantitative estimates based on the medical literature and on the physician's experience, the patient's preferences must be taken into account.[8] Although quantitative assessment of quality of life may be included in many decision and cost-effectiveness analyses, these quantitative approaches are not ideally suited to full consideration of the preferences, attitudes, and individuality of a single patient.

The physician must be cognizant of the benefits, risks, and costs of various options and be an advocate rather than a gatekeeper in advising an individual

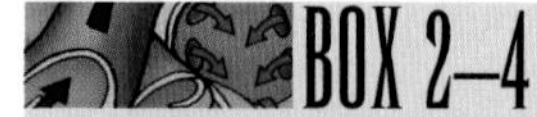

BOX 2–4

Grading of Recommendations in Clinical Guidelines—Three Different Classification Systems

A. American College of Cardiology/American Heart Association guidelines for the appropriateness of various tests and procedures in different clinical settings.

CLASS	DEFINITION
I	Conditions for which there is evidence or general agreement that a given procedure or treatment is useful and effective
II	Conditions for which there is conflicting evidence or a divergence of opinion about the usefulness/efficacy of a procedure
IIa	Weight of evidence/opinion is in favor of usefulness/efficacy
IIb	Usefulness/efficacy is less well established by evidence/opinion
III	Conditions for which there is evidence or general agreement that the procedure/treatment is not useful/effective and in some cases may be harmful

B. Evidence-based cardiology*

Grade A	Level 1 evidence†
Grade B	Level 2–4 evidence†
Grade C	Level 5 evidence†

C. Clinical Evidence‡

Beneficial	Interventions whose effectiveness has been demonstrated by clear evidence from randomized controlled trials and for which harm is likely to be small in comparison with the benefits
Likely to be beneficial	Interventions for which effectiveness is less well established than for those listed under "beneficial"
Tradeoff between benefit and harm	Interventions for which clinicians and patients should compare the beneficial and harmful effects according to individual circumstances and priorities
Unknown effectiveness	Interventions for which data are currently insufficient or of inadequate quality
Unlikely to be beneficial	Interventions for which lack of effectiveness is less well established than for those listed under "likely to be ineffective or harmful"
Likely to be ineffective or harmful	Interventions whose ineffectiveness or harmfulness has been demonstrated by clear evidence

*Adapted from Yusuf S, Cairns JA, Camm AJ, et al (eds): Evidence-Based Cardiology. London, BMJ Publishing Group, 1998, p xxvi.
†See Box 1–6.
‡Adapted from Barton S (ed): Clinical Evidence, Issue 5. London, BMJ Publishing Group, 2001, p xiv.

patient. In conjunction with the patient and the family, it is the physician's responsibility to help set priorities and make recommendations. Although physicians also have a responsibility to recognize the limits and restrictions of society and have a collective duty to try to influence societal priorities,[9, 10] the physician's responsibility to the individual patient is paramount.[11] In an era of capitation and financial incentives to reduce unnecessary testing and treatment, physicians must be careful to not underuse effective and worthwhile tests and treatments. It is also the physician's responsibility to be sure that the patient and family are fully informed about the various options so that the ultimate course of action is a collective decision based on the best available quantitative and qualitative information.

References

1. McGinn TG, Guyatt GH, Wyer PC, et al: Users' guides to the medical literature XXII: How to use articles about clinical decision rules. JAMA 2000;284:79–84.
2. Petitti DB: Meta-Analysis, Decision Analysis, and Cost-Effectiveness Analysis, 2nd ed. New York, Oxford University Press, 2000.
3. Meltzer MI: Introduction to health economics for physicians. Lancet 2001;358:993–998.
4. Prosser LA, Stinnett AA, Goldman PA, et al: Cost-effectiveness of cholesterol-lowering therapies according to selected patient characteristics. Ann Intern Med 2000; 132:769–779.
5. Go AS, Rao RK, Dauterman KW, Massie BM: A systematic review of the effects of physician specialty on the treatment of coronary disease and heart failure in the United States. Am J Med 2000;108:216–226.
6. Philips KA, Shlipak MG, Coxson P, et al: Health and economic benefits of increased ß-blocker use following myocardial infarction. JAMA 2000;284:2748–2754.
7. Cabana MD, Rand CS, Powe NR, et al: Why don't physicians follow clinical practice guidelines? A framework for improvement. JAMA 1999;282:1458–1465.
8. McAlister FA, Straus SE, Gyatt GH, Haynes RB: User's guides to the medical literature XX. Integrating research evidence with the care of the individual patient. JAMA 2000;283:2829–2836.
9. Oliver A, Healey A, Donaldson C: Choosing the method to match the perspective: Economic assessment and its implications for health-services efficiency. Lancet 2002; 359:1771–1774.
10. Lopert R, Lang DL, Hill SR, Henry DA: Differential pricing of drugs: A role for cost-effectiveness analysis? Lancet 2002;359:2105–2107.
11. Lo B: Resolving Ethical Dilemmas. A Guide for Clinicians, 2nd ed. Philadelphia, Lippincott Williams & Wilkins, 2000.

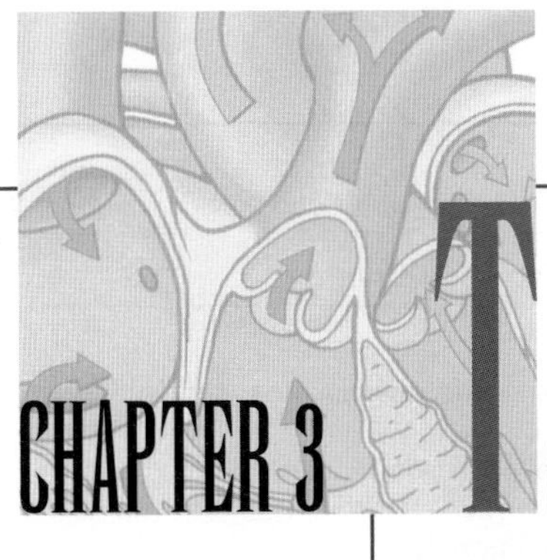

CHAPTER 3 The Clinical Examination

Eugene Braunwald

Since development of the electrocardiograph by Einthoven and the radiograph by Roentgen a century ago, a series of ever more accurate noninvasive and invasive tests have been developed to characterize the structure and function of the cardiovascular system. However valuable these tests may be, they are not inexpensive, are sometimes uncomfortable or hazardous, and can provide conflicting information. The decision to undertake any specialized test of the cardiovascular system must be made in light of the findings on the clinical examination, that is, the history and physical examination.[1, 2] The primary care physician's findings on clinical examination are of the utmost importance in deciding whether specialized testing should be performed, whether continued observation is advisable, whether the advice of a consultant should be sought, or whether the patient can be reassured that serious cardiovascular disease is not present.[3, 4]

Many cardiovascular conditions are part of systemic illnesses, and in conducting the clinical examination, the primary care physician must be aware of three major pitfalls: (1) failure to recognize cardiovascular manifestations in patients with recognized systemic illnesses frequently associated with heart disease, such as congenital heart disease in a patient with Down's syndrome; (2) failure to recognize the presence of an underlying systemic disorder in a patient with recognized cardiovascular disease, such as thyrotoxicosis in a patient with unexplained atrial fibrillation; and (3) failure to recognize the cardiac cause of extracardiac manifestations of cardiac disease, such as severe jaundice in a patient with acute right ventricular failure. Table 3–1 lists a number of abnormalities found during examination of the extremities, skin, eyes, and abdomen that may be observed in patients with cardiovascular disorders.

SYSTEMIC DISORDERS WITH CARDIOVASCULAR MANIFESTATIONS

The noncardiac history and physical examination are of critical importance in a patient with known or suspected cardiovascular disease because of the high frequency of cardiovascular manifestations in many systemic disorders. For example, endocrine abnormalities commonly have important cardiac manifestations, thyrotoxicosis can intensify angina and cause atrial fibrillation and high-output heart failure, myxedema can be responsible for dilated cardiomyopathy and pericardial effusion, and acromegaly often causes dilated and hypertrophic cardiomyopathy. A number of endocrine disorders—Cushing's syndrome, primary hyperaldosteronism, pheochromocytoma, and hyperparathyroidism—may cause hypertension, whereas diabetes may be associated with premature and especially severe atherosclerotic coronary disease. Rheumatoid arthritis may be responsible for constrictive pericarditis, cardiac tamponade, and valvular heart disease, most commonly aortic regurgitation; systemic lupus erythematosus may be associated with mitral regurgitation and pericarditis; and systemic sclerosis may occur with pericarditis, systemic hypertension, pulmonary hypertension, and restrictive cardiomyopathy. Among hematologic disorders, chronic anemia may cause high-output heart failure, polycythemia is associated with an increased risk of clotting, including coronary thrombosis, and hemochromatosis can result in restrictive cardiomyopathy.

A variety of tumors can metastasize to the pericardium and cause cardiac constriction or tamponade,

TABLE 3–1

Noncardiac Physical Findings in Cardiac Disorders

Physical Finding	Cause	Cardiac Condition
General Appearance		
Shaking of body with each heartbeat	Increased stroke volume	Severe aortic regurgitation, third-degree AV block
Weight loss, malnutrition, cachexia	Reduced cardiac output, hypermetabolism	Advanced chronic heart failure
Marked obesity, somnolence, cyanosis	Impaired ventilation, pickwickian syndrome	Cor pulmonale
Long extremities, arm span > height, pubis–foot > head–pubis, arachnodactyly (spider fingers)	Marfan's syndrome	Thoracic aortic aneurysm, mitral valve prolapse
Bones and Skeleton		
Short stature, cubitus valgus, medial deviation of forearm	Turner's syndrome	Coarctation of the aorta, bicuspid aortic valve
Deformities of radius, thumb with extra phalanx	Holt-Oram syndrome	Familial atrial septal defect
Clubbing of digits	Cyanosis	Congenital heart disease, cor pulmonale, pulmonary arteriovenous fistula, infective endocarditis
Severe kyphoscoliosis	Congenital	Cor pulmonale, Marfan's syndrome
Skin		
Bronze pigmentation of skin, loss of axillary and pubic hair	Hemochromatosis	Restrictive cardiomyopathy
Jaundice	Cardiac cirrhosis, hemochromatosis	Congestive heart failure, tricuspid valve disease, chronic constrictive pericarditis
Small, brown, macular lesions on head and trunk	Lentigines	Hypertrophic cardiomyopathy, pulmonary stenosis
Xanthoma, tuboeruptive (extensive surface of extremities), striatum palmare (palmar and digital creases)	Subcutaneous deposits of cholesterol	Premature atherosclerosis
Small, tender, purplish, erythematous skin lesions in pads of fingers or toes	Osler's nodes	Infective endocarditis
Petechiae, especially under nail beds	Splinter hemorrhage	Infective endocarditis
Raised, nontender hemorrhagic lesions in palms or soles	Janeway's lesions	Infective endocarditis
Capillary hemangiomas in skin, lips, nasal mucosa, gastrointestinal tract	Hereditary telangiectasis (Osler-Weber-Rendu disease)	Pulmonary arteriovenous fistula with cyanosis
Eyes		
Exopthalmos and stare	Hyperthyroidism, increased adrenergic tone	High-output heart failure
Ptosis; dull, expressionless face	Myotonic dystrophy	AV block, arrhythmias
Ptosis with external ophthalmoplegia	Kearns-Sayre syndrome	Third-degree AV block
Blue sclerae	Osteogenesis imperfecta	Aortic dilatation, regurgitation, and dissection; mitral valve prolapse
Retinal changes	Arteriolar narrowing	Hypertension
Beading of retinal artery	Hypercholesterolemia	Atherosclerosis
White-centered retinal hemorrhage near optic disk	Roth's spots	Embolization secondary to infective endocarditis
Retinal artery occlusion	Embolus	Atrial fibrillation, mitral stenosis, left atrial myxoma, atherosclerosis of ascending aorta or arch vessels
Cyanosis involving conjunctivae and mucous membranes (central cyanosis)	Arterial desaturation	Intracardiac or intrapulmonary right-to-left shunting
Cyanosis of cool, exposed extremities (peripheral cyanosis)	Impaired perfusion	Heart failure, shock, Raynaud's phenomenon
Abdomen		
Splenomegaly, hepatomegaly, ascites	Severe hepatic congestion	Constrictive pericarditis, tricuspid valve disease
Palpable, enlarged kidney	Polycystic renal disease	Hypertension
Systolic bruit over abdomen	Renal artery stenosis	Hypertension

AV, atrioventricular.

as well as arrhythmias. A number of cardiovascular disorders may occur during pregnancy, including preeclampsia manifested as hypertension, aggravation of symptoms in patients with congenital or valvular heart disease, and primary pulmonary hypertension. Skeletal muscular dystrophies can be associated with various cardiac manifestations, including arrhythmias and dilated and restrictive cardiomyopathies. Chronic renal failure may be associated with pericarditis, systemic hypertension, and accelerated atherosclerosis.

THE HISTORY

Questionnaires and screening histories by nurses or assistants are often quite useful in focusing the physician's questioning, and directed interval histories can frequently be obtained by others, but the first definitive clinical examination should not be delegated by the physician. Important nuances may be appreciated only by the physician, and it is through taking a careful history that physicians can gain their patients' confidence, which is often necessary when agreement must be obtained to undergo complex, uncomfortable, and sometimes risky diagnostic maneuvers and therapeutic interventions.[1]

Initially, when obtaining the history, patients should be encouraged to describe any complaints in their own way, followed by directed interrogation regarding the onset, progression, and timing of symptoms, as well as a description of their aggravating and alleviating conditions. A detailed general medical history, including an occupational, family, and nutritional history, is of critical importance in a patient with known or suspected cardiovascular disease. For example, a history of recent infection, dental extraction, urogenital manipulation, or intravenous drug abuse is vital in the evaluation of patients with known or suspected congenital heart disease or acquired valvular abnormalities because the history may suggest the presence of infective endocarditis. A history of cigarette smoking, hypertension, hypercholesterolemia, or diabetes mellitus and a history of premature vascular disease in first-degree relatives are risk factors for coronary artery disease. Atherosclerosis is usually a diffuse vascular disease, and a history or clinical manifestations of such disease in one arterial bed—coronary, cerebral, renal, aortic, peripheral, or mesenteric—raise the likelihood of its presence in other beds.

When symptoms suggestive of cardiac disease are present, such as dyspnea or chest pain, their aggravation by activity and relief by rest support their cardiovascular origin. Symptoms at rest, of course, do not exclude serious cardiovascular disease because most cardiac arrhythmias, Prinzmetal's angina, and paroxysmal nocturnal dyspnea characteristically occur at rest. The response to therapy is also a critical part of the history. Patients in whom hypertension is first diagnosed and whose blood pressure fails to respond to adequate doses of two different classes of antihypertensive agents may have secondary rather than essential hypertension, whereas failure of the initial administration of appropriate doses of loop diuretics to cause diuresis and improvement in patients with dyspnea and edema should throw some doubt on the diagnosis of congestive heart failure. On the other hand, the diagnosis of angina pectoris is supported when the threshold for exertional chest pain rises in patients receiving beta-blockers or nitrates.

Dyspnea

Dyspnea, an abnormally uncomfortable awareness of breathing,[5, 6] may be caused by a wide variety of cardiac and pulmonary diseases, as well as by anxiety and severe obesity. The mechanisms of dyspnea and distinction among the various causes of this important symptom are described in Chapter 7.

It is useful to separate dyspnea into acute and chronic forms. *Acute dyspnea* occurs in pulmonary edema, pulmonary embolism, pneumonia, asthma, and other forms of airway obstruction. Tachyarrhythmias, acute myocardial infarction, and ruptured chordae tendineae can also cause acute dyspnea in persons who were previously well. *Chronic dyspnea* secondary to cardiac disease is often accompanied by orthopnea, third or fourth heart sounds, and cardiomegaly and usually responds to diuretic therapy. Dyspnea that awakens the patient from sleep and is relieved by sitting upright is characteristic of left ventricular failure (paroxysmal nocturnal dyspnea). In patients with chronic pulmonary disease, nocturnal dyspnea occurs earlier in the night than cardiac dyspnea does, usually immediately on assuming a recumbent position, and it rarely awakens the patient from sleep. It is accompanied and relieved by cough and expectoration. Dyspnea occurring at rest, but not on exertion, and accompanied by sighing respiration is often due to an anxiety state.

Chest Pain or Discomfort

Chest pain is one of the most common complaints faced by primary care physicians and is discussed in detail in Chapter 6. Despite the availability of a number of sophisticated and accurate noninvasive laboratory tests for the evaluation of chest pain, the history remains the cornerstone of diagnosis.[1] Ischemic discomfort is characteristically described as a constricting, squeezing, or burning feeling or as a "heaviness" in the chest. Nonischemic discomfort is more likely to be described as "knifelike"—sharp, stabbing pain that may be brief (seconds) and aggravated by cough or respiration. Alternatively, nonischemic discomfort may be a dull ache lasting several hours. Ischemic discomfort is most commonly retrosternal, in the anterior aspect of the midthorax, and in the arms, shoulders, neck, cheeks, teeth, forearms, and fingers, whereas pain that is localized to the left submammary area or that radiates to above the mandible or to below the umbilicus is not generally ischemic. Ischemic chest discomfort is usually provoked by exercise, excitement, cold weather, a heavy meal, or smoking a cigarette and especially by a combination of these activities. Discomfort that occurs after cessation of exercise or that is provoked by a particular body motion or associated with chest wall tenderness is not generally ischemic.

Effort angina (see Chapters 6 and 25) usually lasts between 3 and 20 minutes. Relief by rest and/or the administration of nitroglycerin is helpful in the diagnosis. Anginal discomfort may be accompanied by exertional dyspnea, which sometimes occurs without chest discomfort as an anginal equivalent. Angina at rest is characteristic of unstable angina (see Chapter 26), is often more severe than exertional angina, is usually described as frank pain, may awaken the patient from sleep (nocturnal angina), and may not be relieved by nitrates. The chest pain of acute myocardial infarction is generally severe and typically persists for more than 30 minutes (see Chapter 27).

The primary care physician should be alert to the combination of chest pain and profuse diaphoresis because these symptoms often signal a serious disorder such as acute myocardial infarction or pulmonary embolism. The chest pain of acute myocardial infarction is frequently accompanied by nausea and vomiting, whereas the combination of chest pain and acute dyspnea occurs in myocardial infarction, pulmonary embolism, pneumothorax, and mediastinal emphysema. The pain of an expanding or rupturing thoracic aortic aneurysm is often severe and persistent and is localized to the interscapular region with radiation laterally and anteriorly (see Chapter 36).

Syncope

The medical history is of critical importance in determining the cause of syncope (see Chapter 10). Vasovagal syncope, the most common cause of syncope, may occur in response to prolonged standing, emotional stress and physical exhaustion, pain, venipuncture, or the sight of blood. Orthostatic hypotension may be precipitated by hypovolemia, dehydration, or the excessive administration of antihypertensive drugs. Syncope secondary to a cardiac arrhythmia (transient ventricular fibrillation or third-degree atrioventricular block) is usually virtually instantaneous in onset. Syncope accompanied by chest pain may occur in massive myocardial infarction. Exertional syncope is characteristic of aortic stenosis and hypertrophic obstructive cardiomyopathy. Syncope of cardiovascular origin is not usually associated with convulsive movements or a postsyncopal confusional state, and consciousness is usually regained promptly.

Edema

Bilateral ankle edema, most prominent at the end of the day, is characteristic of congestive heart failure (see Chapter 8). This diagnosis is strongly supported when edema is accompanied by exertional dyspnea. Cardiac edema is usually preceded by a gain in weight of 5 to 10 lb, is symmetric, and progresses upward from the ankles to the shins, thighs, and genitalia. Cardiac edema that is *not* associated with orthopnea or severe dyspnea may be caused by chronic constrictive pericarditis or tricuspid stenosis. Bilateral ankle edema also occurs in patients with chronic bilateral thrombophlebitis. The presence of periorbital edema favors a renal origin, hypoproteinemia, myxedema, or angioneurotic edema. When the patient reports that edema has been limited to the upper extremities, neck, and face, obstruction of the superior vena cava should be considered. Unilateral edema of an extremity is most commonly caused by thrombophlebitis or lymphatic obstruction, and a history of ulceration and pigmentation of the legs may accompany edema caused by venous disease. When jaundice accompanies edema or when ascites precedes edema, the edema is often of hepatic origin.

Cyanosis

Cyanosis, like edema, is a symptom because it is frequently reported by the patient, as well as a physical finding because it may be noted by the physician. It is a bluish coloration of the skin and mucous membranes and is caused by an increased absolute quantity of reduced hemoglobin (>5 g/dL) in the capillary bed just beneath the surface. It is recognized most readily in the nail beds, lips, and oral mucosa. Cyanosis has two principal causes—central and peripheral (Box 3–1).

Central Cyanosis. In central cyanosis, arterial blood is unsaturated because of a reduced inspired oxygen concentration—as occurs at a high altitude (usually above 10,000 ft)—or because of impaired pulmonary function. It may occur transiently (as in acute extensive pneumonia) or chronically (as in advanced emphysema). Pulmonary edema can reduce oxygen diffusion from the alveoli to the pulmonary capillaries and thereby result in arterial unsaturation and cyanosis. An anatomic shunt in which desaturated venous blood bypasses the pulmonary capillary bed is an important cause of cyanosis. In adults, pulmonary arteriovenous fistulas and congenital cardiac malformations such as Eisenmenger's syndrome and the tetralogy of Fallot (see Chapter 34) are most commonly responsible for right-to-left shunting. Abnormalities in hemoglobin (see Box 3–1), including hemoglobin with an abnormally low affinity for oxygen, are uncommon causes of central cyanosis.

Prolonged central cyanosis, irrespective of its cause, is usually accompanied by clubbing of the digits, that is, selective enlargement of the terminal phalanges of the fingers and toes (Fig. 3–1). Clubbing is *not* usually observed with cyanosis caused by abnormalities in hemoglobin or with peripheral cyanosis. In addition to chronic central cyanosis, clubbing is also frequent in patients with infective endocarditis, lung

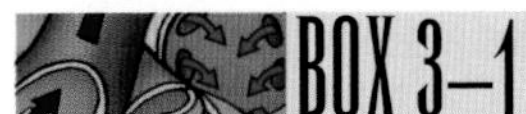

Causes of Cyanosis

CENTRAL CYANOSIS

Decreased arterial oxygen saturation
- Decreased atmospheric pressure—high altitude
- Impaired pulmonary function
  - Alveolar hypoventilation
  - Uneven relationships between pulmonary ventilation and perfusion (perfusion of hypoventilated alveoli)
  - Impaired oxygen diffusion
- Anatomic shunts
  - Certain types of congenital heart disease
  - Pulmonary arteriovenous fistulas
  - Multiple small intrapulmonary shunts
  - Hemoglobin with low affinity for oxygen

Hemoglobin abnormalities
- Methemoglobinemia—hereditary, acquired
- Sulfhemoglobinemia—acquired
- Carboxyhemoglobinemia (not true cyanosis)

PERIPHERAL CYANOSIS

Reduced cardiac output
Cold exposure
Redistribution of blood flow from extremities
Arterial obstruction
Venous obstruction

From Braunwald E: Hypoxia, polycythemia, and cyanosis. In Braunwald E, Fauci A, Kasper D, et al (eds): Harrison's Principles of Internal Medicine, 15th ed. New York, McGraw-Hill, 2001, pp 214–217. Copyright © by McGraw-Hill, Inc. Used by permission of McGraw-Hill Book Company.

cancer, cystic fibrosis, bronchiectasis, and ulcerative colitis.

Peripheral Cyanosis. Peripheral cyanosis is more common than central cyanosis and is caused by reduced blood flow to the extremities, particularly the distal portions; the reduced blood flow results in greater than normal extraction of oxygen from hemoglobin in red cells traversing the capillary bed. Cutaneous vasoconstriction, as occurs with exposure to cold, especially cold immersion, can cause peripheral cyanosis. Blood flow to the periphery is also reduced in heart failure, both acute and chronic, in shock, and with arterial obstruction. Venous obstruction, most commonly caused by thrombophlebitis, can cause cyanosis by dilating the subpapillary venous plexus.

Cough

Although it can be caused by a variety of inflammatory, allergic, and neoplastic disorders of the tracheobronchial tree, cough may be an important manifestation of left ventricular failure and frequently accompanies dyspnea, orthopnea, and paroxysmal nocturnal dyspnea. Cough secondary to left ventricular failure or mitral valve disease is usually dry and often nocturnal. In addition to pulmonary venous hypertension, cough may be caused by other cardiovascular conditions that compress the tracheobronchial tree,[7] including marked enlargement of the left atrium or pulmonary artery (which may also cause hoarseness by compressing the recurrent laryngeal nerve) and thoracic aortic aneurysm. Cough accompanied by frothy, pink sputum occurs in pulmonary edema, whereas yellowish mucoid sputum suggests an infection of the tracheobronchial tree.[8] Hemoptysis most commonly reflects tracheobronchial disease, but it may be seen in four important cardiac conditions—mitral stenosis, pulmonary embolism, pulmonary edema, and pulmonary arteriovenous fistula.

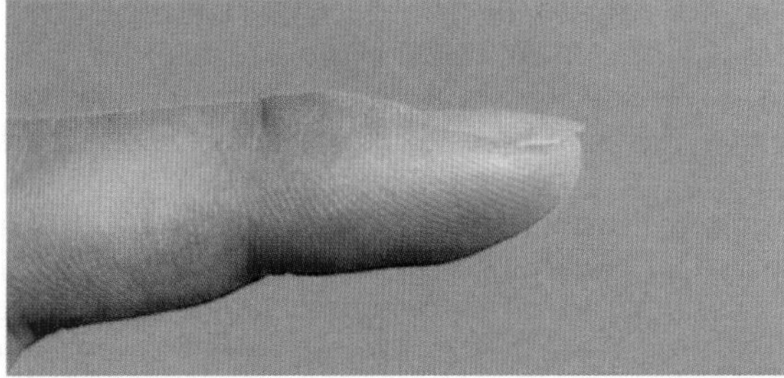

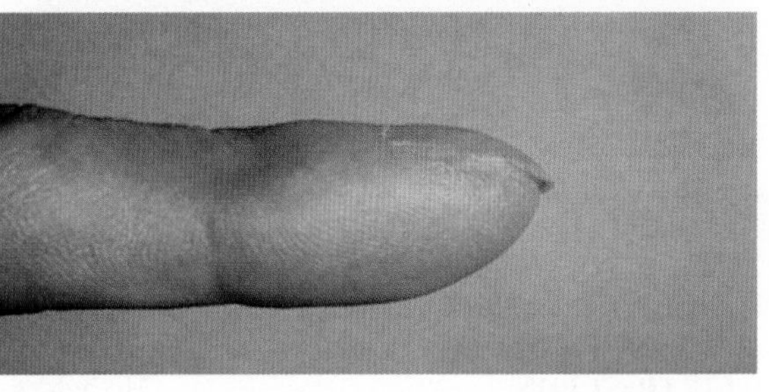

FIGURE 3–1. *A*, Profile of a normal finger. *B*, Profile of a clubbed finger with bulbous enlargement of the terminal phalanx and convexity of the nail bed. (From Mir MA: Atlas of Clinical Diagnosis. London, WB Saunders, 1995, pp 199, 207.)

Fatigue

This nonspecific symptom is present in many cardiovascular and noncardiovascular disorders. Fatigue is an important manifestation of low cardiac output and impaired systemic perfusion in heart failure. It may also be seen in heart failure after excessive diuresis. Profound fatigue is observed in patients with large myocardial infarcts, as well as in those with hypertension who are receiving antihypertensive therapy and their blood pressure has been lowered too rapidly.

Palpitations

A variety of changes in cardiac rhythm or rate can cause palpitations, an unpleasant awareness of rapid or forceful beating of the heart (see Chapter 9). A careful history is often helpful in identifying the cause of the palpitations. An elevated stroke volume, valvular regurgitation, thyrotoxicosis, and both tachycardia and marked bradycardia can all cause palpitations. When patients take their pulse, the rate, when regular, provides a clue to the mechanism underlying the palpitations. In many persons, the cause of palpitations cannot be uncovered despite careful workup, including a 48-hour ambulatory electrocardiogram. Anxiety is often responsible.

Drug-Induced Heart Disease

Cardiovascular manifestations of an adverse reaction to drugs are shown in Box 3–2. The use of legal and illegal drugs is emerging as an increasingly important cause of heart disease. For this reason, it is critical that the primary care physician obtain a careful drug history when evaluating patients with known or suspected cardiovascular disease. For example, quinidine, flecainide, and other class I antiarrhythmic agents may

BOX 3–2

Cardiovascular Manifestations of Adverse Reactions to Drugs

ACUTE CHEST PAIN (NONISCHEMIC)
Bleomycin

ANGINA EXACERBATION
Alpha-blockers
Beta-blocker withdrawal
Ergotamine
Excessive thyroxine
Hydralazine
Methysergide
Minoxidil
Nifedipine
Oxytocin
Vasopressin

ARRHYTHMIAS
Adenosine
Adriamycin
Anticholinesterases
Atropine
Beta-blockers
Daunorubicin
Digitalis
Emetine
Erythromycin
Guanethidine
Lithium
Papaverine
Pentamidine
Phenothiazines, particularly thioridazine
Sympathomimetics
Terfenadine
Theophylline
Thyroid hormone
Tricyclic antidepressants
Verapamil

AV BLOCK
Clonidine
Methyldopa
Verapamil

CARDIOMYOPATHY
Adriamycin
Daunorubicin
Emetine
Lithium
Phenothiazines
Sulfonamides
Sympathomimetics

FLUID RETENTION/CONGESTIVE HEART FAILURE/EDEMA
Beta-blockers
Calcium blockers
Carbenoxolone
Diazoxide
Estrogens
Mannitol
Minoxidil
NSAIDs
Phenylbutazone
Steroids
Verapamil

PERICARDITIS
Emetine
Hydralazine
Methysergide
Procainamide

HYPOTENSION (SEE ALSO ARRHYTHMIAS)
Amiodarone
Calcium channel blockers, e.g., nifedipine

DIURETICS
Interleukin-2
Levodopa
Morphine
Nitroglycerin
Phenothiazines
Protamine
Quinidine
Sildenafil

HYPERTENSION
Clonidine withdrawal
Corticotropin
Cyclosporine
Erythropoietin
Glucocorticoids
Monoamine oxidase inhibitors with sympathomimetics
NSAIDs
Oral contraceptives
Sympathomimetics
Tricyclic antidepressants with sympathomimetics

PERICARDIAL EFFUSION
Minoxidil
Oral contraceptives
Thromboembolism

PROLONGED QT INTERVAL/TORSADES DE POINTES
Amiodarone
Amitriptyline
Chlorpromazine
Diphenylhydramine
Disopyramide
Haloperidol
Ibutilide
Pentamidine
Procainamide
Sotalol
Terfenadine
Trimethoprim-sulfamethoxazole

AV, atrioventricular; NSAIDs, nonsteroidal anti-inflammatory drugs.
Modified from Wood AJ: Adverse reactions to drugs. In Braunwald E, Fauci A, Kasper D, et al (eds): Harrison's Principles of Internal Medicine, 15th ed. New York, McGraw-Hill, 2001.

cause QT prolongation, torsades de pointes, and recurrent syncope (see Chapter 30). Lithium and tricyclic antidepressants may also be responsible for cardiac arrhythmias. Digitalis intoxication can cause atrial and ventricular tachyarrhythmias and atrioventricular block. Disopyramide, beta-adrenergic receptor blockers, verapamil, and diltiazem are cardiac depressants and may exacerbate (or, rarely, induce) congestive heart failure. Excessive ingestion of alcohol can cause a chronic and often fatal form of heart failure (alcoholic cardiomyopathy), and binge drinking can be responsible for acute decompensation, a variety of cardiac tachyarrhythmias, and sudden death. Cocaine can cause myocarditis, coronary spasm, myocardial ischemia, myocardial infarction, and sudden death. Doxorubicin and cyclophosphamide can be responsible for both acute and chronic left ventricular failure, as well as a variety of arrhythmias, whereas 5-fluorouracil can cause angina secondary to coronary spasm.

Assessing Cardiovascular Disability

The history is critical in evaluating cardiovascular disability. The New York Heart Association has proposed four classes ranging from no symptoms on "ordinary" activity to symptoms at rest[9] (Table 3–2). The Canadian Cardiovascular Society Functional Classification provides a similar approach to assessment of the severity of angina.[10] Goldman and associates have developed the so-called Specific Activity Scale based on the estimated metabolic cost of various activities. This scale is a more reproducible and better predictor of exercise tolerance than either of the other two scales are.[11] Regard-

TABLE 3–2

Comparison of Three Methods of Assessing Cardiovascular Disability

Class	New York Heart Association Functional Classification	Canadian Cardiovascular Society Functional Classification	Specific Activity Scale
I	Patients with cardiac disease but without resulting limitations in physical activity. Ordinary physical activity does not cause undue fatigue, palpitations, dyspnea, or anginal pain	Ordinary physical activity such as walking and climbing stairs does not cause angina. Angina with strenuous or rapid or prolonged exertion at work or recreation	Patients can perform to completion any activity requiring ≤7 metabolic equivalents, e.g., can carry 24 lb up eight steps, carry objects that weigh 80 lb, do outdoor work (shovel snow, spade soil), do recreational activities (skiing, basketball, squash, handball, jog/walk 5 mph)
II	Patients with cardiac disease resulting in slight limitation in physical activity. They are comfortable at rest. Ordinary physical activity results in fatigue, palpitations, dyspnea, or anginal pain	Slight limitation in ordinary activity. Walking or climbing stairs rapidly, walking uphill, walking or stair climbing after meals, in cold, in wind, when under emotional stress, or only during the few hours after awakening. Walking more than two blocks on level ground and climbing more than one flight of ordinary stairs at a normal pace and in normal conditions	Patients can perform to completion any activity requiring ≤5 metabolic equivalents, e.g., have sexual intercourse without stopping, garden, rake, weed, roller skate, dance the fox trot, and walk at 4 mph on level ground, but cannot and do not perform to completion activities requiring ≥7 metabolic equivalents
III	Patients with cardiac disease resulting in marked limitation in physical activity. They are comfortable at rest. Less than ordinary physical activity causes fatigue, palpitations, dyspnea, or anginal pain	Marked limitation in ordinary physical activity. Walking one to two blocks on level ground and climbing more than one flight in normal conditions	Patients can perform to completion any activity requiring ≤2 metabolic equivalents, e.g., shower without stopping, strip and make bed, clean windows, walk 2.5 mph, bowl, play golf, and dress without stopping, but cannot and do not perform to completion any activities requiring ≥5 metabolic equivalents
IV	Patients with cardiac disease resulting in an inability to perform any physical activity without discomfort. Symptoms of cardiac insufficiency or anginal syndrome may be present even at rest. If any physical activity is undertaken, discomfort is increased	Inability to perform any physical activity without discomfort—anginal syndrome *may be* present at rest	Patients cannot or do not perform to completion activities requiring ≥2 metabolic equivalents. *Cannot* carry out activities listed above (Specific Activity Scale, class III).

From Goldman L, Hashimoto B, Cook EF, Loscalzo A: Comparative reproducibility and validity of systems for assessing cardiovascular functional class: Advantages of a new specific activity scale. Circulation 1981;64:1227. By permission of the American Heart Association, Inc.

less of the classification used, it is critical to determine whether the patient's disability is stable, increasing, or diminishing over time, which can be ascertained by comparing the symptoms currently elicited by any specific task, such as climbing two flights of stairs, and at some previous time (e.g., 6 months).

PHYSICAL EXAMINATION

Arterial Pressure

The indirect measurement of arterial pressure is described in Chapter 19.

Arterial Pulse

Palpation of the carotid pulse is most useful in assessing the central aortic pulse.[12] In examining this pulse, the right thumb should be applied to the left carotid artery in the lower third of the neck (see Fig. 3–8*C*). The volume, contour, frequency, and regularity of the pulse should be noted.[8] Reduced carotid pulsations occur in shock and other conditions with markedly reduced stroke volume, as well as in carotid atherosclerosis. The carotid pulse is diminished in amplitude and rises more slowly than normal *(pulsus parvus et tardus)* (Fig. 3–2*B*) in patients with fixed, severe obstruction to left ventricular outflow (aortic valvular stenosis, congenital subaortic stenosis). In contrast, the arterial pulse is exaggerated in volume with a sharp rise in conditions in which the stroke volume is augmented, such as aortic regurgitation, arteriovenous fistulas, and other causes of high cardiac output. The pulse rises more rapidly than normal when the arterial tree is inelastic, as occurs in patients with diffuse atherosclerosis and the elderly.

An arterial pulse with two systolic peaks *(pulsus bisferiens)* occurs in patients with isolated aortic regurgitation (see Fig. 3–2*C*), with the combination of aortic regurgitation and stenosis, and with hypertrophic obstructive cardiomyopathy (see Fig. 3–2*D*). A double pulse in which the second peak occurs in diastole *(dicrotic pulse)* (see Fig. 3–2*E*) may occur in normal subjects with reduced peripheral resistance and hypotension (as in high fever), as well as in conditions in which a low stroke volume is ejected into an elastic aorta (heart failure, hypovolemic shock, cardiac tamponade).

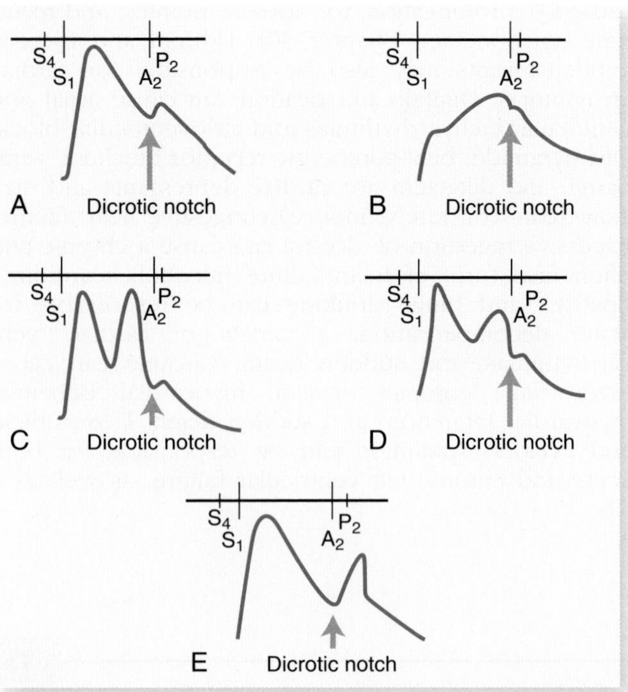

FIGURE 3–2. Schematic diagrams of the configurational changes in carotid pulse and their differential diagnoses. Heart sounds are also illustrated. *A*, Normal. A_2, aortic component of the second heart sound; P_2, pulmonic component of the second heart sound; S_1, first heart sound; S_4, atrial sound. *B*, Anacrotic pulse with a slow initial upstroke. The peak is close to S_2. These features suggest fixed left ventricular outflow obstruction, such as occurs with valvular aortic stenosis. *C*, Pulsus bisferiens with both percussion and tidal waves occurring during systole. This type of carotid pulse contour is most frequently observed in patients with hemodynamically significant aortic regurgitation or combined aortic stenosis and regurgitation with dominant regurgitation. It is rarely observed in patients with mitral valve prolapse or in normal individuals. *D*, Pulsus bisferiens in hypertrophic obstructive cardiomyopathy. It is rarely appreciated at the bedside by palpation. *E*, A dicrotic pulse results from an accentuated dicrotic wave and tends to occur in patients with sepsis, severe heart failure, hypovolemic shock, cardiac tamponade, and aortic valve replacement. (From Chatterjee K: Bedside evaluation of the heart: The physical examination. In Chatterjee K, Parmley W [eds]: Cardiology: An Illustrated Text/Reference. Philadelphia, JB Lippincott, 1991, pp 3.11–3.51.)

Pulsus alternans is a condition in which strong and weak pulses alternate, although they occur with absolute regularity. It is detected best in a more peripheral vessel such as the radial artery and is accompanied by alternations in the intensity of Korotkoff's sounds during indirect sphygmomanometry. Pulsus alternans is often initiated by a premature ventricular contraction and is usually a sign of advanced myocardial failure. Not to be confused with pulsus alternans is *pulsus bigeminus*, in which a premature contraction follows every sinus beat and in which the weak beat follows a shorter interval.

Normally, arterial pressure declines slightly (<10 mm Hg) during inspiration. An exaggerated decline *(pulsus paradoxus)* may be palpable as a diminished arterial pulse during inspiration, but as is the case for pulsus alternans, pulsus paradoxus is more readily detected by sphygmomanometry. It is a key finding in cardiac tamponade but may also be present in chronic constrictive pericarditis, hypovolemic shock, pulmonary embolism, asthma, or other conditions causing unusually wide respiratory swings in intrapleural pressure.

Peripheral Arterial Pulse

In patients suspected of having ischemic heart disease or peripheral arteriosclerosis, bilateral palpation of the common carotid, brachial, radial, femoral, dorsalis pedis, and posterior tibial arteries should be carried out. Diminished or absent pulses suggest obstruction. Systolic bruits are frequently audible at the site of obstruction. The abdominal aorta should be palpated both above and below the umbilicus.

Jugular Venous Pulse

The pressure pulse in the right atrium is reflected in the pulsations of the internal jugular veins. Examination of these veins is best carried out on the right side of the neck, with the patient's head resting on a pillow at an angle at which the skin overlying the jugular vein is just visible at the angle of the mandible.[13, 14] The height of the jugular venous pressure is estimated as the top of the visible proximal vein. It is normally less than 4 cm above the sternal angle, which corresponds to a right atrial pressure of 9 cm (the right atrium being 5 cm below the sternal angle) (Fig. 3–3). When the jugular veins are distended with the patient in a sitting position, venous pressure is markedly elevated (Fig. 3–4). Jugular venous pressure is elevated in right heart failure irrespective of cause, tricuspid valve disease, pericardial constriction, pericardial tamponade, and obstruction of the superior vena cava. In Kussmaul's sign, which typically occurs in constrictive pericarditis and tricuspid stenosis, a paradoxical rise in jugular venous pressure occurs during inspiration because the increased venous return from the reduction in intrapericardial pressure during inspiration cannot be accommodated in the right side of the heart.

The normal jugular venous pattern, which reflects the right atrial pressure pulse, consists of a presystolic expansion, the A-wave, caused by atrial contraction, followed in order by the X descent during atrial relaxation, the X′ descent during early systole, the V-wave during late systole, and the Y descent in early diastole (Fig. 3–5). The A-wave is prominent in conditions in which right atrial emptying is impeded, such as tricuspid stenosis (Fig. 3–6), and in the presence of right ventricular hypertrophy of any cause, including pulmonary hypertension, pulmonic stenosis, and hypertrophy of the interventricular septum in patients with left ventricular hypertrophy. The A-wave is absent in atrial fibrillation (Fig. 3–7). In tricuspid regurgitation, the X′ descent is diminished, and the V-wave and Y descent are unusually prominent (see Fig. 3–7). In tricuspid stenosis, the Y descent is attenuated. In constrictive pericarditis, both the X′ descent and the Y descent are prominent and cause a W-shaped jugular venous pulse. In cardiac tamponade, the X descent is most striking.

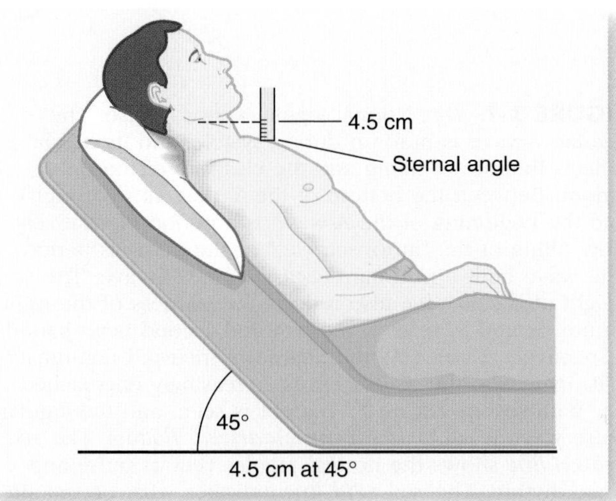

FIGURE 3–3. Venous pressure can be estimated by observing the upper level of internal jugular pulsations above the sternal angle. Pulsations over 4.5 cm at 45 degrees are indicative of elevated right atrial pressure. (From Constant J: Bedside Cardiology, 4th ed. Boston, Little, Brown, 1993, p 71.)

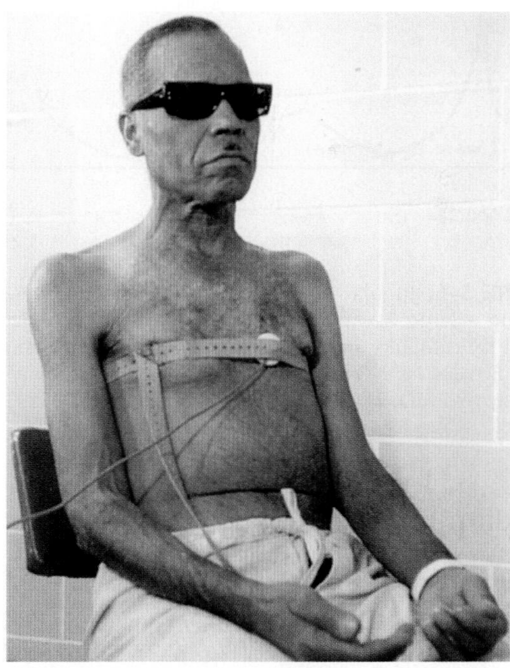

FIGURE 3–4. Visible external jugular venous distention extends to the mandibular level in a seated patient with effusive-constrictive pericarditis. Mean right atrial pressure was 20 mm Hg. (From Fowler NO: Pericardial disease. In Abelmann WH [vol ed]: Cardiomyopathies, Myocarditis, and Pericardial Disease. In Braunwald E [series ed]: Atlas of Heart Diseases, vol 2. Philadelphia, Current Medicine, 1995, pp 13.1–13.16.)

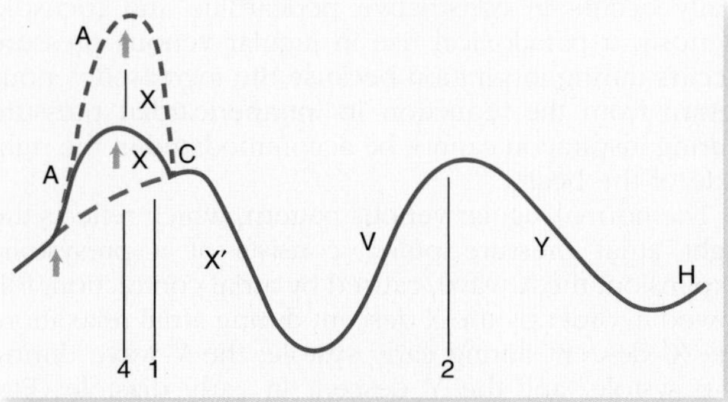

FIGURE 3–5. Jugular venous pulse. The normal contour is shown by the *solid line*. The A-wave *(a)* is absent in atrial fibrillation *(dashed green line)*. The A-wave becomes large or giant when the right atrium contracts against a greater than normal volume of blood, a noncompliant or hypertrophied right ventricle, or a closing or closed tricuspid valve *(dashed blue line)*. *Arrows* indicate the beginning and the end of the A-wave. The *numbers* represent the heart sounds. The fourth heart sound coincides with the peak of the large or giant A-wave. (From Evans TC, Giuliani ER, Tancredi RG, Brandenburg RO: Physical examination. In Giuliani ER [ed]: Cardiology: Fundamentals and Practice, 2nd ed. St Louis, Mosby–Year Book, 1991, pp 204–272. By permission of Mayo Foundation.)

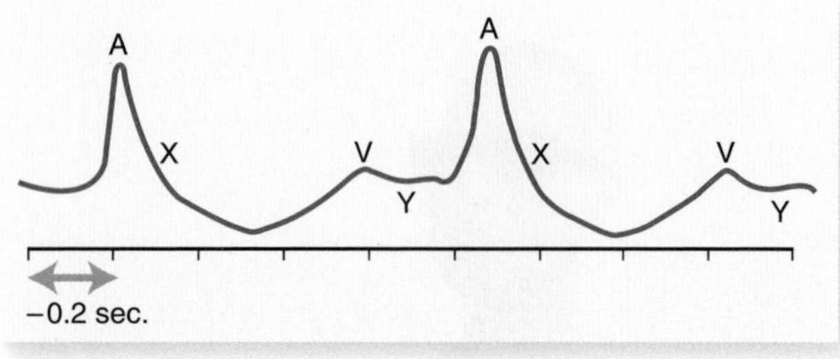

FIGURE 3–6. Jugular venous pulse in tricuspid stenosis showing a large A-wave and a slow Y descent, the latter caused by difficulty in passive filling of the right ventricle. (From Fowler NO: Cardiac Diagnosis and Treatment, 3rd ed. Hagerstown, MD, Harper & Row, 1980, p 52.)

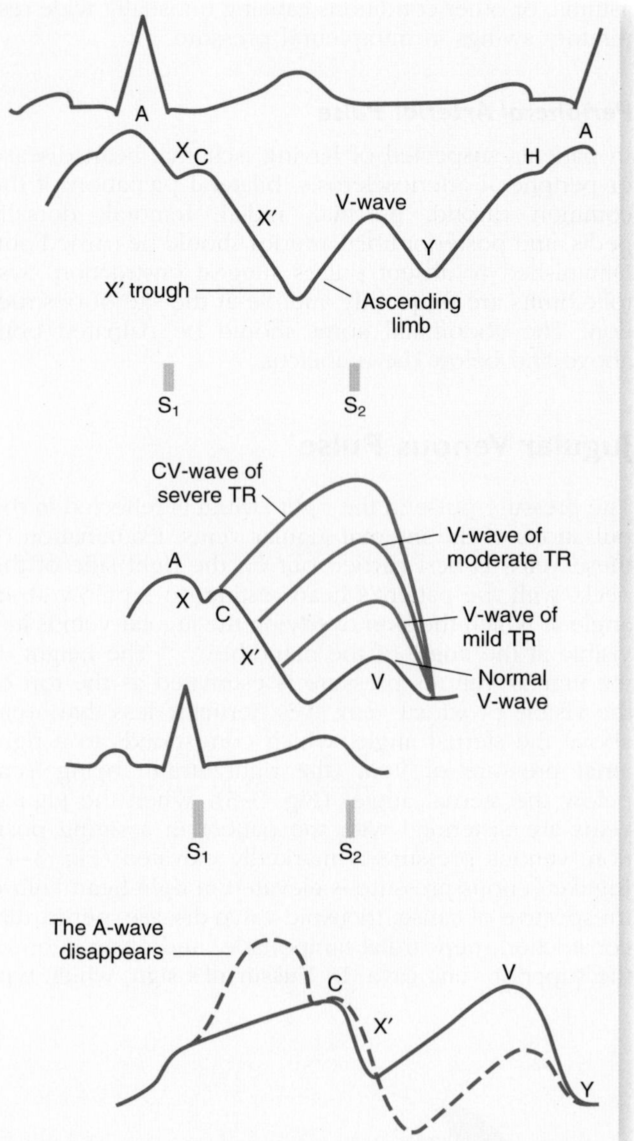

FIGURE 3–7. *Top*, Normal jugular venous pulse. The jugular V-wave is built up during systole, and its height reflects the rate of filling and the elasticity of the right atrium. Between the bottom of the Y descent (Y trough) and the beginning of the A-wave is a period of relatively slow filling of the "atrioventricle," or the diastasis period. The wave built up during diastasis is the H-wave. The height of the H-wave also reflects the stiffness of the right atrium. S_1 and S_2 refer to the first and second heart sounds, respectively. *Center*, As the degree of tricuspid regurgitation (TR) increases, the X′ descent is increasingly encroached on. With severe TR, no X′ descent is seen, and the jugular pulse wave is said to be *ventricularized. Bottom*, The *red broken line* shows the normal jugular venous pulse and sinus rhythm. The *red solid line* indicates what occurs after the development of atrial fibrillation. The dominant descent in atrial fibrillation is almost always the Y descent; that is, it has the superficial appearance of the pulse wave of TR. (From Constant J: Bedside Cardiology, 4th ed. Boston, Little, Brown, 1993, pp 81, 89, 93.)

Cardiac Examination

Inspection and Palpation

The cardiac examination should begin with inspection and palpation of the thorax (Fig. 3–8). Both the fingers and the palm of the hand should be used (Fig. 3–9). The patient should be examined in both the supine and left lateral positions.[2, 12] Timing of precordial movement is aided by simultaneous cardiac auscultation or palpation of the carotid arterial pulse.

Precordial prominence occurs in patients in whom cardiomegaly had developed before puberty. Left ventricular enlargement is suggested by displacement of the apex beat lateral to the midclavicular line and a

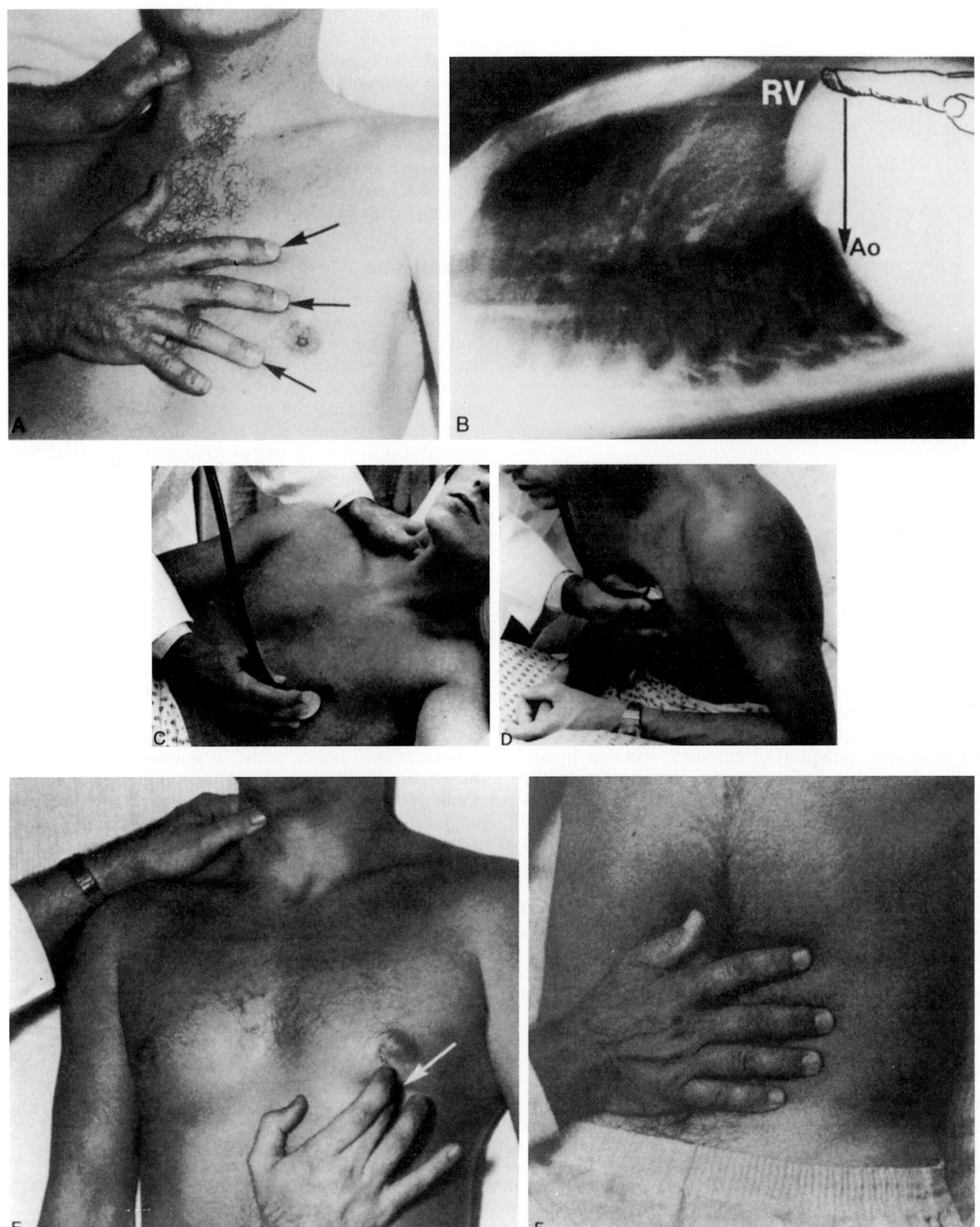

Legend on following page

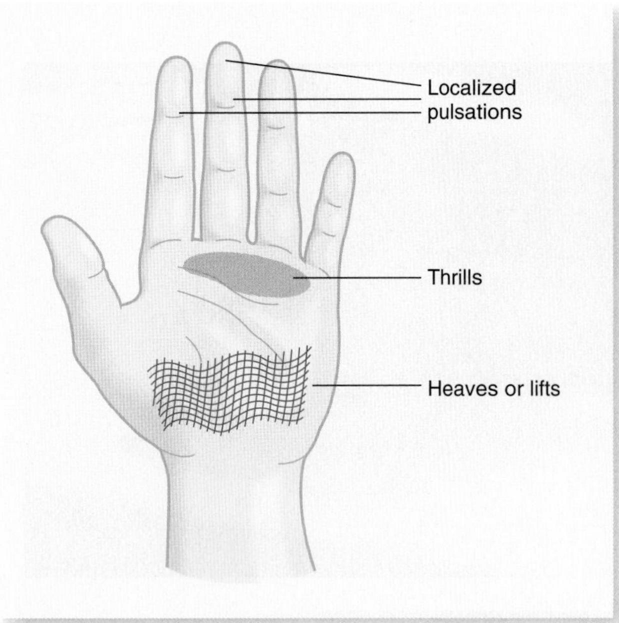

FIGURE 3–9. Although small localized movements are best perceived by the distal tips of the finger pads, thrills are best felt with the distal portion of the palm, and heaves or lifts are best felt with the proximal part of the palm. (From Constant J: Bedside Cardiology, 4th ed. Boston, Little, Brown, 1993, p 128. Reprinted by permission of Lippincott-Raven, Publishers.)

hyperkinetic or sustained, forceful impulse (Fig. 3–10). Left ventricular aneurysm produces a larger than normal area of systolic pulsation of the apex, whereas hypertrophic obstructive cardiomyopathy may cause a double outward thrust during systole. A presystolic apical thrust is palpable, usually with the patient in the left lateral decubitus condition, when the left atrial contribution to ventricular filling is augmented. Such thrust occurs in patients with sinus rhythm and left ventricular hypertrophy of any cause, myocardial ischemia, and myocardial fibrosis.[9] A systolic inward movement is characteristic of constrictive pericarditis.

Right ventricular enlargement or hypertrophy may be detected by a palpable anterior movement in the third or fourth intercostal space in the left parasternal region during systole. When pulmonary hypertension is present, the pulsation extends into the second intercostal space just left of the sternum. A palpable impulse simultaneous with the second heart sound reflects the presence of pulmonary hypertension.

Cardiac thrills are vibratory sensations best appreciated with the flat of the hand (see Fig. 3–9). They are palpable manifestations of loud (grades IV to VI) murmurs with medium- or low-frequency components.

Auscultation

Auscultation should be carried out in a quiet room with the chest fully exposed and the patient in the supine, sitting, and left lateral decubitus positions. The entire region between and including the cardiac apex and second intercostal space at the right sternal margin should be examined. Both the diaphragm (sensitive to high-pitched sounds) and the bell (sensitive to low-pitched sounds) of the stethoscope should be used. Systematic and sequential attention should be directed to the heart sounds and the systolic and diastolic intervals.

Heart Sounds (Figs. 3–11 and 3–12)

The *first heart sound* is produced primarily by closure of the mitral valve; rarely, a second, softer component produced by tricuspid valve closure is audible. The first heart sound is loudest when the mitral valve leaflets are widely apart at the onset of ventricular contraction, as occurs in mitral stenosis or with a short PR interval. *Early systolic sounds* (ejection sounds) are high-frequency events produced by the opening snap of stenotic, albeit mobile aortic or pulmonic valves or by the ejection of blood into a dilated aorta or pulmonary trunk. Mid to late systolic sounds (often termed *clicks*) are most commonly caused by prolapse of the mitral valve, a condition in which the timing and intensity of the sounds are altered by respiration and other maneuvers (see Chapter 11).

The *second heart sound* is caused by closure of the semilunar valves and is heard best in the second left intercostal space along the sternal border. Splitting of the second heart sound is due to asynchronous closure of the valves (Box 3–3 and Fig. 3–13). Normally, the

FIGURE 3–8. *A*, Palpation of the anterior wall of the right ventricle by applying the tips of three fingers in the third, fourth, and fifth interspaces, left sternal edge *(arrows)*, during full held exhalation. The patient is supine with the trunk elevated 30 degrees. *B*, Subxiphoid palpation of the inferior wall of the right ventricle (RV) with the relative position of the abdominal aorta (Ao) shown by the *arrow*. *C*, The bell of the stethoscope is applied to the cardiac apex while the patient lies in a partial left lateral decubitus position. The thumb of the examiner's free left hand is used to palpate the carotid artery for timing purposes. *D*, The soft, high-frequency, early diastolic murmur of aortic regurgitation or pulmonary hypertensive regurgitation is best elicited by applying the stethoscope's diaphragm very firmly to the mid-left sternal edge. The patient leans forward with breath held in full exhalation. *E*, Palpation of the left ventricular impulse with a fingertip *(arrow)*. The patient's trunk is 30 degrees above the horizontal. The examiner's right thumb palpates the carotid pulse for timing purposes. *F*, Palpation of the liver. The patient is supine with knees flexed to relax the abdomen. The flat of the examiner's right hand is placed on the right upper quadrant just below the expected inferior margin of the liver; the left hand is applied diametrically opposite. (From Perloff JK: Physical Examination of the Heart and Circulation, 3rd ed. Philadelphia, WB Saunders, 2000.)

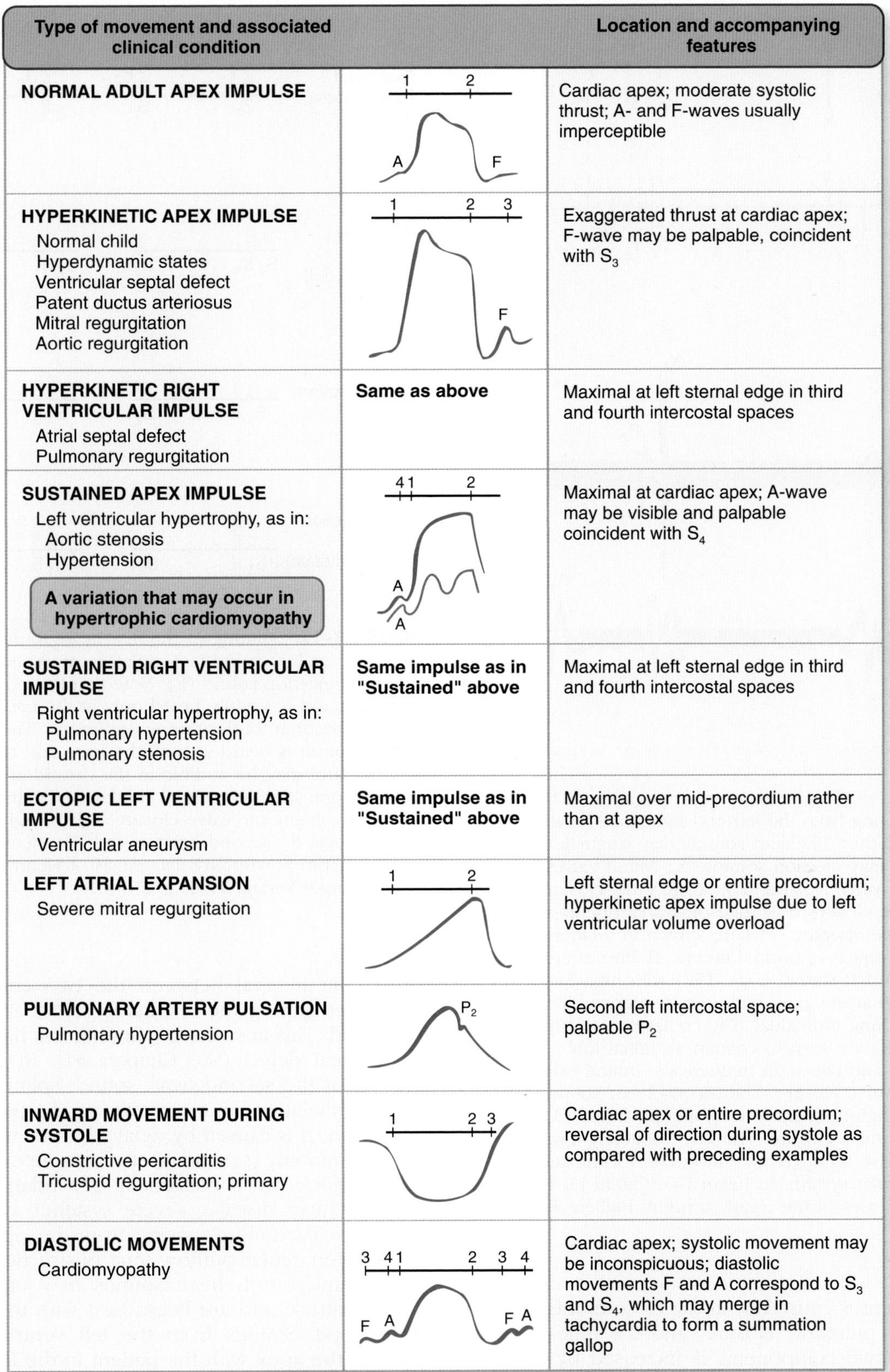

Type of movement and associated clinical condition		Location and accompanying features
NORMAL ADULT APEX IMPULSE		Cardiac apex; moderate systolic thrust; A- and F-waves usually imperceptible
HYPERKINETIC APEX IMPULSE Normal child Hyperdynamic states Ventricular septal defect Patent ductus arteriosus Mitral regurgitation Aortic regurgitation		Exaggerated thrust at cardiac apex; F-wave may be palpable, coincident with S_3
HYPERKINETIC RIGHT VENTRICULAR IMPULSE Atrial septal defect Pulmonary regurgitation	**Same as above**	Maximal at left sternal edge in third and fourth intercostal spaces
SUSTAINED APEX IMPULSE Left ventricular hypertrophy, as in: Aortic stenosis Hypertension **A variation that may occur in hypertrophic cardiomyopathy**		Maximal at cardiac apex; A-wave may be visible and palpable coincident with S_4
SUSTAINED RIGHT VENTRICULAR IMPULSE Right ventricular hypertrophy, as in: Pulmonary hypertension Pulmonary stenosis	**Same impulse as in "Sustained" above**	Maximal at left sternal edge in third and fourth intercostal spaces
ECTOPIC LEFT VENTRICULAR IMPULSE Ventricular aneurysm	**Same impulse as in "Sustained" above**	Maximal over mid-precordium rather than at apex
LEFT ATRIAL EXPANSION Severe mitral regurgitation		Left sternal edge or entire precordium; hyperkinetic apex impulse due to left ventricular volume overload
PULMONARY ARTERY PULSATION Pulmonary hypertension		Second left intercostal space; palpable P_2
INWARD MOVEMENT DURING SYSTOLE Constrictive pericarditis Tricuspid regurgitation; primary		Cardiac apex or entire precordium; reversal of direction during systole as compared with preceding examples
DIASTOLIC MOVEMENTS Cardiomyopathy		Cardiac apex; systolic movement may be inconspicuous; diastolic movements F and A correspond to S_3 and S_4, which may merge in tachycardia to form a summation gallop

FIGURE 3–10. Graphic representation of apical movements in health and disease. The *heavy line* indicates palpable features. A, atrial wave corresponding to the fourth heart sound (S_4), or atrial gallop; F, filling wave corresponding to the third heart sound (S_3), or ventricular gallop; P_2, pulmonic component of S_2. (From Willis P IV: Inspection and palpation of the precordium. In Hurst JW [ed]: The Heart, 7th ed. New York, McGraw-Hill, 1990, p 164. Copyright © by McGraw-Hill, Inc. Used by permission of McGraw-Hill Book Company.)

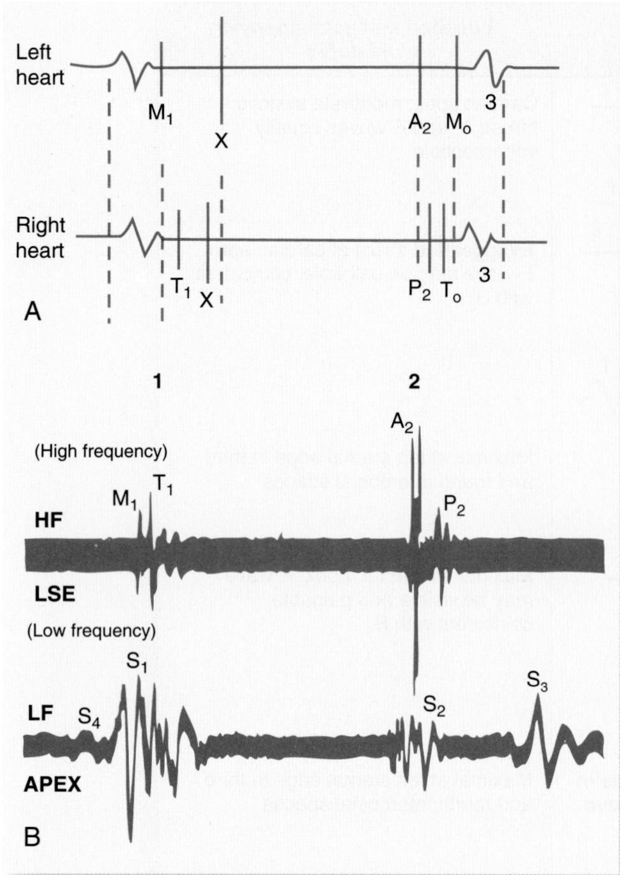

FIGURE 3–11. *A*, Diagrammatic representation of heart sounds originating from the left and right sides of the heart. Fourth (4) and third (3) heart sounds may originate from both sides, as may ejection sounds (X). Mitral valve closure (M_1), tricuspid valve closure (T_1), aortic valve closure (A_2), pulmonic valve closure (P_2), tricuspid valve opening (T_o), and mitral valve opening (M_o) are shown in relation to one another with respect to normal timing. *B*, Phonocardiograms recorded at the left sternal edge (LSE) with high-frequency filters (HF) and at the apex with low-frequency filters (LF) in a normal young individual. The components of the first heart sound (S_1) are seen to contain an initial low frequency (S_4) and two high frequencies—mitral (M_1) and tricuspid (T_1) valve closure. The second heart sound (S_2) contains two high-frequency components—aortic (A_2) and pulmonic (P_2) valve closure. The low-frequency third heart sound (S_3) is also seen. (From Sutton GC: Examination of the cardiovascular system. In Julian DG, Camm JA, Fox KM, et al [eds]: Diseases of the Heart. London, Balliere-Tindall, 1989, p 116.)

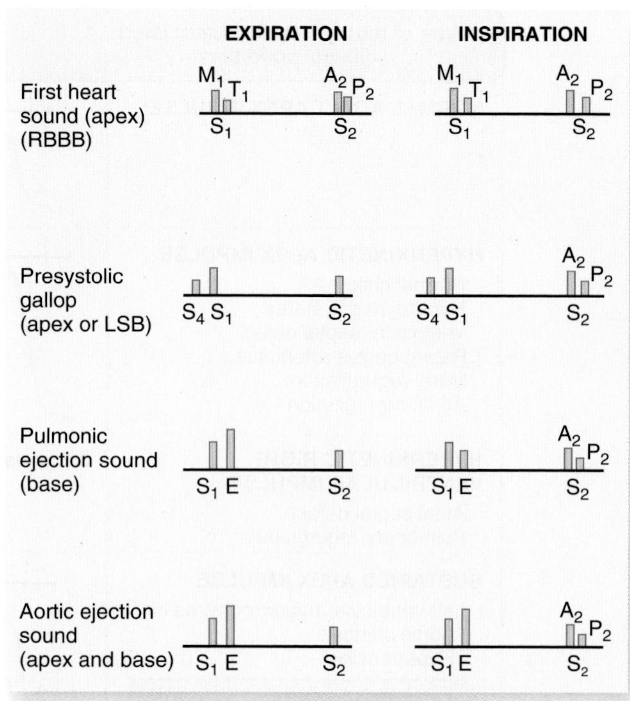

FIGURE 3–12. Splitting of the first heart sound (S_1), presystolic gallop sound (S_4), pulmonary ejection sound, and aortic ejection sound (E). Note that the pulmonary ejection sound is usually heard only at the base of the heart and may become louder during expiration. The aortic ejection sound is heard at both the base and the apex of the heart and may be audible in the carotid area. A_2, aortic valve closure; LSB, left sternal border; M_1, mitral valve closure; P_2, pulmonic valve closure; RBBB, right bundle branch block; S_2, second heart sound; T_1, tricuspid valve closure. (From Fowler NO: Diagnosis of Heart Disease. New York, Springer-Verlag, 1991, p 27.)

first component is caused by aortic closure, the second is caused by pulmonic closure, and the time interval between the two components is increased by inspiration as right ventricular stroke rises and the duration of right ventricular systole increases. A loud first (aortic) component of the second heart sound is present in systemic hypertension, and a loud second (pulmonic) component is heard in pulmonary hypertension. A decision tree for interpreting the second heart sound is presented in Figure 3–14. In *fixed splitting* of the second heart sound, the interval between the two components is unchanged during the respiratory cycle and is usually prolonged. This auscultatory finding is a hallmark of an atrial septal defect (see Chapter 34). In *paradoxical splitting* of the second heart sound, splitting is widest during exhalation and narrows or disappears during inspiration. It is caused by delayed aortic valve closure, most commonly secondary to complete left bundle branch block, but occasionally secondary to chronic ischemic heart disease, severe systemic hypertension, left ventricular failure, pacing from the right ventricle, and left ventricular outflow tract obstruction.

Third and fourth heart sounds may originate from either ventricle and are heard best with the bell of the stethoscope. Sounds from the left ventricle are best heard at the apex with the patient in the left decubitus position, whereas those from the right ventricle are most readily audible along the lower left sternal border in the supine position. The *third heart sound* (see Figs. 3–11 and 3–15) is often heard in normal children and young adults. When present after the age of 40 years, the third heart sound is usually abnormal and caused by altered physical properties of the ventricle or an increased rate

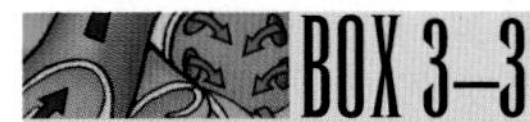

BOX 3–3

Abnormal Splitting of the Second Heart Sound

PERSISTENT SPLITTING

Electrical delay of pulmonary component
- Right bundle branch block
- Left ventricular ectopic beats
- Preexcitation (left ventricular tract)
- Left ventricular pacemaker

Mechanical delay of pulmonary component
- Pulmonary valve stenosis
- Subvalvular pulmonary obstruction
- Large pulmonary embolus
- Right ventricular dysfunction

Decrease in pulmonary vascular impedance
- Dilatation of pulmonary artery
- Atrial septal defect
- After surgical repair of atrial septal defect

Early aortic component
- Mitral regurgitation
- Ventricular septal defect
- Preexcitation (left ventricular tract)

PARADOXICAL SPLITTING

Electrical delay of aortic component
- Left bundle branch block
- Right ventricular ectopic beats
- Right ventricular pacemaker
- Coronary heart disease

Mechanical delay of aortic component
- Aortic valve stenosis
- Hypertrophic cardiomyopathy
- Coronary heart disease
- Patent ductus arteriosus
- Aortic regurgitation

Early closure of pulmonary valve
- Tricuspid regurgitation

From Evans TC, Giuliani ER, Tancredi RG, Brandenburg RO: Physical examination. *In* Giuliani ER, Fuster V, Gersh B, et al (eds): Cardiology: Fundamentals and Practice, 2nd ed. Rochester, MN, Mayo Foundation, 1991, pp 204–272. By permission of the Mayo Foundation.

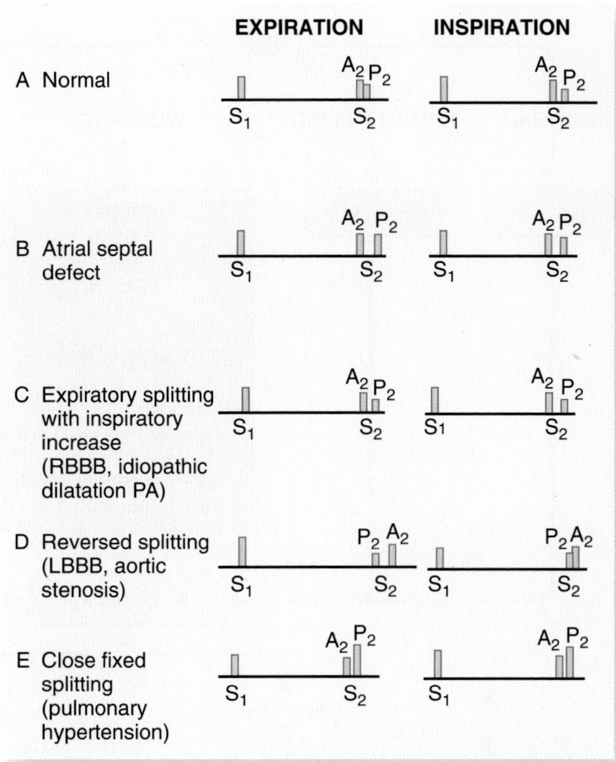

FIGURE 3–13. Demonstration of the relationship of splitting of S_2 to respiration in normal subjects *(A)*, the fixed splitting of S_2 heard in an atrial septal defect *(B)*, expiratory splitting of S_2 with an inspiratory increment as seen in right bundle branch block (RBBB) *(C)*, reversed splitting of S_2 associated with delayed aortic closure—most commonly caused by left bundle branch block (LBBB) *(D)*, and the close but audible and rather fixed splitting of S_2 characteristic of severe pulmonary hypertension associated with idiopathic or thromboembolic pulmonary hypertensive disease *(E)*. A_2, aortic valve closure; P_2, pulmonic valve closure; PA, pulmonic artery; S_1, first heart sound. (From Fowler NO: Diagnosis of Heart Disease. New York, Springer-Verlag, 1991, p 31.)

of ventricular filling in early diastole (Box 3–4). *Fourth heart sounds* may be audible in normal persons after the age of 50 years. Abnormal fourth heart sounds reflect increased ventricular filling during atrial systole and occur in patients with sinus rhythm and ventricular hypertrophy, myocardial infarction, or ischemia (Box 3–5).

Other diastolic sounds include the opening snap of the mitral (rarely the tricuspid) valve. Valves producing this sound are usually stenotic but mobile. The time interval between the second heart sound and the opening snap of the mitral valve varies inversely with the height of the left atrial pressure (see Chapter 32). Opening snaps may be confused with widely split second heart sounds, but the second sound–opening snap interval narrows during inspiration. Early diastolic sounds also occur in patients with chronic constrictive pericarditis, in whom they are known as pericardial *knocks* (Fig. 3–15*C*).

Heart murmurs are discussed in Chapter 11.

Examination of the Chest

Examination of the chest commences with inspection. Severe kyphoscoliosis and a markedly increased anteroposterior diameter may be a cause of cor pulmonale. Patients with chronic bronchitis or emphysema, an important cause of cor pulmonale, may have expiratory wheezing or poor transmission of breath sounds. Rales at the lung bases that do not clear with coughing and

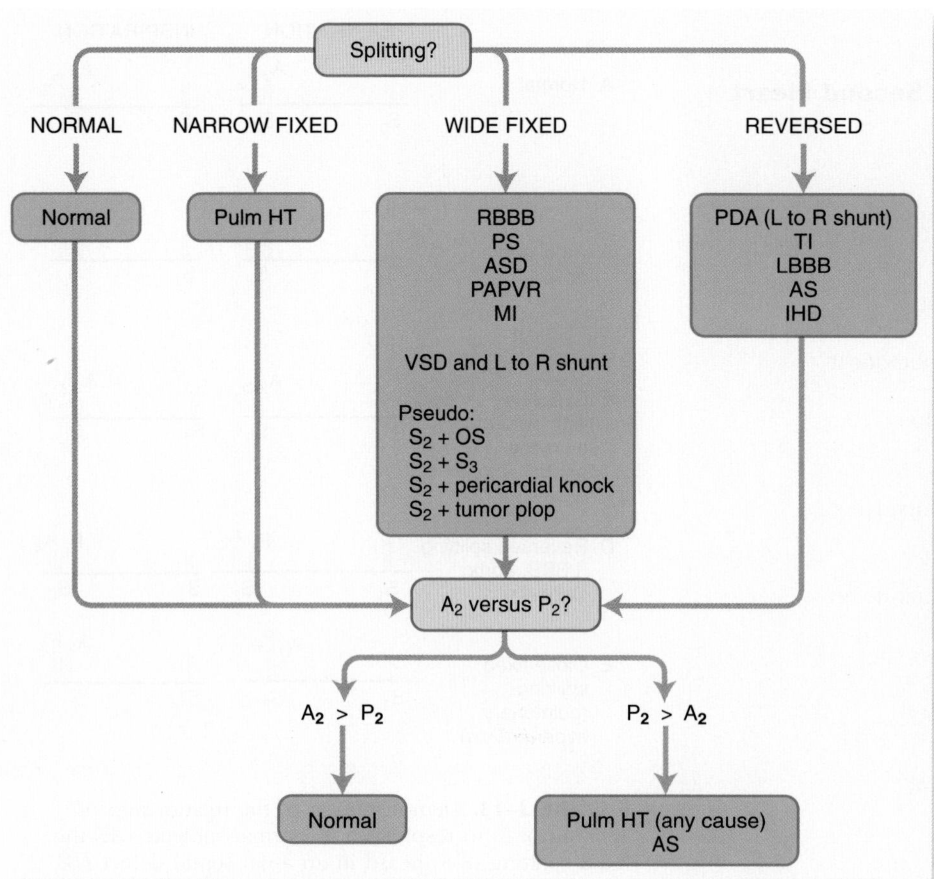

FIGURE 3–14. Decision tree for splitting of the second heart sound (S_2). A_2, aortic valve closure; AS, aortic stenosis; ASD, atrial septal defect; IHD, ischemic heart disease; L to R shunt, left-to-right shunt; LBBB, left bundle branch block; MI, mitral insufficiency; OS, opening snap; P_2, pulmonic valve closure; PAPVR, partial anomalous pulmonary venous return; PDA, patent ductus arteriosus; PS, pulmonic stenosis; Pulm HT, pulmonary hypertension; RBBB, right bundle branch block; S_3, third heart sound; TI, tricuspid insufficiency; VSD, ventricular septal defect. (From Sapira JD: The Art and Science of Bedside Diagnosis. Baltimore, Urban & Schwartzenberg, 1990.)

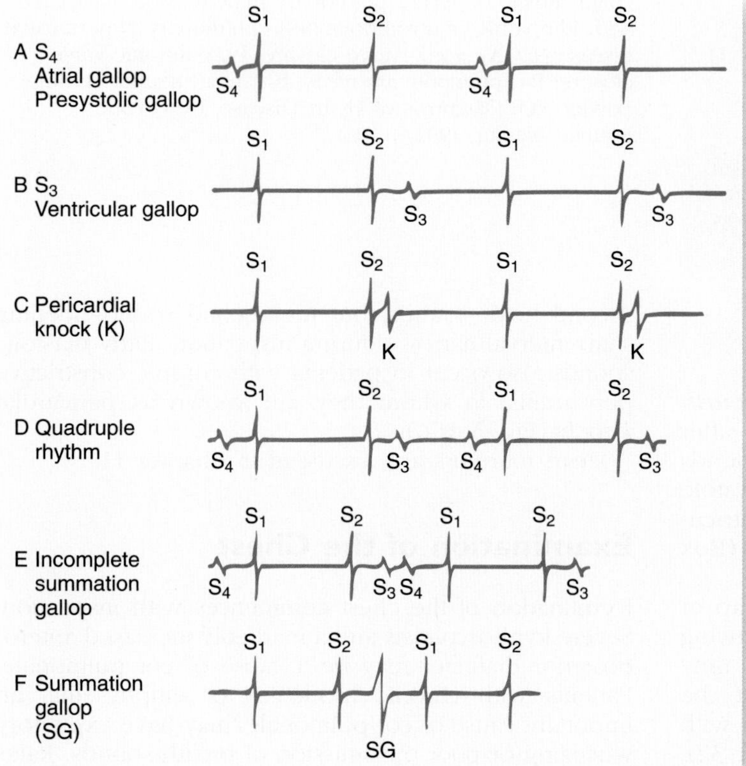

FIGURE 3–15. Diastolic filling sounds. *A*, The fourth heart sound (S_4) occurs in presystole and is frequently called an atrial or presystolic gallop. S_1, first heart sound; S_2, second heart sound. *B*, The third heart sound (S_3) occurs during the rapid phase of ventricular filling. It is a normal finding that is commonly heard in children and young adults but disappears with increasing age. When it is heard in a patient with cardiac disease, it is called a pathologic S_3 or ventricular gallop and usually indicates ventricular dysfunction or atrioventricular valvular incompetence. *C*, In constrictive pericarditis, a sound in early diastole, the pericardial knock (K), is heard earlier and is louder and higher pitched than the usual pathologic S_3. *D*, A quadruple rhythm results if both S_4 and S_3 are present. *E*, At faster heart rates, S_3 and S_4 occur in rapid succession and may give the illusion of a mid-diastolic rumble. *F*, When the heart rate is sufficiently fast, the two rapid phases of ventricular filling reinforce each other, and a loud summation gallop (SG) may appear; this sound may be louder than either S_3 or S_4 alone. (From Shaver JA: Examination of the Heart, Part 4: Auscultation. Dallas, American Heart Association, 1990.)

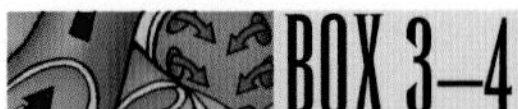

BOX 3–4

Causes of Third Heart Sound (S_3), Ventricular Diastolic Gallop, Protodiastolic Gallop, and Pericardial Knock

Physiologic S_3—children and young adults
- Decreased prevalence with increasing age

Pathologic S_3
- Ventricular dysfunction—poor systolic function, increased end-diastolic and end-systolic volume, decreased ejection fraction, and high filling pressures
- Idiopathic dilated cardiomyopathy
- Ischemic heart disease
- Valvular heart disease
- Congenital heart disease
- Systemic and pulmonary hypertension

Excessively rapid, early diastolic ventricular filling
- Hyperkinetic states
  - Anemia
  - Thyrotoxicosis
  - Arteriovenous fistula
- Atrioventricular valve incompetence
- Left-to-right shunts

Pericardial Knock
- Constrictive pericarditis (pericardial knock)

From Shaver JA, Salerni R: Auscultation of the heart. In Hurst JW (ed): The Heart, 7th ed. New York, McGraw-Hill, 1990, pp 278, 281.

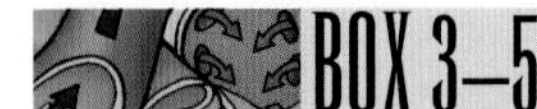

BOX 3–5

Causes of Fourth Heart Sound (S_4), Atrial Diastolic Gallop, and Presystolic Gallop

Physiologic—recordable, rarely audible

Pathologic
- Decreased ventricular compliance
  - Ventricular hypertrophy
    - Left or right ventricular outflow obstruction
    - Systemic or pulmonary hypertension
    - Hypertrophic cardiomyopathy
  - Ischemic heart disease
    - Angina pectoris
    - Acute myocardial infarction
    - Old myocardial infarction
    - Ventricular aneurysm
  - Idiopathic dilated cardiomyopathy
- Excessively rapid late diastolic filling secondary to vigorous atrial systole
  - Hyperkinetic states
    - Anemia
    - Thyrotoxicosis
    - Arteriovenous fistula
  - Acute atrioventricular valve incompetence
- Arrhythmias
  - Heart block

From Shaver JA, Salerni R: Auscultation of the heart. In Hurst JW (ed): The Heart, 7th ed. New York, McGraw-Hill, 1990, pp 278, 281.

signs of pleural effusion are characteristic of heart failure.

Examination of the Abdomen

The liver is usually enlarged in right ventricular failure. When the latter occurs acutely, rapid expansion of the hepatic capsule causes tenderness to palpation in the right upper quadrant. The liver may pulsate in tricuspid valve disease; pulsations are systolic in tricuspid regurgitation and presystolic in tricuspid stenosis. Timing of pulsations is aided by simultaneous auscultation. Firm pressure on the periumbilical region for about 20 seconds causes jugular vein expansion (the abdominojugular reflux) in the presence of right heart failure. Palpation of the abdomen may reveal systolic expansion in patients with an abdominal aortic aneurysm. Splenomegaly is sometimes seen in prolonged, severe right ventricular failure.

References

1. Braunwald E: The history. In Braunwald E, Zipes D, Libby P (eds): Heart Disease, 6th ed. Philadelphia, WB Saunders, 2001, pp 27–44.
2. Braunwald E, Perloff JK: Physical examination of the heart and circulation. In Braunwald E, Zipes, D, Libby P (eds): Heart Disease, 6th ed. Philadelphia, WB Saunders, 2001, pp 45–81.
3. Chizner MA: The diagnosis of heart disease by clinical assessment alone. Curr Probl Cardiol 2001;26:285–380.
4. Clement DL, Cohn JN: Salvaging the history, physical examination and doctor-patient relationship in a technological cardiology environment. J Am Coll Cardiol 1999;33:892–893.
5. Michaelson E, Hollrah S: Evaluation of the patient with shortness of breath: An evidence-based approach. Emerg Med Clin North Am 1999;17:221–237.
6. Mahler DA, Harver A: Do you speak the language of dyspnea? Chest 2000;117:928–929.
7. Irwin RS, Madison JM: Symptom research on chronic cough: A historical perspective. Ann Intern Med 2001;134:809–814.
8. Irwin RS, Madison JM: The diagnosis and treatment of cough. N Engl J Med 2000;343:1715–1721.
9. The Criteria Committee of the New York Heart Association: Nomenclature and Criteria for Diagnosis, 9th ed. Boston, Little, Brown, 1994.
10. Campeau L: Letter: Grading of angina pectoris. Circulation 1976;54:522–523.
11. Goldman L, Hashimoto B, Cook EF, Loscalzo A: Comparative reproducibility and validity of systems for assessing

cardiovascular functional class: Advantages of a new specific activity scale. Circulation 1981;64:1227–1234.

12. Perloff JK: Physical Examination of the Heart and Circulation, 3rd ed. Philadelphia, WB Saunders, 2000.
13. Drazner MH, Rame JE, Stevenson LW, Dries DL: Prognostic importance of elevated jugular venous pressure and third heart sound in patients with heart failure. N Engl J Med 2001;345:574–581.
14. Perloff JK: The jugular venous pulse and third heart sound in patients with heart failure. N Engl J Med 2001;345:612–613.

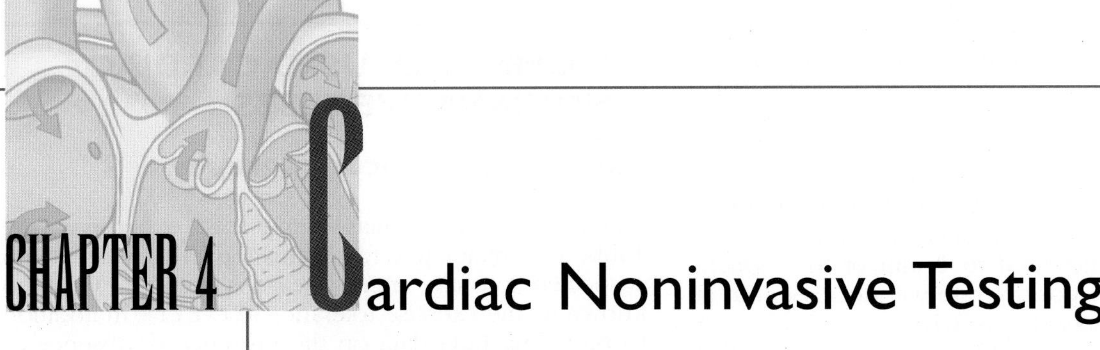

Cardiac Noninvasive Testing

Thomas H. Lee

Noninvasive cardiac tests, including exercise electrocardiography (ECG), echocardiography, and radionuclide tests, can help physicians address several common clinical issues such as the following:

- Does the patient have coronary artery disease?
- Does the patient have severe coronary artery disease that might have a better prognosis if managed with percutaneous coronary angioplasty or coronary artery bypass graft surgery?
- Does the patient have abnormal left ventricular function?
- Does the patient have significant valvular heart disease?

In addition to establishing a diagnosis, cardiac noninvasive tests can also help monitor the effectiveness of therapy and, in some cases, provide reassurance to the patient.

Although cardiac noninvasive tests can enhance the effectiveness of care, they should be used with discretion. The reasons include not only the costs and anxiety associated with the tests themselves, but also the procedures that frequently result from the noninvasive tests. For example, electron beam computed tomography (EBCT) may reveal the presence of coronary artery calcification in an asymptomatic patient who actually has only mild, nonobstructive coronary artery disease. Even though no data document improved outcomes through aggressive intervention in asymptomatic patients with abnormal EBCT results, these patients might undergo exercise testing, coronary angiography, and even coronary revascularization to address the uncertainty created by the abnormal screening test.

Such issues arise frequently for primary care physicians and are exacerbated by the availability of newer screening tests such as EBCT. This chapter therefore describes the following:

1. General principles of test utilization as applied to noninvasive cardiac tests
2. Commonly used cardiac noninvasive tests
3. Strategies for utilization of these tests for common clinical issues

PRINCIPLES OF CARDIAC NONINVASIVE TEST UTILIZATION

Like all tests, cardiac noninvasive tests are imperfect, and an understanding of their "performance characteristics" is an important skill for clinicians. For noninvasive cardiology tests, estimates of "sensitivity" and "specificity" provide a simplistic perspective on the interpretation of test results because these tests rarely provide data in the form of a "yes" or "no" response. "Abnormal" and "normal" test results usually reflect an arbitrary threshold that is applied to quantitative information, such as the amount of ST segment depression seen on ECG during exercise testing. Even when an abnormality is apparently dichotomous, such as the presence or absence of a defect on thallium scintigraphy, classification of that abnormality is often based on subjective interpretation of data.

The tradeoff between the true-positive and false-positive rates associated with various definitions of "abnormal" is readily apparent from exercise ECG data. If the presence of 1 mm of ST segment depression is used to call an exercise test "positive," the test will have high sensitivity for the detection of coronary artery disease, but it will also yield abnormal results in about 23% of patients without coronary artery disease (Table 4–1). If the threshold is increased to 2 mm of ST segment depression, that false-positive rate will decrease, but at the expense of decreased sensitivity.

The example of exercise ECG also demonstrates that the diagnostic performance of tests is influenced by the choice of outcome. Like other noninvasive tests for ischemia, exercise ECG has a much higher sensitivity (about 86%) for detecting three-vessel or left main coronary disease than for milder abnormalities[1] (see Table 4–1). Therefore, even though a test may have an apparently poor sensitivity for detection of one outcome (e.g., the presence or absence of coronary disease), it may have a desirable sensitivity and predictive value for detection of a more severe disease state that is actually of greater interest. On the other hand, when the outcome of interest is severe disease, the most sensitive tests are likely to have a high false-positive rate because of abnormal test results in patients with milder disease.

Ideally, clinicians would be guided in the use of noninvasive cardiac tests by randomized trials in which different testing strategies were compared. However, such trials are rarely performed for several reasons. First, the "outcome" of such trials depends on what clinicians do with the information from a test, and standardization of management strategies that follow from various test results would be logistically and ethically difficult. Second, physicians usually have alternative methods for getting the information that they seek from noninvasive tests, including other tests. Finally, the testing technologies themselves change so rapidly that by the time that the outcomes from use or nonuse of the test could be measured, the findings could be irrelevant to current practice.

COMMONLY USED CARDIAC NONINVASIVE TESTS

Exercise Electrocardiography

The most readily available and least expensive (see Table 4–1) major test for evaluation of a patient with suspected coronary artery disease is exercise ECG, also known as the exercise tolerance test (ETT). In addition to providing ECG data on the presence or absence of ischemia during exercise, this test also addresses several key issues, including

- The patient's functional capacity
- The level of exercise at which ischemia develops
- Whether symptoms such as chest pain with ischemia develop

These data on functional capacity and patient symptoms are critical for the assessment of prognosis, and they influence choices among therapeutic strategies.

Contraindications to exercise testing[2] are listed in Box 4–1. Under proper supervision, mortality can be expected to be less than 1 per 10,000 tests. The most commonly used protocol for exercise testing is the Bruce protocol (see Table 25–1), which increases the grade of elevation and the speed of the treadmill at 3-minute intervals. The protocol begins with the treadmill moving at just 1.7 mph with a 10% incline (stage 1), and just well-conditioned athletes can complete stage 7 (6.0 mph at a 22% incline). Only an approximate correlation is seen between exercise tolerance during treadmill testing and functional classification systems such as the New York Heart Association criteria, the Canadian Cardiovascular Society criteria, and the Specific Activity Scale, but patients are usually considered to be in functional class II if they can complete stage 1 of the Bruce protocol and in class I if they can complete stage 2.

TABLE 4–1

Sensitivity and Specificity of Noninvasive Tests for the Detection of Coronary Artery Disease

Diagnostic Test	Estimated Cost	Sensitivity (Range*)	Specificity (Range*)	Sensitivity for Left Main or Three-Vessel Disease
Exercise electrocardiography	$110	0.68	0.77	.86
Planar thallium imaging	$221	0.79 (0.70–0.94)	0.73 (0.43–0.97)	.93
Single-photon emission computed tomography (SPECT)	$475	0.88 (0.73–0.98)	0.77 (0.53–0.96)	.98
Stress echocardiography	$265	0.76 (0.40–1.00)	0.88 (0.80–0.95)	.94

*Range of sensitivity and specificity reported in individual studies.

Reproduced with permission from Garber AM, Solomon NA: Cost-effectiveness of alternative test strategies for the diagnosis of coronary artery disease. Ann Intern Med 1999;130:719–728.

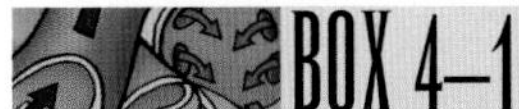

BOX 4–1

Contraindications to Exercise Testing

ABSOLUTE

- Acute myocardial infarction (within 2 days)
- Unstable angina not previously stabilized by medical therapy*
- Uncontrolled cardiac arrhythmias causing symptoms or hemodynamic compromise
- Symptomatic severe aortic stenosis
- Uncontrolled symptomatic heart failure
- Acute pulmonary embolism or pulmonary infarction
- Acute myocarditis or pericarditis
- Acute aortic dissection

RELATIVE†

- Left main coronary stenosis
- Moderate stenotic valvular heart disease
- Electrolyte abnormalities
- Severe arterial hypertension‡
- Tachyarrhythmias or bradyarrhythmias
- Hypertrophic cardiomyopathy and other forms of outflow tract obstruction
- Mental or physical impairment leading to an inability to exercise adequately
- High-degree atrioventricular block

*Appropriate timing of testing depends on the level of risk for unstable angina.
†Relative contraindications can be superseded if the benefits of exercise outweigh the risks.
‡In the absence of definitive evidence, the committee suggests a systolic blood pressure over 200 mm Hg and/or a diastolic blood pressure less than 110 mm Hg.
Adapted from Gibbons RJ, Balady GJ, Beasley JW, et al: ACC/AHA guidelines for exercise testing: A report of the American College of Cardiology/American Heart Association Task Force on Practice Guidelines (Committee on Exercise Testing). J Am Coll Cardiol 1997;30:260–315.

In most patients, the test is "symptom limited"—that is, stopped when fatigue, dyspnea, light-headedness, chest pain, or pain elsewhere in the body (e.g., the legs) develops or when clear evidence of ischemia or arrhythmia is apparent on ECG. In some settings, however, such as in the first days after acute myocardial infarction, the test may be stopped when some pre-specified, low level of exertion has been reached.

With "modified Bruce protocols," the usual purpose of the test is not to push patients to their physical limits but rather to determine whether it is safe for patients to be discharged home. Typically, the first two stages of a modified Bruce protocol are performed at 1.7 mph with a 0% and then a 5% incline, and the third stage is performed at 1.7 mph and a 10% incline. In many laboratories, tests for patients a few days after an acute myocardial infarction are stopped after this third stage. Examples of other settings in which modified Bruce protocols are used include emergency department patients with acute chest pain, patients with potentially unstable arrhythmias or left ventricular dysfunction, and patients with significant valvular disease—in short, patients in whom the safety of a standard exercise test is uncertain, but in whom the results of a test may be useful for management. In such cases, if the patient does not have evidence of ischemia during the first two stages, the ETT may continue as per a standard Bruce protocol until limited by symptoms or ECG abnormalities.

Several drugs can influence ETT results, including digoxin, beta-adrenergic blocking agents, and vasodilators. Guidelines recommend that beta-blockers and other anti-ischemic drugs be stopped about 2 days before exercise testing for the diagnosis and initial risk stratification of patients with suspected coronary disease.[3] Withdrawal of these medications is frequently not practical, and stress testing still is usually abnormal in patients at highest risk for complications.

Alternatives to walking on a treadmill must be considered for patients who cannot do so because of orthopedic or other problems. Bicycle protocols progressively increase resistance and are usually stopped when the patient cannot pedal at least 40 cycles per minute. In subjects unfamiliar with bicycle exercise, the muscles required for such protocols are often not well developed, and tests are stopped at a lower cardiac workload than with treadmill exercise. Advantages of bicycle ergometry include less space requirements and the ability to get ECG tracings with less motion artifact.

Arm crank ergometry protocols, in which patients "pedal" with their arms, increase workloads incrementally at 2- or 3-minute stages. Because the arms of most people have less stamina than their legs, the peak heart rate achieved through such tests is usually only about 70% of that achieved with leg testing.

Interpretation. During and after exercise, the patient's electrocardiogram is monitored to detect evidence of ST segment changes or arrhythmia. Moderate ST segment depression is not necessarily diagnostic of ischemia, particularly if it occurs in the absence of chest pain or if the contour of the ST segment is up-sloping[4] (Fig. 4–1). For this reason, tests are often not stopped at the first instant that ST segment depression becomes apparent.

Because so many types of information are collected during an exercise test, clinicians should specifically note several types of data when reviewing the results of this test:

- *How far did the patient go?* The ability to complete 6 minutes or more of a standard Bruce Protocol indicates a normal work capacity.

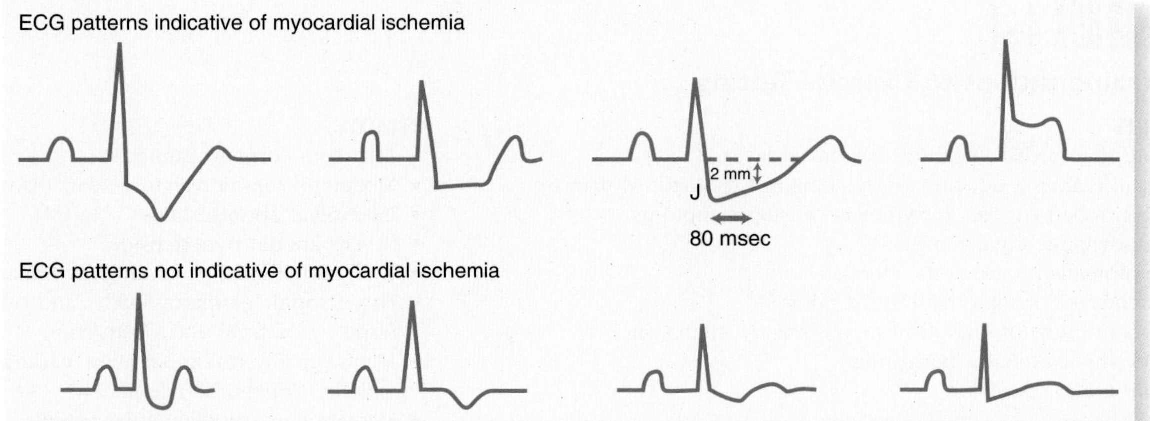

FIGURE 4–1. Electrocardiographic (ECG) criteria suggestive of myocardial ischemia consist of at least 1 mm of J point depression with down-sloping or horizontal ST segments; slowly up-sloping ST segment depression, defined as 2 mm of ST depression measured 80 msec from the J point; and ST segment elevation. Patterns less suggestive of ischemia are included in the second row. (Redrawn from Goldschlager N: Use of the treadmill test in the diagnosis of coronary artery disease in patients with chest pain. Ann Intern Med 1982;97:383–388.)

- *What was the peak rate-pressure product?* Tests may be inconclusive if patients are unable to perform enough cardiac work to provoke ischemia. Multiplication of the peak systolic blood pressure by the peak heart rate provides a rough, but easily calculated index of the heart's work, and tests with a double product that exceeds 18,000 (e.g., peak heart rate of 100, peak systolic blood pressure of 180) are generally considered to be adequate. Beta-adrenergic blocking agents may compromise the ability of a patient to raise the heart rate to a level sufficient to precipitate an ischemic response.
- *Did the patient have symptoms and ECG changes?* The combination of these types of abnormalities is much more likely to be diagnostic of ischemia than either alone.
- *What did the ST segment depression look like?* ST segment depression should persist for at least 0.08 second (two of the little boxes) after the QRS complex for it to be considered significant, and it is much more likely to reflect ischemia if it is horizontal or down-sloping in contour[4] (see Fig. 4–1). The greater the degree of ST segment depression, the more likely coronary disease.
- *Does the patient have any characteristics that might affect the ECG response to exercise testing?* Digitalis and left ventricular hypertrophy can cause resting abnormalities of the ST segment that can be exacerbated by ischemia, even in the absence of coronary disease. Conduction abnormalities such as left bundle branch block or atrioventricular bypass tracts may also lead to false-positive ST segment abnormalities that do not reflect true myocardial ischemia.
- *Did the patient have any abnormal non-ECG responses to exercise?* The normal response to exercise is an increase in heart rate and systolic blood pressure. A decline in blood pressure or failure to increase the rate-pressure product often reflects underlying cardiomyopathy or severe ischemia.

Radionuclide Imaging

Radionuclide imaging is performed with a variety of different tracers, as well as different techniques for capturing images. Much of the early literature on radionuclide imaging was based on simple "planar" images obtained from cameras in standard positions. Today, however, most laboratories use single-photon emission computed tomography (SPECT) to reconstruct anatomic "slices" of myocardium. Positron emission tomography (PET) scanners include multiple rings of stationary detectors that can detect emissions from tracers to describe regional myocardial blood flow; however, PET scanners are more costly, and research has not documented that the additional information either changes or improves management.[5]

In radionuclide imaging, ischemia can be provoked by exercise or pharmacologic agents. Dobutamine is a positive inotropic agent that induces ischemia by increasing myocardial work. Adenosine and dipyridamole are vasodilators that unmask coronary stenoses by increasing flow in nondiseased coronary arteries. As is true with exercise ECG, beta-blockers and other antianginal medications may compromise sensitivity for the detection of coronary artery disease and should be stopped when possible four to five half-lives (about 2 days) before testing.[3]

Interpretation. Two major classes of radionuclide agents are used to assess myocardial perfusion and viability: thallium 201– and technetium 99m–labeled tracers (sestamibi, teboroxime, and tetrofosmin). The initial distribution of these tracers is proportional to myocardial blood flow; "redistribution" images obtained 3 to 4 hours later reflect myocardial viability and are unrelated to flow. A "defect" on an initial scan that

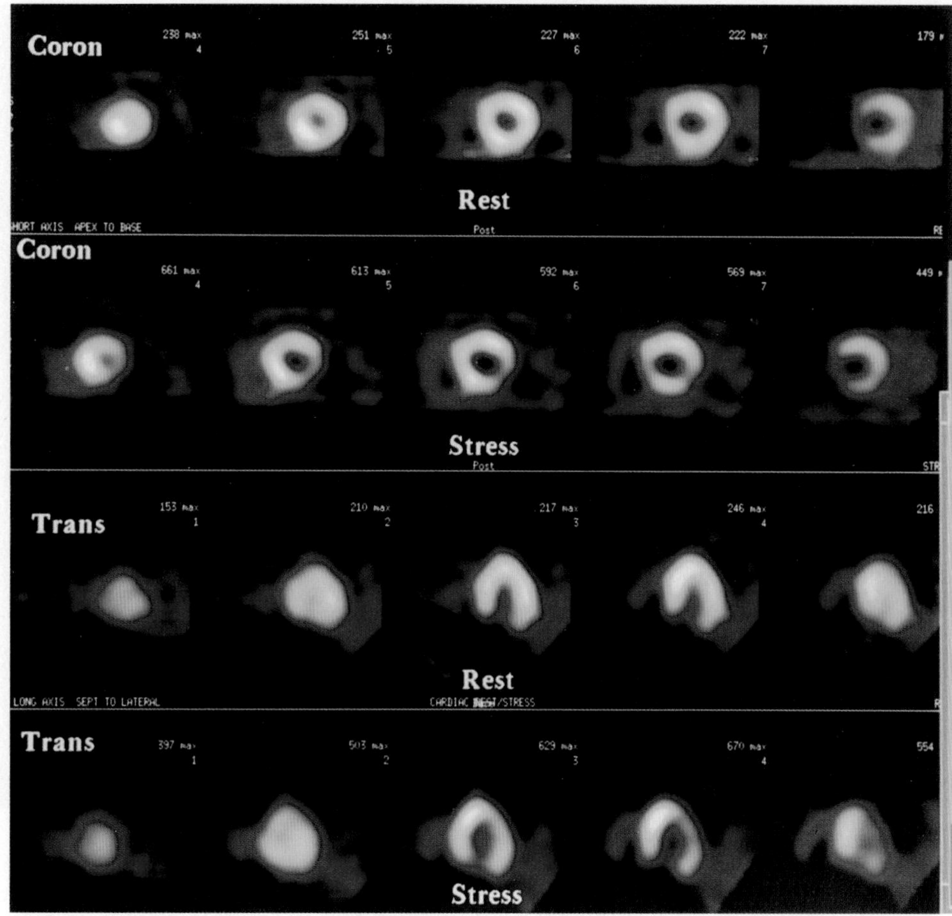

FIGURE 4–2. Myocardial perfusion scan showing moderate ischemia of the inferolateral wall of the left ventricle from the base to the apex with stress (*bottom right* image). With rest, the region that was not perfused during pharmacologic stress receives normal blood flow, and the perfusion defect resolves (third row, *last* image). Coron, coronal view; Trans, transverse view. (Courtesy of Finn Manting, M.D., Ph.D., Director, Nuclear Medicine, Brigham and Women's Hospital, Boston.)

resolves on a later scan is an indicator of myocardium that is threatened but viable (Fig. 4–2). A defect apparent on both scans suggests a region of myocardium that has died, presumably because of myocardial infarction. The diagnostic performance of testing with these agents is similar, so the choice among agents is generally based on the laboratory's preference.

With either planar or SPECT imaging, the sensitivity for detection of coronary artery disease and severe coronary artery disease is greater than with exercise ECG (see Table 4–1). However, published estimates of test performance of radionuclide perfusion imaging are highly variable because of differences in imaging techniques and standards for interpretation. False-positive results are an important problem with SPECT imaging. Apparent perfusion defects can be caused by artifacts (e.g., breast tissue, diaphragm) between the heart and the imaging camera. The experience of the physician reading the scans is especially critical in SPECT imaging, and thus published data on the diagnostic performance of these tests should not be assumed to be valid for all laboratories.

As is true of exercise ECG, radionuclide perfusion imaging is less accurate in women than men. Some data suggest that the better imaging properties of technetium 99m sestamibi may make it a superior agent for evaluation of obese patients or for women with large breasts or breast implants.

Stress Echocardiography

In stress echocardiography, comparisons are made between echocardiographic images obtained at rest and during or immediately after stress (e.g., 1 to 2 minutes after exercise). A test is considered positive if new wall motion abnormalities develop with stress or worsen in a segment that is abnormal at baseline (see Figs. 5–6 and 25–5). Thus, this test provides information on the location and amount of myocardium in jeopardy. In addition, stress echocardiography provides insight into left ventricular and cardiac valve function (see Chapter 5).

Interpretation. Estimates of the diagnostic performance of stress echocardiography vary widely (see Table 4–1), presumably because of differences in patient populations and interpreters of the tests in different studies. Pooled data indicate that exercise echocardiography is less sensitive but more specific than exercise SPECT imaging.[6] The diagnostic performance of dobutamine and dipyridamole stress echocardiography is similar.[7]

Electron Beam Computed Tomography

EBCT, also known as "ultrafast" computed tomography (CT), uses rapid imaging techniques to obtain high-quality cardiac images with little motion artifact.

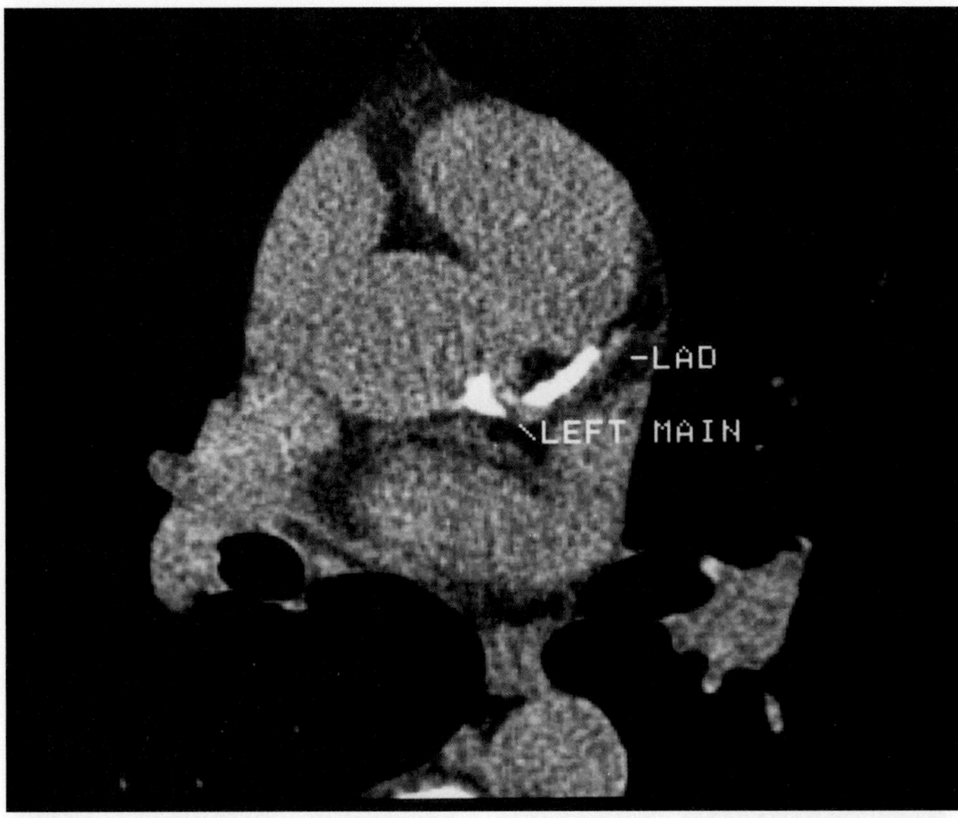

FIGURE 4–3. Cross-sectional view of the heart and great vessels at the level of the left main coronary artery and proximal anterior descending artery. Calcium deposits, in this case heavy, appear as bright white spots. In person with chest pain, a calcium score above 80 predicts 50% coronary stenosis with a sensitivity and specificity of about 84%. Higher calcium scores are more predictive, but no threshold is sufficiently sensitive and specific in asymptomatic patients to be relied on for diagnosis. (Courtesy of Alan Guerci, MD.)

Although these images do not allow assessment of the lumen of the coronary arteries, EBCT can measure the extent of coronary artery calcification, which correlates with the extent of atherosclerosis (Fig. 4–3). The sensitivity for detection of coronary artery disease is as high as 95%; however, the specificity is only 44% to 47%,[8,9] a finding reflecting the high prevalence of coronary calcification and atherosclerosis in patients without obstructive coronary artery disease. The overall predictive accuracy of EBCT is about 70%.[10]

Interpretation of data on the diagnostic performance of EBCT is complicated by variations in the significance of coronary calcification in patients of different ages and by patients' varying clinical risk for coronary disease. In addition, the calcium scores are continuous variables, not categorical yes-no results. Finally, it is not clear that EBCT adds information to what can be gleaned from routine clinical data or risk factors.[11] Thus, an expert panel from the American College of Cardiology (ACC) and the American Heart Association (AHA) concluded that it would not recommend screening EBCT for the diagnosis of obstructive coronary disease.[10] Clinical trials testing the ability of information from EBCT to improve risk stratification and patient management are under way, so the role of this test may evolve in the near future.

Choice of Tests for Coronary Artery Disease

In some patients, the inability to exercise or the presence of baseline ECG abnormalities makes exercise ECG an inappropriate test (Box 4–2). In other patients, the amount and location of myocardium in jeopardy may be a critical clinical issue. In such cases, an imaging technology (either radionuclide or echocardiographic) is the clear first choice. Controversy arises, however, in patients who are reasonable candidates for both exercise ECG and other testing technologies.

As noted in Table 4–1, imaging technologies provide more information than exercise ECG alone does. However, the availability of more information does not necessarily mean that a more expensive test should be the first choice. Other important issues include whether the additional information is likely to change the patient's management in ways expected to improve outcomes. If improved outcomes are likely, yet another issue is the magnitude of the cost required to achieve these improvements.

Two independent cost-effectiveness analyses have indicated that both exercise echocardiography and radionuclide imaging improve outcomes with a cost-effectiveness comparable to that of other accepted medical interventions.[1,12] These analyses reflect the higher specificity of stress echocardiography and higher sensitivity of radionuclide imaging than can be achieved compared with exercise ECG. Stress echocardiography was found to be more cost-effective than radionuclide imaging in these studies, in part because of the lower cost of the test.

Nevertheless, even analyses suggesting that imaging tests can potentially improve the patient's outcomes with reasonable cost-effectiveness do not necessarily mean that they should be adopted as first-line tests for all patients. First, the actual diagnostic performance of

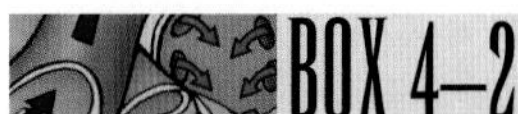

BOX 4–2

Indications for Radionuclide Perfusion or Echocardiography Imaging Instead of Exercise Electrocardiography

- Complete left bundle branch block
- Electronically paced ventricular rhythm
- Preexcitation (Wolff-Parkinson-White) syndrome and other similar electrocardiographic conduction abnormalities
- Patients who have >1 mm of ST segment depression at rest, including those with left ventricular hypertrophy or taking drugs such as digitalis
- Patients unable to exercise to a level high enough to give meaningful results on a routine stress electrocardiogram should be considered for pharmacologic stress imaging tests
- Patients with angina who have undergone previous revascularization, in whom localization of ischemia, establishment of the functional significance of lesions, and demonstration of myocardial viability are important considerations

Adapted from Gibbons RJ, Chatterjee K, Daley J, et al: ACC/AHA/ACP-ASM guidelines for the management of patients with chronic stable angina. A report of the American College of Cardiology/American Heart Association Task Force on Practice Guidelines (Committee on the Management of Patients with Chronic Stable Angina). J Am Coll Cardiol 1999;33:2092–2197.

imaging tests is heavily dependent on physicians' interpretation of the images, which raises the possibility that the information derived from these tests may be less in clinical practice than described in published research. Second, cost-effectiveness analyses based on data derived from patients who actually underwent coronary angiography are of uncertain relevance to lower risk populations, such as those with stable or atypical chest pain. Finally, when resources are limited, investment in more expensive management strategies may not have a high priority even if their cost-effectiveness is attractive.

Because of the higher cost and other limitations of imaging tests, guidelines from the ACC, AHA, and American College of Physicians/American Society of Internal Medicine advocate exercise ECG as the appropriate first test for stable patients with known or suspected chronic angina[2,3,13] (Fig. 4–4). These guidelines express uncertainty about optimal testing strategies in women but conclude that there are "currently insufficient data to justify replacing standard exercise testing with stress imaging when evaluating women."[3]

A "hybrid" approach is to use different testing strategies for patients with varying levels of risk for cardiovascular complications as suggested by the clinical findings, including data from exercise ECG such as through the Duke treadmill score.[14] The Duke treadmill score is calculated as exercise time minus (5 × ST deviation in millimeters) minus (4 × exercise angina), where exercise angina is defined as 0 = none, 1 = nonlimiting, and 2 = exercise limiting. The scores usually range from −25 to +15. These values correspond to low-risk (with a score of +5 or higher), moderate-risk (with scores ranging from −10 to +4), and high-risk (with a score of −11 or lower) categories (Table 4–2). The Duke treadmill score can also be used in the form of a nomogram (Fig. 4–5). Low-risk patients have an excellent prognosis, whereas high-risk patients should usually be considered for aggressive management, including coronary revascularization. In either case, imaging tests are unlikely to change management. However, such tests may be useful in intermediate-risk patients with modest exercise capacity or subtle evidence of ischemia.

Evaluation of Left Ventricular Function and Cardiac Anatomy

The dominant technology for evaluating left ventricular function is echocardiography (see Chapter 5). Echocardiography is a rapidly evolving field, with technical advances including transesophageal echocardiography (TEE), three-dimensional echocardiography, and the use of contrast. An additional innovation likely to have an impact on clinical care is the development of small portable ultrasound devices about the size of an audiocassette player to allow physicians to obtain a qualitative assessment of ventricular and valvular function. Such devices may become important tools to augment the routine examination in emergency departments, intensive care units, and outpatient offices of trained primary care physicians.

Magnetic resonance imaging (MRI) and ultrafast CT are two technologies that can provide three-dimensional images of moving cardiac structures. However, these devices are over 10 times more expensive than ultrasound devices, and the incremental benefit of using MRI and ultrafast CT for many cardiac diagnostic questions is unclear. Radionuclide ventriculography, an alternative to the echocardiogram, provides quantitative estimates of left ventricular function by calculating how much of a radionuclide tracer has been ejected from the left ventricle with each contraction. The radiation exposure is not clinically significant. However, the more precise estimate of left ventricular function than achieved with echocardiography is rarely needed for management decisions, and this test does not provide an evaluation of valvular function. Furthermore, radionuclide ventriculography is more expensive than echocardiography. Therefore, it should usually be considered a second choice to echocardiography.

Assessment of Cardiac Rhythm Disturbances

Although exercise ECG is sometimes used to evaluate whether exercise-induced symptoms are due to arrhythmias, the procedure of choice for patients with known or suspected arrhythmias is long-term ECG monitoring (see Chapters 30 and 31), also known as Holter

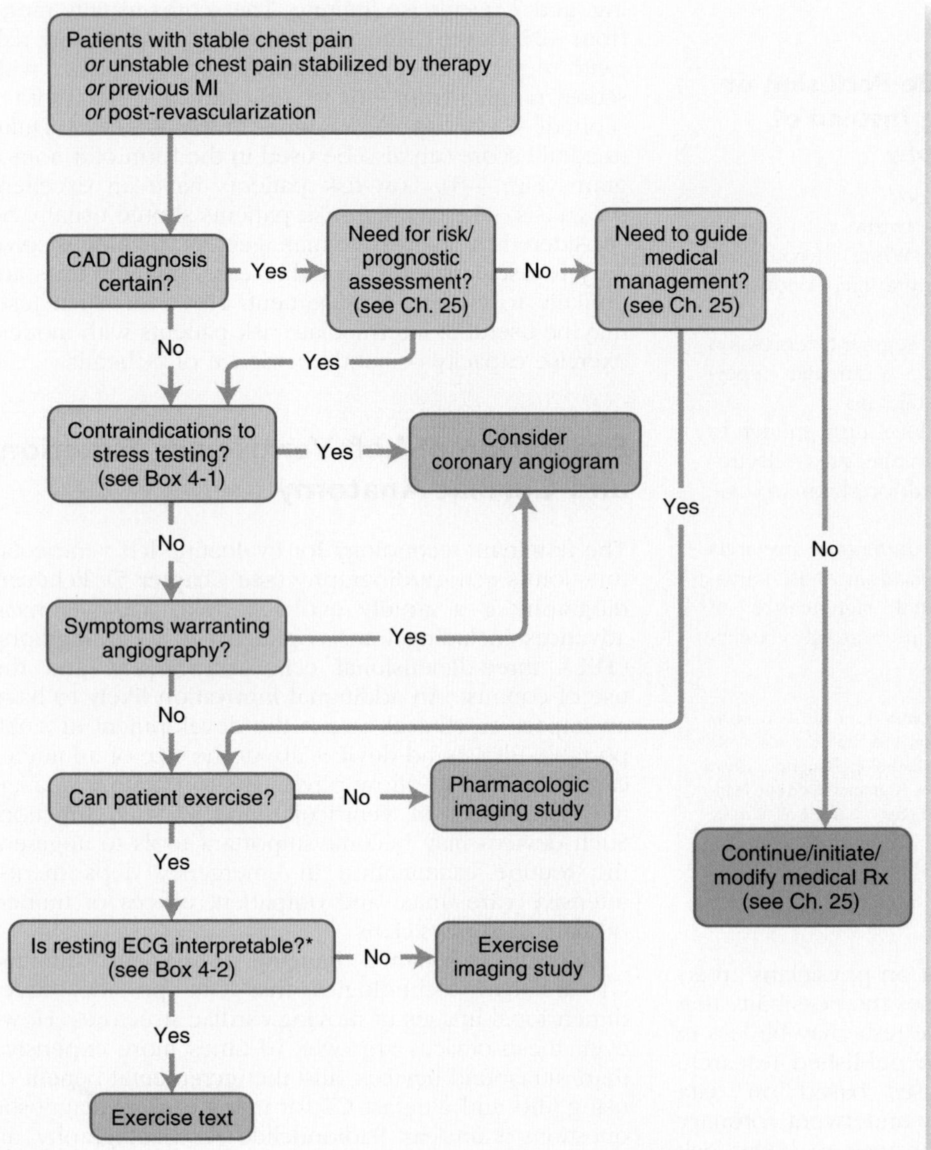

FIGURE 4–4. Exercise testing for the evaluation of patients with suspected ischemic heart disease. *The electrocardiogram (ECG) is interpretable unless preexcitation, electronically paced rhythm, left bundle branch block, or resting ST segment depression greater than 1 mm is present (see Box 4–2). (Also see Figure 25–2.) CAD, coronary artery disease; MI, myocardial infarction. (Adapted from Gibbons RJ, Balady GJ, Beasley JW, et al: ACC/AHA guidelines for exercise testing: A report of the American College of Cardiology/American Heart Association Task Force on Practice Guidelines [Committee on Exercise Testing]. J Am Coll Cardiol 1997;30:260–315. Reprinted with permission from the American College of Cardiology.)

TABLE 4–2

Five-Year Mortality and Prevalence of High-Risk Coronary Disease in 2578 Medically Treated Patients Stratified by Duke Treadmill Scores

Duke Treadmill Score Group (and Score)	5-Year Mortality	Prevalence of High-Risk Coronary Disease		
		2-Vessel or Left Anterior Descending Disease	*2-Vessel and Left Anterior Descending Disease*	*3-Vessel or Left Main Disease*
Low risk (≥+5)	3.1%	10.3%	3.9%	9.5%
Intermediate risk (−10 to +4)	9.5%	14.5%	10%	30.6%
High risk (≤−11)	35.5%	10.7%	9.5%	73.5%

Adapted from Shaw LJ, Peterson ED, Shaw LK, et al: Use of a prognostic treadmill score in identifying diagnostic coronary disease subgroups. Circulation 1998;98:1622–1630.

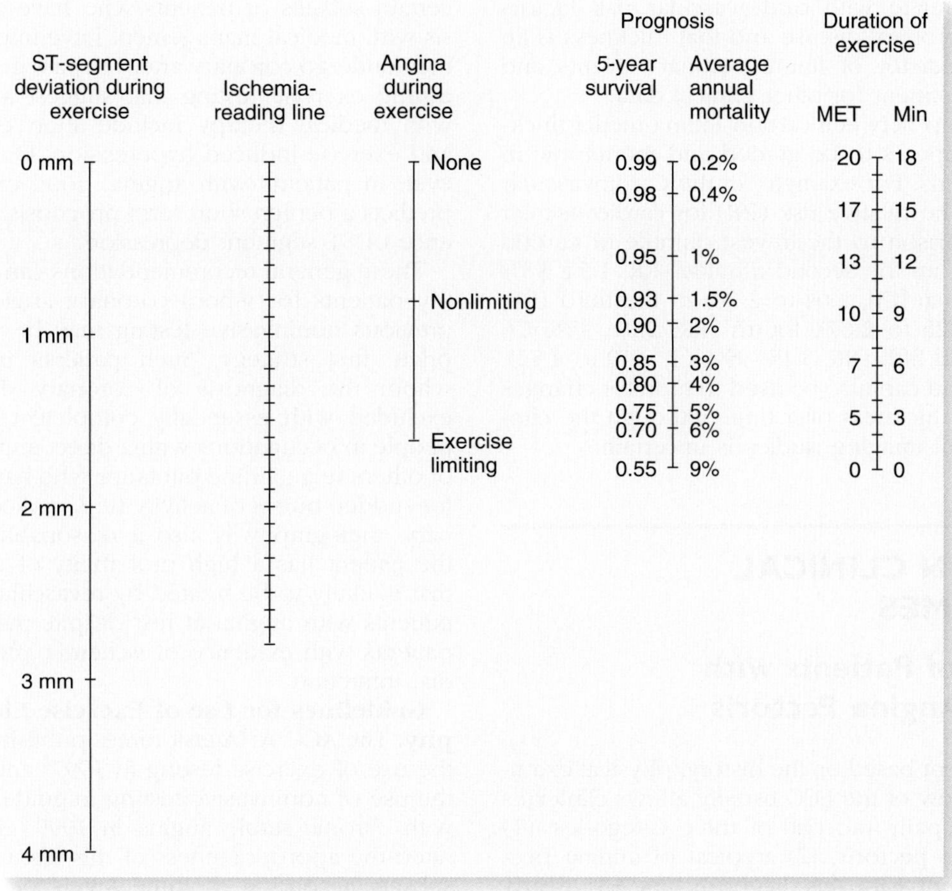

FIGURE 4–5. Nomogram form of the Duke treadmill score to calculate the 5-year cardiovascular survival rate and average annual cardiovascular mortality for patients on the basis of the duration of exercise, ST segment deviation (depression or elevation), and the presence and severity of angina during exercise. To use this nomogram, determine the amount of ST segment deviation detected during exercise testing and mark the vertical line farthest on the left in the corresponding place. Next, mark the third line in the appropriate location that correlates with the nature of any anginal symptoms. Connect these two marks with a straight line and note where they intersect on the second line, which is the ischemia-reading line. Then mark the right-most line to indicate how many minutes of exercise that the patient was able to perform on a standard Bruce protocol. Connect this point with the mark for ischemia. The point at which this line intersects the prognosis line is the result of the Duke treadmill score. (Reprinted, by permission, from Mark DB, Shaw L, Harrell FE Jr, et al: Prognostic value of a treadmill exercise score in outpatients with suspected coronary artery disease. N Engl J Med 1991;325:849–853.)

monitoring. Usually, a recorder the size of a small cassette player records two ECG channels for 24 hours. Newer variations on this technology allow patients to press a button after the occurrence of symptoms, thereby causing the recorder to save the last several minutes of ECG activity. Patients with rare symptoms can wear such an "event recorder" for periods as long as several months.

Assessment of Vasomotor Function

Upright tilt testing can identify patients who have a vasodepressor or neurocardiogenic cause of syncope (see Chapter 10). Patients are strapped to a table in a horizontal position and then tilted upright for 20 to 45 minutes in an attempt to reproduce symptoms, cause syncope, or both. Isoproterenol may be infused to provoke syncope in patients who are asymptomatic after initial testing. Although this test has a high "false-positive" rate for the detection of neurocardiogenic syncope, it can be used to guide therapy in patients with a history of episodes of loss of consciousness.

B-Mode Carotid Ultrasound

This test uses ultrasound to visualize the lumen and walls of the carotid artery. In addition to defining the presence and severity of atherosclerotic plaque, it can provide measurements of the intima-media thickness of the far and near walls of three segments of the carotid circulation—the distal common carotid arteries, the carotid bifurcations, and the proximal 1 cm of the internal carotid arteries. Several research studies have demonstrated that common carotid intima-media thickness scores correlate with cardiovascular risk factors and prevalent coronary disease and that thickness is an independent predictor of future coronary events and stroke after adjustment for other clinical data.[15]

The relationship between carotid intima-media thickness and risk appears to be graded and monotonic in most investigations. For example, in the Cardiovascular Health Study,[16] the relative risk (RR) for cardiovascular events in comparison to the lowest quintile of carotid thickness rose from the second quintile (RR, 1.54; 95% confidence interval [CI], 1.04 to 2.28) to the third (RR, 1.84; 95% CI, 1.26 to 2.67), fourth (RR, 2.01; 95% CI, 1.38 to 2.91), and fifth (RR, 3.15; 95% CI, 2.19 to 4.52). Carotid ultrasound can also be used to monitor changes in intima-media thickness over time, although the clinical role for serial imaging studies is uncertain.

COMMON CLINICAL SYNDROMES

Evaluation of Patients with Suspected Angina Pectoris

Clinical assessment based on the history, physical examination, and review of the ECG usually allows clinicians to classify chest pain into one of three categories: (1) typical of angina pectoris, (2) atypical of angina pectoris but consistent with this diagnosis, and (3) clearly noncardiac chest pain. This categorization is critical to both the decision to order a noninvasive test for ischemia and interpretation of the result. In patients with typical angina, the prevalence of coronary disease is 80% or more, and even a normal test result might not change the assessment of whether the risk for coronary disease is high. In patients whose atypical symptoms suggest a low risk for coronary disease, an abnormal test result might not raise the possibility of coronary disease to a level that warrants coronary angiography or treatment with anti-ischemic medications.

Thus, the primary care physician should have a clear idea of the purpose of noninvasive testing when evaluating patients with suspected coronary disease. The two most common reasons are

- Estimation of the probability of any coronary disease
- Estimation of the probability of severe coronary disease that is associated with a poor prognosis with medical therapy and therefore might warrant revascularization with angioplasty or bypass graft surgery

Noninvasive tests for ischemia are most useful for the *diagnosis* of coronary disease in patients at *intermediate* risk for this diagnosis. In this population, a markedly positive test can essentially establish the diagnosis of coronary disease, whereas a clearly negative result can reduce that possibility to a negligible level.

These tests are also often useful for the evaluation of overall *prognosis* in patients with typical angina in that certain subsets of patients who have a worse prognosis with medical management have improved survival if they undergo coronary artery bypass graft surgery. Signs during exercise testing that suggest a poor prognosis with medical therapy include short exercise duration and exercise-induced hypotension. On the other hand, even in patients with angina, good exercise tolerance predicts a benign short-term prognosis despite the presence of ST segment depression.

These general recommendations can be used to identify patients for whom coronary angiography without previous noninvasive testing may be the most appropriate first strategy. Such patients include those in whom the diagnosis of coronary disease must be excluded with essentially complete certainty, such as people in occupations with a direct impact on the safety of others (e.g., airline pilots) or who have frequent need for sudden bursts of activity (e.g., police officers). Coronary angiography is also a reasonable first test when the patient has a high probability of coronary disease that is likely to be treated by revascularization, such as patients with angina at rest despite medical therapy or patients with evidence of ischemia after acute myocardial infarction.

Guidelines for Use of Exercise Electrocardiography. The ACC/AHA task forces published guidelines for the use of exercise testing in 1997[2] and also addressed the use of noninvasive testing in guidelines for patients with chronic stable angina in 1999.[3] These guidelines rated the appropriateness of this test in various patient subsets according to three levels of appropriateness, including conditions for which or patients for whom it is generally agreed that exercise testing is useful (class I), conditions for which or patients for whom exercise testing is frequently used but opinion differs with respect to its usefulness (class II), and conditions for which or patients for whom it is generally agreed that exercise testing is of little or no usefulness (class III). Within class II, indications were rated IIa if the expert panel thought that the weight of evidence was in favor of usefulness of the test and IIb if the weight of evidence was less well established.

In these guidelines, exercise testing is considered clearly appropriate in patients with an intermediate probability of coronary artery disease (Box 4–3) because of the low likelihood that a test will change the diagnosis in patients with either a low or a high probability of coronary disease based on age and other clinical data. The guideline also provided a framework for qualitative assessment of the probability of coronary disease based on such information (Table 4–3).

The ACC/AHA guidelines note that exercise testing is appropriate in patients with a complete right bundle branch block or less than 1 mm of resting ST depression. They also conclude that cessation of therapy with digoxin or beta-blockers is not necessary before exercise testing, even though these agents can decrease the specificity (digoxin) or sensitivity (beta-blockers) of testing.

The ACC/AHA guidelines did not support the use of exercise testing in any setting to screen apparently healthy individuals or those with chest discomfort not

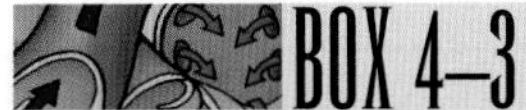
BOX 4–3

Exercise Testing for the Diagnosis of Obstructive Coronary Artery Disease

CLASS I (USEFUL AND RECOMMENDED)

Adult patients (including those with complete right bundle branch block or less than 1 mm of resting ST depression) with an intermediate pretest probability of CAD (see Table 4–3) based on gender, age, and symptoms (specific exceptions are noted in classes II and III)

CLASS IIA (WEIGHT OF EVIDENCE IS IN FAVOR)

Patients with vasospastic angina

CLASS IIB (USEFULNESS AND EFFICACY NOT WELL ESTABLISHED)

Patients with a high pretest probability of CAD by age, symptoms, and gender

Patients with a low pretest probability of CAD by age, symptoms, and gender

Patients with less than 1 mm of baseline ST depression and taking digoxin

Patients with electrocardiographic criteria for left ventricular hypertrophy and less than 1 mm of baseline ST depression

CLASS III (NOT USEFUL OR EFFECTIVE)

Patients with the following baseline electrocardiographic abnormalities:
- Preexcitation (Wolff-Parkinson-White) syndrome
- Electronically paced ventricular rhythm
- Greater than 1 mm of resting ST depression
- Complete left bundle branch block
- Patients with a documented myocardial infarction or previous coronary angiography demonstrating significant disease have an established diagnosis of CAD; however, ischemia and risk can be determined by testing

CAD, coronary artery disease.

From Gibbons RJ, Balady GJ, Beasley JW, et al: ACC/AHA guidelines for exercise testing: A report of the American College of Cardiology/American Heart Association Task Force on Practice Guidelines (Committee on Exercise Testing). J Am Coll Cardiol 1997;30:260–315. Reprinted with permission from the American College of Cardiology.

BOX 4–4

Exercise Testing in Asymptomatic Persons without Known Coronary Artery Disease

CLASS I (USEFUL AND RECOMMENDED)

None

CLASS IIB (USEFULNESS AND EFFICACY NOT WELL ESTABLISHED)

Evaluation of persons with multiple risk factors*

Evaluation of asymptomatic men older than 40 yr and women older than 50 yr
- Who plan to start vigorous exercise (especially if sedentary)

  or
- Who are involved in occupations in which impairment might have an impact on public safety

  or
- Who are at high risk for coronary artery disease because of other conditions (e.g., chronic renal failure)

CLASS III (NOT USEFUL OR EFFECTIVE)

Routine screening of asymptomatic men or women

*Multiple risk factors are defined as hypercholesterolemia (>240 mg/dL), hypertension (systolic blood pressure >140 mm Hg or diastolic blood pressure >90 mm Hg), smoking, diabetes, and a family history of heart attack or sudden cardiac death in a first-degree relative younger than 60 years. An alternative approach is to select patients with a Framingham risk score consistent with at least a moderate risk of serious cardiac events within 5 years.

From Gibbons RJ, Balady GJ, Beasley JW, et al: ACC/AHA guidelines for exercise testing: A report of the American College of Cardiology/American Heart Association Task Force on Practice Guidelines (Committee on Exercise Testing). J Am Coll Cardiol 1997;30:260–315. Reprinted with permission from the American College of Cardiology.

thought to be of cardiac origin (Box 4–4). Furthermore, the guidelines offered only equivocal support (class IIb) for exercise testing of asymptomatic patients with special occupations, those older than 40 years with two or more major risk factors for coronary artery disease, and those older than 40 who are sedentary and about to embark on a vigorous exercise program.

Evaluation of Patients with a Systolic Murmur

In patients with a systolic murmur (see Chapter 11), echocardiography permits visualization of valvular and septal abnormalities via echocardiographic images. Doppler analysis can be used to assess the severity of hemodynamic derangements caused by valvular disease, and the speed of red blood cell flow can be used to estimate the pressure gradient across the aortic valve in patients with aortic stenosis. Doppler analysis can also provide a qualitative (1+, 2+, etc.) description of the severity of mitral regurgitation.

Even if the nature of the valvular abnormality is not in question, echocardiography is useful for assessment of left ventricular function. For patients with mitral or aortic valve regurgitation, progressive dilatation of the left ventricle despite medical therapy with vasodilators should lead to consideration of valvular surgery to prevent irreversible ventricular dysfunction.

Guidelines. The ACC/AHA guidelines on valvular heart disease that were published in 1998 considered echocardiography potentially useful in patients with systolic murmurs unless an experienced observer's physical examination indicated that it was extremely unlikely that the murmur was of organic origin[17] (Box

TABLE 4–3

Probability of Coronary Artery Disease by Age, Gender, and Symptoms

Age (yr)	Gender	Typical/Definite Angina Pectoris	Atypical/Probable Angina Pectoris	Nonanginal Chest Pain	Asymptomatic
30–39	Men	Intermediate	Intermediate	Low	Very low
	Women	Intermediate	Very low	Very low	Very low
40–49	Men	High	Intermediate	Intermediate	Low
	Women	Intermediate	Low	Very low	Very low
50–59	Men	High	Intermediate	Intermediate	Low
	Women	Intermediate	Intermediate	Low	Very low
60–69	Men	High	Intermediate	Intermediate	Low
	Women	High	Intermediate	Intermediate	Low

No data exist for patients younger than 30 or older than 69 years, but it can be assumed that the prevalence of coronary artery disease increases with age. In a few cases, patients with ages at the extremes of the decades listed may have probabilities slightly outside the high or low range. High indicates 90%; intermediate, 10% to 90%; low, less than 10%; and very low, less than 5%.

From Gibbons RJ, Balady GJ, Beasley JW, et al: ACC/AHA guidelines for exercise testing: A report of the American College of Cardiology/American Heart Association Task Force on Practice Guidelines (Committee on Exercise Testing). J Am Coll Cardiol 1997;30:260–315. Reprinted with permission from the American College of Cardiology.

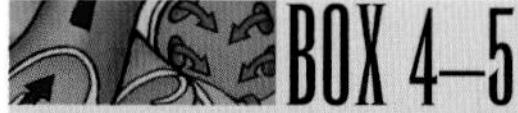

BOX 4–5

Recommendations for Echocardiography in Patients with Cardiac Murmurs

ASYMPTOMATIC PATIENTS

Class I (useful and recommended)

Diastolic or continuous murmurs

Holosystolic or late systolic murmurs

Grade III or greater mid-systolic murmurs

Class IIa (weight of evidence is in favor)

Murmurs associated with abnormal physical findings on cardiac palpation or auscultation

Murmurs associated with an abnormal electrocardiogram or chest radiograph

Class III (usefulness and efficacy not well established)

Grade II or softer mid-systolic murmur identified as innocent or functional by an experienced observer

To detect "silent" aortic regurgitation or mitral regurgitation in patients without cardiac murmurs; then recommend endocarditis prophylaxis

SYMPTOMATIC PATIENTS

Class I (useful and recommended)

Symptoms or signs of congestive heart failure, myocardial ischemia, or syncope

Symptoms or signs consistent with infective endocarditis or thromboembolism

Class IIa (weight of evidence is in favor)

Symptoms or signs probably attributable to noncardiac disease, with cardiac disease not excluded by standard cardiovascular evaluation

Class III (not useful or effective)

Symptoms or signs of noncardiac disease with an isolated mid-systolic "innocent" murmur

From Bonow RO, Carabello B, de Leon AC Jr, et al: ACC/AHA guidelines for the management of patients with valvular heart disease: Executive summary. A report of the American College of Cardiology/American Heart Association Task Force on Practice Guidelines (Committee on Management of Patients with Valvular Heart Disease). Circulation 1998;98:1949–1984. By permission of the American Heart Association, Inc.

4–5). For patients with suspected mitral valve prolapse, the guidelines emphasized that the diagnosis should be made by physical examination and that echocardiography is primarily appropriate for evaluation of mitral regurgitation and ventricular function. Echocardiography was considered appropriate for *excluding* the diagnosis of mitral valve prolapse in patients in whom prolapse had been diagnosed inappropriately.

Syncope

Syncope is often benign, usually easily evaluated without expensive diagnostic testing, but occasionally the first evidence of a life-threatening disorder (see Chapter 10). The most commonly used cardiac tests remain the ECG, which should be performed in all patients older than 40 years and in younger patients with possible cardiac disease, and ambulatory ECG monitoring, which should be considered for patients with suspected cardiac syncope or those without an obvious cause by history or physical examination.[18]

Head-up tilt-table testing can also help diagnose neurocardiogenic syncope and even guide therapy.[18] However, in the absence of a gold standard for the diagnosis of neurocardiogenic syncope, tilt-table testing results must be interpreted cautiously (see Chapter 10).

"Rule Out" (or Find the Source of) Embolic Stroke

Strokes and transient ischemic attacks (TIAs) can result from thrombi, vegetations, or tumors originating in the heart, from paradoxical emboli originating from the venous circulation, or from atheromas in the arterial tree, especially the aorta or the carotid arteries. The noninvasive tests that should be considered in patients who have suffered probable embolic events include echocardiography, ambulatory ECG monitoring, and carotid ultrasound.

Echocardiography is useful for detecting potential sources of cardiac emboli, including left ventricular mural thrombi, mitral valve prolapse, and atrial septal defect (see Chapter 5). Although transthoracic echocardiography (TTE) is widely used in patients who have had embolic episodes, TEE has greater sensitivity for the detection of some important sources of emboli such as thrombi in the left atrial appendage. Even if thrombi are not seen, the detection of "left atrial spontaneous echo contrast"—a swirling, smoky appearance suggesting a low-flow state—correlates with an increased risk for emboli. In addition, TEE provides excellent visualization of atheromas of the aortic arch, which are believed to be the source of emboli in some patients. An algorithm for the use of TTE and TEE in patients with suspected embolic events is presented in Figure 4–6.[19]

Ambulatory ischemia monitoring is often performed to detect periods of atrial fibrillation, which, if present, would suggest this arrhythmia as a contributing factor in the development of cardiac thrombi. Data on the utility of ambulatory ECG in this setting are not available, and use of this test for this purpose was considered equivocal at best (class IIb) in the ACC/AHA guidelines.[20]

The role of carotid ultrasound has been strengthened by research showing that atherosclerotic narrowing of the internal carotid artery at the carotid bifurcation in the neck is a common cause of TIA and stroke. Data from randomized trials indicate that patients with a recent TIA or nondisabling stroke with ipsilateral carotid stenosis benefit from surgery if the stenosis is greater than 50%.[21] Thus, carotid ultrasound is recommended in patients whose neurologic syndrome is consistent with an embolic event in the anterior cerebral circulation.

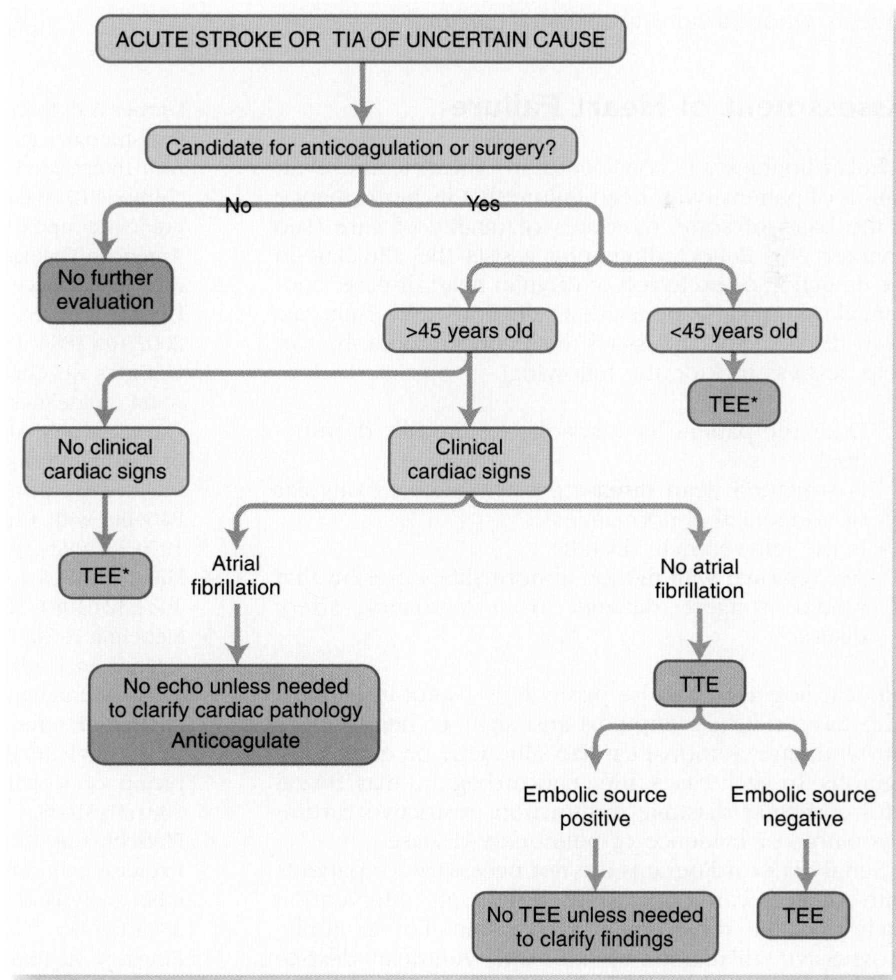

FIGURE 4–6. Algorithm for the use of transthoracic (TTE) and transesophageal (TEE) echocardiography for patients with a suspected cardiac source of emboli. *Because TTE and TEE are complementary, some clinicians may wish to do both. TIA, transient ischemic attack. (Redrawn from DeRook FA, Komess KA, Alabers GW, Popp RL: Transesophageal echocardiography in the evaluation of stroke. Ann Intern Med 1992;117:922–932.)

However, carotid ultrasound for asymptomatic patients, such as those with a carotid bruit, is of unproven value and not routinely recommended. Such patients have an increased risk for cerebrovascular events, but these events are not limited to the distribution of the artery from which the bruit arises. Data on the natural history of asymptomatic carotid artery stenoses were provided by follow-up of patients who were enrolled in the North American Symptomatic Carotid Endarterectomy Trial and who had both symptomatic and asymptomatic lesions in their carotid circulations. The risk of stroke at 5 years was 1.6% annually in those with an asymptomatic stenosis of less than 60% versus 16.2% in those with asymptomatic stenoses of 60% to 99%.[22] However, 45% of the strokes in patients with asymptomatic stenoses were attributable to lacunes or cardiac emboli; thus, the benefit of carotid endarterectomy in this population is uncertain.

The benefit of carotid endarterectomy is likely to be lower in asymptomatic patients than in symptomatic patients, but the surgical complication rates are similar regardless of symptoms. As a result, experts are divided on the role of surgical therapy for asymptomatic patients—and therefore the role of noninvasive testing to detect and measure the severity of asymptomatic carotid stenoses. Some clinicians advocate medical therapy for all patients with asymptomatic disease, whereas others recommend surgery in asymptomatic patients whose lesions are 70% or greater.[23]

Assessment of Heart Failure

Echocardiography is considered so critical to the evaluation of patients with heart failure that its performance is the basis of some measures of quality of care (see Chapter 28). Echocardiography assists the clinician in the detection or exclusion of valvular heart disease, congenital anomalies, pericardial effusion, and ischemic heart disease. Specific issues that echocardiography can help address include the following:

- Does the patient have systolic or diastolic dysfunction?
- Is structural heart disease present, such as valvular or congenital abnormalities?
- Is the left ventricle dilated?
- Are regional wall motion abnormalities present that would suggest damage from coronary artery disease?

Echocardiography can be particularly useful in patients who have clinical symptoms and signs of heart failure but who have a normal cardiac silhouette on chest radiographs. In such cases, the echocardiogram may reveal left ventricular diastolic dysfunction, restrictive cardiomyopathy, or evidence of pulmonary disease.

Serial echocardiograms are not necessary for patients with dilated cardiomyopathy unless an intervention such as valve replacement is possible. For example, progressive dilatation of the left ventricle despite medical therapy warrants consideration of valvular surgery even if the patient is asymptomatic. However, if no such intervention is possible and pharmacologic interventions are being adjusted according to the patient's symptoms and signs, serial echocardiograms are unlikely to influence management.

Evidence-Based Summary

- **Two cost-effectiveness studies[1,12] concluded that exercise echocardiography and radionuclide imaging improve outcomes with cost-effectiveness comparable to that of other accepted medical interventions, but that stress echocardiography was more cost-effective, in part because of the lower costs of the test. However, because the improvement in diagnostic accuracy of imaging technologies is modest, considerable support has been given to a stepwise strategy in which exercise ECG is the initial test in most patients. In this approach, imaging tests are reserved for those with contraindications to exercise ECG testing and for those with intermediate or uncertain risk after exercise ECG testing.[24,25]**

References

1. Garber AM, Solomon NA: Cost-effectiveness of alternative test strategies for the diagnosis of coronary artery disease. Ann Intern Med 1999;130:719–728.
2. Gibbons RJ, Balady GJ, Beasley JW, et al: ACC/AHA 2002 guideline update for exercise testing: A report of the American College of Cardiology/American Heart Association Task Force on Practice Guidelines (Committee to Update the 1997 Exercise Testing Guidelines). Circulation 2002;106:1883–1892.
3. Gibbons RJ, Chatterjee K, Daley J, et al: ACC/AHA/ACP-ASIM guidelines for the management of patients with chronic stable angina. A report of the American College of Cardiology/American Heart Association Task Force on Practice Guidelines (Committee on the Management of Patients with Chronic Stable Angina). J Am Coll Cardiol 1999;33:2092–2197.
4. Hill J, Timmins A: Exercise tolerance testing. Br Med J 2002;324:1084–1087.
5. Siebelink H-MJ, Blanksma PK, Crinjns HJGM, et al: No difference in cardiac event–free survival between positron emission tomography–guided and single-photon emission computed tomography–guided patient management. A prospective, randomized comparison of patients with suspicion of jeopardized myocardium. J Am Coll Cardiol 2001;37:81–88.
6. Fleischmann KE, Hunink MG, Kuntz KM, Douglas PS: Exercise echocardiography or exercise SPECT imaging? A meta-analysis of diagnostic test performance. JAMA 1998; 280:913–920.
7. Pingitore A, Picano E, Varga A, et al: Prognostic value of pharmacological stress echocardiography in patients with

known or suspected coronary artery disease: A prospective, large-scale, multicenter, head-to-head comparison between dipyridamole and dobutamine test. Echo-Persantine International Cooperative (EPIC) and Echo-Dobutamine International Cooperative (EDIC) Study Groups. J Am Coll Cardiol 1999;34:1769–1777.
8. Haberl R, Becker A, Leber A, et al: Correlation of coronary calcification and angiographically documented stenoses in patients with suspected coronary artery disease: Results of 1,764 patients. J Am Coll Cardiol 2001;37:451–457.
9. Shavelle DM, Budoff MJ, LaMont DH, et al: Exercise testing and electron beam computed tomography in the evaluation of coronary artery disease. J Am Coll Cardiol 2000;36:32–38.
10. O'Rourke RA, Brundage BH, Froelicher VF, et al: American College of Cardiology/American Heart Association Expert Consensus document on electron-beam computed tomography for the diagnosis and prognosis of coronary artery disease. Circulation 2000;102:126–140.
11. Detrano R, Wong ND, Doherty T, et al: Coronary calcium does not accurately predict near-term future coronary events in high-risk adults. Circulation 1999;99:2633–2638.
12. Kuntz KM, Fleischmann KE, Hunink MGM, Douglas PS: Cost-effectiveness of diagnostic strategies for patients with chest pain. Ann Intern Med 1999;130:709–718.
13. Ritchie LJ, Bateman TM, Bonow RO, et al: ACC/AHA guidelines for clinical use of cardiac radionuclide imaging. Report of the American College of Cardiology/American Heart Association Task Force on Assessment of Diagnostic and Therapeutic Cardiovascular Procedures (Committee on Radionuclide Imaging), developed in collaboration with the American Society of Nuclear Cardiology. J Am Coll Cardiol 1995;25:521–547.
14. Shaw LJ, Peterson ED, Shaw LK, et al: Use of a prognostic treadmill score in identifying diagnostic coronary disease subgroups. Circulation 1998;98:1622–1630.
15. Greenland P, Abrams J, Aurigemma GP, et al: Prevention Conference V: Beyond secondary prevention: Identifying the high-risk patient for primary prevention: Noninvasive tests of atherosclerotic burden: Writing Group III. Circulation 2000;101:E16–E22.
16. O'Leary DH, Polak JF, Kronmal RA, et al: Carotid-artery intima and media thickness as a risk factor for myocardial infarction and stroke in older adults: Cardiovascular Health Study. N Engl J Med 1999;340:14–22.
17. Bonow RO, Carabello B, de Leon AC Jr, et al: ACC/AHA guidelines for the management of patients with valvular heart disease: Executive summary. A report of the American College of Cardiology/American Heart Association Task Force on Practice Guidelines (Committee on Management of Patients with Valvular Heart Disease). Circulation 1998;98:1949–1984.
18. Sheldon R, Rose S, Ritchie D, et al: Historical criteria that distinguish syncope from seizures. J Am Coll Cardiol 2002;40:142–148.
19. DeRook FA, Komess KA, Albers GW, Popp RL: Transesophageal echocardiography in the evaluation of stroke. Ann Intern Med 1992;117:922–932.
20. Crawford MH, Bernstein SJ, Deedwania PC, et al: ACC/AHA Guidelines for ambulatory electrocardiography: A report of the American College of Cardiology/American Heart Association Task Force on Practice Guidelines (Committee to Revise the Guidelines for Ambulatory Electrocardiography). J Am Coll Cardiol 1999;34:912–948.
21. Albers GW, Hart RG, Lutsep HL, et al: Supplement to the guidelines for the management of transient ischemic attacks. A statement from the Ad Hoc Committee on Guidelines for the Management of Transient Ischemic Attacks, Stroke Council, American Heart Association. Stroke 1999;30:2502–2511.
22. Inzitari D, Eliasziw M, Gates P, et al, for the North American Symptomatic Carotid Endarterectomy Trial Collaborators: The causes and risk of stroke in patients with asymptomatic internal-carotid-artery stenosis. N Engl J Med 2000;342:1693–1701.
23. Kistler JP, Furie KL: Carotid endarterectomy revisited. N Engl J Med 2000;342:1743–1745.
24. Lee TH, Boucher CA: Noninvasive tests in patients with stable coronary artery disease. N Engl J Med 2001;344:1840–1845.
25. Williams SV, Fihn SD, Gibbons RJ: Guidelines for the management of patients with chronic stable angina: Diagnosis and risk stratification. Ann Intern Med 2001;135:530–547.

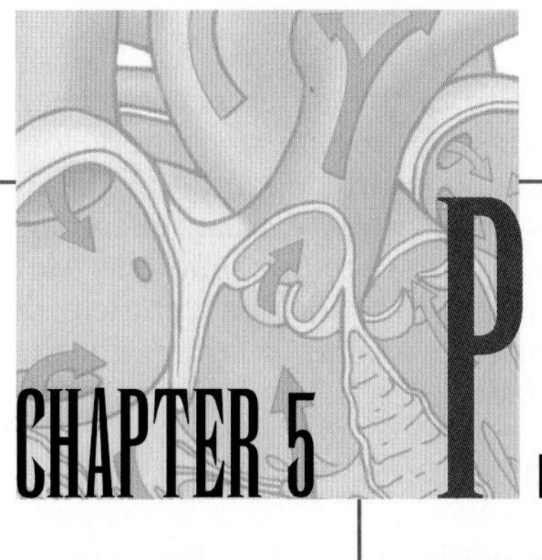

CHAPTER 5 Principles of Echocardiography

Scott D. Solomon

Echocardiography has emerged as one of the most widely used and powerful diagnostic tools available to clinicians. It has gained widespread acceptance because it provides structural, anatomic, and physiologic information about the heart, poses no risk to the patient, and is available in most medical centers.[1] Indeed, echocardiography has become a natural extension to the physical examination in patients with known or suspected heart disease. Nevertheless, as with any widely used test, echocardiography is useful and warranted in some situations and can be inappropriate in others.[2] In addition, the indiscriminate use of even noninvasive diagnostic tests is associated with increased cost to the patient and the health care system. This chapter reviews the basic principles, diagnostic utility, indications, and limitations of echocardiography in the primary care setting.

THE ECHOCARDIOGRAPHIC EXAMINATION

Echocardiography uses high-frequency sound waves (ultrasound) in the range of 2 to 10 MHz to generate images of cardiovascular structures. Ultrasound bounces off interfaces between tissues, and information about depth and intensity from the reflected signal is then used to generate two-dimensional (2-D) images. These "real-time" images are updated continually at a frame rate of at least 30 Hz. In a typical echocardiographic examination, an ultrasound transducer is placed on the patient's chest wall with the patient lying either supine or in the left lateral decubitus position. The use of diagnostic ultrasound has no known risk because it is a completely noninvasive procedure that exposes the patient to no ionizing radiation.

Two-Dimensional and M-Mode Echocardiography

A full echocardiographic examination uses M-mode, 2-D, and Doppler echocardiography. In M-mode echocardiography, a single beam of ultrasound is used to interrogate moving structures in the line of the beam, with depth displayed in the vertical direction and time in the horizontal direction (Fig. 5–1). M-mode echocardiography has for the most part been replaced by 2-D techniques, although it is still used because of its high temporal resolution and remains the preferred method in some clinical settings for making measurements of ventricular wall thickness and cavity size. The main limitation of M-mode echocardiography, however, is that the one-dimensional technique can result in inadvertent off-axis measurements.

2-D echocardiography compiles data from multiple ultrasound beams to form a 2-D planar image (Fig. 5–2). Many echocardiographic measurements are made from 2-D images, and 2-D techniques have become the usual means of assessing left ventricular size and function and valvular morphology. Moving images are recorded on videotape or stored as digital "loops" and archived on a digital server.

Doppler Echocardiography

This technique uses the Doppler principle to assess the velocity of blood flowing within the cardiac chambers. Ultrasound reflected off red blood cells moving either away or toward the ultrasound source will "shift" the frequency, depending on the velocity of the blood flow, which can be calculated from the difference between emitted and reflected ultrasound frequency. The velocity of blood flow within the heart depends on differences in pressure between various cardiac chambers and can be used to calculate pressure gradients (for example, between the left atrium and left ventricle or between the left ventricle and the aorta) with the simplified Bernoulli equation:

$$P = 4V^2$$

where P is the pressure gradient and V is the velocity of blood flow. Calculation of pressure gradients noninvasively has been one of the most important contributions of echocardiography.

Color-flow Doppler is a variation of the Doppler technique in which the velocity of blood flow over a wide area is determined and a color map signifying these velocities is superimposed over a 2-D ultrasound image (Fig. 5–3). Color-flow Doppler has greatly simplified the qualitative assessment of cardiac flow such as valvular regurgitation.

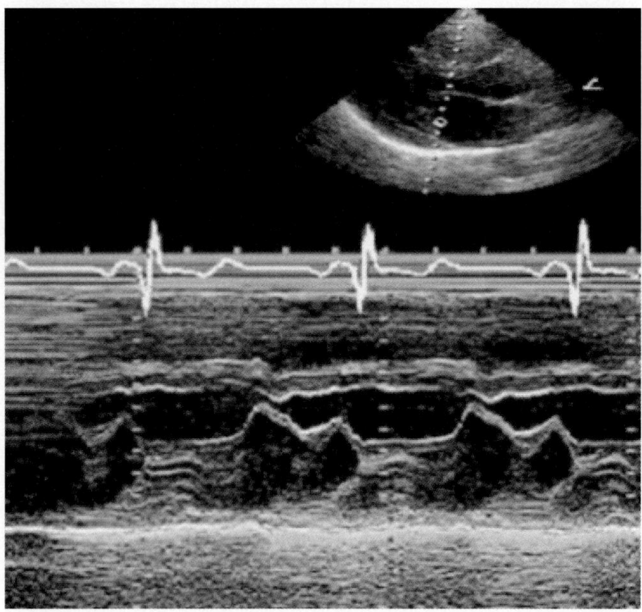

FIGURE 5–1. M-mode echocardiogram.

Technical Factors in an Echocardiographic Examination

Echocardiography can provide diagnostic information in the vast majority of patients in whom it is applied. Nevertheless, echocardiographic image quality—and hence the overall quality of the study—can be affected by a number of factors, including the skill of the operator, the patient's body habitus, the presence of pulmonary disease, and chest wall anatomy. Approximately 5% to 10% of patients have echocardiographic images of such poor quality that an important diagnosis could

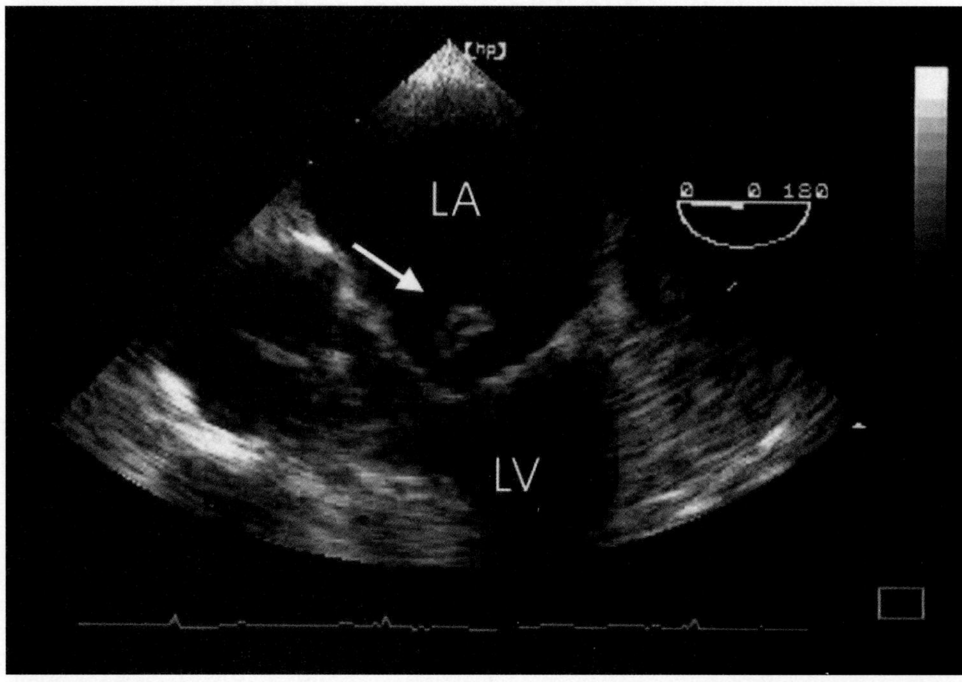

FIGURE 5–2. Transesophageal echocardiogram showing vegetation on the mitral valve. LA, left atrium; LV, left ventricle.

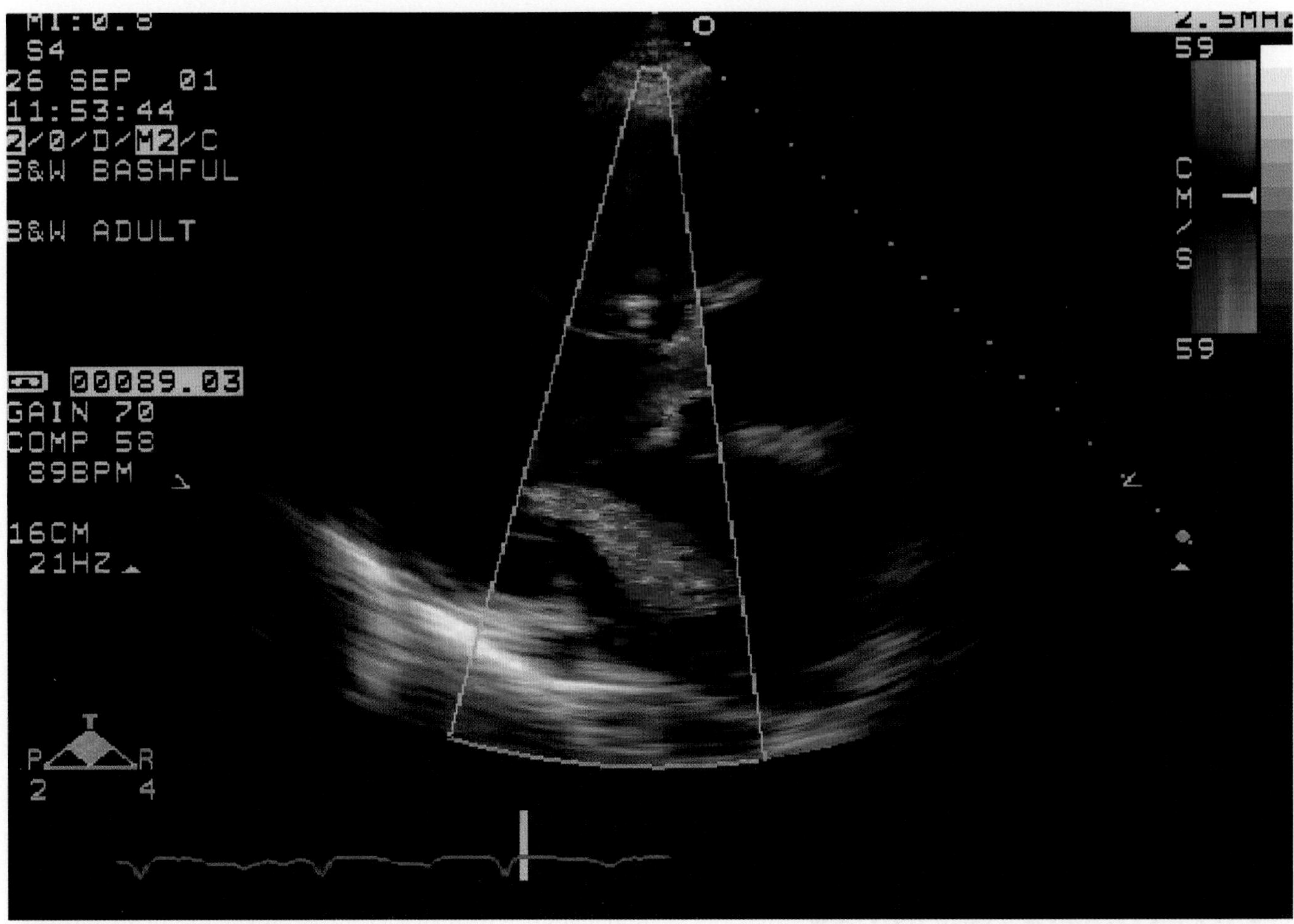

FIGURE 5–3. Color-flow Doppler image of mitral regurgitation.

be missed. Assessment of regional wall motion is particularly sensitive to image quality. Whereas global ventricular function can often be reliably assessed in patients with poor image quality, accurate assessment of regional function can be difficult in such patients. Clinicians should be aware of limitations in study quality that could reduce the ability to make accurate diagnoses.

Echocardiographic examinations in the United States are routinely performed by sonographers and interpreted by cardiologists. The diagnostic accuracy of the test is dependent on the skills of both the individual performing the examination and the interpreting physician. Although standard imaging planes are typically used, echocardiography is not a tomographic technique, and thus the skill of the operator plays a large role in determining which images are available for review. Skillful sonographers may also obtain nonstandard images in situations when they may be valuable, such as in patients with congenital heart abnormalities.

A typical echocardiographic examination involves a number of standard assessments and measurements (Table 5–1), including assessment of left and right ventricular size and function, estimation of the ejection fraction (EF), qualitative assessment of each of the valves, quantitative assessment of any valve stenosis, assessment of the pericardium, and a description of other abnormalities. Most laboratories also report on the technical quality of the examination.

TABLE 5–1

Normal Echocardiographic Values

Measurement	Normal Range (95% Confidence Intervals)
Left ventricular end diastolic diameter	3.5–6.0 cm
Left ventricular end systolic diameter	2.1–4.0 cm
End-diastolic volume, men	62–170 mL
End-diastolic volume, women	55–101 mL
Ejection fraction	55%–75%
Wall thickness (septal)	0.6–1.2 cm
Aortic root diameter	1.4–2.6 cm
Ascending aortic diameter	2.0–3.7 cm
Right ventricular diameter (in the apical view)	2.2–4.4 cm
Left atrium anteroposterior dimension	2.3–4.5 cm
Left atrium length	3.4–6.1 cm

Transesophageal Echocardiography

Transesophageal echocardiography (TEE) is similar in principle to standard echocardiography with the exception that the transducer is located at the end of an endoscopic probe. The esophagus is intubated in a manner similar to that for a gastrointestinal endoscopic examination, and an echocardiographic examination is performed from this unique vantage point. Visualization of posterior cardiac structures—including the atria, mitral and aortic valves, and pulmonary veins—is dramatically improved with the transesophageal approach. In addition, many of the factors that limit the quality of a transthoracic echo, such as obesity and chronic lung disease, do not affect TEE image quality. Nevertheless, some anterior cardiac structures such as the right ventricle, tricuspid valve, and left ventricular apex are better visualized with transthoracic echocardiography (TTE).

TEE is considerably more uncomfortable for the patient than TTE and uses greater resources. Patients typically receive a combination of topical anesthesia combined with conscious sedation, thereby requiring the presence of a suitably trained nurse even for an outpatient examination. Adverse events, including esophageal perforation, aspiration, and pharyngeal trauma, are rare (less than 0.5%). Nevertheless, TEE should be used only in situations in which the appropriate information cannot be obtained with TTE.

Table 5–2 lists current common indications for TEE.

DIAGNOSTIC UTILITY OF ECHOCARDIOGRAPHY

Assessment of Cardiac Structure

Because of its ability to identify blood-tissue interfaces, the primary use of echocardiography is to identify and assess cardiac structure and morphology. Echocardiography is particularly useful in visualizing cardiac chambers, myocardial walls, the cardiac valves, the pericardium, and abnormal structures surrounding the heart. Major abnormalities in cardiac structure, either congenital or acquired, such as after myocardial infarction or in response to valvular heart disease, can easily be identified by echocardiography.

Assessment of Cardiac Size and Function

The size of the left ventricle is an important indicator of the severity of a variety of cardiac diseases. Left ventricular dilatation occurs in most patients with left ventricular dysfunction, whether global (e.g., idiopathic cardiomyopathy) or regional (e.g., myocardial infarction), and is an important predictor of mortality. Left ventricular dilatation also occurs in conditions associated with volume overload, such as mitral or aortic regurgitation, and the size of the left ventricle provides a valuable assessment of the rate of progression of the disease and is often used to guide the timing of cardiac surgery.

A number of methods are currently used to quantify left ventricular size by echocardiography.[3] M-mode or 2-D measurements of cardiac diameter provide a simple but useful measurement of ventricular size, but it is important to recognize that these methods are particularly unreliable in patients with regional left ventricular dysfunction and enlargement and are best used in patients with diseases that affect the heart globally. More accurate estimation of ventricular size requires calculation of a three-dimensional volume from 2-D images. Although a variety of methods for making these estimations exist, those with the highest accuracy generally require manual tracing of the ventricular contours in one or more views.

Assessment of cardiac wall motion is the basis for evaluation of global and regional left ventricular

TABLE 5–2

Indications for Transesophageal Echocardiography

Indication	Advantages over TTE
Improved visualization of abnormalities seen on TTE: Suspected vegetation Suspected thrombus Cardiac mass	TEE offers improved resolution for virtually all structures and findings in the left atrium and surrounding the mitral valve, masses in the left atrium and ventricle (excluding the apical region), and pulmonary veins and pulmonary arteries
Suspected prosthetic valve endocarditis	Improved assessment of prosthetic valves, particularly metallic valves in the mitral position
Assessment of left atrial thrombus	Markedly improved assessment of the left atrial appendage, the most likely location of thrombi
Identification of thrombi in pulmonary arteries	Improved visualization of thrombi in the pulmonary arteries of patients with suspected acute pulmonary embolism Use of TEE in this setting is controversial

TEE, transesophageal echocardiography; TTE, transthoracic echocardiography.

function. Global cardiac function is most commonly assessed on echocardiography by measuring the EF, which is directly calculated from ventricular volumes by dividing the difference between end-diastolic and end-systolic volume by end-diastolic volume. EF is a load-dependent measure of cardiac function rather than a true measure of cardiac contractility. Thus, in conditions in which myocardial afterload is dramatically altered—either increased as in severe aortic stenosis or decreased as in mitral regurgitation—EF might not reliably estimate true myocardial contractility. Nevertheless, EF is the most commonly used method for assessing ventricular function. In adults, an EF over 55% is considered normal. Measurement of EF on repeated examinations can vary by as much as five points in either direction because of both normal biologic variability and measurement variability. Thus, before concluding that a five-point change in EF represents a true change in ventricular function, it is important to compare studies side by side and consider other factors, such as volume status of the patient, that might affect the assessment. EF values over 75% may be seen in high-output conditions, hypovolemic states, severe hypertrophic heart disease, or severe mitral or aortic regurgitation.

Assessment of regional ventricular function is usually more qualitative than assessment of global function is. Although some laboratories use a scoring system for assessment of regional wall motion, more often, regions of the ventricle are simply described as normal, hypokinetic, akinetic, or dyskinetic. Regional wall motion abnormalities that correlate with coronary anatomy are indicative of myocardial infarction or, in some cases, severe myocardial ischemia. Such wall motion abnormalities, however, can also be seen in diseases that affect the heart globally, though not usually in a coronary distribution.

Assessment of Left Ventricular Hypertrophy and Wall Thickness

Conditions that result in chronic pressure overload on the left ventricle—including systemic hypertension, aortic stenosis, and coarctation of the aorta—result in left ventricular hypertrophy that can be accurately measured by echocardiography. Increased ventricular wall thickness (12 mm or greater in an adult) is associated with an increased risk for the development of heart failure and sudden death. Conditions that cause global increases in left ventricular load, such as aortic stenosis or systemic hypertension, generally result in concentric ventricular hypertrophy with wall thickness in the range of 12 to 15 mm. Nevertheless, localized regional hypertrophy, particularly in the outflow tract of the septum, may also be seen in hypertensive heart disease, particularly in elderly patients. This pattern is distinct from that seen in hypertrophic cardiomyopathy, a condition in which left ventricular hypertrophy is unexplained by increased ventricular load (see later and Chapter 29).

Assessment of the Right Ventricle and Pulmonary Pressures

Right ventricular function has important prognostic significance in a variety of conditions, including acute pulmonary embolism, pulmonary hypertension, valvular heart disease, congenital heart disease, heart failure, and myocardial infarction. Conditions that increase pulmonary vascular resistance (acute pulmonary embolism, pulmonary parenchymal diseases, left-sided heart failure) result in acute right ventricular enlargement and failure. Assessment of right ventricular function is usually qualitative because of the lack of generally accepted methods for calculation of right ventricular volume and, hence, EF by echocardiography.

Right ventricular hypertrophy with right ventricular wall thickness greater than 7 mm develops in patients with pulmonary hypertension. Severe pulmonary hypertension leads to flattening of the interventricular septum throughout the cardiac cycle. Pulmonary pressures can be reliably estimated by using the velocity of tricuspid regurgitation to measure the pressure gradient between the right ventricle and atrium and adding this value to an estimate of right atrial pressure.

Assessment of Cardiac Valves

The high temporal and spatial resolution of 2-D echocardiography combined with the utility of Doppler to assess blood flow makes echocardiography an ideal technique for the assessment of valvular lesions (see the section "Valvular Heart Disease" and Chapter 32). In many cases, echocardiography may be the only test needed to determine whether a patient requires cardiac surgery for a valvular lesion, and echocardiography has replaced cardiac catheterization in virtually all circumstances in the initial evaluation of valvular heart disease.

Assessment of the Pericardium

In the absence of pathology, the pericardium itself is not easily visualized by echocardiography (see Chapter 35). Even though pericardial thickening and calcification can often be recognized by echocardiography, these assessments are imprecise and can be very sensitive to equipment settings. Nevertheless, even small pericardial effusions are readily identified by echocardiography, and although pericarditis without effusion could be missed on echocardiography, virtually all clinically important pericardial processes can be diagnosed by this test.

The most clinically significant pericardial process, pericardial tamponade, is characterized by a large pericardial effusion with evidence of impaired cardiac filling, and it can easily be detected or ruled out by echocardiography (see Fig 35–8). Cardiac tamponade, though infrequent in viral pericarditis, is common in patients with malignancy and can occur acutely in patients with aortic dissection, in those with myocardial infarction with ventricular rupture, or in the setting of a cardiac procedure such as pacemaker implantation. True tamponade, or impaired ventricular filling, occurs when pericardial pressure exceeds right or left ventricular filling pressure. Echocardiographic features suggestive of tamponade include diastolic indentation of the right ventricle and significant respiratory flow variation on Doppler echocardiography (the Doppler equivalent of pulsus paradoxus). Although large effusions are more likely to cause tamponade than smaller effusions are, tamponade can also occur in settings of small effusions, especially if right-sided pressures are low or pericardial fluid accumulates rapidly. Conversely, patients with large pericardial effusions who are volume replete may not demonstrate echocardiographic findings of tamponade, but this lack of findings could change rapidly if the balance between pericardial and right-sided pressure changes. Although echocardiography cannot determine the etiology of pericardial effusions, it can be used to assess and monitor the size of an effusion, identify reaccumulation after pericardial drainage, and evaluate patients for constrictive pericardial physiology.

Assessment of Diastolic Function

Diastolic function refers to the ability of the heart to fill during diastole, and patients with diastolic dysfunction have an increased risk of heart failure that is independent of systolic function (see Chapter 28). Direct assessment of diastolic function by echocardiography has been problematic because most Doppler-based parameters of ventricular filling are preload dependent and will vary significantly with relatively minor hemodynamic changes. Nevertheless, some echocardiographic markers of diastolic dysfunction, such as marked shortening of the mitral deceleration time—the time from peak mitral inflow to equilibration of pressure between the left atrium and left ventricle—provide important and prognostic clinical information. A new method of Doppler tissue imaging that measures the rate of myocardial relaxation during diastole has shown promise in assessing diastolic function.[4]

EVALUATION OF PATIENTS WITH SUSPECTED HEART DISEASE

Evaluation of a patient with suspected heart disease begins with a careful history and physical examination (see Chapter 3), and echocardiography can be an important adjunct in patients with appropriate indications (Table 5–3). In general, echocardiography is indicated when the results of the test are likely to provide incremental information and when management of the patient is likely to be altered.

Evaluation of Cardiac Murmurs

Echocardiography is the natural follow-up examination for the evaluation of cardiac murmurs identified on auscultation (see Chapter 11). In addition to assessing both structural and functional abnormalities of cardiac valves, echocardiography is useful in assessing the effect of a valvular lesion on the ventricles and the atria and identifying other concomitant abnormalities.

Because not all murmurs require further evaluation, the decision regarding which patients with murmurs should proceed to echocardiographic evaluation can be difficult and should be based on the timing and severity of the murmur, as well as associated clinical signs and symptoms. Murmurs in patients without cardiac signs or symptoms should be monitored with echocardiography when cardiac pathology is suspected or highly likely (Fig. 5–4). Diastolic murmurs are almost always pathologic and should be assessed by echocardiography. Although systolic murmurs that are thought to be benign do not warrant echocardiographic examination, clear identification of benign murmurs can be difficult even for specialists, and systolic murmurs that are not clearly identified as such should be evaluated at least once in asymptomatic patients. Benign flow murmurs are common during pregnancy and young adulthood, are usually of short duration and low intensity, and are not associated with other abnormal heart sounds or murmurs or other evidence of cardiac pathology. Asymptomatic individuals with a low probability of heart disease but in whom the diagnosis of heart disease cannot be reasonably excluded by a standard physical examination should undergo echocardiography for evaluation of a murmur. Patients with murmurs who have symptoms that are referable to the cardiovascular system—including shortness of breath, syncope, presyncope, heart failure, and chest pain—should always undergo evaluation. Once a murmur has been identified by echocardiography as benign, additional echocardiograms should not be obtained unless significant changes in signs or symptoms occur. Table 5–3 lists the clinical signs, symptoms, and conditions that generally warrant echocardiographic follow-up.

Evaluation of Shortness of Breath

Dyspnea can result from a variety of cardiac and noncardiac conditions (see Chapter 7). Echocardiography is often useful as an adjunct to other tests, such as exercise tolerance testing, when no noncardiac cause of the dyspnea is apparent. Cardiac abnormalities that can lead to dyspnea and be detected by echocardiography include left ventricular dysfunction from any cause; valvular heart disease, including stenosis or regurgitation of either of the left-sided valves; pericardial effusion or constriction; and cardiac masses. Echocardiography can also suggest a noncardiac etiology. Both pulmonary vascular and parenchymal conditions that cause dyspnea can be associated with abnormalities in right ventricular size and function. In particular, acute pulmonary embolism is associated with acute

TABLE 5–3

Common Clinical Signs, Symptoms, or Conditions for Which Echocardiography Is Indicated

Clinical Symptom or Sign	Possible Echocardiographic Findings	Indications for Echocardiography
Clinical Signs		
Systolic murmur	Aortic sclerosis Aortic stenosis Subaortic stenosis Mitral regurgitation Tricuspid regurgitation Pulmonic stenosis Atrial septal defect	Indicated in patients with cardiac symptoms or ECG abnormalities Not indicated when the murmur is clearly identified as innocent or benign by an experienced clinician
Diastolic murmur	Aortic regurgitation Mitral stenosis Atrial septal defect	Indicated for the diagnosis of all diastolic murmurs Not indicated for repeat studies when a definitive diagnosis has previously been made and signs/symptoms have not changed
Continuous murmur	Patent ductus arteriosus	Indicated for all continuous murmurs except when previously diagnosed without change in symptoms or signs
Thrill	Ventricular septal defect	Indicated for evaluation of thrill except when previously diagnosed without change in symptoms or signs
Mid-systolic click	Mitral valve prolapse	Indicated when the diagnosis of prolapse has not previously been made
Third heart sound	Left ventricular dysfunction	Indicated for the diagnosis of a new third heart sound in patients not known to have left ventricular dysfunction
Dyspnea	Left ventricular dysfunction Valvular disease Right ventricular enlargement Right ventricular dysfunction	Indicated for dyspnea in the presence of clinical signs/symptoms of heart disease Not indicated when dyspnea is clearly attributed to a noncardiac cause
Cyanosis	Atrial septal defect with Eisenmenger's physiology Unsuspected congenital heart disease	Indicated for patients with cyanosis not otherwise explained
Cardiomegaly on chest radiograph	Pericardial effusion Cardiomyopathy Left ventricular hypertrophy Congenital heart disease	Indicated for patients with undiagnosed cardiomegaly detected on chest radiograph
Clinical Symptoms		
Syncope	Aortic stenosis Left ventricular dysfunction (predisposes patients to arrhythmia)	Indicated for evaluation of possible aortic stenosis in patients with undiagnosed systolic murmur and syncope Not indicated in patients with clear neurocardiogenic or vasovagal syncope
Chest pain	Regional wall motion abnormalities Right ventricular enlargment and dysfunction Pericardial effusion	Indicated in patients with ECG abnormalities and no previous history of infarction Indicated for the diagnosis of myocardial infarction when standard diagnostic methods are not definitive Indicated for ECG abnormalities suggestive of pericarditis
Conditions		
Supraventricular tachycardia	Atrial septal defect (common with WPW syndrome) Ebstein's anomaly Atrial enlargement	Indicated in patients undergoing electrophysiologic study or ablation or in patients being considered for antiarrhythmic therapy May not be indicated in young patients who have no other symptoms or signs and whose arrhythmia breaks easily
Atrial fibrillation or flutter	Left atrial enlargement Mitral stenosis Mitral regurgitation Left ventricular dysfunction/hypertrophy Pericardial abnormalities	Indicated in patients with new atrial fibrillation or flutter who have not had a recent echocardiogram

ECG, electrocardiographic; WPW, Wolff-Parkinson-White.

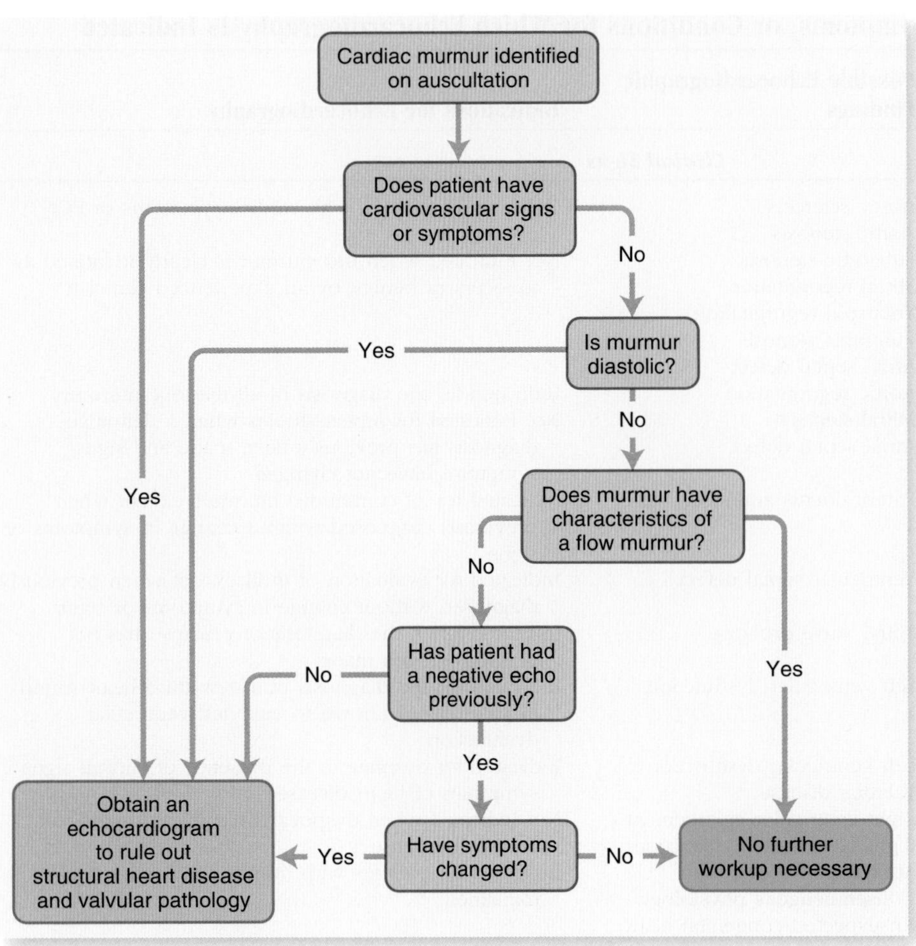

FIGURE 5–4. Diagnostic algorithm for evaluation of cardiac murmurs.

right ventricular enlargement and dysfunction (see later). Exercise echocardiography can provide important functional information in patients being evaluated for dyspnea. Assessment of systolic function during exercise can help determine whether the dyspnea is ischemic in origin.

Evaluation of Syncope, Arrhythmia, and Palpitations

Patients with syncope and other signs or symptoms of heart disease should undergo echocardiographic evaluation to rule out structural heart disease (see Chapters 9 and 10). In particular, patients with syncope who have a previously unevaluated systolic murmur should be assessed for aortic stenosis. Echocardiography is not generally indicated in patients with syncope if a previous recent echocardiogram has not revealed significant heart disease or if symptoms are suggestive of neurocardiogenic or vasovagal syncope. In addition, patients with palpitations attributable to ventricular or atrial premature beats without other documented rhythm disturbances do not require echocardiography in the absence of other indications such as syncope or presyncope.

However, echocardiography is indicated to exclude structural heart disease in most patients with documented arrhythmias, including atrial fibrillation, supraventricular tachycardia, and ventricular arrhythmias. Virtually all patients with supraventricular or ventricular tachycardia should undergo echocardiography before consideration for electrophysiologic study, ablation therapy, or antiarrhythmic therapy. Young patients with documented supraventricular arrhythmia that is easily terminated with vagal maneuvers and who have not had syncope or have no other physical signs and who are not going to undergo ablation therapy may not require echocardiographic evaluation. In patients with atrial fibrillation, echocardiography is used to assess ventricular function and the size of the left atrium and to rule out mitral valve abnormalities. Findings on echocardiography may also guide treatment decisions; for example, assessment of left ventricular function may be relevant in selecting an antiarrhythmic medication.

Assessment of Suspected Endocarditis

The diagnosis of endocarditis is made on the basis of clinical signs and symptoms, including fever, murmur, elevated white blood cell count, and positive blood cultures (see Chapter 33). Echocardiography can be helpful in determining the extent and severity of endocarditis, but it should not be routinely used to establish the diagnosis or to exclude suspected endocarditis.

Vegetations, the characteristic echocardiographic finding in endocarditis, are usually seen as small mobile lesions attached to a valve, but they can be present in other locations in the heart as well. They can sometimes be difficult to distinguish from other types of mobile lesions, including thrombi and fibroelastomas, thus making the clinical scenario extremely important in the diagnosis of endocarditis by echocardiography. Endocarditis most commonly affects the mitral and aortic valves, although the risk of right-sided endocarditis, usually involving the tricuspid valve, is increased in intravenous drug abusers and in patients with indwelling catheters. In addition to identifying and monitoring vegetations, echocardiography can sometimes demonstrate myocardial abscesses, which are most common in the annular region adjacent to the mitral and aortic valves. Myocardial abscess should be suspected in patients with prolongation of the PR or QRS interval on the electrocardiogram (ECG) or in patients with known endocarditis who are not responding appropriately to antibiotic therapy. Because TTE has limited resolution, all but the largest abscesses will be missed, and therefore patients with a high likelihood of having a myocardial abscess should be assessed with TEE. Echocardiography also provides important information on the hemodynamic consequences of endocarditis, including the degree of valvular regurgitation and ventricular function.

In the primary care setting, echocardiography is rarely a first-line test for the diagnosis of endocarditis. Nevertheless, an echocardiogram is reasonable if suspicion of endocarditis is high, as, for example, in a patient with a new murmur who has other signs or symptoms of endocarditis (such as fever or an elevated white blood cell count), even in the absence of positive blood cultures; echocardiography is also useful in patients with a previous history of endocarditis and in those with a prosthetic heart valve and undiagnosed fever.

TTE is a poor screening test in patients with suspected endocarditis. The overall sensitivity of TTE has varied widely in case series but has been estimated at 30% to 90%, with a much higher specificity that has approached the high 90s in some series. Thus, clinicians should never use echocardiography to "rule out" endocarditis. In contrast, the sensitivity of TEE has been estimated to be 88% or greater in multiple series, and its specificity approaches 100%. For this reason, some clinicians advocate proceeding directly to TEE when suspicion of endocarditis is high. Although this strategy would not be cost-effective for most patients, it is reasonable in patients with prosthetic valves who have a high likelihood of endocarditis, in patients with a previous history of endocarditis, in those with prolonged PR or QRS intervals and other signs of endocarditis, and in patients in whom TTE was abnormal but not clearly diagnostic of endocarditis. The incremental value of TEE, however, is minimal in patients with a completely normal transthoracic examination in whom no pathologic regurgitation is seen. TEE is particularly warranted in patients with suspected prosthetic valve endocarditis because the complication rate is so high. Furthermore, prostheses in the mitral position are difficult to visualize on TTE.

Assessment of Cardiac Sources of Emboli

Patients with stroke or transient ischemic attack thought to be embolic in nature are often referred for echocardiography to rule out a cardiac source of embolus. Even though documentation of a cardiac source of emboli can be helpful in the management of patients with stroke or transient ischemic attack, failure to identify a cardiac source does not rule out the possibility that an embolic event originated in the heart. Although embolism originating in the heart is thought to account for up to 30% of ischemic strokes, a variety of heterogeneous cardiac abnormalities can predispose to embolic stroke, including mitral stenosis, valvular calcification, atrial myxoma, akinetic regions after myocardial infarction, aortic plaque, and atrial fibrillation. Identification of these abnormalities may be helpful in determining which type of therapy, including antiplatelet or anticoagulant therapy, may be most appropriate for the patient. Echocardiography to identify a cardiac source of embolus is useful and warranted when the information obtained will help the clinician manage the patient.[5]

The sensitivity and specificity of TTE for the diagnosis of left ventricular thrombi are quite high, between 86% and 95% each, and this test is the best method for diagnosing thrombi in the left ventricular apex, the most likely location of thrombi after myocardial infarction. In addition, TTE can reliably diagnose most large cardiac masses such as myxoma or metastatic tumors, significant valvular abnormalities that might predispose to emboli such as mitral stenosis, valvular or annular calcification, and left atrial enlargement.

A well-performed saline contrast study during standard TTE can reliably diagnose patent foramen ovale in most patients. A patent foramen ovale is present in up to 25% of individuals and can provide a conduit through which thrombi originating on the right side, particularly in the deep veins of the legs, can migrate to the left side of the heart and embolize systemically. Assessment of the interatrial septum is best accomplished with a combination of color-flow Doppler echocardiography to identify flow disturbances suggestive of intra-atrial communication and saline contrast echocardiography. A saline contrast echocardiogram, or "bubble study," involves the systemic injection of agitated saline. Saline bubbles rapidly appear in the right-sided chambers but, in the absence of communication, will be filtered by the lungs and fail to appear in the left side of the heart. However, if an atrial septal defect or patent foramen is present, the bubbles will cross over to the left side of the heart. Although TTE is better for directly visualizing an atrial septal defect or patent foramen, these abnormalities will rarely be missed by a properly conducted saline contrast study on TTE.

Nevertheless, TTE has limited sensitivity, between 39% and 63%, for detection of thrombi in the left atrium and left atrial appendage, the most likely sources of a potential embolus in patients with stroke. In contrast, the sensitivity and specificity of TEE for the detection of an atrial thrombus has been reported to be 99% to 100%.[6] Still, this test should be used only when the information derived will alter a patient's management. Thus, if clear preexisting indications or contraindications for anticoagulation exist, it is difficult to justify the more invasive and resource-intensive TEE, although many clinicians would order TTE for assessment of concomitant cardiac abnormalities. Proceeding directly to TEE is warranted in patients in whom anticoagulation would be considered only if a cardiac source of the embolus were identified or if a suspected abnormality were seen on TTE that could be better visualized on a transesophageal study. Conversely, if a clear cardiac source of embolus were detected on TTE, proceeding to TEE would have limited value.

Evaluation of Acute Chest Pain

Although echocardiography can provide important diagnostic information in patients with acute chest pain (see Chapter 6), the evaluation of symptoms that could represent a myocardial infarction or another cardiac emergency should always be performed in an emergency room or suitable hospital setting, and performance of an echocardiographic examination should never delay appropriate early infarct management. Acute infarction is diagnosed on echocardiography by the presence of a wall motion abnormality in a coronary distribution that does not appear thin and fibrotic. Most often, global ventricular function is reduced in this setting.

In situations in which the ECG is not diagnostic of acute infarction, the echocardiogram can be helpful in distinguishing acute myocardial infarction from other causes of chest pain such as acute pericarditis, pulmonary embolism, or aortic dissection (Table 5–4). For example, the presence of pericardial effusion can be used to diagnose pericarditis in a patient with suggestive symptoms if findings consistent with ischemic heart disease are not detected. When clinical suspicion of acute aortic dissection is high, however, the initial test should be either TEE or computed tomography (CT) because TTE is insensitive for this diagnosis.

TABLE 5–4

Echocardiographic Findings in Patients with Chest Pain

Diagnosis	Echocardiographic Findings
Myocardial infarction	Regional wall motion abnormality in a region of the left ventricle either known to be previously normal or with hypokinesis or akinesis and no associated thinning and fibrosis
Pericarditis	Pericardial effusion, pericardial thickening. Absence of effusion, however, does not rule out acute pericarditis
Pulmonary embolism	In hemodynamically significant pulmonary emboli, right ventricular enlargement, right ventricular dysfunction, and small left ventricular cavity size. Thrombi are occasionally visible in the right atrium, right ventricle, or pulmonary arteries
Aortic dissection	The first 3 cm of the ascending aorta is usually visible with transthoracic imaging, as are parts of the descending aorta. Patients with ascending dissection can have aortic insufficiency, pericardial effusion and tamponade, and pleural effusion

Evaluation of Chronic Chest Pain

The resting echocardiogram is most commonly normal in patients with angina pectoris or stable coronary disease who have not had a myocardial infarction (see Chapter 25). Patients with suspected coronary disease and a normal ECG who do not have abnormalities on physical examination suggestive of left ventricular dysfunction or valvular heart disease do not routinely require echocardiographic examination. In patients with signs or symptoms of left ventricular dysfunction or congestive heart failure or in patients with ECG abnormalities suggestive of previous myocardial infarction, echocardiography is useful for assessment of left ventricular function and for detection of the presence of regional wall motion abnormalities in a coronary distribution consistent with previous infarction. Before revascularization, patients with chronic stable ischemic heart disease should undergo echocardiography to assess left ventricular function and rule out significant valvular disease that could be corrected at the time of surgery.

Evaluation in Suspected Pulmonary Embolism

Pulmonary embolism results in an acute increase in pulmonary vascular resistance and increased right ventricular afterload (see Chapter 38). Although ventilation-perfusion scanning and pulmonary angiography remain the best methods for diagnosis of pulmonary embolism, echocardiography is useful in assessing the hemodynamic severity of this condition.[7] In addition, echocardiography will occasionally demonstrate the presence of thrombi in the pulmonary arteries, right ventricle, or right atrium in patients with pulmonary embolism, but these findings are rare and the location of thrombi in the vast majority of pulmonary emboli is sufficiently distal in the pulmonary tree that they cannot be visualized by echocardiography. Because the signs and symptoms of acute pulmonary embolism are often nonspecific, echocardiography can be useful in

TABLE 5–5

Clinical Conditions in Which Screening Echocardiography Is Indicated in Asymptomatic Patients

Suspected Condition	Clinical Indications for Screening	Echocardiographic Findings
Hypertrophic cardiomyopathy	Patients with a first-degree family relative with hypertrophic cardiomyopathy or sudden death at a young age Patients with unexplained left ventricular hypertrophy on an electrocardiogram	Unexplained ventricular hypertrophy Systolic anterior motion of the mitral value Outflow tract obstruction
Marfan's syndrome	Patients with a first-degree relative with Marfan's syndrome Patients with the classic findings of Marfan's syndrome, including arm span greater than 105% of height, typical facies, severe pectus excavatum, etc.	Dilated aortic root Myxomatous degeneration of the mitral and tricuspid valves
Familial dilated cardiomyopathy	Patients with more than one first-degree relative with a history of cardiomyopathy	Left ventricular dilatation or dysfunction Mitral regurgitation
Patients undergoing potential cardiotoxic therapy (chemotherapy)	Baseline echocardiogram to assess ventricular function Before additional cycles of chemotherapy	Reduced left ventricular function after chemotherapy

distinguishing pulmonary embolism from other diagnoses, including acute myocardial infarction, acute pericarditis, cardiac tamponade, and aortic dissection.

The role of TEE in identifying thrombi in pulmonary embolism is controversial. Although TEE provides better visualization of the pulmonary arteries, this test carries clear risks in acutely ill patients and is not routinely recommended for the evaluation of suspected pulmonary embolism.

Echocardiography in Asymptomatic Patients at Increased Cardiac Risk

Echocardiography is rarely indicated in asymptomatic patients who have no compelling findings on the history or physical examination to suggest the presence of heart disease. Nevertheless, asymptomatic patients who are at risk for specific inherited cardiovascular abnormalities should undergo echocardiography (Table 5–5). Such risks include first-degree relatives of patients with hypertrophic cardiomyopathy, the Marfan syndrome, or familial dilated cardiomyopathy. In patients at risk for familial hypertrophic cardiomyopathy, hypertrophy is usually present by young adulthood, and the likelihood of disease is low in a patient older than 30 years with a negative echocardiogram. Patients with a family history or compelling clinical characteristics of the Marfan syndrome should undergo echocardiographic screening, primarily to evaluate the ascending aorta. In addition, it is generally standard practice for patients about to undergo therapy with a potentially cardiotoxic chemotherapeutic agent such as doxorubicin (Adriamycin) to undergo baseline echocardiographic examination, as well as before additional cycles of chemotherapy. ECG findings that raise the suspicion of heart disease in an asymptomatic patient should be confirmed with echocardiography (Table 5–6).

TABLE 5–6

Electrocardiographic Abnormalities Suggestive of Heart Disease in Asymptomatic Patients

Electrocardiographic Abnormality	Possible Echocardiographic Finding
Pathologic Q-waves	Regional wall motion abnormalities consistent with previous infarction
Right bundle branch block, RSR′ pattern	Atrial septal defect
Left bundle branch block	Regional wall motion abnormality consistent with infarction
Atrial flutter	Pericardial effusion
Atrial fibrillation	Mitral valve abnormalities Left atrial dilatation
Delta wave (Wolff-Parkinson-White syndrome)	Atrial septal defect Ebstein's anomaly
ST segment elevation	Acute myocardial infarction Ventricular aneurysm Acute pericarditis

EVALUATION OF PATIENTS WITH EXISTING HEART DISEASE

Valvular Heart Disease (see Chapter 32)

Aortic Stenosis

Echocardiography has virtually replaced cardiac catheterization as the preferred method for the initial and subsequent evaluation of patients with aortic stenosis. Evaluation of aortic stenosis requires assessment of the valvular gradient, the aortic valve area, left ventricular size and function, and the degree of aortic regurgitation. Valve area is the primary determinant of the severity of aortic stenosis. Although the valve gradient—the difference between aortic and left ventricular pressure—is also an indicator of disease severity, it is a common misconception that the valve gradient consistently increases with the severity of aortic stenosis. Because a gradient is dependent on the ability of the left ventricle to generate pressure, patients with impaired left ventricular function and low cardiac output can have low or minimal gradients despite having significant aortic stenosis. Nevertheless, in a patient with normal ventricular function, a valve gradient over 50 mm Hg signifies significant aortic stenosis.

The aortic valve gradient is determined by application of the Bernoulli equation ($P = 4V^2$) to the peak velocity detected with Doppler. This method can estimate both the peak instantaneous and the mean valve gradient. The peak instantaneous gradient obtained by Doppler is usually approximately 20 mm Hg higher than the peak-to-peak gradient obtained by cardiac catheterization. The aortic valve area is estimated by the continuity principle, in which Doppler flow velocity is measured at a point proximal to the valve, where the cross-sectional area can also be measured, and through the valve, where the cross-sectional area is not known. Because flow in both places is equivalent, the valve area can be calculated. This method is accurate even in patients with decreased cardiac output. An aortic valve area smaller than 0.5 cm^2 is considered critical aortic stenosis; a valve area of 0.5 to 1.0 cm^2 is considered moderate to severe aortic stenosis.

The degree of left ventricular hypertrophy and the functional state of the left ventricle are also important measures in aortic stenosis. Aortic stenosis rarely causes severe left ventricular dysfunction itself, except in patients with long-standing, critical stenosis. In patients with known aortic stenosis, the aortic valve area decreases at a rate of approximately 0.1 cm^2/yr.[8] The decision to operate on patients with aortic stenosis is usually made on clinical grounds and not by echocardiography alone. Although no clear consensus has been reached regarding the frequency of echocardiographic follow-up in patients with aortic stenosis, it is reasonable to obtain repeat echocardiograms in patients with severe aortic stenosis (valve area <0.75 cm^2) yearly or more frequently if symptoms change. Patients with less severe aortic stenosis should probably undergo evaluation every 2 to 3 years unless symptoms suggest a change.

Aortic sclerosis signifies hemodynamically insignificant calcification and thickening of the aortic valve (valve areas >1.5 cm^2). Patients with a history of aortic sclerosis, or a calculated valve area larger than 1.5 cm^2, should undergo echocardiography every 5 years unless symptoms warrant more frequent examination.

Aortic Regurgitation

Chronic aortic regurgitation results in dilatation and, ultimately, dysfunction of the left ventricle. Thus, echocardiography can provide a semiquantitative assessment of the severity of aortic regurgitation and can evaluate the size and function of the left ventricle. Estimation of the severity of aortic regurgitation is made primarily by color-flow Doppler and is based on both the width and the depth of the color-flow Doppler jet (Fig. 5–5). Doppler can also be used to estimate the rate of equilibration between the aorta and the left ventricle, with rapid equilibration being suggestive of elevated end-diastolic pressure and severe or acute aortic insufficiency. Patients with rapid increases in ventricular dimensions, particularly end-systolic dimensions, or deterioration in ventricular function should be considered for valve replacement surgery. Nevertheless, ventricular dimensions and function can remain unchanged for many years in patients with even moderate to severe aortic regurgitation. Thus, patients who are asymptomatic and stable with mild to moderate aortic regurgitation should undergo echocardiography every few years. Patients with severe aortic regurgitation or with evidence of left ventricular dilatation or dysfunction, however, should undergo echocardiography more frequently, perhaps as often as every 6 months. Aortic regurgitation is frequently associated with dilatation of the aortic root.

Mitral Stenosis

Mitral stenosis (see Fig. 32–6) confers an increased risk of pulmonary hypertension, congestive heart failure, and thromboembolism. Echocardiography is used to establish the diagnosis of mitral stenosis and can assess the mitral valve area. The diagnosis of rheumatic mitral stenosis is easily made by the classic findings on echocardiography, which include tethered mitral leaflet tips with relatively pliable leaflets.

The mitral valve area is calculated in a number of ways, including direct planimetry of the valve and by indirect methods such as the pressure half-time method and the continuity method. The pressure half-time method, the most commonly used method to calculate mitral valve area, is based on a regression formula relating the rate of pressure equilibration between the left atrium and the left ventricle to calculate the valve area. Because the velocity of blood flow between the left atrium and the left ventricle as measured by Doppler echocardiography is dependent on the pressure gradient between these two locations, this velocity will reach zero when these pressures equilibrate. It is important to recognize that conditions that increase left ventricular end-diastolic pressure—such as aortic regurgitation and ischemic heart disease—will result in more rapid equilibration of left atrial and left ventricular pressure and may thus overestimate the mitral valve area by this method. In addition to valve area, assessment of left atrial size, right ventricular function, and pulmonary pressure provides extremely useful information in caring for patients with mitral stenosis.

Mitral Regurgitation

Patients with mitral regurgitation have an increased risk of congestive heart failure and endocarditis. Mitral

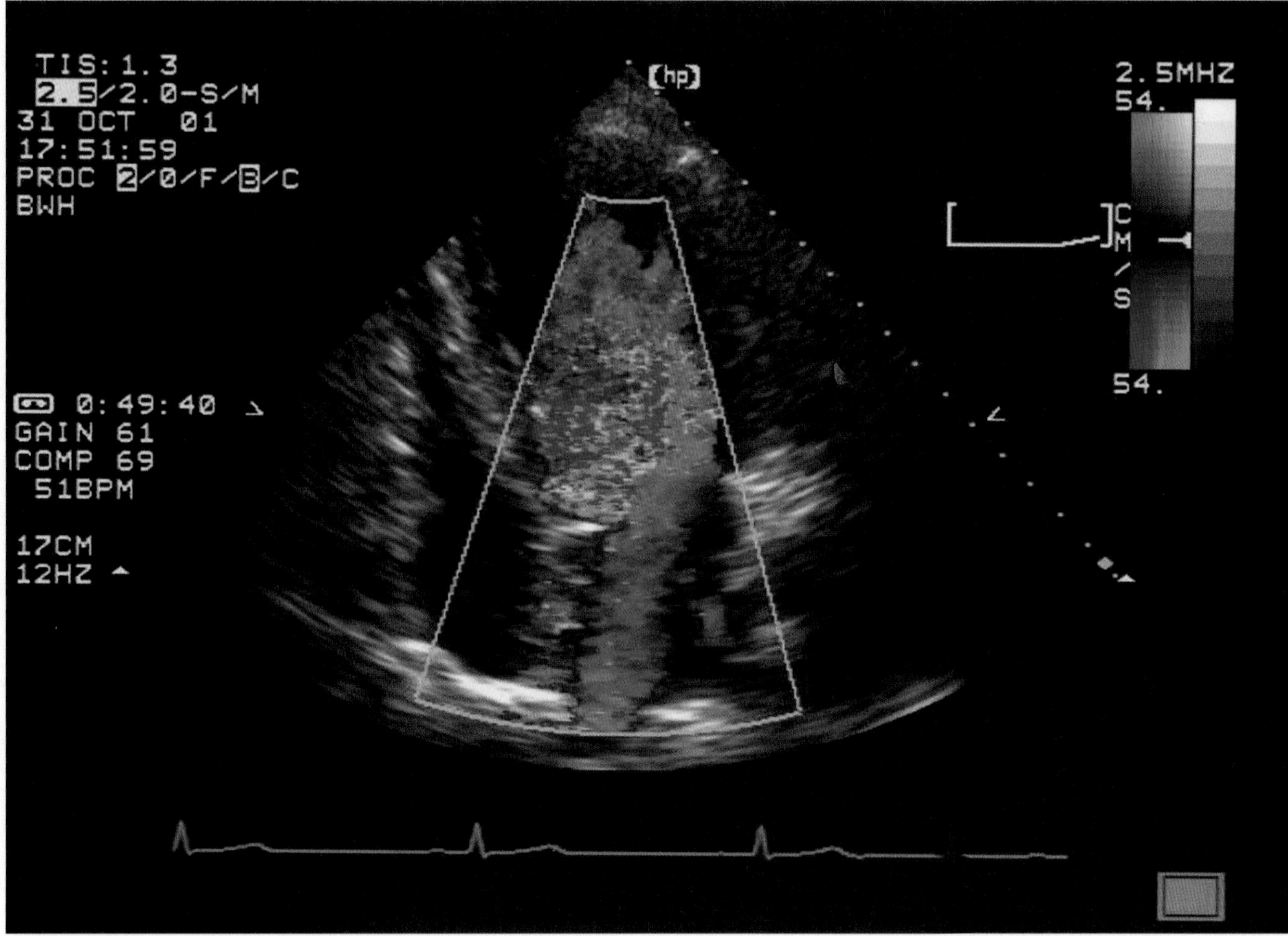

FIGURE 5–5. Color-flow Doppler image of aortic insufficiency.

regurgitation is assessed by color-flow Doppler echocardiography, in which the regurgitant jet can be well visualized as a mosaic-colored plume into the left atrium (see Fig. 5–2). Assessment of the degree of mitral regurgitation is semiquantitative. Determination of the severity of mitral regurgitation is based on the width and depth of the color-flow jet and the presence of flow reversal in the pulmonary veins, which is indicative of severe regurgitation. Assessment of ventricular size and function is an essential part of the evaluation in patients with mitral regurgitation. The EF in patients with moderate to severe mitral regurgitation is generally significantly higher than normal. A decrease in EF from the high-normal to the low-normal range can represent a significant reduction in ventricular contractility in the setting of a marked decrease in afterload.

Patients with mitral regurgitation should undergo repeat echocardiography if the clinical signs or symptoms change. In patients without such changes, repeat echocardiography is not indicated for mild mitral regurgitation. In the absence of a clear consensus regarding how often to study patients with moderate to severe mitral regurgitation and no changing symptoms, it is reasonable to obtain echocardiographic follow-up every 2 to 3 years in such patients, with careful attention to changes in ventricular size and function.

Mitral Valve Prolapse

A rarer disorder than thought previously, true mitral valve prolapse (MVP), in which one or both of the mitral valve leaflets prolapse into the left atrium during systole (see Fig. 32–10), occurs in approximately 2% to 3% of adults and is one of the most overdiagnosed conditions in cardiovascular medicine.[9] Nevertheless, patients with MVP have an increased risk for significant mitral regurgitation and endocarditis. However, the likelihood of clinically important MVP without any physical signs such as a systolic murmur or mid-systolic click is quite low. Therefore, in the absence of physical signs suggestive of this disorder, echocardiography is not indicated for suspected MVP. In particular, echocardiography to rule out MVP in patients with chest pain, palpitations, or other ill-defined symptoms is not warranted. It is reasonable to perform echocardiography in patients in whom MVP has been diagnosed but whose physical examination does not support that diagnosis because a negative examination will make it possible to discontinue the use of antibiotic prophylaxis.

Although most patients with MVP have associated mitral regurgitation, it is possible to have prolapse without clinically important regurgitation; however, these patients probably have an increased long-term risk for mitral regurgitation.

Tricuspid Regurgitation

A small degree of tricuspid regurgitation is common in most adults and does not itself reflect pathology (see Fig. 32–15). Mild tricuspid regurgitation seen on an otherwise unremarkable echocardiographic examination is a normal finding that does not require further evaluation and should not alarm the physician or patient. Echocardiography can identify significant tricuspid regurgitation secondary to elevated pulmonary pressure, acute pulmonary embolism, or conditions that directly affect the tricuspid valve, such as carcinoid.

Dilated and Hypertrophic Cardiomyopathy

Dilated cardiomyopathy is characterized by increased ventricular size and reduced left ventricular function. Although the presence of regional wall motion abnormalities is suggestive of cardiomyopathy of ischemic origin, such abnormalities can be seen in nonischemic cardiomyopathy, and alternatively, global dysfunction can be seen in advanced ischemic heart disease.

Hypertrophic cardiomyopathy is characterized by unexplained ventricular hypertrophy seen on echocardiography.[10] Wall thickness in this disease can typically reach 15 to 40 mm and can be concentric but is more commonly asymmetric (see Fig. 29–4). The characteristic appearance of reversed septal curvature is common in the hereditary form of the disease. The presence of systolic anterior motion of the mitral valve, in which the anterior mitral leaflet is pulled into the left ventricular outflow tract during systole, is common in hypertrophic cardiomyopathy but not necessary for the diagnosis. Outflow tract obstruction is frequent in patients with hypertrophic cardiomyopathy, and an outflow tract gradient may be identified and measured by Doppler techniques. Diastolic dysfunction is common and may be a key abnormality in patients with hypertrophic cardiomyopathy. Doppler tissue imaging has shown promise as a method for assessment of diastolic function by echocardiography.

Abnormalities of the Aorta

Patients with severe dilatation of the ascending aorta are at increased risk for aortic rupture or dissection (see Fig. 36–12). An aortic diameter greater than 2.6 cm at the root or greater than 3.4 cm in the ascending aorta is considered abnormal. Aortic dilatation is common in patients with hypertension, aortic stenosis, or aortic insufficiency. In addition, patients with certain connective tissue disorders such as the Marfan syndrome have an increased risk for aortic dilatation, particularly at the aortic root. An ascending aorta diameter greater than 6.0 cm (or 5.0 cm in patients with the Marfan syndrome) or any aortic diameter that significantly increases over a short period should prompt consideration for surgical repair.

Ischemic Heart Disease

The major use of echocardiography in patients with ischemic heart disease is to determine the presence of regional wall motion abnormalities (see Figs. 25–3 and 25–5) and to assess ventricular function. In patients with ECG abnormalities, the presence of a regional wall motion abnormality on echocardiography can provide confirmation of a previous myocardial infarction.

Exercise Stress Echocardiography

Exercise testing remains the standard means for the provocative assessment and diagnosis of coronary artery disease (see Chapter 4). Over the past 2 decades the addition of imaging procedures to standard exercise testing has increased the sensitivity and specificity of the test in certain clinical situations, particularly in patients with baseline ECG abnormalities.

Although radionuclide-based techniques are most widely used, echocardiographic stress testing is a useful alternative.[11] It is important to recognize that nuclear and echocardiographic stress techniques have fundamental differences. Whereas radionuclide scintigraphy is a perfusion-based technique that directly assesses myocardial blood flow, stress echocardiography evaluates coronary blood flow only indirectly by assessing the effect of exercise on myocardial wall motion. Ischemia is diagnosed on an exercise echocardiogram when a new regional wall motion abnormality develops during exercise (or at peak dose of an inotrope in a pharmacologic stress test). Nevertheless, not all perfusion abnormalities will be manifested as a regional wall motion abnormality on stress testing. Likewise, not all regional wall motion abnormalities are related to perfusion abnormalities.

In a typical exercise echocardiographic examination, 2-D images are obtained at baseline in four views (parasternal long axis, parasternal short axis, apical four chamber, and apical two chamber). The patient then exercises on a standard treadmill, with simultaneous ECG monitoring, until the test is completed. The same criteria used for completion of a standard exercise test are used for an exercise echocardiogram. Postexercise images are obtained within 90 seconds of completion of exercise. Wall motion abnormalities are identified by side-by-side comparison of rest and stress images (Fig. 5–6).

The sensitivity and specificity of exercise echocardiography can be adversely affected by a variety of

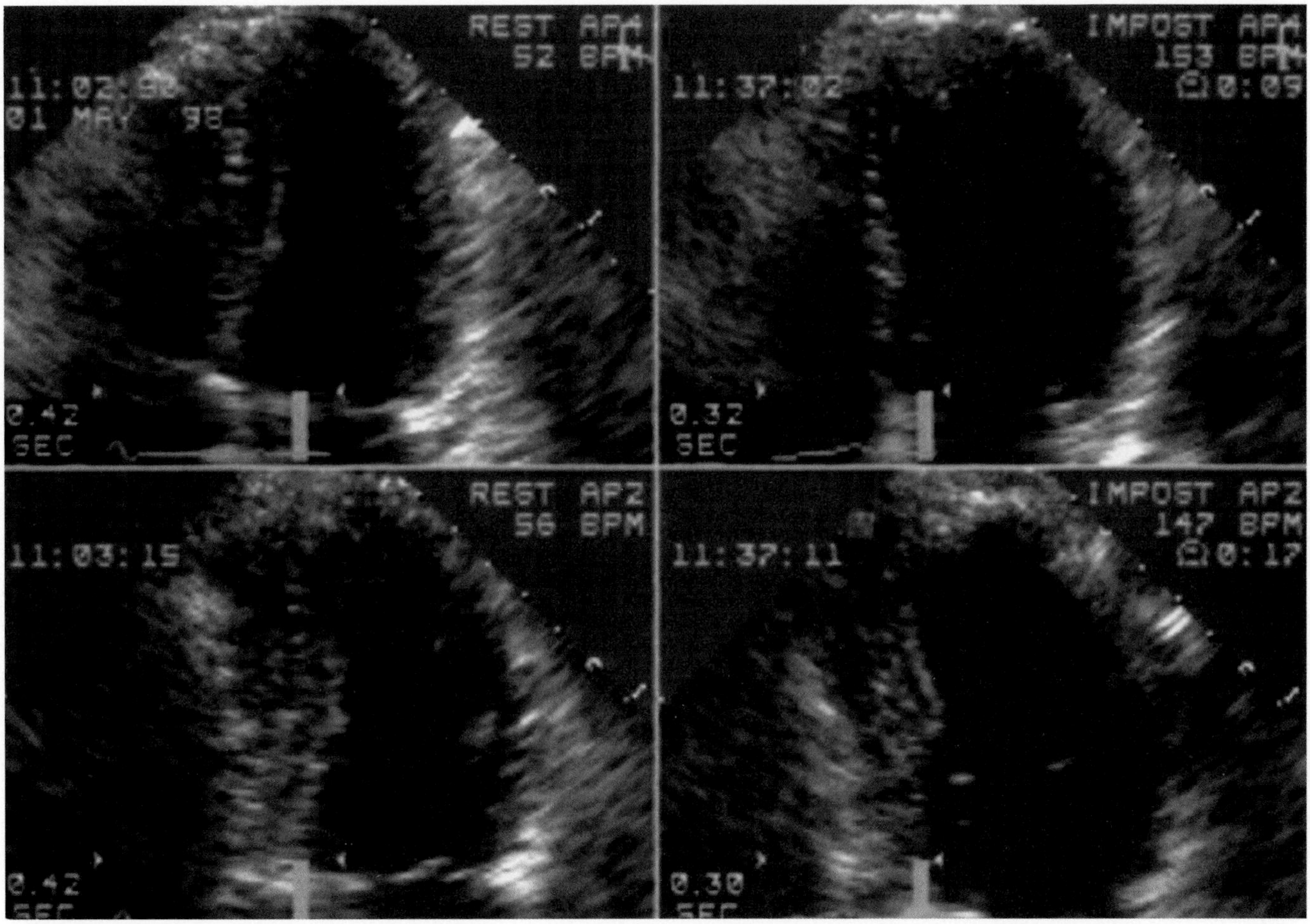

FIGURE 5–6. A stress echocardiogram allows a side-by-side comparison of rest and stress images.

factors, including the presence of baseline regional wall motion abnormalities, poor imaging windows, adequacy of the exercise testing itself, and the presence of bundle branch blocks that result in abnormal myocardial contraction. In addition, interpretation of exercise echocardiograms is subjective and highly dependent on the experience of the reader. Unlike nuclear techniques, no automated methods are available to detect regional wall motion abnormalities. Thus, although the sensitivity and specificity of exercise echocardiography have compared favorably with nuclear techniques in a variety of published reports,[12] these results may not be directly applicable to all centers. In experienced centers, both echocardiographic and nuclear stress testing techniques significantly increase the sensitivity and specificity of standard exercise testing, and most direct comparisons of these techniques have shown similar overall diagnostic accuracy.[13]

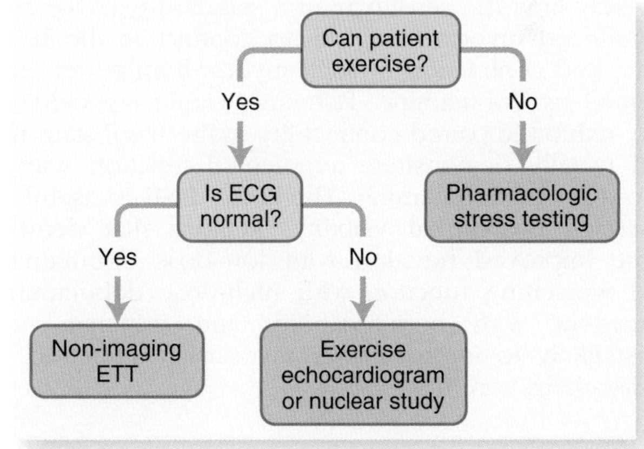

FIGURE 5–7. Diagnostic algorithm for determining when it is appropriate to include imaging with exercise testing. ECG, electrocardiogram; ETT, exercise tolerance testing.

Indications for Exercise Stress Echocardiography

Indications for stress echocardiography are similar to those for nuclear exercise testing. Figure 5–7 presents an algorithm for determining when patients should undergo imaging and pharmacologic exercise testing. Standard ECG exercise stress testing remains the diagnostic test of choice in patients with suspected ischemic heart disease and normal baseline ECGs. However, the reduced sensitivity and specificity of exercise testing in patients with baseline ECG abnormalities can be dramatically improved when combined with cardiac imaging. Still, treadmill stress testing is generally thought to be the preferred method in patients who are capable of exercising. However, in patients who are not capable of exercising, pharmacologic stress testing becomes a necessity.

A number of factors influence the decision regarding which type of imaging test to choose—echocardiographic or nuclear—including the availability of the test and physician expertise in the specific institution. In patients without known coronary disease, stress echocardiography and nuclear stress testing are roughly equivalent in sensitivity and specificity for the detection of coronary disease. In patients with known coronary disease, however, exercise echocardiography may be superior in determining the functional significance of a coronary lesion. In addition, stress echocardiography is useful in determining whether a patient's dyspnea is secondary to ischemia-induced left ventricular dysfunction.

Dobutamine Stress Echocardiography

Dobutamine stress echocardiography (DSE) is a form of pharmacologic stress testing in which the patient receives escalating doses of dobutamine to simulate the physiologic effects of exercise. DSE is indicated in patients who cannot exercise at all or to a level sufficient for a diagnostic study. The usual protocol requires the patient to receive three or four increasing doses of dobutamine starting at 5 μg/kg/min to a maximum of 40 μg/kg/min. If a target heart rate is not achieved, atropine is usually added to the protocol to increase the heart rate. Dobutamine stimulates increased cardiac contractility, as well as systemic vasodilatation, and is thus a good imitator of exercise. In addition, this test is not dependent on patient effort, which itself can severely limit the sensitivity of a standard exercise test.

Infarcted myocardium fails to contract in the basal state, and contraction of such myocardium is not augmented by dobutamine. Ischemic, viable myocardium may exhibit impaired contractility in the basal state but will usually demonstrate augmented function with a low dose of dobutamine. Therefore, DSE is useful in assessing myocardial viability. Regions that demonstrate improved function with low-dose dobutamine and worsening function with high-dose dobutamine, consistent with both viability and ischemia, are most likely to improve after myocardial infarction or revascularization.[14]

Post–myocardial Infarction Status

Patients with reduced left ventricular function after myocardial infarction have an increased risk for death and the development of heart failure. The left ventricular enlargement that can occur after large myocardial infarctions further increases the risk of morbidity and mortality. Thus, assessment of left ventricular size and function after myocardial infarction should be performed routinely. Because a significant amount of myocardial stunning can occur immediately after infarction, residual function after infarction should be assessed in a week or more after hospital discharge.[15] Mitral regurgitation, itself an important prognostic indicator in patients after myocardial infarction, can also be assessed at this time. Because the heart can continue to remodel and enlarge after infarction, regular assessment of ventricular and valvular function is warranted. Major complications of myocardial infarction include rupture of a papillary muscle causing severe mitral regurgitation or rupture of the interventricular septum causing a ventricular septal defect. Both of these complications are characterized by new, loud systolic heart murmurs, and the diagnosis can readily be established by echocardiography.

Congenital Heart Disease in Adults

The most common form of adult congenital heart disease seen in a general primary care practice is atrial septal defect (see Chapter 34). It should be suspected in patients with wide fixed splitting of the second heart sound, unexplained right ventricular enlargement, or signs of pulmonary hypertension. Atrial septal defects are usually assessed with color-flow Doppler. Occasionally, atrial septal defects of the sinus venosus type are difficult to visualize with TTE. Saline contrast examination can be particularly useful in assessing the presence of an atrial septal defect if one is not immediately apparent on standard imaging. TEE can help characterize the location and size of atrial septal defects and can identify other coexisting abnormalities.

TABLE 5–7

Chronic Conditions Requiring Repeated Echocardiographic Examination

Condition	Echocardiographic Parameters to Monitor
Congestive heart failure/ cardiomyopathy	Left ventricular function Mitral regurgitation
Aortic stenosis	Aortic valve area Aortic valve gradient Left ventricular function
Mitral stenosis	Mitral valve area Mitral valve gradient Left atrial size Pulmonary pressures
Mitral regurgitation	Degree of mitral regurgitation Ventricular dimensions Left ventricular function Left atrial size Pulmonary pressures
Aortic regurgitation	Degree of aortic regurgitation Ventricular dimensions Left ventricular function Aortic root dilatation
Congenital heart disease	Identification of anatomy Assessment of left and right ventricular function Assessment of pulmonary pressures

TABLE 5–8

Alternatives to Echocardiography

Modality	Indications	Comparison with Echocardiography
Nuclear sestamibi imaging	Assessment of myocardial perfusion with exercise or during pharmacologic stress	No current robust echo-based perfusion methods Sensitivity and specificity compare well with stress echo for detecting ischemia Usually more expensive than stress echo testing
Nuclear thallium imaging	Assessment of perfusion (see above) largely supplanted by sestamibi imaging Nonfunctional assessment of viability	Lower sensitivity and specificity than sestamibi relative to echocardiography Dobutamine echocardiography provides functional assessment of viability
Nuclear radioventriculography	Assessment of ventricular volumes and ejection fraction	Limited to functional information—no valvular or structural information obtained
Magnetic resonance imaging	Assessment of cardiac function and structure Assessment of myocardial viability after myocardial infarction	Extremely accurate assessment of cardiac size and function Cardiac perfusion and viability studies Cannot be performed in patients with pacemakers or implantable defibrillators Patients are required to hold their breath Imaging can be difficult in patients with atrial fibrillation or arrhythmia
Computed tomography	Aortic dissection	Can be performed quickly Compares well with TEE Advantage for TEE in the region of the aortic arch Requires the use of contrast dye Limited additional functional information obtained

TEE, transesophageal echocardiography.

Echocardiography is likewise indicated in patients in whom congenital heart disease is suspected by virtue of an unexplained murmur (see Fig. 34–5), cyanosis, desaturation, or an abnormal chest radiograph. In patients with known congenital heart disease, echocardiography is indicated at follow-up when signs or symptoms change or to periodically assess left or right ventricular function, valvular function, or pulmonary pressure. The exact interval between follow-up examinations depends on the type and severity of disease. Echocardiography is an excellent technique for imaging vegetations in infective endocarditis (see Fig. 5–2 and Chapter 33).

Chronic Conditions That Require Multiple Examinations

Repeated echocardiographic examination is warranted in patients with chronic progressive conditions in which morphologic changes parallel disease progression (Table 5–7).

ALTERNATIVES TO ECHOCARDIOGRAPHY

Other cardiac imaging technologies can complement or, in some cases, serve as alternatives to echocardiography in appropriate clinical circumstances (Table 5–8). Nuclear techniques incorporating thallium or sestamibi are routinely used to assess perfusion abnormalities in patients with suspected ischemic heart disease. No echocardiographic-based perfusion method is currently approved, although contrast echocardiography may ultimately allow for echocardiography-based assessment of myocardial perfusion. Radioventriculography can be used to assess left ventricular function; it is both reliable and reproducible and is particularly useful for monitoring patients whose EFs are likely to change over time—such as patients receiving chemotherapy. Magnetic resonance imaging (MRI) is rapidly emerging as a viable alternative to echocardiography and can provide high-quality moving images of the heart in patients with poor-quality images on echocardiography. MRI cannot be performed in patients with pacemakers or implantable defibrillators and is difficult to perform in patients who are claustrophobic or have difficulty holding their breath. MRI-based contrast agents can be used to assess myocardial perfusion, and methods to assess cardiac viability are gaining acceptance in the cardiology community. Finally, CT scanning is a reasonable alternative to TEE in patients with suspected aortic dissection (see Chapter 36).

References

1. Feigenbaum H: Echocardiography, 5th ed. Philadelphia, Lea & Febiger, 1994.

2. Cheitlin MD, Alpert JS, Armstrong WF, et al: ACC/AHA guidelines for the clinical application of echocardiography. A report of the American College of Cardiology/American Heart Association Task Force on Practice Guidelines (Committee on Clinical Application of Echocardiography). Circulation 1997;95:1686–1744.
3. American Society of Echocardiography Committee on Standards, Subcommittee on Quantitation of Two-Dimensional Echocardiograms: Recommendations for quantitation of the left ventricle by two-dimensional echocardiography. J Am Soc Echocardiogr 1989;5:358–367.
4. Firstenberg MS, Greenberg NL, Main ML, et al: Determinants of diastolic myocardial tissue Doppler velocities: Influences of relaxation and preload. J Appl Physiol 2001;90:299–307.
5. Kapral MK, Silver FL: Canadian Task Force on Preventive Health Care: Preventive health care, 1999 update: 2. Echocardiography for the detection of a cardiac source of embolus in patients with stroke. CMAJ 1999;161:989–996.
6. Manning WJ, Weintraub RM, Waksmonski CA, et al: Accuracy of transesophageal echocardiography for identifying left atrial thrombi. A prospective, intraoperative study. Ann Intern Med 1995;123:817–822.
7. Solomon SD: Echocardiography in pulmonary embolism. In Goldhaber SZ, Nakano T (eds): Pulmonary Embolism. Tokyo, Springer-Verlag, 1999.
8. Nassimiha D, Aronow WS, Ahn C, Goldman ME: Rate of progression of valvular aortic stenosis in patients > or = 60 years of age. Am J Cardiol 2001;87:807–809.
9. Freed LA, Levy D, Levine RA, et al: Prevalence and clinical outcome of mitral-valve prolapse. N Engl J Med 1999;341:1–7.
10. Maron BJ, Moller JH, Seidman CE, et al: Impact of laboratory molecular diagnosis on contemporary diagnostic criteria for genetically transmitted cardiovascular diseases: Hypertrophic cardiomyopathy, long-QT syndrome, and Marfan syndrome: A statement for healthcare professionals from the councils on clinical cardiology, cardiovascular disease in the young, and basic science. Circulation 1998;98:1460–1471.
11. Stress Echocardiography Task Force of the Nomenclature and Standards Committee of the American Society of Echocardiography: Stress echocardiography: Recommendations for performance and interpretation of stress echocardiography. J Am Soc Echocardiogr 1998;11:97–104.
12. Fleischmann KE, Hunink MG, Kuntz KM, Douglas PS: Exercise echocardiography or exercise SPECT imaging? A meta-analysis of diagnostic test performance. JAMA 1998;280:913–920.
13. Elhendy A, Geleijnse ML, van Domburg RT, et al: Comparison of dobutamine stress echocardiography and technetium-99m sestamibi single-photon emission tomography for the diagnosis of coronary artery disease in hypertensive patients with and without left ventricular hypertrophy. Eur J Nucl Med 1998;25:69–78.
14. Qureshi U, Nagueh SF, Afridi I, et al: Dobutamine echocardiography and quantitative rest-redistribution ^{201}Tl tomography in myocardial hibernation. Relation of contractile reserve to ^{201}Tl uptake and comparative prediction of recovery of function. Circulation 1997;95:626–635.
15. Solomon SD, Glynn RJ, Greaves S, et al: Recovery of ventricular function after myocardial infarction in the reperfusion era. Ann Intern Med 2001;134:451–458.

PART 2

Approach to Common Cardiac Problems

CHAPTER 6 Approach to the Patient with Chest Pain

Lee Goldman

Chest pain is a common symptom that may be caused by a condition as serious as acute myocardial infarction (MI) or as benign as a strained thoracic chest muscle. A patient's concern about chest pain is often unrelated to the severity of the symptom but, instead, related to the possible underlying cause. Similarly, the physician must remember that the intensity of chest pain is often unrelated to the importance of the underlying condition. Many patients with serious coronary artery disease may complain of a vague discomfort rather than severe pain, whereas inflammatory costochondritis may lead to severe pain.

Diagnosis of the cause of chest pain must take into account the chest pain syndrome itself, associated symptoms and signs, and an appreciation for the patient's other general characteristics. For example, the probable cause of burning substernal chest pain will be different in a patient whose pain is associated with diaphoresis and shortness of breath than in a patient whose pain is precipitated by lying flat after a large meal. Furthermore, the same chest pain and associated symptoms would be much more likely to represent coronary artery disease if they were found in a 60-year-old man than in a 20-year-old woman.

Chest pain is one of the most common problems encountered in primary care and is one of the most frequent causes of hospital admission. Coronary artery disease, a leading cause of chest pain, remains the most common cause of death in the United States. Every complaint of chest pain must be taken seriously, but the physician must choose appropriately from among a wide range of diagnostic tests and possible therapeutic trials.[1]

CLINICAL SYNDROMES

Patients who complain of chest pain can quickly be put into one of three general categories: acute chest pain of recent onset, which may be ongoing and persistent; episodic, recurrent chest pain, with each individual episode lasting for minutes rather than hours; or persistent pain, which may continue for hours or even days with variable fluctuation in intensity. By placing an individual patient in one of these three general categories, the physician may focus the evaluation on the various causes of chest pain (Table 6–1).

For some causes such as coronary artery disease, chest pain may be of sudden, new onset, as with an acute MI (see Chapter 27), or it may be recurrent and episodic, as with angina (Table 6–2). When the anginal pain occurs more frequently or at lower levels of stress or even at rest, the episodes suggest unstable rather than stable angina (see Chapters 25 and 26). Other causes of insufficient coronary arterial flow, such as found with valvular aortic stenosis (Chapter 32), hypertrophic cardiomyopathy (Chapter 29), or microvascular angina, also tend to be recurrent and episodic. By comparison, the pain of acute pericarditis (Chapter 35) may be of sudden acute onset, may be recurrent and episodic during the acute phase of pericarditis or during periodic recurrences, or may persist for hours or days as a dull ache.

Among vascular causes, aortic dissection (see Chapter 36) is commonly manifested as severe acute pain with a discrete onset. Much less commonly, patients with chronic aortic dissection may have intermittent episodes

TABLE 6–1

Some Causes of Chest Discomfort

	New, Acute, Often Ongoing	Recurrent, Episodic	Persistent, Even for Days
Cardiac			
Coronary artery disease	+	+	
Aortic stenosis		+	
Hypertrophic cardiomyopathy		+	
Pericarditis	+	+	+
Vascular			
Aortic dissection	+		
Pulmonary embolism	+	+	
Pulmonary hypertension	+	+	
Right ventricular strain	+	+	
Pulmonary			
Pleuritis or pneumonia	+	+	+
Tracheobronchitis	+	+	+
Pneumothorax	+		+
Tumor			+
Mediastinitis or mediastinal emphysema	+		+
Gastrointestinal			
Esophageal reflux	+	+	+
Esophageal spasm	+	+	+
Mallory-Weiss tear	+		
Peptic ulcer disease	+	+	+
Biliary disease	+	+	
Pancreatitis		+	+
Musculoskeletal			
Cervical disk disease		+	+
Arthritis of the shoulder or spine		+	+
Costochondritis	+	+	+
Intercostal muscle cramps	+	+	+
Interscalene or hyperabduction syndromes		+	+
Subacromial bursitis	+	+	+
Other			
Disorders of the breast		+	+
Chest wall tumors			+
Herpes zoster	+		+
Emotional	+	+	+

From Fauci AS, Braunwald E, Isselbacher KJ, et al (eds): Harrison's Principles of Internal Medicine, 14th ed. New York, McGraw-Hill, 1998, p 58. Copyright © by McGraw-Hill, Inc. Used by permission of McGraw-Hill Book Company.

of pain associated with extension of the dissection. Acute pulmonary embolism (Chapter 38) may be associated with severe pain at the time of onset. If the pulmonary embolism leads to pulmonary infarction and irritation of the pleural surface, it may be associated with recurrent episodic pain, especially pain with deep breathing. The pain of pulmonary hypertension and right ventricular strain may be of sudden onset but is more commonly associated with exertion or other stress that leads to increased pulmonary blood flow and hence

TABLE 6–2

Cardiovascular Causes of Chest Pain

Condition	Location	Quality	Duration	Aggravating or Relieving Factors	Associated Symptoms or Signs
Angina	Retrosternal region; radiates or occasionally isolated to neck, jaw, epigastrium, shoulder, or arms—left common	Pressure, burning, squeezing, heaviness, indigestion	<2–10 min	Precipitated by exercise, cold weather, or emotional stress; relieved by rest or nitroglycerin; atypical (Prinzmetal's) angina may be unrelated to activity, often early morning	S_4, or murmur of papillary muscle dysfunction during pain
Rest or unstable angina	Same as angina	Same as angina but may be more severe	Usually <20 min	Same as angina, with decreasing tolerance for exertion or at rest	Similar to stable angina, but may be pronounced. Transient cardiac failure can occur
Myocardial infarction	Substernal and may radiate like angina	Heaviness, pressure, burning, constriction	Sudden onset, 30 min or longer but variable	Unrelieved by rest or nitroglycerin	Shortness of breath, sweating, weakness, nausea, vomiting
Pericarditis	Usually begins over sternum or toward cardiac apex and may radiate to neck or left shoulder; often more localized than the pain of myocardial ischemia	Sharp, stabbing, knifelike	Lasts many hours to days; may wax and wane	Aggravated by deep breathing, rotating chest, or supine position; relieved by sitting up and leaning forward	Pericardial friction rub
Aortic dissection	Anterior of chest; may radiate to back	Excruciating, tearing, knifelike	Sudden onset, unrelenting	Usually occurs in setting of hypertension or predisposition such as Marfan's syndrome	Murmur of aortic insufficiency, pulse or blood pressure asymmetry; neurologic deficit
Pulmonary embolism (chest pain often not present)	Substernal or over region of pulmonary infarction	Pleuritic (with pulmonary infarction) or angina-like	Sudden onset; minutes to <1 hr	May be aggravated by breathing	Dyspnea, tachypnea, tachycardia; hypotension, signs of acute right heart failure, and pulmonary hypertension with large emboli; rales, pleural rub, hemoptysis with pulmonary infarction
Pulmonary hypertension	Substernal	Pressure; oppressive		Aggravated by effort	Pain usually associated with dyspnea; signs of pulmonary hypertension

S_4, fourth heart sound.

From Andreoli TE, Bennett JC, Carpenter CCJ, Plum F: Evaluation of the patient with cardiovascular disease. *In* Cecil Essentials of Medicine, 4th ed. Philadelphia, WB Saunders, 1997, p 11.

increased pulmonary blood pressure in the face of elevated pulmonary vascular resistance.

Pain from pneumonia or pleuritis may be of acute onset at the time of initial pleural irritation, may be recurrent at times of deep breathing or other maneuvers that stretch or irritate the pleura, or may be persistent because of pleural irritation (Table 6–3). Pain from a pneumothorax is usually sudden and acute and then persists until the pneumothorax resolves spontaneously or by treatment. Pain from lung tumors is commonly persistent for days or longer.

Most of the various gastrointestinal (GI) causes of chest discomfort are acute in onset, but many may also be recurrent and episodic. Most GI causes of discomfort can be related to eating, vomiting, or other associated GI signs or symptoms.

Musculoskeletal chest discomfort can be acute and of sudden onset, especially when related to costochondritis, muscle cramps or injuries, or bursitis. Musculoskeletal complaints can also be recurrent and episodic, usually in association with movements that can be directly related to the involved structures. In differentiating recurrent episodic musculoskeletal chest pain from angina pectoris, the relationship to specific movements is vital. Many musculoskeletal problems cause persistent chest discomfort, and this lack of relationship to activity may be an important way to discriminate musculoskeletal chest pain from coronary artery disease.

CAUSES OF CHEST PAIN

Myocardial Ischemia

Myocardial ischemia may be of acute and sudden onset, such as with acute MI, or recurrent and episodic, such as with angina pectoris from atherosclerosis or other causes of coronary stenosis (see Chapters 25 to 27). It may also be seen in patients with normal epicardial coronary arteries but with abnormalities in coronary vascular tone or the coronary microvascular circulation. Coronary ischemia also develops in patients with

TABLE 6–3

Noncardiac Causes of Chest Pain

Condition	Location	Quality	Duration	Aggravating or Relieving Factors	Associated Symptoms or Signs
Pneumonia with pleurisy	Localized over involved area	Pleuritic localized	Usually brief	Painful breathing	Dyspnea, cough, fever, dull to percussion, bronchial breath sounds, rales occasional pleural rub
Spontaneous pneumothorax	Unilateral	Sharp, well localized	Sudden onset, lasts many hours	Painful breathing	Dyspnea; hyperresonance and decreased breath and voice sounds over involved lung
Musculoskeletal disorders	Variable	Aching	Short or long duration	Aggravated by movement; history of muscle exertion or injury	Tender to pressure or movement
Herpes zoster	Dermatomal in distribution	Burning	Prolonged	None	Vesicular rash appears in area of discomfort
Esophageal reflux	Substernal, epigastric	Burning, visceral discomfort	10–60 min	Aggravated by large meal, postprandial recumbency; relief with antacid	Water brash
Peptic ulcer	Epigastric, substernal	Visceral burning, aching	Prolonged	Relief with food, antacid	
Gallbladder disease	Epigastric, right upper quadrant	Visceral	Prolonged	May be unprovoked or follows meal	Right upper quadrant tenderness may be present
Anxiety states	Often localized over precordium	Variable; location often moves from place to place	Varies; often fleeting	Situational	Sighing respirations, often chest wall tenderness

Adapted from Andreoli TE, Bennett JC, Carpenter CCJ, Plum F: Evaluation of the patient with cardiovascular disease. *In* Cecil Essentials of Medicine, 4th ed. Philadelphia, WB Saunders, 1997, p 12.

nonatherosclerotic causes of coronary stenosis, such as may be found with collagen vascular diseases, syphilis, or coronary artery dissection. In addition, myocardial ischemia may be found in patients with congenital anomalies of the coronary arteries, including congenital absence of one or more important coronary arteries, a coronary artery that originates from the pulmonary artery rather than the aorta, or even rarely a coronary arteriovenous fistula. Myocardial ischemia can also occur with totally normal coronary arteries, both anatomically and functionally, if markedly increased oxygen demand is not matched by oxygen supply. For example, myocardial ischemia may develop in patients with valvular aortic stenosis or hypertrophic cardiomyopathy, especially with exercise, because diastolic coronary flow is not adequate to supply the needs of the hypertrophic, stressed myocardium.

When chest pain is caused by an abnormality in the coronary artery, the abnormality may range from total anatomic occlusion to an endothelial or functional defect associated with a normal lumen at the time of coronary arteriography. Sudden, total occlusion of a coronary artery, usually by intrinsic thrombosis but occasionally by embolization, commonly causes acute MI, although it may occasionally be asymptomatic in a patient with an impaired pain response or with adequate, preexisting collateral vessels. In patients with chronic total occlusion, angina pectoris may then develop because the circulation to the affected myocardium via collaterals may be adequate at rest but not during exercise or other stress.

Fixed Coronary Stenoses. These stenoses generally do not impair resting coronary blood flow substantially until they occlude about 70% to 90% of the cross-sectional area of the coronary lumen. However, stenosis of 50% of the luminal diameter, which corresponds to about 70% of the cross-sectional area, is frequently associated with ischemia during exercise or other stress. Because myocardial oxygen extraction tends to be near maximal at all times, increased oxygen supply can be provided only by increased coronary flow. The major determinant of total coronary flow is coronary vascular resistance. The coronary arteries dilate in response to exercise, adrenergic stimuli, and most substances that dilate peripheral arteries. The resulting decrease in coronary resistance permits the increased blood flow that is required to meet the myocardial demands of exercise and stress. In patients with abnormal coronary artery endothelium, vasodilatation may not occur in response to typical vasodilatory stimuli; in some circumstances, paradoxical vasoconstriction may develop. Although impaired coronary vasodilatation may occur in the absence of any evident pathoanatomic abnormalities, it is more common in patients with hypercholesterolemia or those who smoke, and the abnormal reflex may disappear when cholesterol levels are reduced or smoking ceases. Patients with obstructive atherosclerotic coronary disease also commonly have impaired coronary vasodilatation or paradoxical vasoconstriction, sometimes at sites of atherosclerotic stenosis and sometimes in locations in which coronary arteriography does not reveal any gross abnormalities.

Vasoactive substances such as cocaine may lead to inappropriate coronary vasoconstriction and even spasm sufficient to obliterate the coronary lumen and cause severe ischemia or even MI. Patients with Prinzmetal's angina have spontaneous, severe vasoconstriction that may occur at rest, when typical coronary vasodilator stimuli are lacking, or paradoxically with exercise.

Coronary artery emboli may originate from infectious endocarditis, a clot in the left atrium or left ventricle, marantic endocarditis in patients with metastatic malignancies, Libman-Sacks endocarditis, a clot on prosthetic heart valves, or even paradoxical emboli originating in the venous system and shunting to the left side of the heart via a ventricular septal defect, atrial septal defect, or patent foramen ovale.

Acute MI can be caused by any sudden occlusion of a coronary artery ranging from an intrinsic thrombus to an embolus to internal dissection or external compression of a coronary artery.

Acute Myocardial Infarction

Clinical Findings

The pain of acute MI is classically described as constriction, tightness, pressure, or a squeezing discomfort centered in the mid-substernal region and often radiating to the left shoulder, neck, or arm (see Chapter 27). It is classically associated with diaphoresis and may be accompanied by shortness of breath, nausea, or a feeling of impending doom. It typically builds in intensity over a period of 5 to 10 minutes before reaching peak intensity. The pain may begin with exercise or stress, but it most commonly occurs without warning or an obvious immediate precipitating cause. Although acute MI is statistically more likely to occur in the early morning hours, it may happen at any time of day.

Analyses of large numbers of patients evaluated for acute chest pain, however, reveal that many patients do not have these typical findings and many of those without acute MI or even acute myocardial ischemia may have many of the characteristics that are usually thought to be typical of acute ischemia.[1,2] For example, pain that is described as aching, burning, indigestion, or gas is nearly as likely to represent acute MI as pain that is described as pressure, squeezing, tightness, or constriction. Pain is much less likely to represent acute MI if it is described as stabbing or knifelike or as sharp when the term *sharp* is not being used as a synonym for severe but rather to describe the feeling of the pain.

When pain radiates from the chest to the left shoulder, neck, or left arm, the likelihood that it represents acute MI is about threefold higher than when chest pain does not radiate to these locations. It must be remembered, however, that innervation of the thoracic dermatomes is not sufficiently precise for the location or radiation of pain to be considered definitive from a diagnostic perspective. Furthermore, severe pain from any source may stimulate adjacent dermatomes. Therefore, esophageal spasm may cause pain radiation indistinguishable from that of acute MI.

The pain of acute MI may also radiate to the jaw, teeth, right arm, back, or abdomen. Nevertheless, concomitant back pain should raise the possibility of aortic dissection or musculoskeletal causes, whereas radiation to the abdomen should increase suspicion for the various GI causes of acute chest discomfort. The pain of acute myocardial ischemia rarely radiates to the lower part of the abdomen or legs.

Diaphoresis may accompany any discomfort that evokes severe sympathetic stimulation or a parasympathetic response. Diaphoresis tends to be more common in larger, more severe, more obvious MIs, and diagnosis by other means is often easier.

Shortness of breath may accompany acute MI because of concomitant left heart failure secondary to left ventricular dysfunction caused by the myocardial ischemia. Subjective shortness of breath may also develop in patients who are in severe pain or who are anxious or hyperventilating because of the acute pain syndrome.

Physical Examination

Pain is much less likely to represent acute MI if it can be reproduced by localized chest palpation. However, because many patients will have discomfort on vigorous chest palpation, it is critical to determine whether the patient's complaints are truly reproduced by relatively modest chest palpation or whether vigorous chest manipulation is producing a different pain syndrome. The results of physical examination may be totally normal in patients with acute MI unless they have concomitant heart failure or other complications.

Diagnostic Testing

The single most important piece of laboratory information in a patient with possible acute MI is the electrocardiogram (ECG).[1, 2] The ECG will show ST segment elevation or Q-waves not known to be old in about 40% to 45% of patients with acute MI. An additional 30% to 40% of patients will have ST segment depression or T-wave inversion not known to be old on the initial ECG. In patients with such ECG changes and a clinical picture consistent with acute MI, rapid triage to an acute care setting and institution of emergency treatment are mandatory. Cardiac markers provide a definitive diagnosis. The advent of troponin T and troponin I assays has increased the sensitivity for diagnosing acute MI and has led to reclassification of many patients in whom unstable angina was previously diagnosed to what is now considered non–Q-wave, non–ST elevation MI.[3]

For patients with clinical findings that might be consistent with acute MI but might also represent unstable angina pectoris, a combination of clinical factors can be used to estimate the approximate probability of acute MI (Fig. 6–1). Chest pain evaluation units (see later) provide a low-cost, efficient mechanism for a brief, but focused evaluation in such patients.

Angina

Myocardial ischemia (without infarction) that occurs at rest, with less exertion than with previous angina, or for the first time is commonly called *unstable angina* (see Chapter 26). The typical pain of angina resembles that of acute MI, except that it is commonly transient, lasts for minutes, and is relieved by cessation of the precipitating activity or by nitroglycerin.

Angina is commonly induced by any stimulus that increases myocardial oxygen demand, including exertion or emotion (see Chapter 25). It may also be provoked by stimuli that increase peripheral vascular resistance, such as exposure to cold, or that cause selective vasodilatation, such as a heavy meal. In addition, angina may be precipitated by tachycardia from any cause.

In a substantial proportion of patients, symptomatic angina or asymptomatic myocardial ischemia may develop without any previous evidence of increased myocardial oxygen demand, peripheral vasoconstriction or dilatation, or tachycardia. In such situations, intrinsic changes in the coronary arteries themselves, sometimes precipitated by paradoxical responses to stimuli that usually cause coronary arterial vasodilatation, can lead to ischemia.

Whereas most patients complain of chest pain, others may describe an ill-described discomfort or note only shortness of breath or fatigue. The discomfort is usually sufficiently severe to cause the patient to slow down or cease activity. The pain generally persists for no more than 5 to 30 minutes; persistent discomfort may represent acute MI or, in the absence of other evidence of myocardial ischemia, a noncoronary cause. The pain is typically relieved within 5 minutes by sublingual nitroglycerin, which may also delay the onset of pain during exertion. Pain that resolves in less than 1 minute or is precipitated by deep breathing or changes in position is unlikely to be angina.

The chest pain syndrome of myocardial ischemia is similar regardless of whether the cause is intrinsic coronary atherosclerosis or other coronary and noncoronary causes of myocardial ischemia. The underlying cause of the myocardial ischemia is often evident from a careful history and physical examination, although it may occasionally require diagnostic coronary angiography.

Physical Examination

The physical examination is frequently totally normal in patients with acute myocardial ischemia. The ischemia and resulting left ventricular dysfunction may precipitate a third or fourth heart sound or evidence of pulmonary congestion. Papillary muscle ischemia may cause a late systolic mitral regurgitant murmur. Ischemia caused by aortic valvular stenosis or obstructive hypertrophic cardiomyopathy may be accompanied by the typical murmur.

Diagnostic Testing

An ECG during pain will commonly be abnormal in patients with acute myocardial ischemia. Between spon-

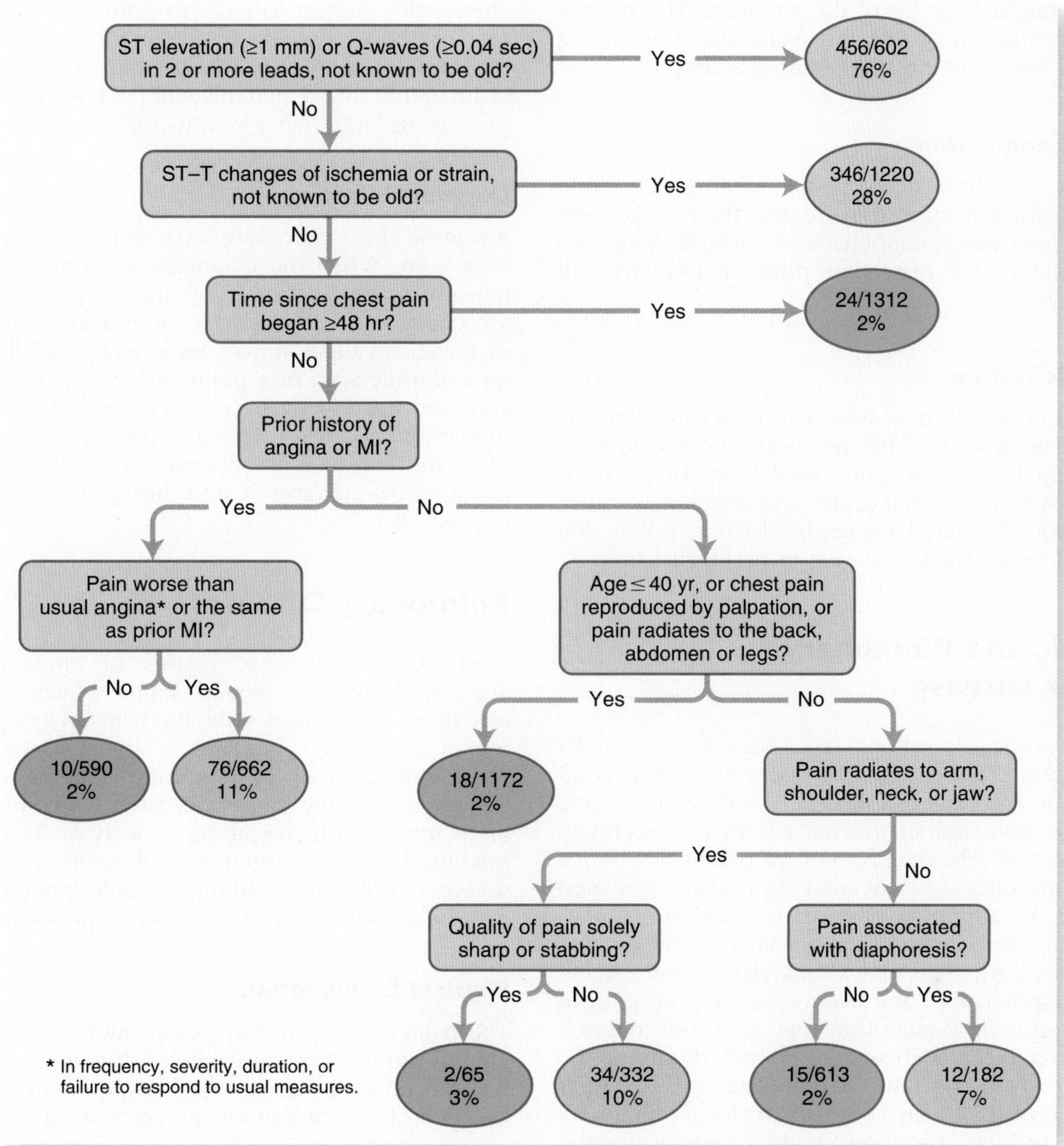

FIGURE 6–1. Flow diagram for estimating the risk of acute myocardial infarction (MI) in emergency departments in patients with acute chest pain. For each clinical subset, the numerator is the number of patients with the set of characteristics in whom an MI developed, whereas the denominator represents the total number of patients with that characteristic or set of characteristics. (Adapted from Pearson SD, Goldman L, Garcia TB, et al: Physician response to a prediction rule for the triage of emergency department patients with chest pain. J Gen Intern Med 1994;9:241–247.)

taneous episodes of discomfort, myocardial ischemia may be precipitated by exercise or pharmacologic maneuvers and be detected by electrocardiography, radionuclide scintigraphy, or echocardiography.

Pericarditis

Pericarditis can cause pain that is acute, episodic and recurrent, or persistent (see Chapter 35). Because the pericardium, except for the inferior parietal surface, is insensitive to pain, most of the discomfort associated with pericarditis is caused by inflammation of the adjacent parietal pleura. Although virtually all pericarditis is inflammatory, infectious causes are commonly associated with more severe pain, whereas noninfectious causes are associated with less pain. In patients with more acute inflammation, irritation of the relatively insensitive pericardium or surface of the heart may cause a persistent pain that can be confused with acute MI when it first begins or with noncardiac causes when it persists.

Depending on the site of pleural and diaphragmatic irritation, the pain may be anterior or upper abdominal or felt in the back or tip of the shoulder. The pain is typically pleuritic and commonly exacerbated by having the patient lean forward in a sitting position.

Physical Examination

Pericarditis is often accompanied by a detectable pericardial friction rub. If sufficient fluid is present to cause pericardial tamponade, typical findings include jugular venous distention, pulsus paradoxus, and hypotension.

Diagnostic Testing

The chest radiograph may show cardiomegaly, whereas an echocardiogram will be the most sensitive test for detecting an increase in pericardial fluid. However, it must be remembered that acute pericarditis may cause pain and an associated pericardial friction rub in the absence of a detectable increase in pericardial fluid.

Systemic and Pulmonary Vascular Disease

An acute aortic dissection (see Chapter 36) usually causes an abrupt onset of severe discomfort that is commonly felt in the center of the chest with an ascending aortic dissection and in the back with a descending aortic dissection. The pain commonly persists for hours, requires substantial doses of analgesics, and is unrelated to exercise, breathing, or changes in position.

Pulmonary emboli (see Chapter 38) can cause acute chest discomfort, sometimes associated with acute hypoxia, hypotension, and even syncope. The pain of an acute pulmonary embolism may be substernal and mimic an acute MI. With smaller emboli, there may be no acute pain at the time of embolization but rather pleuritic pain, which may be caused by focal pulmonary infarction and be associated with a pleural friction rub. Pulmonary hypertension of any cause may produce right ventricular strain and pain similar to angina pectoris.

Physical Examination

The hallmark of acute aortic dissection is asymmetry in blood pressure above and below the site of dissection. An ascending aortic dissection, which may affect all the great vessels and therefore not cause a blood pressure discrepancy, may be associated with retrograde dissection affecting the right coronary artery and hence causing ischemia or infarction in the distribution of that artery, or it may dissect back into the pericardium and cause acute pericardial tamponade with its associated signs and symptoms.

Pulmonary emboli may cause an acute rise in pulmonary vascular resistance and acute right-sided heart failure, often recognized on physical examination by a loud pulmonic second sound. Similar findings are chronically present in patients with long-standing pulmonary hypertension. Focal pulmonary infarction is often associated with a detectable pleural rub at the site of infarction. Many patients will have some evidence of preexisting underlying venous thrombotic disease.

Diagnostic Testing

A routine chest radiograph may show evidence of aortic dissection. When the diagnosis is seriously suspected, transesophageal echocardiography is probably the best screening test. For suspected pulmonary embolism, the diagnostic evaluation may begin with a spiral computed tomographic scan or a pulmonary ventilation-perfusion scan, or the physician may proceed directly to pulmonary angiography. In some patients, documentation of peripheral venous disease may be sufficient for making acute diagnostic and therapeutic decisions (see Chapter 38).

Pulmonary Diseases

Most acute pulmonary causes of chest discomfort are manifested as pleural pain, which is typically described as a sharp stabbing pain related to breathing or coughing. The pain of tracheobronchitis may be described more as a burning discomfort, whereas tumors commonly cause persistent discomfort that is often unrelated to breathing or activity. The pain of a pneumothorax is commonly of acute onset and is severe and disabling, although smaller pneumothoraces may be associated with less severe, persistent pain.

Physical Examination

The hallmark of physical examination is detection of a pleural rub at or near the site of discomfort. In patients with a pneumothorax, focal hyperinflation and the absence of breath sounds are often diagnostic.

Diagnostic Testing

The chest radiograph will commonly detect pulmonary causes of chest discomfort. However, patients with postviral pleurisy may have a normal chest radiograph or minimal atelectasis that may be indistinguishable from the changes found in patients with pulmonary emboli and infarction. In such situations, diagnostic testing to exclude the possibility of pulmonary embolism is often required (see Chapter 38).

Gastrointestinal Conditions

Esophageal pain can be caused by direct irritation of the esophagus, usually by acid reflux from the stomach, or by esophageal obstruction, spasm, or injury. Acid reflux commonly produces a burning discomfort that is exacerbated by alcohol, aspirin, and some foods. The pain is generally relieved promptly by antacids or dairy products and sometimes by other food or water. Acid reflux is usually exacerbated by lying down or by anything that causes eructation, such as swallowing of air. The pain is most often noted in the morning, when the acid is not neutralized by food, or about an hour after eating.

Esophageal spasm, which may be precipitated by acid reflux, frequently causes a deep, visceral pain that may be difficult to distinguish from myocardial ischemia. When severe, the pain of esophageal spasm may radiate to the left arm or shoulder, although such radiation is not typical. Esophageal obstruction from tumor or achalasia is commonly associated with dysphagia, regurgitation of undigested food, or loss of weight. Esophageal injury, such as a Mallory-Weiss tear caused by especially strenuous vomiting, causes acute chest pain.

The pain of a duodenal or gastric ulcer or gastritis typically occurs 60 to 90 minutes after meals, when postprandial acid production is no longer neutralized by food in the stomach. As with acid reflux into the esophagus, it is usually relieved within minutes by antacids or dairy products.

The pain of an ulcer or gastritis is commonly epigastric but often radiates to the substernal area. It will rarely radiate to the neck, shoulder, or arms.

Cholecystitis frequently causes an aching pain, sometimes with colicky spasms, 60 to 90 minutes after a meal. It is more commonly felt predominantly in the right upper quadrant, but epigastric, chest, and even back pain is not uncommon.

The pain of pancreatitis is typically described as a steady aching that may be worsened by eating. The pain of pancreatitis, like that of a posterior penetrating ulcer that irritates the pancreas, commonly radiates to the back.

The presence of a GI abnormality does not guarantee that the chest discomfort is related to it. Hiatal hernia, gallstones, and even ulcers may be asymptomatic. To make the differential diagnosis even more difficult, acid reflux into the esophagus may occasionally precipitate coronary vasospasm, sometimes with resulting myocardial ischemia, as well as esophageal spasm.

Physical Examination

In patients with ulcer disease, gastritis, pancreatitis, or gallbladder disease, careful physical examination will usually reveal epigastric or right upper quadrant tenderness. In patients with esophageal conditions, however, physical examination findings are commonly normal.

Diagnostic Testing

When GI causes of chest discomfort are suspected, the evaluation should include specific tests to assess for possible causes: barium swallow or endoscopy for esophageal disease, an upper GI series or endoscopy for the stomach and duodenum, or ultrasonography, commonly the first test for the gallbladder or pancreas.

In some situations, the difficulty in diagnosing esophageal causes of chest discomfort may warrant a Bernstein test, in which acid is dripped into the esophagus in an attempt to precipitate the patient's typical pain. Esophageal manometry may also be used to document the temporal coexistence of pain and detectable esophageal spasm. However, it is critical that the physician be confident that myocardial ischemia is not the cause of the chest discomfort before ascribing it to esophageal causes.

Musculoskeletal Abnormalities

Chest discomfort may be caused by costochondritis, bursitis, arthritis of the shoulder or spine, cervical disk disease, tendonitis, intercostal muscle cramps, and other abnormalities of the thoracic musculature, skeleton, and nerve roots. Only rare patients will have classic Tietze's syndrome with objective swelling, redness, and warmth over a costochondral joint.

Physical Examination

The pain associated with the various neuromuscular abnormalities may be of acute onset but is often repeatedly precipitated by particular movements, changes in position, or local palpation. Localized palpation of the cervical and thoracic spine, shoulder, pectoral area, and chondrosternal and costochondral junctions is critical for diagnosing or excluding these various syndromes.

Diagnostic Testing

Most neuromusculoskeletal causes of chest pain are diagnosed by physical examination, with subsequent testing required only for potentially serious disk disease or shoulder or joint disease.

Emotional and Psychiatric Conditions

A sensation of tightness or aching in the chest may often accompany emotional and psychiatric conditions, including panic disorder. Commonly, the pain from these emotional conditions persists for 30 minutes or more and is unrelated to exertion or movement. The patient may have other evidence of emotional disorders, and evaluation for possible panic disorder may be very helpful.

Physical Examination

In patients with emotional disorders, the physical examination is typically normal. Chest palpation may reveal various degrees of discomfort but is not usually suggestive of any serious neuromuscular or skeletal abnormality.

Diagnostic Testing

Ascribing severe chest discomfort to an emotional disorder is a diagnosis of exclusion. Patients often require some degree of diagnostic testing to be confident that acute myocardial ischemia is not the underlying cause of the discomfort, especially if other risk factors for coronary disease are present.

EVALUATION OF PATIENTS WITH NEW, ACUTE, OFTEN ONGOING PAIN

In patients with new, acute, ongoing pain, emergency stabilization and treatment often cannot await a definitive diagnosis, and treatment must be instituted on an emergency basis according to clinical judgment (Table 6–4). If the patient has evidence of circulatory collapse or respiratory insufficiency, this emergency treatment (see Chapters 24, 26, and 27) will be critical to maximize the likelihood of a favorable outcome.

Even when the assessment of vital signs indicates that emergency treatment is not required, the history and physical examination should be focused and goal oriented, usually performed simultaneously with an emergency ECG. If the history, physical examination, and ECG suggest possible aortic dissection (see Chapter 36), pulmonary embolism (Chapter 38), or other acute noncoronary conditions, diagnosis and treatment must proceed expeditiously (Figs. 6–2 and 6–3). If the history, physical examination, ECG, or any combination of these assessment tools suggests a potential coronary artery cause, the evaluation must quickly focus on whether urgent reperfusion with either intravenous agents or angioplasty should be pursued (see Chapters 26 and 27).

If the ECG shows ST segment elevation or Q-waves in two or more leads that are not known to be old, the probability of acute MI in the setting of new, acute, often ongoing chest pain is about 75%. If the ECG does not have these changes but shows ST segment depression of 1 mm or more or T-wave inversion suggestive of ischemia in two or more leads and not known to be old, the probability of acute MI is in the 15% to 25% range. Although the probability is somewhat higher in a patient with a more typical history and somewhat lower in a patient with a decidedly atypical history, patients with these ST–T-wave changes and a history of new, acute, often ongoing pain should be considered to have unstable angina until proved otherwise. Treatment generally includes aspirin, intravenous heparin or glycoprotein IIb/IIIa inhibitors, and agents to reduce myocardial oxygen demand (see Chapter 26).

Patients without Major Electrocardiographic Changes

When the chest pain is potentially of coronary cause but the patient does not have ECG changes of ischemia or infarction, further evaluation and treatment may be indicated if the clinical findings are otherwise consistent with acute ischemic heart disease. In addition to multivariate algorithms that have attempted to distinguish patients with a sufficiently high likelihood of acute ischemic heart disease from those with a very low probability (see Fig. 6–1), further observation is generally indicated for patients with clear worsening of a known anginal syndrome, whether the worsening is in terms of the pain's duration, frequency, intensity, or lack of response to rest, nitroglycerin, or interventions that have been successful in the past. For patients without ECG changes and no previous history of ischemic heart disease, those with the highest risk are middle-aged men with typical angina radiating to the neck, shoulder, or arms. However, angina and acute MI may have atypical manifestations, and the physician must always consider the potential risk of inappropriate discharge of a patient with possible new onset of ischemic heart disease.[4]

Intensive Care Units versus Stepdown/Intermediate Care Units

Patients with ECG changes of infarction or ischemia are usually recommended for initial admission to an intensive care unit because of their increased risk for acute complications that will require this level of care[1,5,6] (Table 6–5; Fig. 6–4). Similarly, patients without ECG evidence of ischemia but with two or more other high-risk characteristics (systolic blood pressure below 110 mm Hg, bilateral rales above the lung bases, or clinical worsening of pain known to be due to coronary artery disease) should be admitted directly to intensive care. Patients at low risk (about 4%) of life-threatening complications, such as those without ECG ischemia and with only one high-risk characteristic, are commonly appropriate for admission to a stepdown or intermediate care unit.[1, 5, 6] Very low-risk patients (i.e., none of the high-risk characteristics; <1% risk of life-threatening complications) are appropriate for a stepdown/intermediate care unit, a chest pain evaluation unit (see later), or discharge, depending on their clinical findings and the probability of acute MI or unstable angina.

Chest Pain Evaluation Units

Substantial data indicate that a 6- to 12-hour observation period in a chest pain evaluation unit or a coronary observation unit is an appropriate, cost-effective alternative for very low-risk patients without ECG changes or evident complications but in whom the possibility of new-onset ischemic heart disease is nevertheless sufficiently high to make discharge inadvisable; it is sometimes also appropriate even for patients with clinically unstable angina but no other high-risk features.[1, 5–8] These chest pain evaluation or coronary observation units are generally evaluation areas in the emergency department itself, existing short-stay units

TABLE 6–4

Evaluation of Acute Chest Pain: Excerpts from the Clinical Policy of the American College of Emergency Physicians*

		Action	
Variable	**Finding**	***Rule***[†]	***Guideline***[‡]
Pain	Ongoing, severe and crushing, and substernal or same as previous pain diagnosed as MI	IV access Supplemental oxygen Cardiac monitor ECG Aspirin Nitrates Management of ongoing pain Hospitalizaton	Serum cardiac markers CXR Anticoagulation
	Severe or pressure, substernal or exertional, or radiating to the jaw, neck, shoulder, or arm	ECG	IV access Supplemental oxygen Cardiac monitor CXR Nitrates Management of ongoing pain Hospitalization
	Tearing, severe, and radiating to the back	Large-bore IV access Supplemental oxygen Cardiac monitor CXR ECG	Differential upper extremity blood pressure measurement Aortic imaging Management of ongoing pain Hospitalization
	Similar to that of previous pulmonary embolus	IV access Supplemental oxygen Cardiac monitor ABG/oximetry Anticoagulation/pulmonary vascular imaging ECG	
	Ingestion or burning epigastric	None	ECG
	Pleuritic	None	CXR
Age	Male, >33 yr	None	ECG
	Female, >40 yr	None	Cardiac monitor
Associated symptoms	Syncope or near-syncope	ECG	
	Shortness of breath, dyspnea on exertion, paroxysmal nocturnal dyspnea, or orthopnea	ECG	Hematocrit ABG/oximetry CXR
Medical history	Previous MI, coronary artery bypass graft/angioplasty, cocaine use within last 96 hr, previous positive cardiac diagnostic studies	ECG	
	Major risk factors for coronary artery disease		ECG
Assessment	Unstable angina—new-onset, exertional	See Chapter 26	
	Unstable angina—ongoing or recurrent ischemia	See Chapter 26	
	High clinical suspicion of MI with nondiagnostic ECG	See Chapter 26	
	Acute MI with diagnostic ECG or high clinical suspicion of MI with bundle branch block	See Chapter 27	
	Aortic dissection	See Chapter 36	
	Pericarditis/myocarditis	See Chapters 29 and 35	
	Pulmonary embolism	See Chapter 38	

*Data from the American College of Emergency Physicians: Clinical policy for the initial approach to adults presenting with a chief complaint of chest pain, with no history of trauma. Ann Emerg Med 1995;25:274–299.

[†]A rule is an action that reflects principles of good practice in most situations. In some circumstances a rule does not need to be or cannot be followed; in these situations it is advisable that the deviation from the rule be justified in writing. If a rule is not considered a standard of care at an institution, this fact should be documented as an institutional policy.

[‡]A guideline is an action that may be considered, depending on the patient, the circumstances, or other factors. Thus, guidelines are not always followed, and it should not be implied that failure to follow a guideline is improper.

ABG, arterial blood gases; CXR, chest radiograph; ECG, electrocardiogram; IV, intravenous; MI, myocardial infarction.

Adapted from Lee TH, Goldman L: Evaluation of the patient with acute chest pain. N Engl J Med 2000;342:1190–1191.

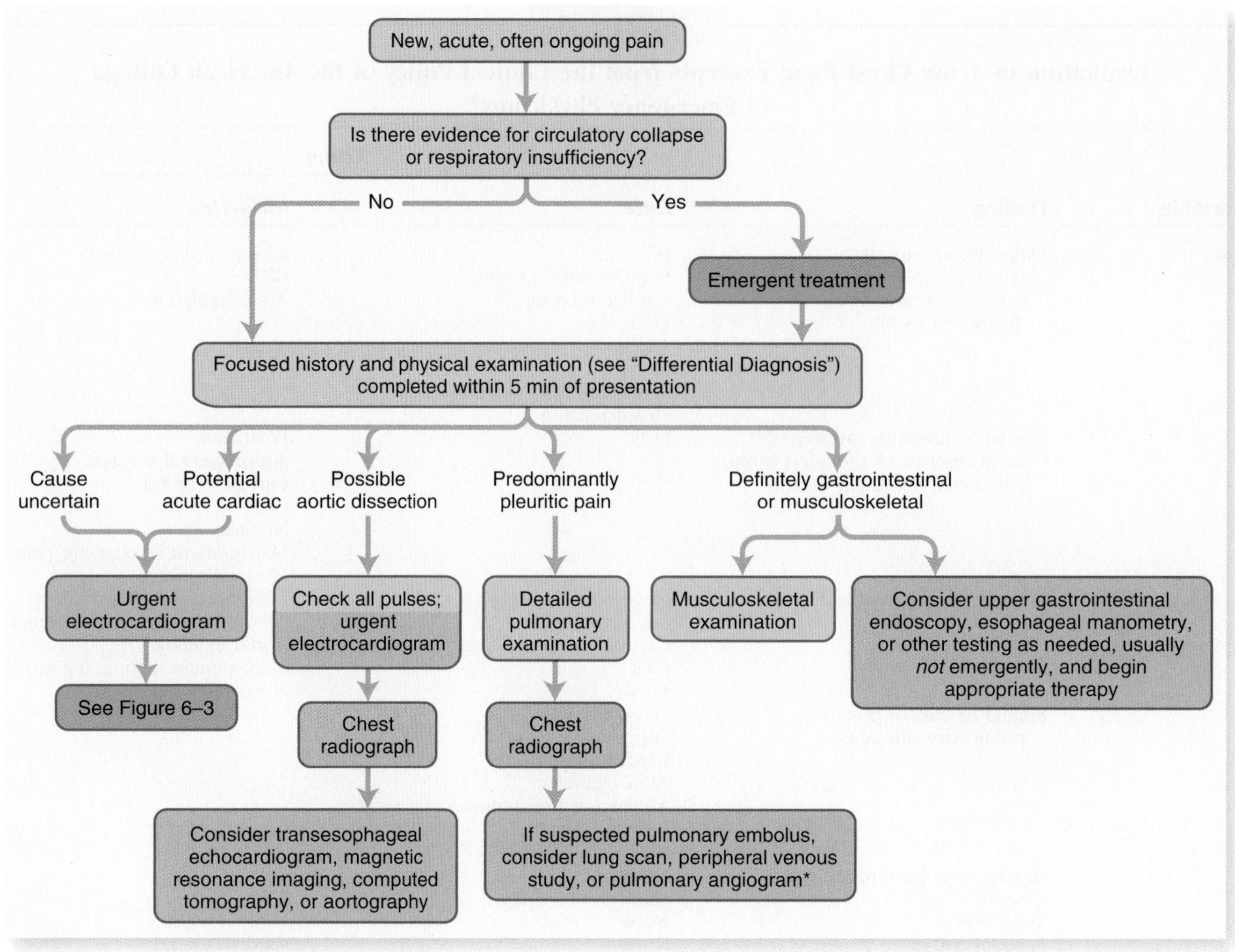

FIGURE 6–2. Diagnostic approach to patients with new, acute, often ongoing chest pain. *Spiral computed tomographic scan should also be considered. (Adapted from Goldman L: Chest discomfort and palpitation. In Fauci AS, Braunwald E, Isselbacher KI, et al [eds]: Harrison's Principles of Internal Medicine, 14th ed. New York, McGraw-Hill, 1998, p 61. Copyright © by McGraw-Hill, Inc. Used by permission of McGraw-Hill Book Company.)

newly equipped with cardiac monitors, or otherwise empty beds newly converted to observation status. These units typically provide continuous ECG monitoring to detect life-threatening arrhythmias. However, nursing services are usually provided at a typical ward level, with the expectation that patients will feed themselves, ambulate to the bathroom on their own, and so on. Patients are generally eligible for admission only if they have a low probability for acute MI, have no other complications or ongoing chest discomfort, have no ischemic ECG changes on admission, and require no intravenous medications, although well-staffed units have also been used for otherwise uncomplicated patients with the clinical diagnosis of unstable angina.

Patients must typically be transferred if any of these findings, recurrent angina, or evidence of acute MI develops. In essence, these units provide the availability of rapid treatment and resuscitation should a life-threatening arrhythmia occur, as well as the rapid institution of appropriate therapy for any evidence of unstable angina or acute MI.

In a number of studies, patients admitted to chest pain evaluation or observation units have rates of acute MI in the 1% to 3% range, with even lower rates of complications potentially requiring intensive care. By providing appropriate monitoring and nursing without the other aspects of intensive care, these units have the same documented safety but costs that are about one third those of a stepdown or intermediate unit. The advent of these units has allowed physicians to have a lower threshold for admitting more patients with complaints that are atypical of acute ischemic heart disease but that make the physician uncomfortable about discharge. The 6- to 12-hour length of stay and lower cost allow more patients to be admitted for observation than previously while still reducing cost as well as the potential morbidity and mortality of inappropriate discharge.

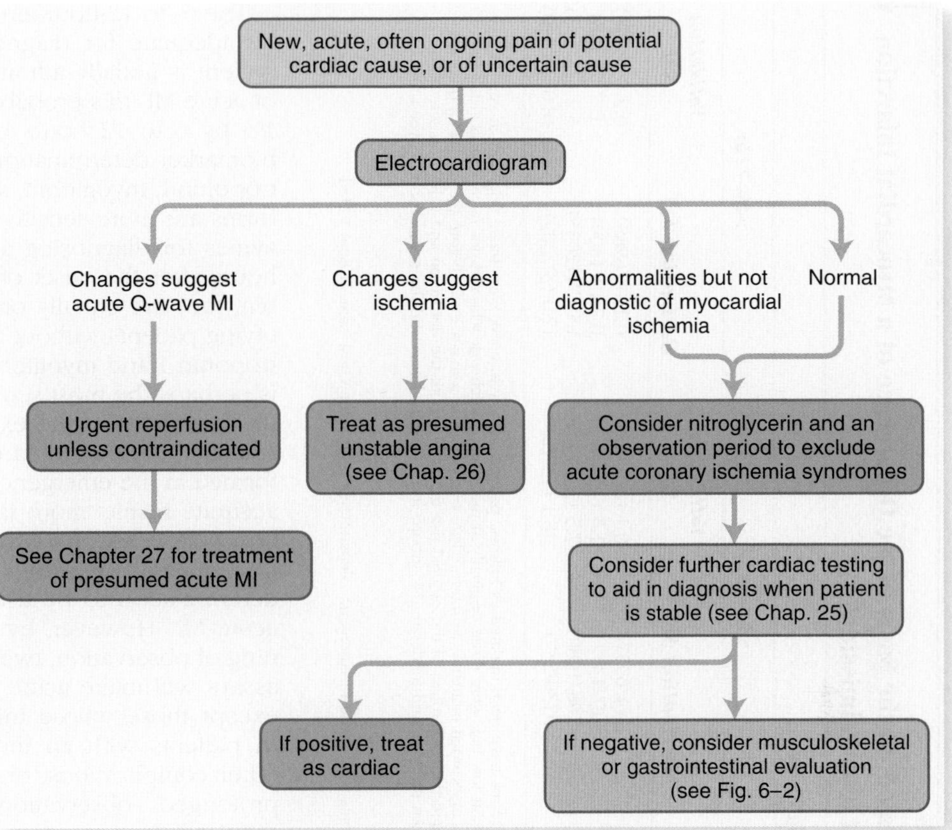

FIGURE 6–3. Diagnostic approach to patients with new, acute, often ongoing pain of potential cardiac or uncertain cause. MI, myocardial infarction. (From Goldman L: Chest discomfort and palpitation. In Fauci AS, Braunwald E, Isselbacher KI, et al (eds): Harrison's Principles of Internal Medicine, 14th ed. New York, McGraw-Hill, 1998, p 62. Copyright © by McGraw-Hill, Inc. Used by permission of McGraw-Hill Book Company.)

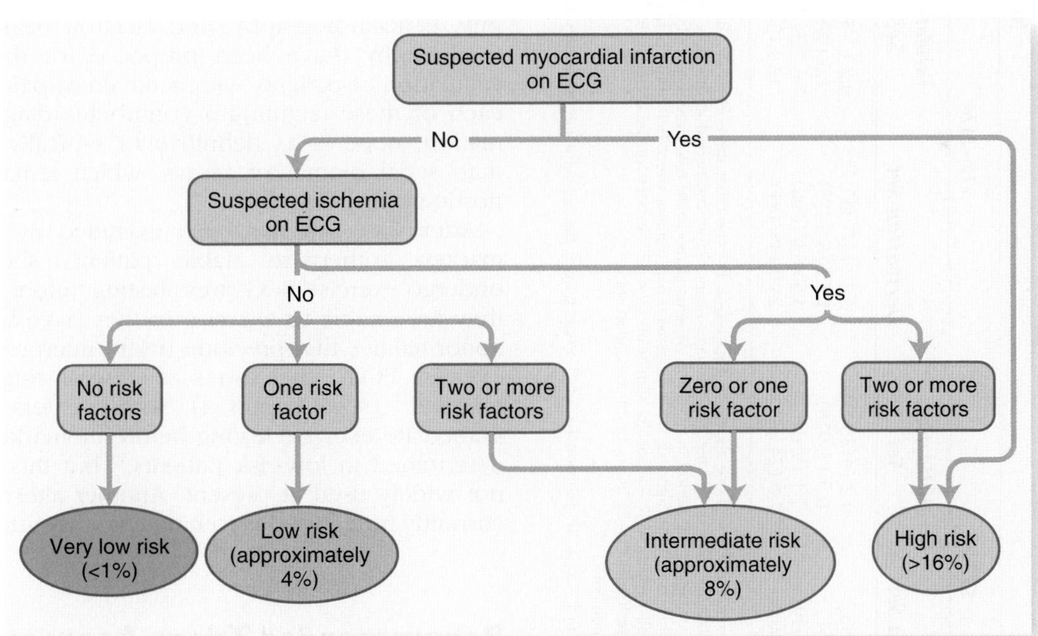

FIGURE 6–4. Derivation and validation of four groups into which patients can be categorized according to the risk of major cardiac events within 72 hours after admission for acute chest pain. The categorization was based on the data available at the time of arrival in the emergency department. Myocardial infarction was suspected if the electrocardiogram (ECG) showed ST segment elevation of 1 mm or more or pathologic Q-waves in two or more leads and if these findings were not known to be old. Ischemia was suspected if the ECG showed ST segment depression of 1 mm or more or T-wave inversion in two or more leads or showed new left bundle branch block and if these findings were not known to be old. Risk factors included systolic blood pressure below 110 mm Hg, bilateral rales heard above the bases on physical examination, and known unstable ischemic heart disease (defined as worsening of previously stable angina, new onset of angina after infarction or after a coronary revascularization procedure, or pain that was the same as that associated with a previous myocardial infarction). (Reprinted, by permission, from Lee TH, Goldman L: Evaluation of the patient with acute chest pain. N Engl J Med 2000;342:1187–1195.)

TABLE 6–5

Rate of New Major Events According to the Original Risk Group and as Updated on the Basis of the Occurrence of a Myocardial Infarction or Intermediate or Major Event after Admission*

	New Major Event							
	≤12 hr		*>12–24 hr*		*>24–48 hr*		*>48–72 hr*	
Risk Group	***Derivation Set***	***Validation Set***	***Derivation Set***	***Validation Set***	***Derivation Set***	***Validation Set***	***Derivation Set***	***Validation Set***
Very low risk	0.1 (5/6188)†	0.2 (4/2596)	0.2 (14/7065)	0.2 (7/3394)	0.1 (4/6957)	0.1 (2/3333)	0.1 (9/6888)	0.2 (6/3288)
Low risk	0.7 (11/1511)	0.5 (5/918)	1.1 (16/1475)	1.0 (9/872)	0.5 (7/1377)	1.3 (11/816)	0.7 (9/1309)	0.7 (5/768)
Moderate risk	2.8 (55/1949)	1.1 (9/845)	3.5 (63/1790)	7.6 (28/367)	4.4 (88/1980)	7.5 (33/439)	3.5 (71/2035)	5.2 (25/483)
High risk	12.1 (125/1034)	7.6 (24/317)	24.9 (45/181)	12.8 (5/39)	12.7 (30/237)	18.1 (13/72)	12.0 (37/309)	18.0 (18/100)

*For the first 12 hours the risk groups correspond to those shown in Figure 6–4. For the other three intervals, the risk groups have been updated as follows: patients at very low risk were those originally at very low or low risk who did not have a myocardial infarction or intermediate or major event before the period in question; patients at low risk were those originally at moderate or high risk who did not have a myocardial infarction or intermediate or major event before the period in question; patients at moderate risk were those who had a myocardial infarction or intermediate event but not a major event before the period in question, regardless of the original risk group; and patients at high risk were those who had a major event before the period in question, regardless of the original risk group. For both the derivation and validation sets, all comparisons between risk groups for all periods were statistically significant ($P < .05$), except for the comparison between the low- and moderate-risk groups in the first 12 hours and the comparison between the moderate- and high-risk groups at more than 12 to 24 hours in the validation set.

†Percentage of patients (number/total number).

Reprinted by permission, from Goldman L, Cook EF, Johnson PA, et al: Prediction of the need for intensive care in patients who come to emergency departments with acute chest pain. N Engl J Med 1996;334:1498–1504.

The 6- to 12-hour length of stay in these units should be adequate for diagnostic purposes. In general, if a patient is initially admitted with a 5% or so probability of acute MI, this probability will be reduced to less than 1% by 6 to 12 hours of sequential ECGs and cardiac biomarker determinations. Assays including troponin T, troponin I, myoglobin, and creatine kinase (CK) MB isoforms are more sensitive than traditional CK-MB isoenzymes for diagnosing acute MI, especially in the early hours after the onset of symptoms; except for myoglobin, they are equally or more specific in terms of identifying patients without acute MI.[9, 10] The combination of troponin I and myoglobin initially and 90 minutes later is perhaps the most sensitive alternative, but it achieves this sensitivity at the expense of somewhat diminished specificity. Point-of-care assays, which can be performed in the emergency department itself, can provide accurate results more rapidly and shorten the observation period.[9] At the current time, no assay or combination of assays is sufficiently sensitive to allow a single determination to be used to exclude the possibility of acute MI. However, by about 6 hours after the beginning of observation, two negative values on any of these assays will make acute MI very unlikely in all patients except those whose initial probability was very high. In patients with an initially higher probability of MI, other complications, or a need for interventions, more prolonged observation or treatment periods are required.

Imaging techniques, including myocardial scintigraphy, echocardiography, and electron beam computed tomography, have been proposed for the diagnostic evaluation of patients with acute chest pain.[11] Although each of these techniques contributes diagnostic information, none is as definitive or typically more rapid than serial biomarker assays, which remain the diagnostic gold standard.[3]

After acute MI has been excluded by cardiac biomarkers, otherwise stable patients should ideally undergo exercise ECG stress testing before discharge. If they are unable to exercise or they have baseline ECG abnormalities that preclude useful interpretation of the exercise ECG, other forms of stress testing are recommended[12] (see Chapter 4). Some centers recommend immediate exercise testing before biomarker assays are determined in low-risk patients,[13] but this approach is not widely used at present. Another alternative that is currently rarely used is routine coronary arteriography.[14]

Recommended Triage Approach

By considering the ECG, a history of previous known coronary artery disease, and evidence of other complications, patients with known or suspected coronary disease as a cause of acute, new, often ongoing pain can quickly be recommended for one of three different in-hospital strategies: coronary intensive care, an intermediate care/stepdown unit, or an evaluation/observation unit (Box 6–1). These recommendations, which are based on both clinical and cost data, provide an

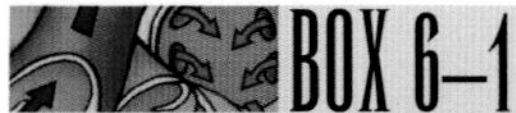

BOX 6–1

Recommended Triage Strategies for Patients with Acute Chest Pain Who Do Not Otherwise Require Intensive Care Because of the Need to Treat Ongoing, Life-Threatening Conditions*

INTENSIVE CARE

1. Major ischemic electrocardiographic changes in two or more leads, not known to be old:
   a. ST elevation of 1 mm or more or Q-waves of 0.04 sec or more *or*
   b. ST depression of 1 mm or more or T-wave inversion consistent with ischemia *or*
2. Any two of the following, with or without major electrocardiographic changes:
   a. Unstable known coronary disease (in terms of frequency, duration, intensity, or failure to respond to usual measures)
   b. Systolic blood pressure below 110 mm Hg
   c. Major new arrhythmias (new-onset atrial fibrillation, atrial flutter, sustained supraventricular tachycardia, second-degree or complete heart block, or sustained or recurrent ventricular arrhythmias)
   d. Rales above the bases

INTERMEDIATE CARE/STEPDOWN UNIT

Patients who do not meet the criteria for intensive care but who either

1. Have one unstable characteristic:
   a. Unstable known coronary disease
   b. Systolic blood pressure below 110 mm Hg
   c. Rales above the bases
   d. Major arrhythmias (new-onset atrial fibrillation, atrial flutter, sustained supraventricular tachycardia, second-degree or complete heart block, or sustained or recurrent ventricular arrhythmias)
2. Have new onset of very typical ischemic heart disease that meets the clinical criteria for unstable angina (see Chapter 26) and that is occurring now at rest or with minimal exertion

EVALUATION/OBSERVATION UNIT

1. Other patients with new-onset symptoms that may be consistent with ischemic heart disease but are not associated with electrocardiographic changes or a convincing diagnosis of unstable ischemic heart disease at rest or with minimal exertion
2. Some patients with known coronary disease whose symptoms do not suggest true worsening but for whom further observation is thought to be beneficial

HOME WITH OFFICE FOLLOW-UP IN 7–10 DAYS TO DETERMINE WHETHER FURTHER TESTING IS NEEDED

Other patients

*Except in patients in whom other serious noncoronary causes of chest pain are being considered, such as possible aortic dissection or pulmonary embolism, the triage will be dictated by the appropriate evaluation for these possible diagnoses.

efficient, high-quality strategy for this often-challenging group of patients.[1]

EVALUATION OF PATIENTS WITH RECURRENT, EPISODIC PAIN

Although patients with recurrent, episodic pain may be having an acute MI superimposed on previous angina, recurrent pulmonary emboli, or even chronic aortic dissection, most patients with this syndrome have less acute conditions for which a complete history and physical examination will be necessary to make the diagnosis (Fig. 6–5). The physician should focus on a description of the pain, what precipitates and relieves it, its location and quality, the patient's age and gender, and other coronary risk factors.

In determining whether the pain is typical, atypical, or highly unlikely to represent coronary ischemia, precipitating factors such as rapid walking, exercise, or sexual activity suggest angina, as does pain that is relieved within several minutes after rest or taking nitroglycerin. By comparison, pain that is precipitated by deep breathing or coughing suggests a pleural or pericardial cause, whereas pain exacerbated by other movements or by palpation is most typical of neuromuscular or skeletal causes.

Physical Examination

The physical examination should be comprehensive and not limited to the cardiopulmonary system. For example, the skin examination should search for xanthelasma and cyanosis. Lymphadenopathy would raise the possibility of a malignancy. The chest wall must be inspected and palpated to search for neuromusculoskeletal causes of chest discomfort. A pulmonary examination should search for evidence of heart failure, pleural rub, or pneumonia. The cardiac examination should include a careful evaluation of possible third or fourth heart sounds, papillary muscle dysfunction, aortic valvular stenosis, or obstructive hypertrophic cardiomyopathy. A pericardial friction rub or increased pulmonic second sound would raise the possibility of pericarditis and pulmonary embolism/pulmonary hypertension, respectively. The abdominal examination is critical for the diagnosis of cholecystitis or pancreatitis and may also be abnormal in patients with peptic ulcer disease.

It is important to emphasize that the same clinical syndrome may have very different implications in individuals with different underlying risk for coronary artery disease based on age, gender, and preexisting hypertension, hypercholesterolemia, smoking status, and other factors. Nevertheless, no single piece of evidence can either diagnose or exclude coronary artery disease, and the physician must be suspicious of a reasonably consistent history in an otherwise low-risk patient, just

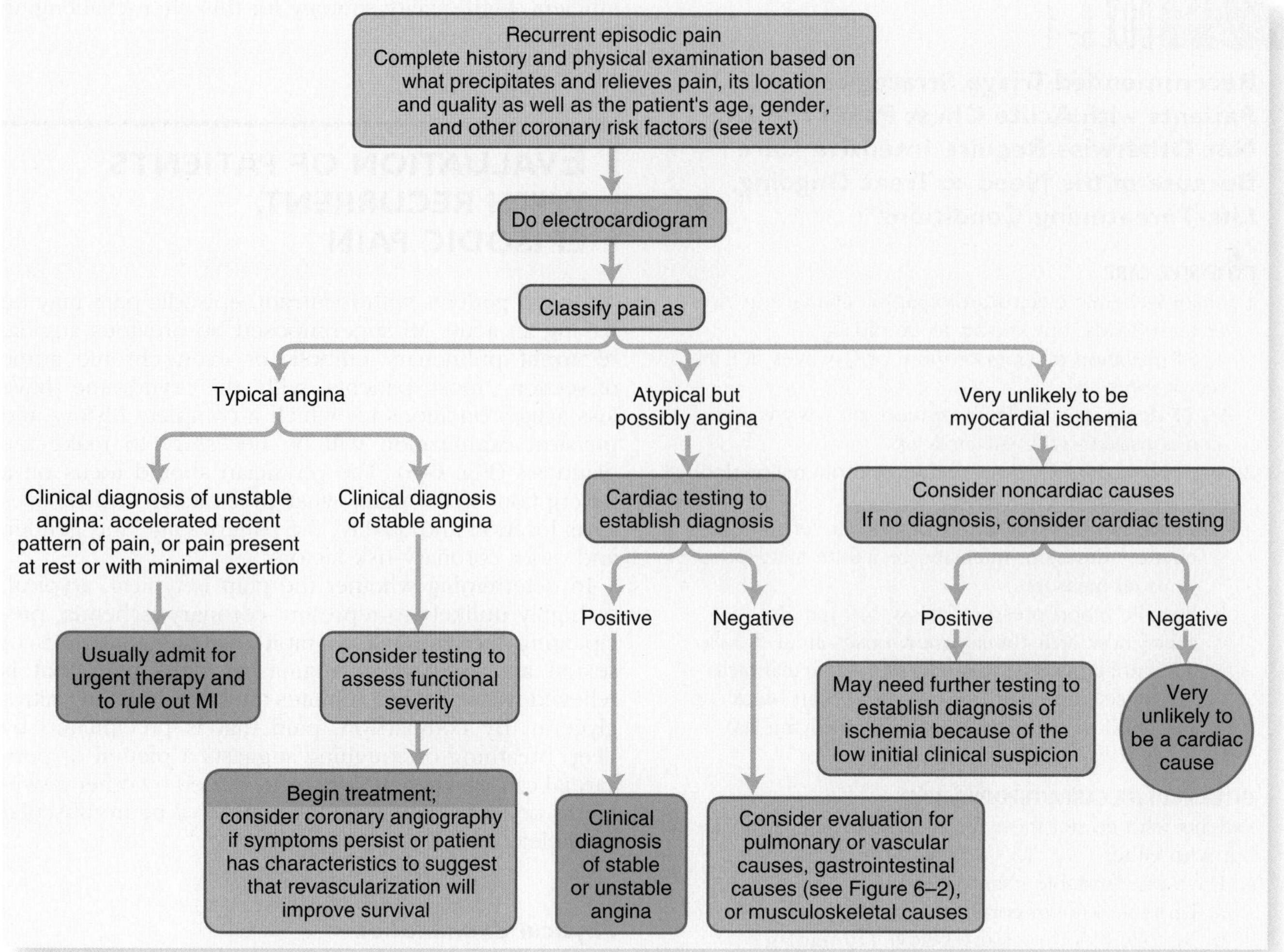

FIGURE 6–5. Diagnostic approach to patients with recurrent, episodic chest pain. MI, myocardial infarction. (From Goldman L: Chest discomfort and palpitation. In Fauci AS, Braunwald E, Isselbacher KI, et al (eds): Harrison's Principles of Internal Medicine, 14th ed. New York, McGraw-Hill, 1998, p 62. Copyright © by McGraw-Hill, Inc. Used by permission of McGraw-Hill Book Company.)

as atypical findings in a high-risk patient demand further evaluation.

Diagnostic Testing

Most patients with recurrent, episodic chest pain caused by myocardial ischemia will have normal ECGs in the intervals between painful episodes, although some may have resting abnormalities or evidence of previous MI. Based on the combination of data from the history, physical examination, and resting ECG, the physician should be able to categorize the pain as typical of angina, atypical but possible angina, or very unlikely to represent angina. In general, these categories correspond to about an 80%, 40%, and 5% probability, respectively, of coronary artery disease if the patient undergoes diagnostic coronary arteriography.

For most patients with recurrent episodic pain, the evaluation can proceed on an ambulatory basis over a period of days or even weeks. However, if unstable angina is suspected, urgent evaluation is indicated, often with hospitalization as described for new, acute chest pain. In patients with new-onset angina that is otherwise stable (see Chapter 26), an ambulatory evaluation is reasonable but should proceed expeditiously (see Chapter 25).

Myocardial ischemia may be detected by typical ECG changes, scintigraphic abnormalities, or wall motion abnormalities on echocardiography (see Chapters 4, 5, and 25). Myocardial ischemia may be precipitated by exercise or by a pharmacologic stress (see Chapter 4). None of these tests are perfect, but they can be integrated with findings from the history and physical examination to evaluate patients with recurrent, episodic chest discomfort (see Figs. 2–5 through 2–7). Although negative test results cannot exclude the possibility of myocardial ischemia in patients with a typical history, the sequence of a negative exercise ECG and perfusion scintigram makes coronary disease very unlikely in a patient with atypical chest discomfort. These negative tests also generally imply a relatively favorable prognosis even if undiagnosed myocardial ischemia is present.

EVALUATION OF PATIENTS WITH PERSISTENT PAIN

When pain persists for hours or even days, it is highly unlikely to be caused by myocardial ischemia in the absence of acute MI. The clinician should suspect musculoskeletal abnormalities, GI diseases, and less commonly, pulmonary disease or pericarditis. The history must be comprehensive, as emphasized under "Evaluation of Patients with Recurrent, Episodic Pain."

Physical Examination

A comprehensive physical examination is mandatory to assess possible musculoskeletal, GI, and pulmonary abnormalities. Careful consideration should be given to any other focal or systemic diseases for which abnormalities in the neck, chest, or upper part of the abdomen may coexist.

Diagnostic Testing

Diagnostic evaluation of persistent pain can be accomplished in the ambulatory setting and rarely requires hospitalization. As directed by the history and physical examination, further testing by chest radiography, upper GI endoscopy, or abdominal ultrasonography should be considered. In some patients, additional testing may be required to reassure the patient that coronary artery disease is not present even though the pain syndrome is highly atypical. In patients with a suggestive history, echocardiography may be useful to evaluate the possibility of pericarditis, although pericarditis and a pericardial friction rub may be present in the absence of increased pericardial fluid or other pericardial abnormalities detectable by echocardiography. Injection of a suspected musculoskeletal source of chest discomfort, such as costochondritis or bursitis, with a local anesthetic may be critical in making the diagnosis.

Careful consideration should be given to the possibility that a patient with persistent pain is suffering from an emotional condition that has previously been undiagnosed or underappreciated. In such patients, this diagnosis of exclusion may require some degree of previous diagnostic testing to exclude other conditions of concern to the patient or physician.

Evidence-Based Summary

- Validated clinical algorithms are available to estimate the probability that a patient with acute chest pain is having an MI (see Fig. 6–1) or complications requiring admission to intensive care (Fig. 6–4).
- The ECG provides the single most important piece of information for the evaluation and triage of patients with acute chest pain.
- Short-stay chest pain evaluation units are a safe, effective, and cost-effective option for patients who are at low risk for acute MI or other serious cardiac complications, but not at low enough risk for the physician to be confident about the safety of immediate discharge.
- Newer cardiac biomarkers (e.g., troponin T and troponin I), especially if measured at the bedside with point-of-care assays, can increase the rapidity of the diagnosis or exclusion of acute MI. Nevertheless, about 6 hours is needed before a physician can feel sufficiently secure to discharge a patient being observed for possible acute myocardial ischemia.

References

1. Lee TH, Goldman L: Evaluation of the patient with acute chest pain. N Engl J Med 2000;342:1187–1195.
2. Panju AA, Hemmelgarn BR, Guyatt GH, Simel DL: Is this patient having a myocardial infarction. JAMA 1998; 280:1256–1263.
3. The Joint European Society of Cardiology/American College of Cardiology Committee: Myocardial infarction redefined—a consensus document of the joint European Society of Cardiology/American College of Cardiology committee for the redefinition of myocardial infarction. J Am Coll Cardiol 2000;36:959–969.
4. Pope JH, Aufderheide TP, Ruthazer R, et al: Missed diagnosis of acute cardiac ischemia in the emergency department. N Engl J Med 2000;342:1163–1170.
5. Reilly BM, Evans AT, Schaider JJ, et al: Impact of a clinical decision rule on hospital triage of patients with suspected acute cardiac ischemia in the emergency department. JAMA 2002;288:342–350.
6. Reilly BM, Evans AT, Schaider JJ, Wang Y: Triage of patients with chest pain in the emergency department: A comparative study of physicians' decisions. Am J Med 2002;112:95–103.
7. Zalenski RJ, Selker HP, Cannon CP, et al: National heart attack alert program position paper: Chest pain centers and programs for the evaluation of acute cardiac ischemia. Ann Emerg Med 2000;35:462–471.

8. Farkouh ME, Smars PA, Reeder GS, et al: A clinical trial of a chest-pain observation unit for patients with unstable angina. N Engl J Med 1998;339:1882–1888.
9. Newby LK, Storrow AB, Gibler WB, et al: Bedside multimarker testing for risk stratification in chest pain units. Circulation 2001;103:1832–1837.
10. Balk EM, Ioannidis JP, Salem D, et al: Accuracy of biomarkers to diagnose acute cardiac ischemia in the emergency department: A meta-analysis. Ann Emerg Med 2001;37:478–494.
11. Ioannidis JP, Salem D, Chew PW, Lau J: Accuracy of imaging technologies in the diagnosis of acute cardiac ischemia in the emergency department: A meta-analysis. Ann Emerg Med 2001;37:471–477.
12. Stein RA, Chaitman BR, Balady GJ, et al: Safety and utility of exercise testing in emergency room chest pain centers. Circulation 2000;102:1463–1467.
13. Amsterdam EA, Kirk JD, Diercks DB, et al: Immediate exercise testing to evaluate low-risk patients presenting to the emergency department with chest pain. J Am Coll Cardiol 2002;40:251–256.
14. deFilippi CR, Rosanio S, Tocchi M: Randomized comparison of a strategy of predischarge coronary angiography versus exercise testing in low-risk patients in a chest pain unit: In-hospital and long-term outcomes. J Am Coll Cardiol 2001;37:2042–2049.

CHAPTER 7

Approach to the Patient with Dyspnea

Richard M. Schwartzstein and David Feller-Kopman

The complaint of "shortness of breath," or dyspnea, afflicts patients both acutely and chronically, is often associated with great discomfort, anxiety, and emotional distress, and may be associated with gradually worsening disability. It may be a sign of only a sedentary lifestyle, or it may portend a potentially life-threatening illness. Everyone, if pushed to the limits of aerobic capacity, will experience shortness of breath. When faced with a patient with dyspnea, the physician has to answer several questions. Two of the most central questions for the primary care physician are whether it is an indication of a pathologic finding or a manifestation of normal physiology and, if the former, whether it is secondary to heart disease or lung disease.

No data are available on the prevalence of dyspnea in the general population, but certain epidemiologic facts suggest that the problem is quite extensive. Coronary artery disease is the leading cause of mortality in the United States, and studies have shown that breathlessness may be a symptom of angina or myocardial infarction. Congestive heart failure (CHF) is the most common reason for hospitalization among Medicare patients, and dyspnea is the most common symptom in patients with chronic CHF. In addition, approximately 25 million people in the United States suffer from asthma or chronic obstructive lung disease; these conditions result in 17 million physician office visits a year, usually for complaints of breathlessness, at a cost of over $10.4 billion.

Given the magnitude of these clinical problems and the central role of dyspnea in the symptoms experienced by patients with heart and lung disease, it is imperative that the primary care physician have a solid understanding of the physiology and qualities of dyspnea and an organized and rational approach to patients with this complaint.

PHYSIOLOGY OF DYSPNEA

Respiratory sensations that are commonly grouped under the term *dyspnea* appear to arise in one of several ways.[1] Primary sensations are associated with increased neural activity within the motor cortex as messages are sent to the ventilatory muscles, within the brain stem respiratory centers under conditions associated with increased "respiratory drive," and from the stimulation of receptors in the lungs, chest wall, and upper airways (Fig. 7–1). In addition, the intensity of dyspnea appears to increase when the efferent or outgoing neural traffic from the brain is dissociated from the afferent or incoming information from peripheral receptors that tells the brain how much the lungs and chest moved and how much airflow was generated.[1]

When a mechanical load is placed on the respiratory system, such as airway obstruction or restrictive lung disease, the motor cortex must increase neural

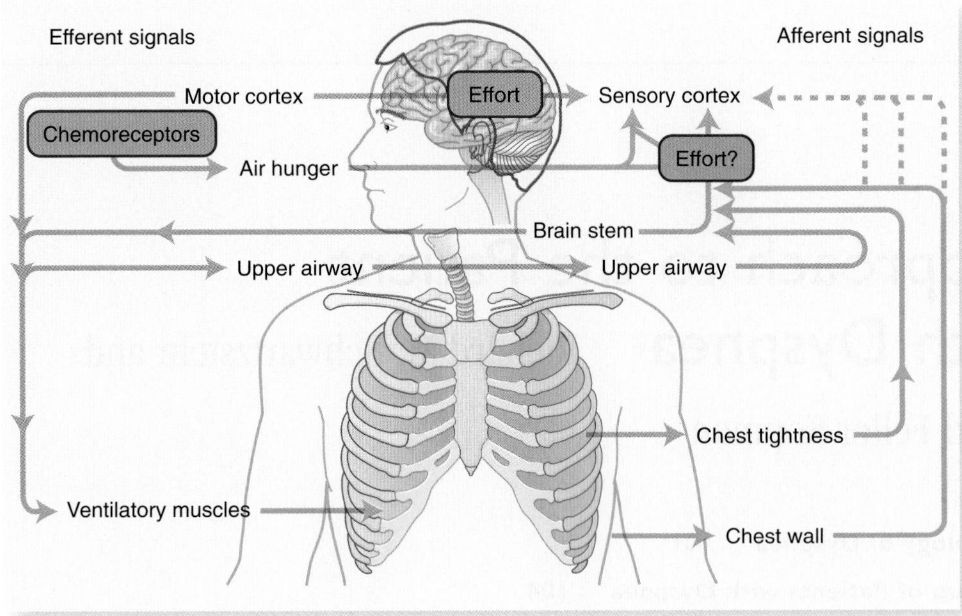

FIGURE 7–1. Afferent and efferent signals that contribute to dyspnea. The sensations that make up "dyspnea" arise from signals within the central nervous system, from chemoreceptors, and from receptors in the lungs, chest wall, and upper airway. Although afferent information from airway, lung, and chest wall receptors most likely passes through the brain stem before reaching the sensory cortex, the *dashed lines* indicate uncertainty about whether some afferents bypass the brain stem and project directly to the sensory cortex. (From Manning HL, Schwartzstein RM: Pathophysiology of dyspnea. N Engl J Med 1995;333:1547–1553.)

discharge to the respiratory muscles to activate the muscles sufficiently to generate appropriate ventilation. The individual is able to perceive the increased neural activity, which is felt as an increased sense of "effort" or "work of breathing." This mechanism also appears to underlie the respiratory discomfort associated with neuromuscular weakness, such as in association with myasthenia gravis.

Impaired motion of the lungs and chest wall, as may be seen in patients with pulmonary fibrosis, kyphoscoliosis, or hyperinflation secondary to obstructive lung disease, adds another dimension to the breathing discomfort in these individuals. The intensity of dyspnea is heightened by the restriction and may produce the sensation of an "inability to get a deep breath" superimposed on a sense of increased effort or work of breathing.[2, 3]

Acute changes in blood gases, such as acute hypoxia or hypercapnia, stimulate the respiratory centers in the brain stem and lead to an increase in ventilation and a sense of respiratory distress. Stimulation of receptors in the lungs may also cause an increase in both ventilation and respiratory discomfort, such as in patients with asthma or pulmonary embolism, although the exact neural pathways that account for these findings have not been fully elucidated. Inhalation of lidocaine or furosemide, drugs that may alter the activity of pulmonary receptors, has been shown to alleviate the dyspnea of bronchoconstriction and resistive loads.[4]

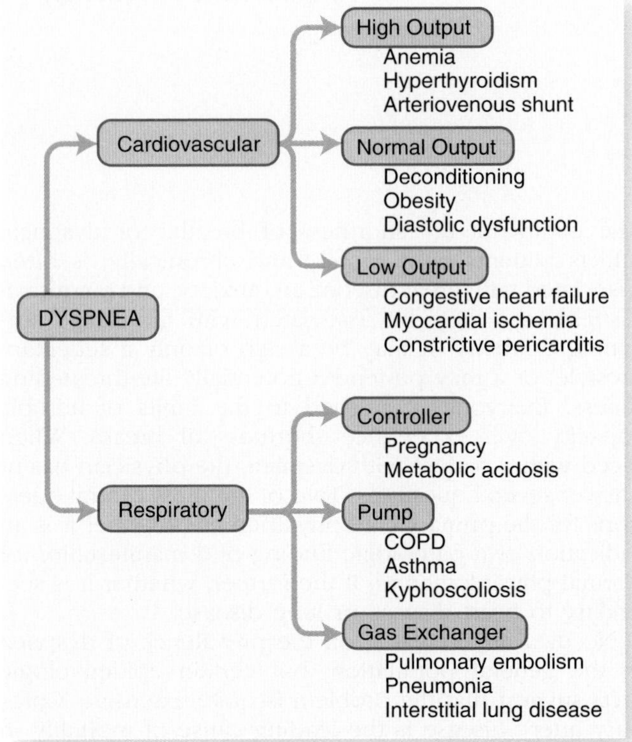

FIGURE 7–2. Clinical pathophysiology of dyspnea. When confronted with a patient with shortness of breath of unclear cause, it is useful to begin the analysis with a consideration of the broad pathophysiologic categories that explain the vast majority of cases. COPD, chronic obstructive pulmonary disease.

Clinical Pathophysiology

When confronted with a patient complaining of dyspnea, one can place the vast majority of individuals into one of two broad categories: cardiovascular dyspnea and respiratory dyspnea (Fig. 7–2).

Cardiovascular Dyspnea

Within the category of cardiovascular dyspnea, one should consider three subsets. Patients with *high cardiac output*—for example, secondary to anemia or shunts—frequently complain of dyspnea with exertion. The exact mechanism underlying this symptom has not been elucidated, but the symptom may reflect either reduced oxygen delivery to tissues or increased vascular pressure necessary to maintain the elevated cardiac output. Individuals with *normal cardiac output*, particularly if they are obese or deconditioned, also have breathlessness with exertion. What ultimately separates the average person from a trained athlete is the level of cardiovascular fitness, which is determined not only by the heart's ability to increase stroke volume and cardiac output during stress but also by the ability of the peripheral muscles to extract and use oxygen, thereby delaying the onset of anaerobic metabolism. An early shift from aerobic to anaerobic processes places added strain on the respiratory system to the extent that greater levels of ventilation are required to compensate for the evolving metabolic acidosis. In addition, the buildup of lactic acid in the muscles may also contribute to breathing discomfort.

Obese patients generally fall into this category unless their obesity is so severe that it causes abnormalities in the pulmonary pump (see later). Individuals with no true physiologic cause for their breathing discomfort, such as those with anxiety or psychogenic dyspnea, might be considered within the category of normal cardiac output.

A special group of patients with cardiovascular dyspnea and normal cardiac output are those with diastolic dysfunction. These patients usually have a stiffened left ventricle and normal cardiac output at rest. With exercise, the heart must increase its rate to a greater extent than stroke volume because of an inability of the left ventricle to dilate. Furthermore, to achieve the cardiac output needed to sustain the metabolic activity of exercise in these patients, left ventricular diastolic pressure must increase, which leads to an elevation in pulmonary capillary pressure and shortness of breath. A similar mechanism is probably responsible for ischemia-induced dyspnea in patients with normal left ventricular systolic function. It is important to note that some patients with myocardial ischemia will not experience chest pain and that dyspnea may be the only sign of acute coronary insufficiency. In these patients, shortness of breath is considered an "anginal equivalent."

The third subset of patients within the category of cardiovascular dyspnea consists of those with *low cardiac output*. Classically, these are patients with compromised left ventricular systolic function or pericardial disease. Forward flow is reduced and the system compensates by increasing filling pressure within the chambers of the heart. As a result, lung water may be increased, as well as pressure within the pulmonary circulation, both of which may lead to dyspnea.

Respiratory Dyspnea

This category can also be divided into three subsets. Patients with disorders of the *respiratory controller*, that is, conditions that result in stimulation of the medullary center that determines the rate and depth of breathing, have a greater neural drive to breathe than would be expected on the basis of the metabolic need for oxygen uptake or carbon dioxide elimination. Common examples of this type of derangement include the dyspnea associated with early pregnancy or with aspirin overdose. In the former, elevated levels of progesterone induce hyperventilation and dyspnea well before the uterus enlarges sufficiently to compromise motion of the diaphragm. In the latter, the direct effect of aspirin on the respiratory centers in the brain stem leads to hyperventilation and, in some cases, a sense of breathing distress. Conditions in which the controller is stimulated are often associated with a sensation of "air hunger" or an "urge or need to breathe."

The second subset of patients with respiratory dyspnea includes those with abnormalities of the *ventilatory pump*. Once the respiratory controller has determined how rapidly and deeply the individual must breathe, neural impulses from the brain must be translated into movement of air into and out of the alveoli. To accomplish this task, one must have a functioning ventilatory pump, which consists of the peripheral nerves connecting the controller to the ventilatory muscles, the muscles of ventilation, the supporting skeleton for these muscles, the pleura that transmits pressure changes generated by the muscles to the lungs, and the airways that serve as a conduit for airflow. Dysfunction of any of these components of the ventilatory pump—for example, spinal cord injury, myopathies, kyphoscoliosis, pleural fibrosis, and airway obstruction—may lead to breathing discomfort, most often associated with an increased sense of effort or work of breathing.

The third and probably most common subset of patients with respiratory dyspnea seen by primary care physicians includes those with abnormalities in the *gas exchanger*, that is, the alveoli and pulmonary capillaries. Ultimately, the goal of the respiratory system is to provide oxygen to the blood and remove carbon dioxide. To achieve this objective, one must have a functioning gas exchanger. Derangements of the gas exchanger generally result in hypoxia or hypercapnia or in increased ventilation to compensate for the ventilation-perfusion abnormalities. A gas exchange problem exists in conditions such as pneumonia, pulmonary edema, pulmonary embolism, asthma, and chronic obstructive pulmonary disease (COPD).

Patients with dyspnea can usually be placed in one or more of these subsets. It is helpful if one can determine that the problem is primarily cardiovascular versus respiratory, although the reality is that many individuals may have a mixed picture. Nevertheless, the practical approach to a patient with breathing discomfort ultimately makes better sense if the pathophysiology has been clarified.

WORKUP OF PATIENTS WITH DYSPNEA

The History (see also Chapter 3)

Definitions of dyspnea have included "difficult, labored, uncomfortable breathing," "an awareness of respiratory distress," "the sensation of feeling air hunger," and "an uncomfortable sensation of breathing." When considering dyspnea, it is important to avoid confusing the symptom, or what a patient describes about the sensations being experienced, with a physical sign, or something that the physician observes, such as a rapid respiratory rate or the use of accessory muscles of ventilation. Common to these definitions is the concept of "discomfort" in the act of breathing. In addition, it is apparent that more than one sensation may be lumped together under the heading of dyspnea.

Physicians can readily conceive different qualities of pain and use the information about the characteristics of pain to focus on the underlying pathology afflicting the patient. For example, a "burning" chest discomfort suggests a gastrointestinal etiology, whereas a "pressure-like" discomfort raises the specter of myocardial ischemia. Formal studies of pain have established that different pain syndromes are characterized by unique sets of phrases and that these phrases can be used to distinguish various types of headache and facial pain.

Physicians, even those in generally good health, commonly experience a variety of pains during their lives—for example, headaches, stomach upset, bruises, and fractures—and thereby develop a vocabulary with which to communicate with their patients. However, they tend to have limited personal experience with dyspnea. In the absence of cardiopulmonary pathology, the only breathing discomfort a doctor may experience is likely to be associated with exercise. Is that sensation the same as what is experienced by a patient with asthma, COPD, pulmonary embolism, CHF, or angina? What information can physicians draw on to construct questions for their patient to elicit the qualities of dyspnea?

Descriptions of Dyspnea

It has now been shown that dyspnea, like pain, is composed of multiple, qualitatively distinct sensations. When presented with a list of phrases used by patients and subjects to describe breathing discomfort, patients with different cardiopulmonary diseases selected unique clusters of verbal descriptors as representative of their dyspnea. Each condition tends to be associated with more than one phrase, some phrases are used to characterize more than one condition, and each condition is associated with a unique set of phrases. These features of the vocabulary chosen by patients suggest that more than one mechanism is probably responsible for dyspnea in a given pathologic state, that different disease states may share common mechanisms for producing respiratory discomfort, and that each condition has a unique set of physiologic factors that produce its particular discomfort.

Studies of the "language of dyspnea" have provided insight into the physiology of respiratory distress for categories of disease and into the specific pathologic conditions causing symptoms in individual patients. Studies to determine the sensitivity and specificity of these tools are under way.[5] There appear to be at least five sensations that can give the physician clues to the underlying diagnosis (Box 7–1).

Questioning the Patient

When obtaining a history of dyspnea, it is important to question the patient about the quality of the breathing discomfort.[6] One should start with an open-ended question designed to elicit the patient's spontaneous verbal response. However, it is not uncommon for the patient

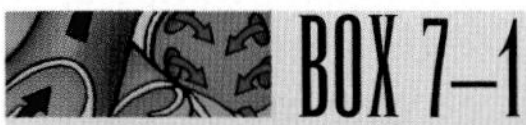

BOX 7–1

The Language of Dyspnea: Association of Qualitative Descriptors and Pathophysiologic Mechanisms of Shortness of Breath

DESCRIPTOR	PATHOPHYSIOLOGY
Chest tightness or constriction	Bronchoconstriction, interstitial edema (asthma, myocardial ischemia)
Increased work or effort of breathing	Airway obstruction, neuromuscular disease, chest wall disease (COPD, moderate to severe asthma, myopathy, kyphoscoliosis)
Air hunger, need to breathe, urge to breathe	Increased drive to breathe (CHF, pulmonary embolism, moderate to severe airway obstruction)
Cannot get a deep breath; unsatisfying breath	Hyperinflation (asthma, COPD) and restricted tidal volume (pulmonary fibrosis, chest wall restriction)
Heavy breathing, rapid breathing, breathing more	Deconditioning

CHF, congestive heart failure; COPD, chronic obstructive pulmonary disease.

to answer with a quizzical expression because this may be the first time that anyone has posed this particular question. Under these circumstances, the next step is to provide the patient with some alternative phrases (Box 7–2) and ask whether one or more phrases describe the sensation that the patient is experiencing. It is also important to ask patients whether they are experiencing different kinds of respiratory discomfort at different times or under different circumstances; a positive response may signify the coexistence of two conditions, with each more prominent at different times—for example, COPD and increased airway reactivity, COPD and CHF, or asthma and deconditioning. Although patients may at first have difficulty describing their sensations, they are often quite adamant that the dyspnea associated with a respiratory infection is different from that associated with walking up the stairs. As noted previously, deconditioning may be the factor that ultimately limits activity in patients with cardiopulmonary disease. Awareness of this fact is critical because the level of deconditioning may be improved with an exercise program independent of the responsiveness of the patient's underlying cardiopulmonary disorder to specific therapy.

In addition to the quality of the dyspnea, the timing of dyspnea and the factors that precipitate episodes of respiratory discomfort are also important to identify. Does the discomfort occur at rest or only with exertion? Is it episodic or continuous? Dyspnea that occurs with exertion may be a manifestation of a variety of disease states that become evident because of the increased metabolic demands of the activity. For example, in a patient with COPD or interstitial lung disease, dyspnea with activity may indicate the development of an acute physiologic change such as bronchospasm or myocardial ischemia, or it may merely reflect the relative cardiovascular conditioning of the individual. Whereas chronic dyspnea at rest usually indicates severe structural lung or heart disease, episodic breathing discomfort at rest invariably indicates an acute derangement that is reversible. Asthma and myocardial ischemia are examples of the latter.

It is also important to identify factors that precipitate the dyspnea and symptoms associated with the respiratory discomfort because they are clues to the cause of the patient's problem. Dyspnea resulting from exposure to fumes, scents, or cigarette smoke is usually the result of constriction of reactive airways in asthma and COPD. Inhalation of cold air may be a trigger for asthma. Hot, humid days with high levels of air pollution typically provoke dyspnea in patients with COPD. Associated symptoms such as pleuritic chest pain and fever may indicate the presence of a respiratory infection or pulmonary embolism, whereas chest pressure, diaphoresis, and nausea along with dyspnea are clues that the patient is suffering from myocardial ischemia.

BOX 7–2

Qualitative Descriptors of Dyspnea

These descriptors may be incorporated into a patient interview when a history of shortness of breath is being elicited. Phrases are grouped into clusters based on studies of the language of dyspnea in normal subjects and patients.

- My chest feels tight.
- My chest is constricted.

- My breathing is heavy.
- I am panting.
- I feel that I am breathing more.

- My breathing requires effort.
- My breathing requires more work.

- I feel that I am suffocating.
- I feel that I am smothering.

- I feel a hunger for more air.
- I cannot get enough air.

- My breathing is shallow.
- I cannot take a deep breath.

Special Forms of Dyspnea

Orthopnea, the presence of dyspnea when lying flat, is classically a sign of CHF. Redistribution of blood volume from dependent portions of the body to the central circulation along with an attendant increase in pulmonary capillary wedge pressure leads to interstitial edema and dyspnea. However, other conditions may also be manifested in this fashion. For example, patients with a paralyzed diaphragm experience breathing discomfort in the supine position because of cephalad displacement of the diaphragm secondary to forces exerted by the abdominal contents. This displacement places a greater burden on the remaining accessory muscles of ventilation, which are responsible for generating negative pleural pressure. When questioning patients about the presence of orthopnea, it is important to ask the following questions:

1. Do you sleep on multiple pillows or in a recliner?
2. Has this condition changed recently?
3. Do you have shortness of breath if you lie flat?

Many patients sleep with their head elevated for reasons unrelated to respiratory sensations—for example, gastroesophageal reflux or chronic cough from postnasal drip—and one should not assume that assumption of this position at night always signifies respiratory discomfort. If any questions remain about the implications of a history of orthopnea, it is useful to challenge the patient during the physical examination by placing the patient in the supine position and observing the respiratory pattern, oxygen saturation, and subjective response.

Nocturnal dyspnea is typically a manifestation of CHF. Paroxysmal nocturnal dyspnea (PND) usually occurs in patients with peripheral edema; reabsorption of interstitial fluid into the circulation during the night leads to increased intracardiac pressure. Depressed left ventricular function secondary to reduced adrenergic activity during sleep may likewise contribute to PND. It is less well known that asthma may also cause nocturnal dyspnea. The etiology of nocturnal asthma is thought to be reflux of acid from the stomach into the esophagus, which triggers a reflex mediated by the vagus nerve and leads to bronchospasm. Intermittent aspiration of gastric contents, a lower level of endogenous steroids, or a trough in the serum level of medications may also play a role in triggering nocturnal asthma in some patients.

Physical Examination

The first part of any physical examination (see also Chapter 3) should be a general assessment of the patient's condition from a distance, what we call the "view from the door." Does the patient appear to be comfortable or in distress? What is the patient's color? Is the patient cyanotic? What position does the patient assume: sitting back easily in the chair or leaning forward with hands braced on the knees or on a table (i.e., the tripod position)? The latter permits the patient to recruit additional chest wall muscles to aid in respiration and, along with large swings in pleural pressure as evidenced by intercostal or supraclavicular retractions, is a good indicator of moderate to severe obstructive lung disease. Breathing with pursed lips is also a fairly typical finding in patients with emphysema because it may decrease breathing discomfort by slowing the breathing rate and reducing hyperinflation, improving oxygenation, and changing transmural pressure across the walls of the airways.

The patient's vital signs offer additional diagnostic clues. Acute dyspnea in association with an increase in the pulse-pressure product, that is, an elevated heart rate and blood pressure, should always raise the possibility of acute myocardial ischemia. A very rapid respiratory rate, usually with a shallow breathing pattern, is most typical of patients with low pulmonary compliance or "stiff lungs," for example, interstitial fibrosis or CHF. *Pulsus paradoxus* refers to the normal fall in systolic pressure seen during inspiration. When exaggerated, that is, greater than 10 mm Hg, it is a clue either to very large negative intrathoracic pressure as seen in patients with severe airway obstruction or to cardiac tamponade (see Chapter 35).

The Chest

Examination of the chest provides additional helpful diagnostic clues. Careful *inspection of the chest* should precede auscultation. Intercostal retractions secondary to intrapleural pressure swings are associated with airway obstruction. The patient's chest wall should be evaluated for symmetry of movement, which is best done by observing the patient from behind. Deformities of the chest wall such as kyphoscoliosis impose a mechanical load on the ventilatory pump. Movement of the lateral aspect of the rib cage during inspiration should be noted. Under normal circumstances, the lateral chest wall moves outward as the diaphragm descends. However, in patients with COPD and marked hyperinflation, the diaphragm is in a flattened position, and contraction of the muscle results in inward motion of the lateral chest wall.

Auscultation of the chest may reveal focal findings suggestive of pneumonia or diffuse findings compatible with asthma, COPD, interstitial lung disease, or CHF. *Rales* are short, high-pitched inspiratory sounds produced by the sudden equalization of pressure in terminal bronchioles as collapsed alveoli pop open. When lungs are "stiff," that is, have reduced compliance because of interstitial inflammation or edema, alveoli tend to collapse at low lung volumes at the end of exhalation. With the next inspiration, the alveoli are reopened and rales are heard. The rales associated with interstitial inflammation and fibrosis are very short, distinct sounds and are often described as "dry rales." In contrast, the rales heard in patients with CHF may have a thicker, slightly gurgling sound and are termed "wet rales." *Rhonchi*, or coarse large airway sounds, are found in patients with increased mucus production. Wheezes, the product of turbulent flow through narrow airways, may be heard in asthma, COPD, and CHF (i.e., "cardiac asthma").

Precordial Examination

Examination of the heart by palpation and auscultation of the anterior of the chest may provide clues about the presence of heart failure and pulmonary hypertension. Lateral displacement of the point of maximal impulse (PMI) suggests left ventricular enlargement. Localization of the PMI to the subxiphoid area is indicative of hyperinflation of the lungs, right ventricular prominence, or both. The latter is typically seen in patients with pulmonary hypertension, and these patients may also have a prominent pulsation over the left second or third intercostal space and a loud pulmonic component of the second heart sound (P_2). If P_2 can be heard at the apex, it should be considered evidence of pulmonary hypertension.

Although a third heart sound (S_3) may be a normal finding in a young person, it is suggestive of elevated left ventricular end-diastolic pressure and the presence of CHF. A fourth heart sound (S_4) is indicative of a stiff or hypertrophied left ventricle, often seen in patients with long-standing hypertension or hypertrophic cardiomyopathy. Interstitial edema may develop and cause exertional dyspnea in these patients. The presence of a holosystolic murmur at the apex, particularly with radiation to the axilla, is indicative of mitral regurgitation. Patients with this finding and exertional dyspnea should be evaluated further for possible exercise-induced CHF.

Extremities

Examination of patients with dyspnea should include a careful inspection of the extremities. Cyanosis is found in patients with at least 5 g/dL of desaturated hemoglobin (individuals with severe anemia will not appear cyanotic even with very marked degrees of hypoxia). The presence of peripheral edema may indicate right ventricular dysfunction or local venous insufficiency. If the edema is due to increased pressure in the right side of the heart, one should also see elevation of the jugular venous pulse and, in some cases, an enlarged, congested liver. Peripheral edema secondary to local factors in the legs may be associated with deep venous thrombosis and pulmonary emboli. Calf pain with dorsiflexion of the foot is suggestive of deep venous thrombosis, as is a palpable cord. However, one must remember that 50% of patients with deep venous thrombosis have a normal physical examination. Finally, although clubbing of the nails is found in patients with congenital heart disease and right-to-left shunts, pulmonary arteriovenous fistulas, lung cancer, interstitial fibrosis, and chronic inflammatory conditions of the lung, it is *not* associated with COPD alone.

Walking with the Patient

In the evaluation of a patient with exertional dyspnea, a formal cardiopulmonary test (described later) can provide very useful diagnostic information. However, even in the office setting, it is possible to glean important data by observing the patient walk in a corridor or up stairs. Is the patient able to perform more physical work than reported in the interview? How distressed does the patient appear? How quickly does the patient recover on stopping? At the point that the patient asks for a rest, is the complaint primarily of fatigue, leg discomfort, or breathlessness? Auscultation of the chest at the end of the walk may reveal rales or wheezes that were not present at rest. If a pulse oximeter is available, the presence of desaturation with walking indicates a gas exchange abnormality.

Laboratory Evaluation

Patients being evaluated for dyspnea, the cause of which is not previously known or evident from the history and physical examination, should have a *chest radiograph*. An enlarged heart and redistribution of blood flow to the apices of the lung may indicate mild CHF, and the shape of the cardiac silhouette will provide important clues regarding the cause of the heart failure. Patients with COPD may have large lung volumes secondary to gas trapping from early collapse of airways. Approximately 90% of patients with interstitial lung disease will have abnormal findings on chest radiographs at the time of clinical examination. Radiographic findings of pneumonia may precede the physical findings on examination. Pulmonary embolism may be suggested by the presence of atelectasis or a small pleural effusion, although most patients with pulmonary embolism have a normal chest film.

In patients with subacute or chronic dyspnea and possible cardiac dysfunction or pulmonary hypertension, an *echocardiogram* can provide much useful information (see Chapter 5). The contractile status of the ventricles is easily determined, as is competency of the cardiac valves. In addition, an estimate can be made of pulmonary artery pressure, which if elevated, may be an indication of left ventricular failure, severe parenchymal lung disease, or occult pulmonary vascular disease. Finally, the pericardium can be viewed to evaluate for pericardial effusion or an infiltrative process.

Assessment of cardiovascular dyspnea should always include a *hematocrit* to eliminate anemia as the explanation for shortness of breath. In general, a hematocrit above 30% is unlikely to explain moderate to severe dyspnea.

Oxygen saturation, or the percentage of hemoglobin saturated with oxygen, has virtually become the "fifth vital sign." The ready availability of pulse oximeters and their ease of use have made them a mainstay of emergency departments and inpatient units, and they are now beginning to appear in the office setting as well. A low oxygen saturation (i.e., below 90%) may immediately suggest to the primary care physician that the patient probably has a major problem with gas exchange. One must be cautious, however, in the setting of a relatively normal oxygen saturation that one does not dismiss the patient's shortness of breath as an insignificant issue. Assessment of oxygen saturation during walking may reveal desaturation even in a patient with a normal resting value. This combination of findings, normal oxygen saturation at rest and significant desaturation with activity, is indicative of processes that lead to destruction of lung tissue (emphysema, pulmonary fibrosis), pulmonary vascular disease, or the acute development of interstitial edema (i.e., CHF).

Interpretation of resting oxygen saturation is further complicated by the physiology of oxygen binding to hemoglobin. Because of the sigmoid shape of the hemoglobin-O_2 association/dissociation curve, oxygen saturation is relatively insensitive to changes in the arterial partial pressure of O_2 (Pao_2) above 60 to 65 mm Hg. Consequently, a patient's Pao_2 may drop by 10 to 15 mm Hg with relatively little change in O_2 saturation. This problem is further complicated by the presence of hyperventilation. When a patient hyperventilates, as often occurs during an acute asthma attack or pulmonary embolism, $Paco_2$ drops and Pao_2 rises. The gas exchange abnormality—reflected by the alveolar-arterial O_2 difference (PAO_2–Pao_2), which is calculated with Pao_2 and $Paco_2$ values obtained from measurement of arterial blood gas (Fig. 7–3)—remains abnormal, but O_2 saturation may be completely normal. Thus, one may be fooled by a patient who has normal O_2 saturation yet a very abnormal PAO_2–Pao_2 value and a very deranged gas exchanger. Additional problems arise with measurement of O_2 saturation by a pulse oximeter when an abnormal hemoglobin is present, for example, carboxyhemoglobin found with carbon monoxide

$$P_{A_{O_2}} = F_{I_{O_2}}(P_{ATM} - P_{H_2O}) - \frac{Pa_{CO_2}}{R}$$

$P_{A_{O_2}}$ = Partial pressure of oxygen in the alveolus

$F_{I_{O_2}}$ = Inspired concentration of oxygen, e.g., at sea level, breathing "room air," the $F_{I_{O_2}} = 0.21$

P_{ATM} = Atmospheric pressure in mm Hg

P_{H_2O} = Vapor pressure for fully saturated air (approximately 47 mm Hg)

Pa_{CO_2} = Partial pressure of carbon dioxide in arterial blood

R = Respiratory quotient (generally assumed to be 0.8 for individuals on a typical diet)

FIGURE 7–3. Alveolar gas equation. Using the alveolar gas equation, one can calculate the partial pressure of oxygen in the alveolus. Then, by knowing the arterial P_{O_2} obtained from a blood gas measurement, the alveolar-arterial oxygen gradient ($P_{A_{O_2}}-Pa_{O_2}$) can be determined. An abnormal gradient indicates a problem with gas exchange, specifically, any cardiopulmonary process that worsens ventilation-perfusion inequalities or impairs diffusion of oxygen into the pulmonary capillary will result in an increase in $P_{A_{O_2}}$–Pa_{O_2}.

poisoning or methemoglobin as seen in patients taking dapsone for the treatment of *Pneumocystis carinii* infection. In these situations, the pulse oximeter will not provide one with an accurate assessment of gas exchange. These abnormal forms of hemoglobin tend to produce O_2 saturation that appears normal even though the ability of the red blood cells to deliver oxygen to the tissues is impaired. Given these limitations, $P_{A_{O_2}}$–Pa_{O_2} should be calculated whenever underlying pulmonary or pulmonary vascular disease is suspected.

Pulmonary Function Testing

Assessment of the ventilatory pump and gas exchanger is further enhanced by the information provided by *pulmonary function testing*. Spirometric testing provides data on airway obstruction. Simple spirometers are now available for use by primary care physicians in their offices, and these devices can be helpful in detecting mild bronchospasm or airway obstruction. Measurement of lung volume must be performed in a formal pulmonary function laboratory and is important in assessing the full extent of COPD, specifically, the degree of hyperinflation and air trapping, which are important criteria for interventions such as lung volume reduction surgery, or in determining whether restrictive lung disease is present, that is, whether total lung capacity is reduced. Respiratory muscle strength is assessed by measurement of maximal inspiratory and expiratory pressure and should be determined if neuromuscular disease is suspected.

The lungs' *diffusing capacity* for carbon monoxide (DLCO) provides insight into the status of the membrane between the pulmonary capillaries and the alveoli. In diseases that result in destruction of lung tissue (e.g., emphysema, pulmonary fibrosis) or inflammation of the pulmonary interstitium, DLCO is reduced. In contrast, patients with mild CHF have an increase in pulmonary vascular blood volume and a mild increase in DLCO.

In the vast majority of cases, the history, physical examination, and elements of the laboratory evaluation outlined earlier will provide an answer to the question of what is causing this patient's respiratory discomfort. In some circumstances, a presumptive diagnosis can be made that leads to a therapeutic trial, for example, a diuretic for subtle volume overload or initiation of bronchodilators for probable intermittent bronchoconstriction. In a small number of cases, however, the answer is still unclear. At this point, a cardiopulmonary exercise test can be extremely helpful.

Cardiopulmonary Exercise Testing

Cardiopulmonary exercise testing incorporates measurements of respiratory and cardiovascular function under conditions of dynamic activity of large muscle groups. By either treadmill or bicycle exercise, the physician assesses a patient's functional capacity and aerobic performance and looks for patterns of physiologic abnormality at the point that the patient is not able to continue to exercise (Box 7–3). The test is particularly useful for patients in whom it is uncertain after preliminary evaluation whether derangements in the cardiovascular or respiratory system are the explanation for the individual's dyspnea.[7]

The major *indications* for cardiopulmonary exercise testing in patients with dyspnea are as follows:

1. To search for an explanation for symptoms whose etiology remains obscure after completing the evaluation outlined previously.

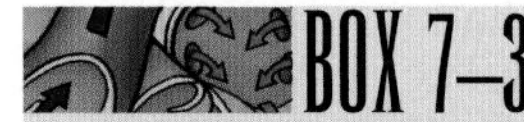

BOX 7–3

Cardiopulmonary Exercise Testing

INDICATIONS

- Evaluate a patient with dyspnea of unclear cause after the history, physical examination, and standard laboratory evaluations fail to yield a diagnosis
- Assess the relative contributions of the cardiovascular and respiratory system to a patient's functional limitation
- Determine the patient's functional capacity

MEASUREMENTS

- Electrocardiogram
- Heart rate
- Blood pressure
- Oxygen consumption
- Carbon dioxide production
- Anaerobic threshold
- Oxygen saturation
- Forced vital capacity and forced expiratory volume in 1 second before and after exercise

2. To determine the relative contributions of cardiac and pulmonary processes to a patient's functional limitation when multiple causes may be present.
3. To determine a patient's functional capacity when there appears to be a discrepancy between the physiologic data and a patient's reported exercise tolerance, that is, when one suspects that the individual should be able to do more than stated.

Exercise testing is particularly helpful for ascertaining whether cardiovascular deconditioning is the major source of a patient's functional limitation and for assessing whether occult myocardial ischemia is the explanation for respiratory distress when the preliminary evaluation is unrevealing. It is not uncommon for individuals who begin to experience respiratory discomfort after activities to alter their lifestyle in ways that reduce the chance that they will become short of breath. Over time, the individual becomes deconditioned and the heart is not able to generate as high a cardiac output, nor are the skeletal muscles of the limbs able to extract and use O_2 as efficiently. Subsequently, the patient experiences dyspnea when performing activities that had been easily accomplished in the past. The response may be to curtail lifestyle even further. A vicious circle is established with diminishing exercise capacity and increasing symptoms (Fig. 7–4).

Not uncommonly, patients attribute this decline in functional status to worsening of their underlying lung or heart disease. Patients with asthma, for example, who report that they are limited by their lung disease have been found in many cases to be deconditioned rather than restricted by fixed airway obstruction or exercise-induced bronchoconstriction. Exercise capacity correlates better with their general level of physical activity than with the severity of their asthma. Patients with severe COPD have also been shown to develop lactic acidosis with minimal activity and to improve their aerobic capacity with an exercise program; that is, their level of conditioning was a major element in their functional limitation. Physicians must be cautious in assuming that all of a patient's dyspnea is due to the underlying pulmonary process.

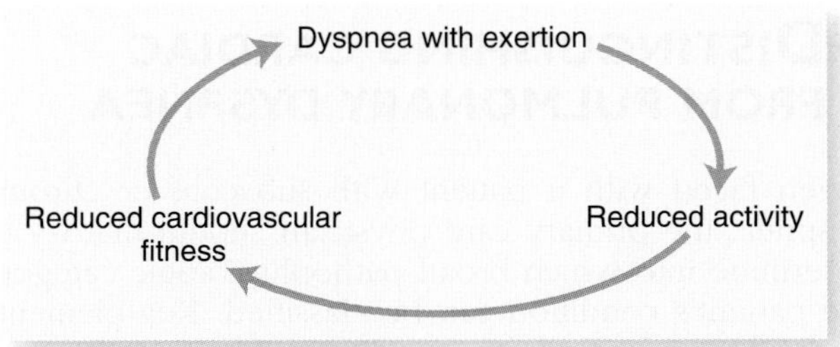

FIGURE 7–4. Cycle of dyspnea and deconditioning. Patients with cardiopulmonary disease commonly experience breathing discomfort with activity. Their response is often to reduce or eliminate activities that produce the shortness of breath. The increasingly sedentary lifestyle results in cardiovascular deconditioning and even greater dyspnea with exertion. The cycle may be repeated many times until the patient experiences trouble performing simple daily activities.

Most exercise testing for patients with a complaint of dyspnea is performed on a treadmill or with a bicycle ergometer. Treadmill testing, to the extent that it more closely reproduces the predominant activity of the individual, or walking, is usually preferable. However, some patients, particularly the elderly, have difficulty coordinating their pace with the machine or have so much anxiety about "falling off" that reliable measurements cannot be made. In these circumstances, an exercise bicycle is used.

Endpoints. The primary endpoints of the test are symptoms, cardiovascular changes, and gas exchange abnormalities. If the patient terminates the test because it is too uncomfortable, one must ask the patient what actually caused him to stop. Observation of the patient during the exercise often provides useful information as one assesses the patient's response. For example, the patient, though complaining of significant distress, may appear quite comfortable with little increase in ventilation or alteration in vital signs, thus suggesting that the individual may be malingering or may have a very low threshold for discomfort after months or years of doing little activity. If the patient states that "shortness of breath" was the reason for stopping the exercise, one should pursue the question further by inquiring about the explicit sensations. As described previously in discussing the language of dyspnea, many sensations are included in the generally used term *shortness of breath*, and these descriptors can give one useful information about the etiology of the symptom. It is useful to ascertain whether the sensation that caused the patient to stop exercising during the test was the same as that felt at home during similar or different conditions. One should also be sure that the patient has stopped because of breathing discomfort rather than leg pain or general fatigue. The latter two symptoms commonly accompany the deconditioned state.

If the patient does not complain of symptoms, the exercise test is stopped when there is evidence that the patient has reached the limits of cardiovascular performance or has signs of possible myocardial ischemia or significant hypoxemia. Cardiac output rises by increasing either stroke volume or heart rate. Achievement of greater than 85% of a patient's predicted heart rate indicates that one is nearing maximal cardiac output. A significant rise or fall in systemic blood pressure, usually with typical changes on the electrocardiogram (ECG), is suggestive of myocardial ischemia and indicates that the test should be terminated. At a minimum, O_2 saturation is monitored with a pulse oximeter to screen for hypoxemia. During the test, multiple *physiologic measurements* are made. As noted previously, respiratory function is monitored with a pulse oximeter and, in many cases, by serial measurement of arterial blood gases and minute ventilation.

If the heart rate reaches greater than 85% of predicted at a low workload, one has evidence that cardiovascular function is contributing to the patient's exercise limitation. As discussed previously (under "Clinical Pathophysiology"), cardiovascular limitations may occur in the setting of both "normal" myocardial function (e.g., deconditioning) and abnormal function (e.g., heart failure). In a patient with well-functioning myocardium, cardiac output is increased by a combination of stroke volume and heart rate, with a preference toward stroke volume. As the limits of stroke volume are reached, further increases in cardiac output require a rising heart rate. Thus, as the pulse approaches the predicted maximum for the individual, one also has an indication that maximal cardiac output is being reached. However, patients in whom acute myocardial ischemia develops may have shortness of breath because of associated elevations in pulmonary capillary pressure before achieving this high a heart rate. Decreases in blood pressure, which may result from failure of cardiac output to rise in the presence of exercise-induced peripheral vasodilatation, may be caused by myocardial ischemia and accompanied by typical ECG changes.

The *anaerobic threshold*, that is, the level of O_2 consumption above which the body begins to use anaerobic metabolism to support its energy needs during exercise, can also be measured during the exercise test. Total body oxygen consumption is determined by the quantity of O_2 delivered to the tissues and the fraction of that oxygen that can be extracted by the tissues. O_2 delivery is primarily dependent on the patient's hemoglobin, the percentage of hemoglobin saturated with O_2, and cardiac output. The ability of tissues to extract O_2 is related to the density of capillaries in the tissue and the biochemical status of the cell, that is, whether the mitochondria and enzymes are primed to use O_2. In a deconditioned person, the heart has a reduced ability to increase cardiac output, which limits O_2 delivery, and the muscles are not in an optimal biochemical state to extract and use O_2. Consequently, the anaerobic threshold is reached at lower workloads than in a well-conditioned athlete. If the anaerobic threshold is low, metabolic acidosis develops as the body produces lactic acid, a byproduct of anaerobic metabolism. This acid load poses an additional stress to the respiratory system because the respiratory system must compensate for the anaerobic metabolism by increasing ventilation, which may drive the patient to an early ventilatory limit.

Patterns of Abnormality. In assessing a patient's response to an exercise test, one looks for patterns of abnormality (Box 7–4). Patients with impaired cardiovascular function (other than acute ischemia) as the primary explanation for the exercise limitation will have high heart rates at low workloads. Metabolic acidosis will occur early during exercise; that is, patients have a low anaerobic threshold. In addition, maximal oxygen consumption is well below that predicted for their age and size. The ventilation achieved during exercise, on the other hand, will not reach the maximal level that can be achieved by the respiratory system. As noted previously, patients with myocardial ischemia demonstrate ECG changes, abnormal hemodynamic responses, or new rales on examination during exercise.

Patients with a respiratory cause of their exercise limitation have a maximal ventilation that reaches or exceeds the predicted value, a significant decline in oxygen saturation (<90%), or a rise in the dead space–to–tidal volume ratio. The heart rate does not reach 85% of the predicted maximum, the anaerobic threshold is in the normal range, and the ECG does not show ischemic changes.

Interpretation of exercise tests must consider the patient's motivation to perform the test and the ability to tolerate uncomfortable sensations. The staff supervising the test should encourage the patient to give maximal effort and should note whether it was achieved.

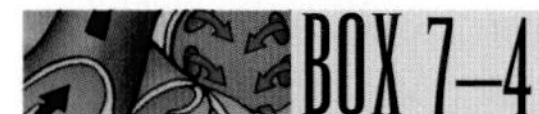

Patterns of Abnormality in Cardiopulmonary Exercise Testing

CARDIOVASCULAR LIMITATION

- Heart rate ≥85% of predicted maximum
- Low anaerobic threshold
- Reduced maximal oxygen consumption
- Drop in blood pressure with exercise
- Arrhythmias or ischemic challenges on ECG
- Does not achieve maximal predicted ventilation
- Does not have significant desaturation

RESPIRATORY LIMITATION

- Achieves or exceeds maximal predicted ventilation
- Significant desaturation (<90%)
- Stable or increased dead space–to–tidal volume ratio
- Development of bronchospasm with falling FEV_1
- Does not achieve 85% of predicted maximal heart rate
- No ischemic ECG changes

Note: All features will not be present in a particular case, and elements of both cardiovascular and respiratory causes of shortness of breath may be present. Look for the predominant pattern in assessing the etiology of the patient's exercise limitation.

ECG, electrocardiogram; FEV_1, forced expiratory volume in 1 second.

DISTINGUISHING CARDIAC FROM PULMONARY DYSPNEA

When faced with a patient with subacute or chronic dyspnea, the primary care physician should first try to determine into which broad pathophysiologic category the patient's condition can be classified. Key elements in the history include the quality of the sensation and the timing and precipitating factors for the symptom. Patients with CHF generally report a sense of air hunger, not being able to get enough air, or having an increased urge to breathe. Patients with COPD and interstitial lung disease complain primarily of increased work or effort of breathing, whereas patients with asthma relate a sense of chest tightness and constriction or a feeling of not being able to get a deep breath. Although patients with intermittent myocardial ischemia may also experience chest tightness or heaviness, these patients have more of a "painful" aspect to the chest discomfort.

Both cardiac and pulmonary causes of dyspnea are precipitated by exercise. However, an onset of symptoms in association with cold air, inhalation of fumes, or respiratory infections generally points toward a pulmonary origin. Nocturnal dyspnea is a strong clue to the presence of CHF, especially if peripheral edema is present. Such patients usually achieve relief within several minutes on assumption of an upright position, redistribution of intravascular fluid, and a decrease in pulmonary capillary wedge pressure. However, nocturnal breathlessness may also be a manifestation of asthma and usually occurs as a result of gastroesophageal reflux or a trough in levels of medications. Cough is often present with asthma, and the symptoms are not as quickly relieved in the upright posture.

After a comprehensive history and physical examination, an empirical trial of therapy is often an appropriate way to try to establish the diagnosis. For example, if dyspnea is relieved by diuretic therapy that induces weight loss of 2 kg or more, the diagnosis of heart failure is supported. Alternatively, improvement in or elimination of respiratory distress after the institution of a beta-agonist inhaler is strong evidence of the presence of airway reactivity in asthma or COPD.

When additional testing is required, the chest radiograph, two-dimensional echocardiogram with Doppler imaging, and pulmonary function tests provide important data. The classic findings of a large heart, upper zone vascular redistribution, increased vascular markings, and pleural effusions point toward the diagnosis of CHF. A completely normal chest radiograph in a patient with intermittent dyspnea suggests the possibility of myocardial ischemia. Patients with COPD typically have evidence of hyperinflation and loss of normal pulmonary vascular markings, whereas those with interstitial lung disease have reduced lung volume and increased interstitial lines. The presence of a normal-sized heart and the absence of pleural effusions can often distinguish the latter group from patients with CHF.

Pulmonary function tests in patients with CHF typically show low normal or mildly reduced lung volumes (total lung capacity, functional residual capacity, and vital capacity), and such patients may have concomitant mild airway obstruction (reduced forced expiratory volume in 1 second [FEV_1] and maximal mid flow). The diffusing capacity in mild CHF is normal or slightly increased as a result of the increased pulmonary vascular volume associated with elevated pulmonary capillary wedge pressure. In the presence of pulmonary edema, the diffusing capacity is reduced. This finding of a normal to elevated diffusing capacity in mild CHF may be helpful in distinguishing these patients from those with interstitial fibrosis, who also demonstrate low lung volumes and increased interstitial markings on chest radiographs but have reduced diffusing capacity. Patients with COPD and asthma typically have airway obstruction with normal to elevated lung volumes and often have evidence of air trapping with an increased residual volume–to–total lung capacity ratio.

Figure 7–5 provides an overview of an algorithm for the evaluation of a patient with shortness of breath. If the diagnosis is still uncertain despite the considerations discussed previously, cardiopulmonary exercise testing may be indicated. Box 7–4 summarizes the patterns of abnormality on exercise testing that can assist one in distinguishing cardiac from pulmonary dyspnea.

Dyspnea in Patients with a Normal Physical Examination and Physiologic Testing

It is not uncommon for patients with dyspnea to have a normal physical examination, chest radiograph, ECG, echocardiogram, and pulmonary function tests. At this point, the possibility of psychogenic dyspnea and malingering should be considered. Patients with psychogenic dyspnea include those with anxiety disorders; such patients tend to hyperventilate and view the increased ventilation as distressing. Typically, these patients have evidence of a respiratory alkalosis with low arterial carbon dioxide pressure (Pa_{CO_2}) and a normal $P_{AO_2}-Pa_{O_2}$ difference. The designation psychogenic dyspnea also includes patients who have become hypersensitive to respiratory sensations, usually after long periods of reduced physical activity. These individuals now experience the increased ventilation associated with even mild exercise as a distressing and, in their minds, abnormal sensation. Finally, some persons may complain of symptoms in an effort to gain Workers' Compensation or some other benefit. The cardiopulmonary exercise test and arterial blood gas measurements are generally quite effective at ruling out organic disease in these patients.

SPECIAL CONSIDERATIONS

Dyspnea in the Emergency Department

The approach to a patient with acute respiratory distress still includes the basic physiologic principles, essentials of history taking, and physical examination outlined previously. However, this group of patients, in addition to dyspnea, usually have symptoms such as chest pain, cough, or fever, and the differential diagnosis for shortness of breath is somewhat different (Box 7–5).

Cardiac disease, especially acute ischemia, leads the list of conditions to be considered in a patient with acute dyspnea and risk factors for coronary artery disease. Acute myocardial infarction or unstable angina is frequently associated with diaphoresis, nausea, and chest discomfort in addition to dyspnea. Physical examination may reveal an increase in pulse and blood pressure, bibasilar rales, elevated jugular venous pulsation, and S_3 or S_4 gallop. Ischemic changes on ECG are diag-

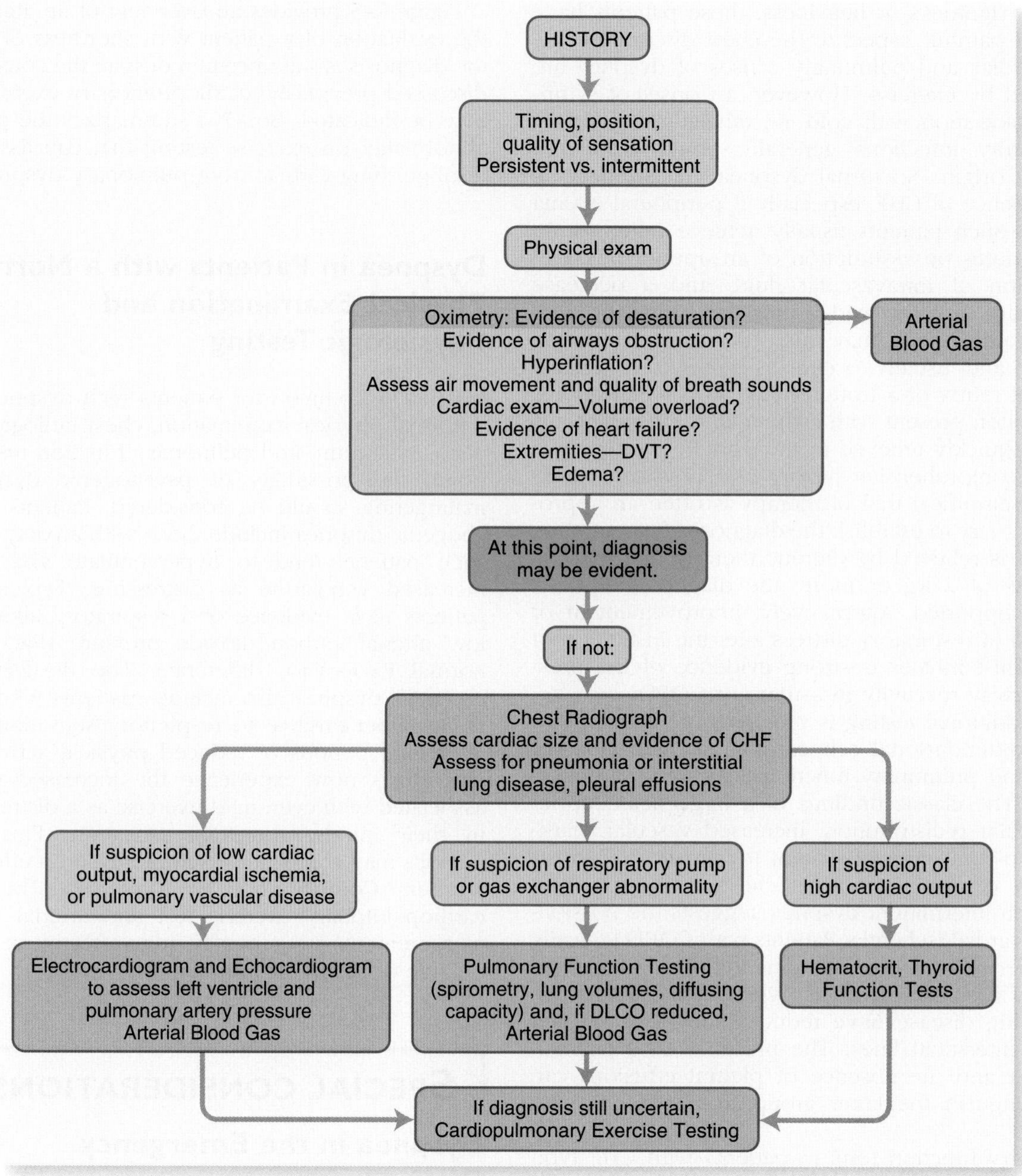

FIGURE 7–5. Algorithm for the evaluation of a patient with dyspnea. The pace and completeness with which one approaches this framework depend on the intensity and acuity of the patient's symptoms. In a patient with severe, acute dyspnea, for example, an arterial blood gas measurement may be one of the first laboratory evaluations, whereas it might not be obtained until much later in the workup of a patient with chronic breathlessness of unclear cause. A therapeutic trial of a medication, for example, a bronchodilator, may be instituted at any point if one is fairly confident of the diagnosis based on the data available at that time. CHF, congestive heart failure; DVT, deep venous thrombosis; DLCO, diffusing capacity of the lung for carbon monoxide.

nostic, as is the response to nitrate therapy. Cardiac tamponade is a much less common cause of acute dyspnea but may be seen in patients with pericarditis or malignant pericardial effusions and after chest injuries.

Respiratory system derangements associated with acute dyspnea include infections, airway obstruction, pulmonary emboli, and pneumothorax. Acute bronchitis and pneumonia are generally associated with cough, sputum, and fever and may impair gas exchange, as well as increase airway resistance. Obstruction of the upper airway, as is seen with anaphylaxis and foreign body aspiration, is often accompanied by stridor, an inspiratory sound produced by turbulent flow through a narrowed larynx or trachea as the internal diameter of the upper airway is diminished during inhalation. Additional signs of upper airway obstruction include

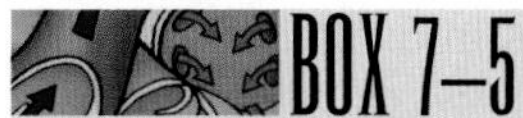 BOX 7–5

Causes of Acute Dyspnea

CARDIAC

- Myocardial ischemia
- Congestive heart failure
- Hypertensive urgency or emergency
- Cardiac tamponade

PULMONARY

- Drug overdose with hyperventilation (e.g., aspirin, ethylene glycol)
- Acute bronchitis
- Pneumothorax
- Pulmonary embolism
- Upper airway obstruction

tongue swelling, drooling, and dysphonia. Acute lower airway obstruction, such as asthma, may be seen with acute respiratory infections or after exposure to cold air or allergens.

Acute pulmonary emboli should be considered in all patients with acute dyspnea. Classic risk factors for venous thrombosis include long periods of immobilization or lower extremity trauma, as well as an underlying hypercoagulable state, as can be seen in patients with malignancy. Additional risk factors include a family history of venous thromboembolism, smoking, obesity, the use of oral contraceptives, the peripartum period, and the presence of CHF. Pleuritic chest pain is frequently present, and the ECG may demonstrate sinus tachycardia, anterior T-wave inversions, or evidence of right ventricular strain. Right ventricular dilatation on echocardiography and typical changes on pulmonary ventilation-perfusion scintigraphy are also helpful in making the diagnosis. It should be recalled that normal arterial blood gas values do not exclude the presence of an acute pulmonary embolism in a patient who otherwise has a history consistent with the condition. Approximately 10% of patients with a pulmonary embolism will have a normal PAO_2–PaO_2.

The combination of acute dyspnea and pleuritic chest pain should also raise the possibility of a pneumothorax. Spontaneous pneumothoraces may be seen in tall, thin individuals, who often have small blebs at the apices of the lung. Patients with asthma have a somewhat increased risk of spontaneous pneumothorax, as do individuals with *P. carinii* pneumonia. One must also consider this diagnosis in patients with chest trauma and acute shortness of breath.

In the emergency department setting, one must frequently initiate therapy based on incomplete data while simultaneously continuing to evaluate the patient. In a patient with COPD, for example, the superimposed diagnosis of CHF may be difficult to confirm from the physical examination and chest radiograph. The destruction of lung tissue associated with emphysema reduces the findings of rales and S_3 gallop on chest examination and may obscure vascular redistribution and increased interstitial markings on the radiograph. If the clinical story is suggestive of CHF, it is appropriate to simultaneously begin treatment of both volume overload and airway obstruction.

Dyspnea and Cough

The presence of cough along with dyspnea is most often a sign of infection, airway reactivity, or interstitial lung disease. The acute onset of cough and dyspnea, especially with associated fever and sputum production, is due almost invariably to acute bronchitis or pneumonia. A chronic productive cough in a patient with dyspnea may be an indication of bronchiectasis or, in a smoker, chronic bronchitis. A history of recurrent respiratory infections, a common occurrence in bronchiectasis, will aid in distinguishing between these two diagnoses. Dyspnea in association with a nonproductive cough is suggestive of asthma or interstitial lung disease. The dyspnea of asthma is often episodic and frequently the consequence of discrete antigenic exposure or environmental stimuli such as smoke, fumes, or cold air. In contrast, the dyspnea of interstitial lung disease is typically associated with exercise, is reproducible with a particular activity, and until the condition becomes severe, is not a problem at rest.

Dyspnea As an Anginal Equivalent

Dyspnea as an anginal equivalent should be suspected in all patients with risk factors for ischemic heart disease, including hypertension, hypercholesterolemia, a positive family history, tobacco use, and especially diabetes. Additionally, the elderly more commonly have "atypical" chest pain or dyspnea as their primary manifestation of cardiac ischemia. The pathophysiology of dyspnea in a patient with cardiac ischemia most likely relates to elevated cardiac filling pressure, which leads to an increase in alveolar and interstitial edema. It is important to realize that this edema can be due to both systolic and diastolic dysfunction inasmuch as treatment of the underlying disease process is different in these conditions.

When dyspnea is associated with wheezing, the primary differential diagnosis in any patient with risk factors for heart disease is between "cardiac asthma" and "bronchial asthma." Symptoms that may indicate a cardiac source include the onset of exertional dyspnea in a patient without underlying lung disease, PND, orthopnea, and edema, as well as a history of exertional dyspnea associated with diaphoresis, nausea, or palpitations. In patients with PND from cardiac disease, cough may be present, but it typically occurs after the development of dyspnea, in contrast to patients with lung disease, who may awaken at night because of a cough that precedes the development of dyspnea. Signs of cardiac disease may include an S_3 or S_4 gallop, especially a transient S_4 that resolves along with improvement in the dyspnea, new-onset arrhythmia, basilar rales, and elevated jugular venous pulsation. A high index of suspicion is required. Because the implications of untreated ischemia are potentially grave, further evaluation should at least include an ECG in all these patients.

Dyspnea and Diastolic Dysfunction

Approximately one third of patients with heart failure suffer from diastolic dysfunction, an abnormality of the left ventricle that leads to elevations in left ventricular end-diastolic pressure with preserved systolic function. Most of these cases are associated with chronic hypertension, aortic stenosis, or primary cardiomyopathy. Patients with diastolic dysfunction commonly have exertional dyspnea. In moderate to severe cases, the dyspnea may be pronounced after the patient walks only 50 to 100 yards. As the metabolic demands of the body increase with activity, the heart attempts to generate greater cardiac output with a combination of a larger stroke volume and higher heart rate. In a relatively stiff or poorly compliant ventricle, however, the result is an increase in left ventricular end-diastolic pressure leading to elevated pulmonary capillary pressure, interstitial edema, and shortness of breath.

In many cases, wheezing will accompany the onset of interstitial edema, and exercise-induced asthma (EIA) may be diagnosed in these patients. In contrast to diastolic dysfunction, however, EIA leads to wheezing and shortness of breath after more intense exercise, and the symptoms often develop after rather than during the exercise. The bronchospasm of EIA is believed to be the consequence of rapid changes in temperature or osmolarity in the airways, both of which require high levels of ventilation that are unlikely to be seen after walking short distances.

Dyspnea in Young Adults

Asthma is a common problem that affects approximately 5% of the population. Consequently, the development of exertional dyspnea in a young, otherwise healthy adult is assumed to be a manifestation of asthma and is treated presumptively with inhaled bronchodilators. When the symptoms do not respond to this therapy, the physician is faced with the prospect of escalating treatment or searching for an alternative explanation for the respiratory discomfort. Frequently, resting lung function and physical examination findings are normal. In the absence of symptoms that are very typical of asthma, especially a sensation of chest tightness with activity[8, 9] that is relieved with a bronchodilator, it is reasonable to stop bronchodilator therapy and perform a methacholine inhalation test to confirm or eliminate the presence of airway reactivity. As many as 80% of patients at a pulmonary unit with normal lung function and dyspnea who failed to respond to empirical treatment with bronchodilators for asthma had a negative methacholine inhalation test.[10] With this information in hand, investigation for alternative causes of dyspnea can begin.

Dyspnea and Hyperinflation

Hyperinflation, or breathing at higher lung volumes than normal, may develop in patients with expiratory airflow obstruction, whether from asthma, COPD, or CHF. Hyperinflation causes dyspnea by increasing demands on ventilatory muscles that are stressed at these lung volumes by their shortened length and by the relative stiffness of the respiratory system.[2, 11] Furthermore, the persistence of positive pressure at the end of exhalation (auto-PEEP), another consequence of hyperinflation, causes an additional load to be imposed on the inspiratory muscles. The presence of hyperinflation may be a more sensitive indicator of airflow obstruction than typical measures such as the FEV_1/forced vital capacity ratio are. The effectiveness of therapeutic interventions such as bronchodilators and continuous positive airway pressure in reducing dyspnea may be the result, in large measure, of their actions on hyperinflation and its physiologic consequences.

IMPLICATIONS FOR THERAPY

If a specific disease process can be identified as the cause of a patient's shortness of breath, one should attempt to reverse the pathologic state and alleviate the individual's breathing discomfort. Bronchodilators are administered for airway obstruction, diuretics and vasodilators are prescribed for CHF, nutritional supplementation is prescribed or blood is transfused in patients with anemia, and supplemental O_2 is given to patients with significant desaturation. However, in many cases the primary disease process may be superseded by other conditions. The physician must not assume that changes in dyspnea are necessarily due to worsening of the underlying problem. One must consider whether the patient has more than one type of dyspnea. Are the sensations qualitatively different in different conditions? Is the dyspnea experienced during respiratory infections the same as that with exercise? Only by considering the possibility of superimposed problems will one be able to find potentially reversible etiologies for the symptoms of many patients with chronic lung disease. In particular, the physician must be sensitive to the role of deconditioning in the deterioration of symptoms of individuals whose lives have become increasingly sedentary over months to years. Yes, the patient may have emphysema, and yes, the COPD may be fairly severe. However, is the COPD actually the reason that the patient is no longer able to do his own shopping? If deconditioning is identified, exercise programs may be of benefit even in patients with marked airway obstruction.

SUMMARY

Dyspnea, or shortness of breath, is a complex symptom composed of multiple, qualitatively distinct sensations. It may result from a range of cardiac and pulmonary pathophysiologic derangements. Attention to the nuances of the history and physical examination will provide considerable insight into the etiology of an individual's breathing discomfort. A focused laboratory evaluation provides the additional information needed to make a diagnosis in most cases. For more complicated cases or when it is suspected that cardiovascular problems, especially deconditioning or myocardial ischemia, are now superimposed on a chronic lung disease, cardiopulmonary exercise testing can be extremely useful.

References

1. Manning HL, Schwartzstein RM: Pathophysiology of dyspnea. N Engl J Med 1995;333:1547–1553.
2. O'Donnell DE, Bertley JC, Chau LKL, Webb KA: Qualitative aspects of exertional breathlessness in chronic airflow limitation. Am J Respir Crit Care Med 1997;155: 109–115.
3. O'Donnell DE, Hong HH, Webb KA: Respiratory sensation during chest wall restriction and dead space loading in exercising man. J Appl Physiol 2000;88: 1859–1869.
4. Nishino T, Ide T, Sudo T, Sato J: Inhaled furosemide greatly alleviates the sensation of experimentally induced dyspnea. Am J Respir Crit Care Med 2000;161:1963–1967.
5. Harver A, Mahler DA, Schwartzstein RM: Use of a descriptor model for prospective diagnosis of dyspnea. Am J Respir Crit Care Med 2000;161:A705.
6. Schwartzstein RM: The language of dyspnea. In Mahler DA (ed): Dyspnea. London, Marcel Dekker, 1998, pp 35–62.
7. Wasserman K, Hansen JE, Sue DY, et al: Principles of Exercise Testing and Interpretation. Philadelphia, Lea & Febiger, 1999.
8. Killian KJ, Watson R, Otis J, et al: Symptom perception during acute bronchoconstriction. Am J Respir Crit Care Med 2000;162:490–496.
9. Binks AP, Moosavi SH, Banzett RB, Schwartzstein RM: "Tightness" sensation of asthma does not arise from the work of breathing. Am J Respir Crit Care Med 2002;165:2–3.
10. Chevalier B, Schwartzstein R: The role of the methacholine inhalation challenge: Avoiding a misdiagnosis of asthma. J Respir Dis 2001;22:153–160.
11. Marin JM, Carrizo SJ, Gascon M, et al: Inspiratory capacity, dynamic hyperinflation, breathlessness, and exercise performance during the 6-minute-walk test in chronic obstructive pulmonary disease. Am J Respir Crit Care Med 2001;163:1395–1399.

CHAPTER 8 Approach to the Patient with Edema

Glenn M. Chertow

Edema of the lower extremities is commonly observed by the primary care physician, and it may reflect a broad spectrum of conditions. The common thread in all causes of edema is elevation of capillary pressure because of either increased venous pressure or impaired lymphatic drainage. The pathophysiology, diagnostic approach, and treatment of the various types of edema, however, are different and depend on their cause. In this chapter, the common causes of edema encountered in primary care practice are described, with a focus on differentiation between systemic edematous disorders (cardiac, hepatic, and renal diseases) and more localized disease. In addition, a practical approach to the differential diagnosis and treatment is presented.

UNILATERAL LOWER EXTREMITY EDEMA

Edema is often considered to be a sign of advanced cardiac, hepatic, or renal disease. However, in primary care practice, *unilateral* lower extremity edema is at least as common as bilateral or generalized edema, and the diagnostic approach and management of these conditions are markedly different[1,2] (Box 8–1).

A key element in the clinical evaluation of unilateral lower extremity edema is the presence or absence of pain. Painful edema points strongly to the presence of deep venous thrombosis (DVT) or a musculoskeletal disorder. DVT may involve both lower extremities, but one leg usually predominates and has clinically apparent leg swelling, erythema, and pain (see Chapter 38). Occasionally, pain is precipitated by dorsiflexion of the foot, the so-called Homans sign. Frequently, a history of trauma or immobility can be elicited. A history of DVT or neoplastic disease, particularly mucin-producing adenocarcinomas of the gastrointestinal tract (e.g., colorectal and pancreatic carcinoma, cholangiocarcinoma), should further heighten suspicion for DVT.

A tape measure is the simplest diagnostic tool for the evaluation of unilateral edema. It should be placed circumferentially around the midcalf at the same distance below the patella on each leg; marking the site may assist in serial examinations. Although normal individuals may have some variability in calf muscle size, asymmetry in circumference in excess of 1 to 2 cm is probably of clinical significance. Doppler examination is a sensitive and specific method for evaluating DVT in the thigh; it is less accurate for determining DVT in the calf. Impedance plethysmography is not commonly used because it is operator dependent and less accurate than venous ultrasonography. Although venography remains the gold standard, its disadvantages include inconvenience, need for radiocontrast, and the risk of inducing venous trauma. In nearly all clinical settings, Doppler has replaced venography as the basis for clinical decisions. A strongly positive serum test for D dimer (a fibrinogen breakdown product) can be used to support the diagnosis of DVT but is not as definitive as a Doppler study.

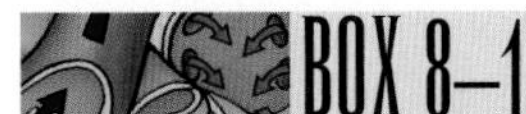
BOX 8–1

Causes of Unilateral Lower Extremity Edema

WITH PAIN
Deep venous thrombosis
Postphlebitic syndrome
Popliteal cyst rupture
Gastrocnemius rupture
Cellulitis
Psoas or other abscess

WITHOUT PAIN
Deep venous thrombosis
Postphlebitic syndrome
Other venous insufficiency
- After saphenous vein harvest
- Varicosities

Lymphatic obstruction/lymphedema
- Carcinoma, including cervical, colorectal, prostate
- Lymphoma
- Retroperitoneal fibrosis
- Sarcoidosis
- Filariasis

The *postphlebitic syndrome* is a relatively common complication after DVT. It is often associated with mild to moderate discomfort and persistent leg swelling and sometimes with pitting edema. Asymmetric painless edema of a lower extremity is often due to chronic venous insufficiency. The latter is increasingly being observed at the site of previous saphenous vein harvest as the number of patients who have undergone coronary bypass surgery grows; this form of venous insufficiency is of little clinical concern unless it causes pain or functional limitation or leads to secondary infection.

Lymphatic obstruction should be considered as a cause of lower extremity edema in patients without a history of trauma or venous system disease. Lymphatic obstruction is most commonly caused by malignant disease in the pelvis or retroperitoneum. Other causes include retroperitoneal fibrosis, either idiopathic or drug related (e.g., methysergide). The diagnosis is usually made by computed tomography with oral and intravenous contrast enhancement.

A *ruptured popliteal (Baker) cyst* is often confused with DVT. It is typically characterized by the relatively rapid development of unilateral leg edema and pain. A subtle clinical clue is the presence of petechiae around and below the lateral malleolus. Gastrocnemius rupture with local hemorrhage may also be confused with DVT and other causes of lower extremity edema. This process can result in significant pain and enlargement of the diameter of the leg, but it rarely results in edema per se. Muscle rupture is best confirmed with magnetic resonance imaging. Skin and soft tissue infections may cause edema and can occasionally be confused with DVT. Cellulitis, usually caused by gram-positive cocci that colonize the skin (e.g., *Staphylococcus, Streptococcus*), can result in unilateral leg swelling, pain with erythema that is often streaky in nature, and systemic signs and symptoms, including fever and leukocytosis.

Treatment of unilateral lower extremity edema depends on its cause. Leg elevation is often helpful, but diuretics should not be used. Anticoagulation is the cornerstone of therapy for DVT (see Chapter 38).

GENERALIZED OR BILATERAL LOWER EXTREMITY EDEMA

In ambulatory individuals, the lower extremities are the predominant site where edema accumulates because of the effects of gravity on hydrostatic pressure. Conversely, in patients who are predominantly supine throughout the day, edema is more uniformly distributed or more localized to the dependent presacral region. Distinct sites of edema (e.g., facial, upper extremity) usually indicate local vascular or lymphatic complications. Generalized edema is the result of systemic sodium retention. The three most common causes are congestive heart failure (CHF), cirrhosis, and the nephrotic syndrome (Table 8–1). Mechanisms of generalized edema include (1) an increase in capillary pressure secondary to an elevation in central venous pressure, as occurs in CHF; (2) primary renal retention of sodium and water, as occurs in primary renal disease; and (3) a reduction in cardiac output that triggers both renal vasoconstriction and activation of the renin-angiotensin-aldosterone system, each of which causes retention of sodium and water.

Heart Failure

CHF secondary to right heart failure caused by left ventricular systolic dysfunction or valvular heart disease (see Chapter 28) is the most common and well-recognized cause of generalized edema. Generalized edema occurs less frequently in patients with diastolic dysfunction. High-output CHF may also be manifested as sodium retention and edema.[2] The most common causes of the latter are anemia, thyrotoxicosis, beriberi, and large arteriovenous fistulas.

Right ventricular failure without preexisting left heart failure also frequently results in severe bilateral lower extremity edema (and occasionally ascites). Acute right ventricular failure occurs most frequently in patients with a massive pulmonary embolism (see Chapter 38) or a large right ventricular infarction, which occurs most commonly with a large inferoposterior myocardial infarction (see Chapter 27). Chronic right ventricular failure (when not secondary to left ventricular failure) occurs in the presence of severe pulmonary hypertension. Frequent causes of the latter are chronic obstructive pulmonary disease, obstructive sleep apnea, chronic pulmonary embolization, and primary pulmonary hypertension. Severe edema is a common feature of chronic constrictive pericarditis (see Chapter 35). Edema

TABLE 8–1

Principal Causes of Generalized Edema: History, Physical Examination, and Laboratory Findings

Organ System	History	Physical Examination	Laboratory Findings
Cardiac	Dyspnea with exertion prominent—often associated with orthopnea—or paroxysmal nocturnal dyspnea	Elevated jugular venous pressure, ventricular (S_3) gallop; occasionally with displaced or dyskinetic apical pulse; peripheral cyanosis, cool extremities, small pulse pressure when severe	Elevated urea nitrogen–to–creatinine ratio common; elevated uric acid; serum sodium often diminished; liver enzymes occasionally elevated with hepatic congestion
Hepatic	Dyspnea infrequent, except if associated with a significant degree of ascites; most often a history of ethanol abuse	Frequently associated with ascites; jugular venous pressure usually normal or low; blood pressure typically lower than in renal or cardiac disease; one or more additional signs of chronic liver disease (jaundice, palmar erythema, Dupuytren's contracture, spider angiomas, male gynecomastia or testicular atrophy, caput medusae); asterixis and other signs of encephalopathy may be present	If severe, reductions in serum albumin, cholesterol, other hepatic proteins (transferrin, fibrinogen); liver enzymes may or may not be elevated, depending on the cause and acuity of the liver injury; tendency toward hypokalemia, respiratory alkalosis; magnesium and phosphorus often markedly reduced if associated with ongoing ethanol intake; uric acid typically low; macrocytosis from folate deficiency
Renal	Usually chronic; associated with uremic signs and symptoms, including decreased appetite, altered (metallic or fishy) taste, altered sleep pattern, difficulty concentrating, restless legs or myoclonus; dyspnea can be present, but is generally less prominent than in heart failure	Blood pressure often high; hypertensive or diabetic retinopathy in selected cases; nitrogenous fetor; periorbital edema may predominate; pericardial friction rub in advanced cases with uremia	Elevation of serum creatinine and urea nitrogen most prominent; also frequent hyperkalemia, metabolic acidosis, hyperphosphatemia, hypocalcemia, anemia (usually normocytic)

S_3, third heart sound.

of cardiac origin is generally accompanied by elevated jugular venous pressure, which is usually detectable on physical examination (see Chapter 3).

Hepatic Cirrhosis

Cirrhosis is the end result of a variety of chronic liver diseases, of which Laënnec's cirrhosis (alcoholic liver disease) is the most common. Edema is a hallmark of decompensated cirrhosis, although the mechanisms of edema formation are still open to debate. Edema of hepatic origin tends to be localized to the lower extremities and the abdominal cavity (ascites), depending on the severity of portal hypertension. Central venous pressure is rarely increased in the absence of concomitant cardiac disease. Other physical findings, such as jaundice and palmar erythema, and abnormal liver function tests can be used to support the diagnosis of cirrhosis.

Nephrotic Syndrome

Nephrotic syndrome is defined as the presence of urinary protein excretion rates in excess of 3.0 g/day, complicated by generalized edema, severe hypoalbuminemia, hypercholesterolemia, and a hypercoagulable state. The hypercholesterolemia involves primarily low-density lipoprotein, which increases the risk of accelerated atherosclerosis. The hypercoagulable state is attributable to renal loss of antithrombin III and other inhibitors of the coagulation cascade and can lead to renal vein thrombosis and pulmonary embolism.

The most common causes of nephrotic syndrome in adults include membranous nephropathy, diabetic nephropathy, focal segmental glomerulosclerosis, human immunodeficiency virus (HIV)-associated nephropathy, diabetic nephropathy, minimal change disease, and multiple myeloma (and other plasma cell dyscrasias, including primary amyloid). Patients with diabetic nephropathy have an increased risk of atherosclerotic vascular complications (e.g., myocardial infarction, stroke) when compared with diabetics without nephropathy. In these patients, it is advisable to use lipid-lowering therapy with 3-hydroxy-3-methylglutaryl coenzyme A (HMG-CoA) reductase inhibitors to lower cholesterol levels. Patients with proteinuria usually benefit from the use of angiotensin-converting enzyme (ACE) inhibitors,[3] angiotensin receptor antagonists, or both classes of drugs.[4] The dose may be titrated to the degree of urinary protein excretion. Some patients with nephrotic syndrome (e.g., approximately 50% of those with membranous nephropathy) will not respond to these agents. Although nonsteroidal anti-inflammatory drugs (NSAIDs) and cyclosporine have been used to reduce proteinuria in selected individuals with nephrotic syndrome, the nephrotoxicity of these agents limits their effectiveness.

Drug-Induced Edema

NSAIDs are the most commonly used agents that promote edema formations.[5] Salt and water retention are primarily due to constriction of the renal microvasculature. In addition to causing edema, NSAIDs can counteract the effects of various antihypertensive agents, including diuretics, and thereby complicate the management of hypertension.

Several commonly prescribed antihypertensive agents have been linked to the development of edema (Box 8–2). The first-generation calcium channel antagonists verapamil, diltiazem, and nifedipine have been reported to cause edema in up to 5% to 10% of patients. The incidence of edema with longer-acting agents such as amlodipine is somewhat lower. Although the exact mechanism or mechanisms are unknown, enhanced renal sodium and water reabsorption related to a reflex sympathetic response and blunting of postural skin vasoconstriction (an effect that limits fluid extravasation when standing) appear most likely. Direct-acting vasodilators used in the treatment of hypertension or CHF, such as hydralazine, minoxidil, and nitroglycerin, may cause edema and require the initiation or intensification of a diuretic regimen. Usually, the edema associated with calcium antagonists and vasodilators (including alpha-adrenergic antagonists frequently prescribed for benign prostatic hypertrophy) can be managed with low to moderate doses of thiazide diuretics, which are also useful adjuncts in the management of hypertension. The concurrent use of ACE inhibitors can reduce the edema caused by calcium antagonists.[6]

Adrenal corticosteroids and sex hormones are two other classes of drugs that promote salt and water retention and edema formation. Hydrocortisone and, to a lesser extent, prednisone and methylprednisolone promote sodium retention via their effects on the aldosterone-sensitive sodium channel in the cortical collecting duct of the nephron. Mild degrees of hypokalemia and metabolic alkalosis may also accompany their use.

BOX 8–2

Drugs Associated with Edema Formation

- Nonsteroidal anti-inflammatory drugs
- Antihypertensive agents
  - Direct arterial/arteriolar vasodilators
    - Minoxidil
    - Hydralazine
    - Clonidine
    - Methyldopa
    - Guanethidine
  - Calcium channel antagonists
  - Alpha-adrenergic antagonists
- Steroid hormones
  - Corticosteroids
  - Anabolic steroids
  - Estrogens
  - Progestins
- Cyclosporine
- Growth hormone
- Immunotherapy
  - Interleukin-2
  - OKT3 monoclonal antibody
- Gene therapy (vascular endothelial growth factor)

APPROACH TO PATIENTS WITH EDEMA

An edematous patient who initially seeks medical care from a primary care physician poses several important challenges. First, it is essential to ensure that the edema is not a sign of a life-threatening condition, such as acute CHF. A careful, directed clinical examination and electrocardiogram are most useful (Fig. 8–1).

The History

The history provides most of the diagnostic clues. Queries should focus on the *five Ds* of edema: distribution (unilateral or bilateral), duration (acute or chronic), degree (severity), dolor (pain), and associated diseases (heart disease, liver disease, renal disease, diabetes, cancer, arthritis, thromboembolism). It should first be determined whether the edema is unilateral or bilateral and, next, whether it is painful or pain free.

Most patients with *unilateral* leg edema should have lower extremity Doppler studies to exclude DVT, unless an alternative diagnosis can easily be established by the history and physical examination. A more extensive evaluation may be required in a patient with a history of abdominal or pelvic malignancy. If the patient has not undergone routine health maintenance checks, a digital rectal examination and bimanual pelvic examination should be performed. If malignancy is suspected as the cause of lower extremity edema, pelvic ultrasonography or computed tomography is usually indicated to investigate possible abnormalities in the retroperitoneal space.

In the presence of *bilateral* edema, a broader differential diagnosis should be entertained, and a detailed history is likely to help narrow the differential. Symptoms of CHF (e.g., exertional dyspnea, orthopnea, paroxysmal nocturnal dyspnea, nocturia) and a history of valvular heart disease or myocardial infarction should be carefully sought because they point to cardiac

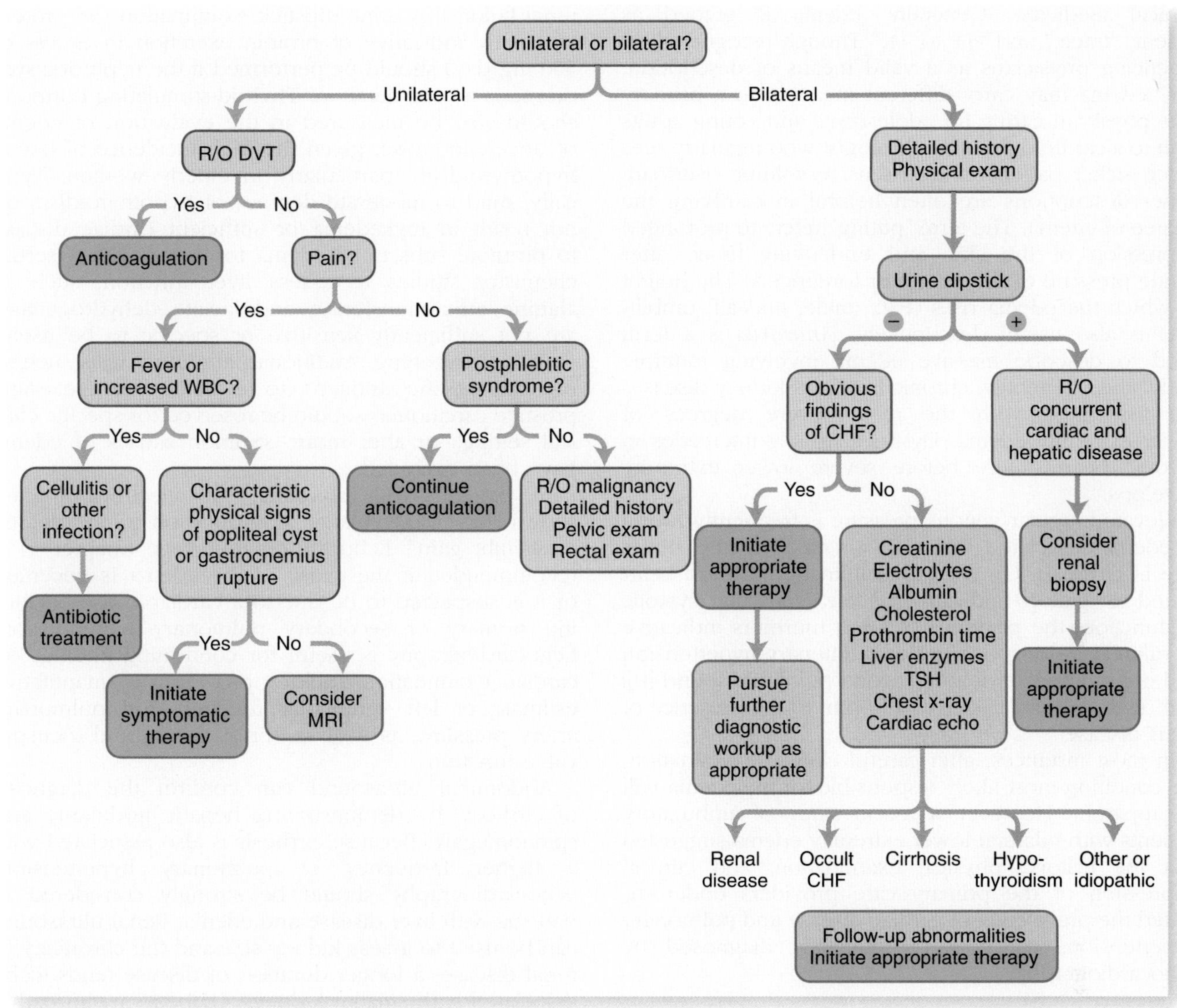

FIGURE 8–1. Diagnostic approach to patients with edema. CHF, congestive heart failure; DVT, deep venous thrombosis; MRI, magnetic resonance imaging; R/O, rule out; TSH, thyroid-stimulating hormone; WBC, white blood cell count.

disease as the probable cause of the edema. Edema may be bilateral and asymmetric as a result of either changes in body position (increased edema on dependent sides) or a combination of factors (e.g., fluid retention secondary to heart failure in the presence of impaired venous drainage unilaterally after harvesting of the saphenous vein).

The duration of edema aids in the differential diagnosis. Long-standing, gradually worsening lower extremity edema is often a sign of chronic heart or liver disease or chronic renal insufficiency. Many causes of nephrotic syndrome (e.g., minimal change disease, focal sclerosis, membranous nephropathy) are typically manifested as sudden edema (often periorbital and elsewhere), and patients can often state the day on which the edema first appeared. The duration of edema can also help differentiate the cause and location of venous and lymphatic obstruction. For example, bilateral edema secondary to retroperitoneal lymphadenopathy will typically lead to gradually worsening edema, whether unilateral or bilateral. By comparison, the edema associated with DVT tends to be more acute in onset.

A history of alcohol abuse or hepatitis or symptoms of active hepatitis (e.g., jaundice, nausea) suggests the possibility of liver disease as a cause of edema. A history of renal disease or a change in the frequency or nature of urinary output (e.g., hematuria, "foamy" urine) suggests a renal cause for the edema. A history of symptoms of thyroid disease should also be elicited. Finally, a detailed drug and dietary history is important for diagnostic clues and also for designing a therapeutic regimen.

Physical Examination

The grading of edema ("degree") is among the most common examples of semiquantitative descriptions in clinical medicine. Generally, edema is graded as absent, "trace," and "1+ to 4+." Though recognized by practicing physicians as a valid means of description, "2+" edema may carry different meaning to a primary care physician caring for adolescents and young adults than to a cardiologist or nephrologist who regularly sees older, sicker patients with extensive volume overload. Other descriptions are often helpful in clarifying the degree of edema. The term "pitting" refers to prolonged depression of the skin and underlying tissue after gentle pressure of the thumb or forefingers. The height to which the edema rises (e.g., ankle, midcalf, umbilicus) is also useful descriptively. *Anasarca* is a term used to describe massive edema involving multiple body sites. Generally, chronic liver and kidney diseases are associated with the most severe degrees of lower extremity edema. Dyspnea usually intercedes in chronic heart failure before severe lower extremity develops.

Elevated jugular venous pressure is frequently found in edema associated with CHF or renal disease but is rare in cirrhosis. On cardiac examination, a third heart sound (S_3 gallop) indicative of left ventricular systolic dysfunction, the presence of heart murmurs indicative of valvular lesions, or signs of pulmonary hypertension and cor pulmonale (a loud second pulmonic sound [P_2] and right ventricular heave) all point to the presence of heart disease.

In most instances, after careful clinical examination, the condition most likely responsible for the edema will be apparent. However, a recent study of ambulatory patients with bilateral lower extremity edema suggested that the history, physical examination, and clinical impression of the primary care providers underestimated the prevalence of cardiac disease and pulmonary hypertension, which were ultimately diagnosed by echocardiography.[7]

Laboratory Studies

After a careful history and physical examination, several screening laboratory studies are advisable (Box 8–3): serum sodium (low values may occur with CHF, cirrhosis, or hypothyroidism), serum albumin (extremely low values [<2.0 g/dL] are seen with nephrotic syndrome; moderate reductions [2.5 to 3.5 g/dL] are often seen with cirrhosis), and serum creatinine (elevated in renal failure). A urine dipstick examination (3+ protein is usually indicative of protein excretion in excess of 500 mg/day) should be performed if the nephrotic syndrome is a consideration. Thyroid-stimulating hormone should also be measured in the evaluation of edema of uncertain cause, given the high incidence of occult hypothyroidism, particularly in elderly women. Typically, mild to moderate degrees of hypothyroidism do not result in myxedema or sufficient cardiac disease to promote substantial edema formation. Other serum chemistry studies to assess liver function, such as alanine aminotransferase and lactate dehydrogenase, are not sufficiently sensitive or specific to be useful on initial screening. Additional laboratory tests such as prostate-specific antigen (to evaluate for metastatic prostate carcinoma) should be reserved for specific clinical settings or after more common causes of edema have been excluded.

In patients with anasarca, the electrocardiogram shows decreased voltage in proportion to the degree of weight gain.[8] Echocardiography (see Chapter 5) is recommended if the cause of the edema is uncertain or it is suspected to be due to a cardiac cause, including primary or secondary pulmonary hypertension. Echocardiography is useful for confirming findings on cardiac examination and for providing a quantitative estimate of left ventricular function and pulmonary artery pressure, as well as aortic, mitral, and tricuspid valve function.

Abdominal ultrasound can confirm the diagnosis of cirrhosis by demonstrating hepatic nodularity and splenomegaly. Because cirrhosis is also associated with a higher frequency of pulmonary hypertension, echocardiography should be strongly considered in patients with liver disease and edema. Renal ultrasound can be used to assess kidney size and the chronicity of renal disease; a longer duration of disease tends to be associated with smaller kidneys. Diabetic nephropathy, amyloid, and HIV-associated nephropathy are exceptions to this rule because affected kidneys tend to be large and to remain so through most of the clinical course.

In primary care practice, bilateral lower extremity edema is usually due to cardiac or pulmonary disease or to venous insufficiency (Table 8–2). Even after complete evaluation, 25% to 30% of patients may have idiopathic edema.[7]

BOX 8–3

Recommended Laboratory Screening Studies for Outpatients with Edema

Serum sodium
Serum albumin
Serum creatinine
Urine dipstick
Thyroid-stimulating hormone

TREATMENT

Patients with chronic or bilateral edema can often be managed on an ambulatory basis with dietary counseling, intensification of oral diuretic therapy, or modification of other medications (e.g., vasodilators), without requiring hospitalization. However, acute worsening of edema may represent progression of the underlying disease state (e.g., the development of myocardial ischemia in the presence of left ventricular dysfunction or the occurrence of spontaneous bacterial peritonitis in the presence of cirrhosis), which should be carefully

TABLE 8–2

Final Diagnoses for 45 Patients with Bilateral Leg Edema after Laboratory Investigation

Diagnosis*	Number (%)
Cardiac diagnosis	
Left ventricular systolic dysfunction	8 (18)
Right ventricular systolic dysfunction	1 (2)
Diastolic dysfunction	4 (9)
Mitral regurgitation	1 (2)
Aortic stenosis	1 (2)
Atrial septal defect	1 (2)
Atrial fibrillation	2 (4)
Pulmonary diagnosis[†]	
Pulmonary hypertension (>40 mm Hg)	9 (20)
Borderline pulmonary hypertension (31–40 mm Hg)	10 (22)
Venous insufficiency	10 (22)
Nephrotic syndrome	1 (2)
Transient renal disease	1 (2)
Proteinuria (>1 g but <3 g/day)	6 (13)
Hypoalbuminemia	1 (2)
Lymphedema	1 (2)
Stenosis of the inferior vena cava	1 (2)
Use of an NSAID (definite)	1 (2)
Use of a corticosteroid or NSAID (probable cause)	6 (13)
Idiopathic (none of the above)	12 (27)

*Patients could have more than one diagnosis.

[†]Nine of these patients also had cardiac diagnoses.

NSAID, nonsteroidal anti-inflammatory drug.

From Blankfield RP, Finkelhor RS, Alexander JJ, et al: Etiology and diagnosis of bilateral leg edema in primary care. Am J Med 1998;105:194.

investigated by clinical and laboratory examination during outpatient evaluation and which might lead to a need for hospitalization.

Dietary Modifications

Sodium restriction is the principal dietary intervention for generalized edema, irrespective of its cause. Sodium restriction may be effective by itself, but it is generally used in conjunction with diuretic therapy.

Daily intake of sodium should be restricted to less than 3 g, a goal that can be accomplished by eliminating the salt shaker from the table. Restriction to below 2 g, which requires the elimination of salt in cooking as well, may be of additional benefit. Further reduction requires foods low in sodium content, but the poor palatability of such a diet makes adherence and maintenance far less likely. It is important to advise patients to avoid the use of canned or other prepared foods, particularly soups and canned vegetables.

Stringent water restriction (<1 L/day) is typically reserved for patients with dilutional hyponatremia associated with advanced CHF or hepatic cirrhosis. Modest water restriction (1 to 2 L/day) may be of some benefit in other cases.

Changes in Body Position

In the supine position, venous pressure in the lower extremities is reduced, and as a result, interstitial fluid is redistributed into the intravascular compartment, where it can be moved away from the edematous site. Like dietary sodium restriction, bedrest in the supine position or prolonged leg elevation can be moderately effective in the treatment of CHF and other edematous states, and these positional changes also enhance the more powerful action of diuretics.

Diuretics

Diuretics (Table 8–3) remain the cornerstone of treatment of edema (Fig. 8–2). Three classes of diuretics are widely used: thiazides, loop diuretics, and potassium-sparing agents.

Thiazides

The thiazide diuretics, alone or in combination with distal tubule or potassium-sparing diuretics, are among the most frequently prescribed drugs, both for the treatment of essential hypertension (see Chapter 19) and in the management of edema. Thiazides are well absorbed, have a peak onset of action between 2 and 6 hours, and have a duration of action between 12 and 24 hours or more, thereby allowing once-daily administration. Like loop diuretics (see later), thiazides are less effective in patients with renal insufficiency.

The site of action of thiazides is the distal convoluted tubule. In contrast to loop diuretics, thiazides exert no effect on the tonicity of the renal medulla and therefore do not impair the capacity to concentrate urine. Patients with renal hypoperfusion from moderate or severe CHF or cirrhosis may have elevated levels of vasopressin, and the use of a thiazide as the only diuretic can lead to hyponatremia.

The recommended dose of thiazide diuretics is now the equivalent of 6.25 to 25 mg/day of hydrochlorothiazide. Higher doses exert marginal natriuretic and antihypertensive effects while increasing the incidence and severity of a variety of metabolic complications, including hypokalemia, hypomagnesemia, hypochloremic metabolic alkalosis, hyperuricemia, and hyperglycemia.

Loop Diuretics

Loop diuretics (e.g., furosemide, bumetanide, ethacrynic acid, and torsemide) are so named because their action is localized to the thick ascending limb of the loop of Henle. The onset of action of loop diuretics is rapid, within 5 minutes when given intravenously and within 30 to 60 minutes when given by mouth. Their duration of action is relatively short (6 to 8 hours, somewhat longer with torsemide), so twice-daily doses are required in most patients for optimal benefit. When compared with thiazide diuretics, loop diuretics are

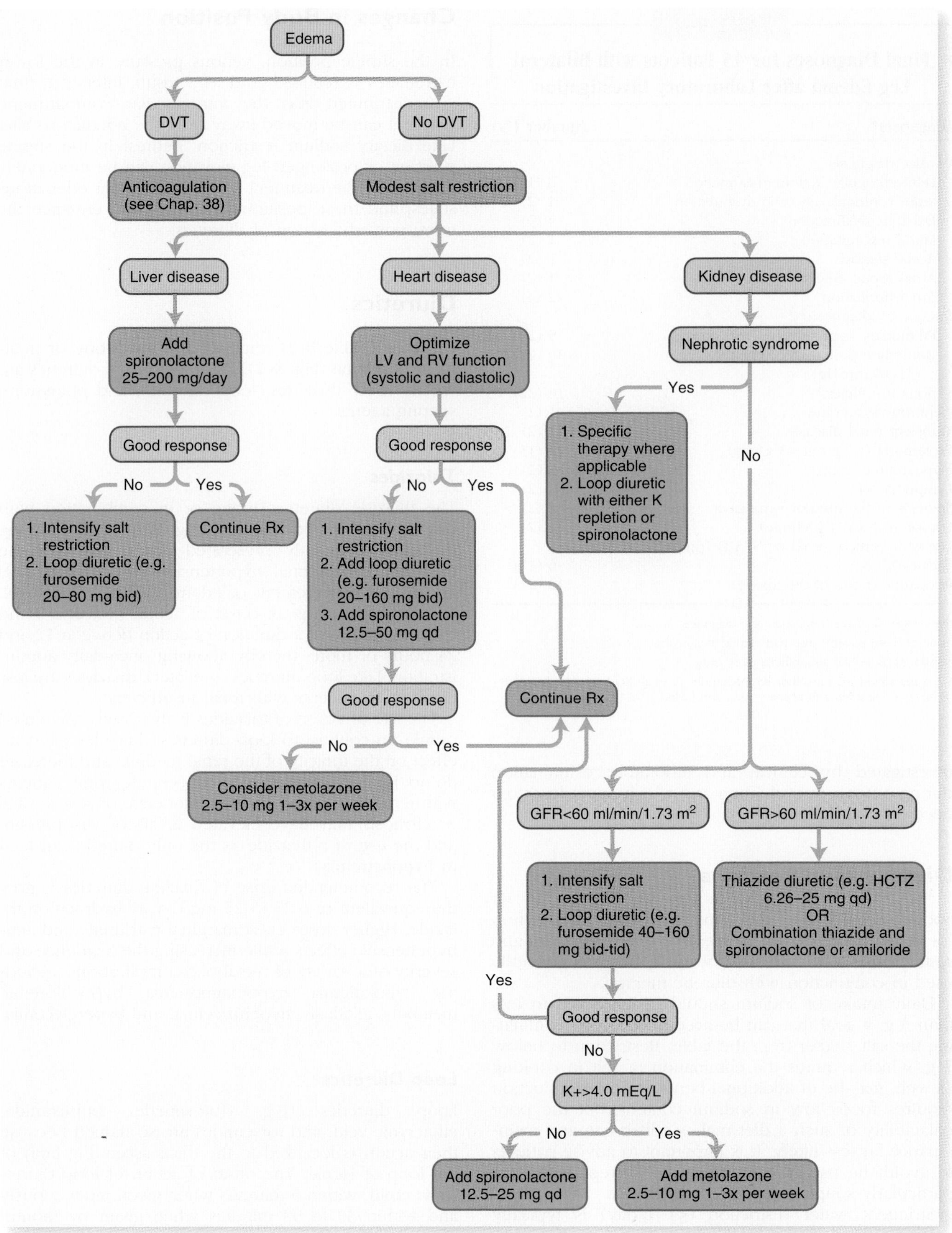

FIGURE 8–2. Therapeutic approach to patients with edema. *Amiloride may be substituted in patients with side effects from spironolactone. DVT, deep venous thrombosis; GFR, glomerular filtration rate; HCTZ, hydrochlorothiazide; K, potassium; LV, left ventricular; RV, right ventricular; Rx, treatment.

TABLE 8–3

Some Commonly Used Diuretic Agents

Drug	Site	Dose	Frequency of Administration	Potency	Comments*
Furosemide	THAL	20–160 mg	Usually bid, qd to qid in some instances	++++	Most commonly used loop diuretic agents; PO dose is 2–3 times the equivalent IV dose; half-life prolonged with renal insufficiency and heart failure
Bumetanide	THAL	1–5 mg	Usually bid, qd to qid in some instances	++++	Higher cost than furosemide but similar therapeutic profile; half-life not prolonged in patients with renal insufficiency
Ethacrynic acid	THAL	50–100 mg	Usually bid, qd to qid in some instances	++++	Highest risk is ototoxicity; occasionally used in patients with allergic reaction to other loop diuretics
Torsemide	THAL	20–100 mg	qd to bid	++++	Longest-acting loop diuretic
HCTZ	DCT	6.25–25 mg	qd	++	Prototype thiazide agent, effective at doses as low as 6.25 mg; half-life prolonged with renal insufficiency and heart failure
Chlorthalidone	DCT	6.25–25 mg	qd	++	Commonly used, similar to HCTZ
Indapamide	DCT	1.25–5 mg	qd	++	Reported to cause less hyperlipidemia than other thiazides
Metolazone	DCT ± PCT	2.5–10 mg	1–3×/wk	+++	Potent agent, distal and proximal tubular activity; effective even at very low GFR
Acetazolamide	PCT	125–250 mg	bid	+	Weak diuretic, leads to hypokalemia and metabolic acidosis; occasionally used in glaucoma and refractory seizure disorders and to alkalinize urine
Spironolactone	CCD	12.5–200 mg	qod to qd	+	Long half-life because of active metabolites; half-life prolonged with renal insufficiency; antidrogen side effects; promotes hyperkalemia and mild metabolic effects; promotes acidosis
Amiloride	CCD	2.5–10 mg	qd to bid	+	Well tolerated; promotes hyperkalemia and mild metabolic acidosis; half-life prolonged with renal insufficiency; preferred over triamterene
Triamterene	CCD	37.5 mg	qd (in combination with HCTZ)	+	Extremely weak diuretic; rarely used
Dopamine	PCT, VASC	0.5–2.5 μg/kg/min	IV drip	++	Promotes natriuresis; may increase renal blood flow; widely used in critically ill patients

*Thiazide class effects: hypokalemia, hypomagnesemia, hyponatremia, hyperuricemia, hypochloremic metabolic alkalosis, hyperglycemia, hypercalcemia, hyperlipidemia. Loop diuretic class effects: hypokalemia, hypomagnesemia, hypochloremic metabolic alkalosis, hypocalcemia, hyperuricemia, hyperglycemia, hypercholesterolemia.

CCD, cortical collecting duct; DCT, distal convoluted tubule; GFR, glomerular filtration rate; HCTZ, hydrochlorothiazide; PCT, proximal convoluted tubule; THAL, thick ascending limb of loop of Henle; VASC, vascular.

more potent (i.e., they promote a larger and more brisk natriuresis) and are better suited for the treatment of edematous disorders. Furthermore, these drugs exert a direct venodilatory effect, which provides additional relief in the acute management of pulmonary edema. However, because of their rapid and powerful diuretic effects, loop diuretics may induce a number of electrolyte abnormalities, including hypokalemia, hypomagnesemia, hypochloremic metabolic alkalosis, and hypocalcemia. Hyperuricemia, hyperglycemia, and hyponatremia occur less frequently than with thiazides.

A low dose of furosemide (e.g., 20 mg/day) is appropriate in patients with edema from CHF despite moderate dietary sodium restriction. Escalating doses (particularly if CHF is accompanied by renal insufficiency) to as high as 320 mg/day (in divided doses) may be required. If symptoms persist despite such large doses, causes of diuretic resistance should be considered (Box 8–4; see also later discussion). Torsemide may provide more reliable gastrointestinal absorption and hence more reliable dosing in patients with advanced CHF.[9]

Diuretics Acting on the Distal Tubule (Potassium-Sparing Diuretics)

Spironolactone, amiloride, and triamterene, the three major drugs in this class, are weak diuretics when administered alone but are valuable in treating edema when used in combination with thiazide or loop diuretics. These agents are effective in augmenting sodium excretion in cases of edema refractory to a single agent, and by their potassium- and magnesium-retentive prop-

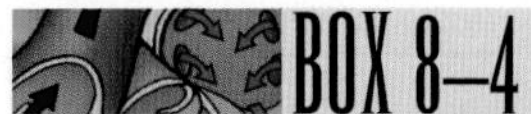

BOX 8–4

Potential Causes of (Loop) Diuretic Resistance

Excessive dietary sodium intake
Profound renal hypoperfusion (e.g., heart failure, cirrhosis, renovascular disease)
Renal insufficiency
Distal nephron hypertrophy with chronic use
Diminished intestinal absorption
Severe hypoalbuminemia
Mineralocorticoid excess

erties, they may abrogate the most serious electrolyte disturbances caused by thiazide or loop diuretic agents when the latter are prescribed alone.

The pharmacokinetics and side effects of this class of diuretics differ considerably; spironolactone may cause gynecomastia and other effects related to its steroid structure, and it has a longer duration of action (24 to 48 hours) than amiloride (12 to 24 hours); the latter is better tolerated. Triamterene is rarely used given its low potency and risk of side effects.

Spironolactone is useful in patients who have edema caused by advanced hepatic cirrhosis and who are in a state of intense stimulation of the renin-angiotensin-aldosterone system. In contrast to loop diuretics, the reduction in plasma volume induced by spironolactone is gradual and less likely to provoke worsening renal function. Moreover, the attenuation of kaliuresis helps prevent exacerbation of hepatic encephalopathy. The major adverse effect of this diuretic class is hyperkalemia, particularly in the presence of renal dysfunction, diabetes, and coadministration of ACE inhibitors and angiotensin receptor antagonists.

When prescribing potassium-sparing diuretics to patients with edematous disorders, the drugs should be started at low doses and gradually escalated to avoid hyperkalemia. In patients with CHF, spironolactone should be considered the potassium-sparing diuretic of choice. When added to a regimen of ACE inhibitors, loop diuretics, and digoxin, low-dose spironolactone (e.g., 25 mg every other day to daily) reduced mortality by 30% in comparison to placebo.[10]

Diuretic Resistance

One or more of the factors listed in Box 8–4 are usually found in patients whose generalized edema cannot be controlled because of resistance to diuretics. The most important of these factors is *excessive dietary sodium intake*. Although most patients with edematous disorders are instructed to limit their sodium intake, the prescription of diuretic agents and the brisk urine output that can ensue after their initiation often provide a false sense of security that leads to liberalization of the diet. This problem can be particularly troublesome with the once-daily use of a short-acting loop diuretic such as furosemide. In this case, patients may have 4 to 6 hours of negative fluid balance, with avid sodium retention during the remainder of the day, thereby leading to recurrent edema. *Severe renal hypoperfusion*, as occurs in advanced CHF, cirrhosis, and renovascular disease and with NSAID therapy, is another cause of diuretic resistance.

Renal insufficiency also often results in diuretic resistance because the reduction in glomerular filtration leads to reduced delivery of drug to the site of action within the tubular lumen. Therefore, progressively higher doses of diuretics are required in patients with advancing renal insufficiency. Oral thiazides (with the exception of metolazone) are generally ineffective in patients with glomerular filtration rates less than 30 to 40 mL/min.

A third common cause of diuretic resistance in the presence of chronic use of a loop diuretic is *hypertrophy of the distal nephron*. The adaptation to a sustained reduction in plasma volume is upregulation of the sodium-retentive effects of the distal nephron. This phenomenon has been confirmed pathologically and serves as the physiologic basis for sequential nephron blockade.

Decreased gastrointestinal absorption of diuretics, as occurs in the presence of bowel wall edema, may further limit active drug delivery. *States of relative mineralocorticoid excess* (including Cushing's syndrome and the pharmacologic use of prednisone or hydrocortisone) may lead to diuretic resistance by increasing sodium reabsorption in the distal nephron. If withdrawal of these drugs is not possible, the addition of amiloride or spironolactone to furosemide may be helpful. Finally, moderate to severe degrees of hypoalbuminemia may impede the response to furosemide therapy.

Diuretic resistance can often be overcome by withdrawal of the offending agents and strict adherence to a low sodium diet or an increase in the dose or frequency of the diuretic administered (to two to four times daily). If these measures are ineffective, sequential nephron blockade, produced by a combination of furosemide or bumetanide with metolazone (5 to 10 mg one to three times per week), may be the most effective means of overcoming diuretic resistance. This combination is particularly effective in patients with chronic exposure to loop diuretics, in whom sodium retention in the distal nephron is enhanced and who are therefore more sensitive to metolazone or another thiazide. In this setting, close monitoring of electrolyte and acid-base status is essential because of the risk of hypokalemia and hypochloremic alkalosis. The addition of amiloride or spironolactone to a loop diuretic may also be extremely effective. The concomitant use of ACE inhibitors may preclude the use of potassium-sparing diuretics because of the risk of hyperkalemia. Occasionally, triple combinations (a loop diuretic, metolazone, and a distal, potassium-sparing diuretic) are used in refractory patients, provided that close monitoring of volume status and plasma chemistry values is possible.

Patients most likely to benefit from continuous intravenous infusion of a loop diuretic are those with chronic exposure to a loop diuretic (e.g., patients with class III and IV CHF) or renal insufficiency. The use of a large bolus dose of furosemide (120 to 240 mg) followed by a continuous infusion (5 to 30 mg/hr) appears to be well tolerated and effective in the treatment of refractory edema.

Administration of albumin is useful in the treatment of edema associated with severe hypoalbuminemia (<2.5 g/dL), including the edema associated with nephrotic syndrome. Delivery of furosemide to the active luminal site of the nephron is reduced in this condition because furosemide is highly protein (albumin) bound. If albumin (12.5 to 25 g) is administered along with furosemide, more of the latter can be delivered to the active site, thereby resulting in augmentation of the diuresis.

In the most extreme cases of diuretic resistance, dialysis may be required for relief of congestive symptoms. Although peritoneal dialysis and hemodialysis have proved effective in individuals with diuretic resistance and edema caused by advanced renal and "cardiorenal" disease, dialysis tends to be extremely poorly tolerated in individuals with advanced cirrhosis and diuretic resistance.

REFERRAL: WHEN AND TO WHOM?

A large majority of patients with edema initially seek medical assistance from their primary care physician, who can implement the strategy outlined previously in a cost-effective manner. Referral to a specialist is advisable for patients in whom the cause of the underlying condition remains obscure or in whom it is far advanced, such as severe CHF. Similarly, patients with chronic liver disease can usually be well managed by generalists, unless and until complications ensue. Patients with edema from nephrotic syndrome or chronic renal failure should be referred to nephrologists.

Patients with edema secondary to DVT do not generally require referral to a specialist unless the episodes are recurrent or they have a strong positive family history, which raises the possibility of an inherited hematologic disorder (e.g., antithrombin III, protein C or S, or factor V Leiden deficiency). Patients suspected of having edema secondary to advanced malignancy (leading to either lymphatic obstruction or a hypercoagulable state) may benefit from chemotherapy, radiotherapy, or debulking procedures, depending on the type and extent of tumor, and they generally warrant consultation with an oncologist.

Evidence-Based Summary

- **Unilateral edema, especially with pain, should prompt a thorough evaluation for thromboembolism. Edema related to systemic disease (cardiac, renal, or hepatic) is usually bilateral.[2]**
- **Cardiac causes of edema, including pulmonary hypertension and obstructive sleep apnea, may be underrecognized solely by relying on the initial history and physical examination. Echocardiography may be a useful adjunct in the differential diagnosis of bilateral edema, especially in older individuals.[7]**
- **Dietary salt restriction is a cornerstone of therapy for most causes of edema. For individuals who fail to respond adequately to dietary salt restriction, a thiazide diuretic (e.g., hydrochlorothiazide, 6.25 to 25 mg/day) is first-line therapy. Loop diuretics (usually in two to three divided doses) are generally more effective for individuals with CHF or renal insufficiency. Spironolactone may be the safest and most effective diuretic agent for persons with ascites and edema related to chronic liver disease, and it appears to improve survival in patients with CHF.[10]**

References

1. Merli GJ, Spandorfer J: The outpatient with unilateral leg swelling. Med Clin North Am 1995;79:435–447.
2. Schrier RW: Pathogenesis of sodium and water retention in high-output and low-output cardiac failure, nephrotic syndrome, cirrhosis, and pregnancy. N Engl J Med 1989; 319:1127–1134.
3. Ruggenenti P, Perna A, Gherardi G, et al: Renoprotective properties of ACE-inhibition in non-diabetic nephro-pathies with non-nephrotic proteinuria. Lancet 1999;354: 359–364.
4. Lewis EJ, Hunsicker LG, Clarke WR, et al: Renoprotective effect of the angiotensin-receptor antagonist irbesartan in patients with nephropathy due to type 2 diabetes. N Engl J Med 2001;345:851–860.
5. Frishman WH: Effects of nonsteroidal anti-inflammatory drug therapy on blood pressure and peripheral edema. Am J Cardiol 2002;89:18D-25D.
6. Pedrinelli R, Dell'Omo G, Melillo E, Mariani M: Amlodipine, enalapril, and dependent leg edema in essential hypertension. Hypertension 2000;35:621–625.
7. Blankfield RP, Finkelhor RS, Alexander JJ, et al: Etiology and diagnosis of bilateral leg edema in primary care. Am J Med 1998;105:192–197.
8. Madias JE, Bazaz R, Agarwal H, et al: Anasarca-mediated attenuation of the amplitude of electrocardiogram complexes: A description of a heretofore unrecognized phenomenon. J Am Coll Cardiol 2001;38:756–764.
9. Murray M, Deer M, Ferguson J, et al: Open label randomized trial of torsemide compared with furosemide therapy for patients with heart failure. Am J Med 2001;111: 513–520.
10. Pitt B, Zannad F, Remme WJ, et al: The effect of spironolactone on morbidity and mortality in patients with severe heart failure. Randomized Aldactone Evaluation Study Investigators. N Engl J Med 1999;341:709–717.

CHAPTER 9 Approach to the Patient with Palpitations

Mark A. Hlatky

Palpitations are common[1, 2] and are defined as an uncomfortable awareness of one's heartbeat. It is important to recognize that although palpitations and arrhythmias are closely related phenomena, they are quite distinct concepts.[2, 3] A patient can have an "uncomfortable awareness" of normal sinus rhythm or sinus tachycardia because of anxiety or a particularly forceful contraction of the heart.[4] Conversely, cardiac arrhythmias may be asymptomatic or may cause symptoms such as dizziness, syncope, shortness of breath, fatigue, or chest pain instead of palpitations. Palpitations and arrhythmias are closely related phenomena, but they are not synonymous.

Cardiac arrhythmias can arise from any form of heart disease or even from a structurally normal heart. Palpitations and arrhythmias may therefore represent anything from a benign, but annoying condition to a foreshadowing of sudden cardiac death. The clinician must have an organized approach to the evaluation and management of a patient with palpitations to establish the diagnosis, prognosis, and therapy efficiently and effectively.

To provide a sound basis for diagnosis and further management, any clinician evaluating a patient with palpitations should address (1) the symptom (palpitations), (2) the functional disturbance (arrhythmia), (3) the substrate (underlying heart disease), and (4) the precipitating factors. By evaluating each of these issues, the physician should be able to base further management on a sound scientific foundation.

PATIENT EVALUATION

Clinical History

A complete history is the first step in the evaluation of palpitations, and it should provide information about all dimensions of the patient's problem (Box 9–1). A complete description of the palpitations should be sought, first by having patients describe the problem in their own words and then through specific questions. Timing is a key element for characterizing palpitations. How long does each episode last? How often do the episodes occur? Are episodes more common at certain times of the day or on certain days of the week? When did the episodes begin to occur? Responses to questions about timing provide information about both the type of the responsible arrhythmia (if any) and the precipitating factors. It is important to ask about the details of the episode, including whether the sensation is brief or prolonged (e.g., "skipped beat," "flip-flop"), whether the heartbeat is regular or irregular ("is it regular like a clock?"), and whether onset and termination of the episode are gradual or abrupt ("like a light switch?"). The physician should help the patient by tapping out examples of a regular or irregular rhythm or have the patient tap out the rhythm that has been experienced. The presence of coexisting symptoms such as lightheadedness, presyncope, chest pain, shortness of breath, and sweating may provide useful information about the probable effects of an arrhythmia on cardiac output and blood pressure.

The circumstances in which the palpitations occur provide clues about the underlying etiology and precipitating factors. In what activities was the patient engaged when struck by palpitations? Mental stress and anxiety may lead to an overawareness of sinus rhythm or may precipitate a cardiac arrhythmia in a patient with an appropriate substrate. Patients who have panic disorders are more aware of their heartbeats, especially when they have sinus tachycardia. Exercise, caffeine, alcohol, and drugs such as cocaine and amphetamines may all precipitate episodes of arrhythmia.

The clinician should also address the likelihood of underlying heart disease and any coexisting medical

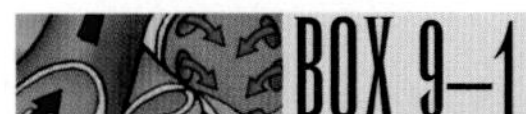

BOX 9–1

Clinical History in Evaluation of Palpitations

SYMPTOMS OF PALPITATIONS

- When did the symptoms first begin?
- Duration of episode
- Frequency of episodes
- Associated chest pain, dyspnea, lightheadedness
- How does an episode start?
- How does an episode stop?

UNDERLYING HEART DISEASE

- Angina, previous myocardial infarction
- Coronary risk factors
- Valvular heart disease
- Congenital heart disease
- Congestive heart failure
- Previous antiarrhythmic therapy

PRECIPITATING FACTORS

- Psychological stress
- Exercise
- Caffeine, alcohol, cocaine, amphetamines
- Thyroid disease
- Anemia, hypoxemia

disorders. Coronary heart disease may be suggested by symptoms of chest pain, a history of previous myocardial infarction, cardiac risk factors (age, gender, smoking, hypertension, hyperlipidemia, diabetes, family history), or the presence of atherosclerosis in other vascular beds. Heart failure may be suggested by shortness of breath or edema. Noncardiac disorders such as anemia, hyperthyroidism, and hypoxemia may lead to tachycardia and symptomatic palpitations.

Physical Examination

Because palpitations are paroxysmal, it is likely that the patient will be between episodes at the time of the physical examination. In these circumstances, the physical examination is aimed at detecting evidence of the presence of underlying heart disease. Cardiac murmurs may be a sign of valvular heart disease (see Chapter 32), congenital heart disease (Chapter 34), or hypertrophic cardiomyopathy (Chapter 29). Signs of heart failure (Chapter 28) such as an S_3 gallop, elevated jugular venous pressure, rales, and peripheral edema are important evidence of serious associated cardiac disease. Carotid or femoral bruits or diminished peripheral pulses provide evidence of atherosclerosis (Chapter 37), thus raising the likelihood of coexisting coronary artery disease.

Observations during a symptomatic attack provide information about the cardiac arrhythmia and its hemodynamic consequences. The rate and regularity of the heartbeat are key findings, and documentation of a possible arrhythmia by electrocardiography is crucial. Physical examination during an episode may provide evidence of atrioventricular (AV) dissociation through intermittent cannon A waves in the jugular venous pulse or variations in the intensity of S_1 (see Chapter 3). The effects of the arrhythmia on perfusion should be evaluated as well. The adequacy of cardiac output and blood pressure can be assessed by the level of consciousness, perfusion of the extremities, and urine output. It is important to recall that patients with ventricular tachycardia may have adequate blood pressure and cardiac output, especially if they are supine.

The Electrocardiogram

The electrocardiogram (ECG) is the single most valuable laboratory study in a patient with palpitations. It provides information about both the arrhythmia and the presence of underlying heart disease. A resting 12-lead ECG should be performed in every patient at the time of initial evaluation, as well as during an episode of palpitations.

ECGs recorded between episodes of palpitations provide evidence regarding the arrhythmia substrate. Particular attention should be paid to the P-wave, PR interval, the presence of either delta waves or abnormal Q-waves, and the QT interval (see Chapter 12). Left or right atrial enlargement increases the likelihood of supraventricular arrhythmias. A short PR interval or delta wave provides evidence for accessory AV pathways that form the substrate for supraventricular tachycardia. Q-waves consistent with myocardial infarction suggest a substrate for ventricular tachycardia. Left or right ventricular hypertrophy suggests underlying structural heart disease. Prolongation of the QT interval may predispose the patient to torsades de pointes or other forms of ventricular tachycardia.

An ECG recorded at the time of symptoms is the definitive diagnostic study to document the presence and type of arrhythmia. Tracings taken during an arrhythmia may be challenging to interpret and may need to be reviewed with a physician experienced in electrocardiography. Computerized ECG interpretation is not sufficiently reliable in the diagnosis of arrhythmias because subtle aspects of the tracing may be missed. The basic principles of arrhythmia evaluation on the 12-lead ECG are simple, and yet application of these principles to interpret tracings may be difficult. Key elements in interpreting an ECG with an arrhythmia are (1) evidence of atrial activity, (2) the relationship between atrial and ventricular complexes, (3) regularity or irregularity, (4) the ventricular rate, (5) width and morphology of the QRS complexes, and (6) duration of the tachycardia (see Fig. 30–1).

Narrow-complex tachycardias (QRS duration <0.10 seconds) indicate that the ventricles are being activated in the usual fashion through the normal conduction system. With rare exception, a narrow-complex tachycardia is supraventricular in origin. An irregular narrow-complex tachycardia without defined P-waves suggests atrial fibrillation (see Fig. 30–3), whereas a regular narrow-complex tachycardia suggests atrial flutter (see Fig. 30–5) or other supraventricular tachycardia. Flutter waves are most visible in the inferior leads (II, III, aVF). AV nodal blockade by increasing vagal tone (e.g., carotid sinus massage) or by pharmacologic means (adenosine, verapamil) may either bring out atrial flutter waves or terminate supraventricular arrhythmias that include the AV node in the reentrant circuit (see Chapter 30).

Wide-complex tachycardia may be due to ventricular tachycardia or to supraventricular tachycardia with aberration. AV dissociation is a highly specific finding for ventricular tachycardia, but not particularly sensitive: the presence of AV dissociation establishes the arrhythmia as ventricular tachycardia, whereas its absence is consistent with either a supraventricular or ventricular origin. In the absence of AV dissociation, careful evaluation of QRS morphology provides additional information on the origin of the arrhythmia (see Fig. 30–1). In uncertain cases, it is safer to assume that wide-complex tachycardia represents ventricular tachycardia until proved otherwise.

DIAGNOSTIC TESTING

After taking a careful clinical history, performing a physical examination, and reviewing the ECG, the physician will have to decide whether further evaluation is necessary and, if so, select the appropriate diagnostic tests. The key issues are (1) establishing which type of arrhythmia (if any) is causing the patient's symptoms and (2) evaluating the risk of death or serious complications. Empiric therapy for palpitations without establishing the type of underlying arrhythmia is unwise because an inappropriate or ineffective drug may be chosen. Antiarrhythmic agents may actually exacerbate arrhythmias and often have significant side effects, so empiric therapy may worsen rather than alleviate the patient's problem. A diagnosis should be established before beginning therapy.

The differential diagnosis of palpitations includes heightened awareness of a normal heartbeat and supraventricular and ventricular arrhythmias. The probability of serious arrhythmias as a source of palpitations is increased in the presence of underlying structural heart disease, which is more likely in older patients. The likelihood of life-threatening ventricular arrhythmia is increased by evidence of previous myocardial infarction or other disease processes that affect the ventricles. Conversely, in younger patients without structural heart disease, the probability of supraventricular arrhythmia is greater, as is the possibility of heightened awareness of isolated premature beats or noncardiac causes of palpitations.

Several series of patients seen in primary care settings (Table 9–1) provide information on the clinical epidemiology of palpitations.[1, 5, 6] A specific arrhythmia was thought to be the cause of palpitations in a minority of patients; atrial fibrillation was the most common cardiac etiology. A cardiac cause of the palpitations was more likely in men, in patients with a previous history of heart disease, in those with an irregular heartbeat, and in patients with a duration of palpitations greater than 5 minutes.[5] Noncardiac disorders, especially panic disorder, were quite commonly the cause of palpitations. Even among patients referred to a cardiology clinic for evaluation of palpitations, about 25% will be found to have nothing more than an awareness of sinus rhythm, and about another 40% will have nothing more serious than extrasystolic beats.[7]

TABLE 9–1

Etiology of Palpitations in Unselected Patients

Reference	No. of Patients	Age (Mean)	% Female	Any Cardiac Disease	Atrial Fibrillation or Flutter
1	762	NA	63	9%	6%
5	190	46	61	43%	15%
6	145	47	57	NA	40%

NA, not available.

Psychological stress, palpitations, and arrhythmias are closely intertwined phenomena. Stress leads to increased levels of catecholamines, which in turn increase the heart rate and contractility. Patients who are particularly anxious, hyperventilating, or suffering from panic attacks may complain of palpitations because of a heightened awareness of sinus tachycardia. The clinician should not, however, simply dismiss symptoms of palpitations in the setting of psychological stress because a wide variety of serious arrhythmias may also be precipitated by increased levels of circulating catecholamines in patients with an underlying arrhythmic substrate.

Documentation of the Arrhythmia

Palpitations and arrhythmias are, by nature, transient phenomena and are hence challenging to document by noninvasive or invasive testing (Box 9–2). Spontaneous arrhythmias may be documented by continuous ambulatory ECG (Holter monitoring) or by intermittent recordings of an ECG during symptoms (event monitors). Arrhythmias may also be provoked by exercise testing or programmed electrical stimulation.

Holter Monitoring

Continuous ambulatory ECG monitoring (also known as Holter monitoring after its developer) is a valuable means of assessing frequent palpitations.[8] The patient has several electrodes placed on the torso, and two or more ECG leads are recorded for 24 hours (see Chapter 4). Correlation between symptoms and the cardiac rhythm is a key feature of ambulatory monitoring, and patients should be instructed to record the time and

TABLE 9–2

Ambulatory Electrocardiography in Evaluating Palpitations

Symptom	Concurrent Rhythm	Interpretation
Present	Sinus rhythm	Symptoms not caused by arrhythmia
Present	Arrhythmia (sustained or not)	Establishes arrhythmia as cause of symptoms
None	Sinus rhythm	Nondiagnostic; further recordings needed
None	Premature atrial or ventricular beats	Nondiagnostic
None	Runs of premature atrial or ventricular beats	Suggestive, but not definitive
None	Supraventricular tachycardia >30 sec in duration	Suggestive, but not definitive
None	Ventricular tachycardia ≥30 sec in duration	Very suggestive of life-threatening arrhythmia

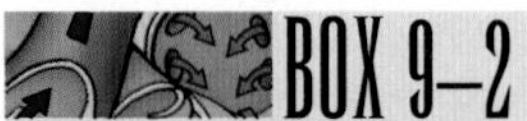
BOX 9–2

American Heart Association/American College of Cardiology Guidelines for Use of Diagnostic Tests in Patients with Palpitations*

AMBULATORY ELECTROCARDIOGRAPHY[9]

Class I: Unexplained palpitations, syncope, or dizziness

Class II: Shortness of breath, chest pain, or fatigue (not otherwise explained)

Class III: Symptoms for which other causes have been identified

ELECTROPHYSIOLOGIC STUDY[10]

Class I:
1. Patients with palpitations who have a pulse rate documented by medical personnel as inappropriately rapid and in whom electrocardiographic recordings fail to document the cause of the palpitations
2. Patients with palpitations preceding a syncopal episode

Class II: Patients with clinically significant palpitations suspected to be of cardiac origin in whom the symptoms are sporadic and cannot be documented. Studies are performed to determine the mechanisms of arrhythmias, direct or provide therapy, or assess prognosis

Class III: Patients with palpitations documented to be due to extracardiac causes (e.g., hyperthyroidism)

ECHOCARDIOGRAPHY[11]

Class I:
1. Arrhythmias with a clinical suspicion of structural heart disease
2. Family history of a genetic disorder associated with arrhythmias
3. Evaluation before an electrophysiologic ablative procedure

Class II:
1. Arrhythmias commonly associated with, but without evidence of, heart disease
2. Arrhythmias requiring treatment

Class III:
1. Palpitations without evidence of arrhythmia
2. Isolated premature ventricular contractions without evidence of heart disease

*Class I: general agreement that the test is useful and indicated; class II: frequently used, but with a divergence of opinion with respect to its utility; class III: general agreement that the test is not useful.

nature of any symptoms carefully in a diary. The test provides much less information in patients who are unable to keep an accurate symptom diary (Table 9–2). If an arrhythmia is recorded at the same time that the patient notes palpitations, a positive link between symptoms and a cardiac arrhythmia is established, and the precise arrhythmia responsible may be identified. Conversely, if typical symptoms occur when the ECG recording shows sinus rhythm, the documented dissociation between symptoms and arrhythmia provides the physician reassurance and a basis for symptomatic management. No useful information is provided by the combination of no symptoms and no recorded arrhythmias. The combination of no recorded symptoms with minor arrhythmias (e.g., premature supraventricular or ventricular beats) also provides little useful information because isolated premature beats are very common in the normal population.[12] Short runs of supraventricular tachycardia or ventricular tachycardia in the absence of symptoms provide suggestive, but not definitive evidence that an arrhythmia may be the cause of the patient's symptoms. These equivocal results of ambulatory monitoring are not usually strong enough evidence to lead to treatment but do suggest the need for further evaluation. Sustained ventricular tachycardia (i.e., 30 seconds or more in duration), even without recorded symptoms, warrants very careful evaluation, usually in consultation with an arrhythmia specialist.

Event Monitors

If palpitations are infrequent, it is unlikely that 24 or even 48 hours of ambulatory ECG monitoring will provide diagnostic information. A convenient alternative is an event monitor, a small portable device that the patient can activate when experiencing symptoms and thus record the ECG for later playback and analysis (see Chapter 10). The smaller size and intermittent recording behavior of this device allow it to be worn or carried for prolonged periods. The information provided is similar to that of continuous ECG recorders. Use of an event monitor requires a conscious patient with the ability to recognize an arrhythmia and activate the device. In patients unable to use the event-recording system, several 24-hour Holter monitors may be needed.

In a study that randomized patients with palpitations to either a Holter monitor for 48 hours or an event monitor for up to 3 months, a recording was made during symptoms in 67% of patients with the event monitor versus 35% of patients with a Holter monitor ($P < .001$).[13] Half of the yield of the event recorder was in the first few days of use, and the remaining events were recorded within 30 days. A cost-effectiveness analysis suggested that use of an event monitor for 2 weeks is the best approach to evaluation of palpitations.[14]

Clinical guidelines recommend an event monitor as the test of choice in patients whose symptoms occur less frequently than every day and who can activate the device if an episode occurs (see Chapter 10).[9] Otherwise, a 24-hour ambulatory ECG is the recommended method of documenting arrhythmias in a patient with palpitations.

Exercise Testing

Exercise testing is helpful in the evaluation of patients who describe having palpitations as a direct result of physical exertion. In some young patients with catecholamine-induced ventricular tachycardia, the arrhythmia may be brought out only by exercise testing. Exercise testing may also be useful in assessing the likelihood that the patient has underlying coronary artery disease.

Electrophysiologic Study

Invasive electrophysiologic (EP) studies have a very high diagnostic yield in patients with suspected arrhythmia, but they should be used only after evaluating palpitations by ambulatory ECG monitoring or an event monitor. Exceptions to this general rule are patients resuscitated from cardiac arrest and patients with other life-threatening symptoms.[10]

EP studies attempt to provoke arrhythmias by the controlled introduction of premature atrial or ventricular beats, which, in patients with the appropriate substrate, can induce a sustained reentrant arrhythmia (see Chapter 30). For example, patients with an accessory AV connection may have inducible AV reciprocating tachycardia, and patients with a previous myocardial infarction may have inducible sustained ventricular tachycardia. Other arrhythmias reliably induced and characterized by EP studies are supraventricular tachycardia and atrial flutter. Each of these arrhythmias occurs with a reentry mechanism in a fixed anatomic substrate, and thus both are ideal for evaluation by EP testing.

EP testing is not as useful in documenting arrhythmias that arise from transient causes, such as ventricular fibrillation resulting from myocardial ischemia or electrolyte disorders. Arrhythmias caused by mechanisms other than reentry are also not reliably induced by EP studies, including torsades de pointes, multifocal atrial tachycardia, and ectopic atrial tachycardia. Very aggressive stimulation protocols may induce nonclinical arrhythmias in some patients. Thus, although EP testing is an extremely valuable laboratory test, it is neither 100% sensitive nor 100% specific in the evaluation of arrhythmias.

The main role for EP testing is to guide therapy in patients with established arrhythmias. Radiofrequency ablation may be used in selected symptomatic patients with Wolff-Parkinson-White syndrome, supraventricular tachycardia, atrial flutter, and certain uncommon forms of ventricular tachycardia (see Chapter 30).[7] EP testing is also useful in evaluating the need for further therapy in patients with nonsustained ventricular tachycardia.[15] Otherwise, the use of an EP study as a purely diagnostic test in patients with palpitations is limited, and clinical guidelines endorse its use only for patients in whom ECG recordings fail to establish a diagnosis.

Assessing Risk Attributable to Arrhythmia

Therapy in patients with palpitations caused by a cardiac arrhythmia is aimed at relief of symptoms and reduction of the risk of serious complications. The risk of the arrhythmia to the patient is jointly determined by (1) the type of arrhythmia responsible for the patient's symptoms and (2) the type and severity of the patient's underlying heart disease, if any.

Atrial Arrhythmias

Atrial arrhythmias do not generally pose a risk of death because transmission of atrial electrical activity to the ventricles is regulated by the AV node. Rapid atrial flutter or atrial fibrillation, for instance, can be conducted directly to the ventricles only when protection of the AV node fails, as in some cases of Wolff-Parkinson-White syndrome or in patients in whom drug therapy accelerates AV nodal conduction (e.g., quinidine or procainamide without an AV node suppressant). Patients with severe underlying heart disease, such as critical coronary artery disease, hypertrophic cardiomyopathy, or heart failure, however, may experience circulatory collapse as a result of myocardial ischemia or loss of effective atrial contraction.

Patients with atrial arrhythmias are also at risk for stroke from emboli. The risk is highest in patients with chronic atrial fibrillation or flutter in whom ineffective atrial contraction leads to stasis and the formation of intra-atrial thrombi, but paroxysmal atrial fibrillation is also associated with an increased risk of stroke. Long-term anticoagulation is generally recommended for all patients with chronic atrial fibrillation (see Chapter 30).[16]

Ventricular Arrhythmia

Patients with ventricular arrhythmias are at increased risk of sudden cardiac death because of the potential for deterioration of the arrhythmia to ventricular fibrillation. Epidemiologic studies in patients with recent myocardial infarction suggest a gradient of increasing risk with increasing complexity of the arrhythmia. The lowest risk category is associated with isolated premature ventricular beats, with somewhat higher risk associated with couplets or triplets of ventricular premature beats; the next higher level of risk is associated with nonsustained ventricular tachycardia (more than three beats but <30 seconds in duration), whereas the highest level of risk is associated with sustained ventricular arrhythmia (>30 seconds or requiring countershock for termination) (see Chapter 30). The frequency of the arrhythmia and the level of complexity jointly establish the risk of death. The greatest information is conveyed by the level of complexity; at any level of complexity, risk increases with more frequent arrhythmias.

The risk posed by ventricular arrhythmias is also determined by the presence and severity of underlying heart disease. Frequent premature ventricular beats are associated with low risk in a young patient with a structurally normal heart[17] but considerably higher risk in an older patient with heart failure or previous myocardial infarction (see Chapter 30). Left ventricular systolic function is particularly important in assessing the risk in patients with ventricular arrhythmia. Patients with normal left ventricular function are generally at low risk, perhaps because they are more able to maintain cardiac output and blood pressure during ventricular tachycardia and perhaps because of the greater difficulty in inducing ventricular fibrillation in a ventricle of normal size and function. Conversely, patients with poor ventricular function are at higher risk in the presence of ventricular arrhythmia, perhaps because the poorer mechanical function of the ventricles may not support adequate cardiac output during ventricular tachycardia or because a dilated and scarred ventricle may be more susceptible to primary ventricular fibrillation. Regardless of the underlying mechanism, the risk of sudden death is inversely proportional to left ventricular function: for any level of ventricular arrhythmia, patients with a lower left ventricular ejection fraction have a worse prognosis. Left ventricular function is such a powerful predictor of outcome that it is reasonable to evaluate the ejection fraction in virtually every patient with a documented ventricular arrhythmia.

Recommended Approach to Diagnosis in the Primary Care Setting

The goals of evaluation in a patient with palpitations are to (1) establish the type of arrhythmia, if any, responsible for the patient's symptoms and (2) evaluate the risk posed by the arrhythmia in light of the nature and severity of any underlying heart disease (Fig. 9–1). All patients should receive a careful history and physical examination, as well as a 12-lead ECG. From this information, the physician should first assess the likelihood of any underlying structural heart disease and the potential risk to the patient. In patients without evidence of structural heart disease, the risk is low, and decisions about further testing may be made solely on the basis of the severity and frequency of symptoms. In patients with structurally normal hearts and either mild symptoms or symptoms consisting of only brief "skipped beats," no further testing is necessary. However, if patients with structurally normal hearts have symptoms frequent enough to require medication for control, the arrhythmia should be documented by an event monitor or ambulatory ECG.

Patients with evidence of structural heart disease or with features suggesting increased risk (e.g., associated presyncope or syncope) should have a 24-hour ambulatory ECG recorded if symptoms occur almost every day or an event monitor if symptoms are less frequent. EP studies should generally be reserved for patients who have documented arrhythmias and who are candidates for specific therapies (e.g., radiofrequency ablation, an implantable cardioverter-defibrillator; see Chapter 30). Patients with clinical evidence of underlying heart disease and documented ventricular arrhythmias should generally undergo echocardiography to evaluate left ventricular function[11] and hence the risk of serious adverse effects from the arrhythmia (see Chapter 5).

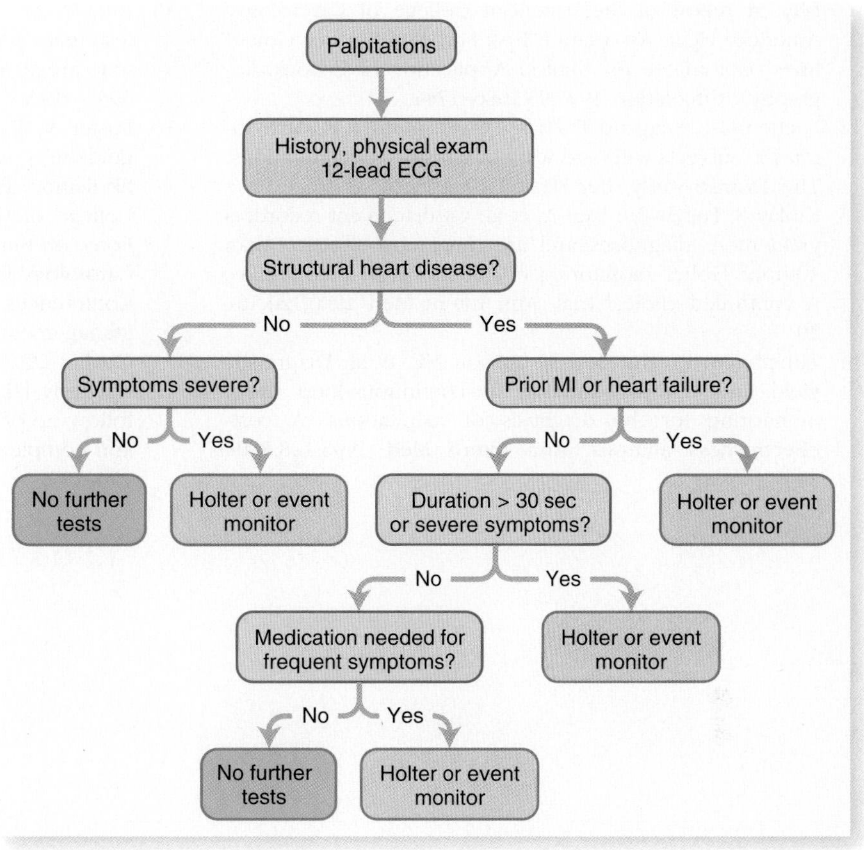

FIGURE 9–1. Diagnostic approach to patients with palpitations. ECG, electrocardiogram; MI, myocardial infarction.

Evidence-Based Summary

- Palpitations are frequent in the general population.
- Palpitations are often due to noncardiac disorders, especially panic disorder.
- The prognosis of patients with palpitations depends on whether an underlying arrhythmia or structural heart disease, or both, are present.
- An event monitor has higher yield than an ambulatory ECG in patients with infrequent palpitations.

References

1. Zwietering PJ, Knottnerus JA, Rinkens PELM, et al: Arrhythmias in general practice: Diagnostic value of patient characteristics, medical history and symptoms. Fam Pract 1998;15:343–353.
2. Barsky AJ: Investigating selected symptoms. Palpitations, arrhythmias, and awareness of cardiac activity. Ann Intern Med 2001;134:832–837.
3. Orejarena LA, Vidaillet H, DeStefano F, et al: Paroxysmal supraventricular tachycardia in the general population. J Am Coll Cardiol 1998;31:150–157.
4. Van der Dose AJW, Antony MM, Ehlers A, Barsky AJ: Heartbeat perception in panic disorder: A reanalysis. Behav Res Ther 2000;38:47–65.
5. Weber BE, Kapoor WN: Evaluation and outcomes of patients with palpitations. Am J Med 1996;100:138–148.
6. Barsky AJ, Cleary PD, Coeytaux RR, Ruskin JN: The clinical course of palpitations in medical outpatients. Arch Intern Med 1995;155:1782–1788.
7. Ehlers A, Mayou RA, Sprigings DC, Birkhead J: Psychological and perceptual factors associated with arrhythmias and benign palpitations. Psychosom Med 2000;62:693–702.
8. Zimetbaun PJ, Josephson ME: The evolving role of ambulatory arrhythmia monitoring in general clinical practice. Ann Intern Med 1999;130:848–856.
9. Crawford MH, Bernstein SJ, Deedwania PC, et al: ACC/AHA guidelines for ambulatory electrocardiography: A report of the American College of Cardiology/American Heart Association Task Force on Practice Guidelines (Committee to Revise the Guidelines for Ambulatory Electrocardiography). J Am Coll Cardiol 1999;34:912–948.
10. ACC/AHA Task Force Report: Guidelines for clinical intracardiac electrophysiological and catheter ablation procedures. A report of the American College of Cardiology/American Heart Association Task Force on Practice Guidelines (Committee on Clinical Intracardiac Electrophysiologic and Catheter Ablation Procedures), developed in collaboration with the North American Society of Pacing and Electrophysiology. J Am Coll Cardiol 1995;26:555–573.
11. Cheitlin MD, Alpert JS, Armstrong WF, et al: ACC/AHA guidelines for the clinical application of echocardiogra-

phy: A report of the American College of Cardiology/American Heart Association Task Force on Practice Guidelines (Committee on Clinical Application of Echocardiography). Circulation 1997;95:1686–1744.

12. Lochen M-L, Snaprud T, Zhang W, Rasmussen K: Arrhythmias in subjects with and without a history of palpitations: The Tromso study. Eur Heart J 1994;15:345–349.
13. Kinlay S, Leitch JW, Neil A, et al: Cardiac event recorders yield more diagnoses and are more cost-effective than 48-hour Holter monitoring in patients with palpitations. A controlled clinical trial. Ann Intern Med 1996;124:16–20.
14. Zimetbaum PJ, Kim KY, Josephson ME, et al: Diagnostic yield and optimal duration of continuous-loop event monitoring for the diagnosis of palpitations. A cost-effectiveness analysis. Ann Intern Med 1998;128:890–895.
15. Buxton AE, Lee KL, DiCarlo L, et al: Electrophysiologic testing to identify patients with coronary artery disease who are at risk for sudden death. N Engl J Med 2000;342:1937–1945.
16. Fuster V, Ryden LE, Asinger FW, et al: ACC/AHA/ESC guidelines for the management of patients with atrial fibrillation: Executive summary: A report of the American College of Cardiology/American Heart Association Task Force on Practice Guidelines and the European Society of Cardiology Committee for Practice Guidelines and Policy Conferences (Committee to Develop Guidelines for the Management of Patients with Atrial Fibrillation). J Am Coll Cardiol 2001;38:1231–1265.
17. Kennedy HL, Whitlock JA, Sprague MK, et al: Long-term follow-up of asymptomatic healthy subjects with frequent and complex ventricular ectopy. N Engl J Med 1985;312:193–197.

CHAPTER 10 Approach to the Patient with Syncope

Wishwa N. Kapoor

Syncope is defined as sudden temporary loss of consciousness associated with loss of postural tone and spontaneous recovery not requiring electrical or chemical cardioversion. Patients with syncope account for 1% to 6% of hospital admissions and up to 3% of emergency department visits. Loss of consciousness is very common in healthy young adults in the community (reported by 12% to 48%), although most do not seek medical attention. Syncope is also a frequent and recurrent symptom in the elderly; in patients in one long-term care institution, 23% reported a history of syncopal episodes sometime during their lifetime.

Previous studies have shown that patients with cardiac causes of syncope have a higher 1-year mortality than do patients with noncardiac or unknown causes of syncope. Most deaths in patients with cardiac causes are sudden. Thus, identifying and treating cardiac causes of syncope are very important issues in the management of patients with syncope.

Primary care physicians are the initial point of contact for most patients with syncope, and several questions need to be addressed: (1) what is the cause of patient's symptoms? (2) how serious is the potential etiology? (3) what tests should be ordered? (4) how rapidly does the workup need to be done? and (5) when should the patient be referred to a subspecialist?

CAUSES OF SYNCOPE

Although syncope has a broad differential diagnosis, the etiologies can be classified into four broad categories (Box 10–1). The first category is neurocardiogenic or neurally mediated syncope, which is loss of consciousness from sudden reflex vasodilatation or bradycardia (or from both). Entities in this group include syndromes such as vasovagal, vasodepressor, situational, and carotid sinus syncope. A neurally mediated reflex mechanism is also implicated in syncope associated with exercise, especially immediately after exercise, in individuals without structural heart disease. Neurocardiogenic syncope may likewise occur with drugs (e.g., nitroglycerin) that decrease venous return to the heart when in an upright position. Syncope with aortic stenosis, hypertrophic cardiomyopathy, supraventricular tachycardia, and paroxysmal atrial fibrillation and that related to pacemakers (i.e., pacemaker syndrome) also appear to result from neurally mediated mechanisms. These entities are grouped under cardiac causes for this review because of a potentially worse prognosis for some and specific treatment considerations in others.

The second broad category is orthostatic hypotension, which may result from age-related physiologic changes, medications, volume depletion, and diseases

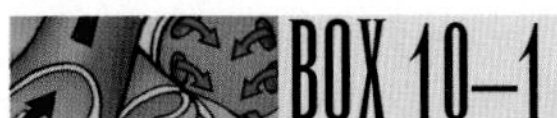
BOX 10–1

Causes of Syncope

NEUROCARDIOGENIC

Vasovagal
Situational
- Micturition
- Cough
- Swallow
- Defecation

Carotid sinus syncope
Neuralgias
High altitude
Psychiatric disorders
Others (exercise, selected drugs)

ORTHOSTATIC HYPOTENSION

NEUROLOGIC DISEASES

Migraines
TIAs
Seizures

DECREASED CARDIAC OUTPUT

Obstruction to flow
- Obstruction to LV outflow or inflow: aortic stenosis, hypertrophic obstructive cardiomyopathy, mitral stenosis, myxoma
- Obstruction to RV outflow or inflow: pulmonic stenosis, PE, pulmonary hypertension, myxoma

Other heart disease
- Pump failure, MI, CAD, coronary spasm, tamponade, aortic dissection

Arrhythmias
- Bradyarrhythmias: sinus node disease, second- and third-degree atrioventricular block, pacemaker malfunction, drug-induced bradyarrhythmias
- Tachyarrhythmias: ventricular tachycardia, torsades de pointes (e.g., associated with congenital long-QT syndrome, acquired QT prolongation), supraventricular tachycardia

CAD, coronary artery disease; LV, left ventricular; MI, myocardial infarction; PE, pulmonary embolism; RV, right ventricular; TIAs, transient ischemic attacks.

BOX 10–2

Causes of Orthostatic Hypotension

PRIMARY

Autonomic failure with multiple system atrophy (Shy-Drager syndrome)

SECONDARY

General medical disorders (e.g., diabetes, amyloidosis, alcoholism)
Autoimmune disease (e.g., Guillain-Barré syndrome, mixed connective tissue disease, rheumatoid arthritis, Eaton-Lambert syndrome, systemic lupus erythematosus)
Metabolic disease (e.g., vitamin B_{12} deficiency, porphyria, Fabry's disease, Tangier disease)
Hereditary sensory neuropathies, dominant or recessive
Central brain lesions, including vascular lesion or tumors involving the hypothalamus and midbrain (e.g., craniopharyngioma, multiple sclerosis, Wernicke's encephalopathy)
Spinal cord lesions
Familial dysautonomia
Aging

DRUGS

Tranquillizers (e.g., phenothiazines, barbiturates)
Antidepressants (e.g., tricyclics, monoamine oxidase inhibitors)
Vasodilators (e.g., prazosin, hydralazine, calcium channel blockers)
Centrally acting hypotensive drugs (e.g., methyldopa, clonidine)
Alpha-adrenergic blocking drugs (e.g., phenoxybenzamine, labetalol)
Ganglion-blocking drugs (e.g., guanethidine, hexamethonium, mecamylamine)
Angiotensin-converting enzyme inhibitors (e.g., captopril, enalapril, lisinopril)
Angiotensin II blockers (e.g., candesartan, losartan, valsartan)

Adapted from Bannister SR (ed): Autonomic Failure, 4th ed. New York, Oxford University Press, 1999.

affecting the autonomic nervous system[1] (Box 10–2). Postprandial syncope occurs especially in the elderly as a result of hypotension after meals. A decline in systolic blood pressure of more than 20 mm Hg after a meal has been reported in up to 36% of elderly nursing home residents and occurs at 45 to 60 minutes in most patients. This decline in blood pressure may rarely lead to symptoms.

The third category is neurologic disorders, which are infrequent causes of syncope. These disorders include transient ischemic attacks (TIA), migraines, and seizures. Syncope secondary to TIAs almost exclusively involves the vertebrobasilar territory. Migraines may be related to involvement of the basilar artery, or syncope may be a response to severe pain. Seizures may be atonic, temporal lobe epilepsy, or unwitnessed grand mal seizures.

The fourth category includes a large group of cardiac etiologies that can be divided into diseases associated with severe obstruction to cardiac output, ischemia, and rhythm disturbances.

Obstruction to Flow

Exertional syncope is a common manifestation of obstruction to flow in which cardiac output is fixed and does not rise with exercise. Structural lesions of either the left or right side of the heart may lead to outflow obstruction and result in syncope (see Box 10–1). The mechanism of exertional syncope in conditions that cause left ventricular outflow obstruction is widely believed to be neurally mediated responses. In these situations, exercise leads to an increase in left ventricular systolic pressure without a corresponding increase in aortic pressure. This discrepancy may result in excessive stimulation of left ventricular mechanoreceptors, which leads to inhibition of sympathetic and activation of parasympathetic tone through cardiac vagal afferent fibers.

Syncope occurs in up to 42% of patients with severe aortic valve stenosis, commonly with or just after exercise. Myocardial ischemia is also often present during syncope (even in patients without coexistent coronary artery disease), but the role of ischemia in causing syncope is not well understood. Syncope is prognostically important in aortic valve stenosis, and patients with aortic stenosis have an average survival of 2 to 3 years after the onset of syncope in the absence of valve replacement.

In patients with hypertrophic obstructive cardiomyopathy (see Chapter 29), syncope, which is reported in up to 30% of such patients, is caused by dynamic pathophysiologic processes that are otherwise similar to what is seen in the fixed obstruction found in aortic valve stenosis. Left ventricular outflow obstruction is worsened by an increase in contractility, a decrease in chamber size, or a decrease in afterload and distending pressure. Thus, the Valsalva maneuver, a severe coughing paroxysm, or specific drugs (e.g., digitalis) may precipitate hypotension and syncope. Ventricular tachycardia is reported in approximately 25% of adult patients with hypertrophic cardiomyopathy and is an important cause of syncope. Predictors of syncope include age younger than 30 years, a left ventricular end-diastolic volume index less than 60 mL/m^2, and nonsustained ventricular tachycardia. Extensive hypertrophy and ventricular tachycardia are associated with a poorer prognosis.

Effort syncope commonly occurs in pulmonary hypertension (up to 30% of patients with primary pulmonary hypertension) and severe pulmonic stenosis. Patients with congenital heart disease (e.g., tetralogy of Fallot, patent ductus arteriosus, and interventricular or interatrial septal defects) can experience syncope with effort or crying as a result of a sudden reversal of a left-to-right shunt and a decrease in arterial oxygen saturation (see Chapter 34). Approximately 10% to 15% of patients with pulmonary embolism have syncope, which is more common in those with massive embolism and greater than 50% obstruction of the pulmonary vascular bed (see Chapter 38). Pulmonary embolism may result in acute right ventricular failure and lead to increased right ventricular filling pressure, decreased stroke volume, decreased cardiac output, hypotension, and subsequent loss of consciousness. Alternatively, activation of cardiopulmonary mechanoreceptors in the setting of increased force of ventricular contraction may be the cause of syncope.

Atrial myxomas may result in obstruction of the mitral or tricuspid valve and lead to symptoms of cardiac failure and rarely syncope. Mitral stenosis may cause exertional syncope as a result of severe obstruction to outflow, but loss of consciousness in patients with mitral stenosis may also be caused by atrial fibrillation with a rapid ventricular response, pulmonary hypertension, or a cerebral embolic event.

Other Organic Heart Disease

Approximately 5% to 12% of elderly patients with acute myocardial infarction initially come to medical attention because of syncope. Loss of consciousness may be due to sudden pump failure resulting in a decline in cardiac output and blood flow to the brain, to rhythm disturbances such as ventricular tachycardia or bradyarrhythmias, or to both mechanisms. Neurocardiogenic reflexes may also be activated by acute inferior infarction or ischemia involving the right coronary artery. In addition, unstable angina and coronary artery spasm have rarely been associated with syncope. Syncope is also a rare manifestation (in 5% or less) in patients with aortic dissection.

Arrhythmias

Tachyarrhythmias reduce the time available for diastolic filling of the ventricles and cause such a marked reduction in stroke volume that cardiac output declines despite the increase in heart rate, especially with atrial fibrillation or ventricular tachycardia, in which an effective atrial kick is lost (see Chapters 30 and 31). The diminished cardiac volume and vigorous ventricular contraction associated with supraventricular tachycardia and paroxysmal atrial fibrillation may also activate cardiac mechanoreceptors and cause neurocardiogenic syncope. Syncope in patients with Wolff-Parkinson-White syndrome may be related to a rapid rate of reciprocating supraventricular tachycardia or to a rapid ventricular response over the accessory pathway during atrial fibrillation.

Sick sinus syndrome includes sinus bradycardia, pauses, arrest, or exit block (see Chapter 31). Supraventricular tachycardia or atrial fibrillation may also occur in association with bradycardia, or atrial fibrillation may be associated with a slow ventricular response (tachycardia-bradycardia syndrome). Syncope is reported in 25% to 70% of patients with sick sinus syndrome.

Ventricular tachycardias (see Chapter 30) generally occur in patients with structural heart disease. Polymorphic ventricular tachycardia (torsades de pointes) may lead to syncope in the setting of syndromes of congenital prolongation of the QT interval (with or without deafness), as well as acquired long QT syndromes, which occur with drugs, electrolyte abnormalities, and central nervous system disorders. Antiarrhythmic drugs, including quinidine, procainamide, disopyramide, flecainide, encainide, amiodarone, and sotalol, are the most common cause of torsades de pointes.

How Often Are Causes of Syncope Assigned?

Studies of consecutive, generally unselected patients indicate a fairly wide range in prevalence of the various causes of syncope[2–6] (Table 10–1). The most common etiologies are neurocardiogenic (vasovagal) syncope, organic heart diseases, arrhythmias, orthostatic hypotension, and seizures. The cause of syncope cannot be diagnosed in a substantial minority of patients, even with the use of event monitoring, tilt-table testing, electrophysiologic (EP) studies, attention to psychiatric illnesses, and recognition that syncope in the elderly may be multifactorial. For example, despite specific diagnostic algorithms or prospective evaluation with newer diagnostic modalities, 14% to 17.5% of patients have unexplained syncope.[4–6] In more recent series, neurocardiogenic syncope remains the most common cause of syncope and accounts for 35% to 58% of cases.

PROGNOSIS AND RISK STRATIFICATION

The 1-year mortality of patients with cardiac causes of syncope has been consistently high and ranges between 18% and 33%. These rates have been higher than those in patients with a noncardiac cause (0% to 12%) and in patients with unknown cause (6%). The incidence of sudden death in patients with cardiac causes was also markedly higher than in the other two groups. Even after adjustments for differences in co-morbid conditions that may affect the prognosis, cardiac syncope remains an independent predictor of mortality and sudden death.

A key issue is whether syncope predisposes to an increased risk of mortality independent of any underlying diseases. Patients who are younger than 60 years and who experience syncope but do not have known cardiovascular or neurologic diseases have rates of mortality, sudden death, stroke, and myocardial infarction similar to those of people without a history of syncope. In patients with advanced heart failure, poor left ventricular function is associated with a high risk of sudden death regardless of the cause of syncope. Among patients with and without syncope, underlying cardiac and noncardiac diseases are associated with increased mortality independent of syncope. In patients older than 45 years, a history of heart failure, a history of ventricular arrhythmias, and an abnormal electrocardiogram (ECG) (other than nonspecific ST changes) predict the occurrence of important cardiac arrhythmias or death during the year after the principal event: in one study, serious arrhythmias or death occurred in 4% to 7% of patients without any of these four risk factors versus 58% to 80% of patients with three or four risk factors.[7]

In summary, these observations indicate that the presence of underlying cardiac disease in patients with syncope predicts a worse prognosis. Every attempt should be made to detect and define any underlying structural heart disease and to treat any cardiac diseases to reduce the probability of mortality and sudden death.

The prognoses of cardiac syncope and neurocardiogenic syncope are different in that neurocardiogenic syncope has an excellent long-term prognosis, although recurrences are common and are a major reason for seeking medical care. Similarly, syncope associated with psychiatric disease does not increase mortality, but 1-year recurrence rates are 26% to 50%.

Among all patients with syncope, the recurrence rate is 34% over 3 years of follow-up. Although recurrences are associated with fractures and soft tissue injury in 12% of patients, they do not predict an increased risk of mortality or sudden death.

TABLE 10–1

Prevalence of Various Causes of Syncope in Major Clinical Series

Cause	Range of Prevalence (%)
Neurocardiogenic	
Vasovagal	8–41
Situational	1–8
Carotid sinus	0–4
Orthostatic hypotension	4–10
Medications	1–7
Psychiatric	1–7
Neurologic	3–32
Cardiac	
Structural heart disease	1–8
Arrhythmias	4–38
Unknown	13–41

Data from references 2 to 6.

DIAGNOSTIC EVALUATION

The history, physical examination, and ECG form the cornerstone of the initial evaluation of patients with syncope and can be used to stratify patients by risk and plan further diagnostic testing.

History, Physical Examination, and Baseline Laboratory Tests

The history and physical examination identify a potential cause of syncope in approximately 45% of patients.

Additionally, organic cardiac diseases causing syncope (e.g., pulmonary hypertension, aortic stenosis, pulmonary embolism) are usually suspected clinically and can then be confirmed by specific testing.

A detailed history regarding events leading to the episode and a description of symptoms during loss of consciousness and after the event are useful in diagnosing specific entities[6,8] (Box 10–3). For example, a history of precipitating factors and the presence of autonomic symptoms may lead to the diagnosis of vasovagal syncope. Similarly, loss of consciousness during or immediately after micturition, coughing, defecation, or swallowing may be diagnosed as situational syncope. Neurologic symptoms of brain stem ischemia concurrent with a brief loss of consciousness suggest TIAs, basilar artery migraines, and subclavian steal syndrome. A detailed drug history may provide clues to possible drug-induced syncope.

Specific findings that are particularly helpful on physical examination include orthostatic hypotension, cardiovascular signs, and an abnormal neurologic examination. Orthostatic hypotension is generally defined as a decline of 20 mm Hg or more in systolic pressure on assuming an upright position. However, this finding is reported in up to 24% of the elderly and is frequently not associated with symptoms. Thus, the clinical diagnosis of orthostatic hypotension should incorporate the presence of symptoms (e.g., dizziness and syncope) in association with a decrease in systolic blood pressure.

Orthostatic hypotension is detected by measuring supine blood pressure and the heart rate after the patient has been lying down for at least 5 minutes. Standing measurements should be obtained immediately and repeated for at least 3 minutes. Sitting blood pressure readings are not reliable for the detection of orthostatic hypotension and should not be used.

Cardiovascular findings may help diagnose specific entities. Differences in pulse intensity and blood pressure (generally >20 mm Hg) in the two arms are suggestive of aortic dissection or subclavian steal syndrome. The cardiovascular examination may also uncover clues suggestive of aortic stenosis, hyper-

BOX 10–3

Clinical Features Suggestive of Specific Causes

SYMPTOM OR FINDING	DIAGNOSTIC CONSIDERATION
After sudden unexpected pain, fear, unpleasant sight, sound, or smell	Vasovagal
Prolonged standing at attention	Vasovagal
Well-trained athlete after exertion (without heart disease)	Vasovagal
During or immediately after micturition, cough, swallowing, or defecation	Situational syncope
Syncope with throat or facial pain (glossopharyngeal or trigeminal neuralgia)	Neurocardiogenic syncope with neuralgia
With head rotation, pressure on the carotid sinus (as in tumors, shaving, tight collars)	Carotid sinus syncope
Immediately on standing	Orthostatic hypotension
Medications that may lead to long-QT syndrome or orthostasis/bradycardia	Drug induced
Associated with headaches	Migraines, seizures
Associated with vertigo, dysarthria, diplopia	Transient ischemic attack, subclavian steal, basilar migraine
With arm exercise	Subclavian steal
Confusion after a spell or loss of consciousness for more than 5 min	Seizure
Differences in blood pressure or pulse in the 2 arms	Subclavian steal or aortic dissection
Syncope and murmur with changing position (from sitting to lying, bending, turning over in bed)	Atrial myxoma or thrombus
Syncope with exertion	Aortic stenosis, pulmonary hypertension, mitral stenosis, hypertrophic obstructive cardiomyopathy, coronary artery disease
Family history of sudden death	Long-QT syndrome, the Brugada syndrome
Brief loss of consciousness, no prodrome, with heart disease	Arrhythmias
Frequent syncope, somatic complaints, no heart disease	Psychiatric illness

Reproduced, by permission, from Kapoor WN: Syncope. N Engl J Med 2000;343:1856–1862.

trophic obstructive cardiomyopathy, pulmonary hypertension, myxomas, and aortic dissection.

Initial laboratory blood tests are not generally abnormal and rarely lead to a diagnosis. Hypoglycemia, hyponatremia, hypocalcemia, and renal failure are found in 2% to 3% of patients, but these abnormalities are frequently suspected clinically and are more often seen in patients in whom seizure rather than syncope is eventually diagnosed.

Approach to Diagnostic Testing

Figure 10–1 shows a diagnostic approach to syncope adapted from guidelines of the American College of Physicians.[2,3,9] Clinical assessment and an ECG are the initial steps in evaluation of patients with syncope. This assessment may lead to a diagnosis or provide suggestive evidence for specific entities (e.g., signs of aortic stenosis or hypertrophic obstructive cardiomyopathy).

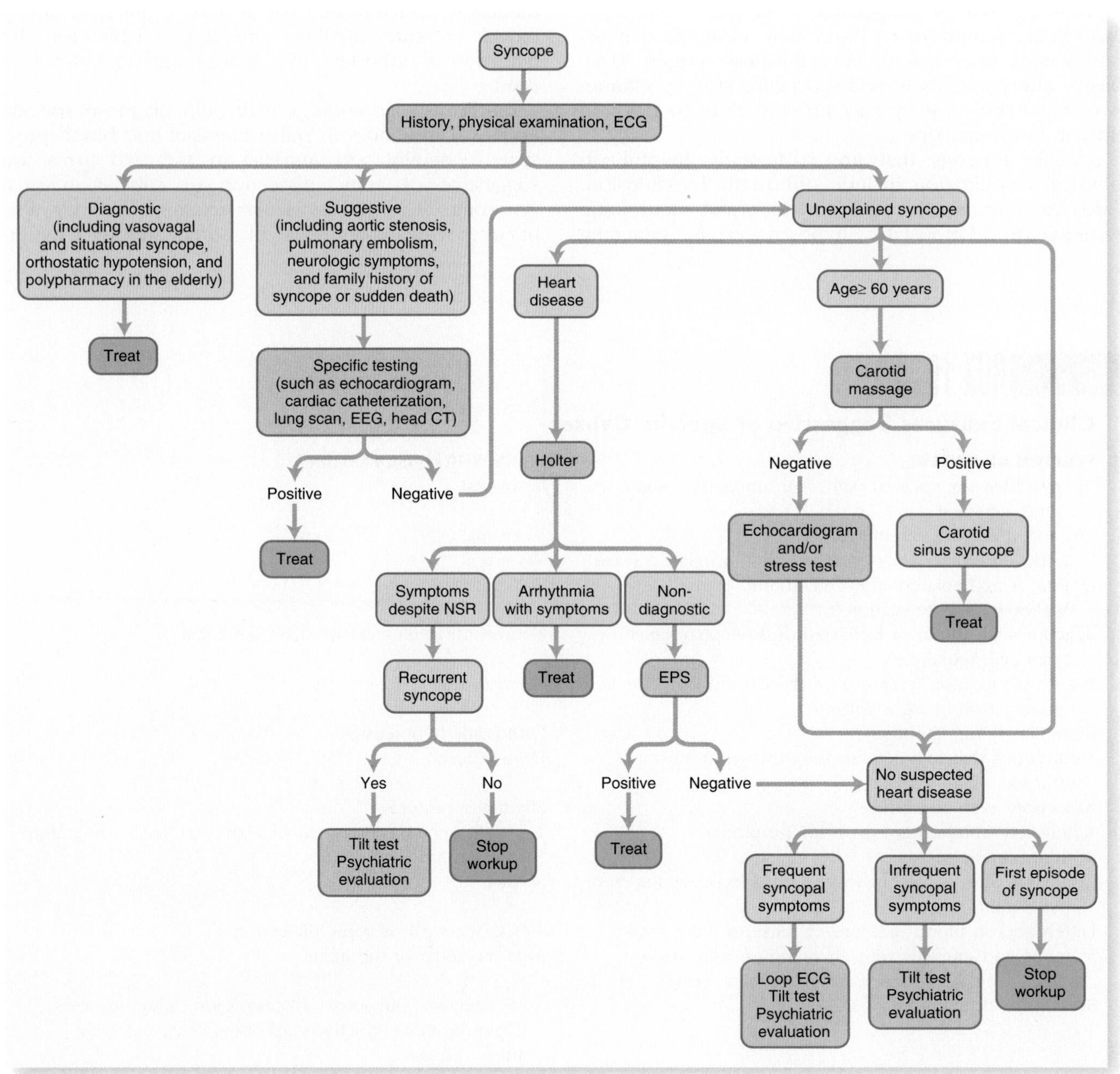

FIGURE 10–1. Diagnostic approach to a patient with syncope. CT, computed tomography; ECG, electrocardiogram; EEG, electroencephalogram; NSR, normal sinus rhythm. (Adapted from Linzer M, Yang EH, Estes NA, et al: Diagnosing syncope. Part 1: Value of history, physical examination, and electrocardiography. The clinical efficacy assessment project of the American College of Physicians. Ann Intern Med 1997;126:989–996; and Linzer M, Yang EH, Estes NA, et al: Diagnosing syncope. Part 2: Unexplained syncope. The Clinical Efficacy Assessment Project of the American College of Physicians. Ann Intern Med 1997;127:76–86.)

These clues can be pursued with further testing to confirm or exclude these conditions as the cause of the patient's syncope. In many patients, however, the initial clinical evaluation does not lead to a specific diagnosis or point to a potential cause of syncope. These patients can be divided into those with structural heart disease or an abnormal ECG and those without either of these findings. Patients with structural heart disease or an abnormal ECG should undergo Holter monitoring (or monitoring in a telemetry unit); if diagnostic arrhythmias are found, treatment can be initiated. Patients with nondiagnostic or negative Holter monitoring but with multiple syncopal episodes can be further evaluated with loop monitoring. Patients with nondiagnostic loop monitoring or those with only one or rare episodes of syncope should undergo EP testing for the evaluation of possible arrhythmic syncope.

In the elderly, cardiac evaluation with echocardiography and stress testing may be needed to determine the presence or absence of heart disease. Carotid sinus syncope is a disorder of the elderly, so carotid massage is a recommended diagnostic test in all patients 60 years or older.

In patients without structural heart disease or an abnormal ECG but with multiple episodes of syncope, tilt-table testing and psychiatric evaluation should be considered early in the investigation (see Fig. 10–1). Loop monitoring may also be considered for detection of arrhythmias in patients with a clinical suspicion of arrhythmic syncope but without known structural heart disease. Patients with one episode of syncope can be monitored closely without further evaluation if the initial clinical evaluation is negative.

Diagnostic tests are discussed in further detail in the following sections.

Cardiovascular Testing

12-Lead Electrocardiogram

An ECG is recommended for all patients with syncope because abnormalities found on the ECG may guide further evaluation or lead to a specific diagnosis. In one study, approximately 50% of patients with syncope had an abnormal ECG, including bundle branch block, old myocardial infarction, and left ventricular hypertrophy. However, causes of syncope are rarely assigned (in less than 5% of patients) on the basis of the ECG and rhythm strip alone because of the transient nature of most arrhythmias.

Prolonged Electrocardiographic Monitoring

Ambulatory monitoring is often difficult to interpret when used for the diagnostic evaluation of patients with syncope because of the rarity of symptoms during monitoring. In studies using more than 12 hours of monitoring, approximately 4% of patients had symptoms concurrently with arrhythmias. In another 17% of patients, symptoms were reported but no arrhythmias were found, thus potentially excluding arrhythmias as the cause of the symptoms. In approximately 79% of patients, no symptoms were reported despite brief arrhythmias in 13%. In the absence of symptoms during monitoring, the finding of only brief arrhythmias or even no arrhythmias does not exclude arrhythmic syncope. Brief arrhythmias are nonspecific and can be found in asymptomatic healthy individuals. Additionally, an absence of arrhythmias on monitoring does not exclude arrhythmic syncope because arrhythmias are episodic and may not be captured during monitoring. In patients with a high pretest probability of arrhythmias, such as brief sudden loss of consciousness without a prodrome, patients with an abnormal ECG, or those with structural heart disease, further evaluation is needed to establish or exclude arrhythmias as a cause of syncope.[10] Holter monitoring for a duration longer than 24 hours is not recommended because the yield of symptomatic arrhythmias is not substantially increased by extending the duration of monitoring to 72 hours.

Long-Term Event Monitoring. External loop ECG monitoring is a noninvasive test that enables patients to be monitored for prolonged periods (such as a month or more). Loop monitors generally use two chest ECG leads that are continuously worn and connected to a small recorder. Loop monitors can be activated after a syncopal episode to record 2 to 5 minutes of the rhythm before activation and 30 to 60 seconds of the rhythm after activation. Tracings can be transmitted via telephone. Loop monitoring is attractive because it provides the capability of electrocardiographic recording during a symptomatic period. Studies of loop monitoring show that arrhythmias with symptoms are found in 8% to 20% of patients. An additional 12% to 27% of patients have symptoms without concurrent arrhythmias. This test is recommended in patients with recurrent syncope when the probability of a recurrent event during the monitoring period is high.

Implantable Loop Event Monitoring. An implantable (inserted subcutaneously) loop recorder with the capability of cardiac monitoring for up to 18 months is now available for use in patients with recurrent, undiagnosed syncope. This type of a device is attractive in patients with infrequent episodes of unexplained syncope. In a randomized trial, prolonged monitoring with an implantable loop recorder was significantly better in establishing an arrhythmic cause of previously unexplained syncope than was a conventional approach using an external loop recorder, tilt testing, and EP testing.[11] This type of monitoring may be used more frequently in the future for difficult-to-diagnose syncope.[12]

Electrophysiologic Testing

EP testing is an invasive modality and often requires hospital admission. EP testing uses electrode catheters and electrical stimulation protocols to determine any cardiac conduction system abnormalities that may be associated with bradyarrhythmias or evidence of tachyarrhythmias as a potential cause of syncope.

Protocols for programmed ventricular stimulation generally include a minimum of three extra stimuli at one ventricular site. More aggressive protocols such as ventricular stimulation at two sites and the use of isoproterenol are associated with high rates of false-positive results.

A major problem with the use of EP testing in syncope is that a large number of findings are nonspecific and difficult to translate into management decisions. Because it is not possible to correlate arrhythmias during EP testing with naturally occurring symptoms, a diagnosis made by EP studies is almost always presumptive. Similarly, a negative EP study does not exclude a diagnosis of arrhythmic syncope. Findings most useful diagnostically in patients with syncope include induction of ventricular tachycardia, a prolonged sinus node recovery time (suggestive of sick sinus syndrome), or a prolonged His-ventricle interval or an infra-His block (suggestive of transient atrioventricular block).

In patients with structural heart disease, an abnormal ECG, or both, the diagnostic yield of EP testing is approximately 50%.[2,3] In patients without structural heart disease, the diagnostic yield is approximately 10%. The structural heart diseases in these studies included coronary artery disease, congenital or valvular heart disease, and cardiomyopathy. Particularly important ECG findings include conduction abnormalities (e.g., bundle branch block), previous myocardial infarction, and evidence of a bypass tract. Bradyarrhythmias are much more likely to be diagnosed in patients with conduction disease on the 12-lead ECG, but the sensitivity as well as specificity of EP studies for detection of bradyarrhythmias is low.

Carotid Massage

Carotid sinus hypersensitivity is detected by carotid sinus massage. Carotid massage is recommended when symptoms are suggestive of carotid sinus syncope (see Box 10–3) and in elderly patients with unexplained syncope.

Carotid massage is generally performed in the supine position and then repeated in the sitting and standing positions if the vasodepressor variety of carotid hypersensitivity is suspected but the supine test is negative. Noninvasive ECG and blood pressure monitoring is needed for interpretation of the results. A positive cardioinhibitory response is defined as a ventricular pause of 3 seconds or longer, and a positive vasodepressor response is defined as a drop in systolic blood pressure of 50 mm Hg or greater. A mixed cardioinhibitory and vasodepressor response can be diagnosed when carotid sinus massage is performed after the cardioinhibitory response is abolished with atropine or atrioventricular sequential pacing. The recommended duration of massage is 5 to 10 seconds on each side of the neck separately. The physician should wait at least 15 seconds between attempts before massaging the second side; simultaneous bilateral massage should never be performed.

Complications of carotid sinus massage include prolonged asystole, ventricular fibrillation, transient or permanent neurologic deficits, and sudden death. Complication rates are extremely low (incidence of neurologic complications <0.2%);[13] however, in patients with cerebrovascular disease, the test should be performed only if all other diagnostic modalities are exhausted and the pretest probability of carotid sinus syncope remains high.

Carotid sinus syncope is diagnosed in patients who are found to have carotid sinus hypersensitivity (a cardioinhibitory or vasodepressor response) and reproduction of spontaneous symptoms during carotid sinus massage. Even if symptoms are not reproduced, carotid sinus syncope remains likely when carotid sinus hypersensitivity is found and (1) spontaneous episodes are related to activities that press or stretch the carotid sinus or (2) the patient has recurrent syncope with an otherwise negative evaluation.

Echocardiogram

An echocardiogram (see Chapter 5) is recommended when the clinical assessment suggests structural cardiac disease as a possible cause of the syncope (e.g., clinical findings of possible aortic stenosis, hypertrophic cardiomyopathy, pulmonary hypertension). Echocardiography in the absence of clinical evidence of structural heart diseases rarely reveals unexpected findings that lead to an etiology of the syncope. Even in patients with known heart disease, the usefulness of echocardiography is low unless obstruction to inflow or outflow is suspected. Echocardiography is not recommended for screening purposes in patients with syncope.

Stress Testing

A stress ECG, myocardial perfusion scan, or echocardiogram (see Chapter 4) is recommended for the evaluation of symptoms with exercise and for the diagnosis of ischemia- or exercise-induced tachyarrhythmias. One of these tests is also recommended for the evaluation of postexertional syncope in patients without clinical structural heart disease. In other patients, the yield of stress testing for the diagnosis of the etiology of syncope is very low (less than 1%). Stress testing is useful as an ancillary diagnostic test for the evaluation of ischemic heart disease in patients with arrhythmic syncope, particularly ventricular tachycardia. In these patients, stress testing, cardiac catheterization, or both are often needed for the management of underlying cardiac disease, as well as for treatment of ventricular arrhythmias.

Upright Tilt Testing

Maintaining the patient in an upright position for a brief duration on a tilt table has become a common means of testing for a predisposition to vasovagal syncope, but the pathophysiologic mechanism of syncope with upright tilt testing is not entirely understood. It is widely accepted that hypotension or bradycardia (or both) during upright tilt testing is equivalent to spontaneous vasovagal syncope. This assumption is supported by the fact that the temporal sequence of blood pressure and heart rate changes during tilt-table testing is similar to that seen with spontaneous syncope. Additionally, the catecholamine release that occurs immediately before tilt-induced syncope is similar to that noted in a spontaneous vasovagal faint.

Upright posture leads to pooling of blood in the lower limbs and thus to decreased venous return. The normal compensatory response to an upright posture is reflex tachycardia, more forceful contraction of the ventricles, and vasoconstriction. However, in individuals susceptible to vasovagal syncope, this forceful ventricular contraction, in the setting of a relatively empty ventricle, may activate the cardiac mechanoreceptors that trigger reflex hypotension or bradycardia. Catecholamine release is also important in precipitating syncope. Catecholamines increase ventricular contraction and may thereby also activate the nerve endings responsible for triggering this reflex. Thus, catecholamines have been used to facilitate positive responses during upright tilt testing.

Tilt testing is generally performed by cardiology services in EP laboratories. The American College of Cardiology Expert Consensus has proposed tilt-testing methods and indications.[14] Box 10–4 shows the general procedures for tilt testing. Testing is performed with a motorized tilt table and footboard support so that position can be changed rapidly. Testing is often performed in a fasting state, and vasoactive drugs (e.g., calcium channel blockers, vasodilators, diuretics) are withheld for approximately five half-lives before testing. It is preferable to measure blood pressure during upright tilt testing noninvasively (e.g., with a blood pressure cuff or digital plethysmography) because invasive intra-arterial catheterization may provoke vasovagal reactions (resulting in a decrease in specificity of the test) and increase the cost and complexity of testing.

Two general types of testing procedures include upright tilt testing alone (passive testing) and tilt testing in conjunction with a chemical agent.[15] Passive tilt testing is rarely used because rates of positive responses appear to be low. The most common methods of testing include a brief period of passive testing followed by chemical stimulation with intravenous isoproterenol or sublingual nitroglycerin.

The sensitivity of tilt testing can be calculated by testing patients with a clinical diagnosis of vasovagal syncope; no other gold standards are available. With this approach, the sensitivity of tilt testing is 67% to 83%. The specificity of most currently used tilt testing protocols approaches 90% with chemical stimulation (either isoproterenol or nitroglycerin). When repeat testing is performed on the same day or days later, reproducibility is 65% to 85%. A patient with an initially negative study will rarely have a positive result on repeat testing. In patients with unexplained syncope, positive responses are reported in approximately 66% with isoproterenol protocols.[15] Results with the use of nitroglycerin appear to be similar.[16]

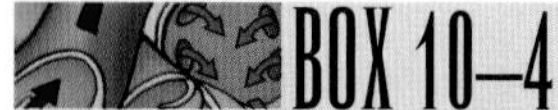

BOX 10–4

Tilt-Table Testing Technique

Laboratory	Quiet, dim lighting, comfortable temperature
	20- to 45-min supine equilibration period
Patient	Fasting overnight or for several hours before the procedure
	Parenteral fluid replacement
	Follow-up studies should be at similar times of the day
Recordings	Minimum of 3 electrocardiographic leads continuously recorded
	Beat-to-beat blood pressure recordings using the least intrusive means
Table	Footboard support
	Smooth, rapid transitions (up and down)
Tilt angle	60 to 80 degrees is acceptable
	70 degrees is becoming most common
Supervision	Nurse or laboratory technician experienced in the tilt-table technique and cardiovascular laboratory procedures
	Physician in attendance or in proximity and immediately available

PROTOCOLS USING ISOPROTERENOL

1. Standard protocol
   Use isoproterenol if drug-free tilt testing is negative (for 30–45 min)
   Return the patient to the supine position
   Begin an infusion of isoproterenol at 1 μg/min
   After 10 min of being supine, retilt for 10 min
   Repeat the procedure until the maximal infusion rate (3 μg/min) is reached
2. Alternative protocol
   Infuse isoproterenol to raise the heart rate by 20% after returning the patient to a supine position
   Retilt once the heart rate is ≥20% of baseline

ENDPOINT OF A POSITIVE TEST

Hypotension or bradycardia and reproduction of symptoms

Adapted from Benditt DG, Ferguson DW, Grubb BP, et al: Tilt table testing for assessing syncope. J Am Coll Cardiol 1996;28:263–275.

Upright tilt testing is recommended in patients with recurrent unexplained syncope in whom cardiac causes have been excluded or are not likely. Women of child-bearing age should undergo a pregnancy test before tilt testing because prolonged hypotension or bradycardia should be avoided in pregnant women. Older patients (>50 years) or patients with a history of ischemic heart disease should also undergo stress testing before tilt testing. In patients with cardiac ischemia, tilt testing should be avoided because hypotension or bradycardia may result in myocardial infarction. Tilt testing is generally contraindicated in patients with cerebrovascular disease.

Neurologic Testing

Skull films, lumbar puncture, radionuclide brain scans, and cerebral angiography do not generally yield diagnostic information for a cause of syncope in the absence of clinical findings suggestive of a specific neurologic process. Electroencephalographic (EEG) studies in patients with syncope have shown that 1% of patients have an epileptiform abnormality; almost all of them were suspected clinically.[17] Treatment based on EEG findings is initiated in only 1% to 2% of patients. Head computed tomographic (CT) scans are rarely useful in assigning a cause of syncope but are needed if subdural bleeding from a head injury is suspected or if a seizure of unknown etiology is suspected as a cause of loss of consciousness.

Psychiatric Assessment

Psychiatric illnesses need to be considered as a cause of syncope, especially in young patients and those who have multiple syncopal episodes as well as other nonspecific complaints. High clinical suspicion of these disorders is needed because they are often missed in medical patients. Disorders that may cause syncope include generalized anxiety and panic disorders, major depression, somatization disorder, and alcohol and substance abuse. Screening instruments for these disorders are available and recommended. The high rate of recurrent syncope in these patients makes detection of these illnesses especially important.

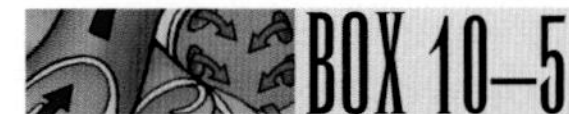

BOX 10–5

Reasons for Hospital Admission in Patients with Syncope

ADMISSION FOR DIAGNOSTIC EVALUATION

- Structural heart disease
  - Known coronary artery disease
  - Congestive heart failure
  - Valvular or congenital heart disease
  - History of ventricular arrhythmias
  - Physical findings of heart disease (e.g., findings of aortic stenosis)
- Symptoms suggestive of arrhythmias or ischemia
  - Associated with palpitations
  - Chest pain suggestive of coronary disease
  - Exertional syncope
- Electrocardiographic abnormalities
  - Ischemia
  - Conduction system disease (e.g., bundle branch block, first-degree atrioventricular block)
  - Unsustained ventricular or supraventricular tachycardia
  - Prolonged QT interval
  - Accessory pathway
  - Right bundle branch block with ST elevation in V_1–V_3 (suggestive of the Brugada syndrome)
  - Pacemaker malfunction
- Neurologic disease
  - New stroke or focal neurologic findings

ADMISSION FOR TREATMENT

- Structural heart disease
  - Acute myocardial infarction, pulmonary embolism, other cardiac diseases diagnosed as causing syncope
- Orthostatic hypotension
  - Acute severe volume loss (e.g., dehydration, gastrointestinal bleeding)
  - Moderate to severe chronic orthostatic hypotension
- Elderly
  - Treatment of multiple coexisting abnormalities
- Discontinuation or modification of doses of offending drug(s)
  - Drugs causing torsades de pointes and long-QT syndrome
  - Drug reaction such as anaphylaxis, orthostasis, bradyarrhythmias

ADMISSION DECISIONS

Most patients who have syncope initially seek care from primary care physicians and can be evaluated and treated as outpatients. Patients should be admitted to the hospital if rapid diagnostic evaluation is deemed necessary, mainly because of concern about serious arrhythmias, sudden death, newly diagnosed serious cardiac disease (e.g., aortic stenosis, myocardial infarction), and new onset of seizure or stroke (Box 10–5). Elderly patients are often hospitalized for rapid evaluation because of concern about asymptomatic underlying heart disease (especially coronary disease) or a fear that recurrent syncope may result in severe injury. No controlled trials have investigated the comparative advantages and disadvantages of managing patients with syncope on an outpatient as compared with an inpatient basis.

REFERRAL TO SPECIALTY CARE

Because syncope has a broad differential diagnosis, multiple consultations are frequently requested for diagnostic evaluation and management. The primary care physician can use the initial clinical assessment to guide the judicious use of specialty services. Specialty consultation can be approached as follows:

History and Physical Examination Leading to Diagnosis of a Specific Cause. Conditions found as causes of syncope can often be treated without any need for consultation. Examples include volume depletion, cough syncope, clinical vasovagal syncope, and neuralgia.

History and Physical Examination Suggesting Specific Entities. In these instances, further testing is generally needed to confirm or exclude the conditions under consideration. The results of specific tests should be obtained before consultation because these results may determine the need for consultation. For example, when aortic stenosis or hypertrophic obstructive cardiomyopathy is being considered clinically, an echocardiogram may be useful to establish or exclude the diagnosis. If the possibility of specific cardiac conditions is still a consideration after appropriate noninvasive testing, cardiology consultation for EP studies or cardiac catheterization may be needed.

Unexplained Syncope. In these situations, the following consultations may be needed:

- If arrhythmias are under consideration clinically (such as in patients with structural heart disease) and Holter and loop monitoring have been nondiagnostic, EP studies may be needed for diagnosis and therapy. Consultation with a cardiac electrophysiologist is recommended in these circumstances.
- If neurocardiogenic syncope is a major consideration, tilt testing is often needed for diagnosis. Consultation with a cardiac electrophysiologist is recommended, although the primary care physician should be able to manage these patients effectively according to the results of testing.

Management Issues. Rarely, patients with syncope have multiple possible etiologies. This situation commonly arises in the elderly, who may have cardiovascular diseases, may be taking multiple medications, and may have orthostatic hypotension. In these situations, the primary care physician should work closely with multiple specialists to coordinate care of the patient.

TREATMENT

Treatment of patients with syncope should focus on treatment of the underlying cause of the symptoms. Bradyarrhythmias commonly require cessation of offending medications, or they may be treated by insertion of a pacemaker (see Chapter 31). Tachyarrhythmias may require antiarrhythmic medication, an implantable cardioverter-defibrillator, or both (see Chapter 30).

Aortic stenosis will require valve replacement (see Chapter 32), whereas hypertrophic obstructive cardiomyopathy may respond to medications (see Chapter 29). Neurologic disease requires specific treatment. For orthostatic hypotension, volume repletion and avoidance of standing after large meals may be helpful.

For the more common neurocardiogenic syncope, treatment can include patient education, tilt training (i.e., repeated frequent tilting until the patient's positive response becomes negative), pharmacologic agents, and dual-chamber pacing. All patients should be instructed on how to prevent episodes by avoiding triggers such as prolonged standing, heat, large meals, fasting, lack of sleep, alcohol, and dehydration. Patients should also be instructed about maneuvers that prevent loss of consciousness, to assume a supine position (or at least to put their head below their heart) on recognizing premonitory symptoms, and to avoid activities that may lead to serious injury.

TABLE 10–2

Commonly Used Drug Therapies for Recurrent Vasovagal Syncope

Therapies	Dose
Beta-blockers	
Atenolol	25–200 mg/day
Metoprolol	50–200 mg/day
Propranolol	40–160 mg/day
Disopyramide	200–600 mg/day
Fludrocortisone	0.1–1 mg/day
Fluoxetine	20–40 mg/day
Paroxetine	10–40 mg/day
Scopolamine patch	1 patch every 3 days
Theophylline	6–12 mg/kg/day

Drug therapy (Table 10–2) should be reserved for patients who have recurrent neurocardiogenic syncope that has not responded to nonpharmacologic measures. The most widely used treatments include beta-blockers or salt in combination with fludrocortisone. Although many recommendations have previously been based on uncontrolled case series, several recent randomized trials provide more helpful data. For example, beta-blockers have been evaluated in several randomized trials. In general, treated patients have fared better than untreated patients.[17–21] Whether some beta-blockers are more efficacious than others is unclear.[21] One trial using paroxetine showed fewer recurrences at 2 years.[22] By comparison, a randomized trial using etilefrine, an alpha-agonist with vasoconstrictor properties, showed no benefit.[23]

Three randomized trials have assessed the efficacy of permanent pacemakers. In one, treatment of patients with severe symptoms (six or more lifetime episodes) and bradycardia on tilt testing showed an 85% reduction in the relative risk of recurrent syncope.[24] Another study showed that 5% of patients in the pacemaker arm experienced a recurrence of syncope versus 61% in the no-pacemaker arm during a mean follow-up of 3.7 years.[25] In the third, permanent pacing was significantly better than atenolol in preventing recurrent events in patients with neurocardiogenic syncope.[26] Thus, pacemakers appear to be the preferred treatment option in patients with severe, recurrent neurocardiogenic syncope and a cardioinhibitory response on tilt-table testing if conservative therapy has not produced a response.

Evidence-Based Summary

- A careful history, physical examination, and ECG can establish a cause of syncope in approximately 50% of patients and are recommended in all patients with syncope.
- Variables useful in risk stratification for the composite outcome of serious arrhythmias or mortality are a history of heart failure, an abnormal ECG, a history of ventricular tachycardia, and age older than 45 years.
- Prolonged monitoring with an implantable loop recorder is preferred over a conventional approach for difficult-to-diagnose syncope.
- EP testing can be useful in patients with structural heart disease or an abnormal ECG because such patients are the type in whom serious arrhythmias are commonly found.
- Patients with syncope and structural heart disease have a worse prognosis than do patients without structural heart disease. Treatment of the underlying cardiac disease is recommended, in addition to identifying and treating the cause of syncope.
- EEGs and head CT scans may provide diagnostic information in patients with symptoms suggestive of seizures or in those with focal neurologic findings. The yield of these tests in other patients with syncope is very low.
- Patients with psychiatric illnesses have higher rates of recurrent syncope than do patients without psychiatric illnesses. Screening plus intervention for psychiatric illness is recommended.
- Neurocardiogenic syncope may respond to conservative therapy (including beta-blockers or paroxetine), but a permanent pacemaker is preferred for recurrent, severe symptoms in patients with a positive tilt test or with bradycardia on prolonged monitoring.

References

1. Mathias CJ, Bannister R (eds): Autonomic failure. In A Textbook of Clinical Disorders of the Autonomic Nervous System, 4th ed. Oxford, Oxford University Press, 1999, pp 428–436.
2. Linzer M, Yang EH, Estes NA, et al: Diagnosing syncope. Part 1: Value of history, physical examination, and electrocardiography. The Clinical Efficacy Assessment Project of the American College of Physicians. Ann Intern Med 1997;126:989–996.
3. Linzer M, Yang EH, Estes NA, et al: Diagnosing syncope. Part 2: Unexplained syncope. The Clinical Efficacy Assessment Project of the American College of Physicians. Ann Intern Med 1997;127:76–86.
4. Ammirati F, Colivicchi F, Santini M: Diagnosing syncope in clinical practice. Implementation of a simplified diagnostic algorithm in a multicentre prospective trial. Eur Heart J 2000;21:935–940.
5. Sarasin FP, Louis-Simonte M, Carballo D, et al: Prospective evaluation of patients with syncope: A population-based study. Am J Med 2001;111:187.
6. Alboni P, Brignole M, Menozzi C, et al: Diagnostic value of history in patients with syncope with or without heart disease. J Am Coll Cardiol 2001;37:1921–1928.
7. Martin TP, Hanusa BH, Kapoor WN: Risk stratification of patients with syncope. Ann Emerg Med 1997;29:459–466.
8. Kapoor WN: Syncope. N Engl J Med 2000;343:1856–1862.
9. Schnipper JL, Kapoor WN: Diagnostic evaluation and management of patients with syncope. Med Clin North Am 2001;85:423–456.
10. Oh JH, Hanusa BH, Kapoor WN: Do symptoms predict cardiac arrhythmias and mortality in patients with syncope? Arch Intern Med 1999;159:375–380.
11. Krahn AD, Klein GJ, Yee R, Skanes AC: Randomized assessment of syncope trial: Conventional diagnostic testing versus a prolonged monitoring strategy. Circulation 2001;104:46–51.
12. Brignole M, Menozzi C, Moya A, Garcia-Civera R: Implantable loop recorder: Towards a gold standard for the diagnosis of syncope? Heart 2001;85:610–612.
13. Davies AJ, Kenny RA: Incidence of complications after carotid sinus massage in older patients with syncope. Am J Cardiol 1998;87:1256–1257.
14. Benditt DG, Ferguson DW, Grubb BP, et al: ACC Expert Consensus Document. Tilt table testing for assessing syncope. J Am Coll Cardiol 1996;28:263–275.
15. Kapoor WN: Using a tilt table to evaluate syncope. Am J Med Sci 1999;317:110–116.
16. Raviele A, Giada F, Brignole M, et al: Diagnostic accuracy of sublingual nitroglycerin test and low-dose isoproterenol test in patients with unexplained syncope. A comparative study. Am J Cardiol 2000;85:1194–1198.
17. Sheldon R, Rose S, Ritchie D, et al: Historical criteria that distinguish syncope from seizures. J Am Coll Cardiol 2002; 40:142–148.
18. Mahanonda N, Bhuripanyo K, Kangkagate C, et al: Randomized double-blind, placebo-controlled trial of oral atenolol in patients with unexplained syncope and positive upright tilt table test results. Am Heart J 1995;130: 1250–1253.
19. Madrid AH, Ortega J, Rebollo JG, et al: Lack of efficacy of atenolol for the prevention of neurally mediated syncope in a highly symptomatic population: A prospective, double-blind, randomized and placebo-controlled study. J Am Coll Cardiol 2001;37:554–559.
20. Ventura R, Maas R, Zeidler D, et al: A randomized and controlled pilot trial of beta-blockers for the treatment of recurrent syncope in patients with a positive or negative response to head-up tilt test. Pacing Clin Electrophysiol 2002;25:816–821.
21. Dendi R, Goldstein D: Meta-analysis of nonselective versus beta-1 adrenoreceptor-selective blockade in prevention of tilt-induced neurocardiogenic syncope. J Am Coll Cardiol 2002;89:1319–1321.
22. Di Girolamo E, Di Iorio C, Sabatini P, et al: Effects of paroxetine hydrochloride, a selective serotonin reuptake inhibitor, on refractory vasovagal syncope: A randomized,

double-blind, placebo-controlled study. J Am Coll Cardiol 1999;33:1227.

23. Raviele A, Brignole M, Sutton R, et al: Effect of etilefrine in preventing syncopal recurrence in patients with vasovagal syncope: A double-blind, randomized, placebo-controlled trial. The Vasovagal Syncope International Study. Circulation 1999;99:1452–1457.
24. Connolly SJ, Sheldon R, Roberts RS, Gent M: The North American Vasovagal Pacemaker Study (VPS). A randomized trial of permanent cardiac pacing for the prevention of vasovagal syncope. Am J Coll Cardiol 1999;33:21–23.
25. Sutton R, Brignole M, Menozzi C, et al: Dual-chamber pacing in treatment of neurally-mediated tilt-positive cardioinhibitory syncope. Pacemaker versus no therapy: A multicentre randomized study. Circulation 2000;102: 294–299.
26. Ammirati F, Colivicchi F, Santini M, for the Syncope Diagnosis and Treatment Study Investigators: Permanent cardiac pacing versus medical treatment for the prevention of recurrent vasovagal syncope: Multicenter, randomized, controlled trial. Circulation 2001;104: 52–57.

CHAPTER 11 Approach to the Patient with a Heart Murmur

Peter J. Norton and Robert A. O'Rourke

The cardiac physical examination is an important feature of any thorough patient evaluation. During both routine physical examination and the evaluation of acutely ill patients, a cardiac murmur is often heard on auscultation, but most murmurs are not associated with cardiac disease. Accordingly, it is essential to be able to differentiate murmurs attributable to cardiac pathology from those caused by accelerated or turbulent flow but not cardiac disease. An accurate understanding of cardiac physiology and its alterations during dynamic auscultation will enable the physician to determine whether the murmur is "innocent" or indicates the presence of valvular, congenital, or other structural heart disease.

Most murmurs are "physiologic" and are commonly related to increases in blood flow velocity. For example, the continuous murmur heard at the left sternal edge in many supine pregnant or lactating women that persists during the Valsalva maneuver is a benign finding. This murmur, known as a "mammary souffle," is due to blood flow through the superficial arteries of the breast. Also, a soft, short mid-systolic murmur heard best in the aortic area in hypertensive elderly patients is usually due to thickening of the aortic leaflets and not to obstruction of the aortic valve. In many such circumstances, assessment of the cardiac murmur often requires little, if any additional diagnostic testing.[1,2]

Similarly, accurate bedside evaluation of a murmur may reveal important cardiac disease.[3] Regardless of the presence or absence of cardiac symptoms, auscultatory findings may direct the examiner to further noninvasive (e.g., echocardiography) or invasive (cardiac catheterization) testing. When a complete evaluation has been completed and the diagnosis of the pathology is certain, appropriate medical or surgical treatment may be instituted. In this chapter we define cardiac murmurs, their auscultatory characteristics, methods for improving the accuracy of their interpretation, and situations in which various degrees of further diagnostic workup are indicated. We emphasize the resulting increase in cost when additional (often unnecessary) testing is ordered.

The traditional auscultatory method of assessing cardiac murmurs has been based on their timing, configuration, location, pitch, intensity, and duration. It is necessary to use this information when making important decisions that are dependent on correct interpretation of cardiac murmurs. As listed in Box 11–1, such decisions include the need for endocarditis antibiotic prophylaxis, the need for antibiotic prophylaxis to prevent recurrent rheumatic fever, the necessity of restricting physical activity, and the need for further cardiac evaluation using various noninvasive or invasive diagnostic techniques. In addition, precise interpretation of an isolated heart murmur is important in

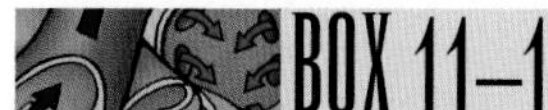

Decisions Dependent on the Correct Interpretation of Heart Murmurs

- Endocarditis antibiotic prophylaxis
- Rheumatic fever antibiotic prophylaxis
- Restriction of activity
- Need for further cardiac evaluation
- Assessment of the risk of noncardiac surgery

determining the risk of noncardiac surgery in a patient with no other evidence of cardiac disease.

MURMUR CHARACTERISTICS

Cardiac murmurs are caused by vibrations set up in the blood stream and the surrounding heart and great vessels as a result of turbulent blood flow that occurs when blood velocity becomes critically high because of high flow, flow through an irregular or narrow area, or a combination of both. Production of murmurs has been attributed to three main factors:

1. High blood flow rate through normal or abnormal orifices
2. Forward flow through a narrowed or regular orifice into a dilated vessel or chamber
3. Backward or regurgitant flow through an incompetent valve, septal defect, or patent ductus arteriosus.

Often, several of these factors are operative.[4,5]

Intensity

The intensity (loudness) of murmurs is usually graded from I to VI. A grade I murmur is so soft (faint) that it can be heard only with great effort, whereas a grade II murmur is faint but can be readily heard. A grade III murmur is moderately loud, and a grade IV murmur is very loud. A grade V murmur is extremely loud and can even be heard when only the edge of the stethoscope is in contact with the chest; it is not heard if the stethoscope is removed from the skin. A grade VI murmur is exceptionally loud and can be heard with the stethoscope slightly removed from contact with the chest.

Experience has shown that systolic murmurs of grade III or higher intensity are more likely to be hemodynamically significant and due to cardiac disease. Systolic thrills are often palpable with murmurs of grade IV or louder intensity. The loudness of the murmur is directly related to the velocity of blood flow across the site of murmur production, and the velocity is determined by the pressure difference that drives the blood across the murmur-producing site. For example, high velocity of flow through a small ventricular septal defect produces a loud systolic murmur, often accompanied by a thrill, whereas large flow at low velocity through an atrial septal defect produces no murmur. The loudness of a murmur as auscultated at the chest wall is also determined by the transmission characteristics of the tissues interposed between the source of the murmur and the stethoscope. Obesity, obstructive lung disease, and the presence of moderate to large pericardial or pleural effusions will diminish the intensity of a murmur, whereas a thin body habitus or severe weight loss will augment it.

Frequency

The frequency (pitch) of a murmur is also directly related to the velocity of blood flow at the site of the murmur's origin.[6] The low-velocity flow caused by a small pressure gradient across a stenotic mitral valve causes a low-pitched rumbling murmur, whereas the large diastolic pressure gradient across a regurgitant aortic valve results in a high-pitched murmur. Sometimes, the frequency components of the same systolic murmur will vary at different sites of auscultation. Often, the systolic murmur of aortic stenosis or sclerosis sounds higher pitched at the apex than at the base. Some murmurs may have an unusual musical quality, including the diastolic murmur of a ruptured or retroverted aortic leaflet and the systolic "whoop" or "honk" of mitral valve prolapse.[3]

Timing and Configuration

The *timing* of a heart murmur relative to the cardiac cycle and its configuration are important considerations. Separation of systole and diastole is usually easy because systole is considerably shorter at normal heart rates. However, with tachycardia, the relative duration of diastole shortens and the two intervals become similar. During tachycardia, the auscultator can usually time the murmur by simultaneous palpation of the carotid artery or relate it to the second heart sound (S_2), which is generally the louder sound at the base. With S_2 defined, murmurs can be accurately identified as occurring in systole or diastole. When sinus tachycardia is present, carotid sinus pressure may temporarily slow the heart rate and enable differentiation of systole from diastole. When premature contractions are occurring, the initial sound after the compensatory pause is the first heart sound (S_1).

The *configuration* of a murmur may be crescendo, decrescendo, crescendo-decrescendo (diamond shaped), or plateau. The precise time of onset and time of cessation of a murmur attributable to cardiac pathology depend on the point in the cardiac cycle at which an adequate pressure difference between two chambers appears and disappears (Fig. 11–1). *Systolic* murmurs are generally classified as holosystolic (pansystolic) murmurs or mid-systolic (systolic ejection) murmurs. Certain other murmurs may not begin until mid or late systole, particularly those caused by papillary muscle dysfunction, and they are called "late systolic" murmurs.

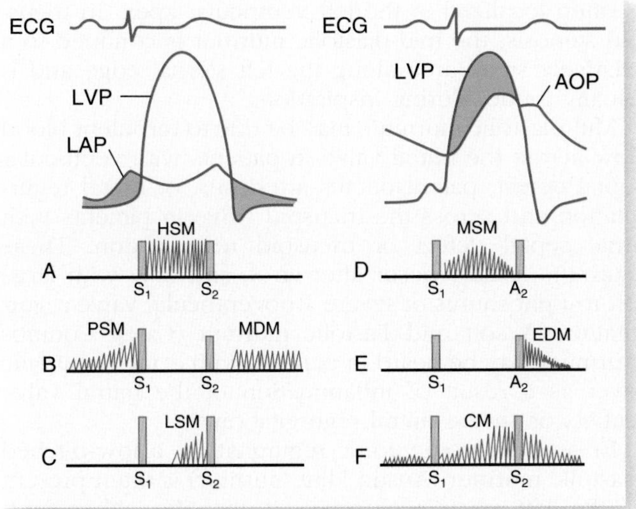

FIGURE 11–1. Schematic representation of the major types of abnormal murmurs and the associated pressure recordings. A_2, aortic second sound; AOP, aortic pressure; CM, continuous murmur; ECG, electrocardiogram; EDM, early diastolic murmur; HSM, holosystolic murmur; LAP, left atrial pressure; LSM, late systolic murmur; LVP, left ventricular pressure; MDM, mid-diastolic murmur; PSM, presystolic murmur; S_1, first heart sound; S_2, second heart sound. (From Crawford MH, O'Rourke RA: Curr Probl Cardiol 1977;1:11.)

The murmur of mitral valve prolapse also commonly occurs in the latter half of systole.

Diastolic murmurs are usually divided into early high-pitched diastolic murmurs, such as those caused by aortic or pulmonic regurgitation; mid-diastolic murmurs, such as those caused by blood flow across a stenotic mitral or tricuspid valve; and presystolic murmurs, which occur for the same reason in patients with a gradient between the atria and ventricle and in sinus rhythm. A continuous murmur can usually be separated from a systolic plus a diastolic murmur because it begins in systole and continues through S_2, where it peaks into diastole.[2,6]

Holosystolic (pansystolic) murmurs are generated when blood flows between chambers that have widely different pressures throughout systole, such as the left ventricle and either the left atrium or right ventricle. The pressure gradient occurs early in contraction and lasts until relaxation is almost complete. Therefore, holosystolic murmurs begin before aortic ejection and at the area of maximal intensity; they begin with S_1 and end after S_2. Holosystolic murmurs are caused by mitral and tricuspid regurgitation, ventricular septal defects, and certain aortopulmonary shunts. Although the typical high-pitched murmur of mitral regurgitation usually continues throughout systole, the murmur may vary in configuration. The murmur of tricuspid regurgitation resulting from pulmonary hypertension is holosystolic and frequently increases during inspiration. Not all patients with mitral or tricuspid regurgitation or a ventricular septal defect have holosystolic murmurs, and changes in murmur intensity with various maneuvers described later in this chapter are often useful for their correct interpretation.[2,6]

Mid-systolic (systolic ejection) murmurs, often crescendo-decrescendo or diamond in shape, occur when blood is ejected across the aortic or pulmonic outflow tracts. The murmur starts shortly after S_1, when ventricular pressure rises sufficiently to open the semilunar valve. As ejection increases, the murmur is augmented, and as ejection declines, it diminishes. The murmur ends before ventricular pressure falls enough to permit closure of the aortic or pulmonic leaflets. In the presence of normal semilunar valves, an increased flow rate as occurs in states of elevated cardiac output (e.g., fever, thyrotoxicosis, anemia, and pregnancy), ejection of blood into a dilated vessel beyond the valve, or increased transmission of sound through a thin chest wall may cause this murmur. Most benign "innocent" murmurs in children and young adults are mid-systolic because of high velocity and originate from either the aortic or pulmonic outflow tracts. Valvular or subvalvular obstruction to either ventricle may also cause such a mid-systolic murmur, with the intensity being related to the velocity of blood flow across the obstructed area.

The murmur of *aortic stenosis* is the typical left-sided mid-systolic murmur of heart disease. Sclerosis of the aortic leaflets without a left ventricular–aortic systolic pressure gradient often causes a similar murmur. If the aortic valve is heavily calcified, the aortic closure sound (A_2) may be soft or inaudible; as a result, the length and configuration of the murmur are more difficult to determine. Mid-systolic murmurs also occur in patients with mitral regurgitation or, less frequently, tricuspid regurgitation from papillary muscle dysfunction. Such mitral regurgitation murmurs are commonly misinterpreted as aortic stenosis or sclerosis, particularly in elderly patients.

The patient's age and the site of maximal murmur intensity are useful in determining the significance of mid-systolic murmurs.[7] Thus, in a young adult with a thin chest and a high velocity of blood flow, a faint or moderate mid-systolic murmur heard only in the pulmonic area usually has no clinical significance, whereas a louder murmur in the aortic area may indicate congenital aortic stenosis. In elderly patients, pulmonic flow murmurs are rare, but aortic systolic murmurs are common and may be due to aortic valve sclerosis, valvular aortic stenosis, or aortic dilatation. Mid-systolic aortic and pulmonic murmurs are intensified by various maneuvers as indicated later in the section "Specific Maneuvers." Echocardiography is often necessary to separate a prominent and exaggerated benign mid-systolic murmur from one caused by congenital or acquired aortic valve stenosis.[4,6]

Early systolic murmurs are less common; they begin with S_1 and end in mid systole. In large ventricular septal defects with pulmonary hypertension and small muscular ventricular septal defects, the shunting at the end of systole may be insignificant, with the murmur limited to early systole. An early systolic murmur is often due to tricuspid regurgitation occurring in the absence of pulmonary hypertension. This murmur is common in drug addicts with active or previous infective endocarditis, in whom a tall regurgitant right atrial V-wave reaches the level of the normal right ventricular pressure in late systole; thus, no pressure difference or murmur occurs in late systole. In patients with acute mitral regurgitation and a large V-wave in a nondilated left atrium, a loud early systolic murmur is often heard that decreases in late systole as the pressure difference between the left ventricle and the left atrium diminishes.

Late systolic murmurs are soft or moderately loud, high-pitched murmurs at the left ventricular apex; they start well after ejection and end before or at S_2. These murmurs are probably caused by ischemia or infarction of the mitral papillary muscles or by dysfunction of these muscles as a result of left ventricular dilatation. They may be heard only during angina but are commonly present in patients with myocardial infarction or dilated cardiomyopathy. Late systolic murmurs in patients with mid-systolic clicks are the result of late systolic mitral regurgitation caused by prolapse of the mitral leaflet or leaflets into the left atrium.[2,3]

Early immediate diastolic murmurs begin with or shortly after S_2 when the associated ventricular pressure drops sufficiently below that in the aorta or pulmonary artery. The high-pitched murmurs of aortic regurgitation or pulmonic regurgitation secondary to pulmonary hypertension are generally decrescendo, consistent with the rapid decline in the volume or rate of regurgitation during diastole. Faint, high-pitched murmurs of aortic regurgitation are often heard only when the diaphragm of the stethoscope is held firmly over the left midsternal border while the patient sits, leans forward, and holds a breath in full expiration.[2,5,6] The diastolic murmur of aortic regurgitation is enhanced by acute elevation of arterial pressure such as occurs with multiple maneuvers discussed in the section "Specific Maneuvers." The diastolic murmur of pulmonic regurgitation without pulmonary hypertension, such as may occur with congenital heart disease, endocarditis, or other diseases directly affecting the pulmonic valve (e.g., carcinoid syndrome), is low to medium pitched. The onset of this murmur is slightly delayed because the regurgitant flow is minimal at closure of the pulmonic valve, when the reverse pressure gradient responsible for the regurgitation is minimal.[6]

Mid-diastolic murmurs usually originate from the mitral and tricuspid valves, occur during early ventricular filling, and are due to a relative disproportion between valve orifice size and diastolic blood flow velocity. Such murmurs may be quite loud despite only slight atrioventricular valve stenosis when blood flow is normal or increased. Conversely, the murmur may be faint or inaudible at rest despite severe stenosis if cardiac output is very low. When the obstruction is marked, the diastolic murmur is longer; its duration is more reliable than its intensity for indicating the severity of valve stenosis.[2,5,6]

The low-pitched, mid-diastolic murmur of mitral stenosis usually follows an opening snap. It is best detected with the bell of the stethoscope placed over the site of the left ventricular impulse with the patient turned to the left side. The murmur of mitral stenosis is often localized to the left ventricular apex. In tricuspid stenosis, the mid-diastolic murmur is confined to a relatively small area along the left sternal edge and is usually louder during inspiration.

Mid-diastolic murmurs may be due to turbulent blood flow across the mitral valve in patients with ventricular septal defect, patent ductus arteriosus, or mitral regurgitation and across the tricuspid valve in patients with atrial septal defect or tricuspid regurgitation. These murmurs usually occur after an S_3 and only with large left-to-right shunts or severe atrioventricular valve regurgitation. A soft mid-diastolic murmur (Carey Coombs murmur) may be heard in patients with acute rheumatic fever as a result of inflammation of the mitral valve leaflets or severe mitral regurgitation.[1,3]

In severe chronic aortic regurgitation, a low-pitched diastolic murmur (Austin Flint murmur) is often present at the left ventricular apex; it may be either mid-diastolic or presystolic. This murmur originates at the anterior mitral valve leaflet when blood flow simultaneously enters the left ventricle from both the aortic root and the left atrium.[2,5,6]

Presystolic murmurs begin during the period of ventricular filling that follows atrial contraction and therefore occur in sinus rhythm. They are usually due to mitral or tricuspid stenosis. These murmurs are low pitched and usually crescendo in configuration, with peak intensity reached at the time of a loud S_1. A presystolic murmur is related to the atrioventricular valve gradient, which may be augmented by right or left atrial contraction. It is often present in patients with tricuspid stenosis and sinus rhythm. A right or left atrial myxoma may occasionally cause either mid-diastolic or presystolic murmurs, similar to tricuspid or mitral stenosis.[2]

Continuous murmurs arise from high- to low-pressure shunts that persist through the end of systole and the beginning of diastole. Thus, they begin in systole, peak near S_2, and continue into all or part of diastole. A patent ductus arteriosus causes a continuous murmur when the pressure in the pulmonary artery is much below that in the aorta. The murmur is louder when systemic arterial pressure is raised and softer when it is lowered. When pulmonary hypertension is present, the diastolic portion may disappear. Surgically produced connections such as a subclavian-pulmonary artery anastomosis result in murmurs similar to that of a patent ductus arteriosus. Continuous murmurs may result from a congenital or acquired systemic arteriovenous fistula, coronary arteriovenous fistula, anomalous origin of the left coronary artery from the pulmonary artery, and communications between an aortic sinus of Valsalva and the right side of the heart. Continuous murmurs may also occur in patients with a small atrial septal defect and high left atrial pressure. In addition, continuous murmurs may be due to abnormal blood flow patterns in constricted systemic or pulmonary arteries. As examples, a continuous murmur in the back may occur with coarctation of the aorta, and pulmonary embolism may cause continuous murmurs in partially occluded vessels.[2,5,6]

Continuous murmurs may result from rapid blood flow through a tortuous bed in nonconstricted arteries, as occurs within the bronchial arterial collateral circulation in patients with severe pulmonary outflow obstruction and cyanosis. The "mammary soufflé," a physiologic murmur heard over the breasts during late pregnancy and early postpartum, may be systolic or continuous. The innocent cervical venous hum is a continuous murmur that is usually heard over the medial aspect of the right supraclavicular fossa with the patient upright. It is generally louder during diastole and can be immediately abolished by digital compression of the ipsilateral internal jugular vein. Transmission of a loud venous hum to the left infraclavicular area may result in an incorrect clinical diagnosis of patent ductus arteriosus.[3]

Location and Radiation

The location on the chest wall where the murmur is best heard and the areas to which it radiates can be helpful in identifying the cardiac structure from which the murmur originates. The location and radiation of a murmur of aortic stenosis are influenced by the direction of the high-velocity jet within the aortic root. In valvular aortic stenosis, the murmur is usually maximal in the second right intercostal space, with radiation into the neck. In supravalvular aortic stenosis, the murmur is generally loudest even higher, with greater radiation to the right carotid artery. In hypertrophic cardiomyopathy, the mid-systolic murmur is generated within the left ventricular cavity, is usually loudest at the lower left sternal edge and apex, and radiates little, if at all to the neck. By contrast, the murmur of mitral regurgitation is most often loudest at the cardiac apex. It may radiate to the left sternal border and base of the heart when the posterior mitral leaflet is involved or to the axilla or back when the anterior leaflet is more seriously affected. In the latter case, the regurgitant blood is directed toward the posterior left atrial wall. However, the location and radiation of a murmur are multifactorial and determined by its site of origin, its intensity, and the duration of blood flow, as well as by the physical characteristics of the chest. For example, in elderly patients, the murmur of aortic stenosis is often loudest at the left ventricular apex.

DYNAMIC CARDIAC AUSCULTATION

Attentive cardiac auscultation during dynamic changes in cardiac hemodynamics (Box 11–2) often enables a careful observer to deduce the correct origin and significance of a cardiac murmur. Maneuvers for evaluating heart murmurs during dynamic cardiac auscultation include respiratory variation, the Valsalva maneuver, exercise, postural changes, pharmacologic agents, changes in intensity after a premature beat, and transient arterial occlusion.[7–10]

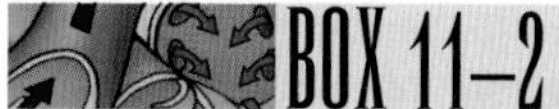
BOX 11–2

Maneuvers Used to Change the Intensity of Cardiac Murmurs

- Respiratory variation
- Valsalva maneuver
- Exercise
- Postural changes
- Changes after a premature contraction
- Pharmacologic interventions
- Transient arterial occlusion

Specific Maneuvers

Respiratory Variation

Normal inspiration decreases intrathoracic pressure and thus increases venous return to the right side of the heart and dilatation of the pulmonary circulation. As right ventricular volume increases, so does stroke volume, partly because of the Frank-Starling mechanism and partly because of lessened impedance to right ventricular ejection. Respiratory changes in systemic flow are most prominent in the sitting or standing position, when venous return is normally lower. In the supine position, venous return is higher, and the changes with inspiration are less marked. Therefore, it is useful to observe auscultatory changes during inspiration with the patient in both the supine and seated positions. If normal respiration does not produce the expected changes in the intensity of murmurs or sounds, the patient should be directed to take slightly deeper breaths. However, maximal inspiration should be avoided because it can result in a partial Valsalva maneuver with possible opposing hemodynamic results.

Respiration is the best maneuver for differentiating between cardiac murmurs originating in the right and left sides of the heart. Inspiration will accentuate most auscultatory events originating in the right side of the heart, including the murmurs of tricuspid and pulmonic valve regurgitation or stenosis, each of which will become louder during inspiration. Insignificant mid-systolic murmurs across the pulmonic outflow tract will also increase in intensity. Conversely, expiration causes a decrease in lung volume by placing the heart closer to the anterior chest wall, and pulmonary venous flow is augmented as well. Therefore, left-sided murmurs originating at the mitral or aortic valve are usually loudest during expiration and diminish or are unchanged with inspiration.

Variations in the normal splitting of S_2 during inspiration often provide an important clue to the presence of heart disease, particularly in patients with a mid-systolic murmur. Normal splitting of A_2 and P_2 may be widened by late activation of the right ventricle, such as occurs with prolonged ventricular contraction because of a right ventricular pressure load (e.g., pulmonic stenosis), or by delayed pulmonic valve closure because of reduced impedance of the pulmonary vasculature (e.g., idiopathic dilatation of the pulmonary artery). In patients with left-to-right shunting through an atrial septal defect, pulmonary vascular impedance may be decreased to the point where augmented venous return during inspiration will not affect right heart flow or stroke volume. In this case, inspiration produces little, if any additional separation between the two components of S_2, and it remains widely split and results in the so-called fixed splitting of S_2 that occurs in patients with atrial septal defect in addition to the mid-systolic pulmonic murmur that is present.[4,5]

Careful evaluation of the timing of the two components of S_2 during respiration can be quite helpful in assessing the significance of a murmur. The aortic component of S_2 may appear early when resistance to left ventricular ejection is decreased, as occurs with mitral regurgitation and ventricular septal defect. By contrast, late aortic valve closure may cause the aortic component of S_2 to occur after the pulmonic component during expiration. Thus, maximal splitting occurs during expiration and results in reversed (paradoxical) splitting of S_2. Prolonged left ventricular ejection such as occurs with severe aortic stenosis may produce reversed splitting of S_2. Reversed splitting of S_2 in a patient with a loud, late-peaking mid-systolic murmur at the base usually indicates very severe aortic stenosis.

Valsalva Maneuver

The Valsalva maneuver is a useful method for determining the probable cause of various cardiac murmurs. The maneuver is a two-part process consisting of a straining period followed by a relaxation period, each of which has importance in characterization of heart murmurs.[7,9]

The Valsalva maneuver is performed by having the patient forcefully attempt to exhale against a closed glottis after taking a normal breath. The examiner should place a hand on the patient's abdomen to be sure that the muscles are tightening. An alternative method is to have the patient exhale into a manometer to maintain a level of 40 mm Hg or greater for the duration of the maneuver. When the Valsalva maneuver is performed, intrathoracic pressure will be elevated considerably, thus increasing both end-systolic and end-diastolic ventricular pressure. The pulmonary vasculature is emptied into the left atrium and left ventricle, and a small initial rise in systemic arterial pressure is generated. Subsequently, venous return to the right side of the heart is inhibited by the higher intrathoracic pressure, right and left ventricular output declines, and cardiac output and systemic blood pressure decrease.

The Valsalva maneuver is usually performed for about 10 seconds while the examiner listens to intensity changes in heart murmurs. The maneuver should be discontinued after 10 seconds to prevent symptoms (e.g., syncope) from the reduced cardiac output and blood pressure. The maneuver briefly decreases myocardial blood flow and should not be used in patients with known myocardial ischemia or recent infarction. Most cardiac murmurs and sounds diminish in intensity during the Valsalva maneuver because of the decreased ventricular filling and cardiac output.

The murmur of mitral valve prolapse is one of only two murmurs that will increase in intensity or duration with the Valsalva maneuver. The decease in left ventricular volume during straining causes earlier mitral leaflet prolapse in systole, which usually increases the length and often the intensity of the systolic murmur. Occasionally, a musical "whoop" will be induced by the Valsalva maneuver.[3]

The murmur of hypertrophic cardiomyopathy is the only other murmur that will increase in intensity with the Valsalva maneuver. The degree of left ventricular outflow tract narrowing from abnormal motion of the anterior mitral leaflet toward the hypertrophic interventricular septum varies with left ventricular volume. When the volume is diminished, as during the strain phase of the Valsalva maneuver, the outflow tract pressure gradient increases and the murmur is louder. Though highly specific, not all patients with hypertrophic cardiomyopathy will exhibit an increase in mid-systolic murmur intensity with the Valsalva maneuver.

During release of straining, the second phase of the Valsalva maneuver, intrathoracic pressure returns to normal, and right and then left ventricular filling and cardiac output are suddenly augmented. The delay in filling between the right and left heart chambers often aids in the differentiation of murmurs of right and left heart origin. Murmurs generated in the right side of the heart usually return to baseline intensity soon after release of straining, within one to four heartbeats. Left-sided murmurs often require 5 to 10 cardiac cycles to return to baseline intensity. Thus, in patients with aortic or mitral valve stenosis or regurgitation, a ventricular septal defect, or other left-sided lesions, the intensity of the murmur decreases during straining and gradually returns to baseline during relaxation. In patients with tricuspid or pulmonic stenosis or regurgitation, the murmur will also soften during straining, but its intensity will return to baseline almost immediately on release of the Valsalva maneuver. This response is observed in most young patients with innocent mid-systolic heart murmurs.

Exercise

All forms of exercise increase the heart rate and cardiac output and may be clinically useful in differentiating various heart murmurs. However, it is impractical for hospitalized, uncooperative, or deconditioned patients to perform many types of dynamic exercise. Thus, isometric exercise in the form of sustained handgrip is often used during cardiac auscultation in the office or at the bedside. Usually, the patient is instructed to squeeze the examiner's finger or another object such as a rolled towel as tightly as possible with one or both hands while auscultatory changes are assessed. In more precise studies, the use of a calibrated dynamometer can measure the amount of force applied to the handle. The patient should be instructed to breathe normally and to squeeze only with the forearm so that the chest remains relaxed and a simultaneous Valsalva maneuver does not confuse the results. A minimum of 60 to 90 seconds usually elapses before a significant heart rate and blood pressure response is noted. Sustained handgrip rapidly increases the heart rate, cardiac output, and both systolic and diastolic arterial pressure, with a quick return to baseline values after cessation of the maneuver. Although isometric exercise causes a smaller increase in heart rate and cardiac output than isotonic exercise does, blood pressure increases are usually greater with handgrip exercise. When the effort expended exceeds 50% of the subject's maximal voluntary contraction, a substantial increase in systemic vascular resistance is noted, as well as an increase in heart rate, cardiac output, and arterial pressure.[7,9]

The rise in systemic arterial pressure during isometric exercise augments the systolic pressure gradient between the left ventricle and left atrium or right ventricle, and the murmurs of mitral regurgitation and ventricular septal defect increase in intensity. The late systolic murmur of mitral valve prolapse is usually louder during handgrip. The increased aortic diastolic blood pressure increases the murmur of aortic regurgitation. Murmurs of aortic stenosis and hypertrophic cardiomyopathy usually soften or are unchanged during handgrip because of the higher aortic pressure.

Because myocardial oxygen demand is increased with isometric exercise, ischemia of the papillary muscles may result in patients with coronary artery disease. New murmurs of mitral regurgitation may be heard during handgrip but are rarely associated with chest pain. However, patients with acute or recent myocardial infarction should not undergo isometric exercise.

Handgrip exercise is an excellent maneuver for assessing patients with rheumatic mitral valve disease. Systolic murmurs of mitral regurgitation and the diastolic rumble of mitral stenosis will be accentuated by the elevated blood pressure and tachycardia during handgrip.

Postural Changes

Cardiac auscultation of a patient only in the supine position fails to use important information that can be obtained about heart murmurs from changes in position. Postural changes are particularly useful for differentiating the mid-systolic murmur of valvular aortic stenosis or aortic sclerosis from that associated with hypertrophic cardiomyopathy or mitral valve prolapse.

When the patient assumes the upright position, venous return diminishes because of gravitational pooling, thereby decreasing ventricular filling pressure. Stroke volume declines and causes a reflex rise in heart rate and systemic vascular resistance. Most heart murmurs soften with these hemodynamic changes, a response similar to that observed with the Valsalva maneuver, which also decreases ventricular filling pressure. Exceptions are the systolic murmurs of hypertrophic cardiomyopathy and mitral valve prolapse; they often become louder and longer when the patient is sitting or stands as a result of the smaller left ventricular volume. Pulmonic mid-systolic flow murmurs are usually softer when the patient stands but will get louder during inspiration in the upright position, similar to most right-sided heart murmurs.[7,9]

Cardiac auscultation while the patient squats rapidly from the upright position is a useful diagnostic maneuver. Squatting is an effective way to assess the physiologic changes of increased ventricular filling volume. During squatting, patients should rest on their heels with the hips flexed laterally. With the physician sitting throughout the examination, the patient can be auscultated immediately on reaching the standing and squatting positions with a minimum of effort.

During squatting, compression of the femoral arteries causes mean aortic pressure to rise abruptly and remain at a level higher than at rest. In addition, reflex bradycardia is observed. Venous return to the heart is augmented as a result of the increased pressure in the legs and abdominal cavity. For patients unable to perform the squatting maneuver because of age or musculoskeletal disease, the examiner can passively bend the patient's knees toward the abdomen ("jack-knifing") while in the supine position and produce similar physiologic and auscultatory changes as during squatting.

Right heart volume and flow are augmented by the increase in venous return during squatting. As left-sided pressures increase, so do the murmurs of mitral regurgitation, ventricular septal defect, and aortic regurgitation. The larger left ventricular volume and higher arterial pressure reduce any aortic outflow pressure gradient in hypertrophic cardiomyopathy, thus diminishing the mid-systolic murmur. In addition, by the same mechanism, the late systolic murmur of mitral valve prolapse will be softer and the systolic click-murmur complex will often begin later in systole closer to S_2.

Changes in murmur intensity during standing may become more evident when the patient stands abruptly from the squatting position. Thus, auscultation during standing, squatting, and then standing again may produce diagnostic changes in murmur intensity. An example is the mid-systolic murmur of hypertrophic cardiomyopathy, which usually becomes louder during standing, much softer during squatting, and still louder when the patient stands again.

All four of the previously described methods for altering the intensity of cardiac murmurs depend on normal autonomic nervous function for inducing the changes in hemodynamics responsible for the auscultatory results. Therefore, in patients with heart failure and other conditions that affect autonomic nervous function, the usefulness of these maneuvers for determining the etiology of heart murmurs is diminished.

Changes after a Premature Contraction

Variations in murmur intensity in the first beat after a premature beat can provide important information on the cause of the murmur. During the compensatory pause, right and left ventricular filling is increased and aortic and pulmonic diastolic pressure declines, thus enhancing stroke volume and promoting forward blood flow. Moreover, ventricular function will be augmented after a premature beat because of the increase in end-diastolic ventricular volume (Frank-Starling effect). Similar hemodynamic responses usually occur in patients with atrial fibrillation and are due to changing R-R intervals and varying cardiac cycle length.[7,9]

Mitral regurgitation murmurs do not generally change in intensity after a long cardiac cycle. Although left ventricular end-diastolic flow and forward flow are each greater after a premature beat and the regurgitant flow across the mitral valve early in systole is also enhanced, the increase in mitral regurgitant flow after a premature beat is primarily confined to the period of isovolumic contraction when the aortic valve is still closed. During the latter half of systole after the aortic valve opens, the regurgitant volume is actually lessened while the forward stroke volume is greater. The net result is little change in mitral regurgitant flow in the beat after a long cardiac cycle and thus no apparent change in murmur intensity.

The increased ventricular filling and decreased aortic impedance accentuate turbulent flow across a stenotic or sclerotic aortic valve. Systolic murmurs of aortic stenosis or sclerosis are louder in the first beat after a premature beat. In aortic stenosis at the valvular, supravalvular, and discrete subvalvular levels, the systolic pressure gradient across the left ventricular outflow tract increases after the extrasystolic beat, and the systolic murmur intensifies. The systolic murmur of hypertrophic cardiomyopathy is more variable, although it usually gets louder. Insignificant pulmonic and mid-systolic murmurs and the murmur of pulmonic stenosis are also louder after premature beats.

In examining a patient with atrial fibrillation or premature beats, the effect of changing cycle length on murmur intensity can be useful for differentiating between the systolic murmurs of mitral regurgitation and left ventricular outflow tract turbulence. In addition, no active patient participation is required, and the results are not dependent on normal function of the autonomic nervous system.

Pharmacologic Maneuvers Used to Change the Intensity of Cardiac Murmurs

In the past, many drugs have been used to aid in the correct identification of heart murmurs by modifying cardiovascular hemodynamics. They have been used less commonly in recent years because of the advent of other maneuvers and the emergence of two-dimensional (2-D) and Doppler echocardiography. The most common drug still used for this purpose is amyl nitrite, the volatile ester of nitrous acid. It is administered by inhalation and works very rapidly; its important hemodynamic effect occurs in the first 10 to 30 seconds after inhalation for two to three rapid, deep breaths.[7,9]

Amyl nitrite is a potent vasodilator that causes an immediate decline in systemic arterial pressure within 15 seconds after inhalation, but it has a duration of only about 30 seconds. Left ventricular size decreases and left ventricular ejection is enhanced. Reflex tachycardia develops within 30 to 60 seconds after inhalation, thus increasing cardiac output.

The most common clinical use of amyl nitrite is in differentiating systolic murmurs of aortic and mitral origin. In the first 15 seconds after inhalation, the rapid decline in arterial pressure increases forward flow. The mid-systolic murmurs of aortic stenosis or sclerosis will increase in intensity as a result of increased turbulence in the left ventricular outflow tract. The murmur of hypertrophic cardiomyopathy will become louder as well. Left-sided regurgitant systolic murmurs such as mitral regurgitation become shorter and softer, particularly in the last half of systole. Because of the decrease in aortic diastolic pressure, amyl nitrite diminishes the murmur of aortic regurgitation.

Blood flow to the right side of the heart is increased with the use of amyl nitrite, which augments right-sided murmurs. Thus, systolic murmurs of tricuspid regurgitation will be louder. The diastolic murmur of tricuspid stenosis is augmented by the tachycardia and enhanced cardiac output. The murmur of pulmonic stenosis and insignificant pulmonic flow murmurs are increased as well. Inhalation of amyl nitrite is useful in differentiating between the low-pitched diastolic murmur of mitral valve stenosis and the Austin Flint mitral diastolic murmur heard in severe aortic regurgitation. Amyl nitrite reduces regurgitant flow across the aortic valve (because of the decline in blood pressure and systemic vascular resistance), thereby lessening the intensity of the Austin Flint murmur. In contrast, mitral valve stenosis murmurs are louder with amyl nitrite, particularly during the tachycardia response.

Though relatively safe, amyl nitrite should be given only to a patient in the supine position and is contraindicated for use in patients with severe aortic stenosis or unstable angina pectoris.

Transient Arterial Occlusion

The maneuvers described in the preceding sections are traditional additions to the routine cardiac examination that can be used to help delineate various auscultatory findings. However, the usefulness of these maneuvers may be limited in some instances. Active patient participation may be difficult to obtain because of musculoskeletal disease or altered mental status. Some patients unintentionally perform two maneuvers with opposing hemodynamic effects at the same time. For example, patients frequently perform the Valsalva maneuver during sustained handgrip exercise or when squatting.

Thus, in 1985 a new maneuver was developed that does not require drug administration or patient participation.[8] Transient arterial occlusion is performed by placing sphygmomanometers around the upper portions of both arms and inflating the cuffs simultaneously to 20 to 40 mm Hg above the patient's systolic blood pressure for 20 seconds. Aortic pressure is not increased by this maneuver, but aortic impedance is. Transient arterial occlusion reliably augments the left-sided regurgitant murmurs caused by aortic regurgitation, mitral regurgitation, and ventricular septal defect. When com-

TABLE 11–1

Sensitivity and Specificity of Maneuvers for the Identification of Systolic Murmurs

Maneuver	Response	Murmur	Sensitivity (%)	Specificity (%)
Inspiration	↑	Right sided	100	88
Expiration	↓	Right sided	100	88
Valsalva maneuver	↑	Hypertrophic cardiomyopathy	65	96
Squat to stand	↑	Hypertrophic cardiomyopathy	95	84
Stand to squat	↓	Hypertrophic cardiomyopathy	95	85
Leg elevation	↓	Hypertrophic cardiomyopathy	85	91
Handgrip	↓	Hypertrophic cardiomyopathy	85	75
Handgrip	↑	Mitral regurgitation and VSD	68	92
Transient arterial occlusion	↑	Mitral regurgitation and VSD	78	100
Amyl nitrite	↓	Mitral regurgitation and VSD	80	90

VSD, ventricular septal defect.

Modified from Lembo NJ, Dell' Italia LJ, Crawford MH, et al: Bedside diagnosis of systolic murmurs. N Engl J Med 1988;318:1572–1578.

pared with squatting, transient arterial occulsion was a better method for increasing the intensity of left-sided regurgitant lesions and resulted in fewer false-positive diagnoses (Table 11–1). Furthermore, this maneuver has a sensitivity equal to that of sustained handgrip exercise or inhalation of amyl nitrite for the detection of left-sided regurgitant murmurs. Importantly, this maneuver can be applied to almost all patients and is a reproducible technique that is easy to perform.

Systematic Dynamic Auscultation

When performing a cardiac examination, the observer should systematically use various maneuvers to test possible murmur etiologies. Some maneuvers are more sensitive and specific than others (see Table 11–1). A logical, efficient approach to patients with a cardiac murmur will often enable the physician to reach a reasonable conclusion about the importance of the murmur in question.

Initial auscultation will reveal whether a murmur occurs during systole or diastole. The next step should always be to listen carefully during respiration because it is very specific for identifying right- or left-sided murmurs.

The right-sided systolic murmurs of tricuspid regurgitation and pulmonic stenosis will both increase in intensity during inspiration with the patient in the upright position. Classically, the tricuspid regurgitant murmur is holosystolic and heard at the lower left sternal edge, whereas the murmur of pulmonic stenosis and the insignificant pulmonic flow murmur are mid-systolic, crescendo-decrescendo in shape and loudest at the left upper sternal edge.

Systolic murmurs that are not augmented or decrease with inspiration are left sided in origin. The application of dynamic auscultation for distinguishing murmurs of mitral regurgitation, ventricular septal defect, valvular aortic stenosis or sclerosis, hypertrophic cardiomyopathy, and mitral valve prolapse is often useful. Murmurs of hypertrophic cardiomyopathy and mitral valve prolapse become louder or longer during the Valsalva maneuver, and the murmurs of both diminish or become shorter during squatting.

Several useful maneuvers can be used to differentiate the murmurs of mitral regurgitation and ventricular septal defect from aortic valvular disease.[7,9] The presence of occasional premature beats or atrial fibrillation may lead to relatively easy differentiation of valvular aortic stenosis from mitral regurgitation. Murmurs caused by flow across a normal or obstructed semilunar valve become louder with the inhalation of amyl nitrite, whereas those of mitral regurgitation and ventricular septal defect become softer. Transient arterial occlusion and sustained handgrip exercise will augment murmurs of mitral regurgitation and ventricular septal defect; the systolic murmur of valvular aortic stenosis changes little, if at all. The presence of an aortic ejection sound, a soft or absent A_2, reversed splitting of S_2, and a fourth heart sound (S_4) are additional clues to the diagnosis of aortic valve stenosis.[2,5,6]

If initial auscultation reveals a diastolic murmur, it usually indicates cardiovascular pathology. Thus, the physician should be certain that the auscultatory finding is definitely present because it has important implications for further diagnostic evaluation, antibiotic prophylaxis, and possible restriction of activity. As with systolic murmurs, the initial evaluation should be careful auscultation during respiration inasmuch as augmentation of a diastolic murmur during inspiration indicates a right-sided origin and either tricuspid stenosis or pulmonic regurgitation. Diastolic murmurs that soften during inspiration and are louder during expiration are due to either mitral stenosis, aortic regurgitation, or possibly an Austin Flint murmur. Diastolic murmurs that return to baseline intensity in the first few cardiac cycles after release of a Valsalva maneuver are usually of right-sided etiology; later return to baseline intensity implies a left-sided origin. Discrimination between the murmurs of mitral stenosis and aortic regurgitation can be difficult at times despite the fact that the murmurs are usually of different pitch, different diastolic timing, and maximal at different auscultatory sites. Both diastolic murmurs are increased with handgrip and squatting, and both are attenuated in the upright position. Although inhalation of amyl nitrite will enhance the diastolic murmur of mitral stenosis and will soften the diastolic murmur of aortic regurgitation, correct interpretation of diastolic and continuous murmurs is usually established by Doppler echocardiography.

OTHER FACTORS IN THE CLINICAL ASSESSMENT

Symptoms or No Symptoms

An important consideration in a patient with a cardiac murmur is the presence or absence of symptoms that may be related to the cause of a heart murmur detected on cardiac auscultation. For example, symptoms of syncope, anginal chest pain, or congestive heart failure in a patient with a mid-systolic murmur will usually result in a more aggressive approach than in a patient with a similar mid-systolic murmur who has none of these symptoms. It is likely that the patient will have at least a 2-D echocardiographic assessment with Doppler flow velocity recordings to rule in or rule out the presence of significant aortic valve stenosis. A history of thromboembolism or possible infective endocarditis will probably also result in a more extensive workup. The presence of systemic embolism in a patient with a cardiac murmur is an indication for 2-D echocardiographic assessment of the cardiac chambers and valves for evidence of thrombosis or vegetations and Doppler echocardiographic flow velocity measurements for detection of valvular stenosis or regurgitation. In patients with mitral valve disease, particularly when atrial fibrillation is present, transesophageal echocardiography may be necessary to demonstrate the presence of left atrial thrombus or vegetations.

In patients with cardiac murmurs and clinical findings suggestive of endocarditis (e.g., fever, petechiae, positive blood cultures, hematuria), 2-D echocardiography with Doppler flow velocity imaging is again indicated. In some cases in which the infection involves the mitral valve or an infected valve prosthesis is suspected, transesophageal echocardiography may be necessary to determine the presence or absence of vegetations and abscesses.

Conversely, many asymptomatic children and young adults with grade II/VI mid-systolic murmurs and no other cardiac physical findings need no further cardiac workup after the initial history and physical examination.[11] A particularly important group is the large number of *asymptomatic* elderly patients, many with systemic hypertension, who have mid-systolic murmurs from sclerotic aortic valve leaflets or from flow into tortuous, noncompliant great vessels, or from both mechanisms. Such murmurs must be distinguished from murmurs caused by mild to severe valvular aortic stenosis, which is prevalent in this age group. The absence of left ventricular hypertrophy on the electrocardiogram (ECG) and a normal chest radiograph are reassuring and less costly than routine echocardiography.[11]

Other Physical Findings

The presence of other physical findings, either cardiac or noncardiac, may provide important clues to the significance of a cardiac murmur.[2] For example, a right-sided mid-systolic murmur probably represents tricuspid regurgitation without pulmonary hypertension in a heroin addict who has fever, petechiae, Osler's nodes, and Janeway lesions. In addition, the diastolic murmur of aortic regurgitation and the mid to late systolic murmur of mitral valve prolapse are common in patients with Marfan's syndrome. A soft systolic murmur at the apex is more likely to indicate mitral regurgitation from coronary artery disease in a patient with uncontrolled systemic hypertension and tuberous xanthomas.

Associated cardiac findings frequently provide important information concerning cardiac murmurs. Fixed splitting of S_2 during inspiration and expiration in a patient with a grade II/VI mid-systolic murmur in the pulmonic area and left sternal border probably indicates an atrial septal defect. Left ventricular dilatation on precordial palpitation, elevated jugular venous pressure, and bibasilar pulmonary rales favor the diagnosis of mitral regurgitation in a patient with a grade II/VI holosystolic murmur at the cardiac apex. A slowly rising, diminished arterial pulse suggests severe aortic stenosis in a patient with a grade II/VI mid-systolic murmur at the upper intercostal spaces.

Electrocardiogram and Chest Radiograph

Although echocardiography usually provides more specific and often quantitative information concerning the significance of a heart murmur and may be the only test needed, the ECG and chest radiograph are often already obtained and readily available. The absence of ventricular hypertrophy, atrial dilatation, arrhythmias, conduction abnormalities, previous infarction, and evidence of active ischemia on ECG provide useful negative information at a relatively low cost when the murmur is probably insignificant. The presence of abnormal findings on the ECG such as ventricular hypertrophy or a previous myocardial infarction will usually lead to more extensive evaluation, including 2-D and Doppler echocardiography.

Posteroanterior (PA) and lateral chest radiographs often yield qualitative information concerning cardiac chamber size, pulmonary arterial blood flow, pulmonary venous blood flow, and cardiac calcifications in patients being assessed with cardiac murmurs. When abnormal findings are present on chest radiographs, 2-D and Doppler echocardiography is commonly performed. Normal PA and lateral chest radiographs, as well as a normal ECG, are likely in patients with insignificant mid-systolic cardiac murmurs, particularly in younger age groups, in females, and when the murmur is less than grade III in intensity.[12] Many of these asymptomatic patients may need neither an ECG nor a chest radiograph when a careful cardiac examination indicates an insignificant vibratory mid-systolic heart murmur and no abnormal cardiac or noncardiac findings.

Echocardiography (see also Chapter 5)

Echocardiography is an important method for assessing the significance of various cardiac murmurs in certain patients by the accurate noninvasive imaging of cardiac structures and function and the direction and velocity of flow within cardiac chambers and vessels.[4–6] The presence of abnormal valvular motion and morphology may be indicated by 2-D echocardiography, but it does not usually indicate the severity. By applying the Doppler effect, the direction of shift in ultrasound frequency is used to determine the direction of flow of the red cells in relation to the transducer. The direction of flow is displayed as a spectral velocity profile, with the profile oriented toward the transducer for blood coming toward it and away from the transducer for blood flowing away from it.

The direction of flow can also be depicted by using color coding of velocity shapes within the cardiac chambers, with the color red depicting blood flow toward the transducer and the color blue indicating blood flow moving away from the transducer. Not only can the direction of flow of the red cells be assessed, but red blood cell velocity can also be measured. This velocity information can be used to quantify flow and measure pressure within cardiac chambers. By using the modified Bernoulli equation ($P = 4V^2$), the peak instantaneous velocity across the region *(V)* can be converted to the peak instantaneous pressure gradient *(P)* across it. The area of a valve can be calculated to assess the severity of stenosis by using the rate of velocity decrease (pressure half-time) or by incorporating the flow through the valve (continuity equation). Thus, the extent of valvular stenosis can be accurately quantitated by measuring the increase in Doppler velocity across the valve. With the Doppler principle, valvular regurgitation and intracardiac shunts can be semiquantitated by showing the extent of abnormal velocity jet into the receiving chamber.

Although 2-D echocardiography and color Doppler flow imaging can provide important information in patients with cardiac murmurs, they are not necessary tests for all patients with cardiac murmurs and usually add little but expense to the evaluation of asymptomatic patients with short grade I to grade II mid-systolic murmurs, otherwise normal physical findings, and no history suggestive of cardiac disease.[11–13]

It is important to consider that many recent studies indicate that with the improved sensitivity of Doppler ultrasound devices, valvular regurgitation may be detected through the tricuspid and pulmonic valves in a very high percentage of young healthy subjects and through left-sided valves in a variable, but lower percentage.[14–17] In a recent study of 200 healthy Japanese subjects, mitral regurgitation could be detected by Doppler in up to 45% of individuals, tricuspid regurgitation in up to 70%, and pulmonic regurgitation in up to 88% even though these patients were healthy, had no cardiac auscultation evidence of heart disease, and had normal ECGs.[15] "Normal" aortic regurgitation is encountered much less frequently, and its incidence increases with increasing age (Fig. 11–2). Thus, echocardiographic interpretations of mild or trivial (physiologic) valvular regurgitation may lead to the echocardiographic diagnosis of cardiac disease in patients with no clinical heart disease.

The valvular regurgitation signal in healthy subjects is usually localized to the immediate proximity of the valve leaflet coaptation site and is much less widely distributed in the receiving chamber than in groups of patients studied with pathologic valve regurgitation. Various criteria have been developed for the diagnosis of "physiologic" valvular regurgitation of the tricuspid, mitral, or pulmonic valves that when detected at the level of the leaflets, is a normal finding.[14] Unfortunately, a gray zone where normal meets abnormal is encountered, as well as variations in the prevalence of observed valvular regurgitation in specific patient populations. An incorrect diagnosis of abnormal regurgitation ("echocardiographic heart disease") may be less frequent if such tests are not routinely ordered in asymptomatic patients with insignificant short mid-systolic murmurs who have no other evidence of cardiac

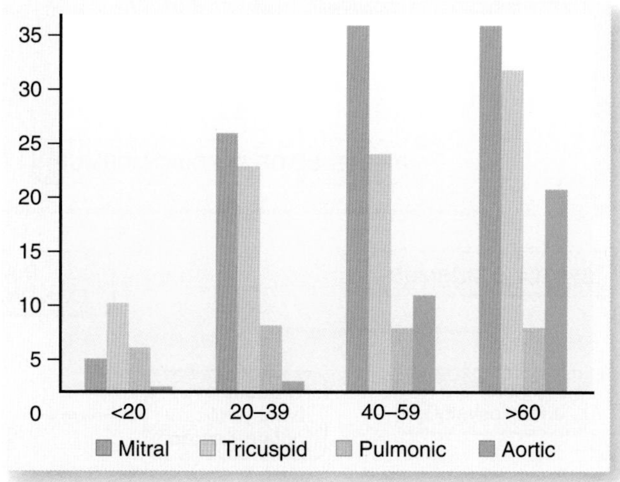

FIGURE 11–2. Percent incidence of mitral, tricuspid, pulmonic, and aortic regurgitation by Doppler echocardiography in clinically normal subjects according to age from younger than 20 to older than 60 years. (Modified from Choong CY, Abascal VM, Weyman J: Prevalence of valvular regurgitation by Doppler echocardiography in patients with structurally normal hearts by 2-dimensional echocardiography. Am Heart J 1989;117:636–642.)

disease by physical examination. General recommendations for performing 2-D and Doppler echocardiography in patients with heart murmurs are listed in Box 11–3. Of course, individual exceptions to these indications may exist. For example, an asymptomatic 60-year-old with a short grade II mid-systolic murmur and ECG evidence of left ventricular hypertrophy may require echocardiography to determine the presence of valvular aortic stenosis.

Cardiac Catheterization

Cardiac catheterization can provide important information on the presence and severity of valvular obstruction, valvular regurgitation, and intracardiac shunting. It is not necessary in most patients with cardiac murmurs and normal echocardiograms, but it provides added information in some patients in whom the echocardiogram has established the presence of significant heart disease as the cause of the cardiac murmur. Cardiac catheterization with coronary arteriography to assess the presence of coronary disease is performed routinely in most adult patients 35 years and older who are being considered for cardiac surgery to correct either valvular or congenital heart disease.

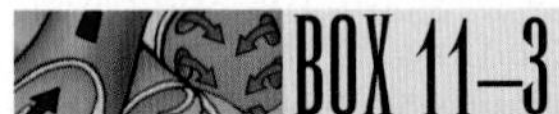

BOX 11–3

Indications for Echocardiography in Patients with Cardiac Murmurs

- Symptoms or signs consistent with congestive heart failure, myocardial ischemia, or syncope
- Symptoms or signs consistent with infective endocarditis or thromboembolism.
- Any diastolic or continuous murmur
- All holosystolic and late systolic murmurs
- Any mid-systolic murmur of grade III or louder intensity
- Additional abnormal physical findings on cardiac palpation or auscultation

Approach to the Patient

The evaluation of a patient with a heart murmur may vary greatly, depending on many of the considerations discussed earlier, including the intensity of the cardiac murmur, its timing in the cardiac cycle, its location and radiation, and its response to various physiologic maneuvers. Also of importance are the presence or absence of cardiac and noncardiac symptoms and whether other cardiac or noncardiac physical findings suggest that the cardiac murmur is clinically significant. The skill and confidence of the cardiac auscultator, the relative cost of various diagnostic approaches, and the accuracy and reliability of additional tests in the laboratory where they are performed are likewise important factors. One systematic approach to patients with a heart murmur is depicted in Figure 11–3. This algorithm is particularly applicable to children and adults younger than 40 years.

Patients with definite diastolic heart murmurs or continuous murmurs not attributable to a cervical venous hum or a mammary soufflé during pregnancy are candidates for 2-D and Doppler echocardiography. If the results of echocardiography indicate significant heart disease, cardiac consultation is generally obtained. An echocardiographic examination is also recommended for patients with apical or left sternal edge pansystolic or late systolic murmurs, for patients with mid-systolic

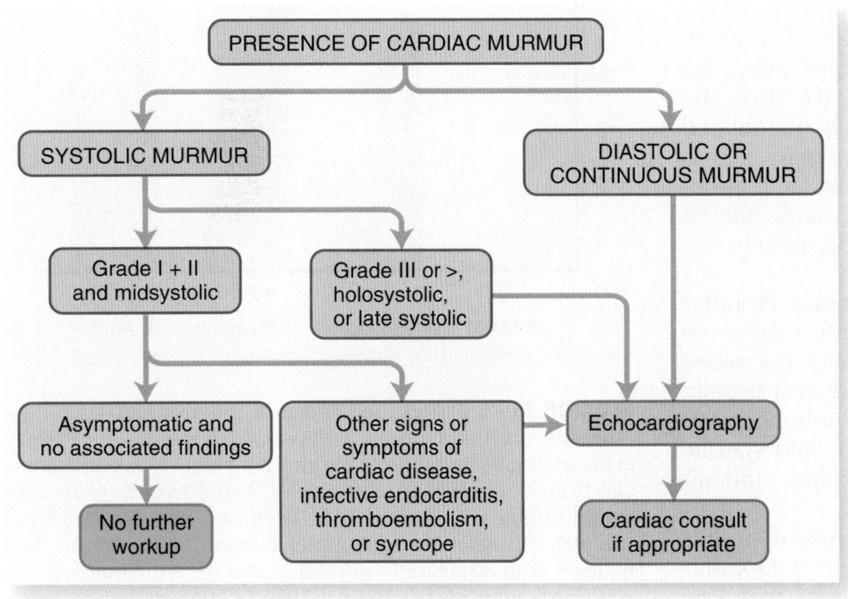

FIGURE 11–3. A schematic approach to the workup of a patient with a cardiac murmur according to whether the murmur is probably innocent or secondary to cardiac pathology. This algorithm is particularly relevant to children and adults younger than 40 years, and echocardiography is recommended before cardiac consultation.

murmurs that are grade III or higher in intensity, and for patients with softer *systolic* murmurs in whom dynamic cardiac auscultation suggests a definite cardiac diagnosis (e.g., hypertrophic cardiomyopathy). The suggested approach is to proceed with 2-D and Doppler echocardiography, with cardiac consultation if abnormal results are obtained.[11–13]

More specifically, further cardiac evaluation, including echocardiography, cardiac consultation, or both, is recommended when the intensity of a systolic murmur increases during the Valsalva maneuver, becomes louder when the patient assumes the upright position, and decreases in intensity when the patient squats. These responses during dynamic auscultation suggest the diagnosis of either hypertrophic cardiomyopathy or mitral valve prolapse. Additionally, further cardiac assessment is indicated when a systolic murmur increases in intensity during transient arterial occlusion, becomes louder during sustained handgrip exercise, or does not increase its intensity in the cardiac cycle either after a premature ventricular contraction or after a long R-R interval in patients with atrial fibrillation. The diagnosis of mitral regurgitation or ventricular septal defect is likely.

In many patients with grade I/II mid-systolic murmurs, an extensive workup is not necessary, particularly in children and young adults who are asymptomatic, have an otherwise normal cardiac examination, and have no other physical findings associated with cardiac disease. These patients do not have any need for routine echocardiography or other tests that increase the cost of health care delivery. However, echocardiography is indicated in certain patients with grade I/II mid-systolic murmurs, including those with symptoms or signs consistent with infective endocarditis or thromboembolism and those with symptoms or signs consistent with congestive heart failure, myocardial ischemia, or syncope. Echocardiography usually also provides an accurate diagnosis in patients with other abnormal physical findings on cardiac palpitation or auscultation, the latter including specific changes in the intensity of the systolic murmur during certain physiologic maneuvers as described earlier. When the diagnosis is in doubt in asymptomatic patients after auscultation, the presence of an abnormal ECG or chest radiograph usually leads to echocardiography (Fig. 11–4). In elderly asymptomatic patients with limited functional activity, echocardiography will distinguish patients with soft mid-systolic aortic murmurs caused by aortic sclerosis from those with valvular aortic stenosis.

Although 2-D and Doppler echocardiography are important tests for those with a moderate to high likelihood that a cardiac murmur is clinically important, it must be re-emphasized that trivial, minimal, or physiologic valvular regurgitation, especially that affecting the mitral, tricuspid, or pulmonic valves, is detected by color flow imaging techniques in many otherwise normal patients, including many who have no heart murmur at all. This drawback must be considered when using echocardiographic results to guide decisions

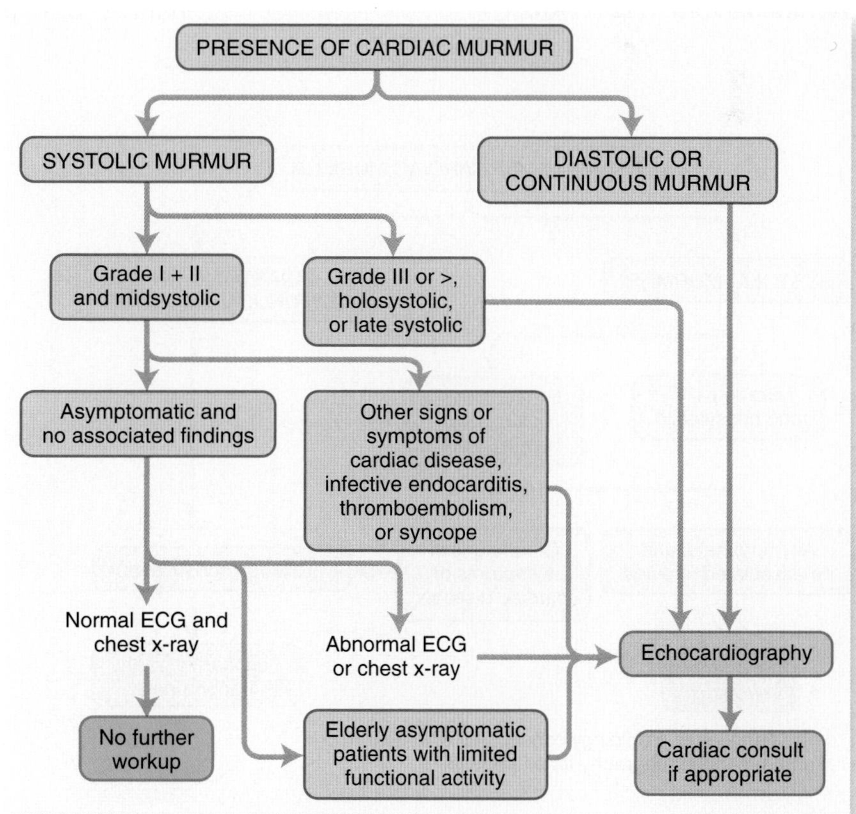

FIGURE 11–4. An alternative "echocardiography-first" approach to the evaluation of a heart murmur that also uses the results of the electrocardiogram (ECG) and chest radiograph in asymptomatic patients with soft mid-systolic murmurs and no other physical findings. This algorithm is useful in patients older than 40 years, in whom the prevalence of coronary artery disease and aortic stenosis as the cause of systolic murmurs increases.

regarding asymptomatic patients in whom echocardiography was used to assess the clinical significance of an isolated heart murmur. In such cases, physiologic cardiac function may be interpreted as pathologic and result in unnecessary testing or therapy.[11]

A cardiac consultation *without additional cardiac testing* costs considerably less than routine echocardiography and is an alternative method for assessing the significance of a cardiac murmur when the primary physician believes that further evaluation is necessary (Fig. 11–5). The relative cost depends on whether the cardiac consultation includes the ordering of a large number of additional tests for many patients who have no underlying cardiac disease. This alternative approach may be most useful in the evaluation of children with loud innocent vibratory systolic murmurs and in adults with insignificant, but loud mid-systolic murmurs during high blood flow states such as pregnancy or severe anemia. It may also be the better approach for asymptomatic patients who are elderly and have short, faint, mid-systolic murmurs resulting from flow across thickened aortic leaflets, such as commonly occur in patients with hypertension; these murmurs often differ from those caused by valvular aortic stenosis or significant mitral regurgitation. If the cardiac consultant orders echocardiography for all patients referred for evaluation with heart murmurs, it is clearly not cost-effective. The absence of left ventricular hypertrophy on the ECG and the presence of normal cardiac size without pulmonary venous congestion on a chest radiograph may aid in the evaluation of an asymptomatic elderly patient with an insignificant short soft mid-systolic murmur without the need for more costly cardiac consultation and echocardiography (Fig. 11–6).

COST CONSIDERATIONS

Very few data are available on the cost-effectiveness of various approaches to patients undergoing medical evaluation because of the presence of a cardiac murmur. Optimal auscultation by well-trained examiners who can recognize an insignificant mid-systolic murmur with confidence during dynamic cardiac auscultation as indicated results in less frequent use of expensive additional testing to define murmurs that do not indicate cardiac pathology. Unfortunately, cardiac auscultation is less emphasized in medical and post-graduate medical training than in previous years because of the more popular high-tech tests that are available for assessing patients with suspected or definite cardiac disease.

The relative cost of a cardiac consultation, PA and lateral chest radiographs, an ECG, Doppler and 2-D echocardiography, and cardiac catheterization without coronary arteriography is indicated in Figure 11–7. When needed, cardiac consultation alone is relatively inexpensive, but many patients with heart murmurs being referred for cardiac consultation have chest radiographs, ECGs, and 2-D and Doppler echocardiograms recorded routinely before or after the consultation visit. Thus, if a cardiac consultation routinely results in the ordering of echocardiography and other noninvasive tests, the accumulated cost is greater than if cardiac consultation is obtained only for patients with echocardiographic evidence of heart disease as the cause of a cardiac murmur.

Because direct availability of echocardiography to primary care physicians is an alternative strategy to

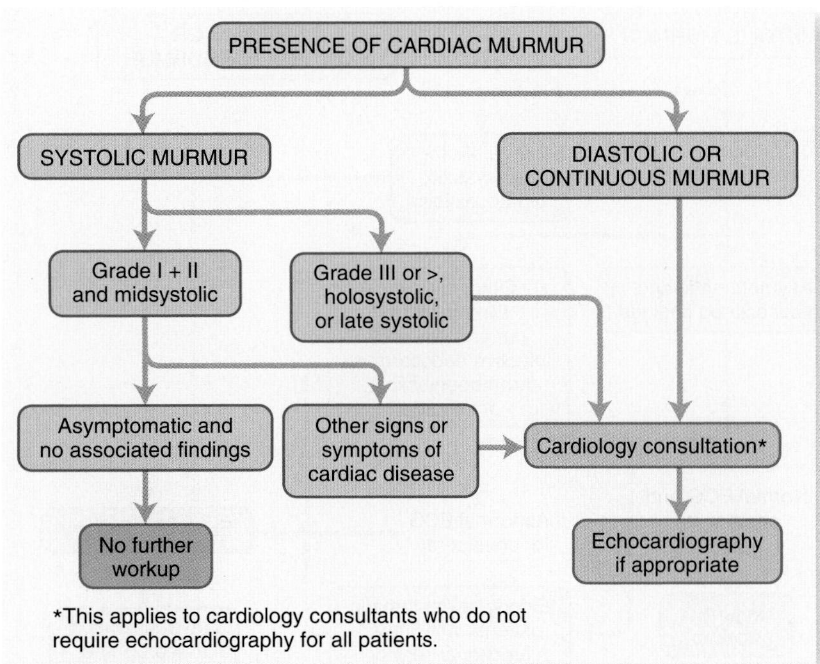

FIGURE 11–5. This schematic approach for assessing patients with heart murmurs recommends cardiac consultation rather than the echocardiogram as the initial step in those with an increased likelihood of having cardiac disease. This approach is particularly useful in situations in which the cardiac consultant does not order routine echocardiography in all patients referred for evaluation of heart murmurs.

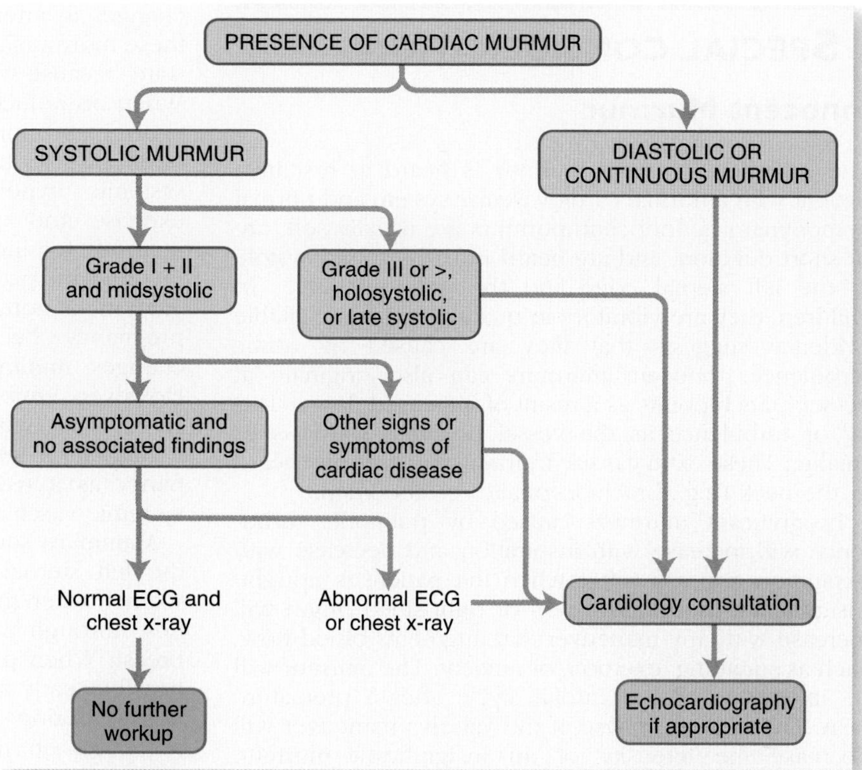

FIGURE 11–6. This modification of the "cardiac consultation–first" approach for the evaluation of heart murmurs uses the results of the electrocardiogram (ECG) and chest radiograph in asymptomatic patients with soft mid-systolic murmurs and no other physical findings. Cardiac consultation is usually obtained for asymptomatic patients who have left ventricular hypertrophy by ECG or have cardiomegaly or pulmonary venous congestion by chest radiography.

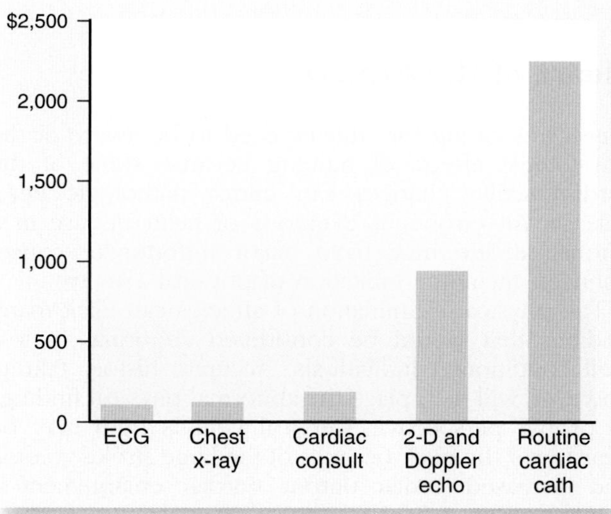

FIGURE 11–7. The relative cost of cardiac evaluation, including laboratory plus interpretation fees for an electrocardiogram (ECG), posteroanterior and lateral chest radiographs, two-dimensional (2-D) and Doppler echocardiography, and cardiac catheterization without coronary arteriography, is compared with the cost of an initial cardiac consultation alone. If the cardiac consultation routinely includes an ECG, chest radiograph, and echocardiogram, it will be less cost efficient than the initial use of 2-D and Doppler echocardiography with further cardiac consultation only if the results are abnormal.

cardiac consultation for evaluation of heart murmurs, Danford and associates[18] used a decision-analysis model to compare the costs of two diagnostic strategies: (1) echocardiography first, with referral to a cardiologist if appropriate, and (2) evaluation of a murmur by a cardiologist and then echocardiography if appropriate. Of the 236 pediatric patients with innocent systolic murmurs in the referral-first group, the pediatric cardiologists ordered an echocardiogram in only 25%. Of those with trivial and significant heart disease, cardiologists ordered an echocardiogram in 53% and 88%, respectively. In the echocardiography-first group, 77% had innocent murmurs, 15% had trivial heart disease, and 8% had potentially significant disease. The echocardiography-first strategy averaged $257 more than the referral-first strategy. Thus, pediatric cardiac consultation appeared to be the preferred approach provided that cardiac consultation costs are moderate, echocardiographic costs are moderate to high, and the rate at which the cardiologists order echocardiography for patients with innocent murmurs is low. In the authors' experience, the percentage of patients undergoing routine echocardiography, if referred to adult cardiologists because of a heart murmur, is much higher. No prospective data are available regarding the cost-effectiveness of the approach indicated in Figures 11–3 to 11–6, but the echocardiography-first approach in patients with clinical indications for further evaluation appears logical at this time.

SPECIAL CONSIDERATIONS

Innocent Murmur

The so-called innocent murmur is heard at rest in a patient with a normal cardiovascular system and normal hemodynamics. Innocent murmurs are usually soft, are of short duration, and are heard in early to mid systole at the left sternal edge and the pulmonic area. In children, they are vibratory in quality, and the available evidence suggests that they are caused by aortic turbulence. Innocent murmurs can also originate at vessel branch points as a result of increased flow velocity or turbulence as the vessel becomes tortuous or smaller. These extra cardiac murmurs are typically heard in the neck (e.g., brachiocephalic) or abdomen.[2,3,7]

Insignificant murmurs caused by pulmonic turbulence will increase with inspiration and decrease with expiration and are softer when the patient is upright. Insignificant murmurs of left- or right-sided origin will increase with any maneuver that augments blood flow, such as squatting, exertion, or anxiety. The murmur will be intensified in the cardiac cycle after a premature beat. The straining phase of the Valsalva maneuver will decrease the intensity of an insignificant murmur, whereas isometric handgrip exercise has no effect on the auscultatory findings.

Physiologic maneuvers will help distinguish the murmurs of mitral regurgitation or tricuspid regurgitation from insignificant outflow murmurs, which can sound quite similar. However, differentiating between insignificant and pathologic aortic or pulmonic murmurs is more difficult and is best done by exclusion. Subjects with benign murmurs are usually asymptomatic and have no other physical findings of cardiac disease. The most useful negative auscultatory finding is the absence of an ejection sound because mild to moderate aortic or pulmonic valvular stenosis is usually associated with this finding.

Pregnancy (see also Chapter 15)

It is important to identify women with cardiovascular abnormalities before or during pregnancy so that proper endocarditis antibiotic prophylaxis can be considered during a complicated labor and delivery. This task is more difficult if the initial cardiac examination is done after early pregnancy because the intensity of some murmurs change greatly during the altered hemodynamics of pregnancy. Cardiac output begins to increase during the first trimester, possibly as early as the 10th week, and remains elevated through the third trimester. Simultaneously, systemic vascular resistance falls during the first and second trimesters and is maintained at a lower level, often with a decrease in mean arterial pressure. Circulating blood volume is increased, and an insignificant mid-systolic murmur and a physiologic S_3 are present in most pregnant women.[7,19]

In the nonpregnant state, murmurs of mitral or aortic regurgitation vary in intensity and duration with changes in arterial blood pressure. During pregnancy, these murmurs are often softer than in the nonpregnant state because of reduced systemic vascular resistance. When no reduction in the intensity of aortic and mitral regurgitant murmurs occurs during pregnancy, it is often due to the onset or exacerbation of maternal systemic hypertension. Bilateral maximal handgrip exercise and transient arterial occlusion are useful methods for increasing left-sided regurgitant murmurs in pregnant patients. Patients with either mitral regurgitation or aortic regurgitation usually do well during pregnancy because the physiologic hemodynamic changes minimize the volume of regurgitant flow. However, antibiotic endocarditis prophylaxis is indicated. The murmurs of mitral stenosis and tricuspid regurgitation generally become louder during pregnancy as a result of changes in cardiac output and systemic vascular resistance.

Mammary soufflé is a continuous murmur heard at the left sternal edge in many pregnant or lactating women when the patient is supine. It results from blood flow through the superficial mammary arteries of the breast. When present, this continuous murmur can be heard as early as the second or third trimester and can persist during lactation. The Valsalva maneuver has no effect on the mammary soufflé, thus serving to differentiate it from the continuous murmur of a venous hum, which disappears during the Valsalva maneuver. Assuming an upright posture will cause the mammary soufflé to fade or disappear. The schematic approaches to assessment of cardiac murmurs depicted in Figures 11–3 to 11–6 pertain during pregnancy as well.

Heart of the Athlete

Physicians caring for athletes need to be aware of the physiologic effects of training because some of the cardiovascular changes can mimic pathologic heart disease. An erroneous diagnosis of heart disease in a normal athlete may have major unfortunate consequences, including limitation of physical activity.

The physical examination of athletes can elicit many findings that would be considered abnormal in less well conditioned individuals. Accurate history taking, however, will help place the abnormal physical findings in proper perspective. Cervical venous hum may be heard over the neck because of the large stroke volume and increased cardiac output. Cardiac enlargement is manifested as a displaced apical impulse or right ventricular lift. The presence of an S_3 is usually due to rapid filling of the left ventricle in early diastole. Approximately half of all athletes will have an audible S_4 for unknown reasons.[7]

Murmurs are very common in this population. They are usually insignificant mid-systolic murmurs caused by the increased stroke volume. Rarely, a mid-diastolic low-pitched murmur occurs as a result of the augmented blood flow across the atrioventricular valves. Having the patient assume an upright posture will cause a decrease or disappearance of both systolic and diastolic murmurs. The approach to the assessment of murmurs indicated in Figures 11–3 to 11–6 also applies to this group.

Mitral Valve Prolapse (see also Chapter 32)

Mitral valve prolapse is defined as the systolic posterior movement of one or both mitral valve leaflets into the left atrium, and it often results in mitral regurgitation. Mitral valve prolapse occurs when left ventricular volume falls below a certain critical level during systole. The hallmark finding on physical examination is a mid-systolic click; it may or may not be followed by a late systolic murmur. The timing of the auscultatory findings during systole can be altered by various maneuvers, with the response often indicating a definite diagnosis.[1,3,7] Unfortunately, despite the skill of the examiner, auscultative detection of mitral valve prolapse is difficult. In one small study of 100 patients, the sensitivity of cardiac examination performed by faculty cardiologists in detecting mitral valve prolapse was only 55%; however, the specificity was very high.[11]

Maneuvers that modify left ventricular end-diastolic volume will affect the timing of a click-murmur during systole. Interventions such as the Valsalva maneuver or assuming an upright posture will decrease left ventricular volume and cause the critical volume at which prolapse occurs to be achieved earlier in systole; as a result, the click-murmur complex moves closer to S_1. Submaximal isometric handgrip exercise also moves the click-murmur complex to an earlier point in systole because the associated tachycardia reduces left ventricular volume and increases contractility.

Maneuvers that increase either left ventricular volume or afterload will move the click-murmur complex to a later point in systole. Therefore, bradycardia, such as induced with beta-blocker therapy, will increase left ventricular volume, and the systolic clicks or murmur moves towards S_2. Rapid squatting increases aortic pressure and afterload and enhances venous return. Thus, left ventricular volume is enlarged, and the click-murmur complex begins later in systole. It is particularly useful to have the patient stand up rapidly from the squatting position because this action markedly reduces left ventricular volume and moves the click-murmur complex to a much earlier point in systole.

Systolic clicks are not necessarily specific for mitral valve prolapse, and some patients with prolapse have a mid-systolic click or clicks without a late systolic murmur. Systolic clicks can mimic a split S_1 or an early systolic ejection sound. An important physical finding is movement of the click with maneuvers because ejection sounds and a split S_1 never occur in mid or late systole. Changes in systolic timing of the murmur during various maneuvers are important when mitral valve prolapse occurs with only a systolic murmur and no click. This finding is often seen in patients with mitral valve prolapse.

The authors recommend 2-D and Doppler echocardiography for all patients with definite or suspected mitral valve prolapse, not only to confirm the diagnosis, which the echocardiogram will fail to detect in up to 10% of clinically certain cases, but more importantly to assess left atrial size, left ventricular size and function, the extent of mitral leaflet redundancy, and the presence and severity of mitral regurgitation. The risk of complications, including infective endocarditis, thromboembolism, and subsequent need for mitral valve surgery, correlates with the severity of the echocardiographic findings.

The late systolic murmur of hypertrophic cardiomyopathy can be confused with the murmur of mitral valve prolapse, although patients with hypertrophic cardiomyopathy rarely have mid-systolic clicks. Both murmurs have a similar response to changes in posture, squatting, and standing. The Valsalva maneuver is the useful method to differentiate between the two conditions. In hypertrophic cardiomyopathy, the murmur is markedly louder during the straining phase of the Valsalva maneuver, whereas in mitral valve prolapse, the murmur is longer but not usually louder and sometimes softer. More reliable is variance in the murmur after a premature beat; it is much louder in hypertrophic cardiomyopathy, but unchanged in mitral valve prolapse. Additionally, transient arterial occlusion will reliably increase the intensity of mitral regurgitant murmurs in mitral valve prolapse but has little effect on the murmur of hypertrophic cardiomyopathy. Doppler and 2-D echocardiography will confirm the correct diagnosis.

Evidence-Based Summary

- Careful and accurate cardiac auscultation forms the cornerstone of the diagnostic evaluation of a patient with a cardiac murmur. Most patients who have associated abnormal cardiac findings and those with symptoms suggesting cardiovascular disease undergo 2-D and Doppler echocardiography.
- Cardiac consultation is appropriate when the echocardiographic findings are abnormal or as an alternative first approach when the murmur is probably significant.
- Many asymptomatic patients with grade I/II mid-systolic murmurs and no associated abnormal cardiac findings need no further diagnostic testing after the history and physical examination.
- When the primary physician is uncertain about the significance of a cardiac murmur after careful auscultation, including the use of physiologic maneuvers to alter its intensity, two alternatives are initial cardiac consultation and echocardiography with subsequent cardiac consultation, if appropriate. If the consultant is likely to order echocardiography in most patients sent for further evaluation, an echocardiogram requested by the primary physician and referral only if the echocardiogram is abnormal may be the most cost-effective approach.

References

1. Abrams J: Synopsis of cardiac physical diagnosis. Boston, Butterworth, 2001.
2. O'Rourke RA, Braunwald E: Physical examination of the cardiovascular system. In Kasper DL, Braunwald E, Fauci AS, et al (eds): Harrison's Principles of Internal Medicine, 15th ed. New York, McGraw-Hill, 2004 (in press).
3. Harvey WP: Cardiac pearls. Dis Mon 1994;20(2):45–116.
4. O'Rourke RA, Shaver JA, Silverman ME: The history, physical examination, and cardiac auscultation. In Fuster V, Alexander RW, O'Rourke RA, et al (eds): Hurst's The Heart, 10th ed. New York, McGraw-Hill, 2001.
5. Shaver JA: Cardiac auscultation: A cost-effective diagnostic skill. Curr Probl Cardiol 1995;20:441–530.
6. Braunwald E, Perloff JK: Physical examination of the heart and circulation. In Braunwald E, Zipes DP, Libby P (eds): Heart Disease, 6th ed. Philadelphia, WB Saunders, 2001.
7. Grewe K, Crawford MH, O'Rourke RA: Differentiation of cardiac murmurs by auscultation. Curr Probl Cardiol 1988;13:699–721.
8. Lembo NJ, Dell'Italia LJ, Crawford MH, et al: Diagnosis of left-sided regurgitant murmurs by transient arterial occlusion: A new maneuver using blood pressure cuffs. Ann Intern Med 1986;105:368–670.
9. Lembo NJ, Dell'Italia LJ, Crawford MH, et al: Bedside diagnosis of systolic murmurs. N Engl J Med 1988; 318:1572–1578.
10. Tavel ME: Cardiac auscultation: A glorious past—but does it have a future? Circulation 1996;93:1250–1253.
11. Shry EA, Smithers MA, Mascette AM: Auscultation versus echocardiography in a healthy population with precordial murmur. Am J Cardiol 2001;87:1428–1430.
12. Attenhofer Jost CH, Turina J, Mayer K, et al: Echocardiography in the evaluation of systolic murmurs of unknown cause. Am J Med 2000;108:614–620.
13. Roldan CA, Shively BK, Crawford MH: Value of the cardiovascular physical examination for detecting valvular heart disease in asymptomatic subjects. Am J Cardiol 1996;77:1327–1331.
14. Choong CY, Abascal VM, Weyman J: Prevalence of valvular regurgitation by Doppler echocardiography in patients with structurally normal hearts by 2-dimensional echocardiography. Am Heart J 1989;117:636–642.
15. Sahn DJ, Maciel BC: Physiological valvular regurgitation: Doppler echocardiography and the potential for iatrogenic heart disease. Circulation 1988;78:1075–1077.
16. Yoshida K, Yoshikawa J, Shakudo M: Color Doppler evaluation of valvular regurgitation in normals. Circulation 1988;78:840–847.
17. Kostucki W, Vandenbossche J-L, Friart A, et al: Pulsed Doppler regurgitant flow patterns of normal valves. Am J Cardiol 1986;58:309–313.
18. Danford DA, Nasir A, Gumbiner C: Cost assessment of the evaluation of heart murmurs in children. Pediatrics 1993;91:365–368.
19. McAnulty JH, Morton MJ, Ueland K: The heart and pregnancy. Curr Probl Cardiol 1988;13:589–665.

CHAPTER 12 Approach to the Patient with Asymptomatic Electrocardiographic Abnormalities

Leonard I. Ganz

Because of the ubiquity of the electrocardiogram (ECG) in clinical practice and the relatively high prevalence of ECG abnormalities, patients with unexpected ECG findings are frequently encountered.[1] Much of what is known about the importance of asymptomatic ECG abnormalities is derived from the Framingham Study and other epidemiologic studies in which asymptomatic, presumably healthy patients were enrolled, had screening ECGs, and then were monitored longitudinally.[2] This chapter focuses on the prognostic significance and recommended evaluation of frequently encountered ECG abnormalities. The primary focus is on ECGs obtained routinely or for screening purposes in patients without signs, symptoms, or suspicion of heart disease.

SCREENING ELECTROCARDIOGRAMS

Although screening ECGs are frequently obtained, data supporting this practice are limited. For any screening test to be useful, abnormal findings need to have prognostic significance and lead to a change in management that will improve outcome. When looked at another way, the clinical utility of a screening ECG depends on its sensitivity and specificity, as well as the pretest probability of clinically significant heart disease (see Chapters 1 and 2). As described later, a screening ECG is rarely the initial method by which clinically significant cardiovascular disease is identified in patients without symptoms or signs. A screening ECG can provide a baseline for comparison with subsequent ECGs if symptoms or signs of cardiovascular disease develop in the future, but few if any data support this use. Screening ECGs are also frequently obtained as part of the preoperative evaluation (see Chapter 14), a practice that is not specifically addressed in this chapter.

At present, the U.S. Preventative Services Task Force does not recommend a screening ECG as part of the periodic health examination in the general population.[3] The American College of Physicians and the Canadian Task Force on the Periodic Health Examination share this opinion.[4,5] However, an American College of Cardiology/American Heart Association Task Force recommends a screening ECG in patients older than 40 years and in other specific situations[6] (Box 12–1).

ELECTROCARDIOGRAPHIC ABNORMALITIES

ECG abnormalities can be divided into those related to heart rhythm and the conducting system and those related to myocardial structure and function. Each abnormality has a precise definition, and its prevalence and prognostic significance help guide appropriate evaluation and follow-up.

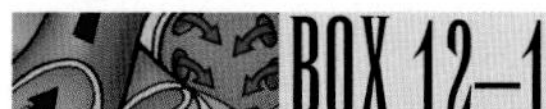

BOX 12–1

American College of Cardiology/American Heart Association Task Force Recommendations for Screening Electrocardiograms in Patients with No Apparent Heart Disease

CLASS I (RECOMMENDED)

- Persons older than 40 yr who are undergoing a physical examination
- Before administration of drugs that have a high incidence of cardiovascular effects (e.g., chemotherapeutic agents)
- Before exercise stress testing
- Persons in occupations that require high cardiovascular performance (e.g., firefighters, police officers, astronauts) or that affect public safety (e.g., pilots, bus/truck drivers, air traffic controllers, railroad engineers, critical process engineers)

CLASS II (UNCERTAIN)

- Evaluation of competitive athletes

CLASS III (NOT RECOMMENDED)

- Persons younger than 40 yr with no extenuating circumstances as described above

Adapted from Schlant RC, Adolph RJ, DiMarco JP, et al: Guidelines for electrocardiography. A report of the American College of Cardiology/American Heart Association Task Force on Assessment of Diagnostic and Therapeutic Cardiovascular Procedures (Committee on Electrocardiography). J Am Coll Cardiol 1992;19:473–481.

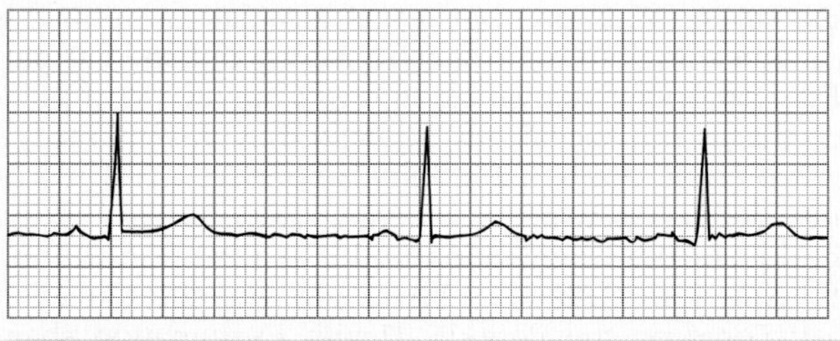

FIGURE 12–1. This rhythm strip (lead II) reveals asymptomatic sinus bradycardia at 46 beats per minute in a healthy young woman.

Abnormalities in Heart Rhythm and the Conducting System

Sinus Bradycardia (Fig. 12–1) (see Chapter 31)

Definition. Sinus bradycardia is defined as a sinus rate less than 60 beats per minute, but changing the definition to a sinus rate of less than 50 beats per minute has been proposed.

Prevalence. Sinus bradycardia is very common and is a normal variant in healthy adults. Resting heart rates in the 50s or even the mid to high 40s are not uncommon in young, athletic adults because of high vagal tone.

BOX 12–2

Causes of Sinus Bradycardia

Sick sinus syndrome
Hypervagotonia
Medications (beta-blockers, calcium channel blockers, digoxin, antiarrhythmic drugs)
Hypothyroidism
Acutely increased intracranial pressure (Cushing's reflex)

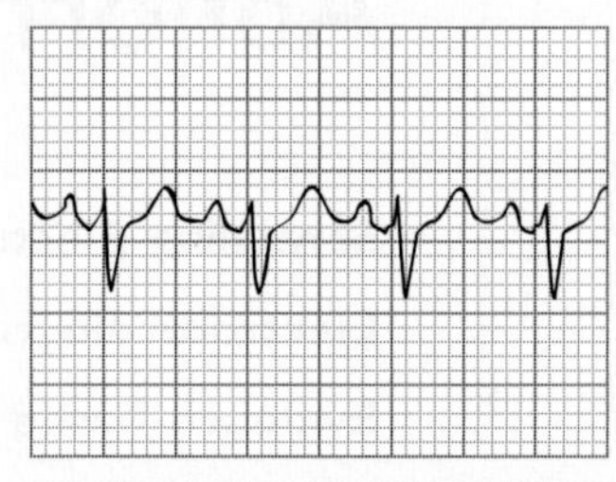

FIGURE 12–2. This rhythm strip (lead II) reveals sinus tachycardia at 115 beats per minute caused by exacerbation of asthma in a young male.

Prognostic Significance. In the absence of symptoms, sinus bradycardia probably has no prognostic significance, although it can be the first sign of early sick sinus syndrome.

Evaluation. Ask the patient about symptoms referable to bradycardia (e.g., syncope, near-syncope, fatigue, poor exercise capacity, lightheadedness). Symptoms may be subtle, particularly in the elderly. Some specific causes of sinus bradycardia are treatable (Box 12–2), but in the absence of symptoms, no specific treatment is necessary, even for sick sinus syndrome.

Follow-up. No specific follow-up is recommended for patients with asymptomatic sinus bradycardia.

Sinus Tachycardia (Fig. 12–2) (see Chapter 30)

Definition. Sinus tachycardia is defined as a sinus rate over 100 beats per minute, but resting sinus rates over 90 beats per minute are unusual in healthy adults. Sinus tachycardia is usually a physiologic response to some perturbation (Box 12–3). The heart rate must, of course, be considered in the context of the clinical setting. If no underlying cause of resting sinus tachycardia can be identified, inappropriate sinus tachycardia may be present.

Prevalence. Sinus tachycardia is very common.

Prognostic Significance. The prognostic significance depends on the underlying cause of the sinus tachycardia.

Evaluation. Identify the underlying cause of the tachycardia.

Follow-up. If inappropriate sinus tachycardia is present, treatment with a beta-blocker is indicated, even in asymptomatic patients, because of the risk of tachycardia-induced cardiomyopathy.

Sinus Arrhythmia (Fig. 12–3)

Definition. Sinus arrhythmia is defined as variability in the sinus rate, generally indicative of high vagal tone. The pattern tends to be respirophasic, with an increase in rate during inspiration and a decrease during expiration. Brief sinus pauses, reflective of hypervagotonia, are also not uncommon in young, healthy patients.

Prevalence. Sinus arrhythmia is very common and is a normal variant in young, healthy patients.

Prognostic Significance. Sinus arrhythmia has no known prognostic significance.

Evaluation. None is needed.

Follow-up. Follow-up is not required.

BOX 12–3

Causes of Sinus Tachycardia

Exertion
Fever
Pain
Anxiety
Hypovolemia
Hypoxia
Bleeding
Anemia
Hyperthyroidism
Pheochromocytoma
Drug intoxication
Heart failure/cardiomyopathy

Ectopic Atrial Rhythm (Fig. 12–4)

Definition. An ectopic atrial rhythm is a rhythm in which a non–sinus node atrial focus overtakes the sinus node. If the rate is bradycardic, the rhythm is a reflection of sinus node dysfunction ("sick sinus syndrome"). If the rate is tachycardic, the rhythm is a form of supraventricular tachycardia (SVT, see later).

Prevalence. Ectopic atrial rhythm is relatively common.

Prognostic Significance. This rhythm probably does not have any prognostic significance.

Evaluation. With ectopic atrial bradycardia, the patient should be evaluated for symptoms of sick sinus syndrome (see Chapter 31). Symptomatic patients generally benefit from permanent pacemaker implantation. Patients with ectopic atrial tachycardia should be evaluated for symptoms such as palpitations and lightheadedness. Frequent or incessant SVT can cause a cardiomyopathy ("tachycardia-induced cardiomyopathy").

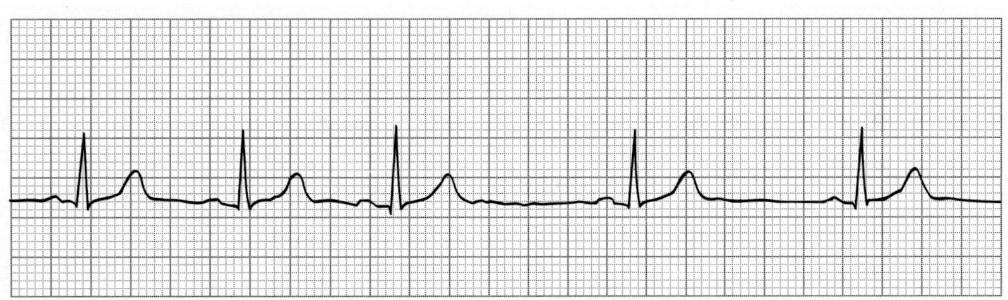

FIGURE 12–3. This rhythm strip (lead II) reveals benign sinus arrhythmia in a healthy young patient.

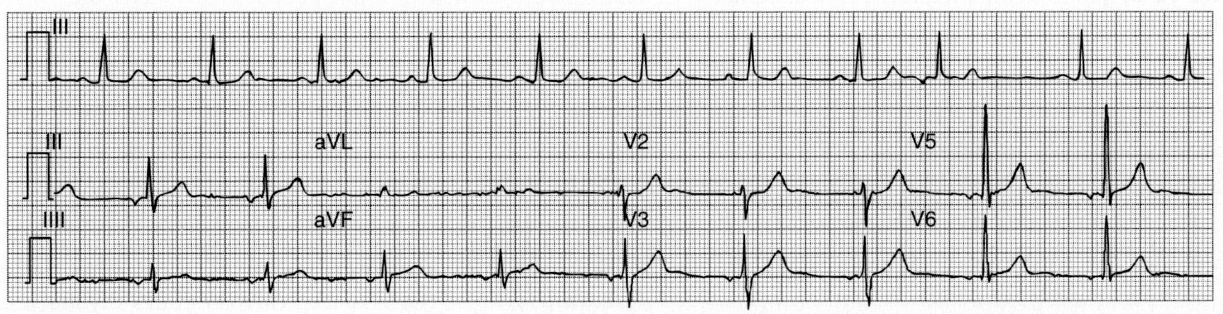

FIGURE 12–4. An ectopic atrial rhythm is present in this patient with sick sinus syndrome. P-waves are inverted in the inferior leads.

Follow-up. Screen for symptoms referable to bradycardia or tachycardia; surveillance for tachycardia-induced cardiomyopathy is recommended.

Junctional Rhythm (Fig. 12–5)

Definition. A junctional rhythm is a rhythm in which an atrioventricular (AV) junctional focus overtakes the sinus node. As with ectopic atrial rhythms, a junctional bradycardia is a reflection of sinus node dysfunction ("sick sinus syndrome"), whereas a junctional tachycardia is a form of SVT.

Prevalence. Junctional rhythms are relatively common.

Prognostic Significance. An asymptomatic junctional rhythm may have no prognostic implications or may be a prelude to symptomatic sick sinus syndrome.

Evaluation. With junctional bradycardia, the patient should be evaluated for symptoms of sick sinus syndrome. Symptomatic patients generally benefit from permanent pacemaker implantation (see Chapter 31). Patients with junctional tachycardias should be evaluated for symptoms such as palpitations and lightheadedness. Frequent or incessant SVT can cause a cardiomyopathy ("tachycardia-induced cardiomyopathy").

Follow-up. Screen for symptoms referable to bradycardia or tachycardia; surveillance for tachycardia-induced cardiomyopathy is indicated if junctional tachycardia persists or recurs frequently.

Premature Atrial Complexes (Fig. 12–6) (see Chapter 30)

Definition. Premature atrial complexes (PACs) are early beats from a non–sinus node atrial origin.

Prevalence. PACs are common.

Prognostic Significance. The prognostic significance of PACs is minimal; they may be associated with atrial fibrillation (AF) or other SVTs.

Evaluation. No specific workup or treatment is necessary in the absence of symptoms.

Follow-up. Follow-up is not necessary.

Premature Ventricular Complexes (Fig. 12–7) (see Chapter 30)

Definition. Premature ventricular complexes (PVCs) are early beats of ventricular origin.

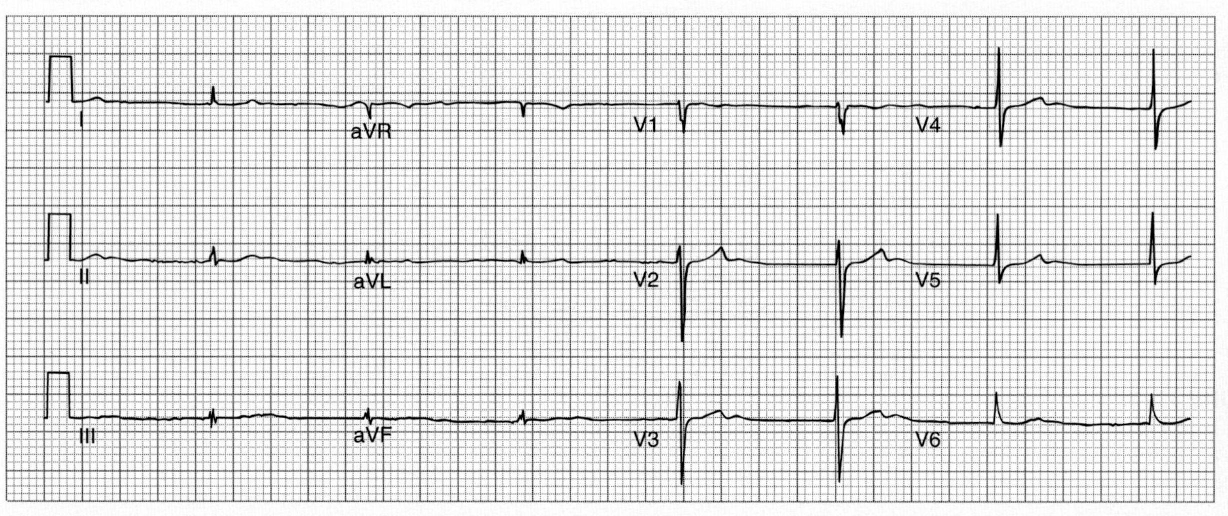

FIGURE 12–5. Junctional bradycardia is a manifestation of sinus node dysfunction in this patient. No P-waves are evident in any lead.

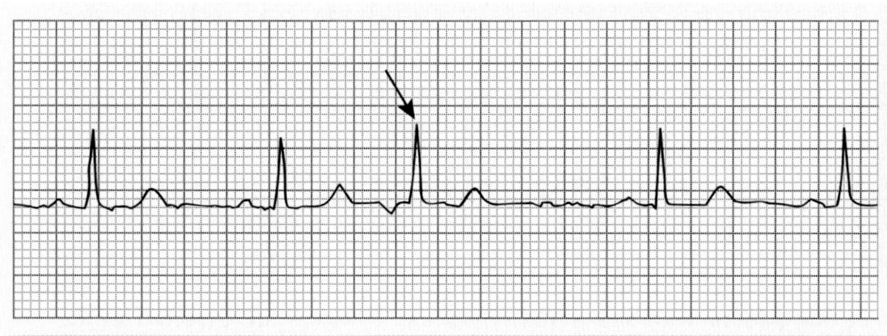

FIGURE 12–6. A premature atrial complex (PAC) is seen (*arrow*) in this rhythm strip (lead II). Note that the premature P-wave is inverted, indicative of a non–sinus node origin. After the PAC is a physiologic pause before the next sinus P-wave.

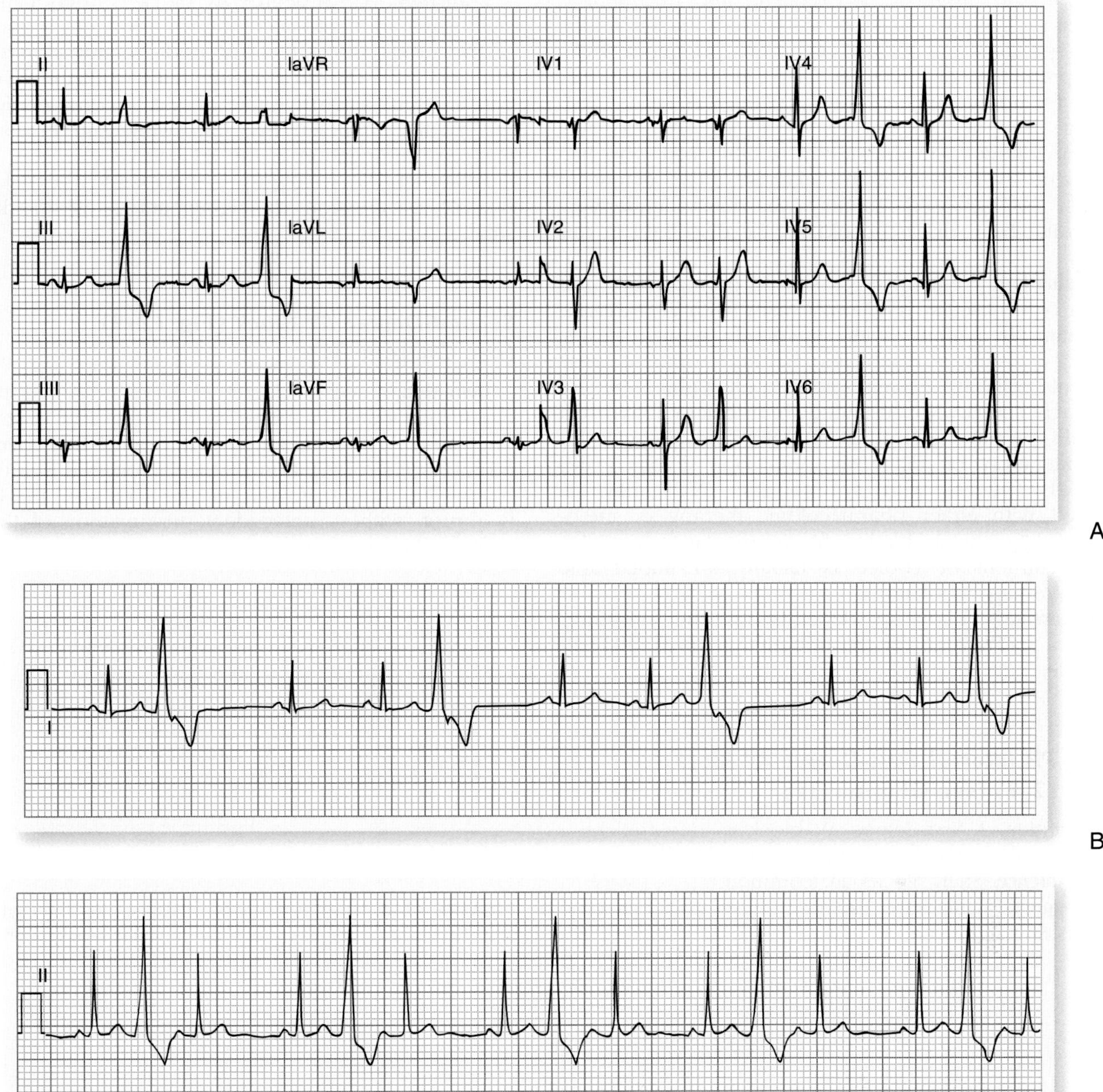

FIGURE 12–7. *A,* Frequent premature ventricular complexes (PVCs) in a bigeminal pattern are noted on this tracing. The QRS morphology has a left bundle branch block (LBBB) pattern and an inferior axis, which suggests an origin in the right ventricular outflow tract (RVOT) in this patient with a structurally normal heart. *B,* Ventricular trigeminy is apparent in this lead II rhythm strip. A physiologic pause follows each PVC. *C,* Ventricular trigeminy is present in this lead II rhythm strip. The PVCs are termed "interpolated" because no pause occurs after the PVC.

Prevalence. PVCs are relatively common. PVCs originating from the right ventricular outflow tract are not uncommon in young, healthy patients with structurally normal hearts (Fig. 12–7*A*).

Prognostic Significance. The prognostic implications of PVCs depend on the presence and severity of any underlying structural heart disease. In population studies, frequent PVCs are associated with increased cardiovascular mortality, but the increased mortality is probably due largely or entirely to associated underlying structural heart disease. Ventricular bigeminy (see Fig. 12–7*A*) or trigeminy (Fig. 12–7*B*) does not necessarily imply a worse prognosis than isolated PVCs do, except in patients with structural heart disease. Most PVCs are followed by a compensatory pause. Those that are not are called interpolated PVCs (Fig. 12–7*C*) and have the same prognosis. In patients with right ventricular outflow tract PVCs and no structural heart disease, the prognosis is excellent, and treatment is necessary only if symptoms are present. In the setting of a previous myocardial infarction, frequent PVCs are predictive of increased mortality; data are less clear for nonischemic cardiomyopathies. A report from France revealed increased cardiovascular mortality during follow-up in apparently healthy men who had frequent PVCs induced by exercise.[7] The extent to which this increased mortality was due to underlying structural heart disease could not be discerned in this study.

Evaluation. Frequent PVCs should prompt an evaluation of ventricular function, usually with an echocardiogram. In patients with structurally normal hearts, exercise testing is reasonable because some of these patients will have exercise-induced idiopathic ventricular tachycardia. Nonsustained ventricular tachycardia should prompt referral to an electrophysiologist for consideration of diagnostic electrophysiologic (EP) studies. Patients with symptomatic PVCs may be treated with either pharmacologic therapy or radiofrequency catheter ablation; for ventricular tachycardia, the treatment of choice is usually an implantable cardioverter-defibrillator.

Follow-up. Follow-up depends on the presence, nature, and severity of the underlying structural heart disease.

Long PR Interval: First-Degree AV Block (Fig. 12–8) (see Chapter 31)

Definition. A first-degree AV block is identified by a PR interval longer than 200 msec (one "big" box).

Prevalence. Such blocks are common.

Prognostic Significance. First-degree AV blocks have no prognostic significance.

Evaluation. A first-degree AV block is rarely clinically significant, so it seldom requires evaluation. In patients taking drugs that affect AV nodal conduction (beta-blockers, non-dihydropyridine calcium channel blockers, digoxin, antiarrhythmic drugs), reconsideration of the medical regimen may be justified in those with marked prolongation of the PR interval.

Follow-up. No follow-up is necessary; the risk and rate of progression to higher grade AV block are small.

Second-Degree AV Block (Fig. 12–9) (see Chapter 31)

Definition. A second-degree AV block is an intermittent block in conduction between the atria and ventricles. The Mobitz I (Wenckebach) pattern is characterized by progressive prolongation of the PR interval before the block (Fig. 12–9*A*). In the Mobitz II pattern, the block is abrupt, without antecedent prolongation of the PR interval (Fig. 12–9*B*).

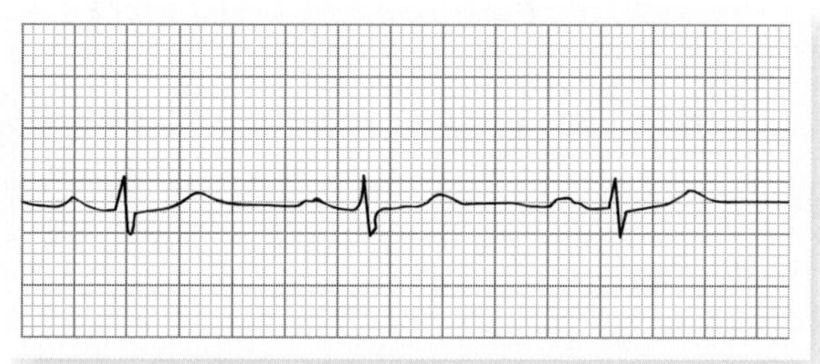

FIGURE 12–8. The PR interval is 240 msec in this rhythm strip (lead II). A first-degree atrioventricular block is present.

A

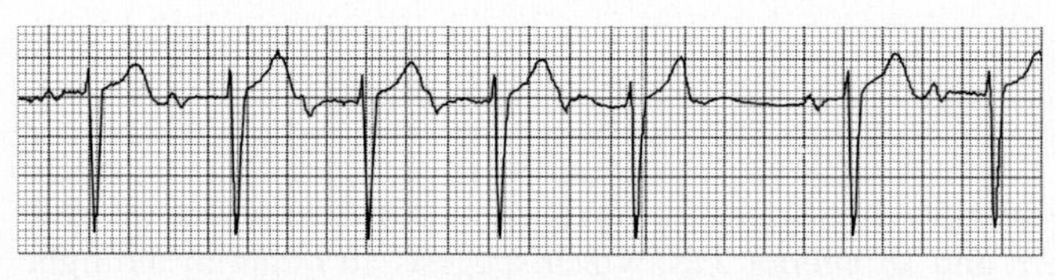

B

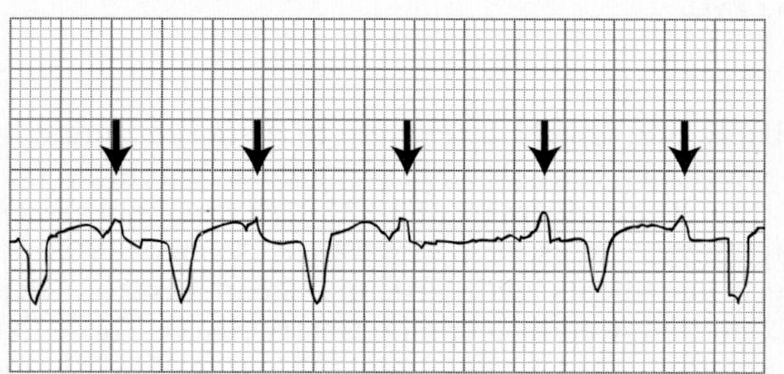

FIGURE 12–9. *A,* The PR interval increases until a P-wave is blocked in this rhythm strip (lead V_1). The QRS complexes are narrow. This defect is a Mobitz I (Wenckebach) second-degree atrioventricular (AV) block, probably at the AV node. *B,* The PR interval is constant before the blocked P-wave in this patient with a Mobitz II second-degree AV block. Note the widened QRS complex. This patient had a bifascicular block (right bundle branch block with a left anterior fascicular block), thus suggesting advanced His-Purkinje system disease.

Prevalence. A second-degree AV block is uncommon.

Prognostic Significance. Such blocks probably have an increased risk of progression to a third-degree AV block.

Evaluation. Some patients with a second-degree AV block require urgent evaluation and treatment, generally with a permanent pacemaker (Box 12–4). If the Mobitz I pattern is present and the QRS complexes are "narrow," the block is at the level of the AV node, and referral/treatment is necessary only in symptomatic patients. Potential symptoms include fatigue, lightheadedness, syncope (see Chapter 10), near-syncope, and poor exercise capacity. Drugs that affect AV conduction (beta-blockers, non-dihydropyridine calcium channel blockers, digoxin, antiarrhythmic drugs) should be reduced in dose or discontinued. In patients with a Mobitz I pattern and a bundle branch block, however, a significant fraction will have a block at the infranodal level rather than the AV nodal level and be at risk for progression to a complete heart block; these patients should be referred to a cardiologist. If the Mobitz II pattern is present, the level of block is probably in the bundle of His or below (i.e., infranodal). In this case, urgent referral/treatment may be necessary, even in asymptomatic patients, because of the risk of progression to higher grade heart block.

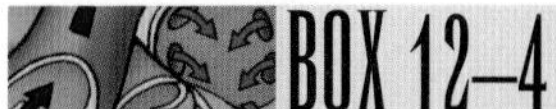

BOX 12–4

Indications for Emergency Evaluation in Patients with Second- and Third-Degree AV Block

History of syncope or near-syncope
Hypotension
Ventricular rate <50
Initial diagnosis of third-degree AV block, unless
- The rate is >50 *and*
- The patient is asymptomatic *and*
- The ORS complex is narrow (i.e., block as at the AV nodal level)

Second-degree AV block with
- A wide QRS complex (bundle branch block) *or*
- A Mobitz II pattern

AV, atrioventricular.

Follow-up. Follow-up depends on the level of the heart block.

Third-Degree AV Block (Fig. 12–10) (see Chapter 31)

Definition. Third-degree AV block is compete absence of conduction between the atria and ventricles. The P-waves and QRS complexes are dissociated, with the atrial rate faster than the ventricular rate.

Prevalence. The prevalence of this abnormality is low.

Prognostic Significance. A third-degree AV block is associated with increased risk of mortality if untreated.

Evaluation. Most patients with a complete AV block should receive a permanent pacemaker (see Chapter 31). The urgency of evaluation and initiation of treatment, as with a second-degree AV block, depends on the level of block, as well as the ventricular escape rate (see Box 12–4). In general, all patients with a complete AV block should be evaluated by a cardiologist or cardiac electrophysiologist. In some patients with a block at the AV nodal level, discontinuation of medications that contribute to the block may alleviate the condition. Young patients with congenital heart block should generally receive permanent pacemakers in their late teen years, even if they are asymptomatic. In acquired complete AV block, indications for permanent pacing include symptoms, an infranodal site of the block, or a ventricular rate less than 40 beats per minute while awake.

Follow-up. Patients treated with pacemakers should receive regular follow-up, ideally in a dedicated pacemaker clinic. Rare patients who do not receive permanent pacemakers should be monitored closely for the development of symptoms or another indication for pacemaker implantation.

Atrial Fibrillation and Atrial Flutter (Figs. 12–11 and 12–12) (see Chapter 30)

Definition. In AF, no organized atrial electrical activity is present; fine fibrillatory waves appear on the ECG (Fig. 12–11). The ventricular rate is generally rapid and irregular. Atrial flutter is associated with a macroreentrant circuit, generally in the right atrium, that inscribes sawtooth flutter waves (Fig. 12–12). The ventricular rate is typically regular and a consistent fraction of the atrial

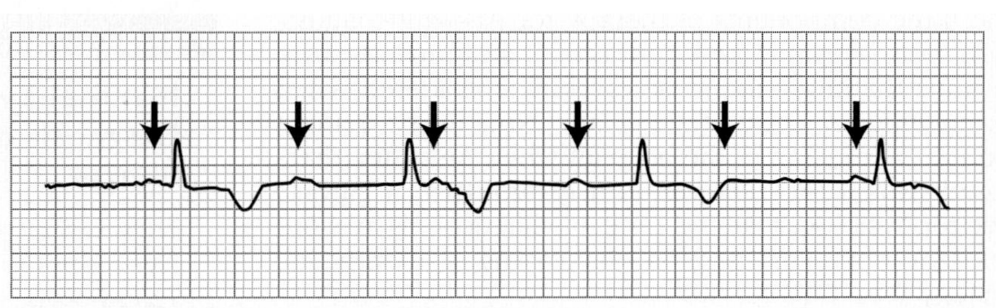

FIGURE 12–10. A complete (third-degree) atrioventricular block is present in this rhythm strip (lead II). Note that the P-wave rate is regular and faster than the QRS rate, but the two are not related to each other. *Arrows* denote the P waves.

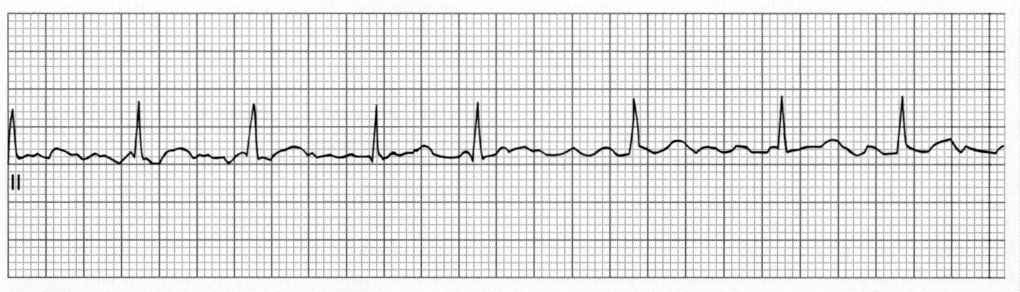

FIGURE 12–11. Atrial fibrillation with a controlled ventricular response (80 beats per minute) was noted in this patient who complained of fatigue and decreased exercise capacity. Note the coarse fibrillation with irregularly irregular QRS complexes in this rhythm strip (lead II).

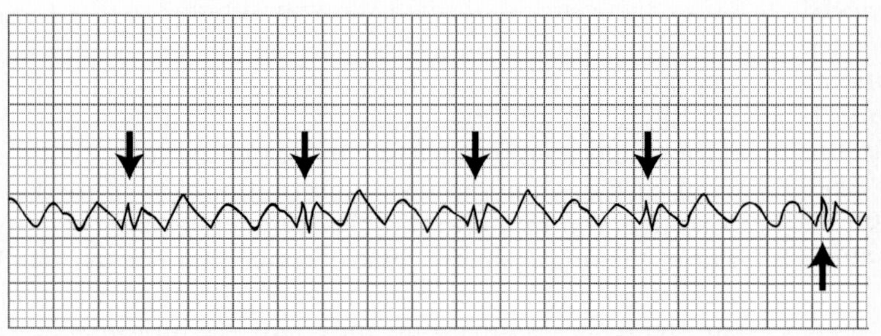

FIGURE 12–12. Atrial flutter with 4:1 atrial-to-ventricular conduction is present in this asymptomatic patient. Note the sawtooth flutter waves, best seen in the inferior leads, and the perfectly regular QRS interval (*arrows*).

rate. Typical atrial flutter frequently conducts 2:1 to the ventricles, for a ventricular rate on the order of 150 beats per minute.

Prevalence. AF is common, with the incidence increasing with age and in association with other cardiovascular disease. AF is far more common than atrial flutter, but some patients have both AF and atrial flutter. When AF occurs in relatively young patients (<60 years of age) in the absence of obvious precipitants, it is called idiopathic or lone AF.

Prognostic Significance. Patients with AF have higher cardiovascular mortality than patients without AF do. Whether this worse prognosis is due entirely to the underlying cardiovascular disease or whether AF itself confers additional mortality remains controversial.

Evaluation. Whenever AF is first diagnosed, the physician should look carefully for signs or symptoms of other conditions that frequently accompany AF (Box 12–5).[8] Even if no co-morbidities are apparent, the diagnosis of AF mandates a thorough evaluation (Box 12–6). The three components of therapy for AF—anticoagulation,[9] rate control, and restoration and maintenance of sinus rhythm—should be carefully considered when formulating a therapeutic plan. Not every patient requires admission to the hospital when AF is first diagnosed (Box 12–7). Referral to a cardiologist or cardiac electrophysiologist at the time of diagnosis is reasonable for obtaining help in developing a therapeutic strategy (see Chapter 30).

Follow-up. The intensity of follow-up depends on the symptoms, as well as the course of therapy elected.

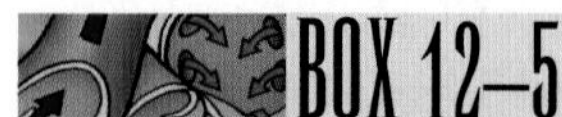

BOX 12–5

Conditions Frequently Associated with Atrial Fibrillation and Atrial Flutter

Hypertension
Coronary artery disease
Valvular heart disease
Cardiomyopathy (dilated, infiltrative, hypertrophic, etc.)
Peripheral vascular disease
Cerebrovascular disease
Diabetes mellitus
Pulmonary embolus
Chronic obstructive pulmonary disease
Pulmonary hypertension
Hyperthyroidism
Alcohol/drug intoxication ("holiday heart")

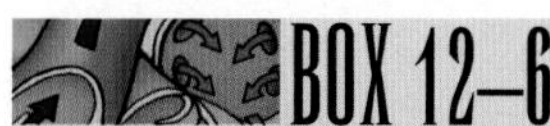

BOX 12–6

Minimal Evaluation after the Initial Diagnosis of Atrial Fibrillation or Atrial Flutter

Thorough history and physical examination
Electrocardiogram
Transthoracic echocardiogram
Thyroid testing

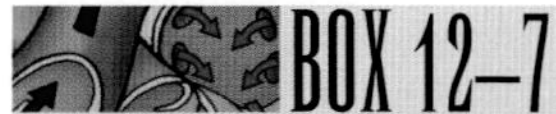

Indications for Hospital Admission with an Initial Diagnosis of Atrial Fibrillation or Atrial Flutter

Significant symptoms or hemodynamic intolerance, which underscores an urgent need to control the ventricular rate or restore sinus rhythm

High risk for thromboembolic complications (e.g., previous transient ischemia attacks or strokes, prosthetic value, mitral valve disease, etc.)

To facilitate prompt cardioversion

Concomitant condition that mandates admission (acute myocardial infarction, acute pulmonary embolus, acute transient ischemic attack or stroke, thyroid storm, etc.)

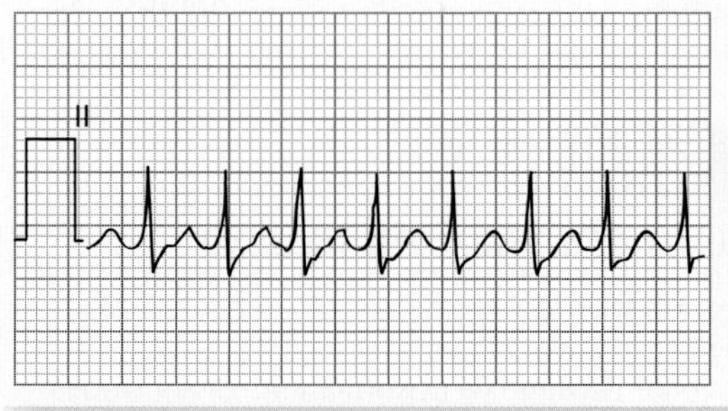

FIGURE 12–13. A supraventricular tachycardia (SVT) is present in this patient with palpitations and lightheadedness. This tachycardia is narrow complex, regular, and rapid (190 beats per minute).

Patients treated with warfarin need to have careful follow-up, ideally by a dedicated anticoagulation practice. Patients who take antiarrhythmic drugs require extremely thorough follow-up because of the risk of adverse effects with these agents.

Supraventricular Tachycardia (Fig. 12–13) (see Chapter 30)

Definition. SVT is defined as a rapid, regular rhythm. QRS complexes are generally narrow, but aberrant conduction can cause a wide-complex tachycardia. The pattern may be paroxysmal or incessant.

Prevalence. SVT is relatively common.

Prognostic Significance. The prognostic implications of SVT are minimal in the absence of Wolff-Parkinson-White (WPW) syndrome (see later).

Evaluation. Patients with SVT should be screened for symptoms such as palpitations and lightheadedness. If vagal maneuvers do not terminate the SVT, the patient should be sent to an emergency department for intravenous medication to terminate the arrhythmia (see Chapter 30). Frequent or incessant SVT can cause a cardiomyopathy ("tachycardia-induced cardiomyopathy").

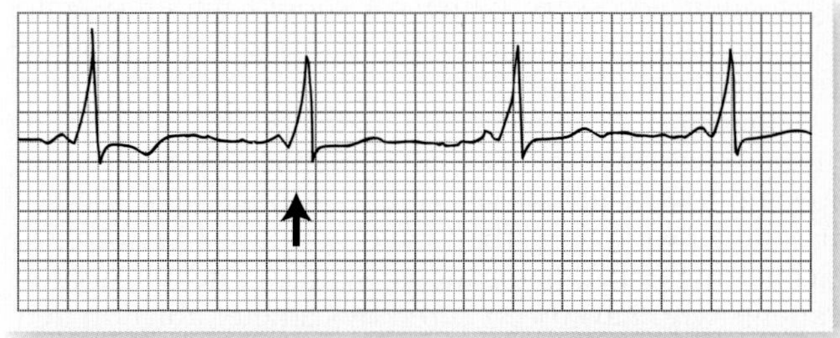

FIGURE 12–14. The Wolff-Parkinson-White pattern is present. The PR interval is short, and the QRS complex has a slurred upstroke (delta wave; *arrow*) because of ventricular preexcitation.

Follow-up. Patients with SVT are generally symptomatic and should be referred to a cardiologist or cardiac electrophysiologist.

Short PR Interval with a "Delta" Wave, Including Wolff-Parkinson-White (Ventricular Preexcitation) Syndrome (Fig. 12–14)

Definition. When an accessory pathway capable of anterograde conduction is present, the result is a short PR interval and a QRS complex that has a slurred upstroke (delta wave). This finding is the WPW ECG pattern (see Chapter 30). Patients with the WPW ECG pattern and paroxysmal SVT are said to have WPW syndrome.

Prevalence. The prevalence of the WPW ECG pattern is about 1 to 3 per 1000.[10] Not all of these patients will ever have symptoms.

Prognostic Significance. WPW syndrome carries a small risk of sudden cardiac death.

Evaluation. Patients with WPW syndrome are at risk for symptomatic AV reentrant tachycardia, a form of paroxysmal SVT involving the accessory pathway. More importantly, however, patients with WPW syndrome are at risk for sudden death related to extremely rapid ventricular rates during AF or atrial flutter. Fortunately, sudden death is very rarely the first manifestation of WPW. Most patients who are asymptomatic at the time of diagnosis remain asymptomatic; with aging, some will even lose the capacity for anterograde accessory pathway conduction. In general, most patients with no symptoms referable to tachyarrhythmia (palpitations, syncope, near-syncope) are not generally evaluated further or treated, whereas patients with symptomatic WPW syndrome should usually undergo EP studies and radiofrequency catheter ablation. The proper management of asymptomatic patients in high-risk occupations (pilots, bus drivers, elite athletes, etc.) remains controversial; many advocate EP studies for risk stratification, with catheter ablation if appropriate. Because of these complexities, patients in whom a WPW ECG pattern or syndrome is newly diagnosed should be referred to a cardiac electrophysiologist for evaluation. Patients with right-sided accessory pathways should undergo echocardiography to exclude the possibility of Ebstein's anomaly (see Chapter 34).

Follow-up. Asymptomatic patients in whom no further evaluation or therapy is planned do not require specific follow-up; these patients should seek medical attention promptly if they have symptoms referable to tachyarrhythmias (palpitations, syncope, near-syncope). Patients who have been cured by catheter ablation generally require one follow-up visit (to verify absence of the accessory pathway on ECG) and can then be instructed to seek attention if symptoms recur.

Short PR Interval without a "Delta" Wave, Including the Lown-Ganong-Levine (LGL) Syndrome (Fig. 12–15)

Definition. This abnormality is defined as a PR interval less than 120 msec but without a slurred upstroke of the QRS complex (i.e., no "delta wave") (Box 12–8). Patients with a short PR interval and paroxysmal SVT in the absence of ventricular preexcitation are said to have Lown-Ganong-Levine syndrome. In the past, this syndrome was thought to be caused by an accessory pathway that bypassed part or all of the AV node. A more likely explanation is that many or all of these patients have "enhanced AV nodal conduction" and SVT. As with any biologic phenomenon, the PR interval is short in some patients and long in others (first-degree AV block). In the absence of ventricular preexcitation (WPW syndrome), it is not clear whether patients with a short PR interval are any more prone to SVT than other patients.

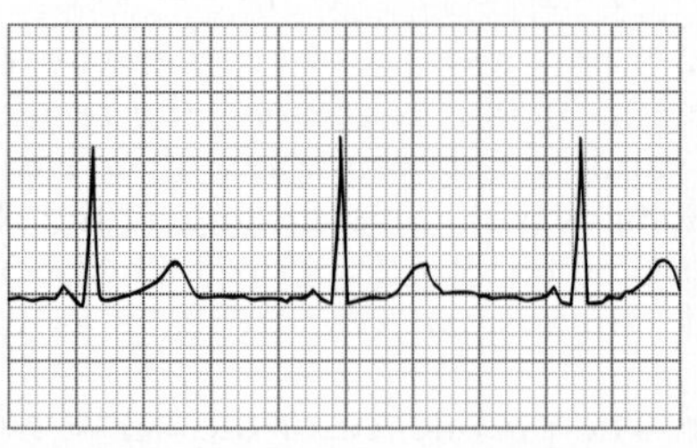

FIGURE 12–15. The PR interval is short in this healthy young patient. The patient had never had symptoms suggestive of supraventricular tachycardia.

Prevalence. A short PR interval without a delta wave is relatively common.

Prognostic Significance. This abnormality probably has no prognostic significance.

Evaluation. Evaluation is not needed in the absence of symptoms.

Follow-up. No specific recommendations have been proposed.

Left Axis Deviation/Left Anterior Fascicular Block (Fig. 12–16)

Definition. Left axis deviation is defined as a QRS frontal-plane axis between −30 and −90 degrees. For a

BOX 12–8

Causes of a Short PR Interval

Catecholamine effect
Preexcitation syndrome
Junctional rhythm (with isorhythmic dissociation)
Pregnancy
Childhood/adolescence
Enhanced atrioventricular nodal conduction
Fabry's disease
Duchenne's muscular dystrophy
Friedreich's ataxia
Pompe's disease

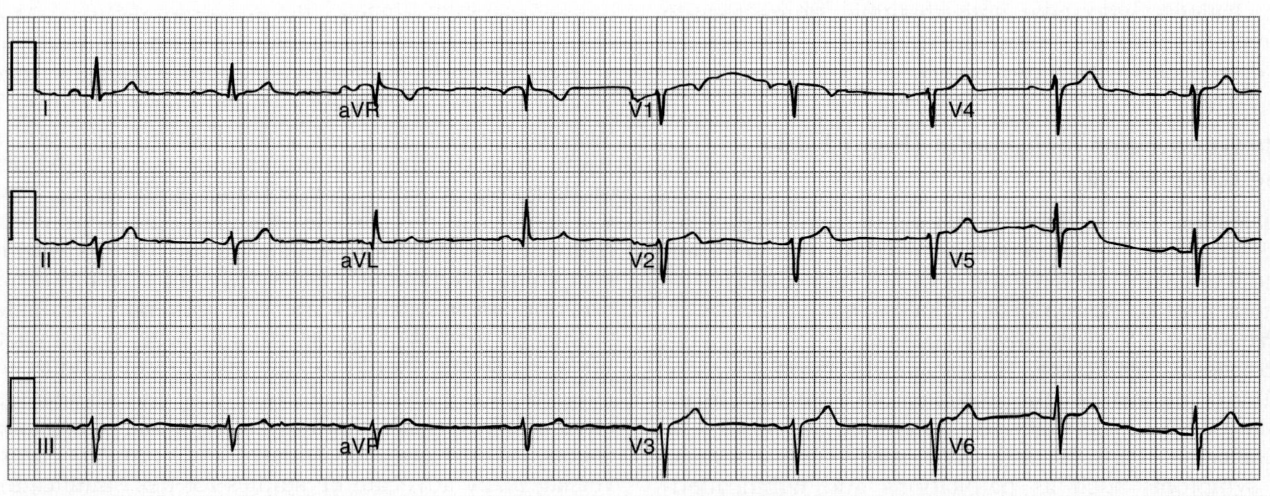

FIGURE 12–16. Left anterior fascicular block (LAFB). Note the left axis (S-wave greater than the R-wave in lead II); small R- and large S-waves in leads II, III, and aVF; and only a minimally widened QRS complex. Delayed R-wave progression across the precordium is common in LAFB.

left anterior fascicular block (LAFB), the axis is between −45 and −90 degrees, small R-waves are present in the inferior leads, and the QRS duration is less than 120 msec.

Prevalence. These abnormalities are common.

Prognostic Significance. An increased risk of cardiovascular mortality may be seen in asymptomatic patients, but the absolute risk remains small.

Evaluation. No specific evaluation is required in absence of symptoms suggestive of cardiovascular disease.

Follow-up. No specific follow-up is advised.

Right Axis Deviation/Left Posterior Fascicular Block (Fig. 12–17)

Definition. Right axis deviation is defined as a QRS frontal-plane axis between +90 and −90 degrees (+270 degrees); axes between +180 and −90 degrees are considered extreme (right) axis deviation. For a left posterior fascicular block (LPFB), the axis is between +90 and +180 degrees, small Q-waves and prominent R-waves are present in the inferior leads, small R- and deep S-waves are present in leads I and aVL, and the QRS duration is less than 120 msec.

Prevalence. These abnormalities are uncommon.

Prognostic Significance. Asymptomatic patients may have an increased risk of cardiovascular mortality, but the absolute risk remains small.

Evaluation. No specific evaluation is needed in the absence of symptoms suggestive of cardiovascular disease.

Follow-up. No specific recommendations have been proposed.

Right Bundle Branch Block (Fig. 12–18*A* and *B*)

Definition. A right bundle branch block (RBBB) is defined as a QRS duration longer than 120 msec, with a secondary R-wave (R′) in lead V_1 (Box 12–9). Note that the QRS axis is normal unless a concomitant LAFB or LPFB is present. A bundle branch block does not imply complete absence of conduction; rather, conduction is slowed relative to the other bundle branch. In incomplete RBBB (IRBBB), the QRS morphology is similar, but the QRS duration is less than 120 msec (see Fig. 12–18*B*). An rSR′ pattern in lead V_1 with a normal QRS width may be seen as a normal variant in healthy young patients.

Prevalence. In the Framingham study, the prevalence of RBBB on the initial screening ECG was 0.3%. The incidence of new RBBB increased with age, with the peak incidence of new cases per year found in subjects 60 to 69 years of age. In the Framingham study, the prevalence of RBBB was higher in men than women. Overall, the cumulative incidence of RBBB in the Framingham and other epidemiologic studies is on the order of 1.6%. The prevalence of IRBBB is considerably higher.

Prognostic Significance. It remains uncertain whether isolated RBBB carries with it an increased mortality independent of associated structural heart disease. IRBBB probably poses no risk other than a higher risk for complete RBBB.

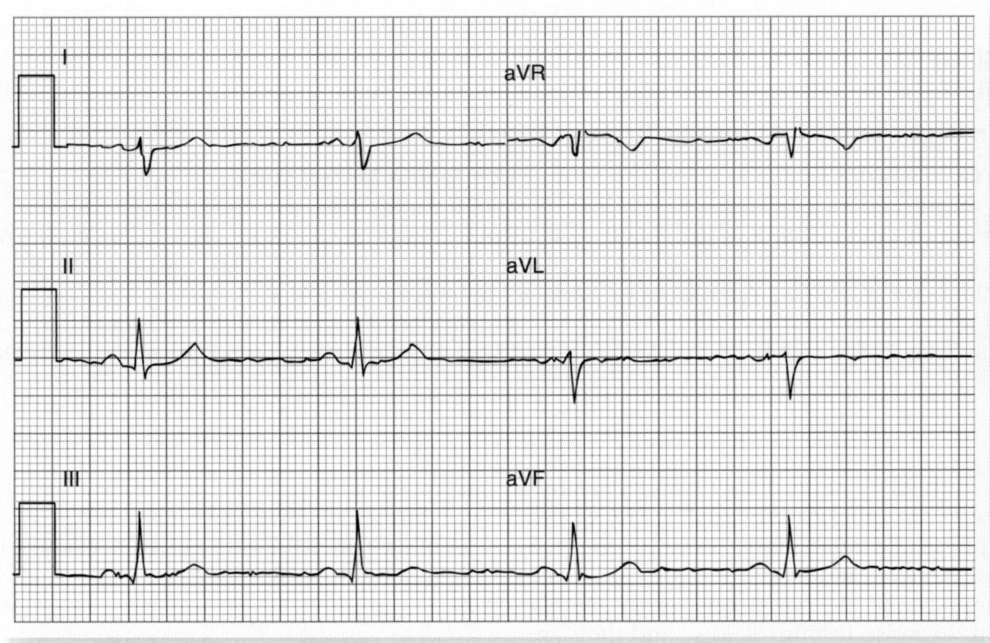

FIGURE 12–17. Left posterior fascicular block (LPFB), limb leads only. Note the right axis (S-wave greater than the R-wave in lead I), with small R-waves and deep S-waves in leads I and aVL and small Q-waves with dominant R-waves in the inferior leads. Sinus bradycardia is also present.

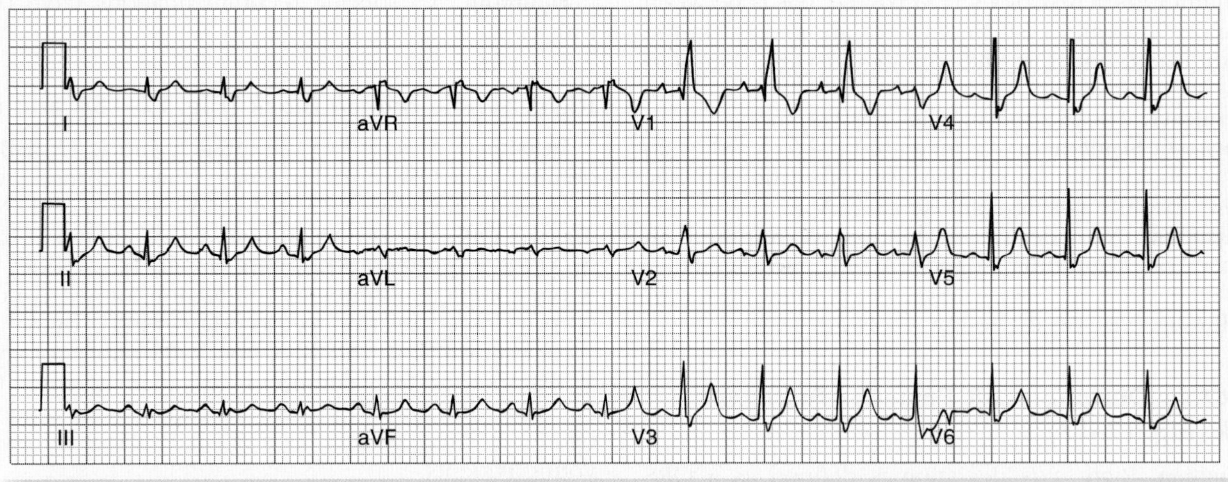

A

B

FIGURE 12–18. *A,* Right bundle branch block (RBBB). Note the rsR′ complex in lead V_1, with a QRS duration longer than 120 msec. Wide S-waves are present in leads I, aVL, and V_6. *B,* Incomplete RBBB (IRBBB). An rSR′ is present in lead V_1, but the QRS width is less than 120 msec. In this case, the QRS width is less than 100 msec, and this is a normal variant.

BOX 12–9

Criteria for Right and Left Bundle Branch Block

RIGHT BUNDLE BRANCH BLOCK

QRS duration >120 msec
Secondary R-wave (R′) in V_1, with R′ larger than the initial R-wave
Interval from the onset of the QRS complex to its peak >50 msec in V_1
Wide S-wave in leads I, aVL, and V_6

LEFT BUNDLE BRANCH BLOCK

QRS duration >120 msec
Broad, frequently a notched R-wave in leads I, V_5, and V_6
Interval from the onset of the QRS complex to its peak >50 msec in V_5 and V_6
Absence of Q-waves in leads I, V_5, and V_6
ST- and T-wave directed opposite to the major QRS deflection

Evaluation. As with AF, bundle branch blocks are frequently associated with other cardiovascular disease, so the history and physical examination should be oriented in this direction. If signs and symptoms of cardiovascular disease are absent, the yield on further testing (echocardiogram, exercise testing) is low, and they are not generally necessary. Even in association with a fascicular block (bifascicular block) or a fascicular block and a first-degree AV block (trifascicular block), the risk of progression to complete AV block is very low in asymptomatic patients, so neither prophylactic pacing nor further evaluation is indicated.

Follow-up. Follow-up is not necessary in the absence of structural cardiac disease.

Left Bundle Branch Block (Fig. 12–19)

Definition. A left bundle branch block (LBBB) is defined as a QRS duration longer than 120 msec, with terminal forces directed to the left (see Box 12–9).

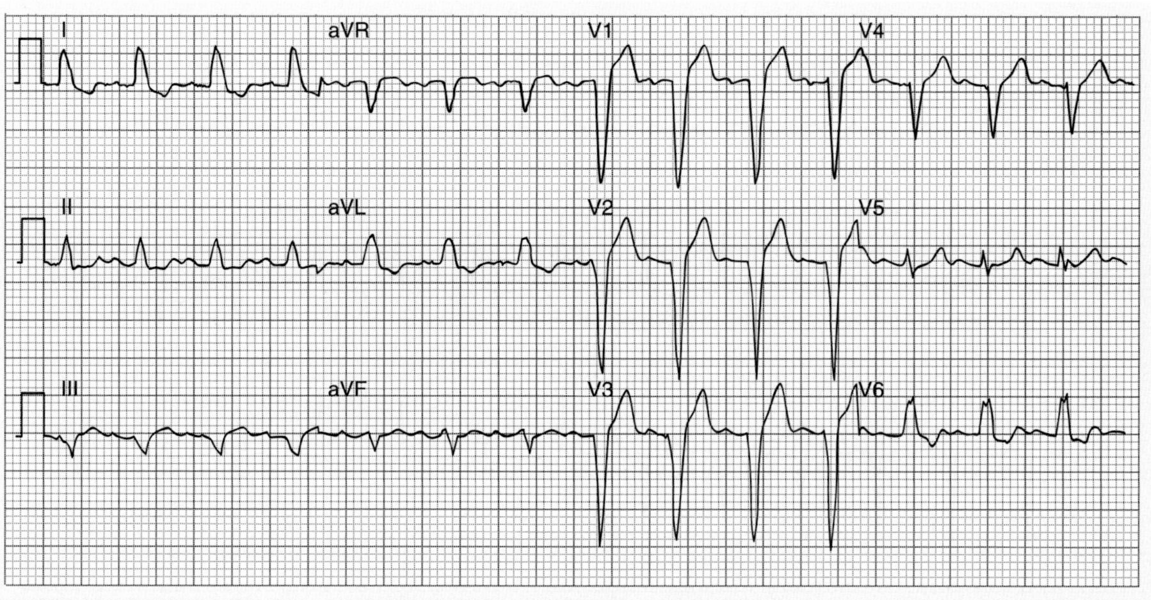

FIGURE 12–19. Left bundle branch block (LBBB). Note the broad, notched R-wave in lead I, with a QRS duration longer than 120 msec.

Prevalence. The prevalence and cumulative incidence of LBBB in the Framingham study were similar to those of RBBB, on the order of 0.3% and 1.4%, respectively. As with RBBB, the incidence of LBBB increases with age. LBBB was more common in men in the Framingham study, but other epidemiologic studies have shown the opposite.

Prognostic Significance. LBBB is associated with increased mortality.[11]

Evaluation. As with RBBB, LBBB frequently accompanies other cardiovascular disease. In addition, LBBB may be the initial sign of cardiomyopathy, especially when it occurs in combination with low limb lead voltage. Thus, even if no other signs or symptoms of cardiovascular disease are present, the initial diagnosis of LBBB should trigger an evaluation of left ventricular function with an echocardiogram or cardiac nuclear medicine study. An assessment for ischemia should be performed if left ventricular dysfunction is noted, even in the absence of symptomatic angina.

Follow-up. Follow-up is not needed in patients without structural cardiac disease.

Bifascicular Block (Fig. 12–20)

Definition. The infrahissian conducting system consists of three fascicles: the right bundle, the left anterior fascicle, and the left posterior fascicle. The two left fascicles together make the left bundle. Whereas bifascicular block frequently refers to an RBBB with an LAFB or LPFB, LBBB can properly be considered a bifascicular block as well. A trifascicular block refers to either of these combinations with a first-degree AV block.

Prevalence. The prevalence of LBBB was described earlier. RBBB with LAFB is uncommon, and RBBB with LPFB is rare.

Prognostic Significance. As with bundle branch blocks, bifascicular blocks generally occur in patients with other cardiovascular disease. The prognostic significance of bifascicular block, independent of the accompanying cardiovascular disease, is uncertain. The risk of progression to complete AV block is very low.

Evaluation. The evaluation should focus on possible signs and symptoms of hypertension and other cardiovascular disease. The recommended evaluation is similar to that for LBBB. The physician should inquire about symptoms attributable to bradycardia (lightheadedness, syncope, near-syncope, etc.). EP studies and permanent pacemaker implantation are not necessary in the absence of symptoms.

Follow-up. Follow-up depends on any underlying structural heart disease.

QT Prolongation (Fig. 12–21) (see Chapter 30)

Definition. The QT interval must be corrected for the heart rate; Bazett's formula is used most commonly, although admittedly, this formula is relatively imperfect at slow or fast heart rates:

QTc = QT ÷ square root of RR

where RR = the interval between R waves in milliseconds. Computerized ECG machines calculate the QTc automatically. Normal QTc values are less than 0.410 second for females and under 0.390 second for males. Diagnostic criteria for congenital long QT syndrome (LQTS) include a QTc over 460 in females and over 450 in males.[12]

Prevalence. The prevalence of congenital LQTS is extremely low. Mild QT prolongation is not uncommon,

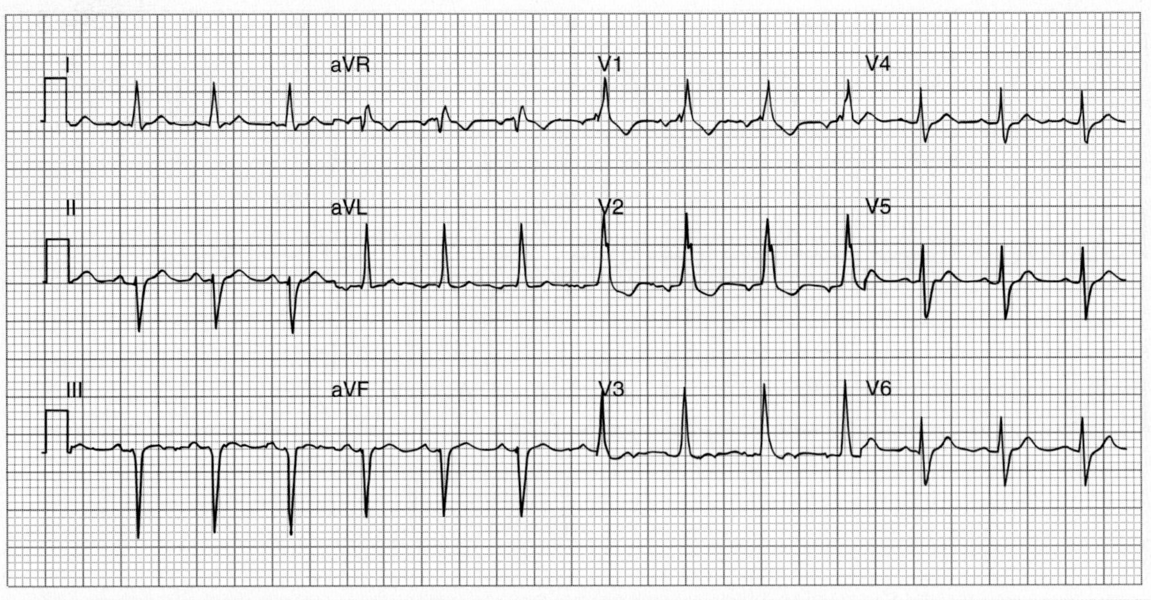

FIGURE 12–20. Bifascicular block with a right bundle branch block and a left anterior fascicular block.

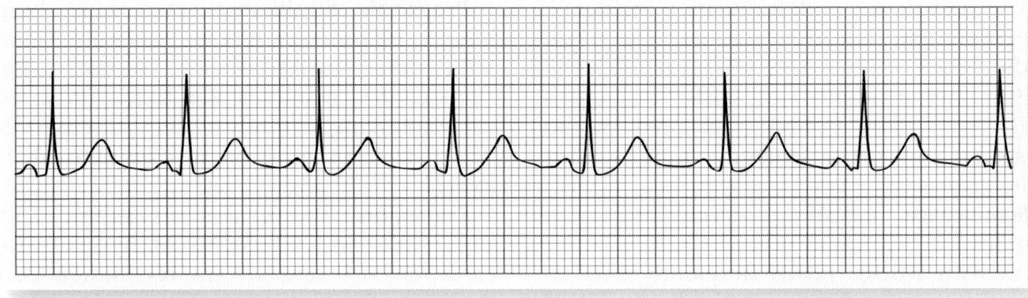

FIGURE 12–21. Marked QT prolongation in a patient with congenital long QT syndrome (LQTS) and recurrent syncope. The QTc is 0.60 second.

particularly in patients taking multiple medications or with multiple co-morbidities.

Prognostic Significance. In population studies, mild QT prolongation has not been reproducibly linked to increased mortality. Patient with LQTS are clearly at risk for sudden cardiac death.

Evaluation. Patients with congenital LQTS (see Chapter 30) are typically identified during childhood or adolescence, and epilepsy is frequently misdiagnosed initially. A history of syncope, particularly with exertion, sudden cardiac death, or congenital deafness in the patient or the family suggests possible congenital LQTS, even if the ECG is borderline. All first-degree relatives of patients with congenital LQTS should be screened. Acquired LQTS is generally due to medications that directly prolong the QT interval (Box 12–10), especially when combined with agents that inhibit the metabolism of QT-prolonging drugs (Box 12–11). Patients with congenital LQTS or those treated with class IA or class III antiarrhythmic drugs should be told to avoid the drugs on this list. Because of the risk of torsades de pointes ventricular tachycardia, patients with suspected congenital LQTS should be referred to a cardiac electrophysiologist (see Chapter 30).

Follow-up. Patients treated with QT-prolonging antiarrhythmic drugs require extremely careful follow-up to minimize the proarrhythmic and other risks of these agents. Concomitant follow-up by a cardiologist or cardiac electrophysiologist is reasonable in these patients.

Abnormalities in Myocardial Structure/Function

Q-Waves (Fig. 12–22)

Definition. Significant Q-waves are generally considered to be at least 40 msec wide (one “small” box) in at least two contiguous ECG leads (see Fig. 12–22*A* and *B*).

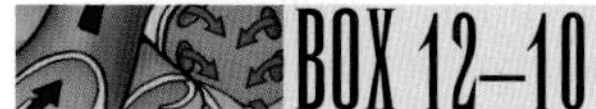

BOX 12–10

QT-Prolonging Medications

Class IA antiarrhythmic drugs
- Procainamide
- Quinidine
- Disopyramide

Class III antiarrhythmic drugs
- Sotalol
- Dofetilide
- Ibutilide
- Amiodarone

Tricyclic antidepressants
- Imipramine
- Desipramine
- Amitriptyline
- Trazodone

Phenothiazines
- Chlorpromazine
- Thioridazine
- Perphenazine
- Fluphenazine
- Trifluoperazine

Haloperidol

Antibiotics/antifungals/antivirals
- Erythromycin, clarithromycin, and other macrolide antibiotics
- Trimethoprim-sulfamethoxazole
- Antimalarials
- Pentamidine
- Amantadine

Probucol

Note: Terfenadine, astemizole, and cisapride all prolong the QT interval but have been withdrawn from the market. A frequently updated drug list may be found at www.torsades.org or www.care.org.

BOX 12–11

Drugs That Inhibit the Metabolism of QT-Prolonging Drugs

Antifungals
- Ketoconazole
- Metronidazole
- Itraconazole

Serotonin reuptake inhibitors
- Fluoxetine
- Fluvoxamine
- Sertraline

Grapefruit juice

Calcium channel blockers (dihydropyridines)
- Nifedipine
- Nicardipine
- Felodipine

Protease inhibitors
- Ritonavir
- Indinavir
- Saquinavir

Note: Frequently updated drug lists may be found at www.torsades.org or www.care.org.

Prevalence. Detection of a clinically silent myocardial infarction (MI) with a screening ECG is unusual. In the Framingham study, 23% of ECG-documented MIs were initially detected on biennial ECGs.[13] Of the unrecognized MIs, 53% were in fact clinically silent; in the other patients, previous symptoms consistent with MI could be elicited. It is important to keep in mind that the presence of inferior Q-waves is somewhat insensitive and nonspecific for previous inferior infarction. Extremely common are "small" or insignificant Q-waves (see Fig. 12–22*B*). More than half of normal adults will have a small Q-wave in a least one of the inferior leads. Small Q-waves are even more common in the left precordial leads of normal adults; these waves reflect normal early septal activation (see Fig. 12–22*B*).

Prognostic Significance. Patients with clinically unrecognized MI are at significant risk for cardiovascular events and mortality.

Evaluation. Given the advances in management of patients with chronic coronary artery disease over recent years, patients with ECG evidence of clinically silent, previous MI should be evaluated as aggressively as those with clinically manifested MI (see Chapter 27). A possible wall motion abnormality should be assessed with an imaging study (echocardiogram or nuclear study). If a previous MI is confirmed, assessment for ischemia should follow. In the absence of signs or symptoms of acute ischemia/infarction, this evaluation can be performed on an elective, outpatient basis.

Follow-up. Further evaluation and treatment are dependent on the extent of left ventricular dysfunction and the level of ischemia, as well as the treatment strategy chosen. If no evidence of left ventricular dysfunction or coronary ischemia is documented, no specific follow-up is necessary.

Poor R-Wave Progression across the Precordium (Fig. 12–23)

Definition. In general, the R-wave should increase in amplitude from V_1 to V_4 or V_5. The amplitude of the R-wave usually exceeds that of the S-wave by lead V_3 or V_4. Potential causes of abnormal R-wave progression across the precordium are listed in Box 12–12.

Prevalence. Poor R-wave progression is relatively common.

Prognostic Significance. The prognostic implications depend on any underlying structural heart disease.

Evaluation. If the ECG cannot be explained by lead placement or the presence of a fascicular block, an echocardiogram is useful to screen for structural heart disease.

Follow-up. Follow-up depends on the underlying structural heart disease.

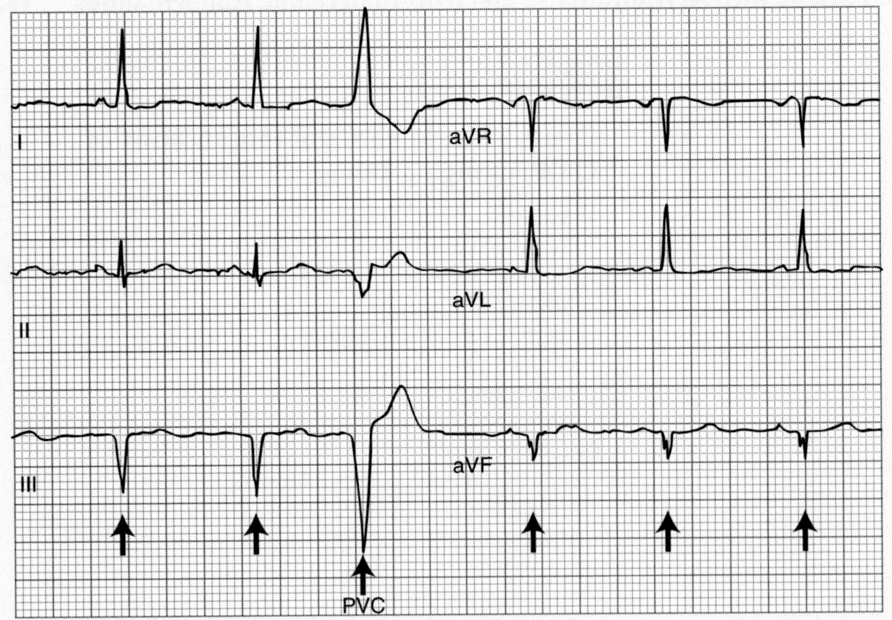

A

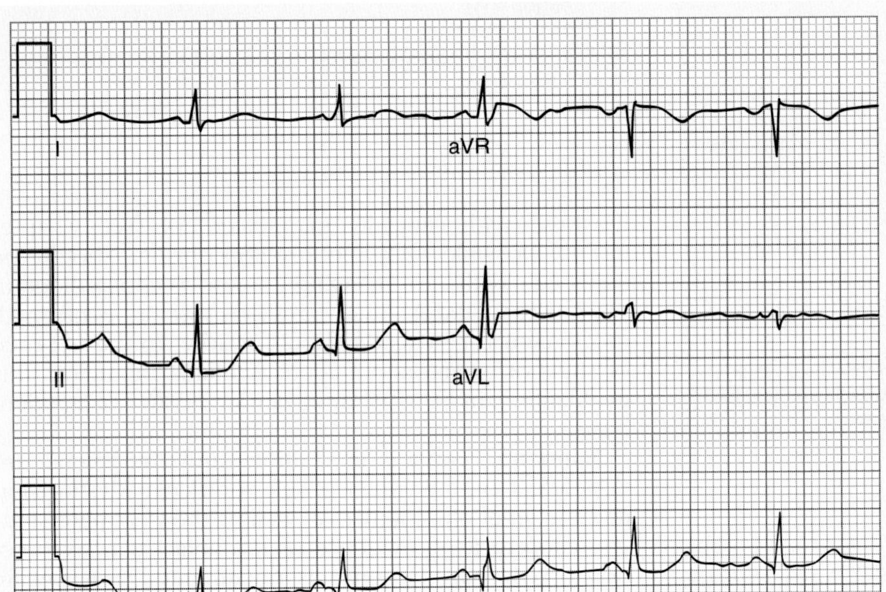

B

FIGURE 12–22. *A,* Pathologic Q-waves (*arrows*) are present in leads III and aVF and reflect a previous myocardial infarction. The Q-waves are more than 40 msec wide. Note the "small" Q-wave in lead II and the single premature ventricular contraction (PVC). *B,* Insignificant Q-waves are present in leads II, III, and avF in this healthy young man. Note how narrow the Q-waves are.

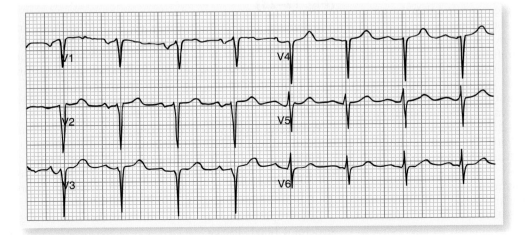

FIGURE 12–23. Poor R-wave progression is present across the precordium in this patient because of previous anterior myocardial infarction. Low QRS voltage is also seen in the limb leads.

Left Ventricular Hypertrophy (Fig. 12–24)

Definition. A number of ECG criteria for left ventricular hypertrophy (LVH) exist. The Romhilt-Estes criteria are probably used most commonly, particularly by computerized ECG interpretation algorithms (Box 12–13). The correlation between LVH by ECG criteria and as diagnosed on echocardiography, the gold standard, is limited.

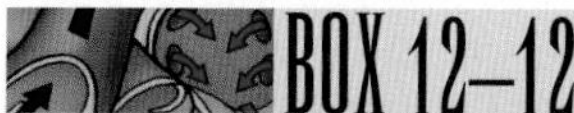
BOX 12–12

Causes of Delayed R-Wave Progression across the Precordium

Previous anterior or anterolateral myocardial infarction
Left anterior fascicular block
Left posterior fascicular block
Lead placement error
Dextrocardia
Right ventricular hypertrophy
Chronic obstructive pulmonary disease

Prevalence. The prevalence of LVH depends on the population screened and the criteria used. Hypertension (see Chapter 19) and aortic stenosis (see Chapter 32) are frequently accompanied by LVH. It is estimated that the prevalence of LVH with repolarization abnormalities (see later) in asymptomatic, apparently healthy patients is on the order of 1%.[14] Estimates of the sensitivity and specificity of the Romhilt-Estes scoring criteria are 30% and 95%, respectively. If the true prevalence in the population being studied is less than 10%, however, more false-positive than true-positive results will occur. The QRS amplitude is higher in younger and thinner patients. Voltage suggestive of LVH is not

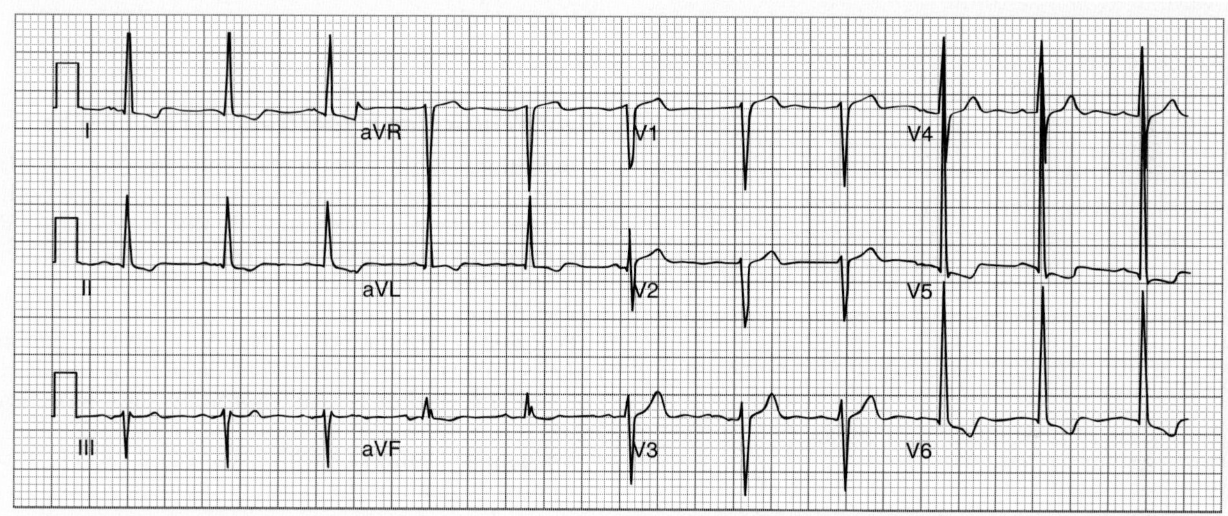

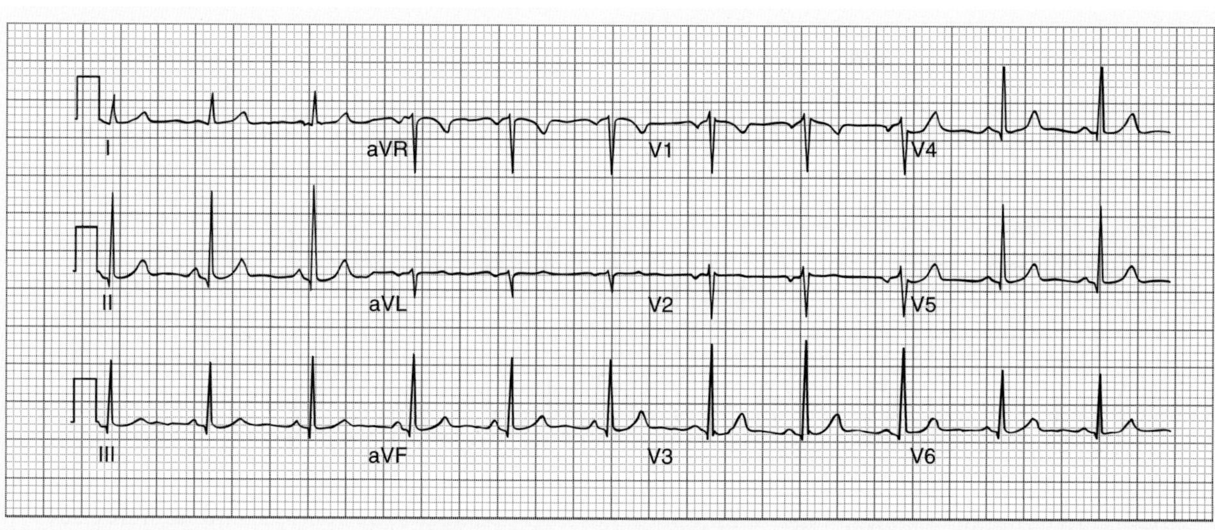

FIGURE 12–24. *A,* Voltage criteria for left ventricular hypertrophy (LVH) (leads I, V_5, and V_6) and QRS widening are present. Repolarization abnormalities are apparent in leads I, aVL, V_5, and V_6. *B,* Voltage criteria for LVH are present in lead II, along with left atrial abnormality, but repolarization abnormalities are absent.

uncommon in young, thin healthy patients, thus making the ECG diagnosis of LVH especially problematic in this population.

Prognostic Significance. Patients with ECG criteria of LVH have a higher risk for cardiovascular events and mortality. When both voltage and repolarization abnormalities are present (LVH-repol) (see Fig. 12–24*A*), the risk is quite high. Isolated voltage criteria for LVH (LVH-voltage) (see Fig. 12–24*B*) may not carry an increased risk beyond that of the (usual) accompanying hypertension.

Evaluation. Echocardiography is reasonable if LVH is present by ECG because echocardiographic confirmation of LVH may modify the therapeutic plan. Some studies have shown regression of LVH with aggressive antihypertensive treatment, particularly with angiotensin-converting enzyme inhibitors. Evaluation for underlying coronary artery disease is reasonable in patients with accompanying ST or T-wave abnormalities if LVH is confirmed echocardiographically. Patients with unexpected, striking LVH, unusual patterns of LVH, or LVH in the absence of hypertension should be screened echocardiographically for the presence of aortic stenosis (see Chapter 32), hypertrophic cardiomyopathy, and dilated cardiomyopathy (see Chapter 29). Prominent ECG voltage may also be seen in patients with WPW syndrome because of the anomalous ventricular preactivation.

Follow-up. The underlying condition determines the need for follow-up.

BOX 12–13

Romhilt-Estes Criteria for Left Ventricular Hypertrophy

R-wave or S-wave in any limb lead ≥2.0 mV* *or*		3 points
S-wave in V_1 or V_2 *or*		
R-wave in V_5 or V_6 ≥3.0 mV*		
Left ventricular strain pattern		
Digitalis absent		3 points
Digitalis present		1 point
Left atrial abnormality		3 points
Left axis deviation (axis ≥ −30 degrees)		2 points
QRS duration >0.09 msec†		1 point
Intrinsicoid deflection in V_5 or V_6 ≥50 msec†		1 point
Total points: ≥5	LVH	
4	Probable LVH	

*At the usual standardization (10 mm/mV), two "big" boxes (10 mm) = 10 mV.
†At the usual paper speed (25 mm/sec), one small box = 40 msec; one "big" box = 200 msec.
LVH, left ventricular hypertrophy.
Adapted from Chou T-C: Electrocardiography in Clinical Practice, 4th ed. Philadelphia, WB Saunders, 1996.

Right Ventricular Hypertrophy (Fig. 12–25)

Definition. Right ventricular hypertrophy (RVH) is extremely difficult to diagnose by ECG. It can both be confused with and coexist with RBBB. Clues to RVH include right axis deviation and an R-wave greater in amplitude than the S-wave in lead V_1.

Prevalence. RVH is rare.

Prognostic Significance. Because RVH generally reflects substantial structural cardiopulmonary disease, the risk of cardiovascular morbidity and mortality is high.

Evaluation. Patients with suspected RVH should undergo evaluation for cardiopulmonary disease; an

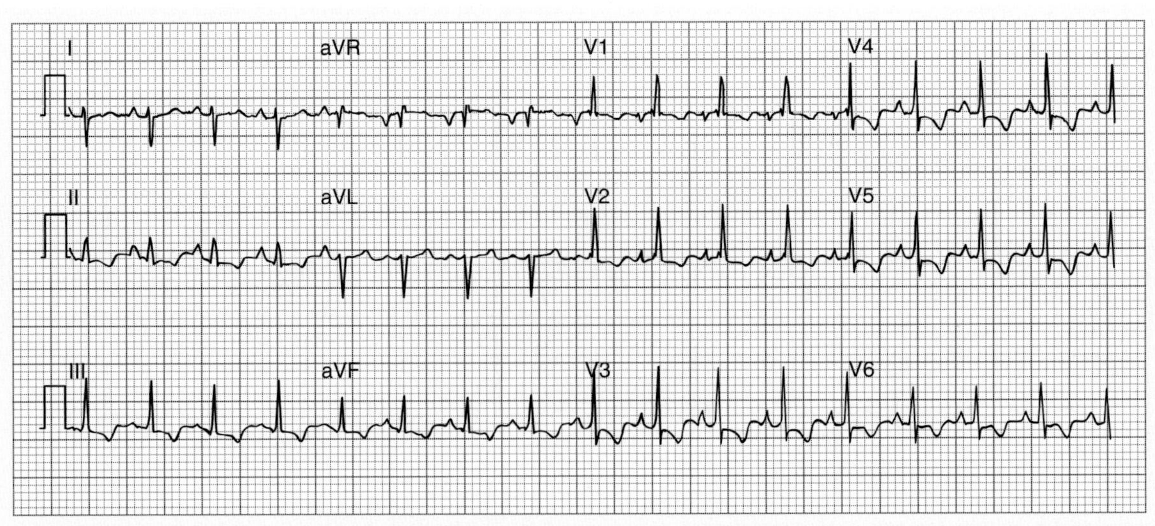

FIGURE 12–25. Right ventricular hypertrophy in a young woman with primary pulmonary hypertension. Note the right axis deviation, right atrial abnormality (prominent initial component of the P-wave, seen best in leads II and V_2), and R greater than S in lead V_1.

echocardiogram is generally the first step. Potential causes of RVH include congenital heart diseases (e.g., tetralogy of Fallot, the Eisenmenger complex, atrial septal defect, pulmonic stenosis; see Chapter 34), primary pulmonary hypertension, cor pulmonale, chronic obstructive pulmonary disease, and pulmonary embolism (see Chapter 38).

Follow-up. Follow-up depends on the underlying structural heart disease.

Low QRS Voltage (Fig. 12–26)

Definition. Definitions of low QRS voltage vary. One common definition is a QRS amplitude less than 0.7 mV (7 small boxes) in all limb leads or less than 1.0 mV (10 small boxes, 2 large boxes) in all precordial leads.

Prevalence. Low QRS voltage is relatively common and is also seen with pericardial effusions (see Chapter 35) or infiltrative cardiomyopathies (see Chapter 29).

Prognostic Significance. The prognostic significance of low QRS voltage depends on the underlying cause (Box 12–14).

Evaluation. Patients should be screened for potential underlying causes of low QRS voltage with an echocardiogram, thyroid testing, and other tests.

Follow-up. Follow-up depends on the underlying cause.

ST Segment and T-Wave Abnormalities (Figs. 12–27 and 12–28)

Definition. Abnormalities of the ST segment include ST depression and ST elevation (see Fig. 12–27*A* to *C*). Abnormalities of T-waves include T-wave inversion, biphasic T-waves, and T-wave flattening (see Fig. 12–28*A* to *C*). Abnormalities of the ST segment and T-wave have a broad differential diagnosis (Box 12–15); for this reason, the term "nonspecific" is frequently used.

Prevalence. Population studies have suggested that the prevalences of T-wave inversion and ST segment depression are approximately 4% and 1% to 2%, respectively, in apparently healthy patients.[15] The prevalence of less specific ECG abnormalities (e.g., T-wave flattening) is uncertain. T-wave inversion in two or more right precordial leads, frequently called a persistent juvenile T-wave pattern (see Fig. 12–28*B*), is not uncommon in healthy young females.

Prognostic Significance. Population studies have suggested that the relative mortality risk conferred by T-wave inversion or ST segment depression in apparently healthy persons is approximately 2; the absolute risk remains quite low, however. The prognostic importance of T-wave flattening is unknown, but it is probably of lower prognostic significance than frank inversion is.

Evaluation. In patients for whom no other explanation for ST depression or T-wave inversion is evident, evaluation for coronary ischemia is reasonable. In the

BOX 12–14

Causes of Low QRS Voltage

Pericardial effusion
Myocardial infarction
Cardiomyopathy
Hypothyroidism
Obesity
Sarcoidosis
Amyloidosis
Chronic obstructive pulmonary disease
Anasarca

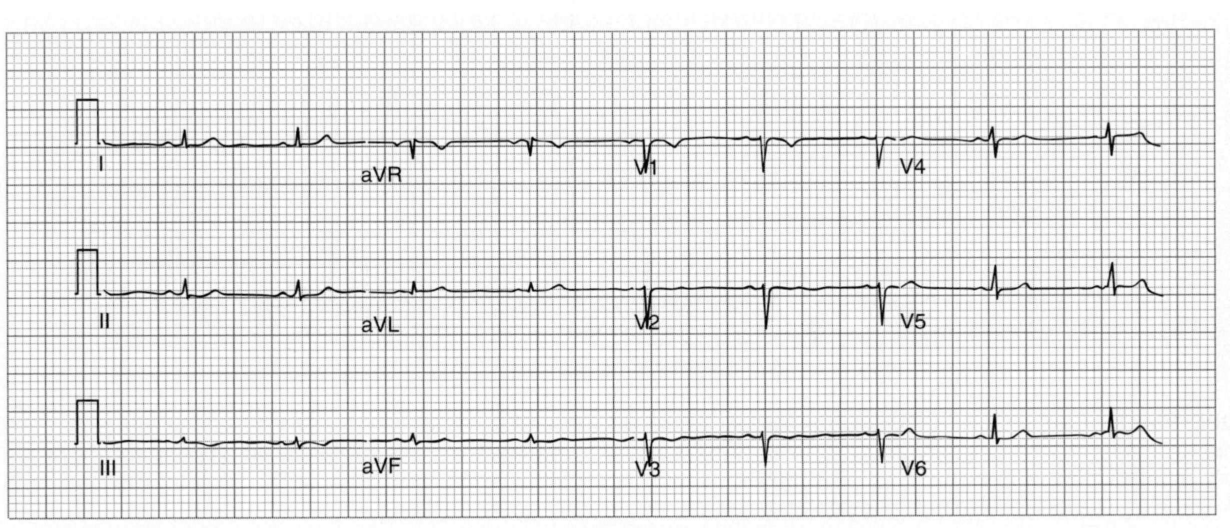

FIGURE 12–26. Low QRS voltage is present in both the precordial and limb leads in this 46-year-old healthy woman. An echocardiogram was normal. No cause was determined for the low QRS voltage.

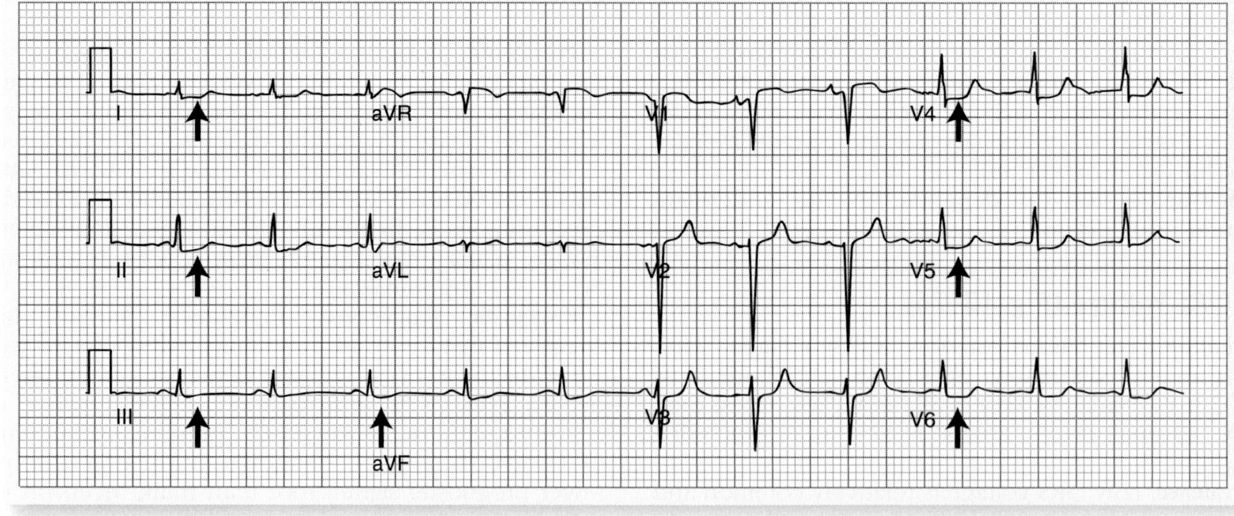

A

B

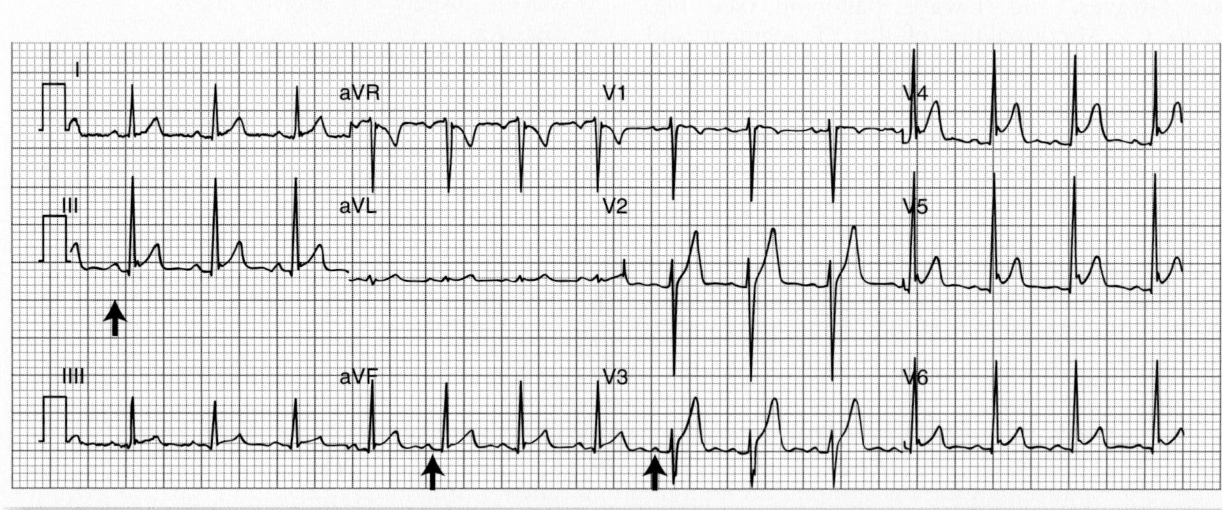

C

FIGURE 12–27. *A,* ST segment depression is evident in the inferolateral (I, II, III, aVF, V_4 to V_6) leads in this patient with chronic hypertension and coronary artery disease. *B,* ST segment elevation is present in this healthy young man as a result of early repolarization, a normal variant. This finding is most apparent at lower heart rates. *C,* ST segment elevation as well as PR segment depression (*arrows*) is apparent in this patient with acute pericarditis.

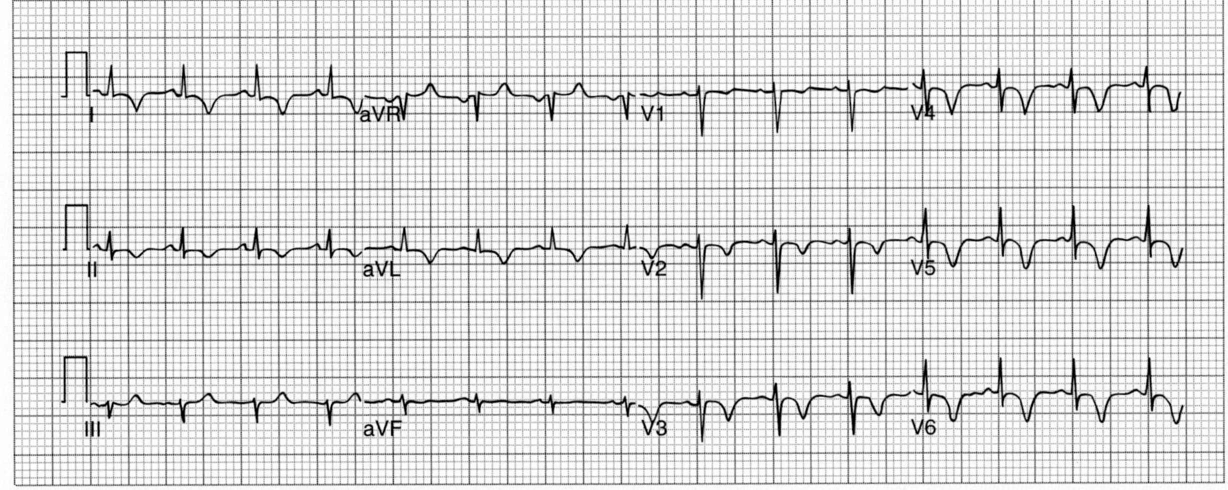

A

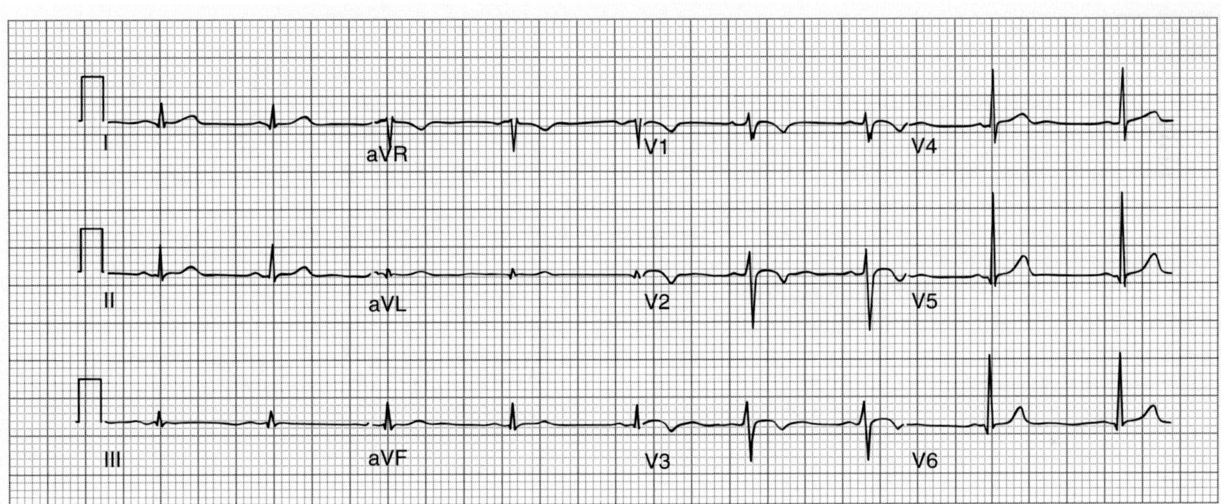

B

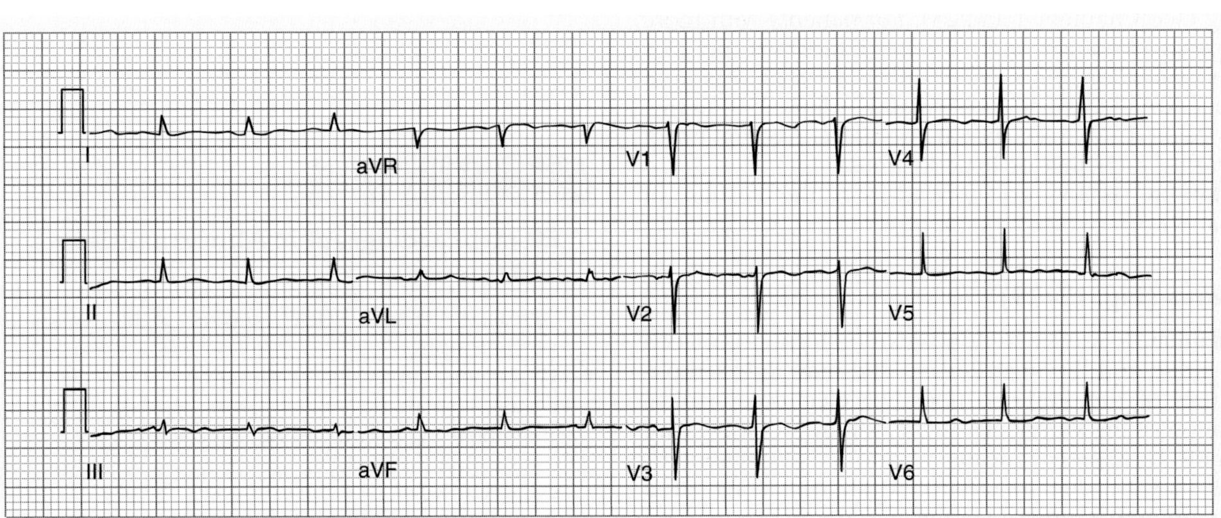

C

FIGURE 12–28. *A,* Diffuse T-wave inversion in the anterolateral leads of a patient with coronary artery disease. *B,* T-wave inversion in leads V_1 to V_3 in a healthy 20-year-old woman with a persistent juvenile T-wave pattern. *C,* Diffuse flattening of the T-waves in a patient with hypertension, diabetes, and coronary artery disease. *Continued*

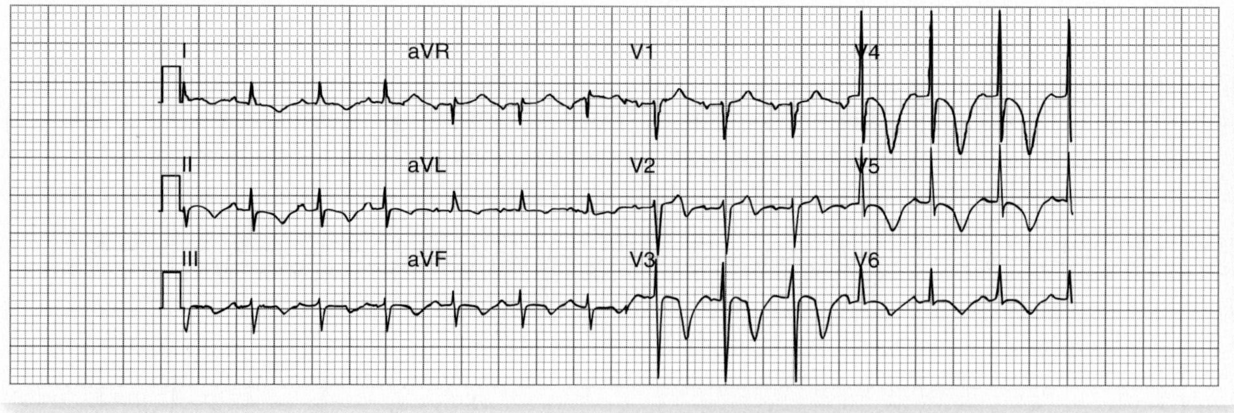

FIGURE 12–28. (*Continued*) *D*, "Neurologic T-waves" in a patient with intracerebral hemorrhage. Note the deep, symmetrically inverted T-waves and prolonged QTc.

BOX 12–15

Causes of ST Segment and T-Wave Abnormalities

Myocardial ischemia/injury
Pericarditis
Electrolyte abnormalities
Left ventricular hypertrophy
Intraventricular conduction delay/bundle branch block
Drug effects (digitalis, antiarrhythmic drugs, etc.)
Long QT syndrome
Stroke/neurologic catastrophe

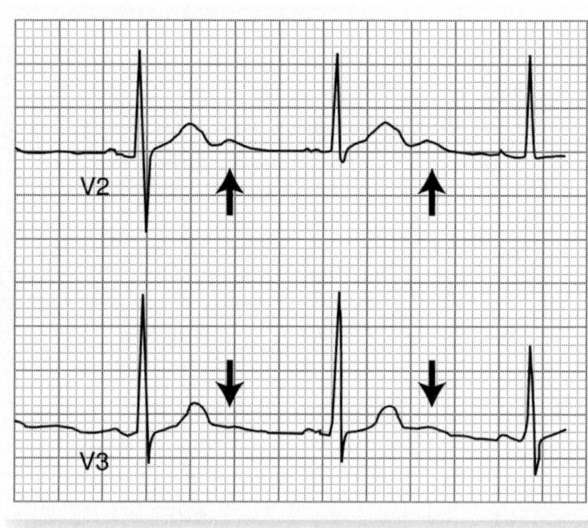

FIGURE 12–29. Prominent U-waves are evident (*arrows*) in leads V_2 and V_3 in this healthy young patient.

absence of acute symptoms or ST segment elevation, this evaluation can be done nonurgently with stress testing (see Chapters 4 and 25). For patients with more nonspecific findings (e.g., T-wave flattening), no particular evaluation is necessary unless one has reason to suspect an electrolyte abnormality (diuretic therapy, etc.). Peaked T-waves should prompt consideration of myocardial ischemia or hyperkalemia.

Follow-up. Follow-up depends on the results of evaluation.

U-Waves (Fig. 12–29)

Definition. U-waves are a positive deflection between the T-wave and the next P-wave and may reflect repolarization of the Purkinje fibers or electromechanical relaxation of the ventricular myocardium.[16] U-waves are generally best seen in leads V_2 and V_3. Prominent U-waves may be due to electrolyte abnormalities, drug effects, ischemia, and LQTS.

Prevalence. U-waves are relatively common.

Prognostic Significance. Prognostic implications depend on the underlying cause.

Evaluation. Screen for electrolyte abnormalities if clinically indicated; screen for LQTS.

BOX 12–16

Electrocardiographic Abnormalities in Athletes

Increased voltage (left and/or right ventricular hypertrophy)
ST segment depression or elevation
T-wave inversion
Incomplete right bundle branch block
Sinus arrhythmia
Sinus bradycardia
Junctional bradycardia
First-degree AV block
Second-degree AV block, Mobitz I

AV, atrioventricular.

Follow-up. No follow-up is necessary in the absence of an identifiable cause.

Athlete's Heart and Hypertrophic Cardiomyopathy (Fig. 12–30)

Definition. A variety of ECG abnormalities have been reported in apparently healthy, highly trained athletes[17] (Box 12–16), including signs of LVH and RVH, as well as marked ST segment and T-wave abnormalities. ST depression, T-wave inversion, and ST elevation (as a result of early repolarization) have been described. The primary differential diagnosis is with hypertrophic cardiomyopathy (see Chapter 29). Sinus arrhythmia, sinus bradycardia, junctional bradycardia, first-degree AV block, and Mobitz I second-degree AV block are common as a result of hypervagotonia.

Prevalence. ECG abnormalities are common, particularly in endurance athletes; hypertrophic cardiomyopathy is uncommon.

Prognostic Significance. The presence or absence of structural heart disease determines the prognostic significance.

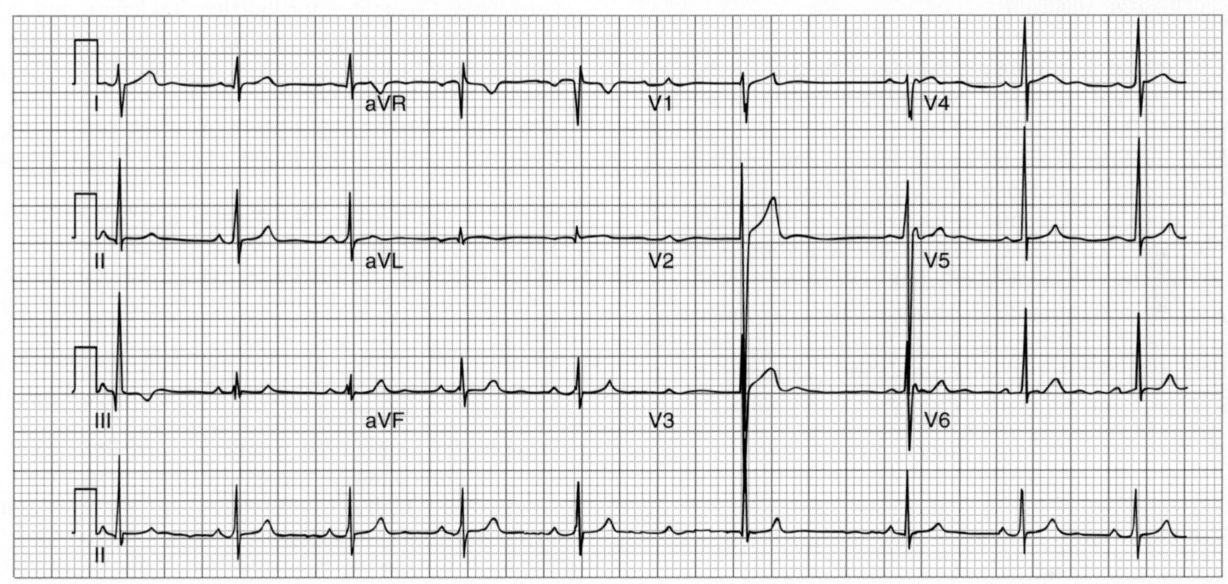

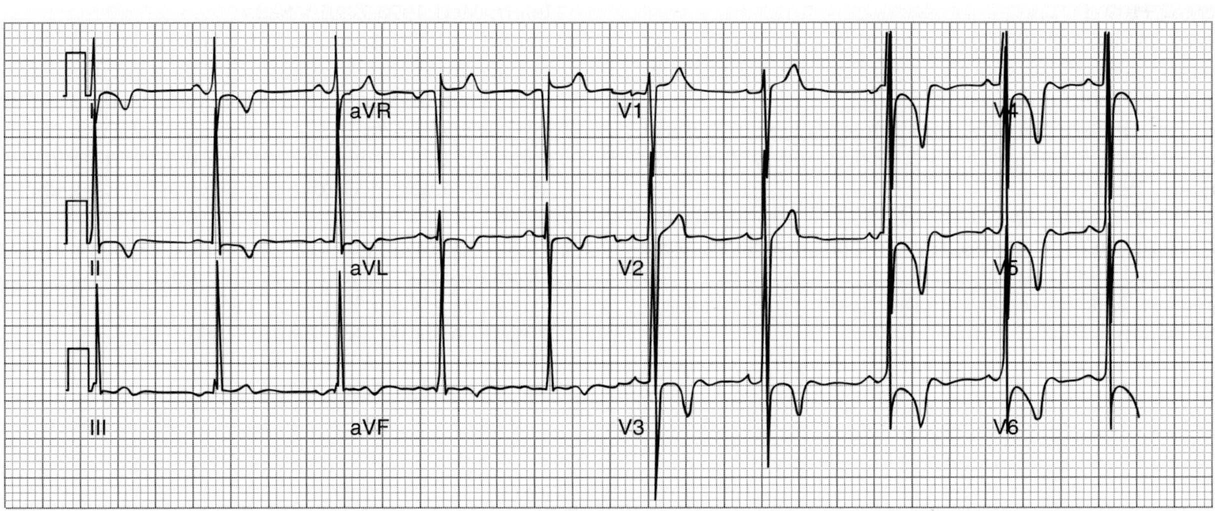

FIGURE 12–30. *A,* Electrocardiogram (ECG) recorded in an asymptomatic 18-year-old basketball player. Although the QRS voltage is consistent with left ventricular hypertrophy (S-wave in V_2 >3 mV), an echocardiogram suggested only mild, physiologic hypertrophy. In the rhythm strip, note the blocked P-wave and junctional escape beat (sixth QRS complex from the left), indicative of high vagal tone. The patient had no symptoms suggestive of bradycardia. *B,* ECG recorded in a 19-year-old athlete. Note the striking QRS voltage, as well as the marked ST segment and T-wave abnormalities. Evaluation led to a diagnosis of hypertrophic cardiomyopathy.

Evaluation. Differentiation between a physiologic hypertrophy induced by athletic training (i.e., "athlete's heart") and hypertrophic cardiomyopathy can be extremely difficult, even with echocardiography and other imaging studies. Referral to a cardiologist is recommended. Asymptomatic bradycardia does not require evaluation, although vagally mediated (i.e., bradycardia induced) AF can occur.

Follow-up. Follow-up depends on the presence or absence of hypertrophic cardiomyopathy or other structural heart disease.

Evidence-Based Summary

- Unfortunately, few data exist regarding the optimal management strategy in patients with "unexpected" ECG abnormalities.
- ECG findings must be considered in the context of potential symptoms (e.g., palpitations, fatigue, syncope) and accompanying conditions (e.g., LVH secondary to hypertension or aortic stenosis), as well as the risk of mortality (e.g., LQTS, Q-waves).
- Among common ECG abnormalities, guidelines are best established for atrial fibrillation, particularly with respect to anticoagulation (see Chapter 30).

References

1. Kannel WB: Contributions of the Framingham study to the conquest of coronary artery disease. Am J Cardiol 1988;62:1109–1112.
2. Ashley EA, Raxwal VK, Froelicher VF: The prevalence and prognostic significance of electrocardiographic abnormalities. Curr Probl Cardiol 2000:25:1–72.
3. U.S. Preventative Services Task Force: Guide to Clinical Preventative Services, 2nd ed. Baltimore, Williams & Wilkins, 1996.
4. Sox HC Jr, Garber AM, Littenberg B: The resting electrocardiogram as a screening test. A clinical analysis. Ann Intern Med 1989;111:489–502.
5. Canadian Task Force on Periodic Health Care: Available at www.ctfphc.org.
6. Schlant RC, Adolph RJ, DiMarco JP, et al: Guidelines for electrocardiography. A report of the American College of Cardiology/American Heart Association Task Force on Assessment of Diagnostic and Therapeutic Cardiovascular Procedures (Committee on Electrocardiography). J Am Coll Cardiol 1992;19:473–481.
7. Jouven X, Zureik M, Desnos M, et al: Long-term outcome in asymptomatic men with exercise-induced premature ventricular depolarizations. N Engl J Med 2000;343:826–833.
8. Fuster V, Ryden LE, Asinger RW, et al: ACC/AHA/ESC guidelines for the management of patients with atrial fibrillation: Executive summary: A report of the American College of Cardiology/American Heart Association Task Force on Practice Guidelines and the European Society of Cardiology Committee for Practice Guidelines and Policy Conferences (Committee to Develop Guidelines for the Management of Patients with Atrial Fibrillation). J Am Coll Cardiol 2001;38:1231–1265.
9. Albers GW, Dalen JE, Laupacis A, et al: Antithrombotic therapy in atrial fibrillation. Chest 2001;119(Suppl): 194–206.
10. Hiss RG, Lamb LE: Electrocardiographic findings in 122,043 individuals. Circulation 1962;25:947–961.
11. Fahy GJ, Pinski SL, Miller DP, et al: Natural history of isolated bundle branch block. Am J Cardiol 1996;77:1185–1190.
12. Schwartz PJ, Moss AJ, Vincent GM, Crampton RS: Diagnostic criteria for the long QT syndrome: An update. Circulation 1993;88:782–784.
13. Margolis JR, Kannel WB, Feinleib M, et al: Clinical features of unrecognized myocardial infarction—silent and symptomatic: Eighteen year follow-up: The Framingham study. Am J Cardiol 1973;32:1–7.
14. Kannel WB, Gordon T, Castelli WP, Margolis JR: Electrocardiographic left ventricular hypertrophy and risk of coronary artery disease: The Framingham study. Ann Intern Med 1970;72:813–822.
15. Kannel WB, Anderson K, McGee DL, et al: Nonspecific electrocardiographic abnormality as a predictor of coronary heart disease: The Framingham Study. Am Heart J 1987;113:370–376.
16. Surawicz B: U wave: Facts, hypotheses, misconceptions, and misnomers. J Cardiovasc Electrophysiol 1998;9:1117–1128.
17. Foote CB, Michaud GF: The athlete's electrocardiogram: Distinguishing normal from abnormal. In Estes NAM III, Salem DN, Wang PJ (eds): Sudden Cardiac Death in the Athlete. Armonk, NY, Futura, 1998.

CHAPTER 13 Approach to the Patient with Cardiac Enlargement

Patrick T. O'Gara

At autopsy, the weight of the heart ranges from 280 to 340 g in adult men and from 230 to 280 g in adult women. The heart increases in size and weight with age, a process that is more pronounced in men. In clinical practice, the first clue to the presence of cardiomegaly is usually provided by the radiologic examination, but it may also be suggested by findings on physical examination. When the adult heart is viewed in the posteroanterior (PA) projection, it generally measures 12 cm from base to apex, 8 to 9 cm in the transverse direction, and on lateral films, 6 cm in the anteroposterior (AP) direction. In some patients, cardiac enlargement may be the first sign of previously undiagnosed cardiac disease, so this finding should prompt a careful search for the cause of the enlargement based on an integrated assessment of the key features of the history, physical examination, and other findings on laboratory examination.

Physical Examination

Observation of the chest wall, palpation of the cardiac impulse, and percussion of the lateral border of cardiac dullness provide a first approximation of heart size, position, and shape[1] (see also Chapter 3). The left ventricular apex beat should not fall outside the midclavicular line or more than 10 cm to the left of the midsternal line and should occupy an area not more than 3 cm in diameter or lower than the fifth intercostal space. Any further leftward or downward displacement or enlargement of the apical impulse usually signifies an increase in heart size. Although the characteristics of the apex beat are best appreciated by palpation with the patient in the left lateral decubitus position, the location of the apex should always be ascertained with the patient supine and the trunk elevated to approximately 30 degrees.

The location and character of the apex beat are also dependent on the size, configuration, and thickness of the thoracic cage, which must be taken into account when estimating cardiomegaly. Tall, asthenic individuals with a thin chest wall tend to have a vertically oriented heart, the lateral border of which may extend only a few centimeters from the midline. However, the apical impulse is well transmitted through the chest wall and may appear unusually prominent. The opposite occurs in short, muscular, or obese persons. Patients with chronic obstructive lung disease and a barrel chest deformity with a flattened diaphragm tend to have displacement of the cardiac impulse—in this case, the right ventricle—into the subxiphoid area. In such patients, left-sided cardiac enlargement can be very difficult to appreciate, but when the signs of left ventricular enlargement are apparent on physical examination, the true enlargement is usually quite severe. Conversely, in patients with pectus excavatum or a straight back deformity with loss of the normal dorsal spine kyphosis and a reduced AP chest diameter, the left ventricular apex beat can be displaced laterally in the absence of true cardiac enlargement. The presence of these two deformities can be confirmed on clinical examination.

Chest Radiography

Enlargement of the heart may first be detected as an incidental finding on a chest radiograph that is obtained for the evaluation of other processes.[2] Cardiomegaly on chest radiography is commonly defined by a cardiothoracic ratio of 0.50 as measured on the PA film. The widest transverse dimension of the cardiac silhouette is compared with the maximal width of the thoracic cage (Fig. 13–1). Assessment of relative cardiac size is less accurate on films obtained in the AP projection because of magnification artifact. Alterations in lung volume also detract from the reliability of this estimate. The cardiothoracic ratio is falsely elevated when lung volumes are low, as during exhalation, and may be misleadingly small with hyperinflation, as occurs in emphysema. Both pectus excavatum and straight back syndrome can exaggerate the size of the cardiac silhouette and increase the cardiothoracic ratio on the PA projection (Fig. 13–2). Relative cardiac volume can be estimated by measuring the long axis (L) and short axis (S) on the frontal view and the AP diameter (D) on the lateral view (Fig. 13–3). The calculation is made as follows:

$$\text{Relative cardiac volume (mL/m}^2\text{ BSA)} = L \times S \times D \times K$$

L, S, K, and *D* are expressed in centimeters; the constant *K,* the enlargement factor, is related to the distance between the x-ray tube and the film and is 0.42 for the usual 6-ft film; and BSA is body surface area. Values exceeding 490 mL/m² in women and 540 mL/m² in men denote definite cardiac enlargement. Other imaging methods (echocardiography, computed tomography [CT], magnetic resonance imaging [MRI]) that are more accurate than the plain chest radiograph are avail-

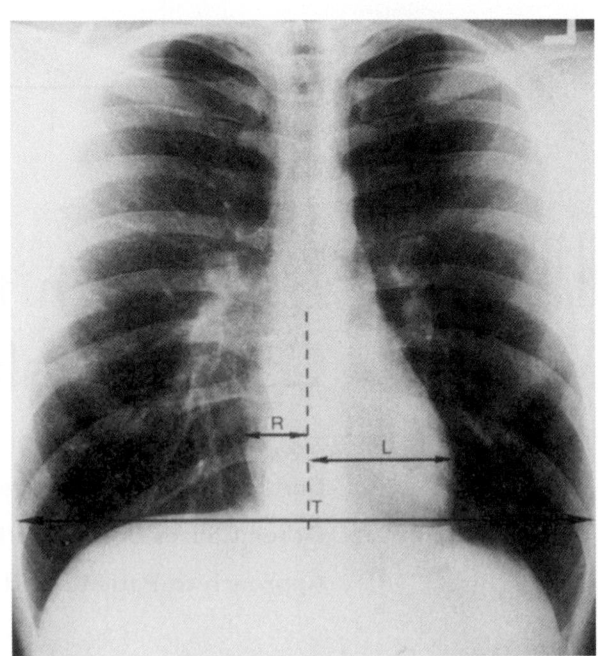

FIGURE 13–1. Measurement of heart size. Transverse cardiac diameter = R + L. Cardiothoracic ratio = (R + L)/T. (From Rubens MB: Chest x-ray in adult heart disease. In Julian DG, Camm AJ, Fox KM, et al [eds]: Diseases of the Heart, 2nd ed. London, WB Saunders, 1996, p 258.)

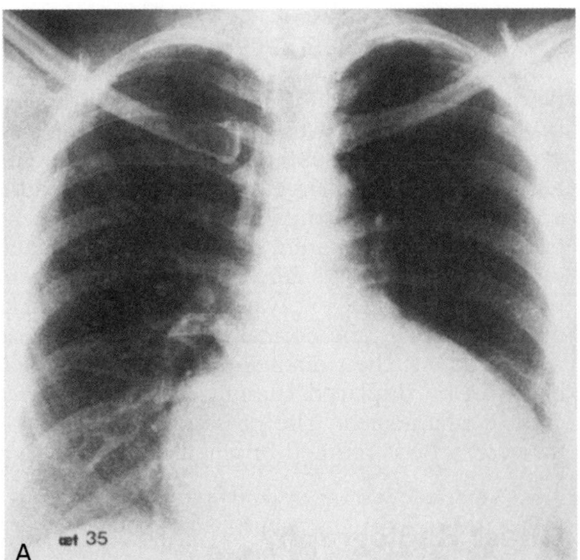

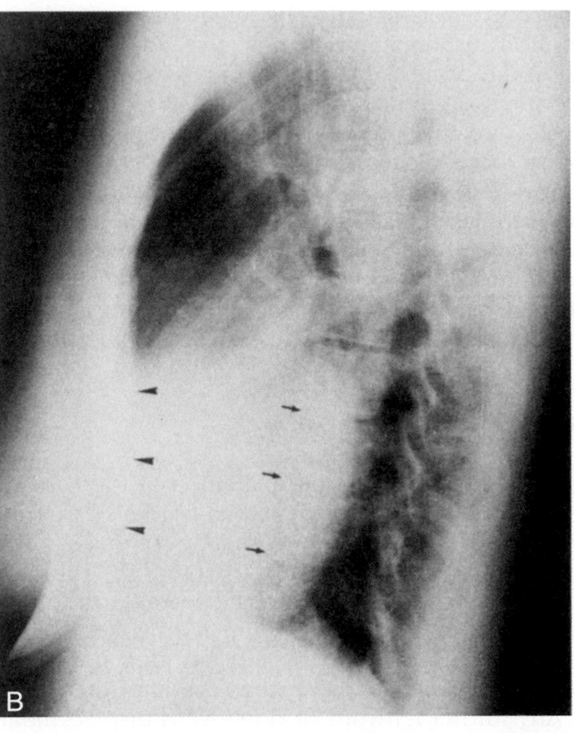

FIGURE 13–2. Straight back syndrome. *A,* On the frontal film, the heart appears markedly enlarged. *B,* The lateral film shows that the dorsal spine is straightened, the thoracic anteroposterior diameter is decreased, and the heart is compressed between the sternum (*arrowheads*) and spine (*arrows*). (From Rubens MB: Chest x-ray in adult heart disease. In Julian DG, Camm AJ, Fox KM, et al [eds]: Diseases of the Heart, 2nd ed. London, WB Saunders, 1996, p 260.)

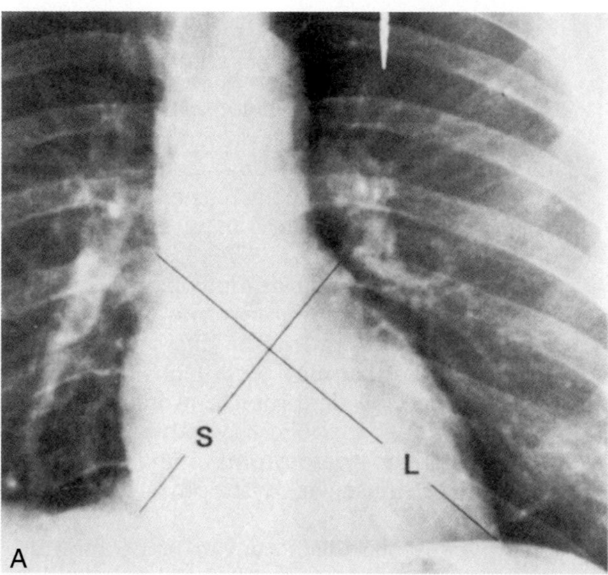

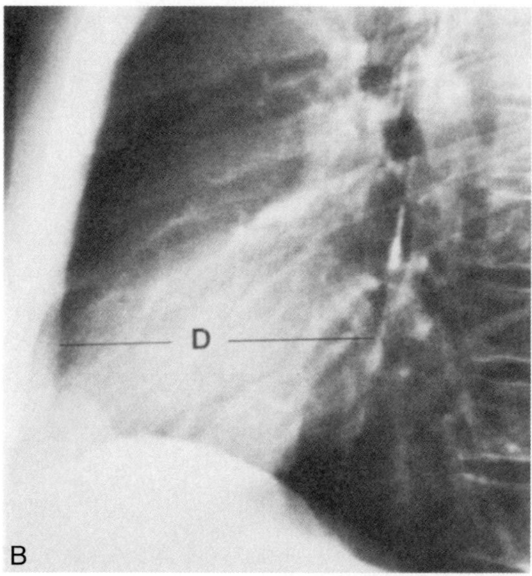

FIGURE 13–3. Measurement of relative cardiac volume. *A,* Frontal projection. The long axis of the heart (L) is measured from the break in the right cardiac contour, where the superior vena cava joins the right atrium, to the apex of the heart. The short diameter (S) extends from the right cardiophrenic angle to the junction of the left atrial and pulmonary artery segments. This line is roughly perpendicular to the long axis. *B,* Lateral view. The widest anteroposterior dimension of the cardiac silhouette constitutes the depth of the heart (D). If the posterior border of the heart cannot be clearly identified, the anterior margin of the barium-filled esophagus can be used as the boundary for this measurement. (From Baron MG: Radiological and angiographic examination of the heart. In Braunwald E [ed]: Heart Disease, 3rd ed. Philadelphia, WB Saunders, 1988, p 151.)

able for the measurement of cardiac size and for monitoring changes.

Differential Diagnosis

The list of disorders associated with cardiomegaly is long, but it can often be pared substantially by careful attention to the history and physical examination. In most patients, additional testing can be pursued thereafter in a focused, hierarchical, and cost-effective manner. A pathoanatomic approach to the differential diagnosis, based on the actual structures shown to be enlarged, is a useful starting point (Box 13–1).

CARDIAC CHAMBER ENLARGEMENT

The normal radiographic anatomy of the heart and the location of the four chambers and great vessel are shown in Figure 13–4.

Left Ventricle

On physical examination, dilatation of the left ventricle is evidenced by leftward and downward displacement of an enlarged apex beat. The PA radiograph also shows such displacement (Fig. 13–5*A*). The enlarged left ventricle may extend posterior to displace the esophagus posteriorly on the lateral view (Fig. 13–5*B*). Enlargement of the left ventricle is especially well seen on the left anterior oblique view (Fig. 13–6*A*).

Left ventricular dilatation occurs in response to the chronic volume overload that accompanies significant mitral or aortic regurgitation, conditions readily identified by their characteristic murmurs (see Chapters 11 and 32); their severity can be estimated by the presence of associated symptoms or additional findings on physical examination, such as a thrill, third heart sound, or pulmonary rales. Unusual causes of left ventricular volume overload in adults include a previously unrecognized patent ductus arteriosus, ventricular septal defect, and arteriovenous fistula, malformations that are usually recognizable by their auscultatory findings. Volume overload and left ventricular dilatation are also observed in high–cardiac output states, such as those associated with anemia and thyrotoxicosis, and in conditions that cause high stroke volume, such as chronic severe sinus bradycardia or complete heart block.

As it attempts to compensate for the reduction in cardiac output resulting from impairment in contractile performance in response to any injury or process, the left ventricle dilates. Ischemic damage (myocardial infarction) is the most common cause of contractile impairment. A previous history of myocardial infarction or the presence of pathologic Q-waves on the electrocardiogram (ECG) suggests an ischemic origin of the enlargement. An anterior or apical infarction, which is

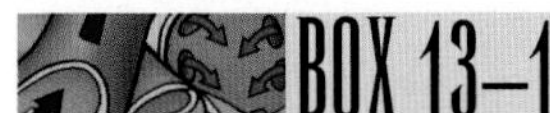

Cardiac Enlargement: Differential Diagnosis

Left ventricle
- Chronic volume overload
  - Mitral or aortic regurgitation
  - Left-to-right shunt (PDA, VSD, AV fistula)
- Cardiomyopathy
  - Ischemic
  - Nonischemic
- Decompensated pressure overload
  - Aortic stenosis
  - Hypertension
- High-output states
  - Severe anemia
  - Thyrotoxicosis
- Bradycardia
  - Severe sinus bradycardia
  - Complete heart block

Left atrium
- LV failure of any cause
- Mitral valve disease
- Myxoma

Right ventricle
- Chronic LV failure of any cause
- Chronic volume overload
  - Tricuspid or pulmonic regurgitation
  - Left-to-right shunt (ASD)
- Decompensated pressure overload
  - Pulmonic stenosis
  - Pulmonary artery hypertension
    - Primary
    - Secondary (PE, COPD)
  - Pulmonary veno-occlusive disease

Right atrium
- RV failure of any cause
- Tricuspid valve disease
- Myxoma
- Ebstein's anomaly

Multichamber enlargement
- Hypertrophic cardiomyopathy
- Acromegaly
- Severe obesity

Pericardial disease
- Pericardial effusion with or without tamponade
- Effusive constrictive disease
- Pericardial cyst, loculated effusion

Pseudocardiomegaly
- Epicardial fat
- Chest wall deformity (pectus excavatum, straight back syndrome)
- Low lung volumes
- AP chest radiograph
- Mediastinal tumor, cyst

AP, anteroposterior; ASD, atrial septal defect; AV, arteriovenous; COPD, chronic obstructive pulmonary disease; LV, left ventricular; PDA, patent ductus arteriosus; PE, pulmonary embolism; RV, right ventricular; VSD, ventricular septal defect.

associated with Q-waves in the precordial leads, may also render the left ventricular impulse dyskinetic on palpation. Occasionally in such patients, the chest radiograph reveals an angulated distortion of the left heart border suggestive of the presence of a left ventricular aneurysm (see Fig. 13–6*B*).

Dilated cardiomyopathy[3] (see Chapter 29) causes not only left ventricular but also generalized cardiac dilatation (Fig. 13–7*A*). Whereas most patients with nonischemic, dilated cardiomyopathy do not have an identifiable cause, the history and physical examination should focus on processes that are most commonly responsible or that may be potentially reversible. Clues to toxic (alcohol, doxorubicin [Adriamycin]), infectious (myocarditis), metabolic (hypothyroidism, hemochromatosis, pheochromocytoma), and genetic (familial, Duchenne's muscular dystrophy) origins should be sought.

Left ventricular dilatation can also complicate the late stages of pressure overload from long-standing, uncorrected, and severe aortic stenosis or systemic hypertension. In their earlier stages, these conditions lead to concentric left ventricular hypertrophy that may not be associated with obvious enlargement of the heart. Thus, although the cardiac impulse in pressure overload hypertrophy may be vigorous, enlarged, and sustained on physical examination, it is not usually displaced and the cardiac silhouette on chest radiographs may be normal despite the presence of ECG evidence of left ventricular hypertrophy. Over time, replacement fibrosis, wall thinning, and progressive systolic dysfunction develop and lead to cardiac dilatation, a low-output state, and clinical heart failure. Left ventricular enlargement may then become evident.

Left Atrium

Enlargement of the left atrium cannot usually be appreciated on physical examination. Rarely, the systolic expansion of the left atrium can be palpated as a mid- or late-systolic lift in patients with severe mitral regurgitation. Radiologic enlargement of the left atrium is suggested by several signs: (1) a prominent, convex upper portion of the left heart border (see Figs. 13–7*B* and 13–9*A*); (2) posterior displacement of the barium-filled esophagus on the lateral projection (Fig. 13–8); (3) a "double density" near the right heart border (representing the left atrial wall) (Fig. 13–9*A*); (4) posterior and superior displacement of the left main stem bronchus (Fig. 14–9*B*); and (5) splaying of the carina beyond 75 degrees.

The left atrium commonly enlarges in the presence of conditions that elevate left ventricular diastolic pressure. Such conditions include left ventricular pressure or volume overload (or both) and left ventricular systolic or diastolic dysfunction as progressively higher left atrial pressure is required to fill the failing ventricle. In chronic mitral regurgitation, in which the volume load is directed into the left atrium, this chamber can attain massive proportions. A thin-walled, capacious left

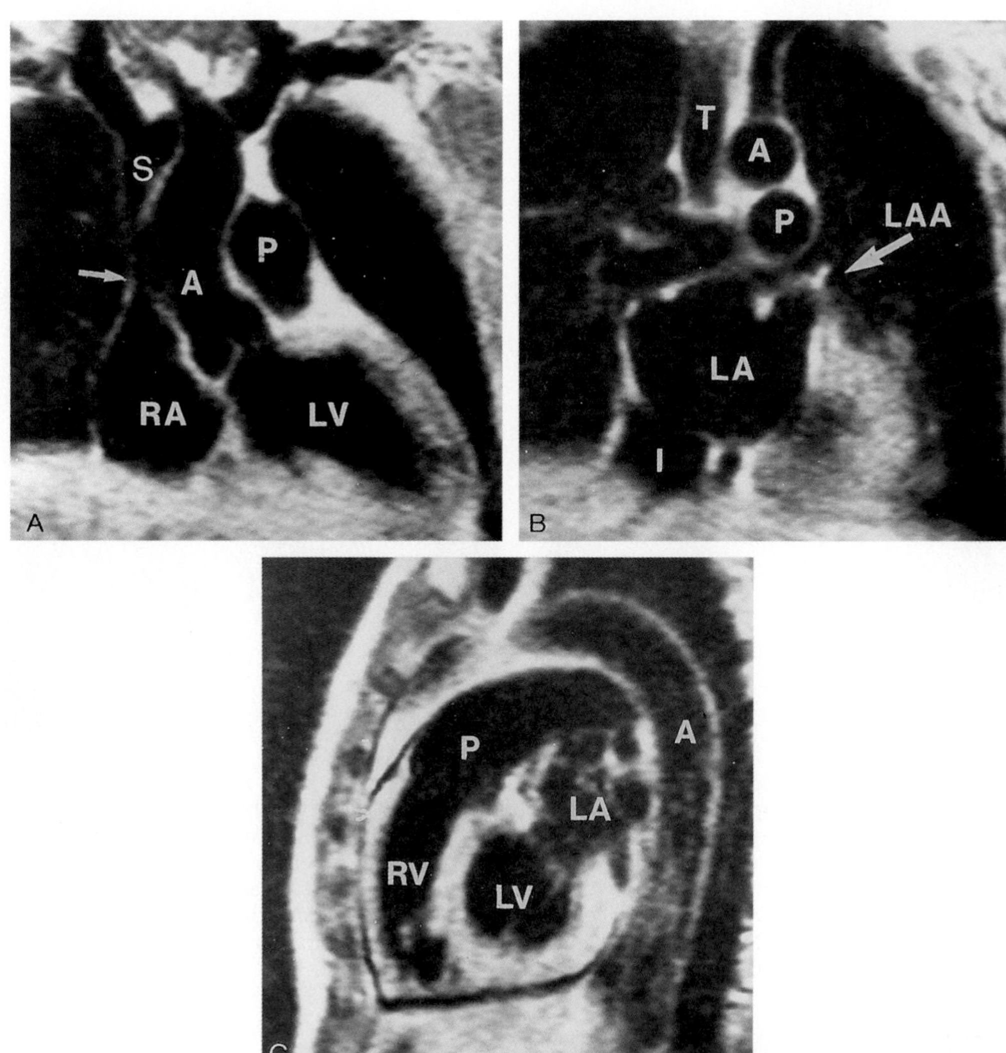

FIGURE 13–4. Normal radiographic anatomy depicted by magnetic resonance imaging. *A*, Coronal section at the level of the aortic valve. The right border of the cardiac silhouette is formed by the superior vena cava (S) and the right atrium (RA). The *arrow* indicates the cavo-atrial junction. The lower portion of the left cardiac border is formed by the left ventricle (LV). A, ascending aorta; P, main pulmonary artery. *B*, Coronal section at the level of the left atrium (LA). The upper portion of the left cardiac border is formed by the ascending aorta, main pulmonary artery, and left atrial appendage (LAA, *arrow*). I, inferior vena cava; T, trachea. *C*, Sagittal section near the midline. The right ventricle (RV) forms the anterior surface of the heart, abutting the sternum. The main pulmonary artery extends upward and posteriorly from the ventricle. The posterior border of the heart is formed by the left atrium and left ventricle. (From Baron MG: Radiology of the heart. In Bennett JC, Plum F [eds]: Cecil Textbook of Medicine, 20th ed. Philadelphia, WB Saunders, 1996, p 181.)

atrium can accommodate a large volume load without much increase in pressure.

The left atrium can enlarge independently of the left ventricle in the presence of obstruction to mitral inflow, as in mitral stenosis (see Fig. 13–7*B*) or, less commonly, left atrial myxoma. The former can usually be identified by the characteristic auscultatory findings, but rarely, it is “silent” and identifiable only by echocardiography. In general, the left atrium enlarges to a greater extent with significant mitral regurgitation than with mitral stenosis (see Fig. 13–9). Radiographic or echocardiographic calcification in the wall of an enlarged left atrium signifies a chronic process usually associated with organized mural/endocardial thrombi.

Right Ventricle

Enlargement of the right ventricle on physical examination is suggested by a prominent parasternal impulse that is medial to the left ventricular apex beat. Sometimes, the right ventricle enlarges so much that it occupies the entire precordial area and the left ventricle cannot be palpated because it has been displaced posteriorly. Under this circumstance, tricuspid murmurs may be incorrectly identified as mitral in origin unless care is taken to examine the neck veins and identify the changes characteristic of tricuspid valve disease (see Chapters 3 and 32) and to listen

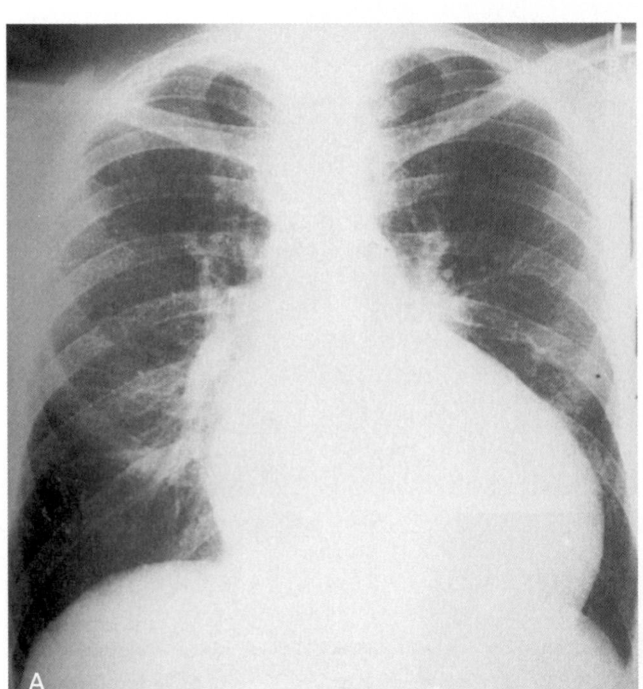

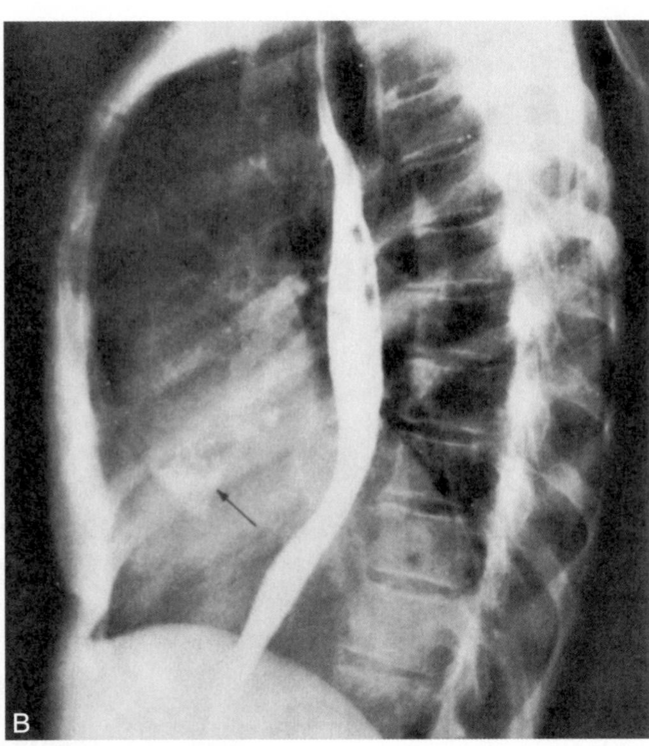

FIGURE 13–5. *A*, Gross left ventricular enlargement in congestive cardiomyopathy. A frontal film shows a convex left heart border with a downwardly displaced apex. Note the redistribution of blood flow and bilateral basal interstitial lines. *B*, Lateral view of dilatation of the left ventricle in aortic valve disease. The left ventricle is markedly enlarged and extends posterior to the esophagus. The aortic valve is densely calcified (*arrow*). The indentation on the anterior midesophageal wall is caused by the moderately dilated left atrium. No evidence of mitral valve disease was evident. (*A*, From Rubens MB: Chest x-ray in adult heart disease. In Julian DG, Camm AJ, Fox KM, et al [eds]: Diseases of the Heart, 2nd ed. London, WB Saunders, 1996, p 275. *B*, From Baron MG: Radiological and angiographic examination of the heart. In Braunwald E [ed]: Heart Disease, 3rd ed. Philadelphia, WB Saunders, 1988, p 145.)

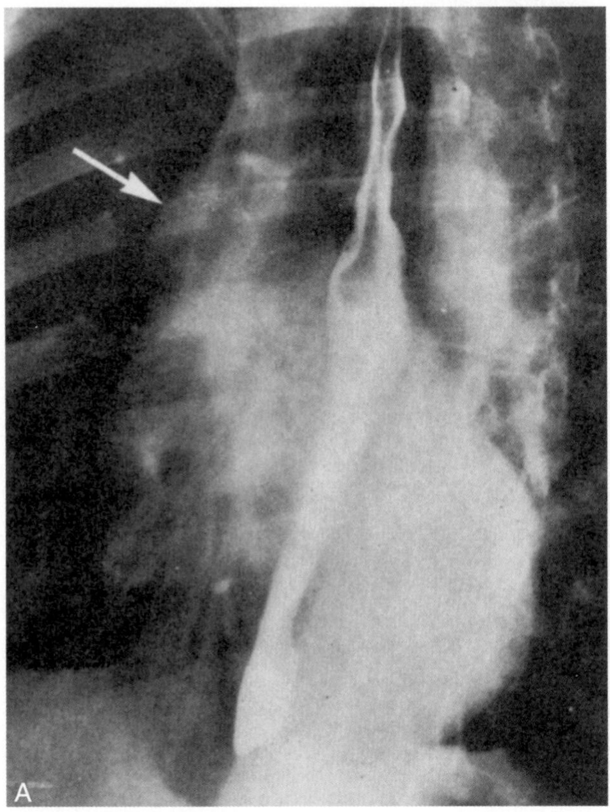

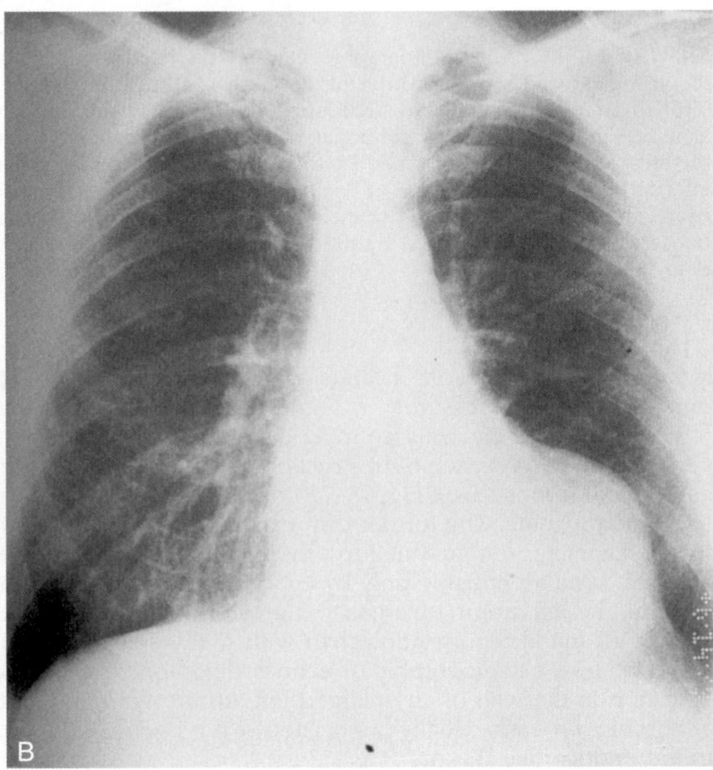

for changes in the murmurs with inspiration. In patients with barrel chest deformity, an enlarged right ventricle may be directed inferiorly and the impulse will best be appreciated in the subxiphoid area. Other signs of right heart failure may also be present, such as ascites or edema.

Right ventricular enlargement can be difficult to detect on chest radiographs. An increase in the transverse dimension of the cardiac silhouette on the PA film, along with concave upward displacement of the lower left heart border (Fig. 13–10), may also signify right ventricular enlargement but is much less specific. The lateral view is especially helpful because the enlarged right ventricle encroaches on the upper retrosternal space (Fig. 13–11*A*).

The most common cause of right ventricular enlargement is left ventricular failure or mitral stenosis with chronic elevation of pulmonary venous and arterial pressure leading to right ventricular systolic dysfunction. In patients with left-sided cardiac abnormalities of sufficient severity to cause right ventricular enlargement, clinical and radiographic signs of pulmonary congestion are usually evident. When such signs are absent, primary lesions in the pulmonary parenchyma and pulmonary vascular bed should be sought (e.g., primary pulmonary hypertension).

The right ventricle can also enlarge as a result of the chronic volume overload associated with an atrial septal defect (see Chapter 34) or from tricuspid or pulmonic valve regurgitation. Tricuspid regurgitation is most

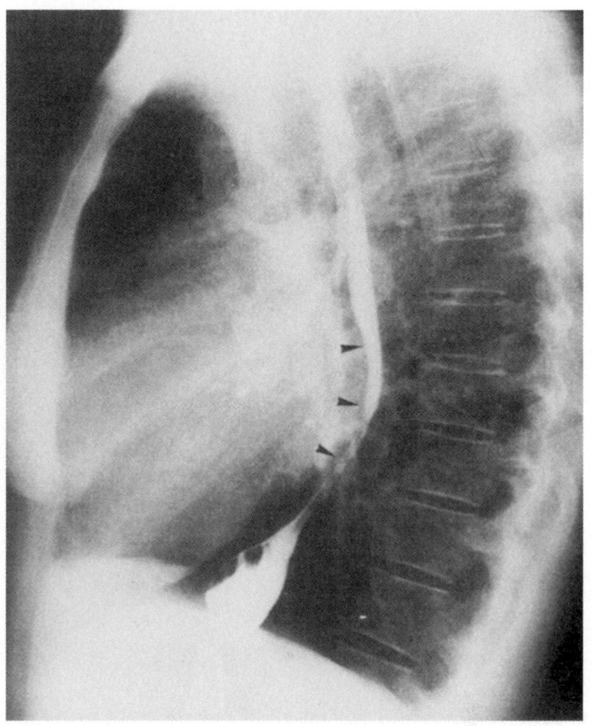

FIGURE 13–8. Left atrial enlargement with mitral stenosis. The body of the left atrium is displacing the barium-filled esophagus posteriorly (*arrowheads*). (From Rubens MB: Chest x-ray in adult heart disease. In Julian DG, Camm AJ, Fox KM, et al [eds]: Diseases of the Heart, 2nd ed. London, WB Saunders, 1996, p 272.)

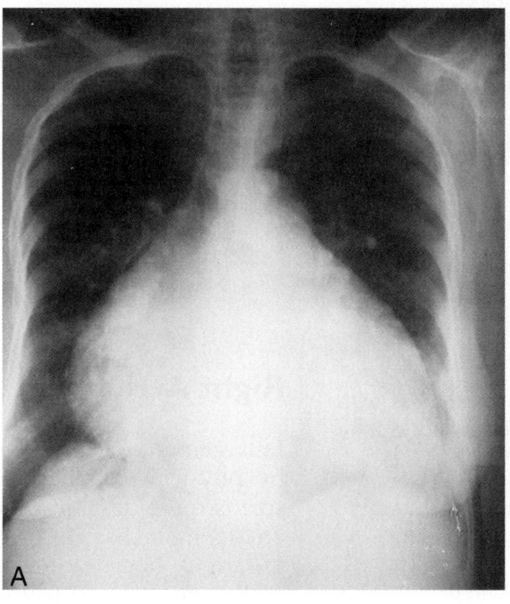

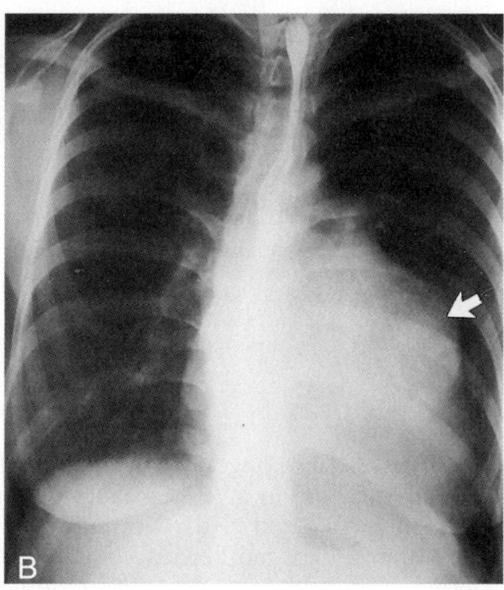

FIGURE 13–7. *A*, Dilated cardiomyopathy. Diffuse dilatation of the heart is present in this woman with systemic lupus erythematosus. *B*, Mitral stenosis. The left atrial border is prominently convex (*arrow*). The aorta is small in this 19-year-old patient with mitral stenosis. (From Steiner RM, Levin DC: Radiology of the heart. In Braunwald E [ed]: Heart Disease, 5th ed. Philadelphia, WB Saunders, 1997, pp 226, 227.)

FIGURE 13–6. *A*, Left ventricular enlargement, left anterior oblique view. The cardiac silhouette is enlarged downward, to the left, and posteriorly, indicative of dilatation of the left ventricle. The ascending aorta is widened (*arrow*). *B*, Left ventricular aneurysm. A localized bulge can be seen on the left heart border. (*A*, From Baron MG: Radiological and angiographic examination of the heart. In Braunwald E [ed]: Heart Disease, 3rd ed. Philadelphia, WB Saunders, 1988, p 150. *B*, From Rubens MB: Chest x-ray in adult heart disease. In Julian DG, Camm AJ, Fox KM, et al [eds]: Diseases of the Heart, 2nd ed. London, WB Saunders, 1996, p 275.)

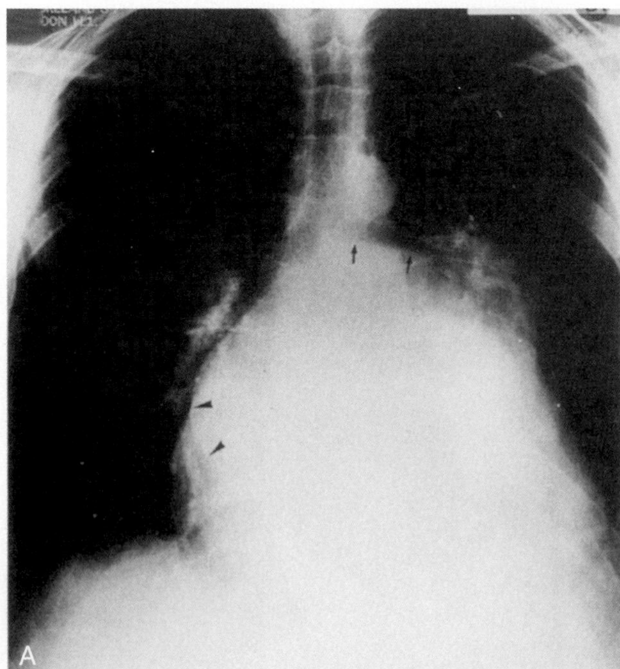

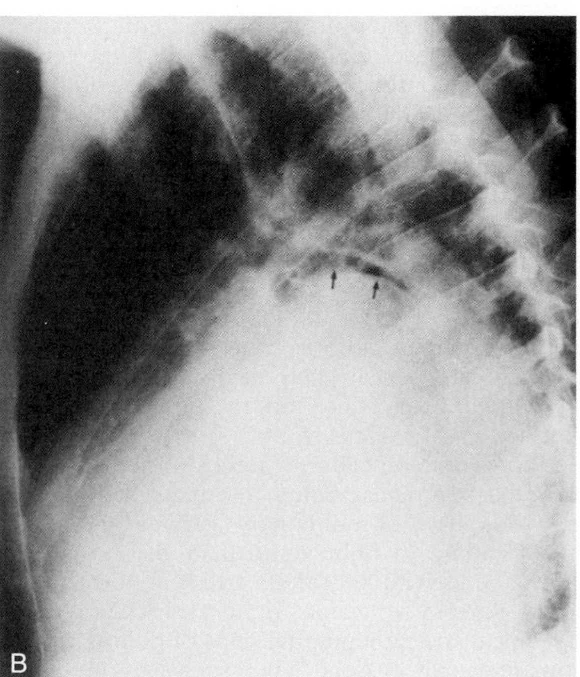

FIGURE 13–9. *A* and *B*, Left atrial enlargement in mitral regurgitation. The body of the left atrium is grossly enlarged and displacing the left bronchus (*arrows*) superiorly and posteriorly. A double density is visible over the right side of the heart (*arrowheads*). (From Rubens MB: Chest x-ray in adult heart disease. In Julian DG, Camm AJ, Fox KM, et al [eds]: Diseases of the Heart, 2nd ed. London, WB Saunders, 1996, p 272.)

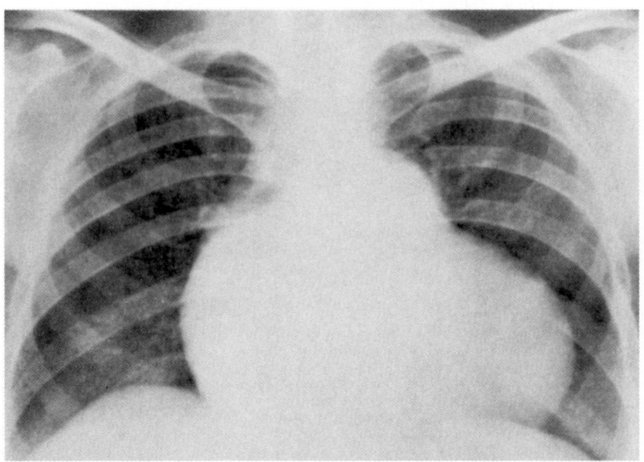

FIGURE 13–10. Congenital pulmonic valvular stenosis with right heart failure in a 38-year-old woman. The shadow of the heart is widened to the left, and the cardiac apex is rounded and elevated because of dilatation of the right ventricle. The tricuspid valve was regurgitant, and the right atrium is markedly enlarged. The main pulmonary artery is dilated, with decreased vascularity of the lungs. (From Baron MG: Radiological and angiographic examination of the heart. In Braunwald E [ed]: Heart Disease, 3rd ed. Philadelphia, WB Saunders, 1988, p 160.)

commonly due to annular dilatation resulting from a gradual and progressive increase in the size of a failing right ventricle. Primary tricuspid regurgitation, however, is seen with endocarditis, carcinoid, anorexiant drugs (fenfluramine-phentermine), myxomatous degeneration, trauma, and rheumatic involvement. Significant pulmonic regurgitation is unusual and typically results from dilatation of the pulmonic annulus in the presence of severe pulmonary hypertension.

Right ventricular pressure overload can also result in right ventricular enlargement. Pulmonary hypertension and uncorrected pulmonic valve stenosis (see Fig. 13–10*A*) are the two important causes. The former can be primary (idiopathic) or secondary to Eisenmenger's syndrome (see Chapter 34), pulmonary thromboembolic disease, or obstructive lung disease (see Chapter 38).

Right Atrium

Enlargement of the right atrium cannot be detected by physical examination. Determination of right atrial size is quite difficult on chest radiographs until marked enlargement has occurred, as suggested by bowing of the right heart border with rightward displacement, well away (>6 cm) from the midline (see Fig. 13–11*B*). Care must be taken to exclude left atrial enlargement as the cause of this displacement. The right atrium enlarges chiefly in the presence of right ventricular failure of any cause, as well as in tricuspid stenosis or regurgitation (see Fig. 13–11*B* and Chapter 32). Ebstein's anomaly of the tricuspid valve (see Fig. 13–11*C* and Chapter 33) and right atrial myxoma are rare causes.

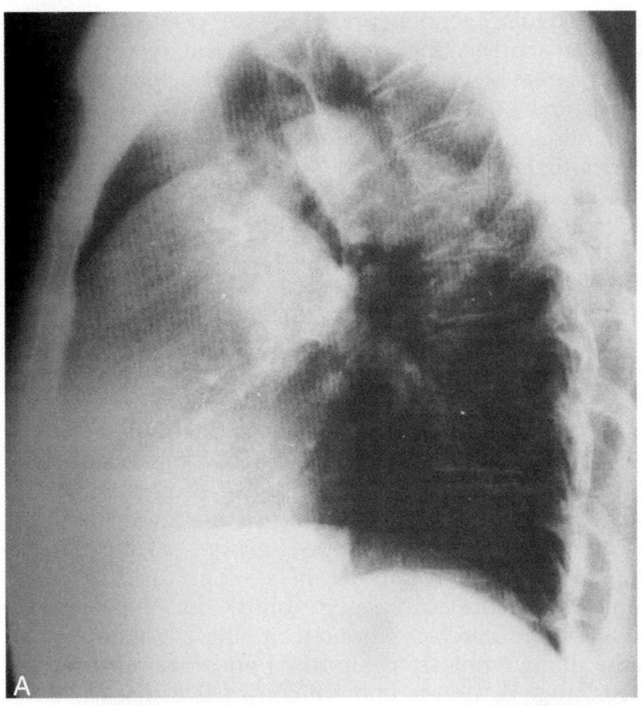

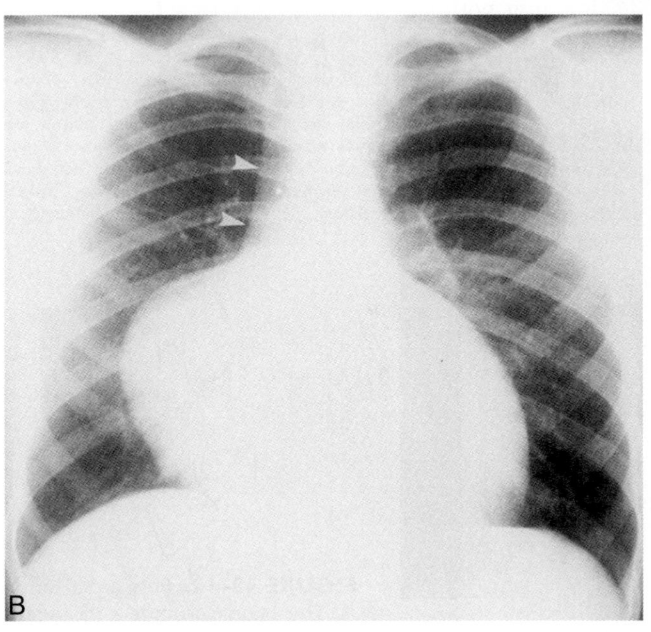

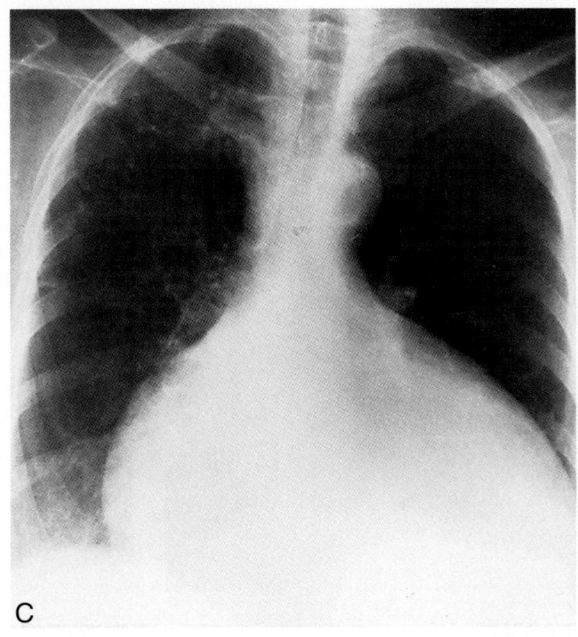

FIGURE 13–11. *A*, Right ventricular enlargement, lateral view, in a patient with primary pulmonary hypertension. Increased contact of the anterior aspect of the heart with the sternum can be seen, and the right ventricular outflow tract is prominent. *B*, Right atrial enlargement in congenital tricuspid stenosis. The right heart border is prominent, and the superior vena cava is dilated (*arrowheads*). *C*, Ebstein's anomaly. The globular cardiac enlargement is due to severe tricuspid regurgitation and right heart enlargement. Pulmonary blood flow is reduced. (*A* and *B*, From Rubens MB: Chest x-ray in adult heart disease. In Julian DG, Camm AJ, Fox KM, et al [eds]: Diseases of the Heart, 2nd ed. London, WB Saunders, 1996, p 271. *C*, From Steiner RM, Levin DC: Radiology of the heart. In Braunwald E [ed]: Heart Disease, 5th ed. Philadelphia, WB Saunders, 1997, p 234.)

OTHER CAUSES OF CARDIAC ENLARGEMENT

Increased Myocardial Mass

The most frequent causes of cardiomegaly secondary to a marked increase in myocardial (predominantly left ventricular) wall thickness are hypertension, aortic stenosis, and hypertrophic cardiomyopathy. The last may be suspected on the basis of the family history, a characteristic heart murmur, and ECG evidence of left ventricular hypertrophy in the absence of aortic stenosis or systemic hypertension.

Patients with marked chronic obesity may also have an increased cardiac size that is greater than that predicted by gender and body surface area. Pathologic studies in such patients have demonstrated both cavity dilatation and eccentric hypertrophy that may occur in the absence of coronary artery disease or hypertension.

Pericardium

Pericardial effusions in excess of 200 mL usually result in cardiac enlargement that can be detected on physical examination or chest radiographs. Although signs of cardiac tamponade (hypotension, pulsus paradoxus, elevated jugular venous pressure) are powerful evidence that cardiac enlargement is secondary to pericardial disease (see Chapter 35), leftward displacement of the lateral border of percussion dullness combined with muffling of the heart sounds may be an early sign of pericardial effusion without tamponade. The history can provide clues regarding a potential cause of pericardial disease (acute infection, neoplasm, irradiation, tuberculosis, uremia, cardiac surgery).

The classic appearance of pericardial effusion on the chest radiograph is that of an enlarged "water-bottle" heart that sits on the diaphragm with effacement of the normal contours of the cardiomediastinal silhouette (Fig. 13–12*A*). On the lateral film, a distinct stripe separating subepicardial fat from subxiphoid fat (epicardial fat pad sign) is a highly specific sign for pericardial effusion (Fig. 13–12*B* to *D*), but it is a relatively insensitive sign and is present in no more than one quarter of patients with this condition. Calcification of the pericardium is present in as many as half of patients with constrictive pericarditis, but the overall size of the cardiac silhouette in these patients is usually normal unless significant pericardial effusion coexists, that is, unless effusive-constrictive disease is present.

Pericardial cysts or loculated effusions are unusual, asymmetric protrusions away from the cardiac border that are typically identified as incidental findings on chest radiographs. They do not equate with cardiomegaly and can be further characterized by echocardiography, CT, or MRI.

Epicardium

Patients with marked obesity, in whom it is difficult to appreciate heart size on physical examination, may display cardiac enlargement on the PA chest film in the absence of chamber dilatation, severe hypertrophy, or pericardial effusion. In these cases, the apparent enlargement is due to a generous epicardial fat pad that extends leftward and inferiorly from the left ventricular apex. Occasionally, the rounded contour of the left ventricular apex can be apparent through the triangular fat pad on the chest radiograph, thus exposing the latter as the cause of the increase in heart size. An analogous increase in epicardial fat also occurs in patients with Cushing's syndrome or those taking large doses of adrenocorticoid hormone. Delineation of epicardial fat as the cause of cardiomegaly usually requires additional imaging with echocardiography or CT.

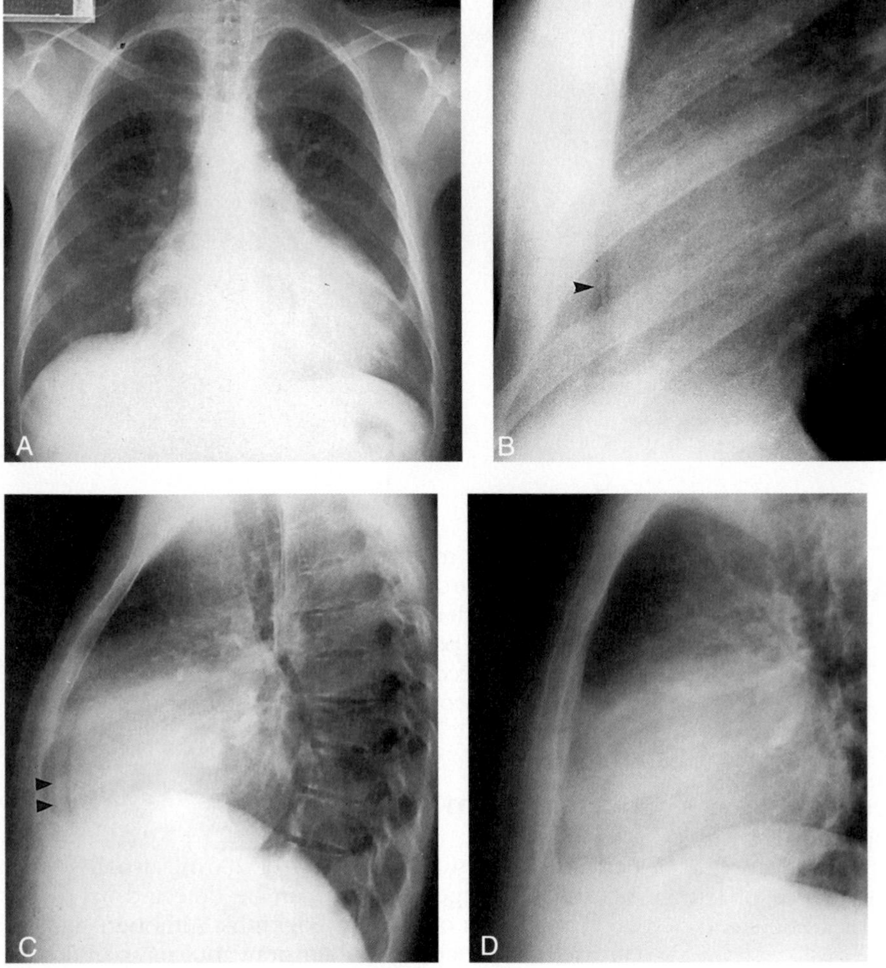

FIGURE 13–12. Pericardial effusion. *A*, The heart assumes a globular shape after the development of pericardial effusion. The normal indentations along the heart borders are effaced, so the cardiac silhouette is smooth and featureless. *B*, Normally, the subepicardial radiolucent fat stripe is separated from the subxiphoid fat by the thin, higher density stripe of pericardial fluid (*arrowhead*). *C*, The pericardial stripe (*arrowheads*) is wider than it is in *B* because of a small pericardial effusion. *D*, A large pericardial effusion is present. (From Steiner RM, Levin DC: Radiology of the heart. In Braunwald E [ed]: Heart Disease, 5th ed. Philadelphia, WB Saunders, 1997, p 234.)

Great Vessels; Mediastinal Structures

The great vessels can enlarge either with or independently from the cardiac chambers, but they are usually distinguishable on the basis of their location, contour, and projection. Expansion of the central pulmonary artery segments can readily be discerned on PA chest films (Fig. 13–13*A*), and it is usually accompanied by right ventricular enlargement. Poststenotic or aneurysmal dilatation of the proximal ascending aorta can sometimes be appreciated on the PA chest film as a rounded bulge along the upper right heart border above the right atrium (Fig. 13–13*B*). Such enlargement may be accompanied by a palpable right upper parasternal pulsation on physical examination. However, enlargement of the great vessels does not result in cardiomegaly per se without an associated abnormality such as left ventricular enlargement secondary to significant aortic regurgitation in the presence of an aneurysm of the ascending aorta.

APPROACH TO PATIENTS WITH CARDIOMEGALY

Because cardiac enlargement may accompany serious heart disease that may adversely affect long-term survival if it is not treated appropriately, it is imperative to delineate its cause and to understand the associated pathophysiologic derangements. Retaking a more directed history can be very useful, especially if the patient was referred for an apparently unrelated problem and the cardiomegaly was detected incidentally. A careful cardiovascular examination, with auscultation in several positions and after provocative maneuvers, may elicit additional clues. An ECG should be obtained routinely. Further evaluation as outlined in the following sections can then be undertaken (Fig. 13–14).

Echocardiography/Doppler (see Chapter 5)

Echocardiography is the most useful initial imaging study and is generally the first test of choice in patients with evidence of cardiac enlargement on physical or radiographic examination. In patients in whom technically adequate studies can be performed, two-dimensional transthoracic echocardiography with Doppler color-flow imaging provides an accurate assessment of chamber dimensions, wall thickness, global and regional ventricular function, valvular morphology and function, great vessel size and orientation, and pericardial characteristics. The technique is safe and reproducible and can also be used to assess the response to any therapies initiated.

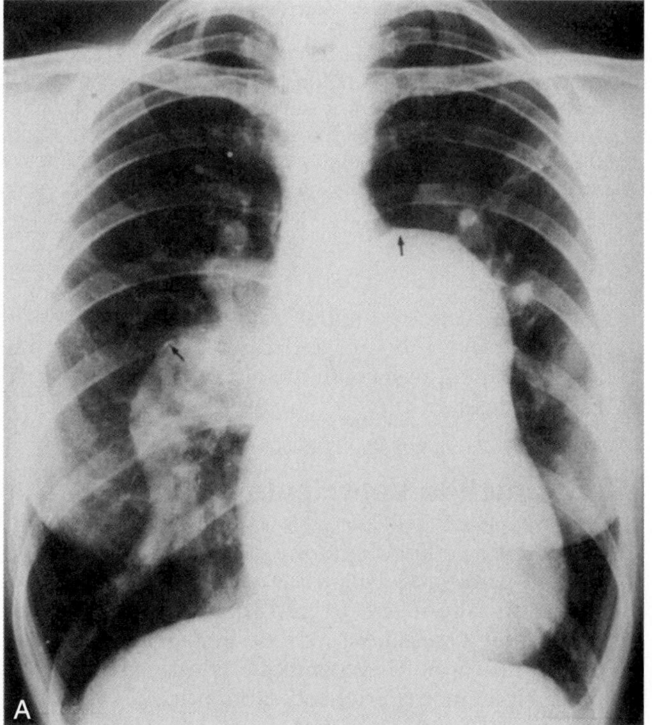

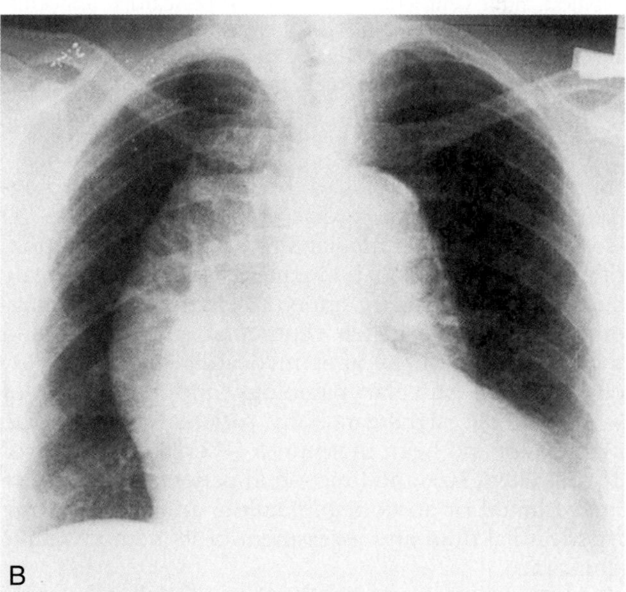

FIGURE 13–13. *A*, Atrial septal defect with Eisenmenger's syndrome. The central pulmonary arteries are enormously dilated, and dramatic peripheral pruning is evident. Pulmonary arterial calcification (*arrows*) indicates severe chronic pulmonary arterial hypertension. *B*, Large aneurysm of the ascending aorta. The descending aorta is diffusely calcified and mildly dilated. (From Rubens MB: Chest x-ray in adult heart disease. In Julian DG, Camm AJ, Fox KM, et al [eds]: Diseases of the Heart, 2nd ed. London, WB Saunders, 1996, pp 266, 276.)

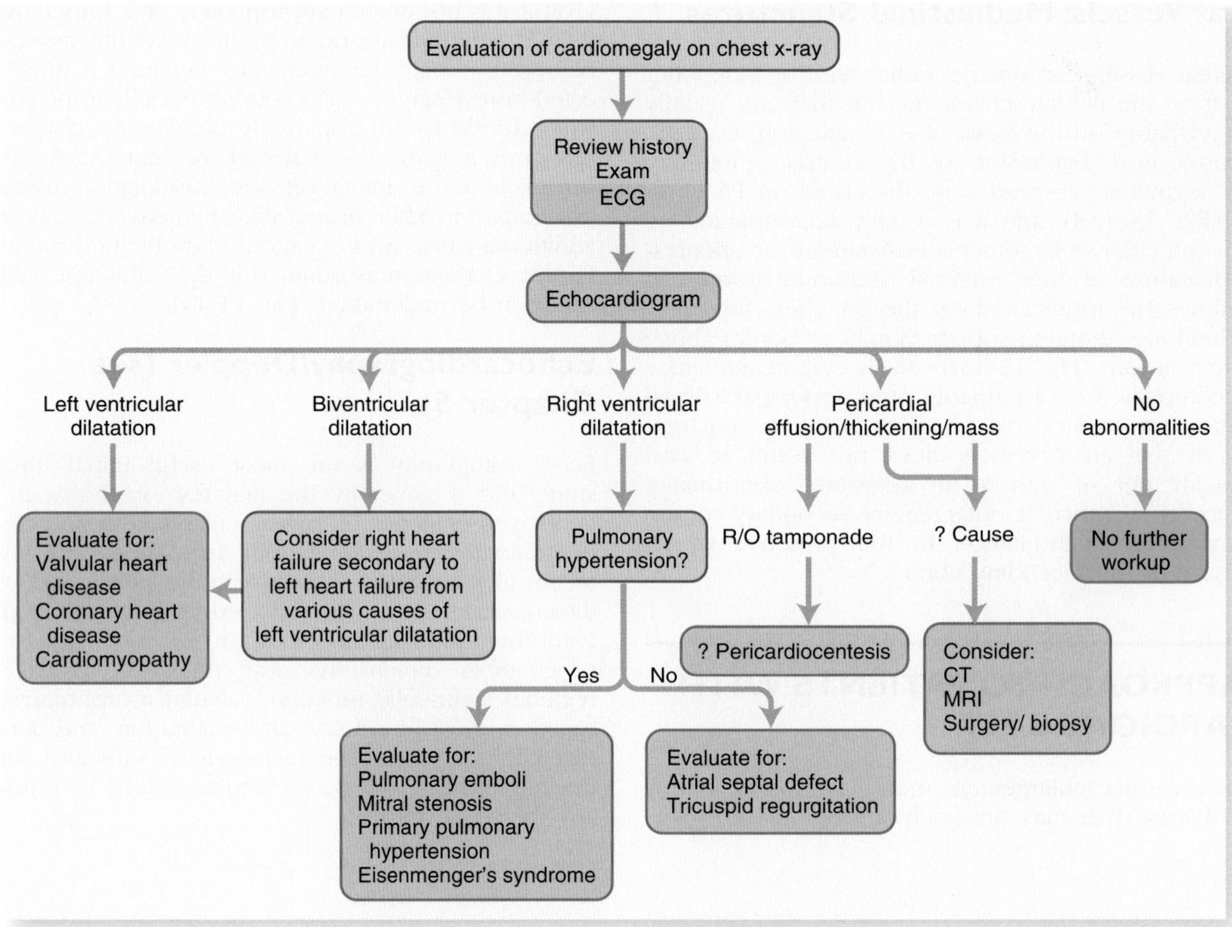

FIGURE 13–14. Approach to a patient with cardiomegaly. When cardiomegaly is found on the chest radiograph, the history and physical examination should be reviewed and an electrocardiogram (ECG) performed before obtaining a two-dimensional Doppler echocardiographic study. Cardiomegaly may be explained by left ventricular dilatation, biventricular dilatation, right ventricular dilatation, or pericardial abnormalities, or it may be found to be spurious on the echocardiogram. Rarely, isolated abnormalities of the atrium, particularly the left atrium, may cause abnormalities on the chest radiograph but will not cause true cardiomegaly. Depending on the echocardiographic findings, further tests can help elucidate the cause of echocardiographically confirmed cardiomegaly. CT, computed tomography; MRI, magnetic resonance imaging; R/O, rule out.

Some clinical examples of the utility of echocardiography in patients with cardiac enlargement include (1) assessment of left ventricular size and systolic function, both global and regional, in patients with cardiomegaly and suspected coronary artery disease; (2) determination of the change in left ventricular size, shape, and function in the weeks after myocardial infarction; (3) delineation of valvular pathology and estimation of its physiologic significance in patients with cardiac enlargement and heart murmurs; (4) serial evaluation of left ventricular size and function in patients with asymptomatic mitral or aortic regurgitation; and (5) detection of pericardial fluid and assessment of its hemodynamic significance.

The images obtained by transthoracic echocardiography are suboptimal in 10% to 15% of patients because of body habitus or chest wall configuration. In such patients, transesophageal echocardiography is a suitable alternative for assessing the cause of the cardiac enlargement. This technique is especially well suited to the study of suspected mitral or aortic valve disease and prosthetic valve function and can be performed safely on an outpatient basis with the aid of light sedation and local anesthesia.

Radionuclide Ventriculography

Radionuclide ventriculography, also known as a MUGA (multiple gated acquisition) or gated blood pool scan, provides an alternative to transthoracic echocardiography for the assessment of left and right ventricular size and function. This technique is safe, accurate, and reproducible in experienced laboratories, but it does entail small exposure to radiation. Left ventricular and right ventricular volumes and ejection fractions and estimates of left ventricular diastolic function can be determined (Fig. 13–15). The technique is especially helpful when investigation of the cause of the cardiac enlargement focuses exclusively on ventricular size and func-

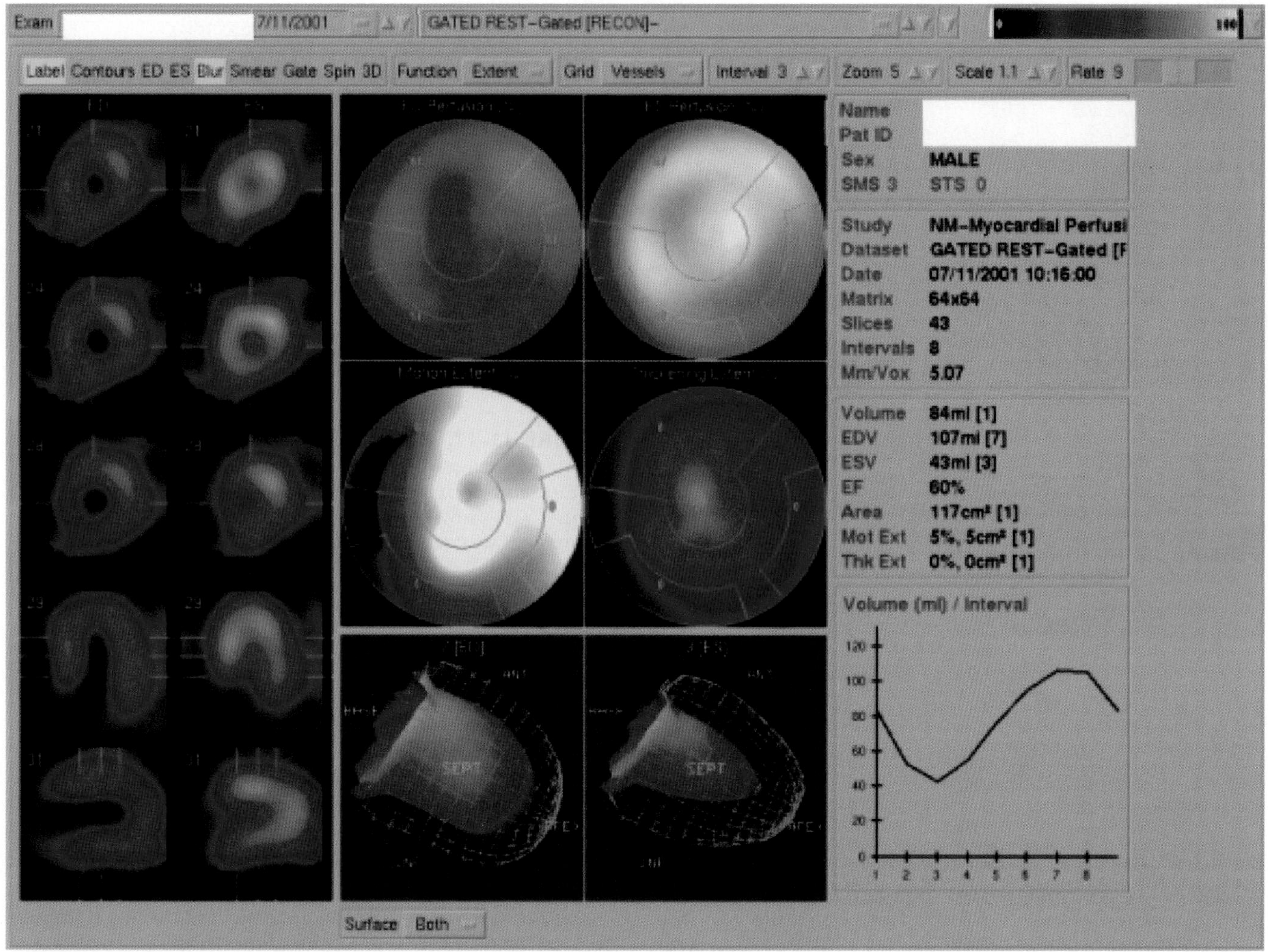

FIGURE 13–15. Technetium Tc 99m sestamibi myocardial perfusion study. The two left columns contain short-axis (top three rows), horizontal long-axis (fourth row), and vertical long-axis (bottom row) end-diastolic (left) and end-systolic (right) images that provide a qualitative assessment of regional left ventricular (LV) function. The bottom middle two panels display a three-dimensional reconstruction of the left ventricle at end diastole and end systole as seen from a right anterior oblique projection. The time-activity curve in the bottom right panel allows quantification of the global LV ejection fraction. (Courtesy of Marcello Di Carli, M.D., Nuclear Medicine Division, Department of Radiology, Brigham and Women's Hospital, Boston.)

tion and not on valvular morphology and function. It is not widely appreciated that the vast majority of nuclear cardiology laboratories perform gated SPECT (single-photon emission computed tomography), in association with radionuclide perfusion imaging (thallium or technetium), to provide an assessment of global and regional left ventricular function in addition to blood flow.[4] In many patients, however, the use of both echocardiographic and radionuclide techniques to evaluate left ventricular function is duplicative and costly.

Computed Tomography

From a clinical perspective, CT scanning may have only a few specific advantages over Doppler echocardiography in the assessment of cardiomegaly.[4] It can provide anatomic information pertaining to chamber dimensions and wall thickness, albeit without simultaneous physiologic or valvular detail and with the disadvantage of requiring exposure to contrast media (to delineate vascular structures) and ionizing radiation. Image quality can be easily affected by patient movement, the presence of intracardiac devices (prosthetic valves, pacemakers), and valvular calcification. Nevertheless, when compared with echocardiography, chest CT scanning provides a better assessment of pericardial thickness (Fig. 13–16), and it is a far more sensitive test for the detection of pericardial calcification.[5] Its wider field of view and superior spatial resolution enhance its value as an appropriate imaging technique for the assessment of great vessel pathology (e.g., suspected aortic dissection or aneurysm [see Fig. 36–5]) and other mediastinal structures (tumor, cyst) that may impart the impression of cardiomegaly on chest films. In most patients with cardiac enlargement, chest CT should be pursued only after careful analysis of the data available from the clinical examination, chest radiograph, and echocardiogram

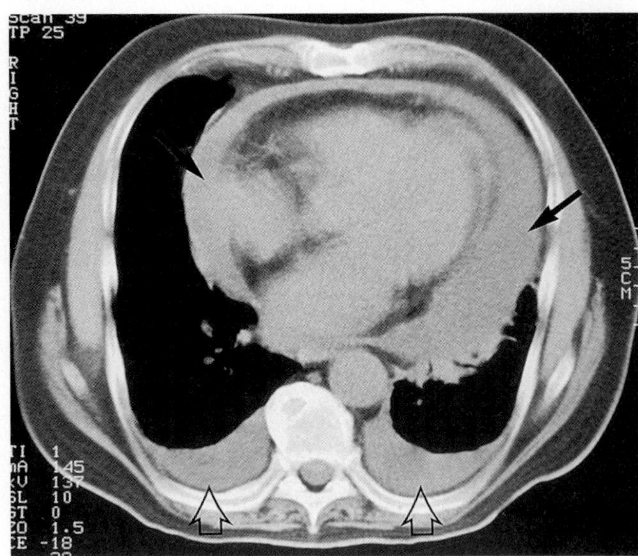

FIGURE 13–16. This chest computed tomographic scan demonstrates a large and circumferential pericardial effusion (*arrows*). Bilateral pleural effusions (*arrowheads*) are also seen.

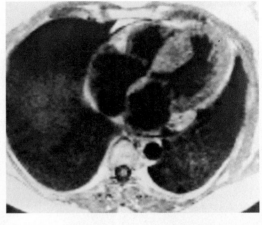

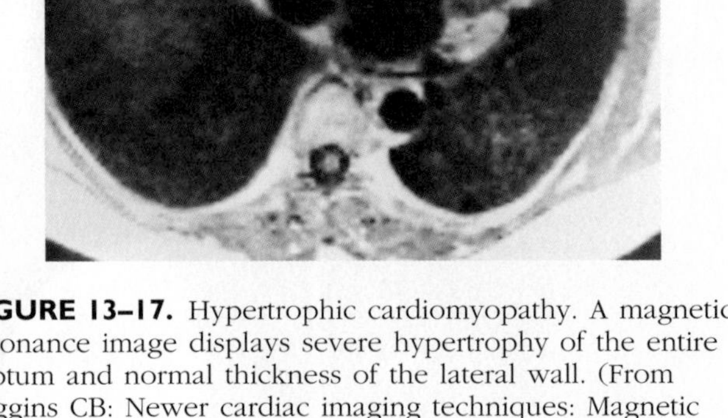

FIGURE 13–17. Hypertrophic cardiomyopathy. A magnetic resonance image displays severe hypertrophy of the entire septum and normal thickness of the lateral wall. (From Higgins CB: Newer cardiac imaging techniques: Magnetic resonance imaging and computed tomography. In Braunwald E [ed]: Heart Disease, 5th ed. Philadelphia, WB Saunders, 1997, p 323.)

and only with a specific question that has been left unanswered, such as pericardial thickness, great vessel appearance, and abnormalities of extracardiac structures.

Magnetic Resonance Imaging

Assessment of cardiac structure and function with MRI is an area of active investigation[5, 6] (Fig. 13–17). Its clinical utility is limited, however, by factors of accessibility and cost. It may be of particular value in patients with cardiac enlargement, in whom cross-sectional imaging of the heart, great vessels, or extracardiac structures is important, but in whom contrast media are contraindicated. In addition, MRI can provide information related to tissue and fluid characteristics that may help in the diagnosis. MRI holds great future promise of becoming the single modality capable of providing critical information regarding myocardial, valvular, pericardial, and coronary arterial anatomy and function in patients with cardiac enlargement.

Exercise Testing

In patients with left ventricular enlargement, exercise or pharmacologic stress testing is most commonly undertaken to screen for the presence of coronary artery disease or to assess myocardial function in those with cardiomegaly. The observations made during provocative testing in patients with cardiac enlargement and left ventricular systolic dysfunction (ejection fraction <0.40) are important determinants of therapy. In particular, demonstration of reversible ischemia in such patients argues for surgical revascularization. Myocardial viability and stress-induced ischemia can be assessed by either myocardial perfusion scintigraphy or stress echocardiography.

Cardiopulmonary exercise testing with measurement of oxygen uptake is a standard feature of the assessment and follow-up of patients with cardiac enlargement and severe heart failure who are under consideration for cardiac transplantation. Exercise-related changes in ventricular dimensions or function as assessed by echocardiography may be helpful in determining the need for surgery in asymptomatic patients with cardiomegaly and mitral or aortic regurgitation.

Coronary Arteriography

The most common indication for coronary arteriography in patients with cardiac enlargement is for delineation of the coronary anatomy when coronary revascularization is being considered. Coronary angiography is also appropriately undertaken as a late step in the evaluation of patients with dilated cardiomyopathy of uncertain cause and in those who are candidates for cardiac transplantation.

Indications for Hospital Admission or Cardiology Referral

Referral to a cardiac specialist should be driven primarily by the clinical context in which the cardiac enlargement is detected. Early consultation should be considered when the cause or significance of the cardiac enlargement is uncertain or when an invasive diagnostic (catheterization/angiography/coronary arteriography) or therapeutic (pericardiocentesis) procedure is being contemplated. In patients with myocardial ischemia, heart failure, arrhythmias, syncope, valvular heart disease, or hypertension, indications for cardiology consultation are based on the responsiveness of the clinical syndrome and are no different in those with and without cardiomegaly.

Long-term follow-up is predicated on the specific diagnosis, the complexity and severity of the patient's illness, and the potential need for cardiac interventions. Once again, the cardiomegaly is usually a reflection of the severity of the underlying condition and not an indication per se for specific intervention.

References

1. Perloff JK: The movements of the heart—percussion, palpitation and observation. In Perloff JK (ed): Physical Examination of the Heart and Circulation, 2nd ed. Philadelphia, WB Saunders, 1990, pp 141–180.
2. Steiner RM: Radiology of the heart and great vessels. In Braunwald E (ed): Heart Disease: A Textbook of Cardiovascular Medicine, 6th ed. Philadelphia, WB Saunders, 2001, pp 237–272.
3. Dec GW, Fuster V: Idiopathic dilated cardiomyopathy. N Engl J Med 1994;331:1564–1575.
4. Hyun IY, Kwan J, Park KS, Lee WH: Reproducibility of Tl-201 and Tc-99m sestamibi gated myocardial perfusion SPECT measurements of myocardial function. J Nucl Cardiol 2001;8:182–187.
5. Higgins CB: Newer cardiac imaging techniques: Magnetic resonance imaging and computed tomography. In Braunwald E (ed): Heart Disease: A Textbook of Cardiovascular Medicine, 6th ed. Philadelphia, WB Saunders, 2001, pp 324–358.
6. Chuang ML, Hibberd MG, Salton CJ, et al: Importance of imaging method over imaging modality in non-invasive determination of left ventricular volumes and ejection fraction: Assessment by two- and three-dimensional echocardiography and magnetic resonance imaging. J Am Coll Cardiol 2000;35:477–484.

CHAPTER 14

Approach to the Patient Undergoing Noncardiac Surgery

Joshua S. Adler and Lee Goldman

Each year, millions of surgical procedures are performed on adults in the United States. The vast majority of patients do not suffer complications from surgery or the anesthetic. Roughly 3% to 10% do suffer serious complications, approximately half of which are cardiovascular in nature. The cardiovascular complications of surgery are more common in patients with underlying cardiovascular disease. Older patients, at increased risk for cardiovascular disease, make up a disproportionate percentage of patients undergoing surgery. As the population ages, an increasing number of older patients are expected to undergo major noncardiac surgery.

There is now substantial consistency among studies that have identified risk factors for cardiac complications of noncardiac surgery and the limited role of preoperative noninvasive cardiac testing. In addition, certain perioperative interventions, most notably beta-adrenergic blocking agents, have been shown to reduce perioperative cardiac morbidity. Several important questions remain, however, regarding the optimal perioperative management of patients with cardiac disease and, in particular, the role of preoperative revascularization.

When the primary care physician's own patient is considered for surgery, collaboration with the surgeon is critical to decide whether the benefits of proceeding with surgery, from both a cardiac and a noncardiac perspective, are outweighed by the risks. In making this decision, the physician must consider not only the morbidity and mortality risks but also the patient's preferences, especially when the surgical procedure is designed to improve quality of life rather than longevity. Much of the needed preoperative cardiac evaluation may already have taken place even before a surgeon was consulted, but additional evaluation may be required once the scope of the planned surgery is understood. If the primary care physician will not be following the patient personally in the hospital after surgery, arrangements should be made for medical consultation for patients who have any chronic medical problems or who are at high risk for cardiac or noncardiac complications of surgery.

When called as a preoperative medical consultant to aid in the care of a patient whom the primary care physician has not followed longitudinally, the primary care physician must quickly determine the severity and stability of the patient's major medical conditions, estimate the patient's risk of cardiac and noncardiac complications of surgery, and recommend further expeditious testing or interventions to reduce risk when appropriate. A collaborative effort with the anesthesiologist and surgeon is essential to manage cardiac disease optimally in the perioperative period. The preoperative consultant must also advise about the timing of surgery, because postponing surgery to address medical problems may reduce the risk of the surgery itself but produce its own risks by delaying a needed operation.

Urgency and Type of Surgery

The urgency of surgery will dictate the speed and extent of the preoperative evaluation and whether there is any potential to delay surgery and, hence, to perform diagnostic tests or institute new therapy. Multiple studies have demonstrated that emergency surgery has a twofold to fivefold increased risk of complications compared with elective surgery.

The type of surgery is very important in helping to establish a baseline risk of cardiac complications (Box 14–1). Differences in the baseline risk reflect differences in the hemodynamic stress of the individual procedures and differences in the prevalence of preexisting severe cardiovascular disease among patients undergoing the procedure.[1,2] The complication rates for procedures performed with local anesthetics and minimal sedation (such as cataract extraction) are very low, primarily because of the short duration and minimal hemodynamic stress during both the procedure and the recovery period. Patients undergoing these procedures generally do not require intensive preoperative evaluation.

Major vascular surgical procedures are associated with the highest risk of complications. This risk is partly attributed to the significant hemodynamic stress of these procedures and partly to a very high prevalence of severe CAD among patients undergoing them. This latter point is complicated by the fact that many vascular surgery patients have such severe functional limitation due to claudication that they are not aware of the symptoms of coronary ischemia in their normal daily activities.

BOX 14–1

Risks of Major Cardiac Complications Associated with Different Types of Surgery*

Highest Risk	(often >5%)[†]
	Aortic surgery
	Peripheral vascular surgery**
High Risk	(2%–5%)
	Thoracic surgery
	Intraperitoneal surgery
Intermediate	(0.51%–2%)
	Orthopedic surgery
	Retroperitoneal surgery
	Head and neck surgery
	Other general surgery
Low Risk	(<0.5%)
	Superficial procedures and biopsies
	Endoscopic surgery
	Transurethral prostate surgery
	Cataract Surgery

*Defined as myocardial infarction, pulmonary edema, cardiac arrest, or cardiac death.

[†]For elective procedures; emergent surgery carries a 2.5-fold higher risk, probably regardless of the type of procedure.

**Mostly because of the high-risk status of the patients rather than because of the stress of the surgery itself.

Based on data from Lee TH, Marcantonio ER, Mangione CM, et al: Derivation and prospective validation of a simple index for prediction of cardiac risk of major noncardiac surgery. Circulation 1999;100:1043–1049 and Eagle KA, Berger PB, Calkins H, et al: ACC/AHA guideline update for perioperative cardiovascular evaluation for noncardiac surgery—executive summary. Circulation 2002;105:1257–1267.

PREOPERATIVE ASSESSMENT OF CARDIAC RISK

An important principle of risk assessment is that of probabilistic decision-making. Risk assessment using this principle begins with a baseline risk, which will generally be the overall cardiac complication rate for a particular procedure at a particular institution. This risk can then be modified by considering an individual patient's clinical data: the history, the physical examination, and the resting electrocardiogram (ECG). The focus of this clinical evaluation is an assessment of the stability and severity of known cardiovascular disease and the identification of any symptoms or signs that may represent previously unrecognized cardiovascular disease. In most patients, an accurate estimate of cardiac risk can be made based on these routine clinical data. In only a small subset of patients will noninvasive or invasive cardiac evaluation significantly alter the clinical risk assessment.

An assessment of the cardiac risks for patients undergoing noncardiac surgery can be made using multifactorial indices.[1,3–5] These indices combine a variety of clinical variables to determine an overall risk of cardiovascular complications including myocardial infarction (MI), cardiac death, pulmonary edema, and important ventricular arrhythmias. The original multifactorial index of Goldman et al[6] and the modification of the original index by Detsky et al[7] have largely been supplanted by the newer index of Lee et al, which is easy to use (Box 14–2) and more accurately discriminates risk in contemporary populations.[1] This new index has already been shown to be accurate in a large series of patients at another hospital (Table 14–1). It must be remembered, however, that more recent experience has been guided by the findings of earlier studies. As a result, very few patients currently undergo

BOX 14–2

Calculation of the Revised Cardiac Risk Index

RISK FACTOR	POINTS
Intrathoracic, intraperitoneal, or infrainguinal vascular surgery	1
History of ischemic heart disease other than in a patient who is asymptomatic after coronary revascularization	1
History of heart failure	1
Insulin treatment for diabetes mellitus	1
Serum creatinine level >2.0 mg/dL	1
History of cerebrovascular disease	1

From Lee TH, Marcantonio ER, Mangione CM, et al: Derivation and prospective validation of a simple index for prediction of cardiac risk of major noncardiac surgery. Circulation 1999;100:1043–1049.

TABLE 14–1

Risks of Major Complications According to the Revised Index of Cardiac Risk in Noncardiac Surgery

		No. of Risk Factors (from Box 14–2)			
	No. of Patients	***0%***	***1%***	***2%***	***≥3%***
Original derivation cohort[1]	2893	0.5	1.3	3.6	9.1
Original validation cohort[1]	1422	0.4	0.9	6.6	11.0
Boersma et al.[5]	1141		1.3	3.1	9.1
Overall weighted average		0.4 (7/1559)	1.2 (27/2284)	4.0 (51/1273)	9.5 (52/550)

From Lee TH, Marcantonio ER, Mangione CM, et al: Derivation and prospective validation of a simple index for prediction of cardiac risk of major noncardiac surgery. Circulation 1999;100:1043–1049.

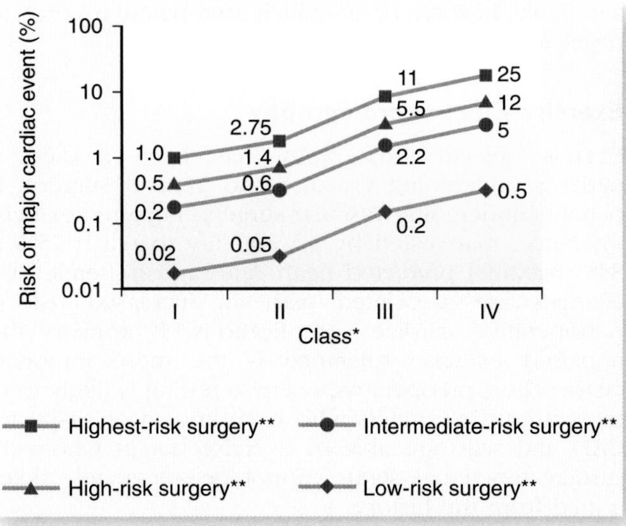

FIGURE 14–1. The risk of cardiac surgery is a combination of the risks of the surgical procedure itself and of the patient's characteristics. The patient's score on a multifactorial risk index (see Box 14–2; see also Table 14–1) can be integrated with the risk of the surgery itself (see Box 14–1) to improve the estimate of risk. *See Box 14–2 and Table 14–1. **See Box 14–1.

elective surgery soon after MI or in the presence of severe aortic stenosis—two characteristics that carried very high risk in earlier series but are present in too few patients in newer series to be identified as statistically significant risk factors despite their continued clinical relevance.

A multifactoral risk index is especially useful to define low risk patients in whom further preoperative testing or treatments are unlikely to be helpful and for providing a risk estimate against which alternative approaches can be compared. The index can also be used in a Bayesian way (for further discussion, see Chapter 2) to modify a baseline risk (Fig. 14–1). In this approach, a low index score decreases a patient's risk, whereas a high score is associated with an increased risk. An intermediate score is generally associated with an unchanged risk. In patients with known cardiovascular disease, a risk index can help guide the perioperative approach but cannot substitute for clinical judgment and disease-specific approaches.

BOX 14–3

Characteristics Defining Patients with Known or Suspected Ischemic Heart Disease

Active-increased risk

History of myocardial infarction or presence of pathologic Q-waves on the electrocardiogram

History of a positive exercise test (or other noninvasive test for ischemia) unless contradicted by a normal coronary arteriogram

Current complaint of chest pain thought to be caused by myocardial ischemia

Past, now inactive and probably not increased risk

After coronary revascularization (coronary artery bypass surgery or angioplasty)—now asymptomatic and no evidence of ischemia on noninvasive testing

Coronary Artery Disease

Coronary artery disease (CAD) is the most important cardiovascular disorder in the evaluation and assessment of patients in the preoperative period. CAD is common in patients undergoing surgery, and the majority of serious cardiac complications are thought to be ischemia-related, particularly MI and cardiac death.[8,9] Most patients at increased risk for CAD-related complications can be identified using routine clinical data (Box 14–3). Patients with none of the listed characteristics are at low risk (<0.5%) for ischemic complications during and after surgery. By contrast, patients with one or more of these characteristics are at a 5- to 50-fold increased risk for ischemic cardiac complications. The combination of the absence of active CAD and a low index score identifies a very low risk group for cardiac complications.

Patients with known or suspected CAD, as a group, have a 4% to 5% risk of perioperative cardiac complications and roughly a 1% mortality for major surgery. A risk estimate in these patients can be further refined through an assessment of the stability and severity of ischemic symptoms and the cardiac functional status. Patients with unstable coronary syndromes, including a recent (within 1 month) MI with evidence of persistent ischemia, unstable angina, or accelerated angina are at particularly high risk. Patients who have had an MI within 6 months before surgery and who have evidence of persistent ischemia are likely to be at higher risk than those without persistent ischemia. In patients with stable ischemic symptoms, the severity may be assessed using a standardized approach that estimates functional status (see Chapters 4 and 25). Patients with class III or IV angina are at substantially increased risk for complications compared with patients with class I or II symptoms. In addition, patients who are able to exercise to increase their heart rate above about 100 beats per minute are at lower risk that those who cannot do so. The majority of patients can be appropriately risk-stratified using this approach and do not require further testing.

For the special case of vascular surgery, the most important independent clinical predictors of cardiac complications have been well defined and mirror the risk factors for patients undergoing other general surgical procedures (Box 14–4).[5,10] Patients with none of these characteristics are at low risk for cardiac complications (<5%). Patients with one or two characteristics appear to be at low risk if treated with perioperative beta-blockers.[5] In patients with three or more characteristics, noninvasive testing may identify a subgroup of patients who are at such high risk as to warrant preoperative coronary revascularization.

BOX 14–4

Clinical Predictors of Cardiac Complications in Vascular Surgery Patients

Increased risk

Age >70 yr
Prior myocardial infarction
Angina pectoris
Heart failure
Prior cerebrovascular accident
Diabetes mellitus

Decreased risk

Beta-blocker therapy

Based on data from Boersma E, Poldermans D, Bax JJ, et al: Predictors of cardiac events after major vascular surgery: Role of clinical characteristics, dobutamine echocardiography, and β-blocker therapy. JAMA 2001;285:1865–1873 and L'Italien GJ, Paul SD, Hendel RC, et al: Development and validation of a Bayesian model for perioperative cardiac risk assessment in a cohort of 1081 vascular surgical candidates. J Am Coll Cardiol 1996;27:779–786.

Preoperative Noninvasive Ischemia Testing

The role of preoperative noninvasive ischemia testing is changing rapidly as newer data support the use of perioperative beta-blockers to reduce risk in patients with known or suspected ischemic heart disease.[5,11–13] Although consensus guidelines[2,14] recommend noninvasive testing for intermediate-risk patients, in the hope of using test results to place them into low-risk or high-risk categories, more recent recommendations limit noninvasive testing to situations in which a patient's risk is unclear because of the inability to exercise or to give a reliable history, or in which preoperative coronary revascularization may be indicated.

Exercise Electrocardiography

Exercise electrocardiography has been studied in patients undergoing vascular and general surgery. In patients undergoing vascular surgery, impaired exercise tolerance, manifested by an inability to reach 75% to 85% maximal predicted heart rate, and ischemic ECG changes are associated with an increased risk of perioperative cardiac complications. It appears that impaired exercise tolerance is the more important factor. Thus, preoperative exercise testing is likely to be most useful in patients who have known or suspected CAD and who are able to exercise but in whom the cardiac functional status cannot be adequately determined from the history.

Dipyridamole-Thallium Scintigraphy

Patients who are unable to exercise because of claudication or orthopedic problems have frequently been referred for preoperative dipyridamole-thallium scintigraphy. Data in patients who were referred for dipyridamole-thallium scintigraphy before vascular surgery demonstrated a sensitivity of at least 90% and a specificity of at least 50% for perioperative cardiac complications.[10] By comparison, data in unselected patients scheduled for vascular surgery found that dipyridamole-thallium scintigraphy was not predictive of cardiac complications. This discrepancy is likely due to a higher prevalence of severe coronary disease among patients referred by their physicians for testing compared with the unselected groups of patients.

Investigators have attempted to identify the subset of patients most likely to benefit from preoperative dipyridamole-thallium scintigraphy, using clinical data as selection criteria for further testing.[10] In patients found to be at low or high risk by clinical data, dipyridamole-thallium scintigraphy does not further refine the risk estimate. Other studies have found that in intermediate-risk patients, thallium redistribution is associated with a higher risk of complications (similar to a high clinical risk), and a normal scan is associated with a lower risk (similar to a low clinical risk). A study of 80 consecutive, unselected, intermediate-risk patients undergoing vascular surgery found that dipyridamole-thallium scintigraphy did not accurately predict risk.[15] Data on the use of dipyridamole-thallium scintigraphy in non-vascular surgery are even more limited.

Echocardiography

Dobutamine stress echocardiography (see Chapter 5) has been studied as a preoperative risk-assessment tool, most recently in consecutive patients undergoing the test before vascular surgery.[5] The presence of one or more regional wall motion abnormalities with stress is associated with a markedly increased risk of cardiac complications.[5] Although more limited, data from non-vascular surgery suggest that dobutamine stress echocardiography may be useful in both intermediate and high-risk patients.[16]

Resting echocardiography is generally not recommended before noncardiac surgery. Nevertheless, resting wall motion abnormalities, left ventricular hypertrophy, and more than mild mitral regurgitation are associated with increased risk, especially in patients who are Class III or IV on the new cardiac risk index.[17] Resting echocardiography is also important for investigating murmurs suspicious for hemodynamically-significant aortic stenosis.

Ambulatory Ischemia Monitoring

Asymptomatic (silent) ischemic ST segment changes are found in roughly 25% of patients with known or suspected CAD who undergo preoperative 24- or 48-hour ambulatory ECGs. The presence of ischemic changes is associated with an increased risk of perioperative cardiac complications. The utility of this test is limited, however, by the requirement for a normal baseline ECG and the 24-hour testing period. The precise role of preoperative ambulatory ischemia monitoring remains undefined.

In contrast to preoperative asymptomatic ischemia, the presence of intraoperative ischemic ECG changes has not been consistently associated with a major increase in perioperative cardiac complications. Intraoperative ischemia monitoring is not recommended for routine use.

Perioperative Management of Patients with Known or Possible Coronary Artery Disease

There are several important issues to consider in the perioperative management of patients with CAD, including medications to reduce risk, the role of preoperative coronary revascularization, the anesthetic technique, and the use of intraoperative and postoperative monitoring.

Anti-ischemia Medications

Patients taking antianginal or other cardiac medications before surgery generally should continue to do so up to and including the day of surgery. Medications also generally should be restarted as soon as possible after surgery.

Two randomized trials with a total of about 450 patients have shown that perioperative beta-blockers reduce the risk of either in-hospital major cardiac complications in high-risk patients identified by stress echocardiography or of adverse outcomes at 1 year in patients with or at risk for CAD by more than 50%.[18,19] Current evidence supports routine perioperative beta-blockers in patients with an increased risk for myocardial ischemia (Box 14–5). The regimens emphasize

BOX 14–5

Eligibility Criteria for Use of Perioperative Beta-Blockers, Unless Clinical Contraindications

CLINICAL CRITERIA[19]

Use beta-blockers in patients with *any* of the following:
- Previous myocardial infarction
- Typical angina
- Atypical angina with positive stress test

or

If the patient has any *two* of the following:
- Age 65 years or older
- Hypertension
- Current smoking
- Serum cholesterol level >240 mg/dL
- Diabetes mellitus

REVISED CARDIAC RISK CRITERIA*

Use beta-blockers in patients with one or more criteria:

High-risk surgical procedure, defined as:
- Intraperitoneal, intrathoracic, or suprainguinal vascular procedure

Ischemic heart disease, defined as:
- History of myocardial infarction
- History of or current angina
- Use of sublingual nitroglycerin
- Positive exercise text
- Q-waves on ECG
- Patients who have undergone PTCA or CABG and who have chest pain presumed to be of ischemic origin

Congestive heart failure, defined as:
- Left ventricular failure by physical examination
- History of paroxysmal nocturnal dyspnea
- History of pulmonary edema
- S_3 or bilateral rales on physical examination
- Pulmonary edema on chest radiograph

Cerebrovascular disease, defined as:
- History of transient ischemic attack
- History of cerebrovascular accident

Insulin-dependent diabetes mellitus

Chronic renal insufficiency, defined as:
- Creatinine level 2.0 mg/dL or greater

*Adapted from Auerbach AD, Goldman L: β-blockers and reduction of cardiac events in noncardiac surgery: Scientific review. JAMA 2002:287;1435–1444.

heart rate control and the importance of preoperative and postoperative, as well as intraoperative, therapy (Table 14–2).

In another randomized trial, mivazerol, an alpha-2 agonist that reduces postganglionic norepinephrine output and modulates sympathetic efferent stimuli from the spinal cord, significantly reduced cardiac death (but not the primary endpoint of MI and all-cause death) in patients with coronary heart disease who underwent noncardiac surgery.[20] In a preplanned subgroup analysis, there was a significant reduction in the primary endpoint of MI and all-cause death as well as cardiac death in 904 patients undergoing vascular surgery.

Mivazerol is not currently available for clinical use. For patients who cannot tolerate beta-blockers, clonidine, which has pharmacologic characteristics similar to mivazerol and can be given orally or via a cutaneous patch, may become a useful alternative.

Delaying Surgery

A decision to delay surgery requires careful consideration of the perioperative cardiac risks associated with proceeding as scheduled, the potential reduction in perioperative risk with delayed surgery, and the risk associated with delaying a necessary surgical therapy. In patients who require emergent lifesaving surgery (such as that for a perforated viscus), there is little potential for delay, regardless of the magnitude of the perioperative cardiac risk. In patients with an unstable coronary syndrome, the perioperative cardiac risk is substantial, and there is significant potential for reducing the risk by delaying surgery until the coronary status is stable. Thus, when feasible, surgery should be delayed in these patients to allow for stabilization of ischemic symptoms and consideration for revascularization.

Coronary Revascularization

The precise role of preoperative revascularization by either coronary artery bypass graft (CABG) surgery or percutaneous transluminal coronary angioplasty (PTCA) is a subject of controversy, due in large part to the absence of controlled studies of patients undergoing preoperative revascularization. Patients who have previously undergone CABG surgery are generally at low risk for cardiac complications of subsequent noncardiac surgery, particularly if the CABG surgery was performed within 5 years of the subsequent surgery. Additional information in patients with angina who have undergone peripheral vascular surgery indicates that those whose angina was treated with CABG surgery had an improved long-term survival compared with those treated with medical therapy.

Results from the Coronary Artery Surgery Study (CASS) demonstrated that patients with coronary artery stenoses of greater than 70% who underwent CABG surgery had a 0.9% mortality with subsequent noncardiac surgery compared with 2.4% for patients treated

TABLE 14–2

Perioperative Beta-Blockers: Agents and Regimens

	Not taking beta-blockers chronically	Taking beta-blockers chronically
Prehospitalization (outpatients) or immediately following admission to hospital	Atenolol 50–100 PO qd OR Bisoprolol 5-10 PO qd	Continue chronic therapy
	Begin as outpatient, up to 30 days prior to surgery	Titrate to heart rate 65 beats/min or lower prior to hospitalization
	Titrate to heart rate of 65 beats/min or lower	
Immediate preoperative period (i.e., in preanesthesia holding area)	Atenolol 5–10 mg IV to reach target heart rate before induction of anesthesia, if needed	Same
Immediate postoperative period	*Patient not taking PO and hemodynamically stable*: Atenolol 5–10 mg IV bid to target heart rate or metoprolol IV to target heart rate	Same
	Patient unstable (i.e., high bleeding risk, or in ICU): Esmolol IV to target heart rate	Same
	Patient taking PO: Resume preoperative beta-blocker at previous dose	
In hospital	Continue preoperative oral beta-blocking agent; titrate to target heart rate	Same
Posthospitalization (outpatient)	Continue preoperative beta-blocker to 30 days postoperatively and taper Consider continuing beta-blocker chronically in appropriate patients, such as those with a history of myocardial infarction, angina, heart failure, or previously unrecognized hypertension	Continue chronic agent

Adapted from Auerbach AD, Goldman L: β-blockers and reduction of cardiac events in noncardiac surgery: Scientific review. JAMA 2002;287:1435–1444.

medically.[21] Patients who survive PTCA appear to receive similar benefits.[22] Noncardiac surgery is hazardous, however, if performed within 2 weeks after a coronary stent procedure because of the high risk of bleeding if anticoagulant medications are continued and of stent thrombosis if they are discontinued.[23] Therefore, it is recommended that noncardiac surgery be delayed at least 4 weeks after a coronary stent procedure. Although these data suggest that patients who undergo revascularization with CABG surgery or PTCA are at low risk for complications with subsequent noncardiac surgery, the magnitude of the risk reduction does not seem to justify the risks of the revascularization procedure itself for patients who are at low risk because the risk of the coronary revascularization procedure itself is in the 1.5% to 2% range.

The 2002 AHA guidelines recommend that angiography and revascularization be predominantly limited to patients who meet the indications for these procedures independent of surgery.[2,24] In such patients, coronary revascularization should generally precede a noncardiac operation, when feasible.

By combining information from studies of risk assessment and beta-blocker therapy,[1,18,19] an updated approach to the perioperative assessment and management of patients with known or suspected coronary disease can be developed (Fig. 14–2). These recommendations emphasize the use of beta-blockers and limit noninvasive testing to situations that would possibly influence a decision regarding preoperative coronary revascularization.[25] With the use of beta-blockers, the large majority of patients with CAD appear to have perioperative risks that are too low to warrant the risks of preoperative coronary revascularization, unless they otherwise meet criteria for CABG or PTCA (see Chapter 25). Patients with unstable angina (see Chapter 26) must be stabilized, if possible, before surgery.

Anesthesia

Neuroaxial blockade, in which local anesthetic medications are used for spinal or epidural anesthesia, may reduce overall postoperative morbidity and mortality.[26] There is no clearly preferred anesthetic technique or combination of anesthetic medications for patients with CAD. Multiple studies have compared the use of different inhalational anesthetic agents and have found no differences in cardiac outcomes. Spinal/epidural anesthesia is associated with peripheral hemodynamic effects similar to those of general anesthesia but it does not cause direct myocardial depression. Opioid-based intravenous anesthetic techniques appear to be associated with greater hemodynamic stability, although they have not been associated with better cardiac outcomes. The choice of anesthetic technique is generally at the discretion of the anesthesiologist and is individualized

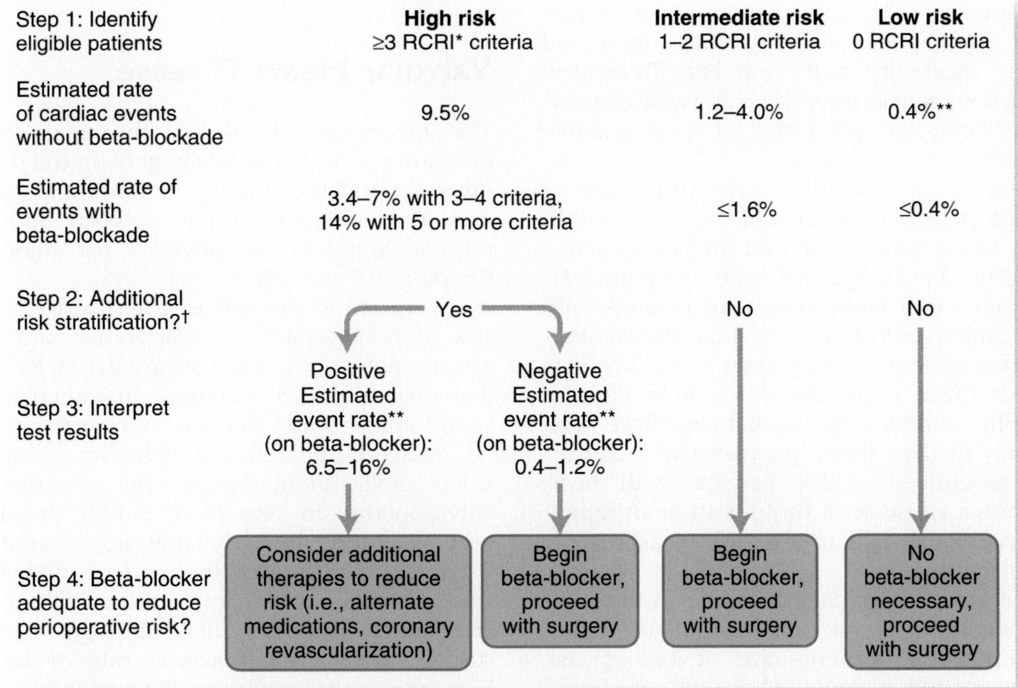

FIGURE 14–2. Perioperative beta-blockers: Patient selection. *RCRI = Revised Cardiac Risk Index; see Box 14–1 and Table 14–1. **Based on data from Boersma E, Poldermans D, Bax JJ, et al: Predictors of cardiac events after major vascular surgery: Role of clinical characteristics, dobutamine echocardiography, and β-blocker therapy. JAMA 2001;285:1865–1873.† Options include dipyridamole thallium scintigraphy, stress echocardiography, exercise electrocardiography, or cardiac catheterization, in appropriate patients. (Adapted from Auerbach AD, Goldman L: β-blockers and reduction of cardiac events in noncardiac surgery: Scientific review. JAMA 2002;287:1435–1444.)

for each patient based on a variety of clinical factors. The medical consultant can provide the anesthesiologist with an accurate cardiac assessment to help the anesthesiologist to choose appropriate individualized anesthesia.

Intraoperative Monitoring

A variety of intraoperative monitoring techniques can be used in patients with CAD, including pulmonary artery catheterization and transesophageal echocardiography. Whether used routinely or in selected patients who receive such catheters as part of their clinical care, pulmonary catheters have not reduced perioperative cardiac complications or improved outcomes.[27–29] The limited data on the use of intraoperative transesophageal echocardiography to detect myocardial ischemia suggest that such monitoring also does not improve outcomes. In practice, the decision to use these monitoring devices is generally left to the anesthesiologist.

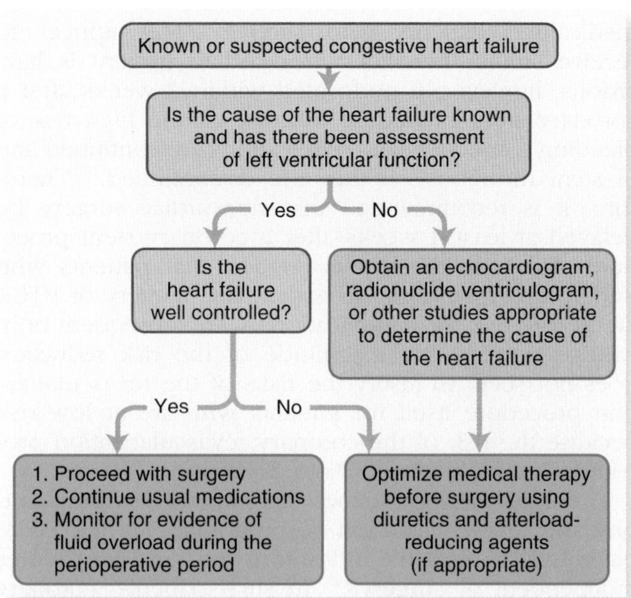

FIGURE 14–3. Preoperative management of a patient with congestive heart failure.

Heart Failure and Left Ventricular Dysfunction

Heart failure and left ventricular systolic dysfunction (see Chapter 28) have been associated with increased perioperative morbidity.[1,4,5] Patients with decompensated heart failure, as manifested by an audible third heart sound, jugular venous distention, or a history of pulmonary edema, are at substantially increased risk of cardiac morbidity and mortality. Decreased ventricular function, as measured by echocardiography, is also an independent predictor of perioperative complications.[5,17]

It is important to determine the underlying cause of heart failure preoperatively because it may have implications for the assessment of risk and for perioperative management (Fig. 14–3). Patients with ischemic cardiomyopathy may be at higher risk than patients with heart failure from hypertension or valvular disease. Furthermore, the perioperative management of medications and intravenous fluids is usually different in patients with hypertrophic cardiomyopathy than in those with dilated cardiomyopathy. Thus, preoperative echocardiography is recommended for patients with heart failure of unknown cause or in those with heart failure who have not previously had an objective measurement of left ventricular function.

Regardless of cause, a guiding principle in the perioperative management of patients with heart failure is that decompensated patients are at higher risk than well-compensated patients. Thus, efforts should be made in the preoperative period to optimize the medical therapy before surgery, which generally will include diuretics and angiotensin-converting enzyme (ACE) inhibitors. Although this strategy is likely to reduce the risk of cardiac morbidity, it has not been studied in randomized clinical trials. Low-dose beta-blocking agents and spironolactone have been shown to reduce morbidity and mortality in patients with severe heart failure. Neither of these two agents have been studied, however, in the perioperative setting for heart failure patients, and thus they are not routinely recommended.

Valvular Heart Disease

The importance of valvular abnormalities in the perioperative period depends largely on the particular valve involved and the severity of the abnormality. In addition, the presence of any valvular abnormality may require antibiotic prophylaxis for endocarditis (see Chapters 32 and 33).

Severe aortic stenosis is associated with the greatest risk of perioperative complications, and patients with symptomatic aortic stenosis appear to be at higher risk than asymptomatic patients. In patients with severe, symptomatic aortic stenosis, noncardiac surgery should be delayed until after a valvular procedure, usually valve replacement surgery but occasionally balloon valvuloplasty, in very ill or elderly patients in whom only short-term hemodynamic improvement is sought.

Limited data suggest that patients with asymptomatic severe aortic stenosis, even those with an aortic valve area less than 1.0 cm^2, may undergo major noncardiac surgery with a complication rate of less than 10%. However, even asymptomatic patients with valve gradients above 40 mm Hg appear to be at increased risk.[17] Noncardiac surgery should be approached cautiously in any patient with aortic valve stenosis.

Patients with mitral stenosis may be at increased risk for perioperative complications, particularly from atrial arrhythmias and congestive heart failure. These patients may benefit from mitral valve surgery or valvuloplasty before noncardiac surgery. In patients with mild mitral stenosis, preoperative control of the heart rate and congestive heart failure should be ensured.

More than mild mitral valve regurgitation imparts excess perioperative risk independent of heart failure or CAD.[17] Preoperative management should focus on controlling congestive heart failure through the use of diuretics and ACE inhibitors or other afterload-reducing agents.

In patients on warfarin because of a mechanical heart valve or atrial fibrillation, the medication should be discontinued preoperatively to allow the International Normalized Ratio (INR) to fall to 1.5 or below, and the patient should be treated with subcutaneous heparin beginning about 12 hours after surgery. If needed, small doses (1 mg subcutaneously) of vitamin K can be given to reduce the preoperative INR more rapidly.[30]

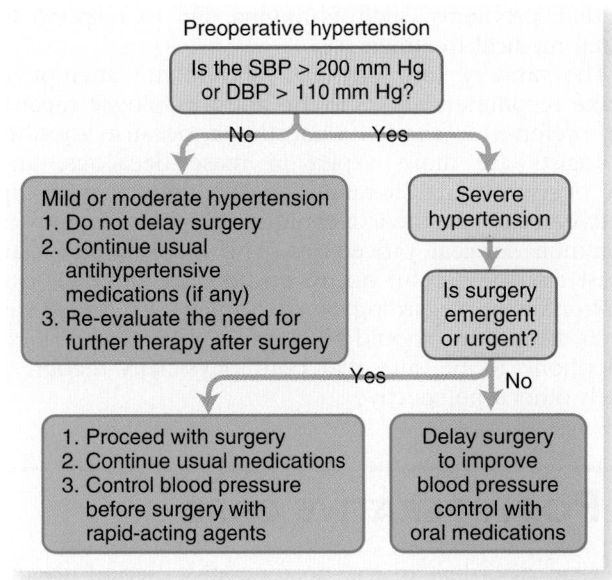

FIGURE 14–4. Preoperative management of a patient with hypertension.

Arrhythmias and Conduction Disease (see Chapters 30 and 31)

Atrial and ventricular arrhythmias have been associated with an increased risk of perioperative cardiac complications. Data have demonstrated that these arrhythmias are frequently associated with structural heart disease, particularly CAD and left ventricular dysfunction. It is likely that much of the perioperative cardiac morbidity in patients with both findings is attributable to the structural heart disease rather than to the rhythm disturbance. Patients with a rhythm disturbance and no evidence of structural heart disease are at very low risk for perioperative cardiac complications. The finding of an arrhythmia on preoperative evaluation should prompt a search for previously unsuspected structural heart disease, particularly if the finding of structural heart disease would alter perioperative management.

Patients with preoperative arrhythmias should receive therapy appropriate for the arrhythmia, independent of surgery. Adequate ventricular rate control should be ensured in patients with atrial fibrillation. Symptomatic supraventricular and ventricular arrhythmias should be treated before surgery. Suppression of asymptomatic arrhythmias before surgery is unlikely to reduce the risk of perioperative cardiac morbidity.

Patients who have indications for permanent pacemaker placement independent of the surgery should generally have the pacemaker placed before elective surgery. For urgent surgery, temporary transvenous pacing should be used during surgery and the perioperative period. Patients who do not meet criteria for permanent pacing, such as those with left bundle branch block, generally do not require temporary pacing during or after surgery.

Hypertension

Preoperative hypertension has been associated with intraoperative blood pressure lability and ECG evidence of ischemia. Patients with severe hypertension, defined as a diastolic blood pressure greater than 110 mm Hg, appear to be at increased risk for perioperative MI and congestive heart failure. Patients with mild or moderate hypertension, however, appear to be at no excess risk for important cardiac morbidity.[31]

Antihypertensive medication should be continued up to and including the day of surgery (Fig. 14–4). In patients with severe preoperative hypertension, it is prudent to delay elective surgery to allow for control of blood pressure for several days. When surgery is urgent, blood pressure should be controlled before the induction of anesthesia, using rapidly acting intravenous antihypertensive agents if necessary. Beta blocking agents and sodium nitroprusside are useful in this setting (see Chapter 19).

In patients with mild or moderate hypertension, surgery need not be delayed. In these patients, the addition of new antihypertensive agents or dosage changes in existing agents during the immediate preoperative period is not likely to reduce the risk of perioperative cardiac complications. When surgery is not scheduled for several weeks, however, it is prudent to try to improve blood pressure control preoperatively.

Role of the Primary Care Physician

The primary care physician should be able to assess and follow his or her own patients through surgery and to serve as a consultant for new patients. The primary care physician should be able to order and evaluate the results of indicated noninvasive tests, but consultation with a cardiologist is recommended when coronary angiography is being considered as a prelude to possible coronary revascularization, and for patients whose cardiac problems, such as angina, fail to respond to usual medical treatment.

The primary care physician should not attempt to make recommendations to the anesthesiologist regarding preferred methods for anesthesia, because anesthesiologists are more expert in these decisions, and an overwhelming literature reveals little relationship between the anesthetic technique and the outcomes of common surgical procedures. The medical physician must also be careful not to engage the surgeon in a written debate regarding the advisability of surgery. Any such discussions should be conducted in person or by telephone to be sure that both physicians recognize each other's perspective.

POSTOPERATIVE CARE

Cardiac disorders in the postoperative period should generally be managed similarly to those in the nonsurgical setting.

Ischemic Heart Disease

Early identification of postoperative MI may alter management and potentially, cardiac outcomes. Serum troponin T or I levels have been shown to be at least as sensitive and somewhat more specific than CK-MB isoenzymes for perioperative myocardial injury. The AHA guidelines advise limiting routine surveillance for perioperative MI to patients with known or suspected CAD.[2] An immediate postoperative ECG and one daily for 2 days is a reasonable strategy.[3] Serum troponin levels should be reserved for patients at high risk for cardiac complications and for those who experience perioperative events suspicious for an MI.

Postoperative ischemia or ST segment changes are a potent predictor of postoperative cardiac complications in high-risk patients.[32] There is the potential that early recognition of postoperative ischemia may allow for rapid treatment and prevention of complications. At present, this strategy has not been evaluated in clinical trials. Postoperative ST segment monitoring is of uncertain benefit and should be used only in high-risk patients in whom it is likely to alter management.

Patients who sustain a perioperative MI have a 15% to 20% in-hospital mortality, and are at substantially increased risk for subsequent MI or cardiac death during the following 10 years. The acute management of perioperative MI or ischemia is similar to the treatment in the nonsurgical setting (see Chapters 26 and 27), with the caveat that the recent surgery may make the bleeding risk of anticoagulation or thrombolysis prohibitive. Once stabilized, most of these patients should undergo noninvasive ischemia testing before discharge. Those with persistent ischemia should be considered for angiography and revascularization.

Patients identified during the preoperative evaluation to have stable CAD should be re-evaluated postoperatively to confirm that medical therapy is optimal and that risk factors for CAD—including hypertension, hyperlipidemia, and tobacco use—have been addressed. Patients without overt CAD preoperatively should be considered for screening for and treatment of coronary disease risk factors during the postoperative period.

Arrhythmias

Postoperative arrhythmias, both ventricular and supraventricular, are often caused by noncardiac problems including infection, abnormalities in serum electrolyte levels, and hypoxia. Management should focus on the identification of the cause of the arrhythmia, either cardiac or noncardiac, and correction of the underlying disorder. Noncardiac causes of rhythm disorders should generally be corrected before attempting cardioversion because the arrhythmia often resolves spontaneously with correction of the underlying cause. When an arrhythmia is associated with hemodynamic compromise, antiarrhythmic medications or electrical cardioversion may be necessary. Correction of the underlying cause remains essential to prevent recurrence of the arrhythmia.

Hypertension

Brief hypertensive episodes are not uncommon in the immediate postoperative period in patients both with and without hypertension preoperatively. Most episodes occur within 1 hour of the end of anesthesia and resolve in a few hours. These episodes most commonly are precipitated by noncardiac problems such as discomfort from the endotracheal tube, pain, hypoxemia, fluid overload, and hypothermia. Treatment directed primarily at these precipitants will usually result in adequate control of blood pressure.

Severe or prolonged hypertensive episodes may require specific antihypertensive therapy, although the exact degree or duration of hypertension for which antihypertensive therapy is of benefit has not been evaluated in clinical trials. A reasonable approach is to treat patients with a diastolic blood pressure above 100 mm Hg or a systolic blood pressure above 200 mm Hg, those whose hypertension does not respond to treatment of precipitants, and those with evidence of myocardial ischemia or cerebral dysfunction. Several intravenous medications are effective in rapidly controlling blood pressure in this setting, including sodium nitroprusside, beta-blocking agents, and calcium channel blocking agents (see Chapter 16).

Heart Failure

Postoperative heart failure usually occurs in the first 2 or 3 postoperative days. Excess fluid administration and myocardial ischemia are the most common precipitating factors. In patients who develop heart failure after surgery, it is important to evaluate for myocardial ischemia or infarction with a 12-lead ECG and cardiac biomarkers (if appropriate), especially in patients with known CAD. Diuretic therapy will usually produce rapid improvement, particularly in patients without concomitant myocardial ischemia.

Role of the Primary Care Physician

The primary care physician should participate actively in the postoperative follow-up of the surgical patient. A daily focused history and physical examination should concentrate on the status of chronic medical problems, the development of possible cardiac signs and symptoms, evidence for local infection or other direct surgical complications, the evaluation of possible deep venous thrombosis, and a careful pulmonary examination to exclude postoperative pneumonia. The medical physician should acquire a good sense of the usual pace of recovery after common surgical procedures and recognize that a patient's failure to demonstrate expected improvement may be a nonspecific sign of an impending important cardiac or noncardiac problem. For example, an otherwise unexplained tachycardia or altered mental status may be the first evidence of postoperative hypoxia, myocardial ischemia, or heart failure. The primary care physician should also help guide the patient's transition to posthospital care, including plans for the titration or adjustment of cardiac medications. Consultation with a cardiologist is recommended for patients who develop postoperative MI or who develop myocardial ischemia, arrhythmias, or heart failure that does not respond to usual measures.

Evidence-Based Summary

- Different types of surgical procedures carry inherently different risks of cardiac complications, independent of the patient's individual characteristics (see Box 14–1).
- The new multifactorial cardiac risk index (see Box 14–2) appears to provide accurate estimates of risk in contemporary elective surgical patients. Although high-risk characteristics, such as a recent MI and severe aortic stenosis, are rarely present in patients currently undergoing elective surgery, they are known risk factors that must be taken into account when present.
- Preoperative, perioperative, and postoperative beta-blocker therapy can reduce the risk of perioperative and subsequent cardiac complications by 50%, or more, in patients who have coronary disease or who are at high risk for it.
- Alpha-2 agonists may be useful in patients who cannot tolerate beta-blockers.
- Given the apparent benefit of perioperative beta-blockers, cardiac noninvasive testing is probably most useful in patients who are at high clinical risk by a multifactorial index, in whom a positive noninvasive test may warrant preoperative coronary revascularization (see Fig. 14–2).
- There is little, if any, correlation between anesthetic technique and cardiac outcomes. Decisions regarding anesthetic technique should be made by the anesthesiologist.
- Preoperative coronary revascularization, using either CABG or PTCA, is associated with about a 1% to 2% peri-procedural mortality and appears to be associated with a lower risk for the subsequent noncardiac surgery. With the advent of beta-blocker therapy, preoperative coronary revascularization probably should be reserved for patients at very high clinical risk (see Fig. 14–2).

References

1. Lee TH, Marcantonio ER, Mangione CM, et al: Derivation and prospective validation of a simple index for prediction of cardiac risk of major noncardiac surgery. Circulation 1999;100:1043–1049.
2. Eagle KA, Berger PB, Calkins H, et al: ACC/AHA guideline update for perioperative cardiovascular evaluation for noncardiac surgery—executive summary. A report of the American College of Cardiology/American Heart Association Task Force on Practice Guidelines (Committee to Update the 1996 Guidelines on Perioperative Cardiovascular Evaluation for Noncardiac Surgery). Circulation 2002;105:1257–1267.
3. Gilbert K, Larocque BJ, Patrick LT: Prospective evaluation of cardiac risk indices for patients undergoing noncardiac surgery. Ann Intern Med 2000;133:356–359.
4. Kumar R, McKinney WP, Raj G, et al: Adverse cardiac events after surgery: Assessing risk in a veteran population. J Gen Intern Med 2001;16:507–518.
5. Boersma E, Poldermans D, Bax JJ, et al: Predictors of cardiac events after major vascular surgery: Role of clinical characteristics, dobutamine echocardiography, and β-blocker therapy. JAMA 2001;285:1865–1873.
6. Goldman L, Caldera DL, Nussbaum, SR, et al: Multifactorial index of cardiac risk in noncardiac surgical procedures. N Engl J Med 1977;297:845–850.
7. Detsky AS, Abrahms HB, McLaughlin JR, et al: Predicting cardiac complications in patients undergoing non-cardiac surgery. J Gen Intern Med 1986;1:211–219.
8. Goldman L, Adler J: General anesthesia and noncardiac surgery in patients with heart disease. In Braunwald E, Zipes DP, Libby P (eds): Heart Disease: A Textbook of Cardiovascular Medicine, 6th ed. Philadelphia, WB Saunders, 2001, pp 2084–2097.
9. Ashton CM, Peterson NJ, Wray NP, et al: The incidence of perioperative myocardial infarction in men undergoing noncardiac surgery. Ann Intern Med 1993;118:504–510.
10. L'Italien GJ, Paul SD, Hendel RC, et al: Development and validation of a Bayesian model for perioperative cardiac risk assessment in a cohort of 1081 vascular surgical candidates. J Am Coll Cardiol 1996;27:779–786.

11. Lee TH: Reducing cardiac risk in noncardiac surgery. N Engl J Med 1999;341:1838–1840.
12. Goldman L: Assessing and reducing cardiac risks of noncardiac surgery. Am J Med 2001;110:320–323.
13. Mathes DD, Stone DJ, Dent JM: Preoperative cardiac risk stratification: Ritual or requirement? J Cardiothorac Vasc Anesth 2001;15:626–630.
14. Palda VA, Detsky AS: for the American College of Physicians Clinical Efficacy Assessment Subcommittee: Guidelines for assessing and managing the perioperative risk from coronary artery disease associated with major noncardiac surgery. Ann Intern Med 1997;127:309–312.
15. de Virgilio C, Toosie K, Ephraim L, et al: Dipyridamole-thallium/sestamibi before vascular surgery: A prospective blinded study in moderate risk patients. J Vasc Surg 2000;32:77–89.
16. Das MK, Pellikka PA, Mahoney DW, et al: Assessment of cardiac risk before nonvascular surgery. J Am Coll Cardiol 2000;35:1647–1653.
17. Rohde LE, Polanczyk CA, Goldman L, et al: Usefulness of transthoracic echocardiography as a tool for risk stratification of patients undergoing major noncardiac surgery. Am J Cardiol 2001;87:505–509.
18. Poldermans D, Boersma E, Bax JJ, et al: The effect of bisoprolol on perioperative mortality and myocardial infarction in high-risk patients undergoing vascular surgery. N Engl J Med 1999;341:1789.
19. Mangano DT, Layug EL, Wallace A, Tareo I: Effects of atenolol on mortality and cardiovascular morbidity after noncardiac surgery. The Multicenter Study of Perioperative Ischemia Research Group. N Engl J Med 1996;335: 1713–1720.
20. Oliver M, Goldman L, Julian DG, et al: Effect of mivazerol on perioperative cardiac complications during noncardiac surgery in patients with coronary heart disease: The European mivazerol trial (EMIT). Anesthesiology 1999;91:951–959.
21. Eagle KA, Rihal CS, Mickel MC, et al for the Coronary Artery Surgery Study (CASS) Investigators and University of Michigan Heart Care Program: Cardiac risk of noncardiac surgery. Influence of coronary disease and type of surgery in 3368 operations. Circulation 1997;96:1882–1887.
22. Hassan SA, Hlatky MA, Boothroyd DB, et al: Outcomes of noncardiac surgery after coronary bypass surgery or coronary angioplasty in the bypass angioplasty revascularization investigation (BARI). Am J Med 2001;110:260–266.
23. Kaluza GL, Joseph J, Lee JR, et al: Catastrophic outcomes of noncardiac surgery soon after coronary stenting. J Am Coll Cardiol 2000;35;1288–1294.
24. Fleisher LA, Eagle KA: Lowering cardiac risk in noncardiac surgery. N Engl J Med 2001;345:1677–1682.
25. Auerbach AD, Goldman L: β-blockers and reduction of cardiac events in non-cardiac surgery: Scientific review. JAMA 2002;287:1435–1444.
26. Rigg JRA, Jamrozik K, Myles PS, et al: For the MASTER Anaesthesia Trial Study Group: Epidural anaesthesia and analgesia and outcome of major surgery: A randomised trial. Lancet 2002;359:1276–1282.
27. Barone JE, Tucker JB, Rassias D, Corvo PR: Routine perioperative pulmonary artery catheterization has no effect on rate of complications in vascular surgery: A meta-analysis. Am J Surg 2001;67:674–679.
28. Polanczyk CA, Rohde LE, Goldman L, et al: Right heart catheterization and cardiac complications in patients undergoing noncardiac surgery: An observational study. JAMA 2001;286:309–314.
29. Sanham JD, Hull RD, Brant RF, Canadian Critical Care Clinical Trials Group: A randomized controlled trial of pulmonary artery catheter use in 1994 high-risk geriatric surgical patients [abstract]. Am J Respir Crit Care Med 2001;163:A16.
30. Kearon C, Hirsh J: Management of anticoagulation before and after elective surgery. N Engl J Med 1997;336:1506–1511.
31. Fleisher LA: Preoperative evaluation of the patient with hypertension. JAMA 2002;287:2043–2046.
32. Landesberg G, Mosseri M, Zahger D, et al: Myocardial infarction after vascular surgery: The role of prolonged, stress-induced, ST depression-type ischemia. J Am Coll Cardiol 2001;37:1839–1845.

CHAPTER 15 Approach to the Woman with Heart Disease, Including During Pregnancy

Pamela Charney and Sandra Wainwright

CORONARY ARTERY DISEASE

Coronary artery disease (CAD) is a major contributor of morbidity and mortality in women (Fig. 15–1), with one third of all deaths in women attributed to CAD.[1] However, both patients and physicians have often not acknowledged the importance of this condition and have incorrectly assumed that CAD is primarily a disease of men. In a national survey of American women, 58% reported that they thought they were more likely to die of breast cancer than CAD, and almost half stated that their physician had not discussed heart disease or its prevention with them. Thus, both women and their physicians underestimate the frequency and seriousness of CAD. This is compounded by the difficulties inherent in diagnosing CAD in women. All forms of CAD (i.e., chronic angina, unstable angina, and acute myocardial infarction) are frequently associated with more atypical symptoms in women than in men.

Physicians' perceptions of a woman's risk for CAD have been shown to be affected by their preconceived biases. In one study, an actress portrayed a woman with chest pain using the same script but different clothes and affect for each of several films. Physicians who observed the video in which the actress described the chest pain with exaggerated emotion predicted that she was less likely to have CAD than did physicians who observed the same actress and script presented in a more businesslike manner. More recently, physicians were recruited to view a video of different actors (black and white women and men) accompanied by the same written information. Physicians were least likely to refer the black woman actress for cardiac catheterization.

Epidemiology and Risk Factors

Epidemiology

CAD is not only the most common cause of mortality in women, but its frequency increases more rapidly with advancing age than does stroke, breast or lung cancer mortality (see Fig. 15–1). In middle-aged (40 to 60 years) populations around the world, men are 2.5 to 4.5 times more likely to die from CAD than are women. Historically, protective effects of estrogen have been suggested as the principal reason why middle-aged women have lower rates of CAD than do men.[2] In older populations, the divergence in CAD prevalence and mortality rates between women and men are markedly reduced and disappear by age 75 years. The Framingham Heart Study noted in white middle-aged patients that clinical CAD occurred about ten years later in women than in men. Furthermore, women presented initially primarily with angina, whereas men presented initially more frequently with acute myocardial infarction.

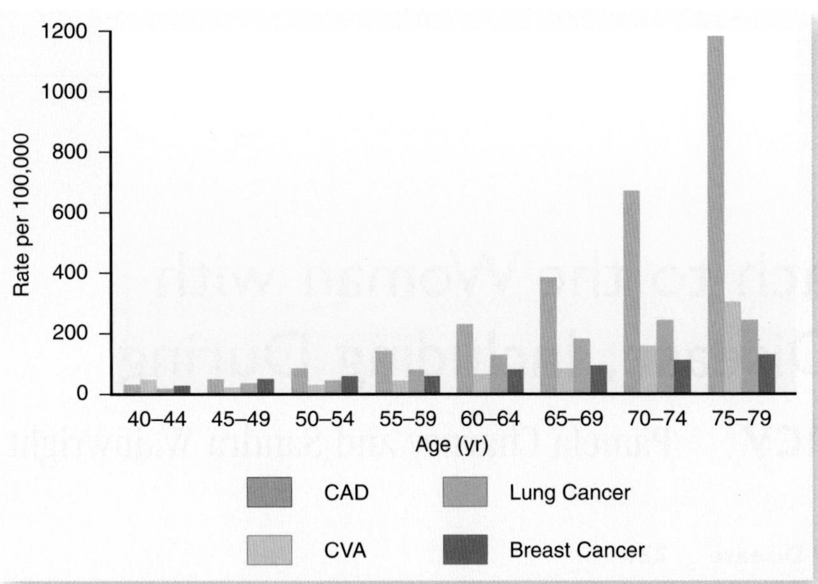

FIGURE 15–1. Age-specific mortality in U.S. women, 1997. (From Wingo PA, Calle EE, McTiernan A: How does breast cancer mortality compare with that of other cancers and selected cardiovascular diseases at different ages in U.S. women? J Womens Health Gend Based Med 2000;9:999.)

Black women develop hypertension, diabetes, and obesity at a younger age than do white women, and black women younger than 55 years have more than twice the incidence of CAD mortality than do white women of the same age. One example of physiologic differences that influence management is that with similar tobacco consumption, black smokers have a slower cotinine clearance and higher serum cotinine levels than do white and Hispanic smokers (see Chapter 21). This observation suggests that black smokers may require pharmacologic aids for tobacco cessation at lower levels of tobacco consumption than white smokers.

Risk Assessment

Results from the Third National Health and Nutrition Examination Survey highlighted the importance of race in the assessment of risk for CAD (Box 15–1). Black and Mexican-American women had higher body mass index (BMI), systolic blood pressure, diabetes, and lower tobacco use than white women of similar socioeconomic status.[3] With increasing age, black and Mexican-American women had a greater prevalence of hypertension than did white women. Smoking rates were also more stable with aging in black and Mexican-American women, whereas they decreased for white women.

The prevalence and impact of individual and multiple risk factors were assessed in the Chicago Heart Association Detection Project in Industry. At the time of enrollment, workers age 40 to 64 years were asked about current tobacco use, blood pressure was recorded and serum cholesterol was determined. About 80% of women participants initially had at least one of these risk factors; two risk factors were found in 34%, whereas all three risk factors were noted in less than 7%. Participants with the most risk factors were at the highest risk of death and high health care costs. Tobacco use was a significantly more important predictor of mortality in women than in men (relative risk 2.85 vs. 1.68, $P < .001$, comparing current smokers with nonsmokers). Women who had fewer risk factors had better long-term cardiovascular outcomes. Thus, women who were *not* current smokers, with blood pressure less than 120/80 mm Hg, total cholesterol less than 200 mg/dL, no history of diabetes or myocardial infarction, and no ECG abnormalities constituted 7% of the cohort at entry. At a mean follow-up of 22 years, however, these women had substantially lower CAD mortality with a relative risk only one fifth of the average.[4]

Clustering of risk factors was also found to be particularly important in women in the follow-up of the Framingham Offspring Study. Seventeen percent of all participants had three of six risk factors (lowest quintile HDL, highest quintile cholesterol, BMI, systolic blood pressure, triglycerides, and glucose). CAD events were associated with three or more risk factors in 48% of women with CAD, compared with only 20% of the men.[5]

Tobacco

Over the last few decades, the percentage of women who smoke has decreased at a slower rate than the percentage of men who do so (see Chapter 21). Although adverse effects of tobacco exposure are dose-related, even with five cigarettes daily or secondhand smoke exposure a woman's risk of CAD increases.[6] Young white women have the highest smoking initiation rates of any gender-racial group and women are less successful than men in tobacco cessation. Fear of weight gain is a major barrier to smoking cessation among women smokers. Tobacco use increases smokers' metabolic rates and most smokers gain weight with smoking cessation. Women smokers are less willing than men to

BOX 15–1

Coronary Artery Disease Risk Factors: Specific Considerations for Women

Tobacco	Young white women have highest initiation rates Women have more difficulty stopping initially and long term Women report fear of weight gain with cessation Weight gain is less while using Wellbutrin
Diabetes	"Female advantage" is lost Gestational diabetes is a risk factor for the subsequent development of diabetes; risk is decreased by regular exercise
Physical activity	Women have less leisure activity, more housework than men Women choose gardening & walking, rather than team sports
Menopause and HRT	Age of menopause is less important than smoking status HRT increases risk of cardiac event and venous thromboembolism, especially at initiation HRT decreases bone fracture rate but also increases gall bladder disease HRT for more than 5 years increases breast cancer risk
Hypertension	It is more common in women and in blacks compared with whites Women with LVH are at higher risk for CAD events than are men ACE and ARB agents are to be avoided in pregnancy Thiazide diuretics decrease fracture rate
Lipids	HDL is most important in women Triglycerides decrease with statins but increase with HRT
Obesity	It is increasingly common in women It carries negative social implications for white women, but not for black or Hispanic women Weight gain after age 18 predicts greater risk of events
Psychosocial issues	Depression and anxiety is more common in women than in men Aggressive pharmacologic treatment after MI improves outcomes
Socioeconomic status	Women are poorer than men and earn less money for similar work Less education and control over work increases CAD event risk

gain weight in order to discontinue smoking. Smoking cessation programs that include counseling and physical activity are more successful in decreasing tobacco use.

Diabetes

Women with diabetes mellitus and those with glucose intolerance without frank diabetes are at a markedly increased risk not only for the development of coronary events but also for mortality if they do develop acute myocardial infarction. Practically speaking, women with diabetes lose the "female protection" from CAD that nondiabetic women enjoy in middle age. Diabetic lipid abnormalities are an example of sex differences in a coronary risk factor. At the time of diagnosis of type II diabetes mellitus, substantial differences between women and men were observed in the United Kingdom Diabetes Study. Women had lower HDL cholesterol concentrations than age-matched diabetic men or nondiabetic women. Subgroup analyses of diabetics within the large HMG-CoA reductase inhibitor (statin) trials have demonstrated benefit from the aggressive treatment of lipid abnormalities among diabetic patients. However, in clinical practice, women generally receive less aggressive management of lipid abnormalities than do men.

Menopause and Postmenopausal Hormone Replacement

Historically, early menopause *without* hormone replacement therapy (HRT) has been considered to be a risk factor for CAD. However, the Nurse's Health Study suggested that the higher rate of coronary events with early menopause could be explained by higher tobacco consumption.[7] Estrogen has been used since 1935 to treat menopausal vasomotor symptoms. A number of trials have shown a beneficial effect of both estrogen and estrogen plus progesterone on lipid profiles, with increased HDL cholesterol, and decreased LDL cholesterol. However, in contrast to statins, HRT *raises* triglycerides and C-reactive protein (CRP) (see Chapter 23).

Several observational studies, including the Nurse's Health Study, have suggested that HRT reduces cardiovascular mortality by about 35%. However, women choosing HRT tend to be healthier, exercise more, weigh less, and avoid tobacco exposure. Actually, several secondary prevention studies with HRT have revealed an increased risk of thromboembolic and coronary disease events soon after HRT is begun. The Heart and Estrogen/Progestin Replacement Study (HERS) trial was a double-blinded study conducted in postmenopausal women with documented CAD who were randomized to a combination of conjugated estrogen plus progestin or placebo.[8] HERS demonstrated that the rate of major coronary events was 52% higher in the hormone treatment group during the first year following randomization. The difference between treatment and placebo arms decreased with follow-up, with only a small number of subjects in years 4 and 5. Similar to other studies, an excess of thromboembolic events occurred soon after HRT was started.

Results from the Women's Health Initiative have been released for hormone replacement therapy. This large, double-blind, randomized trial of postmenopausal women compared conjugated estrogen plus medroxyprogesterone or estrogen alone (only in patients with prior hysterectomy) with placebo. After a mean of 5.2 years' follow-up, the estrogen and progesterone combination arm was stopped because of greater risk of coronary heart disease events, stroke, pulmonary emboli, and breast cancer than decreases in hip fracture or colon cancer (Fig. 15–2).[8a]

As of November 2002, the estrogen-only arm of the trial was still ongoing. However, because endometrial cancer risk increases with duration of exposure to estrogen without progesterone, only women without a uterus are candidates for unopposed estrogen. The Women's Health Initiative results negate the hope that an estrogen-progesterone combination is valuable for the prevention of coronary heart disease. However, there is still a limited role for short-term administration of the estrogen-progesterone combination for relief of severe hot flashes (see Chapter 23).

Physical Activity

Historically, physical activity has been predominantly measured during leisure time. Men report substantially more hours of leisure time activity than do women. Yet women report substantially more physical activity within the home, i.e., housework. Women describe leisure time activities such as gardening and walking, whereas men note participation in group sports. White women report more leisure time activity than do black and Hispanic women.

Physical activity has decreased dramatically with increased industrialization. Whereas prior guidelines stressed the importance of dedicated exercise periods, newer guidelines stress the importance of cumulative activity over the course of the day. This is consistent with promoting increasing activity within daily tasks rather than depending on participation in leisure time activities. After one year in a clinical trial to encourage weight loss through dietary counseling and increasing physical activity, women who increased activity in daily life maintained weight loss more successfully than did women randomized to an aerobics program.

Hypertension (for further discussion, see Chapter 19)

Both elevated systolic and diastolic blood pressures are risk factors for more frequent myocardial infarction, stroke, congestive heart failure, and sudden death. Because life expectancy is greater for women than for men and the prevalence of hypertension increases with advancing age, there are more elderly women than men with hypertension; almost four fifths of women older than 75 years are hypertensive. Black women and men have a higher prevalence of hypertension than their white counterparts at all ages. Left ventricular hypertrophy is a common complication of hypertension and increases the risk of cardiovascular events in women more than it does in men.

There are special considerations when choosing pharmacologic treatment for hypertension in women. Angiotensin-converting enzyme inhibitors and angiotensin receptor blockers, although very effective antihypertensive agents, pose a serious teratogenic risk. Practically, this requires that fertile women who would consider continuing a pregnancy, even if unplanned, be especially vigilant with birth control or switch to another antihypertensive drug, or both. Cough, a common side effect of angiotensin-converting enzyme inhibitors, occurs more frequently in women than in men. Thiazide diuretics are a reasonable first choice in the treatment of hypertension in women and are associated with a lower incidence of hip fracture.

Hypertensive women should be assessed for other CAD risk factors and if any are identified they should be treated aggressively. This includes the use of low-dose aspirin. The advantages of aspirin for *secondary* prevention have been well documented in women and despite the concern that aspirin may increase the risk of hemorrhagic strokes, there is evidence that hypertensive patients receiving daily aspirin have lower overall cardiovascular event rates. A large prospective trial of primary aspirin use in women physicians and nurses is in progress. While these results are awaited, low-dose aspirin (81 mg/day) for primary prevention in hypertensive women should be strongly considered.

Clinical Manifestations

Angina

The diagnosis of angina in women can be particularly challenging.[9] Women generally visit physicians more often than do men and report more symptoms, including chest discomfort. Women present at an older age and are more likely to have associated diabetes and hypertension. They also more often have angina with emotional or mental stress than do men. Women also have more "anginal equivalents," such as dyspnea, fatigue, and weakness, than do men. Women present more frequently with discomfort at atypical sites (arm, jaw, upper abdomen, jaw, and back discomfort vs. substernal discomfort). Older women with CAD often ascribe incorrectly their decreased ability to complete housework to aging. Therefore, regular exploration of a patient's exercise tolerance and considering CAD in the differential diagnosis when there is a decrease in tolerance, are important.

Acute Coronary Syndromes Including Acute Myocardial Infarction

Women with acute myocardial infarction are generally older than men and therefore present with more chronic

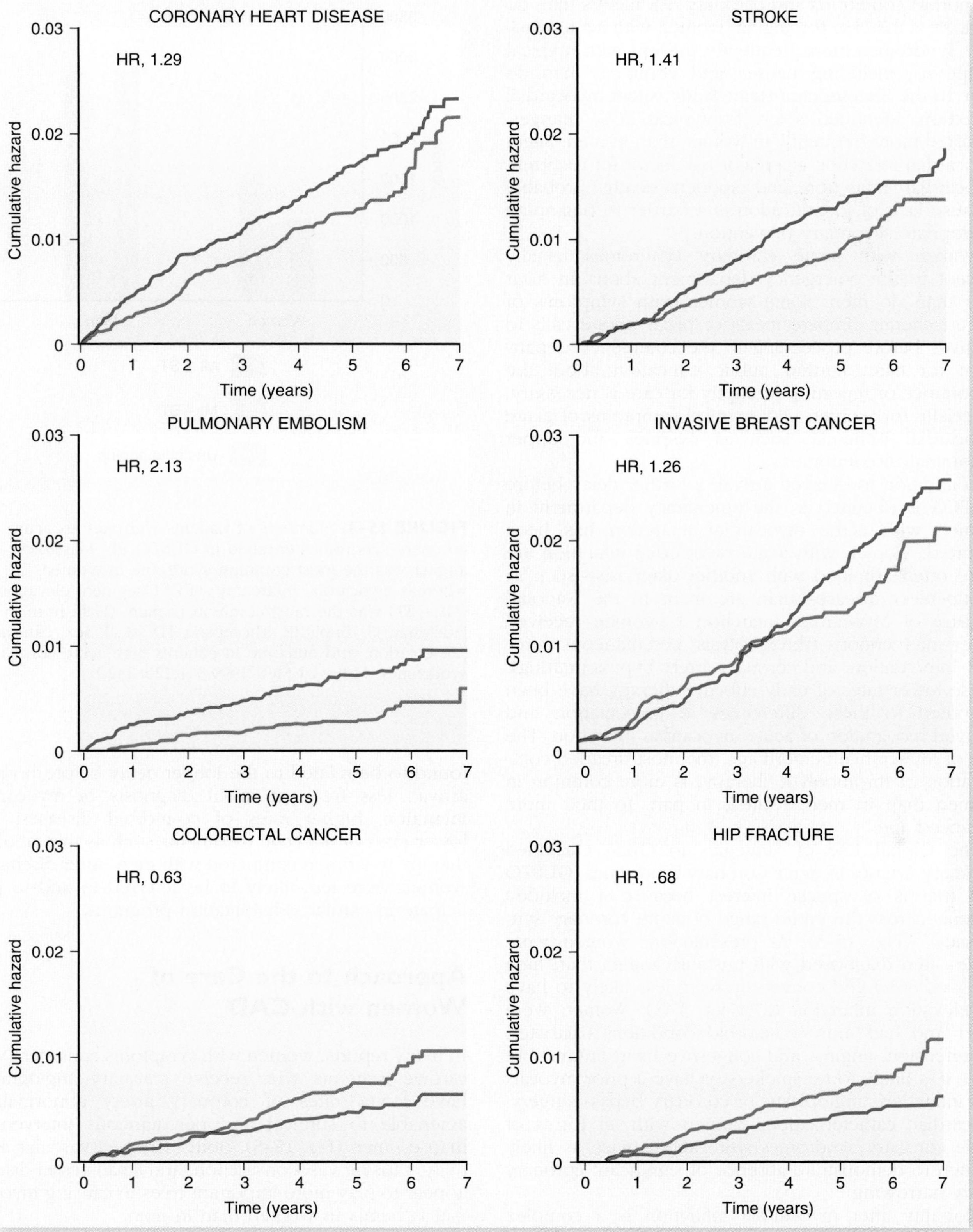

FIGURE 15–2. Kaplan-Meier estimates of cumulative hazards for selected clinical outcomes. *Red line,* estrogen + progestin; *green line,* placebo. HR, hazard ratio. (From Writing Group for the Women's Health Initiative: Risks and benefits of estrogen plus progestin in healthy postmenopausal women: Principal results from the Women's Health Initiative randomized controlled trial. JAMA 2002;288:321–333.)

co-morbid conditions and coronary risk factors than do men. As is the case for angina, women with acute coronary syndromes more frequently present with atypical symptoms, including nausea and vomiting, than do men. In the Framingham Heart Study, silent myocardial infarction, identified solely by typical ECG changes, occurred more frequently in women than in men. Silent myocardial infarction is a major risk factor for recurrent myocardial infarction and sudden death, probably because lack of identification is a barrier to beginning appropriate secondary prevention.

Women with acute coronary syndromes usually present to the emergency department about an hour later than do men. Some women with symptoms of acute ischemia prepare meals or place phone calls to relatives before proceeding to the emergency department for care. Further public education about the importance of reporting promptly for care is necessary, especially for women with atypical symptoms of acute myocardial ischemia, such as dyspnea and upper abdominal discomfort.

In addition to delayed arrival, a further delay before an ECG is obtained in the emergency department in women with acute myocardial infarction has been reported. Women with acute myocardial infarction are more often admitted with another diagnosis—such as peptic ulcer disease—than are men. In the National Registry of Myocardial Infarction I, women received fewer interventions (thrombolysis, percutaneous coronary intervention, and coronary artery bypass grafting). These lower rates of early effective therapy have been attributed to these differences in presentation and delayed recognition of acute myocardial infarction. The rate of intracranial hemorrhage, the most dreaded complication of thrombolytic therapy, is more common in women than in men, related, in part, to their more advanced age.

The Global Use of Strategies to Open Occluded Coronary Arteries in Acute Coronary Syndromes (GUSTO IIb) trial is of special interest because it included patients across the entire range of acute coronary syndromes[10] (Fig. 15–3). At presentation, women were more often diagnosed with unstable angina than men (46% vs. 36%) and conversely were less likely to have ST elevation infarction (27% vs. 37%). Women were older and had more co-morbid conditions (diabetes, hypertension, angina, and congestive heart failure) but were less likely to be smokers or have a prior myocardial infarction, angioplasty, or coronary bypass surgery. At cardiac catheterization, women with all forms of acute coronary syndromes were about twice as likely as men to demonstrate absence of significant coronary artery narrowing.

Mortality after myocardial infarction is a complex interaction between age, co-morbidities, and gender.[11,12] In the Myocardial Infarction Project-II the 30-day mortality rate in women with myocardial infarction was 14% compared with 10% in men. The mortality was about twice as great for women than men aged 30 to 50 years. The difference decreased progressively with advancing age and disappeared between age 75 and 80 years (Fig. 15–4). On multivariate analysis, the differences were

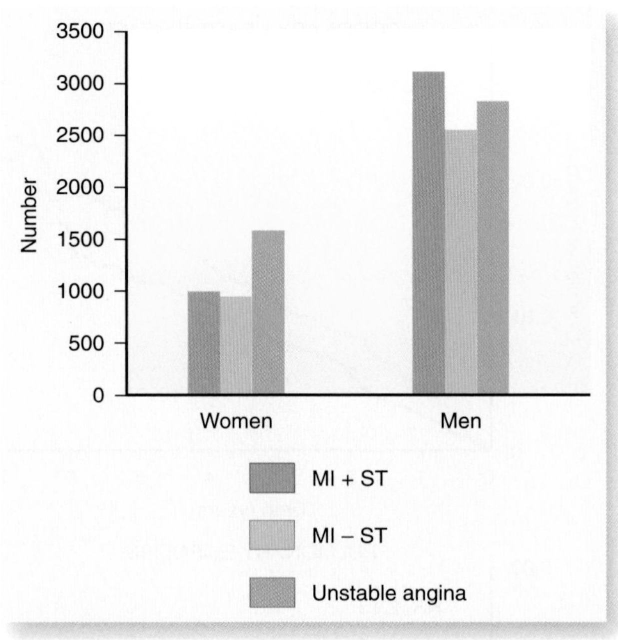

FIGURE 15–3. Numbers of patients with various acute coronary syndromes enrolled in GUSTO IIb. Unstable angina was the most common syndrome in women, whereas myocardial infarction with ST segment elevation (MI + ST) was the most common in men. (Data from Hochman JS, Tamis JE, Thompson TD, et al: Sex, clinical presentation, and outcome in patients with acute coronary syndromes. N Engl J Med 1999;341:226–232.)

found to be related to the longer delay before hospital arrival, less frequent initial diagnosis of myocardial infarction, higher rates of co-morbid diseases, and lower rates of effective treatments such as thrombolytic therapy in women compared with men. After discharge, women were less likely to be referred to and to participate in cardiac rehabilitation programs.

Approach to the Care of Women with CAD

In many reports, women with symptoms consistent with cardiac ischemia who receive coronary angiography have lower rates of coronary artery abnormalities amenable to surgical and percutaneous intervention than do men (Fig. 15–5). Both increased vascular reactivity, causing vasoconstriction, and small vessel disease appear to play more important roles in causing myocardial ischemia in women than in men.

Electrocardiographic exercise stress testing is associated with a higher false-positive rate in women than in men.[13] This is related, in part, to the lower prevalence of CAD in women. In several studies in which ECG exercise stress testing was assessed at different times in the menstrual cycle, lower estrogen levels were associated with more frequent ischemic changes. This is not surprising given that coronary, carotid, and brachial

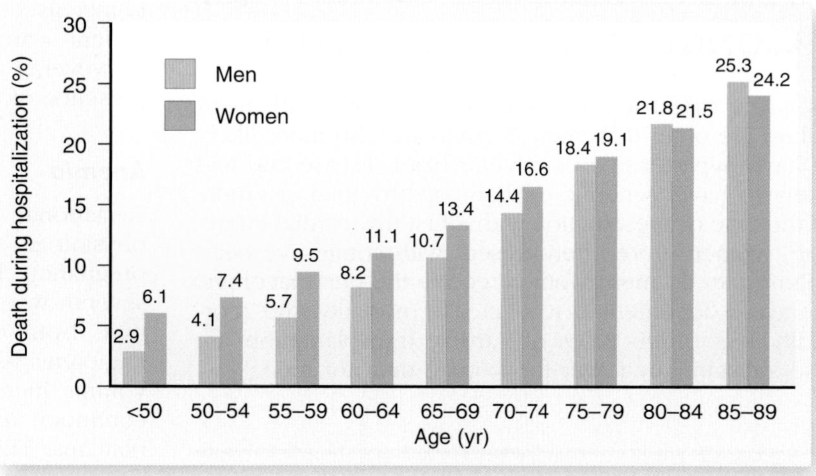

FIGURE 15–4. Rates of death during hospitalization for myocardial infarction among women and men according to age. The interaction between sex and age was significant ($P < .001$). (From Vaccarino V, Parsons L, Every NR, et al: Sex-based differences in early mortality after myocardial infarction. N Engl J Med 1999;341:217–225.)

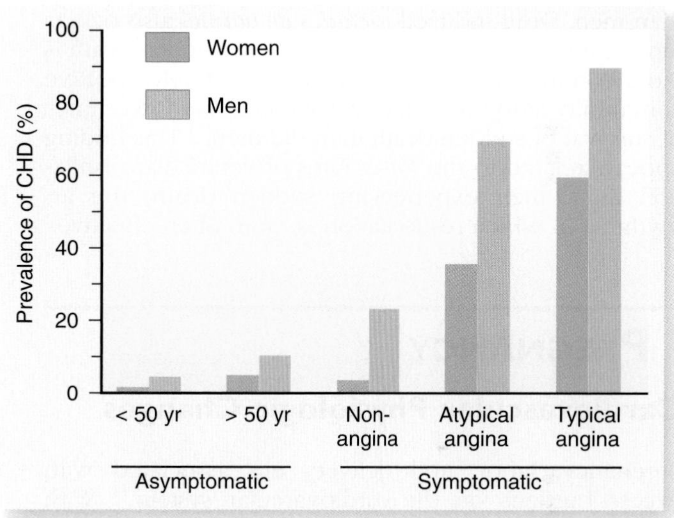

FIGURE 15–5. Prevalence of angiographically documented coronary heart disease (CHD) in men and women according to age and chest pain syndrome. (From Douglas PS: Coronary artery disease in women. In Braunwald E, Zipes DP, Libby P [eds]: Heart Disease, 6th ed. Philadelphia, WB Saunders, 2001, pp 2038–2051. Modified from DeSanctis RW: Clinical manifestations of coronary artery disease: Chest pain in women. In Wenger NK, Speroff L, Pacjard B [eds]: Cardiovascular Health and Disease in Women. Greenwich, CT, Le Jacq Communications, 1993, p 68.)

arterial blood flows have been documented to vary in a similar fashion during the menstrual cycle.

In addition to the higher false-positive rate associated with ECG exercise stress testing in women, the interpretation of myocardial perfusion stress testing utilizing thallium may be complicated in women by the increased attenuation from breast tissue (see Chapter 4). The use of technetium-based (sestamibi) imaging avoids this difficulty. In women who cannot exercise, pharmacologic stress imaging (e.g., dobutamine echocardiography, adenosine myocardial perfusion imaging) are favored when assessing women or staging the severity of CAD in women.

Revascularization

The results of percutaneous coronary intervention are comparable in women and men, except for slightly higher complication rates in women. Women with CAD are referred for surgical cardiac revascularization less frequently than men and their operative mortality is higher. This may be related to their older age at the time of referral, the smaller lumina of their coronary arteries, the higher rates of co-morbid conditions (such as diabetes mellitus) and the greater frequency of emergent or urgent versus elective surgery in women. Postoperatively, women recover more slowly and have higher rates of depression.

Secondary Prevention

Secondary prevention treatment goals for CAD (see Chapter 25) are similar and equally effective in women and men. However, in multiple studies, these interventions have been shown to be used less frequently and treatment goals are reached less often in women. Since HERS, the initiation of HRT in patients with a new diagnosis of CAD is not advised. There is still controversy about whether to continue long-term HRT in women who experience an acute ischemic event.

CONGESTIVE HEART FAILURE

As is the case for CAD, women presenting with heart failure are older than men. Women are also more likely to have hypertensive or valvular heart disease and less likely to have ischemic cardiomyopathy than are men. At the time of presentation with a first myocardial infarction, women more often present with congestive heart failure than do men. Women receive the pharmacologic therapies documented to decrease mortality and morbidity less often. Rates of cardiac transplantation are also substantially lower for women than for men.

ARRHYTHMIAS

Palpitations are reported more commonly by women than men. Drug-induced *torsades de pointes* also occurs more commonly in women. Conversely, sudden death is more common in men than in women. A retrospective community study revealed that women had lower rates of survival of sudden death than did men.[14] This finding appears related to the *lower* rates of ventricular fibrillation in women experiencing sudden death, the arrhythmia in which resuscitation is more often effective.

PREGNANCY

Cardiovascular Physiologic Changes

Pregnancy, labor, and delivery are associated with excess burdens on the cardiovascular system.[15] With improved management, more women with known heart disease are attempting pregnancy. In addition, the number of women choosing pregnancy later in life is increasing. Such women are more likely to have conditions such as hypertension and diabetes, which are not only coronary risk factors, but also independently complicate pregnancy. As corrective surgery for congenital heart disease has improved survival, pregnancy for women with treated congenital disease occurs with increasing frequency. An understanding of the normal cardiopulmonary adjustments during gestation, labor, and delivery is important for patients with heart disease.

During pregnancy cardiac output increases normally to a maximum of 30% to 60% above preconception levels at the end of the second trimester, at which time it plateaus for the remainder of gestation. Both heart rate and stroke volume increase. During the third trimester, as the gravid uterus enlarges, body position can significantly affect cardiac output. In the supine position, the caval compression by the gravid uterus can reduce cardiac output by up to 25%. Turning into the left lateral decubitus position can relieve venocaval compression and restore cardiac output.

Myocardial contractility appears to be unaltered during pregnancy, whereas myocardial oxygen demand is increased. Physical findings in the normal pregnant patient can mimic the findings of heart disease. However, a number of symptoms and signs point to the presence of heart disease (Box 15–2).

Anemia

Gestational anemia is attributed to the normal physiologic responses to the hormonal changes of pregnancy. The blood volume expands as early as the seventh week of gestation, an expansion that results, in part, from estrogen-mediated effects on the rennin-angiotensin-aldosterone axis. The total circulatory volume increases by an average of 50%. This increase continues until the third trimester, at which time it plateaus. This physiologic anemia of pregnancy develops because plasma volume increases more rapidly than does red cell mass. Not surprisingly, the anemia of pregnancy can be more serious in women who were anemic before pregnancy, usually from iron deficiency consequent to menstrual blood loss. Adequate hemoglobin not only protects the mother from blood loss at

BOX 15–2

Cardiovascular Symptoms and Physical Findings in Pregnancy

Symptoms	Fatigue Dyspnea on exertion Decreased exercise tolerance Orthopnea Palpitations
Signs	Increased jugular venous pressure with visible venous waveforms Decreased blood pressure Wide pulse pressure Increased heart rate PMI laterally displaced Peripheral edema
Auscultation	Loud split S_1, loud split S_2 Mammary souffle Suprasternal venous hum Basilar pulmonary rales
Murmurs	Functional murmurs common Pathologic murmurs may decrease
Symptoms & Signs Suggesting Heart Disease	Progressive dyspnea Hemoptysis Exertional syncope, chest pain Cyanosis Loud systolic murmur (Gr. 3/6) Fixed split S_2 Left parasternal heave with loud P_2 (sign of pulmonary hypertension)

delivery but provides oxygen carrying capacity to the developing fetus during pregnancy. Throughout the course of pregnancy, women require daily supplementation of iron to aid both increased maternal and fetal hematopoiesis.

Hemodynamic Changes During Labor and Delivery

In healthy women, the expansion of blood volume during pregnancy compensates for the 500 mL to 1000 mL blood loss that may occur during delivery. During labor, approximately 500 mL of blood may be diverted into the maternal circulation with each uterine contraction. Pain plays an additional role in hemodynamics because it increases heart rate and blood pressure. The cyclic nature of labor with its dynamic effects on cardiovascular loading places a cyclic load on the heart which normally compensates for this load. Complications may arise, however, in the presence of left ventricular hypertrophy, dilatation, or dysfunction. An experienced team of obstetricians, obstetrical anesthesiologists, and cardiologists should guide pregnancy and delivery in patients with overt heart disease.

Preconception Counseling

Identifying medical problems before conception can improve fertility and improve fetal outcome. All women considering pregnancy should avoid tobacco, alcohol, and substance exposure. Because of their serious teratogenic hazards, angiotensin-converting enzyme inhibitors and angiotensin receptor blockers should be discontinued and other antihypertensives substituted early during pregnancy, preferably prior to conception. Women with heart disease in classes III or IV (New York Heart Association Criteria) usually do not tolerate pregnancy well. Either the cardiovascular disease should be dealt with (usually by surgery) or if this is not possible, pregnancy should be avoided in such patients.

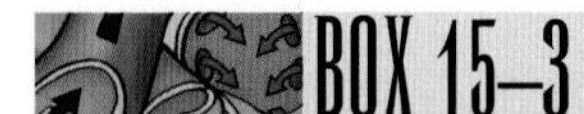

Classification of Hypertension in Pregnancy

Gestational hypertension and/or proteinuria: hypertension and/or proteinuria developing during pregnancy, labor, or the puerperium in a previously normotensive nonproteinuric woman subdivided into
- Gestational hypertension: diastolic blood pressure >110 once or >90 twice, 4 hr apart
- Gestational proteinuria: >300 mg/24 hr or two clean-voided specimens 4 hr apart with 2+ reagent strip (1 g/L)
- Gestational proteinuric hypertension (preeclampsia)

Chronic hypertension and chronic renal disease: hypertension or proteinuria, or both, at the first visit before wk 20 of pregnancy or the presence of chronic hypertension or chronic renal disease diagnosed before, during, or after pregnancy

Unclassified hypertension and/or proteinuria: hypertension and/or proteinuria found either
- At first examination after 20 wk (140 days) in a woman without known chronic hypertension or chronic renal disease.

  or
- During pregnancy, labor, or the puerperium, when information is insufficient to permit classification, is regarded as unclassified during pregnancy and is subdivided into
  - Hypertension (without proteinuria)
  - Proteinuria (without hypertension)
  - Proteinuric hypertension

Eclampsia: the occurrence of generalized convulsions during pregnancy, during labor, or within 7 days of delivery and not caused by epilepsy or other convulsive disorders

From Kaplan NK: Clinical Hypertension. 5th ed. Baltimore: Williams & Wilkins, 1990.

Hypertension in the Pregnant Patient (Box 15–3)

Blood pressure monitoring during pregnancy is most accurate in the sitting position, especially in the third trimester when, as already mentioned, the gravid uterus compresses the inferior vena cava. Blood pressure changes with pregnancy usually include a greater reduction in diastolic than systolic pressure that begins in the first trimester and is most marked toward the end of the second trimester. As women become pregnant at older ages and the criteria for hypertension have broadened (see Chapter 19), the prevalence of hypertension during pregnancy has increased.

Hypertension during pregnancy is defined as a blood pressure greater than 140/90 mm Hg on two occasions.[16] Gestational hypertension, that is, hypertension appearing *after* the twentieth week of gestation in previously normotensive women, occurs in 10% of first pregnancies and resolves post partum. In contrast, coincidental chronic essential hypertension *antedates* pregnancy and is more common in women older than 35 years. Hypertension of any form or cause during pregnancy is a significant risk factor for the development of preeclampsia and intrauterine growth retardation.

The preferred pharmacologic treatment in pregnancy is methyldopa or labetalol. Nifedipine and hydralazine also appear to be well tolerated by mother and fetus. Diuretics are sometimes utilized to manage coexistent hypertension and heart failure, but reduced uteroplacental perfusion is a potential side effect of these drugs.

Preeclampsia is a systemic disorder that is characterized by hypertension with proteinuria.[17] When it is mild, patients should be followed closely with increased rest and antihypertensive therapy. When blood pressure elevation is marked (>160/110 mm Hg) patients should

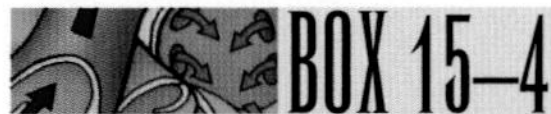
BOX 15–4

Predictors for High Maternal and Fetal Risk in Women with Preeclampsia

Systolic blood pressure ≥160 mm Hg or diastolic blood pressure ≥110 mm Hg
New proteinuria ≥2.0 g per 24 hr (2+ or 3+ on qualitative examination) or decrease in urine volume
New increased serum creatinine level (>2.0 mg/dL)
Platelet count <100,000/L or evidence of microangiopathic hemolytic anemia (e.g., schistocytes or increased levels of lactic acid dehydrogenase and direct bilirubin)
Elevated hepatic enzymes (aspartate aminotransferase or alanine aminotransferase)
Upper abdominal pain (especially epigastric and right upper quadrant)
Headache and other cerebral or visual disturbances
Cardiac decompensation (e.g., pulmonary edema)
Retinal hemorrhages, exudates, or papilledema
Intrauterine growth retardation

Lindheimer MD: Hypertension in pregnancy. Hypertension 1993;22:122–137.

be hospitalized, placed at bed rest, and receive seizure prophylaxis with magnesium sulfate and control of blood pressure with intravenous hydralazine or labetalol. Marked hypertension and new severe proteinuria increase the risk of eclampsia, a convulsive disorder associated with severe maternal and fetal disease (Box 15–4). In cases of severe preeclampsia with uncontrolled hypertension, or frank eclampsia, the cure is termination of the pregnancy, because this removes the nidus of the disease—the placenta.

Acute Myocardial Infarction

Acute myocardial infarction is rare during pregnancy. The highest incidence is during the third trimester in multigravidas older than 35 years. However, fewer than half of such patients evaluated by angiography have been found to have obstructive arterial disease. This suggests that the potential etiologies for myocardial infarction include coronary spasm, coronary artery dissection, cocaine, ergotamine or oral contraceptive use, hypercoagulable states, or collagen vascular disease.

Treatment includes heparin, aspirin, beta-blockers, oxygen, and nitrates. Anticoagulation with unfractionated heparin is preferred (over low molecular weight heparin) because its large molecular weight prevents placental crossing. Anticoagulation therapy can be discontinued 24 hours before induction of labor, or discontinued and reversed with protamine sulfate at the onset of spontaneous labor. Although thrombolytic therapy does not appear to be teratogenic, when administered during the peripartum period, there is an increased risk of maternal hemorrhage. Low-dose aspirin (<165 mg/day) has been shown to be safe in the second and third trimesters.

Peripartum Cardiomyopathy

Peripartum cardiomyopathy, a dilated cardiomyopathy, is a rare and potentially devastating condition that develops between the last month of pregnancy and five months after delivery (see Chapter 29).[18] It is characterized by left ventricular systolic dysfunction in women without other causes for cardiac disease or heart failure, and it is most readily detected by echocardiography. The cause of peripartum cardiomyopathy is unknown, but a viral myocarditis has been proposed. Right ventricular biopsy usually demonstrates myocyte edema, lymphocytic infiltration, necrosis, and fibrosis. Clinical features include dyspnea, weight gain, arrhythmias, and peripheral edema. Chest x-ray shows generalized cardiac enlargement and pulmonary congestion.

About two thirds of women with cardiomyopathy recover, either completely or partially, and the remainder have continued severe heart failure, which is sometimes fatal. Treatment is with diuretics, digitalis, and vasodilators, especially hydralazine, and with anticoagulants. Cardiac transplantation should be considered in patients who do not improve. Subsequent pregnancies should be discouraged.[19]

CONGENITAL HEART DISEASE AND PRIMARY PULMONARY HYPERTENSION

An increasing number of girls with congenital heart disease are surviving to puberty, either with surgical or medical treatment.[20] Patients who are acyanotic without pulmonary hypertension and are in New York Heart Asssociation classes I or II usually tolerate pregnancy well. In women at higher risk, elective induction of labor after fetal maturity has been confirmed should be considered. In those at very high risk (see Box 15–4), early termination of pregnancy should be considered.

As is the case in patients with severe pulmonary hypertension associated with ventricular septal defect (Eisenmenger's syndrome), patients with *primary* pulmonary hypertension do not tolerate pregnancy and experience a mortality as high as 30%. Pregnancy should be avoided or should be terminated early (see Chapter 34).

VALVULAR HEART DISEASE (see Chapter 32)

Physical activity should be restricted in gravid symptomatic patients with valvular heart disease. Prophylactic antibiotic prophylaxis is indicated during delivery. In patients with mitral stenosis, worsening symptoms usually occur during pregnancy due to increased transvalvular blood flow resulting in elevation of pulmonary vascular pressures. Beta-blockers, diuretics and restriction of physical activity are useful, but, if possible, mitral balloon valvuloplasty should be carried out. Rheumatic mitral regurgitation and aortic regurgitation are usually well tolerated during pregnancy. Hydralazine or nifedipine may be used for afterload reduction. If surgery on a regurgitant mitral valve is necessary, the valve should, if at all possible, be repaired, not replaced. Aortic stenosis is rare during pregnancy and is well tolerated unless it is severe (aortic valve area $<1\,cm^2$); the latter should be treated by balloon valvuloplasty or surgery or the pregnancy terminated.

Selection of a Prosthetic Valve

Choice of an appropriate prosthetic valve for women of reproductive capability remains a challenging problem. Bioprosthetic valves do not require anticoagulation, but deteriorate relatively quickly, with replacement in approximately 40% required in women of child-bearing age. Mechanical prostheses are preferred for their excellent durability and better hemodynamic profile than bioprosthetic valves. However, mechanical valves require lifelong anticoagulation. Warfarin may cause an embryopathy and hemorrhage during delivery. Therefore, when anticoagulation is required during pregnancy, for a prosthetic valve (or other indication), heparin should be used during the first trimester to avoid embryopathy and after the 35th week. It should be discontinued when labor commences to avoid hemorrhage. Warfarin may be used between the 13th and 35th weeks.

References

1. Charney P (ed): Coronary Artery Disease in Women: Prevention, Diagnosis and Management. Philadelphia, ACP/ASIM, 1999.
2. Barrett-Connor E: Sex differences in coronary heart disease: Why are women so superior? The 1995 Aneel Jeys lecture. Circulation 1997;95:252–264.
3. Winkleby MA, Robinson TN, Sundquist J, Kraemer HC: Ethnic variations in cardiovascular disease risk factors among children and young adults: Findings from the third national health and nutrition examination survey, 1988–1994. JAMA 1999;281:1006–1013.
4. Stamler J, Stamler R, Neaton JD, et al: Low risk-factor profile and long-term cardiovascular and noncardiovascular mortality and life expectancy: Findings for 5 large cohorts of young adults and middle-aged men and women. JAMA 1999;282:2012–2018.
5. Wilson PWF, Kannel WB, Silbershatz H, D'Agostino RB. Clustering of metabolic factors and coronary heart disease. Arch Intern Med 1999;159:1104–1109.
6. Willet W, Green A, Stampfer M, et al: Relative and absolute excess risks of coronary heart disease among women who smoke cigarettes. N Engl J Med 1987;317:1303–1309.
7. Hu FB, Grodstein F, Hennekens CH, et al: Age at natural menopause and risk of cardiovascular disease. Arch Intern Med 1999;159:1061–1066.
8. Hulley S, Grady D, Bush T, et al: Randomized trial of estrogen plus progestin for secondary prevention of coronary heart disease in post-menopausal women. JAMA 1998;280:605.

8a. Writing Group for the Women's Health Initiative: Risks and benefits of estrogen plus progestin in healthy postmenopausal women: Principal results from the Women's Health Initiative randomized controlled trial. JAMA 2002; 288:321–333.

9. Douglas PS, Ginsburg GS: The evaluation of chest pain in women. N Engl J Med 1996;334:1311–1315.
10. The Global Use of Strategies to Open Occluded Coronary Arteries (GUSTO IIb) Investigators: A comparison of recombinant hirudin with heparin for the treatment of acute coronary syndromes. N Engl J Med 1996;335: 775.
11. Hochman JS, Tamis J, Thompson TD, et al: Sex, clinical presentation, and outcome in patients with acute coronary syndromes. N Engl J Med 1999;341:226–232.
12. Vaccarino V, Parsons L, Every NR, et al: Sex-based differences in early mortality after myocardial infarction. N Engl J Med 1999;341:217–225.
13. Kwok Y, Kim C, Grady D, et al: Meta-analysis of exercise testing to detect coronary artery disease in women. Am J Cardiol 1999;83:660–663.
14. Kim C, Fahrenbruch CE, Cobb LA, Eisenberg M: Out-of-hospital cardiac arrest in men and women. Circulation 2001; 104:2699–2703.
15. Elkayam U: Pregnancy and Cardiovascular Disease. In Braunwald E, Zipes DP, Libby P (eds): Heart Disease, 6th ed. Philadelphia, WB Saunders, 2001, pp 2172–2191.
16. Barton JR, O'Brien JM, Bergauer NK, et al: Mild gestational hypertension remote from term: Progression and outcome. Am J Obstet Gynecol 2001;184:979–983.
17. Walker JJ: Pre-eclampsia. Lancet 2000;356:1260–1265.
18. Pearson GD, Veille JC: Rahimtoola S, et al: Peripartum cardiomyopathy: National Heart, Lung and Blood Institute and Office of Rare Diseases (NIH) workshop recommendations and review. JAMA 2000;283:1183–1188.
19. Elkayam U, Tummala P, Rao K, et al: Maternal and fetal outcomes of subsequent pregnancies in women with peripartum cardiomyopathy. N Engl J Med 2001;344: 1567–1571.
20. Oakely C: Pregnancy and congenital heart disease. Heart 1997;78:12–14.

CHAPTER 16 Approach to the Elderly Patient with Heart Disease

Karen P. Alexander and Eric D. Peterson

The elderly population of the United States is expanding at an unprecedented rate owing to advances in life expectancy and the aging of the baby boomer generation. Currently, 1 in 35 Americans is age 80 years or older; within 50 years, this ratio will be 1 in 12. Manifestations of cardiovascular disease, including coronary artery disease (CAD), heart failure, hypertension, arrhythmias, and valvular heart disease, also increase logarithmically with advancing age. As a result, primary care clinicians will be confronted with a near epidemic of geriatric patients presenting with cardiac disorders, making it vital to understand important age-related differences in the presentation, diagnosis, and treatment of heart disease.[1]

EFFECTS OF AGING ON THE CARDIOVASCULAR SYSTEM

The development of heart disease is influenced by multiple factors including genetics and environmental factors such as smoking, diet, and exercise. As these factors vary among individuals, so does the aging process itself. This heterogeneity of aging results in people with similar "chronologic" age having remarkably different "physiologic" age. Although variable in their time of onset, certain cardiovascular changes are inevitable with advancing age. Atherosclerotic damage to the endothelium occurs over time, resulting in an increased frequency of acute coronary events and strokes. Vessel compliance declines, resulting in a widened pulse pressure and an increased prevalence of systolic hypertension (see Chapter 19). Compliance of the heart chambers also declines owing to ventricular hypertrophy, fibrosis, and other myocardial injuries. On a molecular level, myocardial tissue becomes less responsive to β-adrenergic stimulation, and mitochondria lose capacity to produce adenosine triphosphate (ATP) on demand. Heart valves calcify and lose mobility, leading to valve dysfunction (see Chapter 32). These age-related impairments in cardiac structure and function lead to an increased prevalence of both diastolic and systolic heart failure (see Chapter 28). The conduction system suffers from age-related cell loss and calcification, increasing the elderly individual's risk for brady- and tachyarrhythmias (see Chapters 30 and 31).

GENERAL TREATMENT CONSIDERATIONS IN ELDERLY PATIENTS WITH HEART DISEASE

Whereas some elderly individuals engage in very active, independent lives well into their advanced years, others are frail and have disabling mental or physical illness. Beyond this variability in health and functional status, there is great diversity in the health values of elderly patients. Some consider illness and disability to be inevitable and have no interest in extensive medical or surgical intervention. Recent studies have demonstrated, however, that the majority of very elderly individuals view medical care as an important means of maintaining their health for as long as possible. In addition, many octogenarians, when given a choice, actually prefer *quantity* as opposed to *quality* of life.[2] An individual patient's willingness to take health risks also varies markedly. Some are willing to take high risks to improve symptoms or the odds of long-term survival, whereas others are relatively adverse to risk. Therefore, it is incumbent on physicians not to apply their own health values when deciding how to best treat an individual patient. Instead, the physician should attempt to elicit the elderly patient's treatment goals, while, in turn, providing the patient with the necessary information regarding potential risks and benefits of each treatment option.

Physicians must also understand that many cardiovascular treatment guidelines are based on randomized clinical trials that were performed in selected younger populations and may not apply to their elderly patients. Up to 60% of cardiovascular trials performed before 1990 excluded patients solely based on their age. More than 50% of trials published since 1995 still failed to enroll a single patient age 75 years or older.[3] Age-related physiologic changes make extrapolation of trial results to the elderly potentially misleading. The elderly generally have a decreased volume of drug distribution, less protein binding, and lower hepatic and renal drug clearance. Combined, these differences result in increased drug concentrations and drug potency in the elderly. Pharmacodynamics, or the effects of a drug on its target, are also altered with age. For example, calcification in the conduction system increases an elderly patient's sensitivity to calcium-channel blockers and beta-blockers. Co-morbid illnesses further compromise the safety of specific drugs. For instance, frailty and falling risks can increase the risk for bleeding complications with anticoagulants. Polypharmacy, or the total number of medications prescribed in the elderly, increases the risks for drug-drug interactions. It has been estimated that 25% of older patients have experienced at least one adverse drug reaction, and as many as 10% of all hospital admissions in the elderly are caused by adverse drug reactions.

Physicians also must consider the elderly patient's social and economic situation when formulating appropriate care plans. Transportation issues, which are a major limitation for many elderly, can disrupt close office follow-up. Many elderly patients are on fixed incomes and may not realize or acknowledge that they cannot afford multiple cardiac medications. The health of an ailing spouse can further substantially affect an elderly caregiver's personal health and health decisions. Although addressing these issues can take time, a rare commodity in current primary care practice, it will ensure a more rational and collaborative treatment plan.

HYPERTENSION (see Chapter 19)

Prevalence and Prognosis

About 1 in 4 U.S. adults, or more than 50 million people, have hypertension.[4] Hypertension occurs in 64% of men and 77% of women older than 75 years. Isolated systolic hypertension is more common in the elderly due to increased stiffness and loss of compliance of the medium- and large-compliance arteries. In the elderly, systolic blood pressure and pulse pressure (systolic blood pressure minus diastolic blood pressure) are better than diastolic blood pressure alone as predictors of events such as MI and stroke. A systolic blood pressure over 180 mm Hg is associated with four times the risk of CAD compared with a systolic blood pressure under 120 mm Hg.

Diagnosis and Treatment

Hypertension should be diagnosed in elderly patients based on two measurements under appropriate conditions. Secondary causes of hypertension are much less common in the elderly, except that the prevalence of renal artery stenosis and, hence, renovascular hypertension rises with advancing age. This diagnosis should be considered in elderly patients with difficult-to-control blood pressures, clinical evidence of diffuse vascular disease, worsening renal function, or hyperkalemia as a complication of angiotensin-converting enzyme (ACE) inhibitor therapy. Renovascular hypertension usually results in elevations of both systolic and diastolic pressures, and it is less likely in elderly patients with isolated systolic hypertension.

Diet and lifestyle modifications are efficacious in elderly patients with hypertension,[5] and these modifications are the recommended first step for elderly hypertensive patients. Still, over 80% of elderly patients with hypertension will require pharmacotherapy to achieve adequate control. In an overview of 15 randomized trials of pharmacotherapy in nearly 22,000 patients, treatment of hypertension in the elderly resulted in a significant 16% reduction in overall mortality, a 30% reduction in cardiovascular mortality, and a 40% reduction in cerebrovascular mortality.[6] The overall absolute reduction in cardiovascular morbidity and mortality was 5.2% at 5 years. In fact, the absolute benefit is greater in the elderly than in younger patients due to the higher short-term event rates and higher prevalence of systolic hypertension in the elderly.

Most of the hypertension trials in the elderly have studied diuretics or beta-blockers as first-line agents.[7] Because of the potential for side-effects, particularly orthostatic hypotension, national consensus guidelines recommend starting with half the usual dose and then titrating drugs carefully in the elderly.

CORONARY ARTERY DISEASE

Prevalence and Prognosis

The prevalence of CAD rises in a curvilinear fashion with age in both men and women (Fig. 16–1). Although the frequency of CAD is higher in men than in women in all age groups, most CAD patients older than 75 years are female, because women generally live longer than men. Overall, CAD extracts a disproportionately heavy toll in the elderly in terms of lives lost and medical care costs. Although people 65 years and older constitute 13% of the overall U.S. population, they account for 60% of all myocardial infarctions (MIs) and 88% of all MI deaths. Similarly, persons 75 years and older make up only 5% of the U.S. population, yet they account for 34% of all MIs and 45% of all MI deaths. Medicare patients also account for more than half of all invasive procedures currently performed in the United States (Table 16–1). In total, it has been estimated that the direct cost of coronary care for Medicare patients exceeds 10 billion dollars annually. CAD and its sequelae also have indirect costs, with up to 25% of nursing home patients having CAD as their primary admission diagnosis.[4]

Beyond these overt manifestations of coronary disease, epidemiologic studies have found a very high prevalence of "subclinical" disease in the elderly. For example, the Cardiovascular Health Study performed a series of tests (electrocardiography [ECG], carotid ultrasound, and ankle-brachial blood pressures) among 6000 subjects age 65 years or older. Although one third of these community-dwelling elderly had a prior diagnosis of cardiovascular disease, testing uncovered subclinical disease in another 40% of the remaining asymptomatic patients.[8]

Presentation

The elderly are less likely than younger patients to experience classic chest pain (see Chapter 6) as a symptom of cardiac ischemia.[9] Instead, they may experience vague symptoms of dyspnea, abdominal pain, or fatigue, which may be misinterpreted as normal consequences of the aging process. In one study, patients age 85 years or older with acute MI were less likely to have typical chest pain as compared with those age 65 to 69 years.[9] Another study found that the delay between ECG-documented ischemia and angina during treadmill testing was nearly twice as long in patients older than 70 years as compared with patients younger than 55 years.[10] The elderly may also incorrectly attribute symp-

TABLE 16–1

1998 Estimated In-patients with Cardiovascular Procedures by Age

	Age Group (yr)			
Procedures (thousands)	***<45***	***45–64***	***≥65***	**Total**
Diagnostic catheterization	123	530	638	1291
Angioplasty	60	410	456	926
PTCA	27	235	269	539
Stent	25	168	182	376
All open heart surgery	62	284	382	734
Bypass surgery	14	234	304	553
Permanent pacemakers	—	21	145	166
Implantable defibrillators	—	9	13	22
Heart valves	6	24	45	75

From American Heart Association Heart and Stroke 2000 Statistical Update, www.americanheart.org/statistics/medical.html.

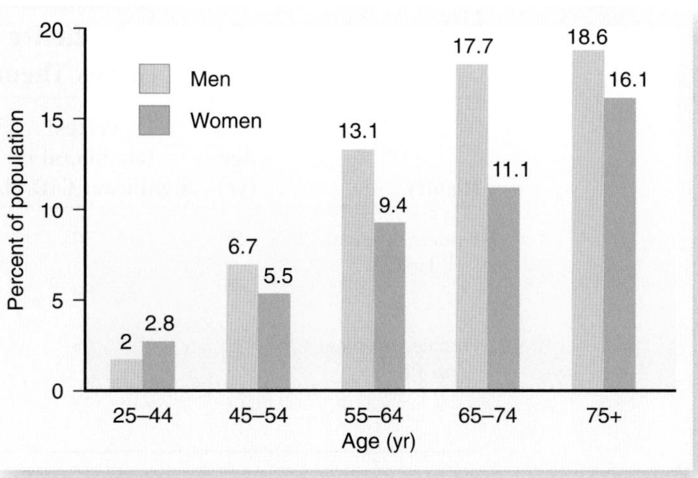

FIGURE 16–1. Prevalence of coronary heart disease by age and sex in the United States from 1988 to 1994. (From American Heart Association: 2001 Heart and Stroke Statistical Update. Dallas, American Heart Association, 2000.)

toms of coronary artery disease to other co-morbid illnesses. Because of the lack of classic angina symptoms (see Chapter 25), decreased mobility, and transportation issues, the elderly with acute coronary events are known to present later than do younger patients. For example, 30% of patients older than 65 years with an acute MI present to an emergency department more than 6 hours after the onset of symptoms.[11]

Elderly patients with an acute coronary event also have a significantly higher morbidity and mortality. In one study, for example, 30-day mortality following ST-elevation MI increased markedly with age (age <65 years = 3.0%, age 65 to 74 years = 9.5%, age 75 to 84 years = 19.6%, and age ≥85 = 30.3%).[12] In a national MI study, the one-year mortality following MI reached 44% in those age 75 years or older.[13] The elderly also have a two- to sixfold higher risk for heart failure, ventricular rupture, stroke, and other morbid events following MI. The very elderly (age ≥75 years) are three times more likely to be discharged to a nursing facility after an acute MI than those age 65 to 69 years.[13]

Diagnostic Evaluation

Asymptomatic Elderly

Given CAD's prevalence and frequently atypical presentation, physicians must have a high index of suspicion when evaluating elderly patients. In terms of primary screening, physicians should evaluate cardiac risk factors as well as symptoms suggestive of cardiovascular disease (see Chapter 18). Blood pressure and lipid screening recommendations should follow the JNC VI and NCEP-ATP-III guidelines, respectively (see Chapters 19 and 20). Obtaining an initial baseline ECG is reasonable in elderly patients even without symptoms, owing to the high prevalence of "silent" MIs in this population (see Chapters 4 and 18). Additional diagnostic testing in the asymptomatic elderly, however, is controversial. Although some would argue that the prevalence of CAD in this population justifies further testing to detect subclinical disease (echocardiography, carotid ultrasound, and the like), most would reserve further testing for those with symptoms (see Chapter 18).[8]

Elderly with Symptoms

In evaluating the elderly symptomatic patient, it is also important to determine the patient's likelihood for CAD based on risk factors and the presenting complaint. As both the positive and negative predictive value of a diagnostic test are altered by disease prevalence (see Chapters 1, 2, and 4), a negative stress test in an elderly patient should not necessarily be interpreted as "ruling out" the diagnosis of CAD. For example, a positive stress test in a 75-year-old woman with typical angina adds little additional information, whereas a negative study still leaves her with more than a 60% likelihood of significant CAD (Table 16–2). Additionally, elderly patients may have difficulty exercising to achieve target heart rates with traditional treadmill protocols. Modified exercise protocols, which have a more gradual increase in exertion (see Table 25–2), can be particularly useful in the elderly. Pharmacologic stress testing can also be considered for the elderly patient who cannot exercise (see Chapters 4 and 25). The diagnostic accuracy of ECG markers of ischemia may be limited in the elderly with baseline ECG abnormalities. In these patients, nuclear perfusion imaging or stress echocardiography may be more accurate (see Fig. 25–2).

Cardiac catheterization can result in vascular injury, bleeding, MI, neurologic events (transient ischemic attacks or stroke), and even mortality. Although advanced age increases these risks slightly, overall, the risk to life remains less than 0.2%, and the risk of other serious adverse events is less than 0.5%, even in those age 75 years or older.[14] Particularly with the elderly, the physician must decide whether information obtained

TABLE 16–2

Influence of Age on Predictive Value of Stress Testing (Bayes Theorem)

History	Age (yr)	Pretest Likelihood of Significant CAD (%)*	Treadmill Test[†]	Post-test Likelihood of Significant CAD (%)
Female, Typical CP	45	30	positive	56
↑ Lipids			negative	16
	75	80	positive	92
			negative	63
Female, Atypical CP	45	5	positive	12
no RF			negative	3
	75	35	positive	62
			negative	18

*Based on CAD Risk Nomogram for predicting significant CAD; [†]Sensitivity of treadmill test = 68%, specificity = 77% (53); CAD = coronary artery disease; CP = chest pain; RF = risk factors.

from a catheterization is likely to change subsequent management. For example, coronary angiography may have limited value in an elderly patient who is not a candidate for coronary revascularization based on medical comorbidities or personal preference.

Treatment

Once the diagnosis of CAD is made, treatment must be individualized for the elderly cardiac patient, taking into account the general treatment consideration outlined above. Nevertheless, it should also be emphasized that the majority of CAD treatment recommendations apply to young and old cardiac patients alike. These treatment recommendations and the evidence supporting them are accessible on professional society websites (www.americanheart.org and www.acc.org) and are summarized at the end of this chapter (see Evidence-Based Summary).

Lipid Lowering (see Chapter 20)

In a randomized trial of simvastatin, 1848 patients age 65 to 70 years had a 34% reduction in subsequent major recurrent coronary events, a reduction that was actually slightly greater than the 28% reduction in the overall study population.[15] In another randomized trial of 1283 patients age 65 to 75 years with an LDL of 115 to 174 mg/dL, treatment with pravastatin resulted in a 32% reduction in major recurrent coronary events in elderly patients following MI compared with a 24% reduction in the overall trial.[16] In a primary prevention study including 6605 patients age 45 to 73 years, those randomized to lovastatin for primary prevention had a 37% reduction in the risk of a coronary event, and the reduction was similar among older and younger patients.[17] To date, however, there are no similar data on patients older than 75 years.

Beta-Blockers (see Chapters 25, 26, and 27)

The major randomized trials of beta-blockers for CAD included few elderly patients. A national Medicare study of more than 45,000 patients found, however, that beta-blocker use was associated with a 14% reduction in mortality among post-MI patients age 65 years or older,[18] a rate of reduction that was about one half what was found in randomized trials in younger patients (see Chapter 27).

Aspirin (see Chapters 25 and 27)

The Antithrombotic Trialists' Group examined the effectiveness of aspirin in more than 14,000 patients age 65 years or older who were enrolled in randomized antiplatelet trials for CAD. The benefits of aspirin were highly significant in reducing death, recurrent MI, or stroke in both younger and older patients (relative risk reduction of 23% for those younger than 65 years vs. 19% for those 65 years or older). Because of their higher baseline risk, the absolute benefit was actually greater in those older than 65 years than in younger patients (absolute risk reduction of 3.3% for those age <65 years vs. 4.5% for those age ≥65 years).[19]

Reperfusion Therapy (see Chapter 27)

Advanced age is a major risk factor for intracranial hemorrhage following thrombolytic therapy and, as such, is often cited as the reason for withholding thrombolytic therapy from otherwise eligible elderly MI patients. Clinicians, however, must understand the relative versus the absolute age-related risk. In one large trial, for example, patients age 70 years or older had a 2.5-fold higher relative risk of intracranial hemorrhage than those younger than 60 years, but the magnitude of absolute risk increase was only 0.3%.[20]

These treatment risks need to be balanced against the potential benefits gained from early reperfusion. In a large meta-analysis, a significant survival advantage for thrombolysis was documented in all patients younger than 75 years (n = 6000). In the oldest subset (age 75 years or older), those receiving thrombolysis had a statistically insignificant 3% lower 30-day mortality when compared with no therapy.[21] A large observational study, however, challenged this assumption. Even after risk adjustment, patients older than 75 years had a higher 30-day mortality with thrombolysis when compared with placebo.[22] However, in a similar analysis looking at longer-term outcomes, the very elderly who received thrombolytic therapy had a statistically significant 16% reduction in mortality at 1 year when compared with those treated with conservative care.[23]

Because of the risks associated with thrombolysis in the elderly MI patient, some have advocated primary angioplasty as an alternative. Observational studies have found that acute primary angioplasty was associated with about a 30% lower 30-day and 1-year mortality compared with conservative care among MI patients age 75 years or older.[24] Although these studies attempted to control for treatment-selection bias, they were not randomized. The only randomized trial addressing age and the benefits of primary angioplasty was conducted in patients with MI complicated by cardiogenic shock. In the overall trial, primary angioplasty significantly reduced mortality compared with a strategy of medical stabilization. However, among patients age 75 years or older, angioplasty was associated with a 41% higher mortality, which was not quite statistically significant.[25] Although not fully resolved, the current consensus is that age alone should not be considered a contraindication to reperfusion therapy, but the choice of reperfusion strategy should be individualized after considering risks and benefits.

Coronary Revascularization

Coronary revascularization, either via percutaneous coronary intervention (PCI) or coronary artery bypass surgery (CABG), has traditionally been used less often in elderly patients. For example, a study of Medicare MI patients in 1992 to 1993 found that octogenarians were nearly five times less likely to receive either PCI or CABG than those age 65 to 69 years.[13] As techniques and patient outcomes have improved, however, these trends are rapidly changing. Currently, 20% of PCI and CABG procedures are performed on those age 75 years or older, whereas more than one half occur in those age 65 years or older (see Table 16–1). To determine whether revascularization is appropriate in an individual elderly patient, clinicians must weigh the risks and potential benefits.

A randomized trial compared invasive therapy, including CABG or PCI as indicated, with medical therapy in patients 75 years of age or older who had chronic angina that was class II or worse.[26] At 6 months, mortality was slightly higher with invasive therapy, and there was no difference in the combined endpoint of death or nonfatal MI. However, patients who received invasive therapy had significantly better exercise tolerance and health status, and they also had a significantly lower likelihood of being admitted for increasing or unstable angina.

Age is certainly an important independent risk factor for periprocedural morbidity (such as stroke and renal failure) and mortality following PCI and CABG (Fig. 16–2).[27, 28] This age-associated risk in procedural mortality is not strictly linear but rather rises more rapidly beyond age 75 years. Additionally, among all age groups, patients undergoing CABG generally have

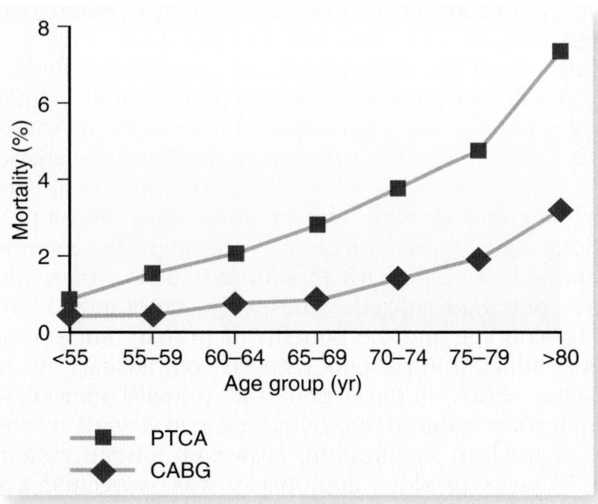

FIGURE 16–2. In-hospital mortality following coronary artery bypass surgery and angioplasty by patient age. National Cardiovascular Network Registry, 1994 to 1998. (From Batchelor WB, Anstrom KJ, Muhlbaier LH, et al: Contemporary outcome trends in the elderly undergoing percutaneous coronary interventions: Results in 7,472 octogenarians. National Cardiovascular Network Collaboration. J Am Coll Cardiol 2000;36:723–730 and Alexander KP, Anstrom KJ, Muhlbaier, LH, et al: Outcomes of cardiac surgery in patients ≥80 years: Results from the National Cardiovascular Network. J Am Coll Cardiol 2000;35:731–738.)

twofold to threefold higher risks than those receiving PCI.[8, 27, 28] After CABG, up to 50% of patients will have small, but measurable, new cognitive impairment at hospital discharge. Although many of these initial impairments improve by 6 months, these cognitive deficits commonly reappear during longer-term follow-up.[29]

Procedural risks must be balanced against potential benefits in terms of prolonged survival, improved functional outcomes, or both. In younger patients, a series of randomized trials have clarified which patients benefit from revascularization (see Chapter 25), but sufficient randomized data are still not available in patients age 75 years or older (Table 16–3). Observational studies, however, suggest that the benefits for older patients are similar to those identified by randomized trials in younger patients. Specifically, elderly patients with one vessel CAD do as well with medical therapy as with revascularization. In contrast, elderly patients with multi-vessel CAD appear to have higher survival rates with PCI or CABG, even after adjusting for baseline prognostic factors. Although better data are required for conclusive recommendations, consensus guidelines for both PCI and CABG conclude that "age alone should not be used as a sole contraindication for consideration of revascularization procedures."[30, 31]

Cardiac Rehabilitation

Multifaceted cardiac rehabilitation programs provide a 20% to 25% reduction in mortality in younger survivors of an MI (see Chapter 22). Participation in these programs also resulted in improved functional capacity, psychological well-being, and overall quality of life. None of these early trials included any patients older than 70 years. In response, several observational studies have specifically looked at the effectiveness of cardiac rehabilitation in elderly populations and demonstrated significant improvements in functional status (e.g., exercise tolerance, treadmill time), similar to what was seen in younger patients. Additionally, patients who participate in comprehensive rehabilitation programs are more likely to adopt healthy lifestyle changes as part of secondary prevention. Most studies have found that cardiac rehabilitation was associated with improvements in functional outcomes and mental health. These improvements appear to be of similar magnitude in both young and older patients, and they are evident even in the very elderly (age 75 years or older). As a result, current consensus guidelines for rehabilitation should be applied to *all* patients, regardless of age.[32]

HEART FAILURE (see Chapter 28)

Prevalence and Prognosis

Heart failure is now the leading cause of hospitalization for Medicare patients, accounting for nearly one million

TABLE 16–3

Representation of Elderly in Revascularization Trials

Trial Name	Comparison	No. Enrolled	Age Exclusion	No. Enrolled ≥75 Years of Age
CASS	CABG-Med	780	age ≤ 65	0
VA	CABG-Med	686	no age	0
European	CABG-Med	767	age < 65	0
RITA	CABG-PTCA	1011	no age	22
EAST	CABG-PTCA	392	no age	36
GABI	CABG-PTCA	359	age < 75	0
CABRI	CABG-PTCA	1054	age ≤ 75	0
BARI	CABG-PTCA	1829	age < 80	109
ACME	PTCA-Med	212	no age	n/a

ACME = Angioplasty compared to Medicine Study; BARI = Bypass Angioplasty Revascularization Investigation; CABRI = Coronary Artery versus Bypass Revascularization Investigation; CABG = coronary artery bypass surgery; CASS = Coronary Artery Surgery Study; EAST = Emory Angioplasty versus Surgery Trial; European = European Coronary Surgery Study; GABI = German Angioplasty versus Bypass Surgery Trial; Med = medical therapy; PTCA = percutaneous transluminal coronary angioplasty; RITA = Randomized Intervention Treatment of Angina; VA = VA Cooperative Study of Coronary Artery Bypass for Stable Angina. From Peterson ED, Alexander KP: Chronic coronary heart disease. In Lewis R, O'Gara P, Parmley W (eds): Adult Clinical Cardiology Self-Assessment Program V. Bethesda, MD, American College of Cardiology Foundation, 2002, pp 21–26.

admissions in the United States each year. Nearly 80% of patients discharged with a new diagnosis of heart failure are age 65 years or older, and 50% are age 75 years or older.[4] Heart failure is second only to hypertension as the leading cause for outpatient evaluations in older individuals, and it accounts for more than 12 million physician visits annually. Given this high resource utilization, heart failure is America's most costly diagnosis, with yearly expenditures exceeding $40 billion.

The ratio of systolic to diastolic heart failure changes with advancing age. Although about 6% of patients younger than 60 years with heart failure have diastolic heart failure, diastolic dysfunction accounts for about 40% of heart failure in patients age 70 years or older and 50% of heart failure in octogenarians (Fig. 16–3). In terms of prognosis, the median survival following the onset of heart failure in the elderly is a little over 2 years, with nearly 80% of elderly heart failure patients dying within 5 years after the onset of heart failure.[4]

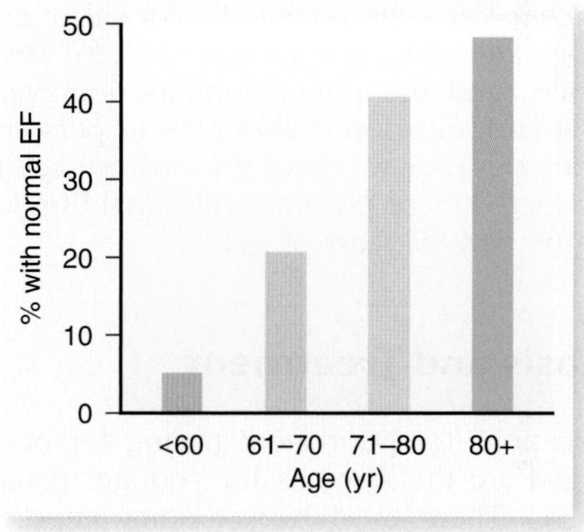

FIGURE 16–3. Incidence of heart failure with preserved systolic function. (From Aronow WS, Ahn C, Kronzon I: Prognosis of congestive heart failure in elderly patients with normal versus abnormal left ventricular systolic function associated with coronary artery disease. Am J Cardiol 1990;66:1257–1259.)

Diagnosis and Treatment

The initial diagnosis of heart failure in the elderly may be challenging due to the gradual onset of nonspecific symptoms. In the elderly, heart failure can manifest as complaints of restlessness, anorexia, or nausea. Even typical symptoms such as cardiac-related fatigue or dyspnea may be attributed to co-morbid illnesses or "old-age" in the sedentary elderly patient. Because of the frequency of diastolic heart failure in this population, it is particularly important to document left ventricular function to guide further diagnostic testing and treatment strategies (see Chapter 28).[33] Ischemia, worsening hypertension, or arrhythmias can cause new onset or worsening heart failure in the elderly. Additionally, increased salt intake or heavy use of nonsteroidal anti-inflammatory drugs (NSAIDs) can worsen fluid retention in the elderly with impaired renal function.

The treatment of heart failure in the elderly is similar to that in younger patients (see Chapter 28) with minor caveats. In an overview of five randomized trials of ACE inhibitors for heart failure, there was no evidence of age-related differences in the known benefit for ACE inhibition in heart failure.[34] ACE inhibitors can increase risks for hyperkalemia in the elderly with borderline renal function.

Digoxin remains a useful adjunct for elderly patients with symptomatic heart failure.[35] Digoxin must be appropriately dosed according to age-adjusted creatinine clearance.

A multidisciplinary team approach to heart failure management can significantly reduce readmission rates and is particularly valuable for the elderly patient who may have difficulty traveling frequently to a physician's office for re-evaluation. The benefit of this team approach comes from patient education and medication adjustments between physician visits. Given the poor prognosis of heart failure in the elderly, it is incumbent upon the physician to initiate discussions regarding end-of-life decisions and preferences when appropriate (see Chapter 17).

ARRHYTHMIAS (see Chapters 30 and 31)

Prevalence

The prevalence of bradyarrhythmias rises rapidly with advancing age owing to age-related degeneration of the conduction system. It is estimated that only 10% of sinus node pacemaker cells remain functional after age 75 years. The elderly also are at higher risk for atrial tachyarrhythmias, and the population-based prevalence of chronic atrial fibrillation is about 2% in persons age 60 to 69 years but rises to about 9% in those age 80 to 89 years. In fact, 70% of patients with atrial fibrillation are between 65 and 85 years of age.[4, 36]

Diagnosis and Treatment

The indications for permanent pacing for bradycardia in the aged are the same as for younger patients (see Chapter 31). There are, however, some important considerations for the management of atrial fibrillation in the elderly.

The risk of stroke associated with atrial fibrillation increases substantially with age. In addition, valvular heart disease, hypertension, and diabetes increase the risk of stroke associated with atrial fibrillation. Regardless of the management for rate control or maintenance of sinus rhythm (see Chapter 30), patients older than 65 years should be considered for warfarin prophylaxis due to their high risk of stroke. Data pooled from five randomized trials comparing warfarin or aspirin with placebo in patients with atrial fibrillation found a 66% reduction in the risk of stroke with warfarin and a 16% reduction with aspirin. Patients with atrial fibrillation who received placebo had about a 4.5% annual rate of stroke.[37] The annual rate of major hemorrhage was about 1% to 2% for the placebo group, 1.3% for the aspirin group, and 2.2% for the warfarin group. Close surveillance of International Normalized Ratio (INR) levels is recommended because of the greater likelihood of bleeding complications in the elderly. Elderly patients with atrial fibrillation who cannot safely receive warfarin should be given aspirin (see Chapter 30).[38]

Atrial fibrillation is also a common cause of heart failure in elderly patients, who often rely on their atrial kick, which can account for up to 20% to 30% of stroke volume in patients with impaired left ventricular function. Some elderly persons tolerate atrial fibrillation because their associated conduction system disease tends to slow the ventricular response and, hence, the heart rate. However, elderly patients with slow atrial fibrillation may have periods of significant bradycardia alternating with periods of tachycardia ("tachy-brady" syndrome) and be difficult to manage medically. These patients often require both AV nodal blocking medications and implantation of a permanent pacemaker (see Chapters 30 and 31).

VALVULAR HEART DISEASE

Prevalence

Systolic murmurs are extremely common in the elderly, with a prevalence of 60% or greater (see Chapter 11). By far, the most common valvular disorder associated with aging is aortic stenosis. In an echocardiographic study of 577 randomly chosen 75- to 86-year-olds, 40% had mild aortic valve disease, whereas another 15% had severe or critical aortic stenosis.[39]

Diagnosis and Treatment

Similar to other cardiovascular complaints, symptoms of valvular heart disease can be difficult to identify in the elderly patient (see Chapter 32). The elderly often present with a lack of energy, weakness, or other heart failure symptoms. The severity of aortic stenosis can be reasonably well assessed in the elderly patient based on the physical examination. Echocardiography is used to confirm valvular heart disease in those with suspicious murmurs (see Chapter 32). Surgery is the mainstay for aortic stenosis, but the risks of valve surgery rise with age. For example, based on the Society of Thoracic Surgery National Database ($n = 108{,}000$), operative mortality following isolated valve surgery ranges from about 3% in those age 60 years or younger to more than 10% in octogenarians. Besides the risk for death, octogenarians undergoing valve surgery face an 8% risk of stroke, a 13% risk of renal failure, and up to a 20% likelihood of prolonged ventilation, all approximately threefold higher than in younger patients.[8] Nevertheless, the elderly generally have the same indications for valve surgery as younger patients, unless comorbidities or patient preferences dictate otherwise. When valve surgery is selected in the elderly patient, bioprosthetic (rather than mechanical) valves are often used to avoid the potential risks of anticoagulation. Aortic balloon valvuloplasty can relieve symptoms for several months, but the nearly universal risk of restenosis markedly limits its clinical utility.

Evidence-Based Summary

1. Lipid lowering appears to be as beneficial in the elderly as in younger patients (see Chapter 20), although data are limited in patients age 75 years or older.
2. Treatment of hypertension (see Chapter 19) using thiazide diuretics or low-dose beta-blockers provides an equivalent proportional reduction, and hence a greater absolute benefit, in the elderly as compared with younger patients.
3. For patients with CAD, aspirin (see Chapter 25) appears to have an equivalent proportional benefit, and hence a greater absolute benefit, in patients older than 65 years compared with younger patients.
4. Recanalization/reperfusion therapy for acute MI in the elderly is probably beneficial. Intravenous fibrinolysis has a significant benefit in patients up to age 75 years. In patients age 75 years or older, the acute risks of fibrinolysis are higher, and the benefits are much less certain. Observational studies support the benefit of primary angioplasty in patients older than 75 years, but randomized controlled trial data are not currently available in this patient population.
5. Elderly patients have high risks of complications after percutaneous coronary interventions and coronary artery bypass surgery. The benefits in patients with indications for these procedures appear to be equivalent to those found in younger persons, and the recommendations are generally similar for elderly as for younger patients.
6. ACE inhibitors for heart failure appear to have equivalent benefits in the elderly as in younger patients.
7. The risk of stroke with atrial fibrillation increases substantially with age. Warfarin prophylaxis is clearly beneficial and should be the standard of care in all patients aged 65 years or older unless contraindicated by substantially elevated risks of bleeding or falling.
8. Patients with valvular aortic stenosis can undergo aortic valve replacement with acceptable risks even in their eighties or nineties, provided they meet criteria for aortic valve replacement and are otherwise in acceptable medical condition.

References

1. Williams MA, Fleg JL, Ades PA, et al: Secondary prevention of coronary heart disease in the elderly (with emphasis on patients ≥75 years of age): An American Heart Association scientific statement from the Council on Clinical Cardiology Subcommittee on Exercise, Cardiac Rehabilitation, and Prevention. Circulation 2002;105:1735–1743.
2. Tsevat J, Cook EF, Green ML, et al: Health values of the seriously ill. Ann Intern Med 1994;122:514–520.
3. Lee PY, Alexander KP, Hammill BG, et al: Representation of elderly persons and women in published randomized trials of acute coronary syndromes. JAMA 2001;286:708–713.
4. American Heart Association. American Heart Association heart and stroke 2001 statistical update. www.americanheart.org/statistics/medical.html. Dallas, American Heart Association, 2001.
5. Whelton PK, Appel LJ, Espeland MA, et al: Sodium and weight loss in the treatment of hypertension in older persons: A randomized controlled trial of nonpharmacologic interventions in the elderly (TONE). JAMA 1998;279: 839–846.
6. Mulrow C, Lau J, Cornell J, et al: Pharmacotherapy for hypertension in the elderly. Cochrane Database of Systematic Reviews. 2000. The Cochrane Library. http://cochrane.co.uk. Accessed June 2001.
7. Tu K, Mamdani MM, Tu JV: Hypertension guidelines in elderly patients: Is anybody listening? Am J Med 2002;113: 52–58.
8. Cheitlin MD, Gerstenblith G, Hazzard WR, et al: Do existing databases answer clinical questions about geriatric cardiovascular disease and stroke? Am J Geriatr Cardiol 2001;10:207–223.
9. Mehta RH, Rathore SS, Radford MJ, et al: Acute myocardial infarction in the elderly: Differences by age. J Am Coll Cardiol 2001;38:736–741.
10. Ambepitiya G, Roberts M, Ranjadayalan K, Tallis R: Silent exertional myocardial ischemia in the elderly: A quantitative analysis of anginal perceptual threshold and the influence of autonomic function. J Am Geriatr Soc 1994;42: 732–737.
11. Sheifer SE, Rathore SS, Gersh BJ, et al: Time to presentation with acute myocardial infarction in the elderly: Associations with race, sex, and socioeconomic characteristics. Circulation 2000;102:1651–1656.
12. White HD, Barbash GI, Califf RM, et al: Age and outcome with contemporary thrombolytic therapy. Results from the GUSTO-I Trial. Global utilization of streptokinase and TPA for occluded coronary arteries trial. Circulation 1996;94: 1826–1833.
13. Alexander KP, Galanos AN, Jollis JG, et al: Postmyocardial infarction risk-stratification in elderly patients. Am Heart J 2001;142:37–42.
14. Bashore TM, Bates ER, Kern MJ, et al: American College of Cardiology/Society for Cardiac Angiography and Interventions Clinical Expert Consensus Document on Catheterization Laboratory Standards. J Am Coll Cardiol 2001;37:2170–2214.
15. Miettinen TA, Pyorala K, Olsson AG, et al: Cholesterol-lowering therapy in women and elderly patients with myocardial infarction or angina pectoris: Findings from the Scandinavian Simvastatin Survival Study (4S). Circulation 1997;96:4211–4218.
16. Lewis SJ, Moye LA, Sacks FM, et al: Effect of pravastatin on cardiovascular events in older patients with myocardial infarction and cholesterol levels in the average range: Results of the cholesterol and recurrent events (CARE) trial. Ann Intern Med 1998;129:681–689.
17. Downs JR, Clearfield M, Weis S, et al: Primary prevention of acute coronary events with lovastatin in men and

women with average cholesterol levels: Results of AFCAPS/TexCAPS. Air Force/Texas Coronary Atherosclerosis Prevention Study. JAMA 1998;279:1615–1622.

18. Krumholz HM, Radford MJ, Wang Y, et al: National use and effectiveness of β-blockers for the treatment of elderly patients after acute myocardial infarction. National Cooperative Cardiovascular Project. JAMA 1998;280:623–629.
19. Antithrombotic Trialists' Collaboration. Collaborative meta-analysis of randomised trials of antiplatelet therapy for prevention of death, myocardial infarction, and stroke in high-risk patients. Br Med J 2002;324:71–86.
20. Maggioni AP, Maseri A, Fresco C, et al: for the Investigators of the Gruppo Italian per lo Studio della Sopravvivenz nell'infarcto Miocardico (GISSI-2). Age-related increase in mortality among patients treated with thrombolysis. N Engl J Med 1993;1442–1448.
21. Fibrinolytic Therapy Trialist's (FFT) Collaborative Group: Indications for fibrinolytic therapy in suspected acute myocardial infarction: Collaborative overview of early mortality and major morbidity results from all randomised trials of more than 1000 patients. Lancet 1994;343:311–322.
22. Thiemann DR, Coresh J, Schulman SP, et al: Lack of benefit for intravenous thrombolysis in patients with myocardial infarction who are older than 75 years. Circulation 2000;101:2239–2246.
23. Berger AK, Radford MJ, Wang Y, Krumholz HM: Thrombolytic therapy in older patients. J Am Coll Cardiol 2000;36:366–374.
24. Berger AK, Schulman KA, Gersh BJ, et al: Primary coronary angioplasty vs. thrombolysis for the management of acute myocardial infarction in elderly patients. JAMA 1999;282:341–348.
25. Hochman JS, Sleeper LA, Webb JG, et al: Early revascularization in acute myocardial infarction complicated by cardiogenic shock. SHOCK Investigators. Should we emergently revascularize occluded coronaries for cardiogenic shock? N Engl J Med 1999;341:625–634.
26. The TIME Investigators. Trial of invasive versus medical therapy in elderly patients with chronic symptomatic coronary-artery disease (TIME): A randomised trial. Lancet 2001;358:951–957.
27. Klein LW, Block P, Brindis RG, et al: Percutaneous coronary interventions in octogenarians in the American College of Cardiology–National Cardiovascular Data Registry. Development of a nomogram predictive of in-hospital mortality. J Am Coll Cardiol 2002;40:394–402.
28. Alexander KP, Anstrom KJ, Muhlbaier LH, et al: Outcomes of cardiac surgery in patients age > 80 years: Results from the National Cardiovascular Network. J Am Coll Cardiol 2000;35:731–738.
29. Newman MF, Kirchner JL, Phillips-Bute B, et al: Longitudinal assessment of neurocognitive function after coronary-artery bypass surgery. N Engl J Med 2001;344:395–402.
30. Smith SC, Dove JT, Jacobs AK, et al: ACC/AHA guidelines for percutaneous coronary intervention (revision of the 1993 PTCA guidelines)—executive summary. A report of the American College of Cardiology/American Heart Association task force on practice guidelines (Committee to revise the 1993 guidelines for percutaneous transluminal coronary angioplasty). Circulation 2001;103:3019–3041.
31. Eagle KA, Guyton RA, Davidoff R, et al: ACC/AHA guidelines for coronary artery bypass graft surgery: Executive summary and recommendations. A report of the American College of Cardiology/American Heart Association Task Force on practice guidelines (Committee to revise the 1991 guidelines for coronary artery bypass graft surgery). Circulation 1999;100:1464–1480.
32. Balady GJ, Fletcher BJ, Froelicher ES, et al: Cardiac rehabilitation programs. A statement for healthcare professionals from the American Heart Association. Available at www.americanheart.org. Accessed July 2001.
33. Williams JF, Bristow MR, Fowler MB, et al: Guidelines for the evaluation and management of heart failure. Available at www.americanheart.org. Accessed July 2001. Dallas, American Heart Association, 1995.
34. Flather MD, Yusuf S, Kober L, et al: Long-term ACE-inhibitor therapy in patients with heart failure or left-ventricular dysfunction: A systematic overview of data from individual patients. Lancet 2000;355:1575–1581.
35. Rich MW, McSherry F, Williford WO, Yusuf S: for the Digitalis Investigation Group. Effect of age on mortality, hospitalizations and response to digoxin in patients with heart failure: The DIG study. J Am Coll Cardiol 2001;38:806–813.
36. Go AS, Hylek EM, Phillips KA, et al: Prevalence of diagnosed atrial fibrillation in adults. National implications for rhythm management and stroke prevention: The anticoagulation and risk factors in atrial fibrillation (ATRIA) study. JAMA 2001;285:2370–2375.
37. Segal JB, McNamara RL, Miller MR, et al: Anticoagulants or antiplatelet therapy for non-rheumatic atrial fibrillation and flutter. Cochrane Database Syst Rev 2001;DC001938 (updated November 29, 2000).
38. Taylor FC, Cohen H, Ebrahim S: Systematic review of long term anticoagulation or antiplatelet treatment in patients with non-rheumatic atrial fibrillation. Br Med J 2001;322:321–326.
39. Lindroos M, Kupari M, Heikkila J, Tilvis R: Prevalence of aortic valve abnormalities in the elderly: An echocardiographic study of a random population sample. J Am Coll Cardiol 1993;21:1220–1225.

CHAPTER 17 Approach to End-of-Life Care for the Patient with End-Stage Heart Disease

Steven Z. Pantilat

THE END OF LIFE

Despite the many treatment advances that permit patients to live longer with a better quality of life, heart disease remains the most common cause of death in the United States. Many Americans have an ideal vision of death in which they die at home surrounded by loved ones, free of pain and other distressing symptoms. The reality, however, is that most Americans die in hospitals, in pain, and alone.[1] It need not be this way. Though death may always be sad, physicians can help dying patients and their families manage symptoms and promote psychosocial well-being. Understanding the limitations of medicine and the inevitability of death can help physicians recognize when attempts to prolong life may no longer be beneficial or desired. In these situations, "end-of-life care" or "palliative care" offers an active, aggressive approach that focuses on the whole patient; it places symptom management, communication about death and dying, and support for the patient and family above attempts at cure.

Research studies have demonstrated that patients and their families have very specific expectations about end-of-life care: having control over their care, controlling pain and other distressing symptoms, completing relationships with loved ones, and receiving ongoing support from their physician.[2] Physicians who provide end-of-life care should be guided by these concerns. Although end-of-life care commonly refers to the treatment of patients who are within weeks or months of dying, the precepts of end-of-life care need not be restricted to patients with such limited prognoses. The principles discussed are appropriate for all patients with advanced heart disease for whom relief of symptoms, communication about illness, and support are important issues.

Discussing End-of-Life Care with Patients

For many physicians, opening the discussion about end-of-life care looms as one of the most difficult tasks in caring for patients with terminal or serious, chronic illness.[3] Many physicians worry that such discussions will cause the patient to lose hope or become angry or depressed. Studies show, however, that most patients want to discuss such issues even if the topic makes them anxious. Despite their desire to talk about death and dying, patients expect their physicians to raise the issue. Helping patients identify *in a timely way* that they

BOX 17–1

Helpful Phrases for Discussing End-of-Life Care

Opening the conversation	"Mr. Johnson, what is your understanding of your heart disease after this last hospitalization?"
Values and goals of care	"When you think about getting sicker, what worries or frightens you the most?"
Prognosis	"I have information about your illness. Some patients want to hear from me directly, and others prefer that I speak with someone else. How do you feel?"
Hope	"When you think about the future, what do you hope for?"
Surrogate decision maker	"If you were to get so sick that you could not talk to me directly, with whom should I speak to help me make decisions about your care?"
Nonabandonment	"I will be your doctor throughout this illness."
Hospice	"It sounds like you think your husband could use more help caring for you at home. Have you considered hospice?"

BOX 17–2

Communicating about End-of-Life Care

- Listen
- Avoid jargon
- Elicit the patient's values and goals of care
- Make empathic statements

are approaching the end of life is critical because this knowledge influences how they make treatment decisions and how they spend their remaining time.

Deciding when to begin end-of-life care discussions with cardiac patients can be difficult, particularly when a patient's clinical status is declining gradually. Four indications for initiating end-of-life discussions are when death is imminent, when patients talk about wanting to die or make inquiries about hospice or palliative care, after a hospitalization for an exacerbation of a chronic illness such as heart failure, or if the physician would not be surprised if the patient were to die in the next 6 to 12 months.[3] These criteria will include many patients with advanced heart disease. For these patients, a follow-up visit after a recent hospitalization presents a particularly good opportunity to inquire about the care provided, the experience of hospitalization, and the patient's desires regarding future care. Physicians can begin these conversations with open-ended questions that establish patients' understanding of their condition and prognosis. For example, "Mr. Johnson, what is your understanding of your heart disease after this last hospitalization?" (Box 17–1).

Physicians can adopt several straightforward strategies to improve end-of-life discussions (Box 17–2). First, physicians should listen more than they speak to encourage patients to share important information. Next, they should avoid jargon and, rather than focusing on specific interventions such as mechanical ventilation or vasopressors, should elicit the patient's values and goals of care. For example, a physician could say, "Mrs. Johnson, when you think about getting sicker, what worries or frightens you the most?" It is also important to remember the emotional nature of these discussions and to seize opportunities for empathic connection. Physicians may respond to patients' anxiety with reassurances that the physician cares about their experience, is willing to discuss difficult issues, and will be present throughout the illness to provide the care that they desire.

Prognosis

Patients with advanced heart disease often think about prognosis, as do their families. Although some patients are reluctant to discuss the issue, many welcome a direct discussion rather than discovering their prognosis in indirect ways. Physicians find discussing prognosis stressful and difficult, and they frequently provide overly optimistic assessments, especially to patients they have known for a long time.[4] Physicians should remember that discussions about prognosis allow patients to plan for the future and make decisions based on more accurate information. When older patients were asked their preferences for cardiopulmonary resuscitation (CPR), half of those who had desired CPR before the discussion, based on their own overly optimistic estimates of survival, changed their preference after being given a more accurate prognosis.[5]

For patients with heart failure, functional status is an excellent predictor of survival.[6] Mortality is 5% to 10% per year, even among patients with class I or II heart failure, and it rises to 50% per year for patients with class IV heart failure (see Chapter 28). Cardiac cachexia, defined as nonintentional, nonedema weight loss of 7.5% of the previous normal weight over a 6-month period, is also an independent predictor of mortality.[7] In one study, the survival rate at 18 months for patients with heart disease and cachexia was 50%, versus 83% for those without cachexia. One challenge of prognostication in advanced heart disease is that these data apply to groups of patients and cannot be applied directly to individuals. The inability to predict survival accurately for an individual patient, however, should not dissuade physicians from discussing prognosis. Patients often appreciate and understand clear explanations in general terms such as, "half of people with a condition like yours will die in the next year." A follow-up statement such as, "I hope you are the person who lives longer than that, and I will do all I can to make sure you are," conveys reassurance while still imparting important information. As patients get closer to death, the provision of general ranges, such as "weeks to months," "days to weeks," or "hours to days," can reasonably convey prognosis as well as the inherent uncertainty.

Another major challenge in discussing prognosis with patients with advanced heart disease is that up to 50% of deaths occur suddenly. The specter of sudden death highlights the need to inform patients and their families of this possibility and to initiate discussions of prognosis early so that both patients and their families can plan for the future.

A final challenge in talking about prognosis is that in some cultures, patients and families consider such discussions inappropriate.[8] For example, the Navajo believe that articulating a bleak prognosis can change the future and make it a certainty. A physician may also encounter families who ask that the patient not be told of the prognosis. One response to such a request is to ask the patient for "informed refusal" by offering the patient the opportunity to decide whether to be given this information. For example, the physician might say, "I have information about your illness. Some patients want to hear from me directly, and others prefer that I speak with someone else. How do you feel?" This question allows patients to embrace or ignore the cultural norm and obtain the amount of information they want.

Hope

Many clinicians worry that discussions of prognosis rob patients of hope. However, sensitive discussions of prognosis need not rob patients of hope but, instead, can focus their hope and illuminate what is most important. Questions such as, "When you think about the future, what do you hope for?" encourage hope and offer insights into the patient's values and goals.[9]

Even patients with limited prognoses have hope, but their hopes change over time. Whereas a patient with advanced heart disease may have hoped to see his newborn grandchild graduate from high school, knowledge of his prognosis might lead him to realize that he can still hope to bequeath to his grandchild the watch he received at his own graduation. A discussion of prognosis could motivate the patient to write a letter that the child could read on receiving the watch at graduation.

Caring for the Family

The family often plays a central role in the care of a patient with advanced heart disease. In addition to supporting the patient, the physician must frequently support the family because the caregiving needs of terminally ill patients often impose many stresses. At the same time that loved ones are providing care and support to the patient, they must often deal with feelings of sadness, guilt, grief, anger, and loss. The care of a terminally ill family member frequently causes financial hardships as well. In one study, nearly a third of families of seriously ill patients reported loss of most or all of their savings and a major source of their income. By maintaining regular and open communication with the family, acknowledging its support of the patient, identifying a spokesperson for the family, conducting family meetings, allowing all to be heard, and providing time to reach consensus, physicians can productively assist the patient's family in a time of overwhelming need.

DECISION MAKING AT THE END OF LIFE

Advance Directives

An advance directive is a written or spoken statement made by a competent adult that is intended to guide medical care, designate a surrogate decision maker, or both if the patient becomes unable to communicate. Advance directives allow patients to project their autonomy into a future time when they may not be able to participate in decision making. Advance directives can be oral statements made to a family member, friend, or physician or written expressions of a patient's wishes such as a Durable Power of Attorney for Health Care (DPOA-HC). Although written advance directives are typically considered a more definitive reflection of a patient's true values and goals, spoken preferences should also be respected. It is important to emphasize to patients that these statements take effect only if they lose the ability to communicate directly with the doctor.

Most patients with serious illnesses want to discuss advance directives. A recent study showed that patients who had discussed advance directives with their primary care physicians were more satisfied with their care.[10] For patients with advanced heart disease, important topics to discuss include code status and preferences regarding hospitalization, intensive care, and mechanical ventilation. In addition, because it is impossible to anticipate all the contingencies that might arise, it is critical for the patient to designate a surrogate who can make decisions regarding care if the patient is no longer able to communicate. The role of the surrogate is to provide substituted judgment, specifically, make decisions the way the *patient* would, *not* the way the surrogate would decide for the patient or himself. A nonthreatening way to initiate a discussion of advance directives and to help the patient choose a surrogate is to say, "If you were to get so sick that you could not talk to me directly, with whom should I speak to help me make decisions about your care?"

Discussion of a patient's preferences regarding specific interventions such as tube feeding and mechanical ventilation should be placed within the context of the patient's overall values and goals for care. Questions such as, "When you think about the future, what do you worry about most?" help identify the patient's primary concerns and can guide discussions about how to avoid fears such as not being able to eat or becoming a prisoner of technology.

Do-Not-Attempt-Resuscitation Orders

Determining a patient's preference for CPR and writing do-not-attempt-resuscitation (DNAR) orders when patients request them is particularly important in advanced heart disease because half of all deaths are sudden. The term DNAR, rather than "do not resuscitate" (DNR), emphasizes that although we attempt CPR, it is usually ineffective. Even though patients who receive CPR after a myocardial infarction or for a ventricular arrhythmia tend to have a more favorable prognosis, with up to a 25% to 50% survival rate to discharge versus a 14% survival rate to discharge for all hospitalized patients needing CPR, those with advanced heart disease and co-morbidities are less likely to survive.[11] Despite this relatively poor outcome for patients with advanced heart disease, one study found that only a quarter of patients hospitalized with severe heart failure expressed a preference to not be resuscitated.[12] Another study demonstrated that patients with end-stage heart failure are less likely to have DNAR orders written than patients with acquired immunodeficiency syndrome, cancer, or stroke who had similar prognoses. Still another study documented that physicians failed to write DNAR orders in nearly half the cases in which the patient or family desired one.[2] These studies emphasize the need to discuss preferences for CPR with all patients with advanced heart disease and to write DNAR orders at the time that they are requested.

It is important to describe CPR in neutral terms and avoid the temptation to obscure our recommendations with either an overly graphic or white-washed description of the procedure. Discussions should include the probability of survival and an explicit recommendation based on the patient's values and goals. Patients with end-stage heart disease may decline CPR because they prefer to die suddenly or at home rather than from progressive pulmonary edema and dyspnea. When properly introduced and put into perspective, discussions of CPR are not merely about an intervention but more about how and where a patient prefers to die.

Ethical and Legal Issues

The same ethical principles that guide all medical care—autonomy, beneficence, nonmaleficence, confidentiality, truth telling, and justice—form the foundation for care decisions at the end of life. As in other areas of medical practice, two or more principles may conflict and require skillful communication and understanding to resolve. When faced with particularly thorny ethical conflicts, physicians can turn to trusted colleagues, institutional ethics committees, books, and journals for guidance.[13]

Futility. In addition to commonly confronted ethical issues such as confidentiality and informed consent, certain ethical considerations take on particular relevance at the end of life. The concept of futility arises when the preferences of the patient or family for an intervention conflict with the physician's willingness to provide it. Such conflicts commonly arise over a patient's or family's requests for interventions, such as hemodialysis or mechanical ventilation, that the physician believes are unlikely to benefit the patient or whose use would violate the physician's own moral code. Although some have argued that any intervention with less than a 1% chance of success should be defined as futile, little agreement has been reached concerning what constitutes a futile intervention. Invoking futility to override a patient's or family's request is symptomatic of a serious breakdown in communication, one likely to cause alienation, anger, and guilt. Instead, physicians should reassess their approach and attempt to seek a mutually satisfactory resolution regarding the decision at hand by means of ongoing discussions with the patient and family.

Withholding and Withdrawing Treatment. An ethical issue that often causes confusion in end-of-life care involves the withholding and withdrawing of life-sustaining interventions. Although withdrawing interventions such as mechanical ventilation, vasopressors, hemodialysis, antibiotics, or artificial nutrition and hydration may feel different from withholding them, these actions are ethically and legally the same.[13] In the Cruzan decision, the U.S. Supreme Court established that patients or their surrogates have the right to refuse any unwanted medical intervention and to request the discontinuation of any intervention, including nutrition and hydration. Respect for the principle of autonomy requires physicians to honor such wishes.

Hastening Death. In striving to relieve pain, physicians may need to prescribe opioids at doses that might depress respiration and hasten death. The ethical concept of "double effect" clarifies that these known, but unintended consequences are acceptable when the overriding goal of an intervention is to relieve suffering and provide comfort. Except in very rare circumstances, it is always possible to relieve suffering without hastening death.

Physician-Assisted Suicide. Patients may also raise the issue of physician-assisted suicide. Although a full discussion of this topic is outside the scope of this chapter, it is important to recognize that such requests are often a cry for help or are symptomatic of unrelieved suffering. In particular, unrelieved pain, caregiver burden, and depression are associated with a desire for assisted suicide.[14] Importantly, half of patients who make such requests later change their minds. Inquiries about pain, depression, and caregiver burden can identify issues that may respond to a physician's interventions. It is critical to remember that assisted suicide is illegal in every state in the United States except Oregon, and legal there only under strict guidelines.

SYMPTOM MANAGEMENT

Patients with advanced heart disease frequently experience distressing symptoms at the end of life.[15] It is important to assess and treat symptoms aggressively to allow patients to focus on completing important tasks and saying goodbye to loved ones.

Pain

Pain is the most common symptom in patients with advanced heart disease. In one study, 78% of patients with heart disease experienced pain in the last year of life.[15] Because pain at the end of life can be severe, patients often require opioids. Unfortunately, patients and physicians are often reluctant to use opioids and therefore do not achieve an acceptable level of pain control. Barriers to good pain control include poor assessment of pain, concern about side effects and addiction, and fear of legal consequences. Attitudes associated with better pain control include believing that the patient has pain, insisting on total pain relief, and prescribing pain medications liberally.

Pain cannot be measured objectively. The only way to know whether a patient is in pain is to ask. Patients with chronic pain can be especially challenging because they no longer have the physiologic changes associated with acute pain such as tachycardia, hypertension, tachypnea, and diaphoresis. Pain scales offer quantitative, reproducible methods for assessing the severity of pain and its response to treatment[16] (Fig. 17–1). The 0 to 10 numeric rating scale offers a quick tool for assessing pain. One can ask the patient, "On a scale of 0 to 10, with 0 being no pain and 10 being the worst pain you can imagine, how much pain are you having now?" An alternative is to ask the patient to choose the most appropriate description of the severity of pain: no pain, mild pain, moderate pain, severe pain, very severe pain, or worst possible pain.

It is also important to determine the cause of the pain (Fig. 17–2). Understanding the etiology may help direct specific treatment. For example, anginal pain might respond better to increased antianginal medications. Neuropathic pain, often described as burning, shooting, or electrical and commonly associated with numbness, responds well to tricyclic antidepressants and anticonvulsants such as gabapentin, clonazepam, and carbamazepine (Table 17–1). However, given the risk of orthostatic hypotension and arrhythmias, it is best to avoid tricyclics in patients with advanced heart disease.

For mild pain, acetaminophen and aspirin can be helpful. Because nonsteroidal anti-inflammatory drugs, including the cyclooxygenase-2 inhibitors, can precipitate exacerbations of heart failure, they should be avoided in patients with advanced heart disease.[17] For moderate or severe pain, opioids are appropriate. Whenever possible, the oral route is preferred because it is easy to administer at home, avoids the risk of infection from needles, and is less expensive for the patient. When using opioids, it is best to begin with low doses and titrate upward to achieve adequate pain control. Equianalgesic dosing charts (Table 17–2) help the physician convert between opioids or from a parenteral to an oral or transdermal route of administration.

Chronic, severe, or anticipated pain should never be treated on an "as needed" basis. Long-acting opioids (such as methadone, sustained-release morphine or oxycodone, or transdermal fentanyl) in combination with short-acting preparations for breakthrough pain (such as immediate-release morphine or oxycodone) offer the best relief in these situations. Tolerance to opioids, defined as a need for increasing doses of an opioid to achieve the same analgesic effect, is uncommon. Typically, a patient's need for higher doses of opioids in response to worsening pain indicates that the disease is progressing. In such circumstances, the best approach is to increase the dose of the opioid to achieve adequate pain control.

Side effects such as sedation, respiratory depression, and constipation are also concerns with opioid use. Sedation typically resolves after 2 to 3 days at the same dose of opioid. For persistent sedation, methylphenidate or dextroamphetamine, 2.5 mg orally in the morning and at noon, can help. A typical dose is 5 to 15 mg/day, not to exceed 40 to 60 mg/day.[18] Concern about respiratory depression may prevent patients from receiving adequate pain control. Although respiratory depression can occur, it is uncommon if

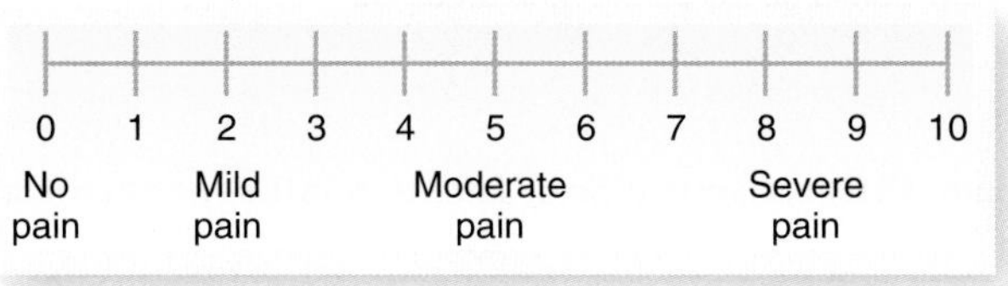

FIGURE 17–1. Numeric rating scale for assessing the severity of pain. See text for an explanation.

TABLE 17–1

Treatment of Neuropathic Pain

Drug	Dose
Tricyclic antidepressants*	
Amitriptyline	10–150 mg orally at bedtime
Nortriptyline	10–150 mg orally at bedtime
Desipramine	10–200 mg orally at bedtime
Anticonvulsants	
Carbamazepine†‡	200 mg orally bid to qid
Clonazepam†	0.5–1.0 mg orally tid
Gabapentin	300–900 mg orally tid

*Begin with the smallest dose because analgesia can often be achieved at doses far below antidepressant doses, thereby minimizing adverse side effects.

†Begin at half the lowest dose and titrate every few days until pain relief is achieved or the maximal dose is reached.

‡Periodically monitor blood counts because the drug can cause bone marrow suppression.

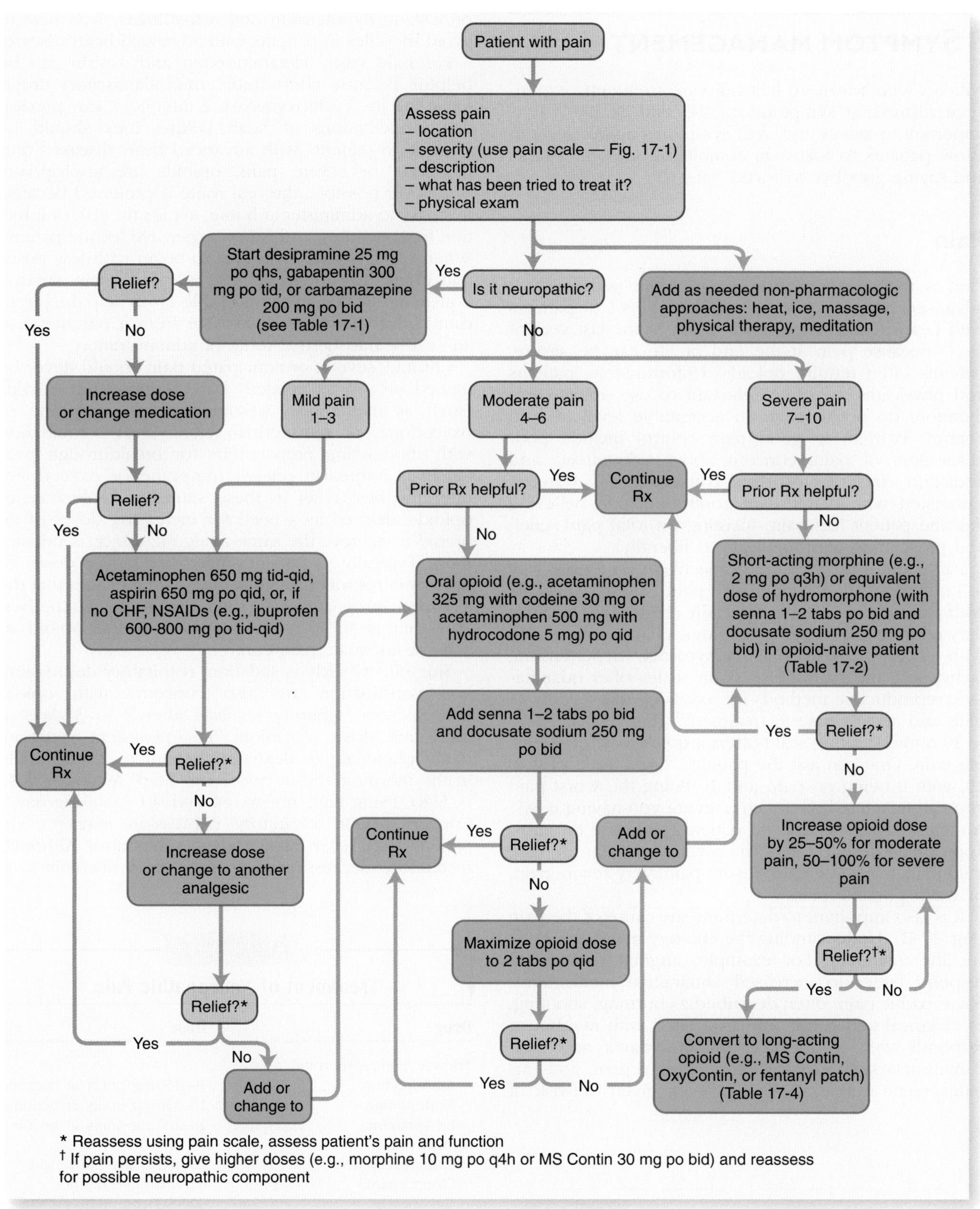

FIGURE 17–2. Algorithm for determining the cause of a patient's pain. CHF, congestive heart failure; NSAIDs, nonsteroidal anti-inflammatory drugs; Rx, treatment.

TABLE 17–2

Equianalgesic Dosing Table

Opioid Analgesic	Equianalgesic Dose (mg)	
	Oral	***Parenteral***
Morphine* (Roxanol, MS Contin)	30	10
Hydromorphone (Dilaudid)	7.5	1.5
Oxycodone (Percocet, OxyContin)	20	—
Methadone (titrate slowly because of long half-life)	20 (acute) 2–4 (chronic)	10 (acute) 2–4 (chronic)
Hydrocodone (Vicodin, Lortab, Norco)	30	—
Codeine (Tylenol with Codeine: No. 2 = 15 mg, No. 3 = 30 mg, No. 4 = 60 mg)	180–200	130
Fentanyl†	—	0.1 (100 µg)
Fentanyl transdermal‡ (Duragesic)	2 : 1 rule§	—

*Most references use a 6 : 1 ratio of intramuscular/intravenous/subcutaneous to oral morphine, but that number is based on single-dose studies. For patients in a steady state, it is more appropriate to use a ratio of 2 : 1 or 3 : 1.

†Oral transmucosal fentanyl is now available for acute, breakthrough pain, but it is not used for routine pain control and therefore no oral equivalents are given.

‡The onset of analgesia is delayed 8 to 12 hours, so pain must be treated for the first 12 hours with other medication. A residual effect occurs after the patch is removed. *Do not* use in opioid-naive patients. Use only for chronic stable pain.

§If the total 24-hour dose of oral morphine is 100 mg, the approximate equianalgesic dose of transdermal fentanyl is 50 µg/hr, or a 2000 : 1 equivalency.

Data from Doyle D, Hanks GWC, MacDonald N: Oxford Textbook of Palliative Medicine. Oxford, Oxford University Press, 1998, pp 331–355; and University of California, San Francisco: Adult Pain Management Guide. San Francisco, University of California, 2002.

treatment starts with a low dose, which is then titrated upward very slowly. Even patients with concomitant pulmonary disease can tolerate low-dose opioids if they are monitored carefully. Unlike sedation, constipation does not resolve with time. Many patients will find constipation worse than pain and stop taking the opioid. Therefore, it is critical to prescribe a bowel regimen for all patients receiving opioids. Senna, a laxative that stimulates the bowel, at doses of 2 tablets or 10 to 15 mL of syrup orally twice a day (not to exceed 8 tablets or 30 mL/day), and docusate sodium, a stool softener, 250 mg orally twice a day, can help prevent constipation. Occasionally, nausea, pruritus, or urinary retention may develop in response to a particular opioid. Lowering the dose or switching to another opioid will often relieve the symptom.

Dyspnea

Dyspnea, the subjective sensation of difficulty breathing, occurs in over 60% of patients dying of advanced heart disease.[15] Treatment approaches for patients with dyspnea are discussed in Chapter 7.

For dyspneic patients with advanced heart disease, the physician should first determine whether the patient desires an evaluation to determine the underlying cause or simply prefers nonspecific treatment directed at alleviating the dyspnea. Pleural effusions or pulmonary edema will develop in many patients dying of heart disease and may respond to specific treatment such as diuretics or thoracentesis. For all patients with dyspnea, oxygen and opioids may provide relief. Oxygen is especially helpful for patients with hypoxemia, but it should be tried in all patients. Some patients will find relief simply by having cool air blow across their face. Although most studies of opioids for the treatment of dyspnea have been conducted in cancer patients, experience suggests that opioids can also be effective in relieving dyspnea caused by heart disease, often at lower doses than those needed for pain relief.

Nausea and Vomiting

Nausea and vomiting are experienced at the end of life by up to 32% of patients with advanced heart disease.[15] Because treatment is best targeted at the mechanism and pathway causing these distressing symptoms, it is helpful to group the causes by mechanism (Table 17–3). Some causes of nausea and vomiting, such as drugs, toxins, and metabolic disorders, stimulate the chemoreceptor trigger zone in the brain. Treatment can be directed at blocking the chemoreceptor trigger zone

TABLE 17–3

Mechanisms and Causes of Nausea and Vomiting

Mechanism/Pathway	Cause
Chemoreceptor trigger zone	Drugs: opioids, digoxin, antibiotics, NSAIDs Metabolic derangements: hypercalcemia, uremia Chemotherapeutic agents
Vagal afferent nerve	Mucosal irritation (candidiasis) Gastrointestinal stretch or enlargement as a result of constipation, gastroparesis, gastric outlet obstruction, bowel obstruction Organ enlargement
Higher cortical structures	Increased intracranial pressure from tumor, bleeding, infection Anxiety
Vestibular apparatus	Movement

NSAIDs, nonsteroidal anti-inflammatory drugs.

receptors for dopamine, serotonin, and histamine. If an opioid is the suspected cause of the nausea and vomiting, changing to another opioid may provide relief. In addition, prochlorperazine, a phenothiazine that blocks dopamine receptors, administered at 10 mg orally or intravenously every 8 hours or 25 mg rectally every 6 hours, is a good initial agent for the treatment of nausea. If no response is seen to this class of drug or if the patient becomes too sedated, a reasonable next step is a trial of haloperidol at a dose of 0.5 to 5 mg orally every 6 to 8 hours.

Mucosal irritation, stretching of the bowel from constipation, obstruction, gastroparesis, or organ enlargement such as hepatomegaly can stimulate vagal afferent nerves that directly trigger vomiting. When possible, the underlying cause should be treated by relieving constipation or bowel obstruction or by stimulating the bowel with a promotility agent. Nasogastric suctioning may provide quick relief for nausea associated with constipation, obstruction, or gastroparesis. Antihistamines may be useful because histamine receptors play a role in this type of nausea. Diphenhydramine, meclizine, and hydroxyzine at 25 to 50 mg orally every 6 hours are good first choices. Diphenhydramine can be given intravenously at the same doses. Benzodiazepines alone are poor antiemetics and may increase the risk of aspiration. Finally, small meals, avoidance of strong odors, and the use of carbonated drinks can help reduce nausea and vomiting.

Depression

Sadness and grief are normal in patients approaching the end of life. Depression is not. Depression is underdiagnosed at the end of life and leads to diminished quality of life, heightened sensation of pain, and requests for hastened death.[14,19] One difficulty in diagnosing depression in terminally ill patients is that the classic vegetative symptoms of anhedonia, poor sleep, decreased appetite, and diminished concentration are often the result of the underlying illness and not depression. Therefore, emotional symptoms such as feelings of guilt, hopelessness, helplessness, and worthlessness are more helpful in determining whether a patient with a terminal illness is depressed.

Depression can be successfully treated in patients approaching the end of life, and clinicians should have a low threshold for initiating therapy. Despite the lack of controlled trials, experts recommend an approach that includes psychotherapy, patient and family education, and medications.[19] Medications that work quickly may be preferred because patients frequently do not have the 6 weeks or more that is often required for selective serotonin reuptake inhibitors (SSRIs) to work. Methylphenidate and dextroamphetamine at starting doses of 2.5 mg orally morning and noon can begin working in as little as 1 to 2 days.[19] Tricyclic antidepressants should be avoided because of the risk of orthostatic hypotension and arrhythmias.

Delirium

Delirium (a state of waxing and waning consciousness combined with confusion, agitation, disturbance of the sleep-wake cycle, anxiety, and disorders of memory, cognition, and behavior) is common in patients with end-stage heart disease and is intensely disturbing to patients and family members.[15] Rapid identification plus treatment of delirium is imperative. Drugs, metabolic derangements, organ failure, and infections can precipitate delirium. In mild cases, simple interventions such as a familiar, well-lit environment, reassuring words from loved ones, and companionship may be sufficient to control delirium. Attention to the choice, use, and dosing of psychoactive drugs such as opioids and benzodiazepines can also ameliorate delirium. When a specific cause cannot be found or the specific etiology reversed, delirium can be treated directly with haloperidol at a dose of 0.5 to 10 mg orally, subcutaneously, intramuscularly, or intravenously every 6 hours.

Benzodiazepines often cause delirium, are ineffective at treating it, and should be avoided.

Death Rattle

A "death rattle," the sound made by air passing over the thin layer of saliva and mucus that forms in the back of the throat when secretions can no longer be cleared, may develop in patients who are within days of death. The rattling sound can be very disturbing to loved ones, although it is difficult to know to what extent it causes the patient discomfort. Death rattle can be eased and possibly prevented if discovered and treated early. Both 1% atropine ophthalmic solution at a dose of 1 to 2 drops sublingually every hour and a 1.5-mg scopolamine patch applied behind the ear every 3 days are effective. It is best to avoid suctioning, which can cause discomfort.

Home Intravenous Inotrope Therapy

Some patients with class III and IV heart failure will continue to have symptoms despite maximal oral therapy. For these patients, intravenous dobutamine or milrinone administered at home may be an option. Some hospice programs and other home care services can provide this therapy.[20] Unfortunately, although home intravenous inotropic therapy can improve symptoms and prevent hospitalization for exacerbations of heart failure, this benefit is associated with higher mortality.[21] Before initiating intravenous inotropic therapy, physicians must inform patients of its risks and benefits. Dobutamine is the more commonly used agent. In general, this therapy should be reserved for patients with refractory symptoms in whom a trial of intravenous dobutamine in the hospital has demonstrated symptomatic relief and improved functional status. Starting doses of intravenous dobutamine range from 2.5 to 5.0 μg/kg/hr (Box 17–3).

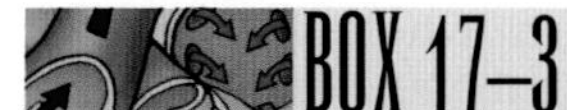

BOX 17–3

Example of Dobutamine Home Infusion Orders

1. Patients must have had previous dobutamine treatment.
2. Patients must meet National Hospice and Palliative Care Organization Medical Guidelines for Non-cancer Diagnoses (2nd ed.) for end-stage heart disease (see Box 17–5).
3. Maintenance infusion rate, frequency, and duration (to be determined by the ordering physician): Dobutamine fixed rate to infuse at •• μg/hr (usual range, 2.5–15 μg/kg/hr): •• continuous or •• days/wk M Tu W Th F Sa Su (circle days) •• number of hours of infusion.
4. Nursing visits daily for 5 days, then 1–2 times per week and as needed.
5. Blood pressure to be checked 30 min after the initiation of infusion. If systolic blood pressure has decreased 10 mm Hg or the reading is <85 mm Hg, call the physician for further orders.

Adapted with permission from Nathan Adelson Hospice, Las Vegas, NV, as published in Cross KL: The use of dobutamine in hospice patients. Am Acad Hospice Palliative Med Bull 2000;1:6–7.

Nutrition and Hydration

As patients approach death, they often stop eating and drinking. Because food has great cultural significance and because feeding expresses caring, love, and affection, it is often difficult for families to accept that their loved one will not eat. Families also worry that not eating or drinking will lead to discomfort and that the patient will "starve to death." In response to poor oral intake, patients or their families may request enteral or parenteral nutrition. These requests typically arise from a sincere hope that nutrition will help the patient recover strength and achieve a better and longer life. Although the efficacy of parenteral nutrition has not been studied in patients with terminal heart disease, studies of patients with cancer, stroke, and dementia do not support these hopes. When these patients become too sick to eat and drink, parenteral nutrition via a nasogastric, gastrostomy, or jejunostomy tube neither prevents aspiration pneumonia nor promotes comfort, weight gain, or prolonged life.[22] Although supplemental nutrition may be useful in selected patients with heart disease, it is unlikely that patients with terminal heart disease who are too ill to eat or drink will have any more benefit from parenteral nutrition than patients with cancer have.

The physician plays an important role in explaining, to both the patient and family, the risks and lack of benefit of tube feeding for patients with end-stage disease. Physicians can redirect the family's desire to provide care toward moistening the patient's mouth and carefully spoon-feeding patients who are still able to eat. One prospective study of patients with cancer demonstrated that the vast majority of terminally ill patients never or only briefly experienced hunger or thirst. For these patients, small amounts of food and water or simply wetting the mouth sufficed to relieve hunger and thirst. Finally, physicians should explain that for patients with terminal heart failure, minimizing fluid may promote comfort by preventing pulmonary and peripheral edema.

PSYCHOSOCIAL SUPPORT AND SPIRITUAL ISSUES

In the setting of powerful technologies and life-prolonging medications, physicians may undervalue the healing power of their presence. Nowhere is that power more evident or necessary than at the end of life.[9] Death is not merely a physiologic event but, more importantly, a psychological, social, and spiritual experience. To provide comprehensive care to dying patients, physicians must not only relieve distressing physical symptoms but also provide psychosocial support and attend to spiritual issues.

Grief

Over 40 years ago, Elizabeth Kübler-Ross described five stages of grief experienced by dying patients. These stages—denial, anger, bargaining, depression, and acceptance—provide a useful framework for understanding the psychological states of patients at the end of life. Though often thought of as a progression, more commonly patients move back and forth between stages, and not every patient will experience each stage. In addition, patients experience the anticipatory grief of losing all their personal relationships at once. Listening, assurance, and personal support, as well as psychotherapy and group support, can be helpful.

Psychosocial Support

Patients with a terminal illness want reassurance that as they approach death, their physician will not abandon them. Nonabandonment is a central obligation of the physician that continues throughout the course of illness. For patients nearing the end of life, statements such as "I will be your doctor throughout this illness" and "I will take care of you, whatever happens," emphasize the durability of the doctor-patient relationship at a time when the patient is most vulnerable and in need of care. Physicians may also consider giving their pager or direct phone numbers to their dying patients or making house calls to reaffirm their commitment to being available to the patient.

In one sense, patients abandon the physician when they die. In response, some physicians may begin to pull away from their dying patients to lessen their own grief and loss. In addition, some physicians mistakenly adopt the stance that "there is nothing more to do" simply because cure is no longer possible. To the contrary, physicians provide many concrete interventions to dying patients in addition to communicating and offering support. Too often, discussions at the end of life focus on what will not be done; however, an emphasis on what will be done is more helpful and sends a more hopeful message to patients and their families.

Growth and Development

Increasingly, death is seen as a stage of growth and development with unique tasks to complete. One important task involves attending to important relationships. One author suggests that to bring closure to these relationships, we must make five statements: "Forgive me," "I forgive you," "Thank you," "I love you," and "Goodbye." Physicians can encourage patients and their families to think about and make these statements. Approaching the end of life also involves discharging personal, professional, and business obligations and effects. Writing a will, giving away possessions, and making funeral and burial arrangements can complete these tasks. Knowing that life is waning focuses some patients on achieving a specific goal such as writing a book, creating a work of art, or establishing a trust or foundation.

Another task involves ensuring a legacy. For many patients, the great fear at the end of life is not about dying, but about never having lived. One way to alleviate this fear is for patients to tell their life stories. Through these stories, patients live on in the hearts and minds of their loved ones. Physicians can encourage patients to write their stories, record them on audiocassette or videocassette, or simply recite them aloud. Looking at photographs creates another opportunity to tell these stories.

Spiritual Issues

It has been said that "there are no atheists in foxholes," and spiritual matters often take on increased importance when the end of life approaches. There is even some evidence that dying patients who are spiritual have less anxiety. Although the implications of such data are not clear, it is certain that many dying patients find comfort in spiritual pursuits and that physicians are not the best-trained professionals to explore these issues. Nonetheless, physicians can ask about spiritual matters and thereby legitimize the issue as an important topic for discussion[9] (Box 17–4). Furthermore, exploration of these issues may require simple listening rather than any specific intervention. When necessary, it can also be helpful to refer patients to their own spiritual advisors and clergy or to a chaplain.

BOX 17–4

Helpful Phrases for Discussing Spirituality

"Where do you draw your strength from?"
"What role does religion or spirituality play in your life?"
"Do you believe in God or a higher power?"
"Are you a religious or spiritual person?"
"Do you pray?"
"Do you attend a synagogue, mosque, temple, or church?"

Adapted from Pantilat SZ: Care of dying patients: Beyond symptom management. West J Med 1999;171:253–256.

Cultural Issues

As with other major life events, there are many cultural issues surrounding death. In addition to the cultural differences already described regarding the desire for prognostic information, preferences regarding involvement of extended family and friends in decision making, the site of death, and traditions after death are all influenced by culture. For example, in one study, Korean Americans were more likely to want to involve their families in decision making than were European Americans. In addition, whereas somber, restrained reactions to death are typical in Western culture, loud cries of anguish and wailing are common in many Middle Eastern cultures. Finally, it is common among Buddhists to want to dress their loved one in new clothes just before death in anticipation of a better journey to a new life, whereas Catholics will typically ask a priest to give the patient the Sacrament of the Sick.

By being curious, asking open-ended questions, and remaining sensitive to differences, physicians can demonstrate their respect for the patient's culture.

HOSPICE

The care, communication, and support that patients with terminal heart disease and their families require can be a daunting task for even the most dedicated physician. Especially as patients become sicker and are no longer able to come to the office for visits, managing symptoms and providing support can be difficult. The best end-of-life care is provided by an interdisciplinary team offering comprehensive care. Nurses, social workers, pharmacists, chaplains, physical therapists, psychiatrists, psychologists, and others can play vital roles in providing comprehensive, holistic care to the patient and family. One way to marshal this type of interdisciplinary care is through hospice.

Although many people think of hospice as a place, hospice is actually a service provided to patients and their families, typically in their homes.[23] To qualify for hospice, patients must meet specific criteria, including a prognosis of 6 months or less, and agree to an exclusively palliative approach to care. Unfortunately, only one quarter of all dying patients use hospice, and most patients are referred to hospice late in their course, with a median survival in hospice of less than 3 weeks.[23] In addition, although heart disease remains the most common cause of death in the United States, patients with heart disease are underrepresented in hospice. Therefore, it is important to consider referring these patients early to hospice, thereby allowing them and their families to take maximal advantage of hospice services. Although identifying patients with advanced heart disease who have a 6-month prognosis can be difficult, the National Hospice and Palliative Care Organization has published guidelines to aid physicians[24] (Box 17–5).

BOX 17–5

National Hospice and Palliative Care Organization

General Medical Guidelines for Determining Prognosis in Selected Noncancer Diseases

I. *The patient should meet all of the following criteria:*
   - A. The patient's condition is life limiting, and the patient and/or family know this
   - B. The patient and/or family have elected treatment goals directed toward relief of symptoms rather than the underlying disease
   - C. The patient has either of the following:
     1. Documented clinical progression of the disease, which may include
        - a. Progression of the primary disease process as listed in the disease-specific criteria (see section II), documented by serial physician assessment, laboratory, radiologic, or other studies
        - b. Multiple emergency department visits or inpatient hospitalizations over the previous 6 mo
        - c. For home-bound patients receiving home health services, documentation of a nursing assessment
        - d. For patients who do not qualify under a, b, or c, documentation of a recent decline in functional status. Clinical judgment is required
     2. Documented recent impaired nutritional status related to the terminal process:
        - a. Unintentional, progressive weight loss >10% over the previous 6 mo
        - b. Serum albumin <2.5 g/dL may be a helpful prognostic indicator but should not be used in isolation from other factors above

II. *In addition to meeting the general guidelines above, the following criteria help identify patients with heart disease who are appropriate for hospice:*
   - A. Intractable or frequently recurrent symptomatic heart failure or intractable angina pectoris with heart failure
   - B. Patients should already be *optimally treated* with diuretics and vasodilators
   - C. Other factors contributing to a poor prognosis: symptomatic arrhythmias, history of cardiac arrest and resuscitation or syncope, cardiogenic brain embolism, or concomitant human immunodeficiency virus disease

Adapted from Medical Guidelines for Determining Prognosis in Selected Non-cancer Diagnoses. The National Hospice Organization. Hosp J 1996;11:47–63.

Patients enrolled in hospice must also have a designated physician who will manage their care. Even if the patient's physician has little experience with hospice, the ideal of nonabandonment endorses the primary care physician's continuing role in caring for the patient. The professional staff of the hospice, including nurses, social workers, and the medical director, can provide guidance regarding specific management issues.

Once enrolled, all medications related to the terminal diagnosis, as well as all durable medical equipment and oxygen, are provided and paid for by hospice. One advantage to hospice care is that provision of these services can be based on need without a qualifying requirement of documented disability. In addition, hospice can provide home health aides for assistance with bathing and personal care, volunteers for companionship and support for caregivers, and bereavement and grief counseling for the family. Hospice can even provide respite care to allow caregivers a few days to rest.

Physicians may be reluctant to discuss hospice for fear of taking away hope, but there are ways of broaching the topic that may be less threatening. One approach involves raising the issue of hospice in the context of providing more help at home: "It sounds like you think your husband could use more help caring for you at home. Have you considered hospice?" In addition, it may be helpful to raise the possibility of hospice early in the course of illness by saying, "I realize this may not be right for you now, but I would like to start us thinking about hospice." Patients and their families may view hospice as giving up.[23] Reassurances of what will be done and of continued care by the physician can alleviate these concerns. Finally, many people associate hospice with imminent death. Late referrals may contribute to this perception. However, the patient need not be at death's door to enroll. In fact, some patients continue to travel and go out while enrolled in hospice. Thus, hospice should not be thought of as a service only for the moribund, but more appropriately for patients with an ultimately terminal illness who no longer desire aggressive attempts at prolonging life.

AFTER DEATH

In addition to the many issues that physicians must address in caring for dying patients, several tasks must be completed after the patient dies.

Death Certificate

The physician must complete the death certificate. Accurate reporting of the cause of death aids the family in understanding the family medical history and obtaining insurance benefits. It also helps maintain public health records. In addition, these data help determine funding and research priorities. Unfortunately, physicians are often unskilled in properly reporting the cause of death. For example, physicians commonly list "cardiopulmonary arrest" as the cause of death. This designation reflects only the common final pathway of death and not the underlying etiology. The physician should be as specific as possible when assigning the cause of death. Causes of death such as "congestive heart failure due to atherosclerotic coronary artery disease" provide more accurate and useful information. In addition, physicians should complete the death certificate in a timely manner so as to not delay the funeral. Such delays can be particularly problematic in cultures that mandate prompt disposition of the body.

Autopsy

Despite advances in medical technology, autopsy remains the gold standard for determining the cause of death and for confirming diagnoses. Studies attest to the continuing value of autopsy in revealing unsuspected diagnoses. Remarkably, in up to 12% of cases, conditions are discovered that could have made a difference in the patient's survival had they been diagnosed during life. These diagnoses are helpful in revealing previously unsuspected family medical histories and may assist physicians in their care of future patients.

Physicians can increase the likelihood of obtaining consent for an autopsy simply by asking. A study comparing families who consented to autopsies with those who did not found that never being asked was an important reason for the autopsy not being performed. Other reasons provided were lack of information about the importance of autopsy and misplaced concern about disfigurement of the body.[25] Families who consented cited the following factors as influencing their decisions: advancement of medical knowledge, understanding of the cause of death, and reassurance that appropriate care was given. Physicians should use these data in discussing autopsy with families.

Care of the Family after Death

Frequently, the physician comes to know the family well in the course of caring for a patient with terminal heart disease, and although the patient dies, the family lives with the grief and memory of the patient and the death. Physicians can provide comfort and support to the family after the death of a loved one. Calling the family several weeks after the death expresses the physician's concern and can lend support. Such contact provides an opportunity for the family to ask questions that no one else can answer about the circumstances of the death or illness. Family members often feel guilty that they did not act quickly enough or provide sufficient care. The physician can reassure the family about these matters. In addition, these calls may identify individuals who are depressed or having complex grief reactions that may require referral to a physician or mental health professional. Physicians can also consider sending a condolence card. Hospice provides these services and typically contacts the family on the 1-year anniversary of the death of the patient, a time that can be especially difficult.

Self-Care

The care of dying patients can be extremely rewarding but also emotionally taxing. It is important to recognize that physicians also experience loss with the death of each patient. Many physicians develop long-standing and intimate relationships with their patients, and their deaths have a profound impact. Physicians must recognize the toll that these deaths can take and make time to process them. Talking with colleagues, friends, or partners about the loss, writing about it, and performing rituals such as saying prayers or planting trees for each death can help physicians deal with the loss. Physicians may also consider attending the funeral or memorial service. Although these actions may not be right in every situation, they can help the physician cope with the loss and bring a sense of closure, especially in cases in which the physician knew the patient well.

Patients' Perspectives on Quality End-of-Life Care

A total of 126 patients maintained on hemodialysis, infected with human immunodeficiency virus, or residing in a long-term care facility participated in open-ended, in-depth, face-to-face interviews about their thoughts regarding advance directives, advance care planning, and patient control at the end of life. The researchers identified five major themes that patients believed were important for ensuring quality care at the end of life:

- Receiving adequate pain and symptom management
- Avoiding inappropriate prolongation of dying
- Achieving a sense of control
- Relieving burden on loved ones
- Strengthening relationships with loved ones

These findings are consistent with several expert panel recommendations regarding end-of-life care.[2]

Shortcomings in End-of-Life Care

The Study to Understand Prognoses and Preferences for Treatment (SUPPORT) has provided the most extensive look at how people die in America. SUPPORT was a two-phase trial conducted at five teaching hospitals in the United States and was designed to improve decision making and the quality of end-of-life care for seriously ill patients. The first phase enrolled 4301 patients with serious illness, including heart failure, with an estimated 50% prognosis at 6 months. Phase 1 lasted 2 years and revealed that for half the patients who requested DNR orders, physicians failed to write them, that half of all DNR orders were written within 2 days of death, and that half of conscious patients had moderate to severe pain in the last 3 days of life. Phase 2 enrolled 4804 similar patients in a randomized trial of an intervention to improve the shortcomings identified in phase 1. The intervention consisted of providing prognostic information to the patient's physician and a nurse who helped facilitate communication. Although the intervention had no effect on care, the SUPPORT study has yielded remarkable insight into the shortcomings of end-of-life care in the Unites States and has spurred countless efforts to improve it.[1]

Symptoms in Patients Dying of Heart Disease

In a retrospective survey of caregivers of 600 adult patients who died of heart disease in Great Britain, the caregivers were contacted about 10 months after their loved one's death and asked to report the patient's symptoms in the last year of life. These data provide the most in-depth picture of symptom burden in patients dying of heart disease. The most common symptom was pain, reported for 78% of patients, followed by dyspnea in 61%, depressed mood in 59%, constipation in 37%, nausea and vomiting in 32%, and confusion in 27%.[15]

Attitudes toward Physician-Assisted Suicide

In a prospective study conducted at six sites across the United States, 988 patients were identified by their physicians as having a significant illness with a survival time of 6 months or less and were asked about their attitudes regarding physician-assisted suicide. A total of 650 subjects were surveyed a second time, 2 to 6 months after the first survey. Overall, 60% of patients supported permitting physician-assisted suicide or euthanasia, even though only 10% had seriously considered requesting either one for themselves. Patients who had depressive symptoms, were more of a burden on caregivers, and had more pain were significantly more likely to have considered physician-assisted suicide. Only half of the patients continued to have an interest in physician-assisted suicide at the follow-up interview.[14]

Home Dobutamine for Refractory Heart Failure

The largest randomized, placebo-controlled trial of outpatient dobutamine found that patients treated with dobutamine experienced symptomatic relief at the risk of excess mortality, a result consistent with what was reported in a review of smaller trials. Similar results were found in a more recent randomized trial that analyzed mortality, hospitalization, and functioning after intermittent, low-dose home dobutamine infusion over a period of 6 months in patients with class III or IV heart failure and ejection fractions of 30% or less. All patients were assessed at weekly clinical visits during the 6 months of the study. All 38 enrolled patients received maximal oral therapy, and 19 were randomly assigned to dobutamine at 2.5 μg/kg/min infused for 48 hr/wk. Overall, no statistically significant differences were noted between the groups in terms of functioning, hospitalizations, or mortality, but a trend toward improvement in the first two outcomes was seen in patients randomized to receive dobutamine. A total of three patients in the control group and five in the dobutamine group died ($P = .91$). The close follow-up may have contributed to the improved outcomes in both groups, although the small number of patients limits the ability to conclude that low-dose intermittent dobutamine infusion is safer. These findings suggest that if successful in relieving a patient's symptoms, intermittent, low-dose home dobutamine infusion might offer a safer alternative to higher dose continuous infusions, although physicians should continue to inform patients that such treatment may shorten their lives.[21]

Evidence-Based Summary

- Do-not-attempt-resuscitation orders are often written very late in the course of care; earlier discussions about prognosis and preferences for care should be encouraged.
- Patients at the end of life often have pain, which is commonly undertreated but can be effectively managed with appropriate therapies.
- Hospice care should be considered earlier in the course of end-stage disease.

References

1. A controlled trial to improve care for seriously ill hospitalized patients. The study to understand prognoses and preferences for outcomes and risks of treatments (SUPPORT). The SUPPORT Principal Investigators. JAMA 1995;274:1591–1598.
2. Singer PA, Martin DK, Kelner M: Quality end-of-life care: Patients' perspectives. JAMA 1999;281:163–168.
3. Quill TE: Initiating end-of-life discussions with seriously ill patients: Addressing the "elephant in the room." JAMA 2000;284:2502–2507.
4. Christakis NA, Lamont EB: Extent and determinants of error in doctors' prognoses in terminally ill patients: Prospective cohort study. BMJ 2000;320:469–472.
5. Murphy DJ, Burrows D, Santilli S, et al: The influence of the probability of survival on patients' preferences regarding cardiopulmonary resuscitation. N Engl J Med 1994;330: 545–549.
6. Nohria A, Lewis E, Stevenson LW: Medical management of advanced heart failure. JAMA 2002;287:628–640.
7. Anker SD, Ponikowski P, Varney S, et al: Wasting as independent risk factor for mortality in chronic heart failure [published erratum appears in Lancet 1997;349:1258]. Lancet 1997;349:1050–1053.
8. Crawley LM, Marshall PA, Lo B, Koenig BA: Strategies for culturally effective end-of-life care. Ann Intern Med 2002;136:673–679.
9. Pantilat SZ: Care of dying patients: Beyond symptom management. West J Med 1999;171:253–256.
10. Tierney WM, Dexter PR, Gramelspacher GP, et al: The effect of discussions about advance directives on patients' satisfaction with primary care. J Gen Intern Med 2001;16: 32–40.
11. Ebell MH, Becker LA, Barry HC, Hagen M: Survival after in-hospital cardiopulmonary resuscitation. A meta-analysis. J Gen Intern Med 1998;13:805–816.
12. Krumholz HM, Phillips RS, Hamel MB, et al: Resuscitation preferences among patients with severe congestive heart failure: Results from the SUPPORT project. Study to Understand Prognoses and Preferences for Outcomes and Risks of Treatments. Circulation 1998;98:648–655.
13. Meisel A, Snyder L, Quill T: Seven legal barriers to end-of-life care: Myths, realities, and grains of truth. JAMA 2000;284:2495–2501.
14. Bascom PB, Tolle SW: Responding to requests for physician-assisted suicide: "These are uncharted waters for both of us. . . ." JAMA 2002;288:91–98.
15. McCarthy M, Lay M, Addington-Hall J: Dying from heart disease. J R Coll Physicians Lond 1996;30:325–328.
16. Jacox A, Carr DB, Payne R, et al: Management of Cancer Pain. Clinical Practice Guideline No. 9. Rockville, MD, Agency for Health Care Policy and Research, U.S. Department of Health and Human Services, Public Health Service, 1994, pp 24–28.
17. Page J, Henry D: Consumption of NSAIDs and the development of congestive heart failure in elderly patients: An underrecognized public health problem. Arch Intern Med 2000;160:777–784.
18. Doyle D, Hanks GWC, MacDonald N: Oxford Textbook of Palliative Medicine. Oxford, Oxford University Press, 1998, pp 331–355.
19. Block SD: Assessing and managing depression in the terminally ill patient. ACP-ASIM End-of-Life Care Consensus Panel. American College of Physicians–American Society of Internal Medicine. Ann Intern Med 2000;132:209–218.
20. Cross KL: The use of dobutamine in hospice patients. Am Acad Hospice Palliative Med Bull 2000;1:6–7.
21. Oliva F, Latini R, Politi A, et al: Intermittent 6-month low-dose dobutamine infusion in severe heart failure: DICE multicenter trial. Am Heart J 1999;138:247–253.

22. Finucane TE, Christmas C, Travis K: Tube feeding in patients with advanced dementia: A review of the evidence. JAMA 1999;282:1365–1370.
23. Lynn J: Serving patients who may die soon and their families: The role of hospice and other services. JAMA 2001; 285:925–932.
24. Medical guidelines for determining prognosis in selected non-cancer diseases. The National Hospice Organization. Hosp J 1996;11:47–63.
25. McPhee SJ, Bottles K, Lo B, et al: To redeem them from death. Reactions of family members to autopsy. Am J Med 1986;80:665–671.

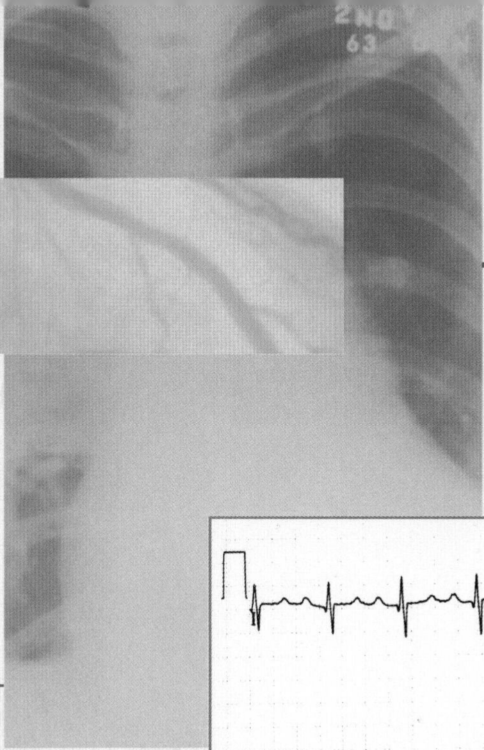

PART 3

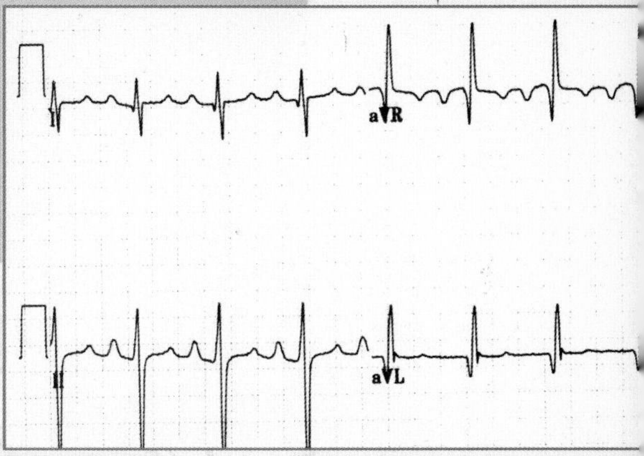

Preventive Cardiology

CHAPTER 18

Screening for Coronary Heart Disease and Its Risk Factors

J. Michael Gaziano

The medical encounter of William Osler's day involved reaction to specific patient complaints. The structure of the medical interview that evolved in the 19th century focused on the chief complaint, and this approach was designed to deal with acute manifestations of diseases. The management strategy was intended to resolve or palliate the acute problem, and little attention was paid to long-term prevention.

In the early part of the 21st century, the health care system is primarily engaged in the management and, just as important, the prevention of chronic illnesses, the consequences of which may take as long as decades to become evident. To prevent subsequent events in patients with overt chronic illnesses or prevent first events in those who do not have such illnesses, we must have a keen awareness of the likelihood that a future event will develop in an individual. Whether in the hospital or in the office, we must now be concerned with not only the immediate complaints of our patients but also the risk of future events. Although the concept of screening would have made little sense to a 19th century physician, it is fundamental to the practice of 21st century medicine.

Coronary heart disease (CHD) is the most common cause of death in the developed world, and by the year 2020, it will be the chief cause of death worldwide. In the United States, about a half million CHD deaths and 1.5 million heart attacks occur annually. Thus, the incidence and prevalence of CHD are high enough to warrant consideration of a screening strategy, and the consequences of undetected disease are important. This chapter considers various issues in screening for CHD as the first step in the assessment and prevention of CHD events.

BASIC PRINCIPLES OF SCREENING

A screening strategy must meet several criteria before its widespread use should be advocated:

1. The test must accurately detect the disease or one of its risk factors at an early stage.
2. The test must also be feasible and safe.
3. The information gained from the screening test must be useful in the assessment and preferably the reduction of long-term risk.
4. The improvements in long-term outcome must be worth the cost of the screening test, as well as the resultant tests and interventions.

Types of Screening

Screening in its broadest sense is the application of some instrument for assessment of the risk of a future health event in an individual with no symptoms. This assessment of future risk can be used to provide the patient with prognostic information, but more importantly, screening is the first step in the prevention of future events. Screening can be divided into three categories that are not mutually exclusive:

First, screening can be used to detect underlying disease in an individual who has no overt manifestations of that disease for the purposes of early intervention. This approach is the one used in much of cancer screening, and it is designed to detect cancer in its early stages so that early intervention can lower the chance of future harmful events. An example is testing stool for occult blood as a way of detecting colon cancer at an early stage and thus increasing the cure rate and ultimately decreasing the risk of death from colon cancer.

Second, we can screen patients for individual risk factors that increase the chance of contracting a disease or having a disease-related event at some point in the future. The goal of this type of screening is to intervene on that single risk factor in appropriate patients. An example of such screening is the detection of hypertension, which may result in the prevention of stroke or heart disease.

Finally, it is possible to use elements of disease detection and risk factor screening to estimate, in a composite fashion, the global or absolute risk for development of a disease or a future event. This type of screening is helpful in providing prognostic information and can be used to direct costly interventions toward those who are most likely to benefit. Specific screening tools for assessment of global risk are available for persons with and without CHD. For example, using the Framingham Heart Study CHD score in a disease-free individual provides a quantitative estimate of that patient's risk for CHD events over the next 10 years.

Disease Burden

Incidence and Prevalence. If a screening test for a disease or one of its risk factors is to have utility in a target population, the rate of the disease in the population must be relatively high. The more common a disease or one of its risk factors, the more likely a screening strategy will be useful. These concepts are captured by the terms *incidence* and *prevalence*. Incidence is the rate of new cases of a given disease or factor. Prevalence is the proportion of individuals with a given condition at a single point in time. Coronary artery disease (CAD) and its risk factors are ideal candidates for screening given their high incidence and prevalence, the associated morbidity and mortality, and their direct and indirect costs.

Estimating Risk. For screening to be useful, the consequences of undetected disease must be important. Measures quantifying the harm of a disease or risk factor include relative risk, absolute risk, and population attributable risk (see Chapter 1). *Relative risk* is the proportional risk in one person or group in comparison to another individual or group. For example, the relative risk of a smoker having a myocardial infarction (MI) is twofold that of a nonsmoker. *Absolute risk* refers to the probability or chance that an event will develop in an individual at some point in the future. *Population attributable risk*, or how much of the population's risk of disease is attributable to a single factor, is driven by the proportion of the public with a given risk factor and the magnitude of the associated risk.

Many factors are in a continuum, so we can assess the population attributable risk against an ideal standard or a low-risk individual on the basis of an arbitrary cut point. Hypertension is an example of such a continuous factor. Other factors are all or nothing, such as cigarette smoking. The distribution of the factor in the population and the shape of the relationship between the factor and the risk of subsequent events help determine the population attributable risk. For example, the shape of the risk curve is linear for hypertension; thus, lowering blood pressure at any level can be of benefit. By contrast, the shape of the curve for obesity appears to be nonlinear. The risks of obesity increase in a nonlinear fashion, with much more risk associated with each pound gained in those who are obese.

Screening Test Characteristics

Rational use of any screening tool requires consideration of the basic principles of test selection and interpretation[1] (see Chapter 1). The *sensitivity* of a test is a measure of the test's ability to detect the disease in the general population. A test with perfect sensitivity detects all the disease in the screened population. In other words, the test has no false negatives. The *specificity* of a test captures the accuracy of a positive test. A test with perfect specificity indicates that it does not produce any false positives. Tests with perfect sensitivity and specificity do not exist. Tradeoffs must often be made when setting a parameter for test positivity.

The *likelihood ratios* of a test change the probability of having disease according to Bayes' theorem. Sensitivity and specificity are reflected in the likelihood ratios. According to Bayes' theorem, the results of a screening test change the probability that a patient will have the disease that the screening test was designed to detect. Multiplication of the pretest probability by the likelihood ratio results in the posttest probability. Pretest odds is the probability that an individual has the disease before application of the screening test. Both positive tests and negative tests have likelihood ratios.

Benefits of Early Detection

Estimating the Impact of Intervention. The impact of an intervention is measured as relative or absolute risk reduction. *Relative risk reduction* is the proportional reduction in risk in comparison to an untreated individual. Often more useful, *absolute risk reduction* permits an estimate of how many lives will be saved or events reduced in a given population. The ability to assess absolute risk enables cost-effective targeting of interventions. This approach of using absolute risk to gauge the level of intensity of an intervention has been adopted by the National Cholesterol Education Program (NCEP)[2] and the sixth Joint National Committee on Prevention, Detection, Evaluation, and Treatment of High Blood Pressure (JNC VI).[3] Guidelines from the NCEP Adult Treatment Panel III adjust treatment cut points and goals according to the level of underlying risk; persons who have known CHD are targeted to receive the most aggressive care (target level of low-density lipoprotein [LDL] cholesterol, 100 mg/dL), those with two or more risk factors but no CHD are targeted with an intermediate level of care (target LDL level, 130 mg/dL), and those with fewer than two risk factors are targeted with the least aggressive care (target LDL level, 160 mg/dL). Similarly, the JNC VI guidelines stratify interventions according to baseline risk. The American Diabetes Association (ADA) has also recommended a tiered approach to management of diabetes.

Primary versus Secondary Prevention. Screening strategies can be applied to those with and without a given disease. Screening of those without known disease is the first step in primary prevention. Screening in secondary prevention is designed to assess and reduce the risk of subsequent events in those with known disease. Many factors that predict a first CHD event also predict subsequent events in patients with known CHD. However, the relative importance of an intervention for primary prevention versus secondary prevention varies. Preventive interventions tend to be more cost-effective in secondary prevention. Because the absolute risk in those with established disease is higher, it is necessary to treat fewer higher risk individuals to save one life than it is to treat lower risk individuals, even if the relative risk reduction is identical in both groups.

Cost Efficacy. Once reasonable estimates of the benefit and risk of any interventions have been established for a given risk factor, cost- and risk-benefit analyses can be helpful in establishing guidelines for intervention. The common currency to compare interventions is the quality-adjusted life-year (QALY) or the disability-adjusted life-year (DALY). Similar to estimates derived from meta-analyses, those from cost- and risk-benefit analyses are dependent on the underlying assumptions for a given analysis. The cost-effectiveness of interventions to prevent heart disease is of particular concern because of the prevalence of CHD and the high cost of treatment with technologically advanced interventions. Several issues in the interpretation of cost analyses must be considered. Analyses of preventive measures have a long time horizon, and thus models are necessarily complex. The consequences of initial assumptions on the prevention of chronic diseases can be much more significant than those of interventions with a short time horizon, such as treatment of acute MI (with a 30-day primary outcome). The estimates used for some of the major assumptions are often based on limited data. The cost-effectiveness of a screening strategy must include all costs of screening, as well as the cost of interventions.

Cost-effectiveness estimates are calculated as the ratio of net costs to the gain in life expectancy and are usually presented as the cost per QALY. Interventions with an incremental cost-effectiveness ratio of less than $40,000 per QALY are comparable to other chronic interventions such as hypertension management and hemodialysis. Those less than $20,000 are very favorable. On the other hand, costs exceeding $40,000 per year of life saved tend to be considered excessive.

Guidelines

Government agencies, professional societies, and health care providers, among others, help define public health policy *and* often provide practice guidelines. The process generally involves assembling a group of experts who assess and summarize the data on a given relationship. The U.S. Preventive Services Task Force (USPSTF)[4] and the Canadian Task Force on Periodic Health Examination (CTFPHE)[5] provide general guidelines on the utility of various screening and treatment strategies for cardiovascular and other diseases. In the United States, detailed guidelines are available for individual risk factors. For example, the NCEP and the JNC provide detailed guidelines for screening and treatment of cholesterol and hypertension, respectively. The American College of Cardiology (ACC) and the American Heart Association (AHA) also provide guidelines for CHD screening and management. The ADA has updated its guidelines for the detection and treatment of diabetes. In many countries where the health care systems tend to be more centralized, individual risk factor guidelines have been combined and synthesized into a composite strategy for CHD primary and secondary prevention.

SCREENING TO DETECT CAD IN THOSE WITHOUT KNOWN DISEASE

A number of diagnostic tests have been developed to confirm the diagnosis of CAD and assess short-term risk in those with symptoms. These tests include the electrocardiogram (ECG), exercise stress testing (EST), nuclear imaging, cardiac catheterization, echocardiography, ambulatory monitoring for rhythm disturbance and ischemia, electron beam computed tomography (EBCT), positron emission tomographic scanning, magnetic resonance imaging, and carotid and peripheral ultrasonography. The utility of many of these tests is clear, and guidelines have been established for their use in specific circumstances. The application of many of these tests is well established in the acute or outpatient setting for persons with symptoms of CHD, such as those with chest pain. These applications are discussed in other chapters (see Chapters 4, 5, and 25). However, the use of these valuable diagnostic tools in persons with symptoms is *not* screening. Two of these tests,

ECG and routine EST, are safe and widely available and are thus considered possible screening tools. In addition, EBCT, another noninvasive test, has received recent attention and is therefore discussed here.

Accuracy of Screening Tests

Electrocardiography. Abnormal ECG findings are associated with an increased risk of serious cardiac events. One study demonstrated relative risks of future cardiac death that ranged from 2.0 to 3.6 for various abnormalities, including Q-waves, ST segment depression, T-wave abnormalities, premature ventricular beats, and left axis deviation. However, data on the sensitivity and specificity of resting ECG in detecting clinically relevant CAD in the general population are limited. One problem is the lack of an ideal gold standard. In the Honolulu Heart Study, the sensitivity for the development of CAD at some point in the future was so low (less than 5%) that resting ECG was considered a useless screening tool.[6] In summary, resting ECG lacks sensitivity, and its utility as a screening test is limited.

Exercise Stress Testing. Several exercise protocols have been designed for asymptomatic persons, and various exercise-related and ECG parameters have been used to determine test outcome. EST is commonly used to assist in the diagnosis of CHD in symptomatic individuals. Guidelines have been developed to define the appropriate use of exercise testing in symptomatic patients.

Several studies have shown that an ischemic EST result in apparently healthy people can identify heightened risk of future MI and sudden death. In the Seattle Heart Watch, the Lipid Research Clinics Coronary Primary Prevention Trial (LRC-CPPT), and the Multiple Risk Factor Intervention Trial (MRFIT),[7–9] abnormal EST results were associated with at least a fourfold higher coronary mortality rate in asymptomatic middle-aged men with elevated baseline levels of CHD risk factors than in similar persons with normal EST results. A recent report confirmed the prognostic utility of EST in 25,927 men with a mean age of 43 years and free of clinical disease who underwent maximal exercise testing during a screening evaluation.[10] Using the endpoint of CHD death, an abnormal maximal EST result yielded relative risks ranging from 8 to 10 in men with coronary risk factors in comparison to similar men with normal test results. Prognostic data on EST are limited in asymptomatic women and the elderly (>75 years). The use of EST in asymptomatic people has been widely criticized because of both a high rate of false-positive test results, especially in low-risk people, and a high rate of false-negative test outcomes. The predictive value of a positive test in an unselected population has been reported to range from 25% to 72%.

Electron Beam Computed Tomography. Calcification within the coronary arterial wall is a marker of atherosclerosis. EBCT uses an electron sweep of stationary tungsten rings to generate radiographic images that can detect small amounts of calcium, which is essentially pathognomonic for coronary atherosclerosis. EBCT has been criticized as being nonspecific when compared with coronary angiography as the "gold standard."[11] In a meta-analysis of 16 published EBCT studies that compared coronary calcium scores with coronary angiographic findings, the weighted average sensitivity was 80.4% and the specificity was 39.9%. A separate meta-analysis reported a pooled sensitivity of 92% and a specificity of 51%, both with narrow confidence intervals.[12] Both meta-analyses noted significant heterogeneity in published studies as a result of differences in study populations and variety in the diagnostic criteria used. In any case, the published literature indicates that EBCT would yield an unacceptably high false-positive rate (because of low specificity) if the test were applied to unselected populations to detect silent CHD. Indeed, one meta-analysis reported that the receiver operating characteristic curve for EBCT demonstrated a diagnostic accuracy in detecting obstructive coronary disease approximately comparable to that of traditional EST.

Benefits of Early Intervention

Screening of asymptomatic patients for CHD for the purpose of directing revascularization procedures is not likely to be cost-effective because no data clearly demonstrate a benefit of angioplasty or bypass surgery in an asymptomatic patient. Although EST and EBCT may have acceptable predictive values in certain circumstances, in particular, in those with multiple risk factors, no data in the general asymptomatic population demonstrate a clear benefit of early intervention in this population. As presented elsewhere, angioplasty in acute coronary syndromes such as acute MI has been shown to be beneficial (see Chapter 27), and coronary bypass surgery has been shown to reduce short- and intermediate-term event rates in those with symptomatic CHD. However, no trials have studied the impact of intervention in asymptomatic individuals with detected CAD. Because of the lack of studies demonstrating benefit, the cost efficiency of a strategy to detect and treat early CAD cannot be determined.

Guidelines and Recommendations

Electrocardiography. The ACC/AHA recommends a single routine ECG for those older than 40 years.[13] Although an ECG may be useful as a baseline and is relatively inexpensive, no data support intervention based on the results of an abnormal ECG. The USPSTF recommends a resting ECG for those with CHD risk factors if the results would alter management or in circumstances of public safety. The American College of Physicians (ACP) does not recommend resting ECG for those with or without evidence of CHD.

Exercise Stress Testing. The USPSTF has advised against routine (i.e., unselected) screening for CHD on grounds that include limited test sensitivity, low predictive value, and high cost of screening and follow-up. The task force advised that noninvasive testing of selected high-risk asymptomatic persons (specifically, those with multiple coronary risk factors) may be indicated when the results can influence preventive intervention decisions (i.e., the use of aspirin or lipid-lowering drugs). Strategies to select patients for such testing were not defined. The ACC/AHA guidelines for exercise testing cautiously advised the use of EST in the evaluation of asymptomatic persons without known coronary disease but with multiple CHD risk factors.[14] A major concern of the ACC/AHA guideline was that noninvasive test results may lead to the inappropriate use of revascularization procedures in asymptomatic persons, a group for whom benefit has not convincingly been established by clinical trials.

In limited circumstances, EST may have utility in asymptomatic persons that could be considered screening. When a patient undergoes surgery for peripheral vascular disease, the likelihood that that individual has CHD is much higher than the that of the average person. The near-term consequences of undetected CHD in a patient undergoing surgery appear to be sufficient to warrant consideration of a noninvasive test to screen for CHD. Those with a negative stress test of any kind are generally deemed safe to proceed with surgery. On the other hand, those with positive studies are often advised to undergo coronary angiography for further risk stratification and intervention if warranted. A second circumstance in which stress testing has been used as a screening tool with an eye toward possible intervention is in individuals who have great responsibility for the lives of others, such as airline pilots. After the age of 50, pilots are advised to have routine EST. Abnormal results are often followed by catheterization and revascularization. A pilot with known CHD must have a normal stress test before being allowed to return to work.

Electron Beam Computed Tomography. Currently, no recommendations regarding the use of EBCT in screening asymptomatic persons have been advocated. An AHA/ACC consensus panel recommended against routine screening of unselected populations.

SCREENING FOR SINGLE RISK FACTORS

Two complementary approaches may be used to reduce the overall population's burden of preventable disease and events: (1) dissemination of general recommendations throughout the population and (2) identification and targeting of higher risk individuals generally through mass screening. The first approach does not require screening. The nationwide public health approach has the advantage of potentially reaching the entire population and promoting modification of the population's overall risk by making modest changes in various behavior in a large segment of the population. The campaigns against cigarette smoking are an example of the public health approach.

Three factors for which screening and subsequent intervention are clearly cost-effective are cigarette smoking, hypertension, and hyperlipidemia. Two additional factors with the potential for intervention and for which the screening test is exceedingly inexpensive are obesity and physical inactivity. Screening for diabetes warrants discussion despite a lack of consensus on the utility of screening the general public.

Screening recommendations are summarized in Table 18–1.

TABLE 18–1

Risk Factors, Screening Tools, and Recommendations for Coronary Heart Disease

Risk Factor	Screening Tool	Recommendations
Cigarette smoking	History	Taking a smoking history and counseling tobacco users to quit are generally recommended by USPSTF
Hypertension	Blood pressure measurement	JNC VI recommends periodic blood pressure measurement
Cholesterol	Total cholesterol, HDL cholesterol, fasting lipid profile	NCEP recommends periodic assessment of the fasting lipid profile for all adults older than 20 yr
Physical activity	History	USPSTF recommends assessment of physical activity and counseling
Obesity	Height and weight	USPSTF recommends height and weight measurement and the use of BMI and/or weight tables to direct interventions
Diabetes	Fasting glucose and oral glucose tolerance test	Careful history and measurement of fasting blood glucose are recommended by the ADA for those with risk factors for diabetes mellitus
Global risk	Framingham CHD risk score, ESC risk tables	Global risk assessment is recommended for anyone considering cholesterol treatment

ADA, American Diabetes Association; BMI, body mass index; CHD, coronary heart disease; ESC, European Society of Cardiology; HDL, high-density lipoprotein; JNC VI, Sixth Joint National Committee on Prevention, Detection, Evaluation, and Treatment of High Blood Pressure; NCEP, National Cholesterol Education Program; USPSTF, U.S. Preventive Services Task Force.

Cigarette Smoking

Disease Burden

Prevalence. In the United States, per capita cigarette consumption rose dramatically in the first half of the 20th century. Over 65% of men born between 1911 and 1920 were smoking by 1945. Cigarette smoking rates have declined from a peak of 42% in 1965 to 25% in 1995, although the rate of decline has been different in men and women. Among men, smoking rates have been cut by almost half, from 52% of the adult male population in 1965 to 27% in 1995. Among women, rates have dropped by only one third (34% of adult women in 1965 to 23% in 1995) because of increasing smoking rates in women younger than 30 years. Smoking rates tend to be higher in blacks, those with lower socioeconomic status, and those with a high-school education or less.

Associated Risk. The Surgeon General's report in 1964 reaffirmed the epidemiologic relationship between cigarette smoking and CHD,[15] and by 1983, the Surgeon General firmly established smoking as a leading avoidable cause of CHD.[16] The Surgeon General's report in 1989[17] presented definitive data from observational case-control and cohort studies, largely among men, demonstrating that smoking increases CHD mortality by 50% and doubles the incidence of CHD and that the risk increases with age. The risk increases linearly with smoking level so that the heaviest smokers have as much as a fivefold higher risk of CHD events than nonsmokers do.

Screening Test

Taking a history during routine office visits is the most important screening test. Certain biochemical tests can be used to confirm the accuracy of self-report, but they are rarely used given the general accuracy of self-reported data. Cigarette smoking is best quantified as the number of packs or cigarettes per day.

Benefit of Intervention

Although large-scale randomized trial data on the reduction in risk associated with smoking cessation as an isolated intervention are limited, observational studies demonstrate that smoking cessation has clear benefits in reducing the risk of CHD. Studies of previous smokers have demonstrated MI and CHD rates comparable to those of nonsmokers 3 and 5 years after cessation, respectively. The benefit is comparable in both low- and high-risk individuals, even in those with established CHD. Half of the estimated 60% reduction in the risk of MI occurs within the first few months after stopping smoking.

Cost Efficacy. The cost efficacy of smoking cessation is generally accepted. The intervention is usually short term and thus low cost. In fact, smoking cessation programs typically cost less than continued smoking. The gains in life expectancy are large and tend to be larger the younger one stops smoking. A 35-year-old male smoker may add 3 years to his life expectancy on cessation. Costs vary depending on the intensity of the intervention and the use of pharmacologic agents. However, given the large gains and short duration of the intervention, costs per QALY are often less than $1000. There is little doubt of the enormous cost-effectiveness of this intervention in primary or secondary prevention.

Guidelines and Recommendations

The USPSTF recommends screening for smoking at every office visit for all adults and adolescents. Although smoking rates are falling in some developed countries, they are stagnant or increasing in the rest of the world. The greatest concern with smoking in the United States is the increasing number of young women, particularly minorities, who are taking up smoking. Tobacco cessation counseling is recommended on a regular basis for all who use tobacco products. Most of those who give up smoking do not use an organized cessation program.

Hypertension (see Chapter 19)

Disease Burden

Prevalence. Data from two national surveys suggest that 30% of American adults are hypertensive and that the prevalence of hypertension is greater in blacks than whites and in men than women; a clear increase in prevalence is noted with older age, and rates increase from 9% in those aged 19 to 24 to 75% in those older than 75 years.

Associated Risk. Elevated systolic or diastolic blood pressure has consistently been associated with an increased risk for CHD. The best estimates for the magnitude of associated risk have been derived from a meta-analysis of nine large, prospective observational studies with more than 400,000 participants who accrued over 4850 CHD events during follow-up.[18] A 7-mm Hg increase in diastolic blood pressure from any baseline blood pressure was associated with a 27% increase in the risk of CHD and a 42% increase in the risk of stroke. The shape of the risk curve is linear.

Screening Test

Screening for hypertension by routine blood pressure measurements is safe, inexpensive, and widely available. The JNC VI defines six levels of blood pressure according to the risk imparted (Box 18–1).

Benefit of Intervention

For patients with malignant hypertension (defined as diastolic blood pressure higher than 115 mm Hg), the benefits of pharmacologic intervention are clear and uncontroversial. Beginning in the late 1960s, a number of randomized trials confirmed the protective effect of treating mild to moderate hypertension, and these early

BOX 18–1

Blood Pressure Levels (mm Hg) as Defined by JNC VI

Optimal	<120/80
Normal	Systolic 120–129 Diastolic 80–84
High normal	Systolic 130–139 Diastolic 85–89
Stage 1 hypertension	Systolic 140–159 Diastolic 90–99
Stage 2 hypertension	Systolic 160–179 Diastolic 100–109
Stage 3 hypertension	Systolic ≥180 Diastolic ≥110

JNC VI, Sixth Joint National Committee on Prevention, Detection, Evaluation, and Treatment of High Blood Pressure.

trial data led to the establishment of treatment guidelines in the 1970s. The most precise estimates of risk reduction have come from recent meta-analyses reporting that lowering diastolic blood pressure by 5 to 6 mm Hg results in a 42% reduction in the risk of stroke and a 14% to 17% reduction in the risk of CHD events. A number of studies have demonstrated the utility of lifestyle interventions in lowering blood pressure, in particular, weight reduction. However, these trials have not generally been powered to demonstrate a reduction in coronary events.[19–22]

Cost Efficacy. The extensive trial data available have permitted ample data on the cost efficacy of intervention. The cost efficacy is clearly favorable for secondary prevention. In general, costs per QALY are below $10,000 for patients with established CHD, even in those with mild elevations in blood pressure. In primary prevention, among persons with a moderate to severe elevation in blood pressure, costs are in the range of $10,000 to $20,000 per QALY. Cost more than doubles for those with mild elevations. The cost of intervention increases with the cost of the medication and can approach an unacceptable range of $100,000 per QALY for higher priced medications. In contrast to the estimates for lipid lowering, cost efficacy decreases with increasing age as anticipated.

Guidelines and Recommendations

General consensus has been reached by the ACP, CTFHE, and USPSTF on widespread screening of hypertension, with screening of adults older than 21 years recommended at least every 2 years. The diagnosis should be confirmed at multiple visits. For an initial blood pressure less than 130/85 mm Hg, JNC VI recommends that blood pressure be rechecked in 2 years. For successively higher levels of blood pressure, more frequent evaluation is recommended. For a person with newly elevated blood pressure, an evaluation to rule out a secondary cause, exclude end-organ damage, and identify cardiovascular risk factors is recommended. No upper age limit has been established for hypertension screening.

Screening efforts in the United States should be intensified because the prevalence of hypertension increases with the age of the population. In the United States, the proportion of hypertensive persons who are managed appropriately has decreased recently, thus reversing a 2-decade trend. Treatment recommendations are presented in Chapter 19.

Hypercholesterolemia

Disease Burden

Prevalence. Based on data from several national surveys, mean age-adjusted cholesterol levels have declined modestly in the United States since the early 1960s. Even with this decline, the latest estimates suggest that half of all American adults aged 20 through 74 years have cholesterol levels greater than 200 mg/dL and that 20% of American adults have cholesterol levels of 240 mg/dL or greater.

Associated Risk. Abundant observational evidence indicates a clear causal link between elevated serum cholesterol and CHD. Specifically, a 10% increase in serum cholesterol is associated with a 20% to 30% increase in the risk of CHD, and elevations earlier in life may be associated with higher increases in risk.

Screening Test

Various tests are available to assess blood lipids. Commonly used screening tests include total cholesterol, high-density lipoprotein (HDL) cholesterol, and a fasting lipid profile.

Benefit of Intervention

Randomized trial data clearly demonstrate a reduction in the risk of CHD with treatment to lower serum cholesterol levels. Meta-analyses of randomized trials have generally shown a reduction in the risk of both fatal and nonfatal CHD in both primary and secondary prevention trials. Treatment aimed at lowering the serum cholesterol level by 10% has been shown to reduce the risk of CHD death by 10% and CHD events by 18%, and treatment for more than 5 years yields a 25% reduction in CHD events. The recently completed large-scale primary and secondary prevention trials using statins confirm these findings and provide reassuring data supporting the conclusion that cholesterol reduction, per se, does not increase the risk of nonvascular mortality. The recent Heart Protection Study demonstrated a benefit of cholesterol lowering in higher risk patients at all levels of LDL cholesterol.[23]

Cost Efficacy. The cost efficacy of nonpharmacologic interventions to lower LDL cholesterol is unclear; however, the cost-effectiveness of screening for and treatment of elevated cholesterol has been explored with several models and the use of various baseline assumptions. Pharmacologic intervention is clearly cost-effective in certain conditions, and the available data permit tailoring of recommendations to the level of baseline CHD risk.

Guidelines and Recommendations

Authorities are in agreement regarding screening in those with cardiovascular disease and the utility of screening for primary prevention. However, some controversy remains regarding the age to begin screening for primary prevention. The NCEP recommends screening for all adults older than 20 years, whereas the ASP and USPSTF recommend screening only for men aged 35 to 65 and women aged 45 to 65. Furthermore, the NCEP recommends measurement of the complete fasting profile for adults. Although triglycerides are a strong marker of future CHD events, their utility in screening is unclear.

Exercise

Disease Burden

Prevalence. Despite widespread interest in exercise in the United States, information on the level of activity in this country is limited. Data from the National Health Interview Survey estimated that 40% of adults exercise regularly (43% of men, 38% of women, and 23% of those older than 65 years), but only 4% to 8% of adults engage in vigorous exercise for 20 minutes or more three or more times per week. The number of adults considered sedentary declined from over 40% to approximately 27% by the early 1990s.

Associated Risk. A number of observational studies have reported an inverse association between work activity level and CHD. Leisure activity has also been consistently associated with a lower risk for CHD. This relationship between activity of any kind and a lower risk for CHD has been confirmed in a number of primary prevention studies. Exercise after CHD events also appears to confer benefit in preventing subsequent events. In a meta-analysis of 27 observational cohort studies of leisure and occupational activity, the risk of a CHD event was almost twice as great in sedentary individuals as in active individuals after controlling for other coronary risk factors.[24] Much more limited observational data strongly suggest a similar inverse relationship in those with known CHD.

Screening

Screening for physical inactivity involves taking a history of physical activity, which should include an assessment of both work-related and leisure activities. In addition, specific barriers can be assessed, including medical limitations to regular physical activity. Fitness can also be assessed by stress testing; however, historical information generally suffices as an initial screening test.

Benefit of Intervention

Although cessation of activity appears to result in an increased risk for CHD, no large-scale, randomized primary prevention trials have been conducted to determine the benefit of exercise intervention in terms of CHD reduction. Physical activity has clear benefit in terms of other cardiovascular risk factors. A physically active lifestyle may increase the level of HDL, reduce the level of LDL and triglycerides, increase insulin sensitivity, and reduce resting blood pressure.

In secondary prevention, cardiac rehabilitation programs with an exercise component tend to report benefit in reducing subsequent events. However, most of these studies have been too small to detect benefit in terms of CHD events or mortality. Pooled data from many of these smaller trials showed a reduction of about 25% in total and cardiovascular mortality.[25]

Guidelines and Recommendations

The USPSTF recommends an assessment of physical activity and counseling to promote physical activity in all patients. The USPSTF and the Surgeon General recommend progression to a level of activity of 30 minutes or more on most days of the week. For secondary prevention, patients should be strongly encouraged to engage in regular exercise. Nurse case managers or structured exercise programs may enhance long-term compliance. For primary prevention, data are lacking on the optimal interventions for increasing physical activity at low cost.

Obesity

Disease Burden

Prevalence. Over 20% of the U.S. population is obese, defined as 20% over the desirable weight, a problem that seems to be more prevalent in women than men. Despite growing awareness of the detrimental health effects of obesity, the proportion of the U.S. population that is overweight has increased steadily over the past 2 decades in both men and women, and the rate of increase is accelerating.

Associated Risk. Although few data would dispute the association of obesity with CHD, the independent status of this risk factor is controversial. Reports on the association of obesity with CHD have been understandably conflicting because of the use of various measures of obesity. Furthermore, the impact of obesity on the risk of CHD may be mediated, at least in part, by other coronary risk factors such as hypertension, dyslipidemia, and glucose intolerance. A review by Hubert[26] that summarized prospective data, largely in men, found an independent effect of obesity after controlling for other risk factors. In the Nurses' Health Study,[27] a greater than threefold risk of fatal and nonfatal CHD was found in those with the highest body mass index (BMI of 29 or higher), as well as an 80% increase in the moderately obese (BMI of 25 to 29), when lipoprotein abnormalities, hypertension, and diabetes were not included in the multivariate model. Whether obesity is associated with a residual increased risk after controlling for hypertension, serum lipoprotein levels, and diabetes (the prevalence of all of which is increased with obesity) remains unclear at this time; however, obesity is clearly associated with CHD and is an important and easily assessed marker of risk.

Screening

Screening for obesity can be achieved at low cost during routine office visits. Periodic height and weight measurements can be used to calculate BMI or can be compared with a table of suggested weights for a given height.

Benefit of Intervention

The effect of weight reduction on the risk of CHD in both primary and secondary prevention remains uncertain because of limited trial data. No large-scale trials of weight reduction as an isolated intervention on which to estimate the benefits of this intervention have been conducted. However, given the improvements in glucose tolerance, blood pressure, and lipoprotein profile that have been clearly documented, general consensus has been reached on the role of weight reduction as part of primary and secondary prevention programs. There is little consensus, however, on the ideal approach to weight reduction. Promoting lifestyle changes to encourage weight reduction or maintenance of body weight has been universally disappointing. Although 30% to 40% of the American population report attempts at weight reduction, failure rates are extremely high. Effective treatment strategies generally involve a multifaceted approach, including dietary counseling, behavioral modification, increased physical activity, and psychosocial support. Without a precise estimate of the benefit and because of substantial variability in intervention strategies, it is impossible to estimate the cost-benefit ratio of this intervention.

Recommendations

The USPSTF and the AHA recommend periodic weight and height measurement for all patients. BMI and the waist-hip ratio can also be used as a basis for intervention.

Diabetes

Disease Burden

Prevalence. In the United States, approximately 15 million persons have diabetes; fully a third of them do not know that they have this disease. These estimates increase with the adoption by the ADA and the World Health Organization of new recommendations revising the definition of diabetes to include those with a fasting plasma glucose level of 126 mg/dL or higher. Approximately 90% of cases are non–insulin-dependent diabetes. Over the past decade, the prevalence of diabetes appears to be increasing, which may be a reflection of increasing BMI.

Associated Risk. CHD is a major complication of both insulin-dependent (IDDM) and non–insulin-dependent (NIDDM) diabetes mellitus. There is little doubt that diabetes causally increases the risk of atherosclerotic disease. By the age of 40, CHD is the number one cause of death in diabetic men and women; a recent survey found that CHD was listed on 69% of the death certificates of a representative national cohort of 14,734 diabetic adults aged 25 to 74. Age-adjusted rates for CHD are two to three times higher in diabetic men and three to seven times higher in diabetic women than in nondiabetics. The onset of clinically apparent CHD in those with IDDM occurs at an early age, with a markedly increased risk by the third decade of life. The risk is related to the duration of the disease, not the age at onset. In the Danish Steno Hospital Study,[28] mortality from MI alone was 12.5% after 35 years of diabetes, regardless of the age at onset. For this reason, individuals with diabetes, irrespective of the presence or absence of other risk factors, must be considered to be at higher risk for CHD.

Screening

Screening for diabetes begins with an assessment of risk factors for diabetes. The diagnosis is made by measuring the fasting plasma glucose level or by the oral glucose tolerance test. The sensitivity and specificity of a fasting blood glucose test vary depending on the threshold set used to define a positive test. A single fasting glucose level of about 140 mg/dL is highly specific (>99%) but has low sensitivity (21% to 75%). A lower level of blood glucose (about 115 mg/dL) greatly improves sensitivity but at the expense of specificity. For this reason, the ADA recommends that the oral glucose tolerance test be used as a secondary screen in persons with an abnormal fasting glucose level (above 115 mg/dL).[29]

Benefit of Treatment

Mounting evidence suggests that maintaining normoglycemia in diabetics may translate to a reduced risk for microvascular (renal and eye) disease; however, data on reduction of the risk for CHD associated with tight glycemic control are scant. In the Diabetes Complications and Control Trial,[30] an apparent reduction in CHD events was observed in patients with IDDM who were assigned to intensive therapy. This finding did not achieve statistical significance, probably because of small numbers of events in this relatively young cohort. Although oral hypoglycemic agents and insulin can improve glycemic control, their role in reduction of the risk for macrovascular complications of NIDDM remains unclear because of scant and conflicting trial data. In addition, treatment of NIDDM with insulin may result in weight gain. Data from the U.K. trial suggest that tight control in type 2 (NIDDM) diabetics may reduce the risk of CHD.

Cost Efficacy. The cost efficacy of screening for and intervening in diabetes is unknown.

Guidelines and Recommendations

The ADA recommends measurement of fasting glucose levels in persons with risk factors for diabetes mellitus, including obesity, a family history, a history of gestational diabetes, or certain higher-risk ethnic backgrounds.[31] The ACP, USPSTF, and CTFPHE all recommend against routine screening in the general population. Refinement of screening, as well as management guidelines for both primary and secondary prevention, must await more trial data. In contrast to people with well-controlled IDDM, those with NIDDM are much more likely to have multiple coronary risk factors than is the case in the general population. Thus, of paramount importance in reducing the risk of CHD in diabetic patients is aggressive modification of associated risk factors, including treatment of hypertension, reduction in serum cholesterol, weight reduction, and increased physical activity.

Novel and Biochemical Genetic Markers

Hemostatic markers, inflammatory markers, novel lipid parameters, cellular adhesion markers, indicators of previous infection, and markers of oxidative stress have all been linked to steps in atherogenesis, thrombosis, and CHD events. These markers include factors such as fibrinogen, homocysteine, lipoprotein(a), tissue plasminogen activator, von Willebrand factor, factor VII, C-reactive protein, and antibodies to oxidized LDL. A number of gene polymorphisms that are associated with various coronary risk factors or directly with cardiovascular events are being explored. Many of these polymorphisms represent promising potential screening tests. However, none meet the necessary requirements for a cost-effective screening strategy. Whether these parameters represent independent risk factors for atherosclerotic disease or are in the causal pathway for other risk factors is not entirely clear. Other risk factors such as cigarette smoking, alcohol consumption, and dyslipidemia appear to alter the levels of various biochemical factors. Additional observational data, as well as interventional trials aimed at altering these factors, will provide valuable information about the role of these factors in the treatment and prevention of atherosclerotic disease. At this point, recommendations for screening with these factors are premature.

SCREENING FOR GLOBAL RISK ASSESSMENT

This section discusses the utility of using both modifiable and nomodifiable risk factor information in a composite fashion to screen for those at high absolute risk of future CAD. Clinical information, including family history, tobacco use, diabetes, gender, age, blood lipids, body weight, and blood pressure, is useful in risk assessment.

Utility of Assessing Absolute Risk

The cost efficacy of any intervention is related to the underlying risk of the preventable disease or event in a given individual or population. A fundamental step in establishing a preventive strategy is assessing an individual's risk for clinically relevant outcomes. Cost efficacy varies according to absolute risk. To illustrate this concept, assume that an intervention reduces the relative risk of dying by 25% in both high- and low-risk patients. Furthermore, assume that a high-risk individual with CHD has a 20% chance of death over the next 10 years whereas a low-risk individual has a 1% chance of death during the same period. To save a life among those at high risk, one would have to treat only 20 patients (4 of whom are destined to die) for 10 years, so a 25% relative risk reduction would result in one life saved (three deaths instead of four). On the other hand, one would have to treat 400 low-risk patients (4 of whom are destined to die) for the same 25% relative risk reduction to yield three deaths instead of four. Thus, the total cost per lives saved is considerably lower in those at higher risk. This concept is the basis for more aggressive intervention strategies in those at higher risk.

Screening Tools

The first step in global assessment is the identification of those with known CHD because they are at high known risk for future CHD events. Any evidence of atherosclerotic disease, including previous MI or stroke, angina, and peripheral vascular disease, greatly increases the risk for subsequent CHD events. Because this type of information is often available from the medical history, screening for active CHD or previous events is recommended as part of the routine medical encounter. The risk of events in these patients is sufficiently high to warrant aggressive secondary preventive interventions for management of hypertension and high cholesterol levels.

Among those without known CHD, several useful tools are available for assessing the overall risk for subsequent disease. Investigators in the Framingham Heart Study have developed tools to assess the risk of cardiovascular events based on age, gender, total or LDL cholesterol level, HDL cholesterol level, systolic and diastolic blood pressure, history of diabetes, and cigarette smoking[32] (Fig. 18–1). Point-based weights are assigned to the presence or level of the various risk factors. Once the points have been assigned and summed, by using a simple table the total point score can be translated to an estimated absolute risk of a CHD event occurring within the next 10 years.

The European Society of Cardiology, in conjunction with several other European medical societies, has also released recommendations for the prevention of heart disease that stratify preventive interventions on the basis of classification of patients as high risk, intermediate risk, or low risk.[33] Those with known CHD constitute the highest risk category because most of these individuals have a greater than 20% chance of subsequent events over the next 10 years. Individuals without known CHD are assessed for the risk of subsequent events by using a modified Framingham risk assessment tool (Fig. 18–2). This tool, presented in a series of easy-to-use charts, allows clinicians to assess the risk of an event over the next 10 years based on age, gender, smoking status, diabetes, cholesterol level, and blood pressure. Those for whom the risk of a primary event exceeds 20% over the next 10 years are recommended for aggressive management of various modifiable risk factors. Those for whom the risk of an event is lower are prescribed a less intense and less costly approach to managing risk factors. The major difference between the Framingham score and the European Society of Cardiology score is the absence of HDL from the European formula. (HDL was omitted because it is not routinely measured in general population screening in some countries.)

Scales are also available for assessing risk in secondary prevention. The Framingham Heart Study investigators developed a scale for those with CHD that was based on the same cardiovascular risk factors used for assessing the 10-year risk for a first CHD event. This scoring system assigns a 2-year risk based on a composite risk score. In addition, a similar approach has been developed to assess the risk of a subsequent stroke. It should be pointed out that these tools only broadly categorize individuals in a limited number of risk strata.

Noninvasive Diagnostic Testing in Global Risk Assessment

Previous experience has shown that clinicians have not readily adopted multiple risk factor assessment tools in clinical practice as a means of maximizing risk assessment. On the other hand, clinicians cannot accurately estimate the risk of a coronary event by intuition. Furthermore, although multiple risk factor models such as the Framingham score improve risk prediction, accuracy is still well below 100%. Noninvasive tests, normally used in symptomatic patients to help diagnose atherosclerotic disease, have been proposed as a means of improving the prediction of clinical events in asymptomatic persons as a guide to targeting aggressive preventive strategies (see Chapter 4).

In patients who have a low pretest probability of an event based on multiple risk factor assessment, noninvasive tests such as ECG, EST, and EBCT are *not* usually helpful in identifying persons at high risk because a positive test does not yield a high enough posttest probability of a future event to justify aggressive application of preventive interventions such as lipid-lowering drugs. Conversely, when the pretest probability is high (e.g., when multiple risk factors or an extremely high level of a single risk factor such as severe hypercholesterolemia is present), a negative noninvasive test result is not generally regarded as sufficient evidence to withhold long-term preventive interventions. Such high-risk patients would be considered candidates for aggressive primary preventive interventions based on risk factor considerations alone. When risk prediction is *intermediate* between these extremes, a noninvasive test could be helpful in refining preventive decision making.

It is uncertain exactly where to set limits for high, low, or intermediate risk for a future cardiovascular event. Cut points should be based on considerations of cost efficacy and will therefore be progressively refined as more data accumulate on the costs and benefits of any screening strategy. With a sensitivity of 85% and a specificity of 75%, a noninvasive test such as EST or EBCT could modify the interpretation of intermediate risk (between 6% and 20% in 10 years) to either high or low risk, depending on test outcome.

Benefits of Intervention

No clinical trials have specifically tested whether a strategy that involves noninvasive testing in asymptomatic patients can stratify risk, target those at highest risk, and improve patient outcomes. However, in the LRC-CPPT, exercise testing was able to identify high-risk patients, and randomized use of lipid-lowering therapy markedly reduced the risk in all subgroups of EST results, but most strikingly in those with abnormal test results. A similar result was found in the MRFIT, in which EST results identified the patient group that experienced the greatest impact of intervention. It is possible that EST, as well as EBCT, if used appropriately in selected patients, could be both clinically effective and cost-effective. Cost-effectiveness data concerning the full range of testing have not been published.

Guidelines

New NCEP guidelines, European guidelines, and AHA advisories each propose that initial risk estimation with one of the available Framingham Heart Study multivariate models should be performed in all asymptomatic adults. American and European cholesterol and blood pressure guidelines encourage physicians to screen all asymptomatic adults for CHD risk factors to assess their overall cardiovascular risk. Clinicians should become familiar with the process of screening patients for a high absolute risk of CHD. First, assessment for existing CHD is important. In those without CHD, counting the number of *major* CHD risk factors is a crude way of assessing global risk. Those with none or one major CHD risk factor and no diabetes can generally be considered low risk. However, if more than one risk factor (smoking, family history, hypertension, diabetes, low HDL) is present, use of one of the available risk assessment tools should be considered. This strategy is recommended by the NCEP for

Step 1

Age		
Years	LDL Pts	Chol Pts
30–34	−1	[−1}
35–39	0	[0]
40–44	1	[1]
45–49	2	[2]
50–54	3	[3]
55–59	4	[4]
60–64	5	[5]
65–69	6	[6]
70–74	7	[7]

Step 2

LDL-C		
(mg/dl)	(mmol/L)	LDL pts
<100	<2.59	−3
100–129	2.60–3.36	0
130–159	3.37–4.14	0
160–190	4.15–4.92	1
≥190	≥4.92	2

Cholesterol		
(mg/dl)	(mmol/L)	Chol pts
<160	<4.14	[−3]
160–199	4.15–5.17	[0]
200–239	5.18–6.21	[1]
240–279	6.22–7.24	[2]
≥280	≥7.25	[3]

Step 3

HDL-C			
(mg/dl)	(mmol/L)	LDL pts	Chol pts
<35	<0.90	2	[2]
35–44	0.91–1.16	1	[1]
45–49	1.17–1.29	0	[0]
50–59	1.30–1.55	0	[0]
≥60	≥1.56	−1	[−2]

Step 4

Blood Pressure					
Systolic (mm Hg)	Diastolic (mm Hg) <80	80–84	85–89	90–99	≥100
<120	0 [0] pts				
120–129		0 [0] pts			
130–139			1 [1] pts		
140–159				2 [2] pts	
≥160					3 [3] pts

Note: When systolic and diastolic pressures provide different estimates for point scores, use the higher number

Step 5

Diabetes		
	LDL pts	Chol pts
No	0	[0]
Yes	2	[2]

Step 6

Smoker		
	LDL pts	Chol pts
No	0	[0]
Yes	2	[2]

Step 7 (sum from steps 1–6)

Adding up the points	
Age	____
LDL-C or Chol	____
HDL-C	____
Blood pressure	____
Diabetes	____
Smoker	____
Point total	____

Step 8 (determine CHD risk from point total)

CHD Risk			
LDL pts total	10-yr CHD risk	Chol pts total	10-yr CHD risk
<−3	1%		
−2	2%		
−1	2%	[<−1]	[2%]
0	3%	[0]	[3%]
1	4%	[1]	[3%]
2	4%	[2]	[4%]
3	6%	[3]	[5%]
4	7%	[4]	[7%]
5	9%	[5]	[8%]
6	11%	[6]	[10%]
7	14%	[7]	[13%]
8	18%	[8]	[16%]
9	22%	[9]	[20%]
10	27%	[10]	[25%]
11	33%	[11]	[31%]
12	40%	[12]	[37%]
13	47%	[13]	[45%]
≥14	≥56%	[≥14]	[≥53%]

Step 9 (compare to average person your age)

Comparative Risk			
Age (years)	Average 10-Yr CHD risk	Average 10-Yr hard* CHD risk	Low† 10-Yr CHD risk
30–34	3%	1%	2%
35–39	5%	4%	3%
40–44	7%	4%	4%
45–49	11%	8%	4%
50–54	14%	10%	6%
55–59	16%	13%	7%
60–64	21%	20%	9%
65–69	25%	22%	11%
70–74	30%	25%	14%

Key	
Color	Relative risk
	Very low
	Low
	Moderate
	High
	Very high

* Hard CHD events exclude angina pectoris

† Total risk was calculated for a person the same age, optimal blood pressure, LDL-C 100–129 mg/dl or cholesterol 160–199 mg/dl, HDL-C 45 mg/dl for men or 55 mg/dl for women, nonsmoker, no diabetes.

Risk estimates were derived from the experience of the Framingham Heart Study, a predominantly Caucasian population in Massachusetts, USA.

FIGURE 18–1. Coronary heart disease (CHD) score sheets for estimating the 10-year risk for CHD according to age, total cholesterol (or low-density lipoprotein cholesterol [LDL-C]), high-density lipoprotein cholesterol (HDL-C), blood pressure, diabetes, and smoking as risk factors. Average risk estimates are based on typical subjects in the Framingham Heart Study, and estimates of idealized risk are based on optimal blood pressure, a total cholesterol level of 160 to 199 mg/dL (or LDL of 100 to 129 mg/dL), HDL-C of 45 mg/dL in men and 55 mg/dL in women, no diabetes, and no smoking. Use of the LDL-C categories is appropriate when fasting LDL-C measurements are available. Pts, points. *Left,* Score sheet for men 30 to 74 years of age. *Right,* Score sheet for women 30 to 74 years of age. (From Wilson PW, D'Agostino RB, Levy D, et al: Prediction of coronary heart disease using risk factor categories. Circulation 1998;97:1837–1847. By permission of the American Heart Association, Inc.)

Step 1

Age		
Years	LDL Pts	Chol Pts
30–34	–9	[–9]
35–39	–4	[–4]
40–44	0	[0]
45–49	3	[3]
50–54	6	[6]
55–59	7	[7]
60–64	8	[8]
65–69	8	[8]
70–74	8	[8]

Step 2

LDL-C		
(mg/dl)	(mmol/L)	LDL pts
<100	<2.59	–2
100–129	2.60–3.36	0
130–159	3.37–4.14	0
160–190	4.15–4.92	2
≥190	≥4.92	2

Cholesterol		
(mg/dl)	(mmol/L)	Chol pts
<160	<4.14	[–2]
160–199	4.15–5.17	[0]
200–239	5.18–6.21	[1]
240–279	6.22–7.24	[1]
≥280	≥7.25	[3]

Step 3

HDL-C			
(mg/dl)	(mmol/L)	LDL pts	Chol pts
<35	<0.90	5	[5]
35–44	0.91–1.16	2	[2]
45–49	1.17–1.29	1	[1]
50–59	1.30–1.55	0	[0]
≥60	≥1.56	–2	[–3]

Step 4

Blood Pressure					
Systolic	Diastolic (mm Hg)				
(mm Hg)	<80	80–84	85–89	90–99	≥100
<120	–3 [–3] pts	0 [0] pts	0 [0] pts	2 [2] pts	3 [3] pts
120–129	0 [0] pts	0 [0] pts	0 [0] pts	2 [2] pts	3 [3] pts
130–139	0 [0] pts	0 [0] pts	0 [0] pts	2 [2] pts	3 [3] pts
140–159	2 [2] pts	2 [2] pts	2 [2] pts	2 [2] pts	3 [3] pts
≥160	3 [3] pts	3 [3] pts	3 [3] pts	3 [3] pts	3 [3] pts

Note: When systolic and diastolic pressures provide different estimates for point scores, use the higher number

Step 5

Diabetes		
	LDL pts	Chol pts
No	0	[0]
Yes	4	[4]

Step 6

Smoker		
	LDL pts	Chol pts
No	0	[0]
Yes	2	[2]

Step 7 (sum from steps 1–6)

Adding up the points	
Age	______
LDL-C or Chol	______
HDL-C	______
Blood pressure	______
Diabetes	______
Smoker	______
Point total	______

Step 8 (determine CHD risk from point total)

CHD Risk			
LDL pts total	10-yr CHD risk	Chol pts total	10-yr CHD risk
≤–2	1%	[≤–2]	[1%]
–1	2%	[–1]	[2%]
0	2%	[0]	[2%]
1	2%	[1]	[2%]
2	3%	[2]	[3%]
3	3%	[3]	[3%]
4	4%	[4]	[4%]
5	5%	[5]	[4%]
6	6%	[6]	[5%]
7	7%	[7]	[6%]
8	8%	[8]	[7%]
9	9%	[9]	[8%]
10	11%	[10]	[10%]
11	13%	[11]	[11%]
12	15%	[12]	[13%]
13	17%	[13]	[15%]
14	20%	[14]	[18%]
15	24%	[15]	[20%]
16	27%	[16]	[24%]
≥17	≥32%	[≥17]	[≥27%]

Step 9 (compare to average person your age)

Comparative Risk			
Age (years)	Average 10-Yr CHD risk	Average 10-Yr hard* CHD risk	Low** 10-Yr CHD risk
30–34	<1%	<1%	<1%
35–39	<1%	<1%	1%
40–44	2%	1%	2%
45–49	5%	2%	3%
50–54	8%	3%	5%
55–59	12%	7%	7%
60–64	12%	8%	8%
65–69	13%	8%	8%
70–74	14%	11%	8%

FIGURE 18–1. *Continued*

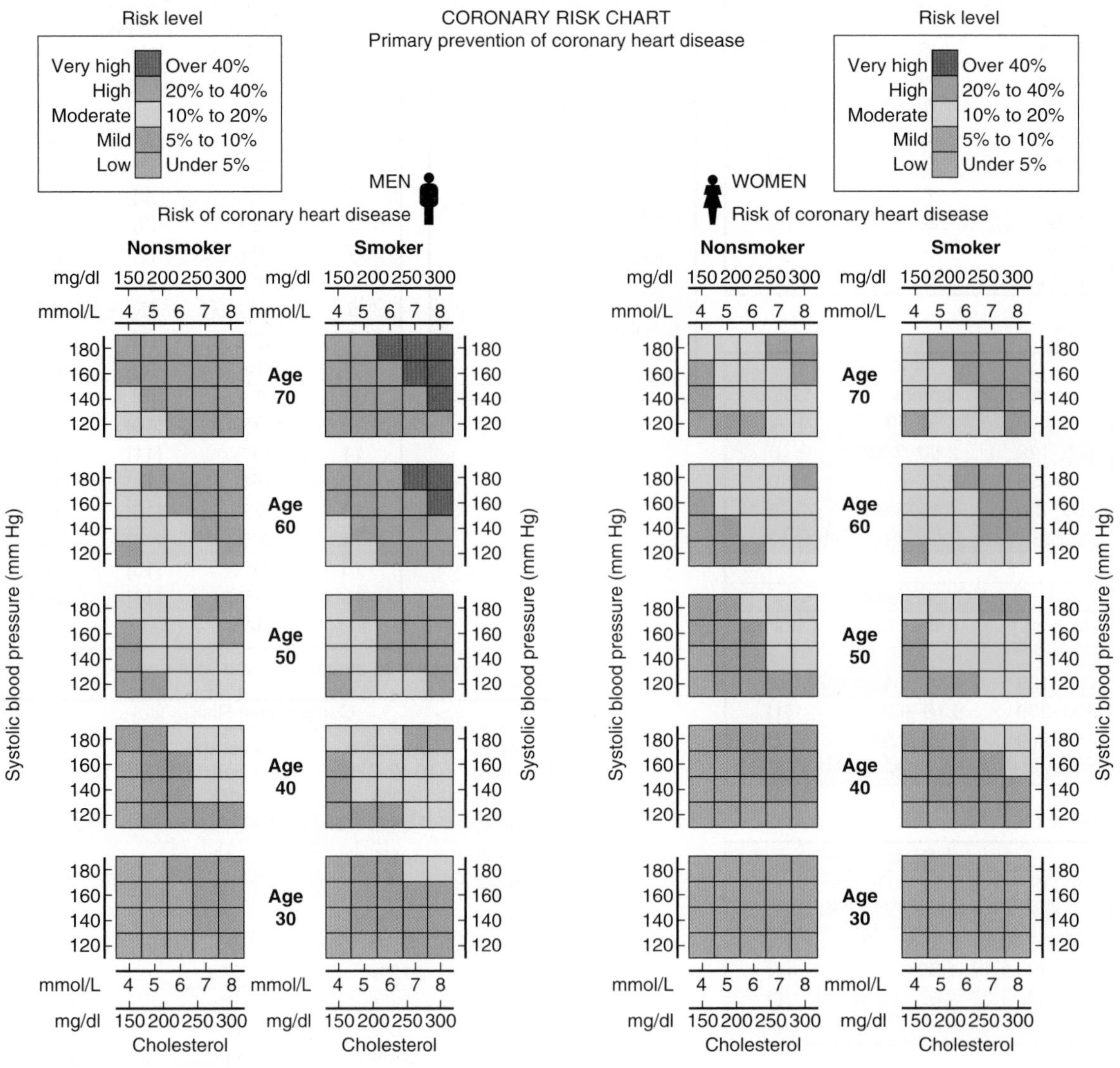

How to use the Coronary Risk Chart for Primary Prevention

The chart is for estimating coronary heart disease (CHD) risk for individuals who have not developed symptomatic CHD or other atherosclerotic disease. Patients with CHD are already at high risk and require intensive lifestyle intervention and, as necessary, drug therapies to achieve risk factor goals.

- **To estimate a person's absolute 10-year risk of a CHD event,** find the table for their gender, smoking status, and age. Within the table, find the cell nearest to their systolic blood pressure (mm Hg) and total cholesterol (mmol/L or mg/dl).
- **CHD risk is higher than indicated** in the chart for those with:
  - Familial hyperlipidemia
  - Diabetes: risk is approximately doubled in men and more than doubled in women
  - Those with a family history of premature cardiovascular disease
  - Those with a low HDL cholesterol. These tables assume HDL cholesterol to be 1.0 mmol/L (39 mg/dl) in men and 1.1 (43) in women
  - Those with raised triglyceride levels>2.0 mmol/L (>180 mg/dl)
  - As the person approaches the next age category.
- **The effect of lifetime exposure to risk factors** can be seen by following the table upwards. This can be used when advising younger people.
- **High risk individuals are defined as those whose 10-year CHD risk exceeds 20% or will exceed 20% if projected to age 60.**
- **To find a person's relative risk,** compare their risk category with that for other people of the same age. The absolute risk shown here may not apply to all populations, especially those with a low CHD incidence. Relative risk is likely to apply to most populations.
- **The effect of changing** cholesterol, smoking status, or blood pressure can be read from the chart.

FIGURE 18–2. Risk assessment tool devised by a European task force on coronary prevention based on cholesterol levels, blood pressure, and smoking status. *Left,* Risk assessment for men. *Right,* Risk assessment for women. (From Prevention of coronary heart disease in clinical practice. Recommendations of the Second Joint Task Force of European and Other Societies on Coronary Prevention. Eur Heart J 1998;19:1434–1503.)

targeting cholesterol reduction in single risk factor intervention guidelines.

As an aid to target preventive strategies, an ACC/AHA consensus document and an AHA conference[34] concluded that EBCT or EST may be used in "selected patients" when the physician determines that the patient is at "intermediate" risk after office-based risk assessment.

Evidence-Based Summary

- Screening plays an important role in the prevention of CAD events. Whereas the use of diagnostic tests is clear in those with known or suspected CAD, the role of screening to detect disease in the asymptomatic general population is limited. Because no data suggest a clear benefit of revascularization in those without symptoms, most guidelines recommend against screening for CAD in the general population. In special circumstances, EST screening may be useful. Certain high-risk individuals such as patients with peripheral vascular disease who are undergoing surgery may warrant screening with an eye toward intervention to reduce short-term risks. Furthermore, in situations of public safety, such as for pilots, screening for quiescent disease can be considered.
- It is evident that screening and subsequent interventions are clearly cost-effective for three single risk factor interventions. Screening for smoking, hypertension, and hyperlipidemia is warranted and generally recommended for all asymptomatic patients at periodic health examinations.
- Screening for obesity and physical activity is very inexpensive and is thus generally recommended despite a lack of clear efficacy of any intervention strategy.
- Screening for diabetes is a bit more expensive because it requires blood testing, although the blood test is cheap and available. Because diabetes is such a potent predictor of subsequent risk and this knowledge is useful in gauging the intensity of other interventions such as hypertension and hypercholesterolemia management, screening of those with risk factors for diabetes mellitus should be considered.
- The use of various screening tools such as the Framingham Heart Study CHD score to assess global risk can be helpful in providing patients with prognostic information regarding their long-term risk of CHD events. In addition, screening for global risk can be very useful in determining the level of aggression for single risk factor intervention.
- Although noninvasive testing has potential utility as an adjunct to other less costly global assessment tools, the use of stress testing and EBCT is *not* recommended in the asymptomatic general population, and the cost efficacy of such tests in various higher risk subgroups is unclear.

References

1. Griner PF, Mayewski RJ, Mushlin AI, Greenland P: Selection and interpretation of diagnostic tests and procedures: Principles and applications. Ann Intern Med 1981;94:557–592.
2. Executive Summary of the Third Report of the National Cholesterol Education Program (NCEP) Expert Panel on Detection, Evaluation and Treatment of High Blood Cholesterol in Adults (Adult Treatment Panel III). JAMA 2001;285:2486–2497.
3. The sixth report of the Joint National Committee on prevention, detection, evaluation and treatment of high blood pressure. Arch Intern Med 1997;157:2413–2446.
4. Report of the U.S. Preventative Services Task Force: Guide to Clinical Preventive Services, 2nd ed. Baltimore, Williams & Wilkins, 1996.
5. Canadian Task Force on the Periodic Health Examination: Canadian Guide to Clinical Preventive Health Care. Ottawa, Canada Communications Group, 1994, pp 649–699.
6. Knutsen R, Knutsen SE, Curb JD, et al: The predictive value of resting electrocardiograms from 12-year incidence of coronary heart disease in the Honolulu Heart Program. Stroke 1988;19:555–559.
7. Bruce RA, Hossack KF, DeRouen TA, Hofer V: Enhanced risk assessment for primary coronary heart disease events by maximal exercise testing: Ten years' experience of Seattle Heart Watch. J Am Coll Cardiol 1983;2:565–569.
8. Gordon DJ, Ekelund LG, Karon JM, et al: Predictive value of the exercise tolerance test for mortality in North American men: The Lipid Research Clinics Mortality Follow-up Study. Circulation 1986;74:252–261.
9. Okin PM, Grandits G, Rautaharju PM, et al: Prognostic value of heart rate adjustment of exercise-induced ST segment depression in the Multiple Risk Factor Intervention Trial. J Am Coll Cardiol 1996;27:1437–1443.
10. Gibbons LW, Mitchell TL, Wei M, et al: Maximal exercise test as a predictor of risk for mortality from coronary heart disease in asymptomatic men. Am J Cardiol 2000;86:53–88.
11. Nallamothu BK, Saint S, Bielak LF, et al: Electron-beam computed tomography in the diagnosis of coronary artery disease: A meta-analysis. Arch Intern Med 2001;161:833–838.
12. O'Rourke RA, Brundage BH, Froelicher VF, et al: American College of Cardiology/American Heart Association Expert Consensus document on electron-beam computed tomography for the diagnosis and prognosis of coronary artery disease. Circulation 2000;102:126–140.
13. American College of Cardiology/American Heart Association: Guidelines for exercise testing: A report of the American College of Cardiology/American Heart Association Task Force on Assessment of Cardiovascular Procedures (Subcommittee on Exercise Testing). J Am Coll Cardiol 1986;8:725–738.
14. Gibbons RJ, Balady GJ, Beasley JW, et al: ACC/AHA guidelines for exercise testing: A report of the American College of Cardiology/American Heart Association Task Force on Practice Guidelines (Committee on Exercise Testing). J Am Coll Cardiol 1997;30:260–315.

15. US Public Health Service: Smoking and Health. Report of the Advisory Committee to the Surgeon General of the Public Health Service. Washington, DC, Government Printing Office, PHS Publication No. 1103, 1964.
16. US Department of Health and Human Services: The Health Consequences of Smoking: Cardiovascular Disease. A Report of the Surgeon General. Washington, DC, Government Printing Office, DHHS Publication No. (PHS) 84–50204, 1983.
17. US Department of Health and Human Services: Reducing the Health Consequences of Smoking: 25 Years of Progress. A Report of the Surgeon General. Washington, DC, Government Printing Office, DHHS Publication No. (CDC) 89–8411, 1989.
18. MacMahon S, Peto R, Cutler J, et al: Blood pressure, stroke, and coronary heart disease. Part 1, Prolonged differences in blood pressure: Prospective observational studies corrected for the regression dilution bias. Lancet 1990;335:765–774.
19. National Conference on High Blood Pressure Education: Report on Proceedings. Bethesda, MD, US Department of Health, Education and Welfare, Public Health Service, National Institutes of Health, US DHEW Publication No. (NIH) 73–486, 1973.
20. Report of the Joint Commission on Detection, Evaluation and Treatment of High Blood Pressure: A cooperative study. JAMA 1977;237:255–261.
21. Collins R, Peto R, MacMahon S, et al: Blood pressure, stroke, and coronary heart disease. Part 2, Short-term reductions in blood pressure: Overview of randomised drug trials in their epidemiological context. Lancet 1990; 335:827–838.
22. Hebert PR, Moser M, Mayer J, et al: Recent evidence on drug therapy of mild to moderate hypertension and decreased risk of coronary heart disease. Arch Intern Med 1993;53:578–581.
23. Heart Protection Study: Findings presented at the American Heart Association meeting, November 2001. See Web site: *http://www.ctsu.ox.ac.uk/projects/hps.shtml.*
24. Berlin JA, Colditz GA: A meta-analysis of physical activity in the prevention of coronary heart disease. Am J Epidemiol 1990;132:612–628.
25. Franklin BA, McCullough PA, Timmis GC: Exercise. In Hennekens CH (ed): Clinical Trials in Cardiovascular Disease: A Companion Guide to Braunwald's Heart Disease. Philadelphia, WB Saunders, 1999, pp 278–295.
26. Hubert HB: The importance of obesity in the development of coronary risk factors and disease: The epidemiologic evidence. Annu Rev Public Health 1986;7:493–502.
27. Rexrode KM, Carey VJ, Hennekens CH, et al: Abdominal adiposity and coronary heart disease in women. JAMA 1998;280:1843–1848.
28. Deckert T, Poulsen JE, Larsen M: Prognosis of diabetics with diabetes onset before the age of thirty one. I. Survival, causes of death, and complications. Diabetologia 1978;14:363–370.
29. American Diabetes Association: Clinical practice recommendations 1999. Diabetes Care 1999;22(Suppl 1):5–19.
30. The effect of intensive treatment of diabetes on the development and progression of long-term complications in insulin-dependent diabetes mellitus. The Diabetes Control and Complications Trial. N Engl J Med 1993;329:977–986.
31. Report of the Expert Committee on the Diagnosis and Classification of Diabetes Mellitus. Diabetes Care 1997; 20:1183–1197.
32. Wilson PW, D'Agostino RB, Levy D, et al: Prediction of coronary heart disease using risk factor categories. Circulation 1998;97:1837–1847.
33. Wood D, DeBacker G, Faergeman O, et al: Prevention of coronary heart disease in clinical practice. Recommendations of the Second Joint Task Force of European and Other Societies on Coronary Prevention. Eur Heart J 1998;19:1434–1503.
34. Smith SC, Greenland P, Grundy SM: AHA Conference Proceedings. Prevention Conference V. Beyond secondary prevention: Identifying the high-risk patient for primary prevention: Executive summary. American Heart Association. Circulation 2000;101:111–116.

CHAPTER 19

Diagnosis and Management of Patients with Hypertension

William J. Elliott and Henry R. Black

High blood pressure (BP), or "hypertension," is a major contributor to the leading causes of morbidity and mortality across the world. When compared with other risk factors for stroke, acute myocardial infarction, and heart failure, hypertension is among the simplest to diagnose and easiest to treat, and (particularly in high-risk individuals) its management is the most cost-effective preventive strategy. Because so much information about hypertension has been derived from clinical trials, many excellent, evidence-based recommendations can be made about its diagnosis and management.[1,2] As a result of its high prevalence (e.g., 24% of adults) in the United States,[3] hypertension ranks first among chronic conditions for which Americans visit a health care provider. Every primary care physician needs to know how to measure BP correctly, how to classify hypertension, and how to assess cardiovascular risk before recommending and implementing a successful therapeutic program. In fact, one of the reasons for the impressive reduction in age-adjusted stroke mortality (≈62%) and coronary heart disease mortality (≈45%) in the Unites States since 1972 is the widespread treatment of hypertension by primary care physicians.

DEFINITION AND CLASSIFICATION OF HYPERTENSION

From 1974 to 1993, hypertension in the United States was defined as a diastolic BP of 90 mm Hg or higher and was classified as "mild, moderate, or severe." Because of burgeoning evidence in support of the importance of systolic readings from both epidemiologic studies and clinical trials (especially those that enrolled *only* patients with elevated systolic BP), the fifth report of the Joint National Committee on Detection, Evaluation, and Treatment of High Blood Pressure (JNC V) changed the classification scheme once in 1993 and again in 1997 (Table 19–1). Both versions allow hypertension to be diagnosed if *either* systolic BP is higher than 140 mm Hg *or* diastolic BP is higher than 90 mm Hg and abandoned the descriptive classifications in favor of a "staging" system similar to that used in oncology.[4] Many thought that the term "mild hypertension" was inappropriate because stage 1 hypertension

TABLE 19–1

Classification of High Blood Pressure

Category	Systolic (mm Hg)		Diastolic (mm Hg)
Optimal	<120	and	<80
Normal	<130	and	<85
High-normal	130–139	or	85–89
Stage 1 hypertension	140–159	or	90–99
Stage 2 hypertension	160–179	or	100–109
Stage 3 hypertension	180	or	110

Adapted from The sixth report of the Joint National Committee on prevention, detection, evaluation, and treatment of high blood pressure. Arch Intern Med 1997;157:2413–2446.

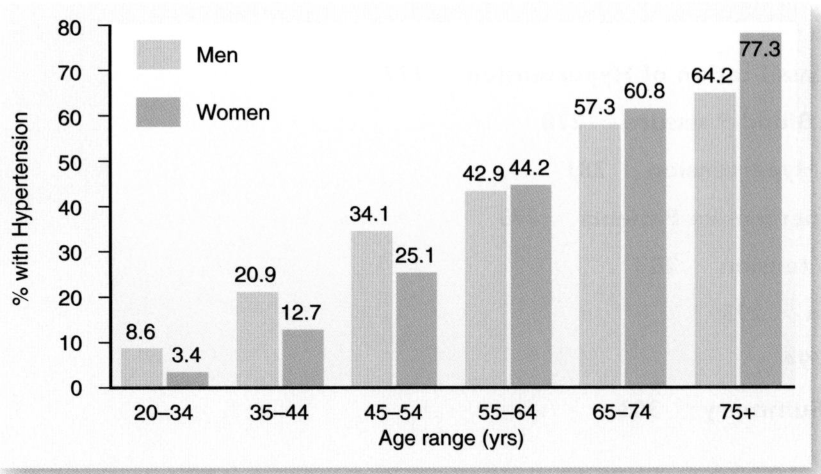

FIGURE 19–1. Age- and gender-specific prevalence of hypertension in the Third National Health and Nutrition Examination Survey (part 1, 1988–1991). In this large epidemiologic study, nearly 180,000 Americans had a blood pressure (BP) measurement taken at their homes by specially trained nurses; hypertension was defined as a BP of 140/90 mm Hg or taking antihypertensive medication. (Adapted from Burt VL, Whelton PK, Roccella EJ, et al: Prevalence of hypertension in the U.S. adult population: Results from the Third National Health and Nutritional Examination Survey, 1988–91. Hypertension 1995;25:305–313).

includes about 70% of those in whom hypertension is diagnosed and accounts for well more than half of the deaths and disability attributed to hypertension. The "cut points" for the stages of hypertension were chosen to reflect roughly equal future cardiovascular risk such that a diastolic reading of 100 mm Hg carries about the same prognostic importance as a systolic reading of 160 mm Hg. When the systolic and diastolic readings for a given patient fall into different stages, the BP is classified in the higher stage. For instance, both 182/94 mm Hg and 142/112 mm Hg would be properly placed in stage 3, the former because of the systolic reading and the latter because of the diastolic elevation. The correct classification of a patient's hypertension is likely to become more important if current proposals are implemented that tie reimbursement of health care providers directly to the absolute risk of the individual being treated.[5]

Although hypertension is more common in older women (Fig. 19–1), the current classification of hypertension is not modified by age or gender. Systolic BP typically increases with age, but diastolic pressure tends to fall in the sixth decade. In large populations older than 55 years, systolic BP is a far better predictor of many important sequelae of untreated or undertreated hypertension. The use of pulse pressure (systolic minus diastolic pressure) has recently generated some enthusiasm, especially in older persons. In the absence of aortic regurgitation, an arteriovenous fistula, and other uncommon conditions, a wide pulse pressure is often a marker for noncompliant and often atherosclerotic arteries. In several epidemiologic studies and clinical trials, pulse pressure was a better predictor of heart failure, myocardial infarction, heart attack, stroke, and all cardiovascular events than either mean arterial or systolic pressure alone.

MEASUREMENT OF BLOOD PRESSURE

Currently, the terminology first introduced by Korotkoff is used: systolic BP is identified when clear and repetitive tapping sounds are heard, and diastolic BP is recorded when the sounds disappear. Exceptions to these general rules are still recognized in patients who have audible sounds even down to 0 mm Hg; in this situation, "muffling" of the sounds (Korotkoff phase IV) is recorded, either in addition to the phase V measurement or as diastolic BP.

Techniques of Measuring Blood Pressure

The proper technique of accurate BP measurement is typically taught very early during medical training but seldom followed thereafter. Many expert panels have made recommendations regarding the methodology of BP measurement,[6] and these recommendations frequently do not agree in all details, but they share several general principles:

- A cuff size appropriate for the patient's arm circumference should be used: a 3-inch-wide cuff in young children, a 5-inch cuff in adults with average arm size, and an 8-inch cuff in obese adults. The deflation rate of the column of mercury should be 2 to 3 mm Hg/sec.
- Multiple measurements should be made on different occasions to decide whether a person should have BP lowered.

BP measurements have much intrinsic variability, and several steps can be taken to minimize this variability, including the following:

- Obtain multiple measurements, especially when the pulse is irregular.
- Center the bladder of the cuff over the brachial artery, with its lower edge within 2.5 cm of the antecubital fossa. Have the subject rest silently and comfortably (with back support if seated) for at least 5 minutes before the measurement.
- Have the patient abstain from drinking caffeine- or alcohol-containing beverages or tobacco use within 30 minutes before a BP measurement.
- Measure BP when the rectum and bladder are not full. Ensure that the arm is supported at the level of the heart.
- Auscultate over the brachial artery with the bell of the stethoscope and exert minimal pressure on the skin. Inflate the cuff 20 mm Hg higher than the pressure at which the palpable pulse at the radial artery disappears. Be sure to use a properly calibrated sphygmomanometer.
- Avoid "terminal digit preference" (more than 20% of measurements ending with a specific even digit).
- Measure BP in both arms initially and in the arm with the higher BP thereafter if the difference is greater than 10/5 mm Hg.

Home Blood Pressure Measurements

The technology for accurate and reproducible BP measurement outside the traditional medical environment has improved greatly over the last 30 years.[7] Many convenient, inexpensive, and relatively accurate devices are now available. Even persons with hearing difficulties, problems with hand-eye coordination, and other disabilities can estimate BP with semiautomatic devices that have digital readouts and printers. Some authorities believe that such devices should be provided to every person with elevated BP, but others are concerned about their use because they have not been commonly used in clinical decision making in clinical trials.

Home BP readings are typically lower than measurements taken in the traditional medical environment (by about 12/7 mm Hg on average[7]), even in normotensive subjects. Home readings tend to correlate better with both the extent of target organ damage and the risk of future mortality than do readings taken in the health care provider's office. Home readings can be helpful in evaluating symptoms suggestive of hypotension, especially if intermittent or infrequent. During treatment, reliable home readings can lower cost by substituting for multiple visits to health care providers. Persons who routinely measure BP at home probably have a better prognosis than those who do not because of both selection bias (they tend to be more interested in their BP than those who refuse to purchase and use a home BP device) and increased social support (when a friend or spouse becomes involved in measurement and overseeing pill-taking and appointment-keeping behavior).

Home BP readings should be interpreted cautiously, carefully, and conservatively. Many of the factors that contribute to BP variability (discussed earlier) are more difficult to control in the home environment, including intrinsic circadian variation, food and alcohol ingestion, exercise, and stress. The possibility that taking BP measurements may become an obsession is a disadvantage. If home readings are taken, the instrument should be calibrated against a standard sphygmomanometer with the use of a Y tube, and the technique of the measurer must be checked. No long-term clinical studies have based all treatment decisions solely on home readings, but several preliminary reports show benefit to supplementing office BP measurements with home readings. The prognosis is better predicted by home readings than by one or two "casual" office BP measurements. Home readings can be a useful adjunct to information obtained in the physician's office, especially when the two are widely disparate. One long-term study has shown that people with much lower home BP readings (than readings in the physician's office) suffer fewer major cardiovascular events than do people who have elevated readings both in the office and at home.

Ambulatory Blood Pressure Monitoring

Extensive research has led to a better definition of the role of frequent, automated BP measurement over a 24-hour period, during a person's usual daily activities (including sleep).[7] These devices will have increased utility in clinical practice in the United States because federal authorities have decided to cover the cost. As a research tool, the advantages and disadvantages of ambulatory BP monitoring (ABPM) have been well documented (Box 19–1), normative values have been proposed, and multiple publications correlating abnor-

BOX 19–1

Advantages and Disadvantages of Ambulatory Blood Pressure Monitoring

ADVANTAGES

Can measure BP many times during a 24-hour period
Measures diurnal variation (BP during sleep)
Measures BP during daily activities
Can identify and diagnose "white-coat hypertension"
No "alerting response"
No placebo effect
Better correlation with target organ damage than noted with other methods of BP measurement

DISADVANTAGES

Cost
Limited availability of equipment
Disruption of daily activities because of noise or discomfort (e.g., sleep quality, need to keep arm flaccid during measurement)
Lack of prospectively defined "normal values" and guidelines for treatment
Lack of long-term prospective studies demonstrating utility in comparison to traditional (and much less expensive) methods of BP measurement

Adapted from Elliott WJ, Black HR: Special situations in the management of hypertension. In Hollenberg NK (vol ed): Hypertension: Mechanisms and Treatment, vol 1. In Braunwald E (series ed): *Atlas of Heart Disease*, 3rd ed. Philadelphia, Current Medicine, 2000, pp 252–274.

BOX 19–2

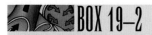

Uses of Ambulatory Blood Pressure Monitoring

DIAGNOSIS AND PROGNOSIS

Evaluation of suspected "white-coat" hypertension
Evaluation of refractory hypertension
Evaluation of circadian patterns of blood pressure

SYMPTOMS

Evaluation of dizziness, presyncope, and syncope
Evaluation of relationship of blood pressure to clinical symptoms

EVALUATION OF ANTIHYPERTENSIVE AGENTS

Evaluation of trough-to-peak ratios (research)
Evaluation of antihypertensive efficacy (research)
Evaluation of the effects of timing of dosing of antihypertensive agents

mal patterns of ABPM and adverse outcomes have appeared. Several "expert panels" have been convened and have defined the special situations in which ABPM is particularly useful (Box 19–2).

Several varieties of ABPM devices are currently available in the United States; those that measure BP indirectly (i.e., without arterial cannulation) use either an auscultatory or oscillometric technique. The former uses a microphone placed over the artery to detect Korotkoff sounds in the traditional fashion, whereas the latter measures biophysical oscillations of the brachial artery. A standardized algorithm is used to compare these oscillations with those observed with a mercury sphygmomanometer: systolic BP is determined directly from the threshold oscillation, mean arterial pressure is estimated, and diastolic pressure is calculated. Both types of monitors are light (<450 g), easy to apply and use, accurate, relatively quiet and tolerable, and powered by two to four small standard batteries. Data from 80 to 120 measurements of BP and pulse are typically stored in a microprocessor and subsequently downloaded into a desktop computer, which then edits the readings and prints the report.

None of the current ABPM devices are completely devoid of problems. Indirect measurement of BP by auscultatory techniques can be confused by ambient noise levels, even if R-wave gating is used (which requires electrocardiographic leads attached to the chest). Oscillometric techniques require that the subject keep the arm straight and flaccid during the measurement, and BP may be uninterpretable if the subject has a tremor. The value of ABPM readings may be enhanced if the subject records a diary of activities, but such diaries are seldom complete.

ABPM routinely measures BP during sleep and has reawakened interest in the circadian variation of pulse and BP. Most normotensive persons and perhaps 80% of those who are hypertensive have at least a 10% lower average BP during sleep than during the daytime. Although blacks and elderly persons appear to have smaller nocturnal drops in BP, an increased risk of cardiovascular events has been seen in several recent studies among individuals with a "nondipping" BP or pulse pattern. The results of several studies have raised the concern that elderly persons with greater than a 20% difference between nighttime and daytime average BP may suffer unrecognized ischemia in "watershed areas" (of the brain and other organs) during sleep if their BP declines below the autoregulatory threshold.

ABPM readings correlate rather well with the prevalence and extent of target organ damage in large groups of hypertensive individuals. Perhaps the most important data demonstrating the value of ABPM come from several studies of cardiovascular endpoints (death, myocardial infarction, stroke, etc.). In the first published study of outcomes in central Italy, ABPM was the best predictor of future cardiovascular events; "nondipping hypertensives" had approximately three times the risk of hypertensives whose BP was at least 10% lower at night than in the daytime. A substudy of the Systolic Hypertension in Europe (Sys-EUR) clinical trial involved 808 patients who had ABPM in addition to the usual clinic BP measurements. In the group randomized to placebo, ABPM was a much better predictor of future cardiovascular events than was the office BP measurement. Furthermore, the risk of a cardiovascular event was higher in patients who did not have a normal nocturnal decline in BP.

White-Coat Hypertension

According to recent studies using ABPM, approximately 10% to 20% of hypertensive Americans have substantially lower BP measurements outside the health care provider's office (so-called white-coat hypertension). The "white coat" itself is unlikely to be the only factor that increases BP. Careful studies originally performed in Italy (and now corroborated elsewhere) show that BP rises in response to an approaching physician who is not previously known to the subject. The acute elevation in BP is apparently less marked if the subject is approached by a nurse.

The clinical consequences and prognostic significance of white-coat hypertension are controversial. One school of thought suggests that if a person has an acute rise in BP as a result of "stress" induced by an approaching physician, similar elevations in BP are likely when other stressful stimuli are encountered. This situation is analogous to exercise-induced hypertension, which is often a precursor to more substantial and more sustained hypertension. A minority view based on more conservative definitions of the "white-coat effect" proposes that some individuals consistently show a similar and marked elevation in BP in response to the health care environment. Several long-term observational studies have shown a much reduced risk of either target organ damage or major cardiovascular sequelae in people with lower BP measured either at home or by 24-hour BP monitoring when compared with measurements taken in the physician's office. Whether the future risk of such individuals for cardiovascular events is similar (or even identical) to that of completely normotensive people is still open to question.

The best treatment of white-coat hypertension is still unresolved. Clearly, these individuals should benefit from lifestyle modifications, which would presumably reduce the probability of progression to sustained hypertension. Complete abstinence from antihypertensive medication in white-coat hypertensives appears unwise. It has been shown that in the long term, the risk of future cardiovascular events does not differ between white-coat and sustained hypertensives, assuming that both were treated with antihypertensive medications. Whether intensive treatment with continuous antihypertensive medication is warranted for only temporary increases in BP is debatable. Antihypertensive drug treatment and the repeated ABPM sessions required to monitor therapy would certainly not be very cost-effective, although perhaps 10% to 20% of hypertensives might be spared the cost of treatment and close follow-up.

EPIDEMIOLOGY OF HYPERTENSION

Despite widespread reliance on randomized clinical trials for incontrovertible evidence on which to base treatment decisions, much of what is known about the prevalence of hypertension and its associated risk for cardiovascular sequelae is based on epidemiologic studies. Some studies (e.g., the National Health and Nutritional Education Surveys [NHANES]) are designed to assess the prevalence of hypertension and the degree to which it is controlled. Other large, well-organized, long-term observational surveys of defined populations (e.g., the Framingham Heart Study) have initially identified individual cardiovascular risk factors and how they are interrelated. Both types of epidemiologic studies are relevant to today's primary care physician. Many primary care physicians are responsible not only for the health of individual patients but also for that of larger groups (or populations) of patients. To assess the compliance of a given physician or practice group with current guidelines (e.g., achieving a BP goal of <140/90 mm Hg in at least 50% of hypertensive patients), chart audits are often performed. Similarly, outcome studies that indicate whether a particular physician or practice has higher or lower hospitalization rates for common medical conditions are becoming more common. Such surveys are very important to today's primary care physician and are often used to assess the "quality of care" delivered.

Several large, representative surveys of the noninstitutionalized civilian U.S. population indicate that BP is nearly normally distributed (Fig. 19–2). Very few persons have BP in excess of 210/120 mm Hg. As a result, the "stage 4 hypertension" of JNC V was removed in JNC VI and incorporated into "stage 3." Similarly, JNC VI has a much greater focus on "high-normal blood pressure" than in previous reports because it is much more common than even stage 2 and 3 hypertension.

The first estimates of how much hypertension predisposes to stroke, heart attack, heart failure, and other cardiovascular events were derived from prospective epidemiologic surveys. Perhaps the most well known of these in the United States is the Framingham Heart Study, in which 5209 healthy men and women were extensively evaluated initially and then monitored over time. After a sufficient number had events, a quantitative estimate of the role that hypertension played in the development of these events could be made after adjusting for the presence of other risk factors (e.g., elevated plasma lipid levels or smoking). This approach firmly established *a strong, positive, and continuous relationship* between BP and stroke or heart attack. No specific threshold separates individuals who will or will not suffer these cardiovascular events. Figure 19–3 summarizes data from many observational studies of BP and either stroke (left panel) or coronary heart disease (right panel). From each panel, it is clear that the risk of an event rises as BP increases; the relative slopes of the lines indicate that elevated BP appears to be a bigger risk for stroke than for coronary heart disease. These data may be somewhat misleading, however, in that they are corrected (or statistically adjusted) for the presence of other risk factors and provide only an estimate of the *relative risk*. For instance, from the left-hand panel it appears that for every 7.5–mm Hg increase in diastolic BP, the *relative risk* of stroke increases by about 50%. The right-hand panel is constructed so that

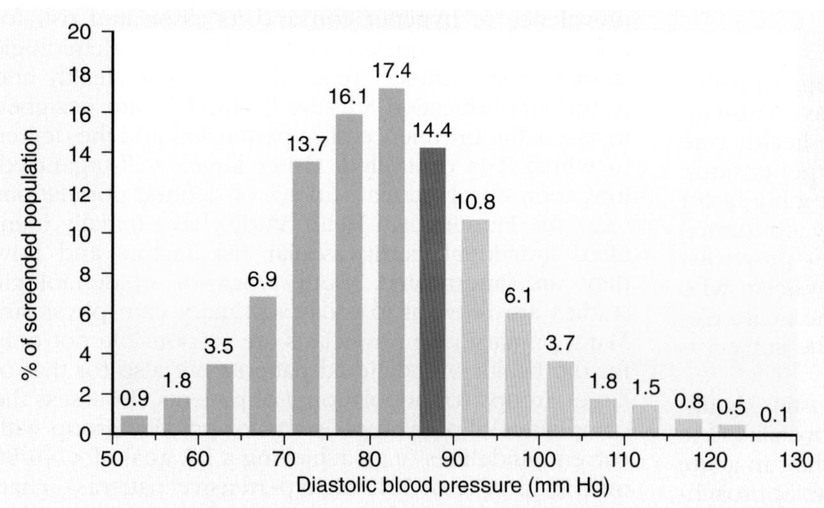

FIGURE 19–2. Distribution of blood pressure values (measured in the home) of a representative sample of about 157,000 untreated, noninstitutionalized, civilian citizens of the United States. Hypertension is present in those with a diastolic blood pressure of 90 mm Hg (*pink bars,* 25.3% of the population); high-normal blood pressure is diagnosed when diastolic pressure is between 85 and 89 mm Hg (*blue bar,* 14.4% of the population). (Adapted from Johansson B, Strandgaard S, Lassen NA: The hypertensive breakthrough of autoregulation of cerebral blood flow with forced vasodilation, flow increase, and blood-brain barrier damage. Circ Res 1974;34:167–171.)

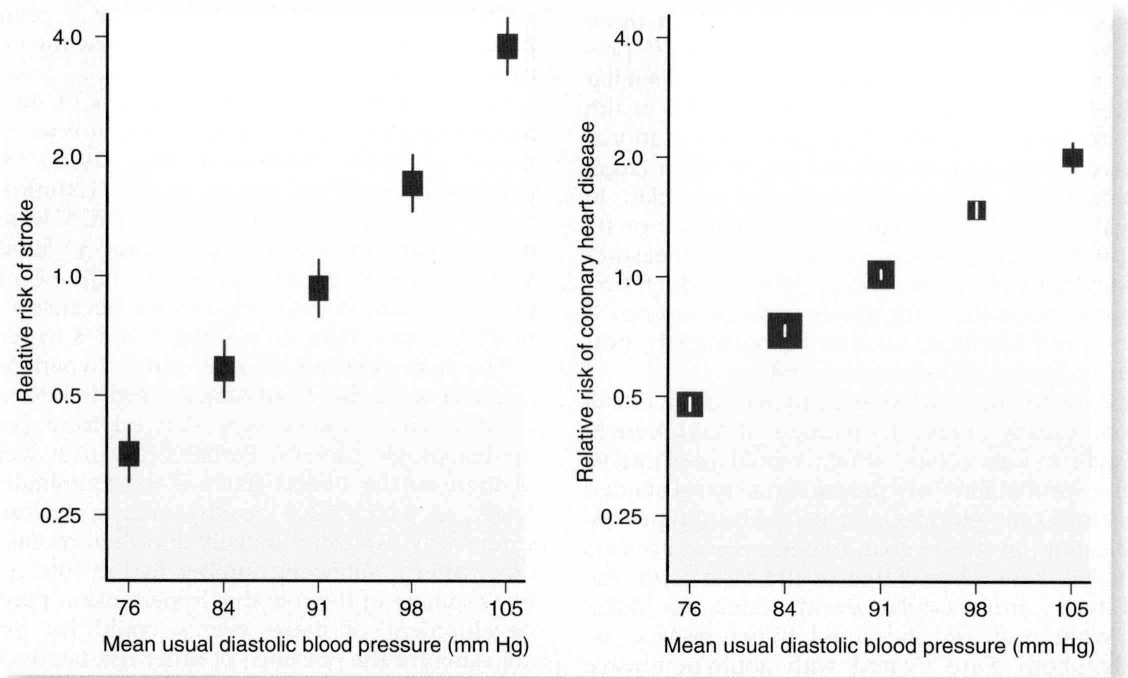

FIGURE 19–3. Relative risk of stroke *(left panel)* and coronary heart disease *(right panel)* estimated from the combined results of several prospective observational studies for each of five categories of diastolic blood pressure (DBP). Estimates of the usual DBP in each baseline DBP category are taken from mean DBP values obtained 4 years after the baseline examination in the Framingham Heart Study. The 95% confidence intervals for the estimates of relative risk are denoted by *vertical lines* in the *left panel.* The *solid squares* in the *right panel* represent the risk of disease in each category relative to the risk in the entire study population; the size of the *squares* is proportional to the number of events in each DBP category. (Redrawn from MacMahon S, Peto R, Cutler J, et al: Blood pressure, stroke, and coronary heart disease. Part I. Prolonged differences in blood pressure: Prospective observational studies corrected for the regression dilution bias. Lancet 1990;335:765–774.)

each "box" on the chart has an area that is proportional to the number of coronary heart disease events at that diastolic BP. This design gives an impression of the *absolute risk* associated with each level of diastolic BP. Even though the *relative risk* of coronary events is highest if diastolic BP is over 105 mm Hg, the greatest number of persons having such events is found in the group with diastolic BP in the 84– to 91–mm Hg range. This paradox is most easily explained by the fact that only a very small fraction of the population is in the highest pressure range, and even though these persons have the highest individual risk, they contribute only relatively few heart attacks to the total seen in the entire population. Conversely, even though the *relative risk* of "high-normal" BP is much smaller than a BP in excess of 105 mm Hg diastolic, many *more* individuals have the lower levels of BP, thereby resulting in a much higher *absolute risk* for the entire population.

These epidemiologic observations have several important consequences for the treatment of individual patients. First, it is clear that increased BP is only a "risk factor"; it affects the probability that a stroke or coronary event will develop in a given person, but it is *not* a *cause* of these conditions. The sensitivity as well as specificity of increased BP is low: not everyone with high BP will eventually have an event, just as, regrettably, not every person with "normal" BP will be spared. Any strategy that attempts to fix a value above which everyone should receive treatment is unlikely to be successful and cost-effective. The strategy recommended in JNC VI (see later) is based on estimates of absolute risk. Persons with modest BP levels and no other risk factors are at such low risk that preventing even one event with therapy would require many thousands to be treated, which places them at risk for adverse events related to the treatment and is wasteful of resources. Conversely, diabetic hypertensives are at such high risk for cardiovascular events that treatment can be justified even if the initial BP is only in the "high-normal" range.

EVALUATION OF HYPERTENSIVE PATIENTS

Four key issues must be addressed during the initial office evaluation of a person with elevated BP readings:

- Documenting an accurate diagnosis of hypertension (see earlier)
- Stratifying the person's risk for cardiovascular disease (according to risk group A, B, or C in JNC VI), which involves (1) defining the presence or absence of existing cardiovascular or renal disease or "target organ damage" related to hypertension and (2) screening for other cardiovascular risk factors that often accompany hypertension
- Assessing whether the person is likely to have an identifiable cause of the hypertension (secondary hypertension) and should have further diagnostic testing for it
- Obtaining information that may be helpful in choosing effective therapy

Documenting the Diagnosis

BP should be measured under relaxed and controlled conditions after appropriate rest (typically 5 minutes) and should be taken by someone whose ability to perform the measurement accurately has been certified. Excellent programs are available that can train, validate, and recertify the competency of individuals performing BP measurements.

To establish the diagnosis of hypertension, an individual should usually have elevated BP measurements documented at least twice at visits separated by a week or more. Each measurement should be an average of two or three readings differing by less than 5 mm Hg from each other and taken a few minutes apart in the seated or supine position. Patients who exhibit wide fluctuations in BP or who are hypertensive at some evaluations but normotensive at others may need additional measurements, either in the office, at home, or by ABPM to confirm that they are indeed hypertensive. In general, treatment should *not* be instituted until the diagnosis is clearly proved. In rare circumstances—such as when stage 3 hypertension or end-organ damage is present—treatment may need to be started after a single set of measurements.

Stratifying Risk for Cardiovascular Disease

Before beginning a treatment program directed at lowering BP, a thorough assessment of the person's risk for cardiovascular disease is warranted. In the JNC VI stratification scheme for risk assessment (Table 19–2), persons with elevated BP are divided into three general categories designated A, B, or C. Individuals in risk group C (19.2% of individuals with either high-normal BP or hypertension in NHANES I[8]) have the highest absolute risk by virtue of either existing cardiovascular or renal disease, target organ damage, or diabetes mellitus. Those in risk group A (9.0% of the at-risk population in NHANES I[8]) have the lowest risk, and most persons in risk group B have an intermediate risk.

Individuals with the highest short-term risk of a stroke or coronary event are those who already have concomitant cardiovascular or renal disease, for instance, a history of a recent transient ischemic attack or previous myocardial infarction. These individuals' BP should be treated promptly, intensively, and to a lower BP goal than in uncomplicated hypertensive persons. The search for evidence of concomitant cardiovascular or renal disease need not be extensive or expensive, however. Ordinarily, a complete medical history, directed physical examination, and a few routine laboratory tests (including an electrocardiogram [ECG], urinalysis, and serum chemistry panel) are sufficient.

Hypertensive persons with target organ damage are at the next highest level of risk for cardiovascular events. Target organ damage encompasses many subclinical features of the physical examination or laboratory tests that indicate the presence of preexisting derangement of structure or function in the eyes, heart, kidneys, or blood vessels related to uncontrolled hypertension. Although these individuals may not as yet have suffered an irreversible event (e.g., stroke) related to hypertension, they are at high risk for these sequelae, and the presence of target organ damage indicates that the hypertension has been present for some time. These

TABLE 19–2

Risk Stratification in Hypertensive Patients and Initial Treatment Recommendations

	Risk Group		
	A	***B***	***C***
No. risk factors	0	≥1 (not DM)	DM
Target organ damage	Absent	Absent	Present
Cardiovascular or renal disease	Absent	Absent	Present
Initial treatment			
High-normal blood pressure	LM only	LM only	LM + drug therapy
Stage 1 hypertension	LM × 12 mo	LM × 6 mo	LM + drug therapy
Stage 2 hypertension	LM + drug therapy	LM + drug therapy	LM + drug therapy
Stage 3 hypertension	LM + drug therapy	LM + drug therapy	LM + drug therapy

DM, diabetes mellitus; LM, lifestyle modification.

Adapted from The sixth report of the Joint National Committee on prevention, detection, evaluation, and treatment of high blood pressure. Arch Intern Med 1997;157:2413–2446.

persons should also receive prompt and intensive effort to lower their BP to a lower than usual BP goal because of their high absolute short-term risk of a cardiovascular event.

Recent data from both epidemiologic studies and clinical trials have shown that diabetic hypertensives have about twice the risk of cardiovascular events as nondiabetic hypertensive persons do, essentially equivalent to the presence of existing cardiovascular disease in a nondiabetic. JNC VI recognized this risk by categorizing all diabetics as risk category C; a similar approach was recently taken by the National Cholesterol Education Program, in which the presence of diabetes was considered a "coronary heart disease equivalent." This major change in strategy—relating risk stratification to treatment—means that a diabetic person with a BP of 130/85 mm Hg or higher should receive antihypertensive drug therapy even though the diagnosis of hypertension is *not* confirmed. This recommendation is perhaps the most striking example of how JNC VI has embraced the concept of treating individual patients according to their *absolute* risk for cardiovascular events and *not* by BP levels alone.

Other cardiovascular risk factors (tobacco use, family history of premature cardiovascular disease) are often found in hypertensive persons, and central obesity, dyslipidemia, diabetes, and hypertension have a tendency to cluster. Because other risk factors tend to be additive (if not multiplicative) in increasing the probability of cardiovascular events, it is important to screen a person with newly diagnosed hypertension for these other risk factors to more accurately estimate the future risk of cardiovascular and renal events. Risk group B (of JNC VI, see Table 19–2) includes any person with one or more risk factors (but not diabetes) who has no concomitant cardiovascular or renal disease or target organ damage. Risk group A is a particularly low-risk group inasmuch as no other risk factors are present. Because the risk in both these groups is substantially lower than that in risk group C, JNC VI recommends drug therapy at the time of diagnosis *only* if stage 2 or 3 hypertension is present. If the hypertension is stage 1, a time-limited duration of lifestyle modification to reach the goal BP is recommended: risk group B should receive 6 months and risk group A 12 months before antihypertensive drug therapy is begun. This recommendation is a further example of how JNC VI espouses treatment based on absolute risk rather than BP level (or relative risk). This approach is expected to improve the cost-effectiveness of antihypertensive drug therapy. Many more risk group A or B persons would need to be treated (at an equivalent cost) to prevent one stroke or heart attack in comparison to those in risk group C.

Even though age is the most important (nonmodifiable) predictor of cardiovascular risk, the risk stratification system recommended in JNC VI is independent of the patient's age. The old adage that it is acceptable to have a "systolic BP less than 100 + age (in years)" is clearly erroneous; good data and a large meta-analysis now show that older persons, even those older than 80 years, benefit greatly by lowering their BP.[9] Similarly, gender is not specifically mentioned in the risk stratification system, except that male gender *is* a cardiovascular risk factor. Therefore, only women are in risk group A.

Considering Secondary Hypertension

More than 95% of Americans with hypertension have no specific cause of their elevated BP (i.e., idiopathic or primary hypertension). It is important, however, to consider the possibility that newly diagnosed hypertension has a specific cause (Box 19–3), for three reasons:

1. BP control is often difficult to achieve in those with secondary hypertension; diagnosing it early is likely to get the BP to goal more quickly.
2. Diagnosis plus remediation of secondary hypertension is particularly important in younger people because it will reduce the future burden of treatment

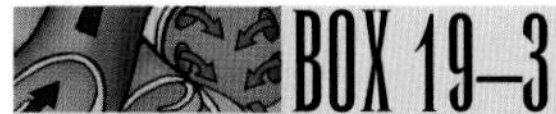

BOX 19–3

Types of Hypertension

- I. **Systolic and diastolic hypertension**
  - A. Primary, essential, or idiopathic
  - B. Secondary
    - 1. Renal
      - a. Renal parenchymal disease
        - (1) Acute glomerulonephritis
        - (2) Chronic nephritis
        - (3) Polycystic disease
        - (4) Diabetic nephropathy
        - (5) Hydronephrosis
      - b. Renovascular
        - (1) Renal artery stenosis
        - (2) Intrarenal vasculitis
      - c. Renin-producing tumors
      - d. Renoprival
      - e. Primary sodium retention (Liddle's syndrome, Gordon's syndrome)
    - 2. Endocrine
      - a. Acromegaly
      - b. Hypothyroidism
      - c. Hyperthyroidism
      - d. Hypercalcemia (hyperparathyroidism)
      - e. Adrenal
        - (1) Cortical
          - (a) Cushing's syndrome
          - (b) Primary hyperaldosteronism
          - (c) Congenital adrenal hyperplasia
          - (d) Apparent mineralocorticoid excess (e.g., licorice ingestion)
        - (2) Medullary: pheochromocytoma
      - f. Extra-adrenal chromaffin tumors
      - g. Carcinoid
      - h. Exogenous hormones
        - (1) Estrogen
        - (2) Glucocorticoids
        - (3) Mineralocorticoids
        - (4) Sympathomimetics
        - (5) Tyramine-containing foods and monoamine oxidase inhibitors
    - 3. Coarctation of the aorta
    - 4. Pregnancy-induced hypertension
    - 5. Neurologic disorders
      - a. Increased intracranial pressure
        - (1) Brain tumor
        - (2) Encephalitis
        - (3) Respiratory acidosis
      - b. Sleep apnea
      - c. Quadriplegia
      - d. Acute porphyria
      - e. Familial dysautonomia
      - f. Lead poisoning
      - g. Guillain-Barré syndrome
    - 6. Acute stress, including surgery
      - a. Psychogenic hyperventilation
      - b. Hypoglycemia
      - c. Burns
      - d. Pancreatitis
      - e. Alcohol withdrawal
      - f. Sickle cell crisis
      - g. After resuscitation
      - h. Postoperative
    - 7. Increased intravascular volume
    - 8. Alcohol and drug use
- II. **Systolic hypertension**
  - A. Increased cardiac output
    - 1. Aortic valvular insufficiency
    - 2. Arteriovenous fistula, patent ductus arteriosus
    - 3. Thyrotoxicosis
    - 4. Paget's disease of bone
    - 5. Beriberi
    - 6. Hyperkinetic circulation
  - B. Rigidity of aorta
- III. **Iatrogenic hypertension**

Adapted from Kaplan NM. Systemic hypertension: Mechanisms and diagnosis. In Braunwald E, Zipes DP, Libby P (eds): Heart Disease: A Textbook of Cardiovascular Medicine, 6th ed. Philadelphia, WB Saunders, 2001, p 946.

(both in cost of medication and follow-up, adverse effects of therapy, and quality of life). For some secondary causes, specific and potential curative therapy is available.

3. Routine consideration of secondary causes when the diagnosis of hypertension is first made will ensure that at least once during the person's lifetime a potential diagnosis will be entertained and the pros and cons of further testing critically evaluated. This process is discussed in detail later.

Guiding Therapy

Many of the nearly 90 antihypertensive agents currently available in the United States differ in BP-lowering efficacy in various situations. It is often helpful to discuss these potential confounders of treatment with the patient in an effort to "individualize" treatment according to the patient's specific dietary, medical, and personal considerations. For example, diuretics and calcium antagonists are more effective than angiotensin-converting enzyme (ACE) inhibitors and angiotensin II receptor blockers (ARBs) when dietary sodium is excessive. JNC VI now recommends treating hypertension and a concomitant illness/condition with a specific antihypertensive drug when that drug has been shown in clinical trials to improve cardiovascular morbidity and mortality. Thus, even though ACE inhibitors had not been routinely recommended as initial therapy for uncomplicated hypertensives, if the patient has heart failure because of impaired systolic function, an ACE inhibitor would be expected to not only lower BP but also provide the impressive benefits seen in many long-term studies in every New York Heart Association (NYHA) class of heart failure. Finally, some patients are particularly fearful of specific potential adverse effects of certain antihypertensive drugs, such as male sexual dysfunction. If this information is known to the physician, effort may be taken to attempt to avoid medications with a high incidence of this particular problem.

Medical History

In addition to assessing the risk for cardiovascular and renal disease, a careful drug, environmental, and nutritional history should be obtained during the initial evaluation of a hypertensive patient and intermittently during subsequent management. It is particularly important to ascertain whether the patient is taking any drug (by prescription or over the counter) or substance that might elevate BP (Box 19–4). Of particular concern are nonsteroidal anti-inflammatory drugs (NSAIDs), which are widely available over the counter and are not recognized as "drugs" by many patients. Sympathomimetic amines (once commonly found in weight loss, cold, and allergy preparations) have been associated with both increased BP and a risk of intracerebral hemorrhage and stroke. Hypertensive persons should avoid both NSAIDs and sympathomimetic amines and attempt to obtain relief of pain with acetaminophen and relief of the symptoms of nasal congestion with antihistamines, if possible. When these agents are ineffective, short-term use of the usually proscribed drugs may be condoned, but with the recognition that BP control is likely to be suboptimal during and immediately after their consumption.

Oral contraceptive pills containing estrogens and progestins may raise BP in some women, although this adverse effect is much less common with the lower doses in common use today. If a woman with newly diagnosed hypertension uses these pills, discontinuation for 6 months and observation of BP may allow a decision to be made about whether the pills are the cause of the hypertension. Conjugated estrogens (with or without progesterone), typically given for postmenopausal hormone replacement therapy, do not raise BP. Hypertensive women receiving hormone replacement do *not* need to alter this preventive therapy for osteoporosis.

Other prescription drugs can either elevate BP or interfere with certain antihypertensive agents. Of the former, cyclosporine, erythropoietin, corticosteroids, cocaine, and theophylline are perhaps the most widely recognized. Of the latter, monoamine oxidase inhibitors, NSAIDs, and tricyclic antidepressants are the most common. It is important to ascertain whether a hypertensive patient has taken any of these agents, as well as several other illicit drugs (e.g., phencyclidine). Some chemical elements, particularly lead and chromium, may elevate BP long after exposure; questioning about these and other environmental toxins may sometimes be helpful.

A focused dietary history is very important because the most effective lifestyle modifications involve limiting calories, sodium, or both. Both dietary salt and saturated fat intake can be estimated from an informal survey of dietary habits and preferences. Many processed foods, "fast foods," "diet foods," condiments, and snack items are very concentrated, often-unrecognized sources of salt. Now that most of these items bear labels attesting to their high salt content, many patients are more easily able to choose healthier foods. A sensible target (now validated in several clinical trials, most recently the Dietary Approach to Stop Hypertension [DASH]—sodium substudy[10]) is 100 mEq (2.4 g or 2400 mg) of sodium per day; this goal can usually be achieved if the high salt items mentioned earlier are avoided and the patient does not add salt, either at the table or while cooking. Occasionally, it is useful (and relatively inexpensive in comparison to formal dietary counseling) to have the patient collect a 24-hour urine sample to assay for sodium, particularly when the patient claims to be avoiding salt but the physician is suspicious. Although not all hypertensive patients will experience a reduction in BP with a low salt diet or an increase in BP with a high salt diet, individuals who are salt sensitive will benefit from reducing dietary sodium. In general, African Americans, the elderly, the obese, and diabetic patients are more likely to be "salt sensitive" and have a BP that will be more responsive to dietary salt restriction.

The nutritional history should also include questions about consumption of saturated fat, dairy product intake, and whether any mineral or vitamin supplements are being used. Because obesity is a major problem for many hypertensive patients, caloric intake, eating patterns, and changes in weight should be included in the history. Weight loss remains the most successful of all the lifestyle modifications for hypertension and should be part of the therapeutic plan in all overweight hypertensives from the outset.

BOX 19–4

Substances That Can Raise Blood Pressure (Partial List)

Nonsteroidal anti-inflammatory drugs (including the newer COX-2 inhibitors celecoxib and rofecoxib)
Corticosteroids
Sympathomimetic amines
Oral contraceptive hormones
Methylxanthines (including theophylline and caffeine*)
Cyclosporine
Erythropoietin
Cocaine
Nicotine†
Phencyclidine (PCP)

*Short duration (minutes to hours).

†Very short duration (seconds to minutes).

COX-2, cyclooxygenase-2; PCP, phenylcyclohexyl piperidine ("angel dust").

Social History

Although alcohol in moderation (one or two usual-sized drinks—less than 24 oz of beer, 8 oz of wine, or 3 oz of distilled spirits) protects against coronary heart disease, excessive alcohol intake (four or more drinks per day) raises both BP and all-cause mortality. In some patients, reducing or stopping alcohol ingestion can have very salutary effects on BP. Consuming tobacco has both acute and chronic adverse effects on BP. Smoking a single cigarette raises BP and the heart rate acutely (within seconds to minutes) because of nicotine's stimulation of catecholamine secretion. This effect disappears in about 15 minutes, so BP should be measured at least 15 to 30 minutes after the most recent cigarette is extinguished. Chronic tobacco abuse roughly doubles the long-term risk of coronary disease and has an even larger effect on peripheral arterial disease (including renovascular hypertension). Inquiry about tobacco abuse and advice to discontinue it should be part of every encounter with a health care professional. Tobacco's permissive effect on cardiovascular disease, not to mention carcinogenesis, should be sufficient motivation for most patients to stop smoking.

Hypertensive patients should also be questioned about a sedentary lifestyle and whether they are willing and able to engage in regular physical activity. Even limited aerobic exercise, including brisk walking for 30 minutes three times weekly, can reduce BP and the risk of all-cause and cardiovascular mortality. Snoring, daytime sleepiness, and other clinical features of sleep apnea, especially in obese hypertensives, should lead to consideration of a formal evaluation for this under-appreciated and underdiagnosed form of secondary hypertension. Although reducing stress has not frequently been shown in clinical trials to lead to lowering of BP, questions about the home and work environment can address psychosocial issues—such as lack of social support, transportation, or financial resources—that might occasionally raise BP or complicate plans for follow-up.

In addition, the medical history should carefully ascertain the patient's previous experience with and attitudes toward antihypertensive drugs and be sensitive to cultural factors or health beliefs that could hinder diagnostic or therapeutic plans.

Physical Examination

The "directed" physical examination of a hypertensive patient should pay special attention to weight, target organ damage, and features consistent with secondary hypertension. It should focus on items that were suggested by the medical history.

- The pattern of fat distribution should be noted. Android obesity (waist-to-hip ratio >0.95) is associated with increased cardiovascular risk, whereas gynecoid obesity (waist-to-hip ratio <0.85) is not. Android obesity is a feature of the syndrome of insulin resistance, sleep apnea, "the deadly quartet" (hypertension, dyslipidemia, and impaired glucose tolerance in addition to obesity), and glucocorticoid excess states. Recently, expert panels have focused on waist measurement (at the umbilicus) alone. Men whose waist is over 100 cm (40 inches) and women whose waist is greater than 88 cm (34 inches) are at increased risk. Measurement of hip circumference and the waist-hip ratio adds little to the simpler waist measurement.[11]
- Funduscopic examination is important in assessing the duration and severity of hypertension. The presence of hypertensive retinopathy (grade 1, arterial tortuosity and silver wiring; grade 2, arteriovenous crossing changes ["nicking"]; grade 3, hemorrhaging or exudates; grade 4, papilledema) provides definitive evidence of target organ damage.
- The neck should be examined for an enlarged thyroid gland, abnormalities of the venous circulation (e.g., jugular venous distention, abnormal or "cannon" a-waves), and carotid bruits.
- The chest should be auscultated for evidence of heart failure or bronchospasm; the latter would make beta-blocker therapy relatively contraindicated.
- The heart should be carefully examined for cardiomegaly, murmurs, and extra sounds.
- Abdominal examination is a very important part of the "directed" physical examination because the search for abdominal bruits is one of the most cost-effective ways to screen for renovascular hypertension. All four abdominal quadrants and the back should be auscultated, typically by using the pulse at the wrist as the synchronizing stimulus. Diastolic or continuous bruits are common in renovascular hypertension, but systolic bruits in young and especially thin hypertensive subjects may not be indicative of renal artery stenosis. Abdominal masses can sometimes be palpated in patients with pheochromocytoma or polycystic kidney disease.
- The groin and legs should be examined for evidence of peripheral arterial disease, which is often manifested as bruits, absent or decreased pulses, and abnormal hair growth patterns. Edema can be a sign of heart failure or renal disease and can be exacerbated by high doses of dihydropyridine calcium antagonists.
- The neurologic examination need not be extensive in a hypertensive patient with no history of cerebrovascular disease, but it should be complete if a history of stroke or transient ischemic attack is present.
- The patient's skin should be carefully examined for café-au-lait spots (suggesting neurofibromatosis and possible pheochromocytoma), acanthosis nigricans (suggesting insulin resistance), and xanthomas at tendons or xanthelasma (indicating dyslipidemia). Other skin signs suggesting pheochromocytoma (axillary freckles, ash-leaf patches, port-wine stains in the trigeminal distribution, adenoma sebaceum) are uncommon except in patients with phakomatoses.
- The many physical signs associated with other secondary causes should be sought if the medical history is suggestive. Signs of Cushing's syndrome

(purple striae, moon facies, dorsocervical fat pad, atrophic skin changes) or thyroid disease (abnormal Achilles reflexes, hair quality, and eye signs) are typically difficult to ignore.

Laboratory Testing

In most hypertensive patients, only a few inexpensive and simple laboratory tests are needed as part of the initial evaluation. In selected patients, however, more extensive testing is not only appropriate but also necessary to avoid missing secondary hypertension and delaying proper treatment. Laboratory tests recommended for all hypertensive persons can be divided into those that are performed to assess risk, establish cause, screen for important common diseases, and finally, guide the choice of initial therapy.

For uncomplicated hypertensive patients whose history and physical examination do not suggest a secondary cause, the simple battery of tests in Box 19–5 is all that is needed. A lipid profile and fasting glucose levels are indicated in hypertensive patients because of the high prevalence of the association of these risk factors with hypertension. The presence of diabetes mellitus or additional risk factors not only requires institution of therapy for these conditions but also indicates substantially increased cardiovascular risk, thus requiring more intensive therapy for hypertension and closer follow-up. Recent clinical trials in diabetics have also demonstrated the specific benefits of certain types of antihypertensive drug therapy, particularly ACE inhibitors and ARBs, so any regimen intended for a diabetic hypertensive should include a member of these classes of drugs.

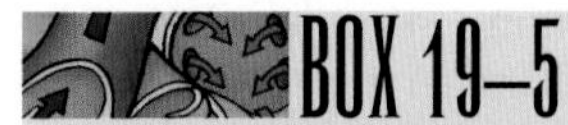
BOX 19–5

Laboratory Tests Appropriate for All Patients with Newly Diagnosed Hypertension

ASSESSING RISK
Lipid profile (including total cholesterol, HDL cholesterol, and triglycerides)
Serum glucose (preferably fasting)
Serum creatinine
Urinalysis (both dipstick and microscopic)
12-Lead electrocardiogram

ESTABLISHING CAUSE
Serum potassium
Serum creatinine
Urinalysis (both dipstick and microscopic)
?Thyroid-stimulating hormone (with further reflex testing, if indicated)

SCREENING FOR COMMON ASYMPTOMATIC DISEASES
Complete blood count
Serum calcium

GUIDING THERAPY
Lipid profile (including total cholesterol, HDL cholesterol, and triglycerides)
Serum glucose (preferably fasting)
Serum creatinine

HDL, high-density lipoprotein.

Routine measurement of serum creatinine and a complete urinalysis are recommended for three reasons. First, urinalysis is useful in assessing risk because hypertensive patients with renal impairment, proteinuria, and even microalbuminuria have a worse prognosis. Second, urinalysis may help identify hypertension secondary to chronic renal disease, which is characterized by proteinuria and typically an active sediment. Renal impairment (elevated serum creatinine) with a normal urinary sediment may be a valuable clue suggesting renal artery stenosis with ischemic nephropathy. Third, knowledge of the serum creatinine level guides therapy because loop diuretics are routinely needed and are more effective than thiazide diuretics when creatinine clearance is less than 30 mL/min.

An ECG may provide important, but limited information in most hypertensive patients. Although it may identify an occasionally important dysrhythmia or even an unsuspected old myocardial infarction, its biggest role is in screening for left ventricular hypertrophy (LVH), which is an objective measure of both the severity and duration of elevated BP. Despite a sensitivity of only 10% to 50% (depending on which criteria are used in its interpretation) in the Framingham Heart Study, ECG evidence of LVH was associated with an approximately threefold increase in incidence of cardiovascular events. LVH detected by echocardiogram appears to be an even better predictor of future events. Echocardiography is not recommended for routine evaluation because of cost and the high intrinsic variability of a single echocardiogram.

Because hypothyroidism is a subtle cause of remediable hypertension, especially in the elderly, a thyroid-stimulating hormone assay may be helpful. Serum calcium is useful in evaluating hyperparathyroidism and is often included in automated chemistry panels. It is not necessary to measure plasma renin activity to screen for secondary causes of hypertension, determine prognosis, or guide therapy. However, this test is useful in the diagnosis of mineralocorticoid excess states such as primary hyperaldosteronism.

SECONDARY HYPERTENSION

Clues to the presence of secondary hypertension are often provided by a carefully obtained medical history. Many patients with primary hypertension report an isolated elevated BP reading or two some time in their 20s and 30s that was not reproducible or sustained until at least a decade or more later. Their BP gradually rises until it reaches a threshold level, and then hypertension is diagnosed. In contrast, patients with an identifiable secondary cause of hypertension usually have a very different history. Instead of a gradual onset of elevated BP, they typically have a relatively abrupt onset of hypertension and are generally initially seen at a higher stage and with considerable target organ damage. The onset of elevated BP at ages younger than 30 or older than 50 years should alert the clinician to the possibility of secondary hypertension. Thus, the history of the patient's initial manifestation of hypertension should be carefully documented. At what age was the BP first elevated? How high was the pressure? Were all previous readings within the normal range? Was it discovered during a routine office visit, or did the patient have clinical problems related to BP elevation or related target organ damage?

Because patients with secondary hypertension typically do not respond to antihypertensive drug therapy as well as patients with primary hypertension do, the history of the patient's response to treatment must be ascertained. Which drugs were used and at what doses? Did the patient's BP respond initially and then become resistant? A positive answer to this question is frequently found in patients with primary hypertension in whom secondary hypertension later develops, particularly atherosclerotic renovascular disease.

The response to specific drugs may also offer important clues to the presence and type of secondary hypertension. Were ACE inhibitors or ARBs particularly effective, as might be expected in unilateral renovascular disease? Did one of these agents precipitate a significant, but reversible rise in serum creatinine (after use of the drug was stopped), as often occurs with renovascular disease? Was the response to an alpha-adrenoceptor blocker impressive but a beta-adrenoceptor blocker raised the BP, as is sometimes seen with pheochromocytoma? Did even low doses of a thiazide or thiazide-like diuretic precipitate hypokalemia unresponsive to an ACE inhibitor or ARB (with or without potassium supplementation), as is commonly seen in excess mineralocorticoid states? Was an ACE inhibitor or an ARB nearly totally ineffective in lowering BP, as often occurs with excess mineralocorticoid states?

Laboratory Testing for Secondary Hypertension

All types of secondary hypertension are unusual in the general hypertensive population. When interpreting test results in a given patient, bayesian analysis (which incorporates the pretest probability of finding disease; see Chapter 2) is therefore more important than the sensitivity of the test (i.e., the percentage of persons with disease who have a positive test). The medical history, physical examination, and routine laboratory studies can be used to identify hypertensive patients with a higher likelihood of having a particular kind of secondary hypertension. The cost-effectiveness of testing for secondary hypertension is greatly enhanced by subjecting only individuals with a high pretest probability of disease (on clinical grounds) to more intensive investigation.

When the initial evaluation suggests that a patient might have secondary hypertension, establishing or excluding that particular diagnosis by properly selecting further tests is important, especially in patients with difficult-to-control hypertension. The choice of tests and the order in which they should be performed depends not only on the pretest probability of disease but also on safety, availability, local expertise with the test, and its cost.

Renovascular Hypertension

Patients with renovascular hypertension often have stage 3 hypertension with considerable target organ damage at initial evaluation, and they are at risk of losing renal function from ischemic nephropathy.[12] Atherosclerotic renal artery stenosis accounts for 80% to 90% of cases, with the remainder being due to fibromuscular dysplasia. Vasculitis, arterial bands and other forms of extrinsic compression of the renal arteries, and trauma account for a small percentage of cases. Fibromuscular dysplasia consists of two distinct forms of arteriopathy and is found mostly in young white women (10 to 25 years old) with very high BP; it is particularly well treated with angioplasty. Atherosclerotic renal artery stenosis is a disease of older people, many of whom had easily controlled primary hypertension and then refractory hypertension developed after the age of 55. Many of these people have evidence of atherosclerotic disease in other vascular beds (carotids, coronaries, and peripheral arteries), and many are (or were) heavy cigarette smokers. Though more common in white persons, renovascular hypertension can also develop in African Americans, and the identifying characteristics are very similar. A simple, but relatively accurate "clinical prediction rule" can estimate the pretest probably of renovascular disease based on clinical information gathered at the initial evaluation[13] (Table 19–3).

Diagnostic Testing

The goal of laboratory testing in patients suspected of having renovascular hypertension is to not only demonstrate the presence of renal artery stenosis but also determine that the lesion or lesions discovered are in fact the cause of the patient's hypertension.[12] Before testing, however, it is useful to have a discussion with the patient regarding the possible results. If a patient is unsuitable for or unwilling to have surgery (e.g., should the renal artery be damaged during percutaneous transluminal renal angioplasty), further investigation is probably unwarranted. Recent data from The Netherlands and the Mayo Clinic suggest that continued medical therapy (including ACE inhibitors and ARBs) may be as useful in the long term as revascularization, thus suggesting that only patients with uncontrolled hypertension need to be evaluated. A guide to the selection of screening tests, based on the pretest probability of disease, is shown in Figure 19–4. Tests used to screen persons at moderate risk for renovascular hypertension

TABLE 19–3

Clinical Prediction Rule for Estimating the Probability of Renovascular Hypertension*

Clinical Characteristic	Never Smoked	Current or Former Smoker	Points (Sum from Left Side)	Probability of Renovascular Hypertension (95% CI)
Age (yr)			5	<2 (0–5)
20–29	0	0	6	3 (1–8)
30–39	1	4	7	5 (2–10)
40–49	2	8	8	8 (3–12)
50–59	3	5	9	11 (5–20)
60–69	4	5	10	15 (7–28)
70–79	5	6	11	25 (14–40)
Female gender	2	2	12	37 (18–55)
ASCVD	1	1	13	47 (28–65)
Hx HTN for 2 yr	1	1	14	62 (40–80)
BMI <25 kg/m^2	2	2	15	72 (46–84)
Abdominal bruit	3	3	16	80 (62–86)
Serum creatinine (mg/dL)			17	87 (72–92)
0.5–0.75	0	0	18	89 (78–95)
0.75–1.0	1	1	19	90 (82–97)
1.0–1.2	2	2	20	90 (92–100)
1.2–1.65	3	3		
1.7–2.2	6	6		
2.3	9	9		
Hypercholesterolemia (>250 mg/dL or receiving treatment)	1	1		

*The sum of the point score (from the left of the table) is compared with the column at the right (labeled Points) to estimate the probability or renovascular hypertension. ASCVD, signs, symptoms, or clinical evidence of atherosclerotic cardiovascular disease; BMI, body mass index (weight in kg/[height in cm]^2); Hx HTN, history of hypertension.

Adapted from Krijnen P, van Jaarsveld BC, Steyerberg EW, et al: A clinical prediction rule for renal artery stenosis. Ann Intern Med 1998;129:738–740.

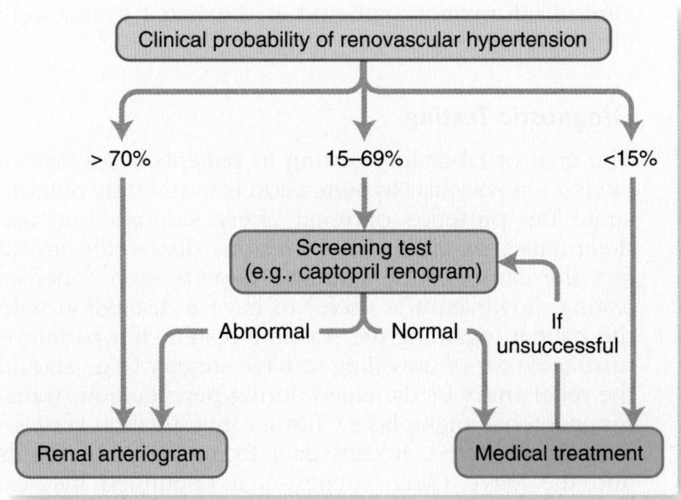

FIGURE 19–4. Algorithm for testing for renovascular hypertension. Based on the pretest probability of disease (perhaps most easily accomplished with the "clinical prediction rule"; see text), moderate-risk individuals (i.e., with a pretest probability of renovascular disease of ~15% to 69%) may have a screening test initially and then angiography if the test is positive. High-risk individuals (with a pretest probability perhaps exceeding 70%) may proceed directly to angiography because a negative screening test would most likely be a false negative. The choice of initial screening test depends on local availability and expertise in interpreting the results, as well as cost. (Adapted from Mann SJ, Pickering T: Detection of renovascular hypertension, state of the art, 1992. Ann Intern Med 1992;117:845–853.)

are based on either biochemical or imaging techniques (Table 19–4).

Two newer imaging modalities deserve special attention. Visualization of the renal arteries by ultrasound with quantification of flow by Doppler measurements is widely available, but the utility of the test varies greatly. When an experienced, dedicated technician examines a properly prepared patient, the sensitivity

TABLE 19–4

Screening Tests for Renovascular Hypertension

	Sensitivity (%)	Specificity (%)	Invasive?	Availability	Cost* ($)
Biochemical Tests					
Serum potassium	~70	~5	No	Widespread	12–25
Plasma renin activity	~80	~60	No	Variable	35–105
Captopril challenge test	60–70	~80	No	Widespread	90–250
Renal vein renin activity ratio	~75–90	~80	Yes: F vein	Variable	1500–2000
Imaging Tests					
Rapid-sequence intravenous pyelography	74	80–86	A or F vein	Widespread	250
Renal scintigraphy (^{99m}Tc-DTPA)	74	77	A vein	Widespread	200
Renal scintigraphy with captopril (or enalaprilat); ^{99m}Tc-DTPA or MAG3	85	90	A vein	Most major medical centers	250
Intravenous DSA	80	88	A vein	Variable	500
Intra-arterial DSA	95	99	F artery	Limited	1000
Standard angiography	>99	>99	F artery	Widespread	3000
Duplex ultrasound of renal arteries	Operator dependent (50–99)	Operator dependent (50–99)	No	Highly variable	600
Magnetic resonance imaging	Perhaps ~90	Perhaps ~90	No	Limited	2500

*Costs vary over time and from institution to institution. These figures are approximate and derived from purveyors at RUSH-Presbyterian-St. Luke's Medical Center, Chicago, in 2001.

A, antecubital; DSA, digital subtraction angiography; DTPA, diethylenetriamine pentaacetic acid; F, femoral; MAG3, mercaptoacetyltriglycine (mertiatide).

and specificity of the test are well in excess of 90%, and the cost is reasonable. Unfortunately, in obese patients and those with much intestinal gas, the test is much less useful, and the rate of localization of the renal arteries is only about 60%. In some centers, however, this modality has emerged as the screening test of first choice. Magnetic resonance angiography (with gadolinium enhancement) will probably be the test of choice shortly; it is very accurate (with images approaching the quality of a standard angiogram) and noninvasive, and the patient needs no specific preparation. These advantages are currently outweighed by the limited availability and the very high cost.

In many centers, the screening test of choice is captopril scintigraphy. Only ACE inhibitor and ARB therapy needs to be stopped before performing the test, and adverse reactions from the single dose of captopril are rare. Some centers perform a captopril scan about an hour after the baseline scan (without captopril), which doubles the cost but may make it more convenient for the patient. In many centers with a low prevalence of positive scans, investigations stop after an initially normal captopril scan. A "captopril-induced change in the renogram" (especially a change in the distribution of tracer between kidneys) predicts successful BP lowering after revascularization. Most centers use ^{99m}Tc-DTPA (a radioisotope of technetium chelated to diethylenetriamine pentaacetic acid), but the more expensive MAG3 (mercaptoacetyltriglycine [mertiatide]) is more accurate in detecting bilateral renal artery stenosis. When digital subtraction angiography from a femoral arterial approach is followed by angioplasty and stenting (especially when the lesion is ostial), the technical success rate for opening a stenosed renal artery is in excess of 95%. Screening of high-probability patients with captopril scintigraphy, followed by angioplasty and stenting, has the most positive cost-effectiveness ratio; if the pretest probability of renovascular disease is higher than 30%, the process has been alleged to *reduce* overall monetary costs!

Pheochromocytoma

Patients with pheochromocytoma are nearly always symptomatic when initially evaluated. They usually have "spells" or paroxysmal symptoms that are typical for each patient, spaced by hours or sometimes months. Some patients recognize "triggers" (eating, pain, postural changes, urination) that precipitate an attack. Hypertension is most commonly sustained, but exacerbated during a paroxysm. The most common symptoms include headache, diaphoresis, and palpitations, but other symptoms, particularly anxiety, weakness, and tremulousness, are also frequently found. The pattern of symptoms is often a clue to the predominant hormone secreted by the tumor: norepinephrine-secreting tumors most commonly produce pallor, whereas flushing is more characteristic of those secreting epinephrine.

Diagnostic Testing

Diagnostic testing for pheochromocytoma generally involves two steps: demonstrating that excess catecholamines are being produced and then localizing the tumor.[14] Currently, multiple possibilities may be used to implement each step[15] (Table 19–5).

Because of generally lower cost, simpler handling procedures, and wider availability, we prefer 24-hour urinary collections for total catecholamines, vanillylmandelic acid, and metanephrines. Measuring catecholamine levels in plasma samples is also occasionally useful, particularly in conjunction with pharmacologic testing with clonidine or glucagon. Because clonidine testing normally reduces both plasma norepinephrine levels and BP, it is generally preferred over glucagon stimulation, but the latter may be necessary in persons with repeatedly normal plasma values. After demonstration of overproduction of catecholamines, a T2-weighted magnetic resonance scan is probably the most readily available and useful imaging test because the pheochromocytoma tissue "lights up" with this technique. A nuclear scan using meta-iodobenzylguanidine (MIBG) may also be helpful, especially when a metastatic tumor is suspected. Computed axial tomography may be more sensitive than magnetic resonance imaging in detecting small tumors, but it is probably less specific. Surgery to remove the tumor should be attempted after a suitable period of alpha-adrenergic blockade; occasionally, a beta-blocker is also required, but it should be added only *after* alpha-blockade is established. Although most patients do not have a hereditary-familial cause of their pheochromocytoma, skin examination and screening for other tumors (related to multiple endocrine neoplasia syndromes) are recommended (see earlier).

Mineralocorticoid Excess States

The symptoms of these forms of secondary hypertension that may be useful to the clinician are related to hypokalemia.[16] Typically, muscle weakness, cramps, polyuria, and even nocturia are prominent, although many who are incidentally hypokalemic at initial examination are free of these complaints. Target organ damage is typically less severe and less extensive than often seen with similar levels of BP in primary hypertension. Most patients (about 50% to 60%) with this syndrome have a benign adrenal adenoma that secretes aldosterone autonomously; some (30% to 50%) have bilateral (idiopathic) adrenal hyperplasia. Rarer causes include adrenal carcinomas, glucocorticoid-suppressible hyperaldosteronism, and licorice ingestion. Recent research has shown that both glycyrrhizic acid (the active agent in licorice) and its hydrolyzed product glycyrrhetinic acid inhibit peripheral (e.g., intrarenal) 11-beta-hydroxysteroid dehydrogenase (the enzyme responsible for inactivation of cortisol to cortisone). Such inhibition leads to excessive mineralocorticoid action of cortisol, which then has clinical manifestations similar to those of hyperaldosteronism.

TABLE 19–5

Diagnostic Tests for Pheochromocytoma

	Advantage	Disadvantage	Availability	Cost* ($)
		Biochemical Tests		
24-hr urinary catecholamines, VMA, and metanephrines	Integrates production over time	Time lag between order and results	Widespread	50–150 or higher
Spot urinary metanephrine/creatinine ratio	Quicker assay than 24-hr collection; useful after a "spell"	Limited experience with normal values	Widespread	100 or higher
Plasma catecholamines	Useful during a "spell"	Special collection, handling needed	Limited	90–160
Plasma metanephrines	Useful during a "spell"	Special collection, handling needed	Limited	200
Clonidine suppression test	Safer than glucagon	Expertise needed	Limited	500 and higher
Glucagon stimulation test	Useful "final test"	Expertise needed	Limited	1000 and higher
		Localization Tests		
CAT scan	Widely available	Contrast often needed	Widespread	800–1500
Magnetic resonance imaging (esp. T2 weighted)	Higher specificity than a CAT scan	May miss smaller tumors	Limited	900–2000
^{131}I-MIBG	Very useful for metastatic tumors	2 days between injection and scan	Limited	1000 and higher
Abdominal ultrasound		Nonspecific test	Widespread	200
Adrenal venous sampling	Used only as a "last resort"	Expensive, invasive, special expertise needed	Limited	5000 and higher

*Costs vary over time and from institution to institution. These figures are approximate, as cited at RUSH-Presbyterian-St. Luke's Medical Center, Chicago, in 2001.

CAT, computed axial tomographic; MIBG, meta-iodobenzylguanidine; VMA, vanillylmandelic acid.

Diagnostic Testing

A low serum potassium level discovered as part of the routine evaluation of a hypertensive patient may be the only clue that a mineralocorticoid excess state is present. Hypokalemia, especially a serum level less than 3.2 mEq/L, when not secondary to diuretic therapy, indicates that mineralocorticoid excess hypertension is likely. Hypertensive patients who become hypokalemic with low-dose (<25 mg/day of hydrochlorothiazide or 12.5 mg/day of chlorthalidone) diuretic therapy and whose serum potassium stays below normal (<3.5 mEq/L) despite either potassium supplementation or concomitant use of drugs that inhibit the renin-angiotensin-aldosterone system (ACE inhibitors or ARBs) may have mineralocorticoid excess hypertension.

Three major steps are necessary in the diagnostic evaluation of primary hyperaldosteronism: (1) demonstrating autonomous overproduction of mineralocorticoids, (2) distinguishing between the several causes, and (3) monitoring the chosen therapy.[17] The single best test for identifying patients with normal renal function and primary aldosteronism is measurement of 24-hour urinary aldosterone excretion during salt loading. An excretion rate greater than 14 µg of aldosterone in 24 hours after 3 days of salt loading (>200 mEq/day) distinguishes most patients with primary aldosteronism from those with essential hypertension. Classically, all drugs that interfere with the renin-angiotensin-aldosterone system are discontinued for at least a week before this urine collection. Because a substantial number of patients with primary aldosteronism do not initially have hypokalemia, the plasma aldosterone-renin ratio has been used to define the appropriateness of plasma renin activity for the circulating levels of aldosterone. Some authorities recommend this calculation as an initial screening tool. Direct genetic testing of DNA or a dexamethasone challenge test can diagnose glucocorticoid-suppressible hyperaldosteronism.

Although some authorities recommend a number of hormonal tests to differentiate aldosterone-producing adrenal adenomas from bilateral adrenal hyperplasia, we typically perform a thin-cut (every 5 mm) adrenal computed tomographic (CT) scan instead. It is noninvasive, and essentially all adenomas larger than 1.5 cm in diameter can be identified. The sensitivity of high-resolution CT scanning for adenomas exceeds 90%, probably somewhat better than iodocholesterol scintigraphy. Adrenal venous aldosterone assays are very expensive and risky in inexperienced hands and are needed only rarely, such as when the biochemical findings are highly suggestive of an adenoma but the thin-cut CT scan is not diagnostic.

Chronic medical therapy is indicated in patients with adrenal hyperplasia, in patients with adenoma who are poor surgical risks, and in those with bilateral adrenal adenomas that may require bilateral adrenalectomy. Typically, potassium-sparing diuretics and calcium antagonists are most useful. In most patients, surgical excision of an aldosterone-producing adenoma reverses the hypertension and biochemical defects. One year postoperatively, about 70% of patients are normotensive, but 5 years postoperatively, only half remain so. The restoration of normal potassium homeostasis is usually permanent. Patients undergoing surgery should receive drug treatment for at least 8 to 10 weeks, both to decrease BP and to correct metabolic abnormalities. These patients have a significant potassium deficiency that must be corrected preoperatively because hypokalemia increases the risk of cardiac dysrhythmias during anesthesia.

Other Forms of Secondary Hypertension

The clinician should inquire about symptoms characteristic of sleep apnea, thyroid disorders, hyperparathyroidism, and Cushing's syndrome because these conditions may be associated with hypertension that responds to specific therapy directed at the primary disease. Physical examination is generally sufficient to exclude acromegaly and coarctation of the aorta, especially if the peripheral pulses are palpated (to search for radial-femoral artery pulse delay). A BP measurement in the thigh is recommended for all young persons with newly diagnosed hypertension to exclude this possibility; an echocardiogram can identify about 95% of aortic coarctations through the first 8 cm of the descending aorta.

PATIENT EDUCATION

The initial evaluation of a hypertensive patient is not complete until the clinician or health educator provides adequate education and advice about the problem and its impact on the patient's prognosis. Patients should understand that

- Hypertension is not a disease, but rather a pathophysiologic condition that increases the likelihood of a cardiovascular or renal complication; not everyone with hypertension will inevitably be affected.
- BP measurements vary, and those taken in the health care provider's office should usually carry the greatest importance because we know the most about their prognostic significance. Self-measurement of BP can be very useful in monitoring and understanding day-to-day fluctuations, but it is not usually sufficient to determine therapy.
- Although hypertension is rarely cured, it can almost always be successfully treated.
- Systematic introduction of both lifestyle modifications and drug therapy, if needed, is the most effective approach to lowering BP and reducing the risk of cardiovascular problems.
- If medications are needed to control hypertension, most patients will require them lifelong unless substantive changes are made in the patient's lifestyle.
- Patients should know their BP and their BP goal and be strongly encouraged to take their medications as directed and keep follow-up appointments.

MANAGEMENT

Successful management of hypertension requires a major commitment from the patient, the health care provider, and the health care system. The patient must continue to take what could be a costly medication with potential side effects and see a physician frequently for an asymptomatic condition in the belief that these measures will reduce the risk of a major complication or even death. The physician must help the patient achieve the goal BP and maintain surveillance of this and other cardiovascular risk factors. The health care system must agree to fund both physician and pharmacy benefits, with the realization that many people require treatment for many years before one serious adverse event is prevented.

Lifestyle Modification

Nearly all hypertension guidelines recommend nutritional-hygienic measures to control BP despite the absence of clinical trial data demonstrating that these modalities significantly reduce cardiovascular morbidity and mortality. There is, however, good public health rationale for advocating weight loss, dietary salt restriction, and other nonpharmacologic methods as preventive, adjunctive, and (occasionally) definitive treatment of hypertension. In multicenter clinical trials involving overweight subjects, weight loss is the most effective single modality that reduces BP in the short term. Dietary salt restriction to about 90 to 100 mmol (2000 to 2400 mg) of sodium per day is also effective in lowering BP. A more significant effect was observed in the sodium arm of the DASH study.[10] In this recently published trial, low (vs. high) salt content reduced BP by 6.7/2.5 mm Hg in the control diet and by 3.0/1.6 mm Hg in the DASH diet. All these differences were statistically significant, as were comparisons between both intermediate and high salt diets. Recidivism may be a problem with these recommendations, however, and long-term adherence to such programs is uncommon in many clinics. Also recommended are alcohol restriction to one to two drinks per day, tobacco avoidance, major exercise (three to six times weekly), caffeine reduction (if excessive), and supplements of potassium, calcium, or magnesium (if a deficiency state is present).

In the Treatment of Mild Hypertension Study (TOMHS), a vigorous program of lifestyle modification, executed by experts with very motivated participants, was shown to be inferior to antihypertensive drug therapy *plus* lifestyle modification in both reducing BP and preventing overall cardiovascular events.[18] Because of difficulty in sustaining initial efforts at lifestyle modification alone, many patients and most clinicians prefer a strategy that adds effective antihypertensive drug therapy even earlier than JNC VI would recommend, particularly when initial efforts at weight loss and sodium restriction are unsuccessful or not sustained.

Choice of Initial Drug Therapy

Initial Antihypertensive Drug Therapy for "Uncomplicated Hypertensives"

At the time that JNC VI was written, only diuretics or beta-blockers, or both, had been used in clinical trials in otherwise uncomplicated hypertensives, and they had demonstrated an improvement in prognosis in comparison to long-term treatment with placebo. Because it is no longer ethical to give *only* placebo in long-term morbidity and mortality studies in hypertensive patients, we will probably *never* have data with newer classes of drugs showing superiority over placebo, except perhaps in some situations (stage 1 isolated systolic hypertension or high-normal patients in risk group B, for example). Nonetheless, several recently published large studies indicate that differences across different classes of antihypertensive agents in the prevention of cardiovascular events are small (if indeed they exist at all).

The only obvious exception to this suggestion is initial treatment with an alpha-blocker, which was associated with an increased risk of cardiovascular events (mostly heart failure) in the Antihypertensive and Lipid-Lowering (Treatments to Prevent) Heart Attack Trial (ALLHAT).[19] Although systolic BP was higher by 3 mm Hg (137 vs. 134 mm Hg) in the 9067 hypertensive patients randomized to doxazosin than in the 15,268 initially receiving chlorthalidone, the investigators in this trial implicated the initial drug rather than the differential BP lowering resulting from it as the reason for the differences in prognosis observed.

Currently, the proper role of calcium antagonists as initial treatment of hypertension is controversial. One meta-analysis that included most of the clinical trials using this type of drug (even those with previously published results that were not intended as "outcome trials") concluded that calcium antagonists were significantly less effective in preventing myocardial infarction and heart failure than other initial treatments were (ACE inhibitors, diuretics, or beta-blockers, lumped together).[20] The prospective meta-analysis of studies collected under the auspices of the World Health Organization/International Society of Hypertension came to a slightly different conclusion and suggested that a more valid comparison of calcium antagonists and other antihypertensive agents could be made only after several of the long-term studies that are currently under way have completed their follow-up.[21] In both meta-analyses, calcium antagonists were superior to standard care (diuretics, beta-blockers, or both) in the prevention of stroke, though not as effective in the prevention of myocardial infarction. All-cause mortality was not different in either analysis. Several of the larger studies have shown very significant cardiovascular benefits, compared with placebo, with treatment regimens that began with a calcium antagonist.

Nationwide pharmacy dispensing data indicate that hypertensive American patients are now receiving more ACE inhibitors than calcium antagonists. Many physicians have been favorably impressed with recent hypertension trials that included an ACE inhibitor. In most of them, the ACE inhibitor was at least as good, if not significantly better than a regimen without an ACE inhibitor (e.g., the Heart Outcomes Prevention Evaluation [HOPE] Study).[22] The definitive answer to whether an ACE inhibitor is as good or better than a diuretic (or a dihydropyridine calcium antagonist) will probably come from the ALLHAT study, which randomized more than 42,000 hypertensive patients to chlorthalidone versus lisinopril versus amlodipine (and originally doxazosin; see earlier).

Most health care providers working in cost-sensitive clinical environments nowadays are exhorted to use the least expensive initial drug that will lower BP. In many circumstances, this drug is a low-dose thiazide or thiazide-like diuretic. Our approach to the choice of antihypertensive drug therapy for patients with uncomplicated hypertension without an explicit reason to choose a specific drug is shown in Figure 19–5.

Initial Antihypertensive Drug Therapy for "Complicated Patients"

For the first time, JNC VI formally recognized that many hypertensive people begin treatment too late, after the development of cardiovascular disease or other medical conditions that may be positively affected by specific antihypertensive drug therapy.[1] JNC VI divided these situations into "compelling conditions" and "clinical conditions." In the former, a specific class of antihypertensive drug should be prescribed if clinical trials showed that the class of drug reduces morbidity or mortality for that condition. Thus, for a hypertensive person with systolic heart failure, an ACE inhibitor will not only lower BP but also reduce clinical events and hospitalization. In Table 19–6 are shown other examples of antihypertensive drugs that have demonstrated benefit in improving prognosis in conditions commonly seen in hypertensives. In addition, some absolute and relative contraindications to specific antihypertensive drugs limit

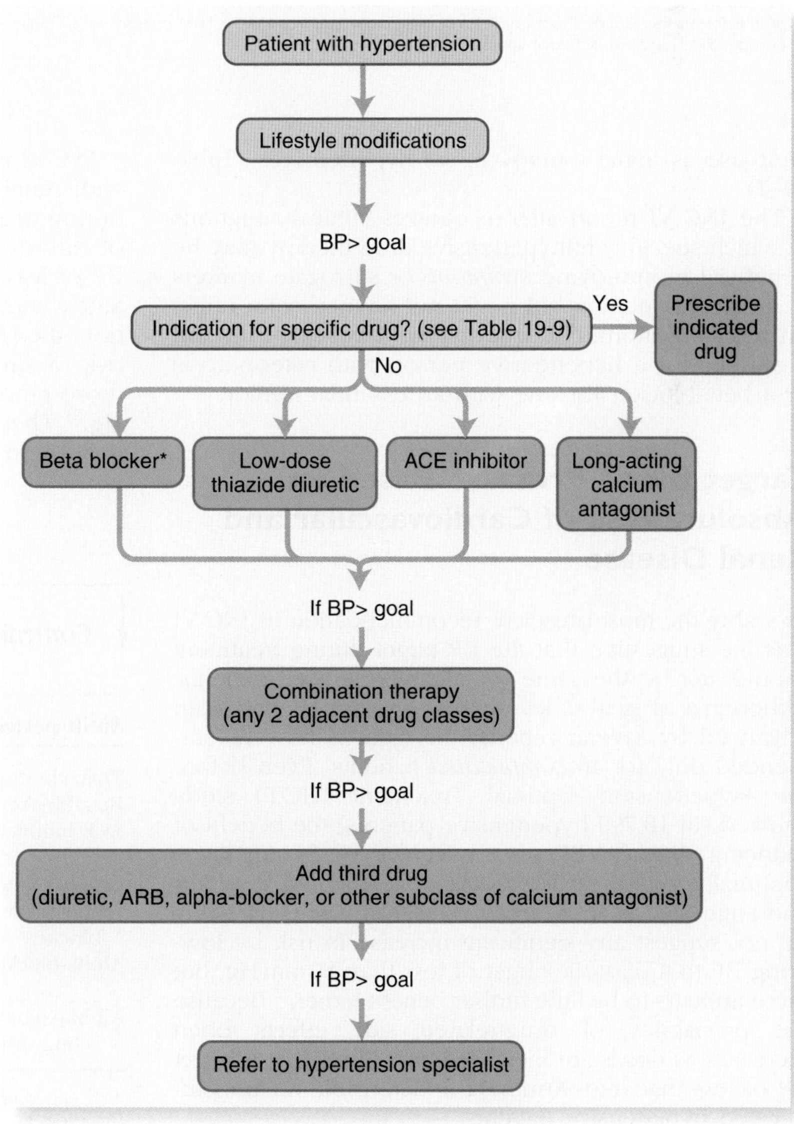

FIGURE 19–5. Proposed algorithm for choosing initial antihypertensive drug therapy for patients without a reason to select a specific treatment. *An initial beta-blocker is not recommended for hypertensive patients older than 60 years. The combination of a diuretic and a calcium antagonist may lower blood pressure (BP), but it has not yet been shown in clinical trials to reduce morbidity and mortality in hypertensive persons. ACE, angiotensin-converting enzyme; ARB, angiotensin II receptor blocker.

TABLE 19–6

Compelling Conditions for Which Specific Antihypertensive Drug Therapy Has Reduced Morbidity and Mortality in Clinical Trials

Compelling Condition	Indicated Therapy	Clinical Trial(s)
Post–acute coronary syndrome	Beta-blocker	Norwegian Timolol Survival Study, BHAT, others
With left ventricular dysfunction or heart failure	ACE inhibitor	SAVE, others
Heart failure	ACE inhibitor, then beta-blocker	CONSENSUS, many others; MERIT-HF, many others
Left ventricular dysfunction	ACE inhibitor	SOLVD, others
Type 1 diabetes with renal dysfunction	ACE inhibitor	Captopril Cooperative Study Group
Renal impairment with proteinuria	ACE inhibitor	GISEN, others
Established vascular disease	ACE inhibitor	HOPE[29]
Type 2 diabetes with 1 additional risk factor	ACE inhibitor	HOPE[29]
Type 2 diabetes with renal dysfunction	ARB	IDNT, RENAAL
Post-stroke/TIA	ACE inhibitor ± diuretic	PROGRESS
Isolated systolic hypertension	Diuretic or dihydropyridine calcium antagonist	SHEP, Syst-EUR, Syst-China

ACE, angiotensin-converting enzyme; ARB, angiotensin II receptor blocker; BHAT, Beta-Blocker Heart Attack Trial; CONSENSUS, Cooperative New Scandinavian Enalapril Survival Study; GISEN, Gruppo Italiano di Studi Epidemologici in Nefrologia; HOPE, Heart Outcomes Prevention Evaluation; IDNT, Irbesartan Diabetic Nephropathy Trial; MERIT-HF, Metoprolol Extended-Release Randomized Intervention Trial in Heart Failure; PROGRESS, Perindopril Protection against Recurrent Stroke Study; RENAAL, Reduction of Endpoints in NIDDM with Angiotensin II Antagonist Losartan; SAVE, Survival and Ventricular Enlargement; SHEP, Systolic Hypertension in the Elderly Program; SOLVD, Studies of Left Ventricular Dysfunction; Syst-China, Systolic Hypertension in China; Syst-EUR, Systolic Hypertension in Europe; TIA, transient ischemic attack.

their use as initial therapy in *all* hypertensives (Table 19–7).

The JNC VI report also recognizes clinical situations in which specific antihypertensive drug therapy may be beneficial in improving *symptoms* or surrogate markers of another condition but might not have a major effect on reducing morbidity or mortality. Two examples are a diuretic for a hypertensive person with osteoporosis or a beta-blocker for one with an essential tremor.

Target Blood Pressure Based on Absolute Risk of Cardiovascular and Renal Disease

Probably the most prescient recommendation in JNC VI was the suggestion that the BP target during treatment should *not* be the same for all hypertensive patients. Although a BP goal of less than 140/90 mm Hg had been advanced by several reports, this goal is now recommended only for *uncomplicated* patients. Even before the Hypertension Optimal Treatment (HOT) study showed (in 18,790 hypertensive patients) the benefit of reducing diastolic BP to an average of 84 mm Hg to "optimally reduce cardiovascular risk," the JNC VI report had suggested such a target. Data from the HOT study do not suggest any significant increase in risk by lowering BP to a diastolic target of less than 80 mm Hg, but there appears to be little further benefit either.[22] Because the probability of drug-related side effects often increases as doses are increased, it is likely that a target BP of less than 140/90 mm Hg is defensible for uncomplicated hypertensive patients.

JNC VI recommended that diabetic patients and those with renal impairment should have a lower BP target during treatment than individuals at lower absolute risk of cardiovascular and renal events. JNC VI suggested a BP of less than 130/85 mm Hg, and at least two important clinical trials have since corroborated this suggestion: the HOT study's 1501 diabetics showed the lowest risk of stroke, heart attack, or cardiovascular death in those randomized to a diastolic BP of less than 80 mm Hg.[23] These data have led to more recent recommendations from several expert panels to lower diabetics'

TABLE 19–7

Contraindications to Specific Antihypertensive Drug Classes (see JNC VI)

Antihypertensive Drug Class	Contraindication
Thiazide diuretic	Allergy
Beta-blocker	Asthma
ACE inhibitor	Angioedema secondary to ACE inhibitor, pregnancy
Calcium antagonist	Allergy
Angiotensin II receptor blocker	Pregnancy, renal artery stenosis
Alpha-blocker	Orthostatic hypotension with frequent falls
$Alpha_2$-agonist (centrally acting drug)	

ACE, angiotensin-converting enzyme; JNC, Joint National Committee on the Detection, Evaluation, and Treatment of High Blood Pressure.

goal BP to less than 130/80 mm Hg. The second clinical trial to demonstrate the benefit of a lower BP target for diabetics was the United Kingdom Prospective Diabetes Study (UKPDS) No. 38.[24] Over 8.4 years of follow-up, 1148 type 2 diabetics randomized to two different BP goals (<150/85 mm Hg or <180/105 mm Hg) did much better if treated to the lower goal.

Those responsible for health care financing expressed initial concern that the lower BP goal recommended for diabetics would require more antihypertensive medications and more visits to health care providers and may therefore not be justified economically. Cost analyses taken directly from the UKPDS clinical trial, as well as from an economic analysis of U.S. epidemiologic and clinical trial data for older (>60 years) diabetics treated to a goal of less than 130/85 mm Hg versus leaving the target BP at less than 140/90 mm Hg, showed that the lower BP goal impressively reduces the risk of expensive cardiovascular events, including stroke, heart attack, heart failure, and renal replacement therapy. Consequently, the incremental cost-effectiveness ratio for the lower BP goal is negative (meaning that more intensive treatment reduces cost).

Clinical trial data (from both HOPE and the African American Study of Kidney Diseases [AASK]) suggest that an ACE inhibitor is a good initial choice for diabetic patients or those with renal impairment. In the HOPE trial, an impressive morbidity and mortality benefit was seen in diabetic patients randomized to ramipril, which the authors attributed more to the ACE inhibitor than to the approximately 3/2–mm Hg difference in BP between the groups[22]; that conclusion remains to be proved. The Irbesartan Microalbuminuria (IRMA 2) study recently reported that an ARB can protect type 2 diabetic patients with microalbuminuria (urinary albumin excretion between 30 and 300 mg/day) from progressing to frank proteinuria (>300 mg/day of proteinuria) in a dose-dependent fashion.

JNC VI recommended the lowest BP target (<125/75 mm Hg) for hypertensive individuals with renal impairment and proteinuria less than 1 g/24 hr. However, this recommendation was not supported by data from the second randomization in the AASK trial, according to a preliminary report.

Constructing a Regimen

Because most hypertensive patients will require more than a single drug to achieve the more intensive treatment goals recently recommended, one probably needs to worry less about the initial choice of therapy (see Fig. 19–5) than choosing appropriate combinations of drugs to achieve the goal BP. The initial choice should be based on the clinician's assessment of which potential complication of hypertension poses the greatest risk to the individual patient. For example, a diabetic should always have an ACE inhibitor (or an ARB) as part of the regimen, and thus it should be the initial choice. A hypertensive patient with coronary heart disease should begin with a beta-blocker or ACE inhibitor; a person at highest risk of stroke should start with a diuretic or calcium antagonist.

One of the attractive features of Figure 19–5 is that after an initial treatment is found not to lower BP to goal, an appropriate choice for a second-line agent is found adjacent to the initially chosen drug. Another option is to recommend a diuretic as the most versatile of the second-choice agents because a diuretic has been used in this role in several successful long-term outcome studies.

It is important to recognize that the ideal drug regimen would have many characteristics. In addition to lowering the BP to goal, the regimen should be able to be administered once daily without regard to meals, be relatively inexpensive, cause few adverse effects (and perhaps even result in fewer side effects than seen with single-drug therapy), and be widely available in all pharmacies and benefits plans. Some of the newer fixed-dose combination products have several of these attributes; those combining a dihydropyridine calcium antagonist and an ACE inhibitor, for instance, cause less pedal edema than a calcium channel blocker alone does.

Follow-up and Drug Withdrawal

JNC VI also recommended a visit schedule for follow-up of individuals with hypertension (Table 19–8). This schedule pertains to untreated or previously undiagnosed hypertension and does not address the common issue of how frequently a hypertensive person should see the health care provider. Many experienced clinicians believe that at minimum, semiannual visits are needed for most hypertensive patients to confirm the adequacy of BP control, maintain surveillance about weight and other modifiable risk factors, review and renew prescriptions, and sustain motivation for lifestyle modification and medication compliance. Every 3 months might be even more appropriate.

When BP is not at goal, most clinicians ask the patient to return at much shorter intervals; 1 month is probably sufficient for most patients. Weekly visits for dose titration are probably too frequent because most popular antihypertensive agents have long serum elimination half-lives. Once-daily antihypertensive agents require at least 5 days of administration before achieving a reasonable steady-state plasma level, and achieving a stable pharmacodynamic effect typically takes twice as long. After the BP target is achieved, the visits may be spaced less frequently.

Although JNC VI recommended "step-down therapy" for hypertensive patients whose BP has been effectively controlled for at least 1 year, more recent data question the wisdom of that advice. Some currently used antihypertensives have been available for decades, and once patients are maintained on a stable regimen that they can tolerate, it might not be useful to step treatment down if retitration to goal is often needed.

Management in Special Circumstances

Aside from patients who have a "special indication" for a particular antihypertensive drug (see Table 19–6),

TABLE 19–8

JNC VI Recommendations for Follow-up Based on Initial Blood Pressure Measurements in Adults

Initial Blood Pressure (mm Hg)*		
Systolic	***Diastolic***	***Follow-up Recommended***†
<130	<85	Recheck in 2 yr
130–139	85–89	Recheck in 1 yr, and provide/reinforce information about lifestyle modifications
140–159	90–99	Recheck within 2 mo, and provide/reinforce information about lifestyle modifications
160–179	100–109	Evaluate or refer to source of care within 1 mo
180	110	Evaluate or refer to source of care immediately or within 1 wk, depending on the clinical situation

*If the systolic and diastolic categories are different, follow the recommendations for the shorter time of follow-up (e.g., adults with a blood pressure of 160/86 mm Hg should be evaluated or referred to a source of care within a month).

†The schedule for follow-up may be modified according to reliable information about past blood pressure measurements, other cardiovascular risk factors, target organ damage, or any combination of these factors.

Adapted from The sixth report of the Joint National Committee on the Prevention, Detection, Evaluation, and Treatment of High Blood Pressure. Arch Intern Med 1997;157:2414–2446.

hypertensive patients with increased cardiovascular risk require more attention from the primary care physician. These individuals are typically hypertensive patients with older age, diabetes, pregnancy, impending surgery, refractory hypertension, renal impairment, or hypertensive crisis.

Older Patients with Hypertension

For many years it was controversial whether older hypertensive persons should be treated with antihypertensive drug therapy. This question has now been answered with a resounding affirmative inasmuch as clinical data in older patients demonstrate the overwhelming benefit of treatment for essentially all important endpoints, including all-cause mortality. Many recent trials in older hypertensive patients show that successfully lowering BP is probably more important than which drug is initially used to lower it.

Because many of the early clinical trials in hypertension excluded patients older than 74 years by design, little evidence was available to show that individuals older than 75 benefit from antihypertensive drug therapy. Some have argued that the lack of such evidence should preclude antihypertensive drug therapy in older hypertensive people. Recently, a meta-analysis that included all 1870 patients older than 80 years enrolled in eight clinical trials has shown that substantial and significant reductions in stroke, cardiovascular events, coronary heart disease events, and heart failure accrue in persons older than 80 who are given antihypertensive medications.[9]

Diabetic Patients with Hypertension

JNC VI acknowledged the special role of diabetes in increasing cardiovascular risk (see Table 19–2) and recommended that all diabetic patients be treated to a lower BP goal than those at lower risk (<130/85 mm Hg, see earlier). The challenge in attaining this goal (or perhaps even lower, <130/80 mm Hg, as recommended by the American Diabetes Association) is substantial. Most surveys of BP control in large groups of patients (e.g., in response to the Healthcare Employer Data Information Set [HEDIS]) have shown much worse control of BP in diabetic subjects than in nondiabetics, even when an equivalent target BP (<140/90 mm Hg) is used.

For patients who begin more than 15/10 mm Hg over their goal BP, the National Kidney Foundation's consensus statement recommends an ACE inhibitor and a diuretic (thiazide or thiazide-like diuretic if the serum creatinine is <1.5 mg/dL or a loop diuretic if higher). If these drugs are insufficient to achieve the BP goal, the National Kidney Foundation recommends the sequential addition of a long-acting calcium antagonist (the non-dihydropyridine type is preferred over the dihydropyridine type), a beta-blocker (or an alpha-beta-blocker) if the pulse is 84 beats per minute or higher, the other type of long-acting calcium antagonist (if the pulse is <85 beats/min), and finally an alpha-blocker. If this strategy does not achieve the goal BP, referral to a hypertension specialist may be helpful.

These recommendations were made before the release of the results of three clinical trials that showed effectiveness of an ARB for type 2 diabetic hypertensive patients with albuminuria. The American Diabetes Association now recommends an ARB as first-line therapy for type 2 diabetes.

Pregnant Patients with Hypertension

Over the last few decades, hypertension has been seen more commonly in pregnant women, perhaps because obstetricians are more aware of the short- and long-term risks of elevated BP. In few other situations does only an elevated BP (in the absence of target organ damage) routinely precipitate hospitalized bedrest and the institution of both lifestyle modification and drug therapy. When hypertensive women become pregnant, the primary care physician must work in close collaboration with the obstetrician. Although chronic hypertension (before pregnancy) increases both maternal and fetal risk, it seldom increases the risk of preeclampsia or eclampsia.[25]

Management of hypertension during pregnancy is challenging because many of the drugs generally used in therapy are either contraindicated or a potential threat to the mother or fetus. Diuretics, which are often the preferred first-line therapy for nonpregnant hypertensives, are generally avoided during pregnancy (unless the woman had been taking them before conception) because of the risk of oligohydramnios. ACE inhibitors and ARBs are contraindicated in pregnancy in view of the risk of renal and other fetal malformations. Nitroprusside is contraindicated because of its metabolic transformation to cyanide, which is very toxic to the fetus.

Most physicians caring for hypertensive pregnant women fall back on time-tested and traditional antihypertensive drug therapy, which usually includes, in order, methyldopa, hydralazine, a beta-blocker (typically labetalol in the United States), and then perhaps a calcium antagonist. These agents have the advantage of many years of use and, in the case of methyldopa, outcome studies showing no increased risk of either fetal or maternal morbidity or mortality.

Hypertensive Patients with Impending Surgery

The American Society of Anesthesiologists recognizes uncontrolled hypertension as a risk factor for perioperative and postoperative morbidity and mortality. Accordingly, most hypertensive patients receive closer scrutiny when elective surgery is planned; occasionally, the procedure must be postponed to achieve better BP control (typically <160/95 mm Hg). Because of the large armamentarium of intravenous antihypertensive drugs, however, even emergency operations can usually be performed without incident related to hypertension because most anesthesiologists are very well acquainted with intraoperative antihypertensive therapy.

Inasmuch as major surgery (often vascular surgery) carries a high risk of postoperative complications in hypertensive patients with unrecognized heart disease, preoperative cardiac testing of hypertensive patients well before the planned operation is often considered. Much has been written about the proper sequence of such tests; in our center and in some of the recent literature, dobutamine echocardiography has become the favored test. For individuals who show no wall motion abnormalities and whose tests are not otherwise suggestive of major coronary disease, short-term treatment with a beta-blocker is recommended.

Patients with Refractory Hypertension

Although definitions of what formally constitutes "refractory hypertension" vary (usually BP >140/90 mm Hg despite two or three appropriately chosen antihypertensive drugs in proper doses[26]), general agreement has been reached regarding treatment and evaluation of these patients. The more common causes of refractory hypertension are listed in Box 19–6. A small fraction of these patients have white-coat hypertension. If ABPM is unavailable, home BP monitoring may be used to detect this cause.

Most physicians believe that the primary reason for refractory hypertension is failure of the patient to take the medications as prescribed. Patients may not be adherent to their treatment regimen over time for many reasons (see Table 19–8), some of which can be discovered by the physician. Inspecting pill bottles for dates of dispensation and performing pill counts, a telephone call to the pharmacist to ascertain the number of refills during the previous year, and using simple clinical measurements (e.g., heart rate and orthostatic BP readings in patients supposedly taking a beta-blocker or an alpha-blocker, respectively) can be very useful.

All too often, BP control is compromised by other drugs that the patient may be taking (see Boxes 19–4 and 19–6). NSAIDs, including the cyclooxygenase-2 inhibitors, are probably the most common offenders, but corticosteroids, cyclosporine, nicotine, caffeine, and erythropoietin can also raise BP. Effort to reduce exposure to these medications can be attempted, but many times the therapeutic effects of these other medications are more important than their BP-raising effects, and additional antihypertensive drug therapy must be given.

Secondary hypertension is much more common in patients with refractory hypertension. In our clinic, renovascular disease is approximately three times more common in referred patients who have refractory hypertension than in the self-referred population, even after controlling for differences in initial BP. Pheochromocytoma and mineralocorticoid excess states are less common causes of refractory hypertension. The most common successful intervention for patients with resistant hypertension in our clinic is modification of the drug regimen. Adding or switching to an appropriate diuretic (a thiazide if the glomerular filtration rate [GFR] is 50 mL/min or higher or a loop diuretic if the GFR is less than 50 mL/min) and adding an alpha-blocker are the most frequent alterations.

Hypertensive Patients with Renal Impairment

Chronic renal impairment may be either a cause of hypertension or a sequela of undertreated hypertension. Patients with hypertension and chronic renal impairment differ in two important ways from those with normal renal function: their doses of renally excreted antihypertensive drugs should be reduced (or less commonly, the frequency of administration should be reduced) in comparison to patients with preserved renal function. Those with renal impairment should also have a lower BP target, especially because reduction in BP may be the most important intervention to prevent or delay the onset of dialysis or renal transplantation.

ACE inhibitors play a special role in the management of hypertension in patients with renal impairment. Although many patients have a modest rise in serum creatinine during the first few weeks after starting an ACE inhibitor, this increase should not generally be of concern unless it is more than 25% higher than the baseline measurement (i.e., before the ACE inhibitor). ACE

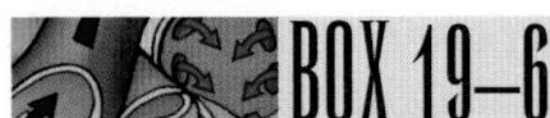

BOX 19–6

Common Causes of "Resistant Hypertension"

PSEUDORESISTANT HYPERTENSION

"White-coat" hypertension (clinic responder)

NONADHERENCE TO ANTIHYPERTENSIVE THERAPY

Dietary indiscretion regarding salt, ethanol, or other dietary stimuli
Poor adherence to drug treatment because of
- Side effects of antihypertensive agents
- Excessive cost of medication(s)
- Inconvenient or inappropriate dosing schedules
- Organic brain syndrome (e.g., impairment of memory, forgetfulness)

Poor understanding of the importance of taking pills as directed
- Inadequate patient education
- Instructions not understood
- Lack of continuing, consistent primary source of medical care

DRUG-RELATED CAUSES

Inadequate doses of antihypertensive drugs
Inappropriate combinations of antihypertensive drugs (e.g., clonidine + methyldopa)
Rapid metabolism (e.g., rapid acetylators of hydralazine)
Drug-drug interactions
- Nonsteroidal anti-inflammatory drugs
- Sympathomimetic agents (e.g., nasal decongestants, appetite suppressants, cocaine, caffeine)
- Oral contraceptive pills (more of a problem with older, high-dose agents)
- Corticosteroids
- Licorice (and similarly flavored chewing tobacco)
- Cyclosporine/tacrolimus
- Erythropoietin
- Cholestyramine (or other resin-binding agents taken simultaneously with antihypertensive drugs)
- Antidepressants (monoamine oxidase inhibitors, some tricylics [venlafaxine])
- Rebound hypertension after abrupt discontinuation of centrally acting drugs, beta-blockers, or occasionally, calcium antagonists

ASSOCIATED MEDICAL CONDITIONS

Tobacco use (especially cigarette smoking during the 15 min before blood pressure measurement)
Increasing weight (and obesity)
Chronic pain
Intense, acute vasoconstriction (e.g., Raynaud's phenomenon)
Insulin resistance/hyperinsulinemia
Anxiety-induced hypertension, hyperventilation, and/or panic attacks

SECONDARY HYPERTENSION

Renovascular hypertension
Chronic renal impairment
Sleep apnea
Pheochromocytoma
Mineralocorticoid excess states

VOLUME OVERLOAD

Excessive sodium intake
Progressive renal damage and impairment (e.g., hypertensive nephrosclerosis)
Fluid retention because of direct (or indirect) vasodilators (e.g., minoxidil)
Inadequate or inappropriate diuretic therapy

Adapted from the sixth report of the Joint National Committee on Prevention, Detection, Evaluation, and Treatment of High Blood Pressure. Arch Intern Med 1997;157:2413–2446.

inhibitors are not usually considered agents of first choice for many African American patients with hypertension and renal impairment (perhaps because of their greater incidence of cough, angioedema, or both), but in the recent AASK disease trial, the ACE inhibitor and perhaps the beta-blocker were *more* effective in preventing death, dialysis, and renal transplantation than the calcium antagonist was. These data suggest that an ACE inhibitor (or an ARB if cough is a sequela) should be part of the antihypertensive drug regimen for hypertensive patients with renal impairment.

Evidence to answer the question of which BP target should be achieved in hypertensive patients with renal impairment is still being gathered in prospective clinical trials. JNC VI recommended less than 130/85 mm Hg for the goal BP of patients with renal impairment and a still lower target of less than 125/75 mm Hg for those with 1 g or more of proteinuria. Many clinical studies have shown that proteinuria is a marker for established cardiovascular disease and a risk factor for future cardiovascular events (including not only renal failure but also stroke, myocardial infarction, and heart failure, especially in diabetics).

Patients with Hypertensive Crises

The term *hypertensive crisis* tends to blur the distinction between what was formerly called "hypertensive emergency" (typically defined as "very high BP with evidence of acute target organ damage") and "hypertensive urgency." The major important difference between the two conditions is the rapidity and setting of their treatment. Hypertensive emergencies are best treated in a hospital (usually in the intensive care unit) with a short-acting, rapidly reversible, intravenously administered antihypertensive drug. Hypertensive urgencies may be routinely treated in an outpatient setting with any of a number of oral antihypertensive agents, including captopril, labetalol, or clonidine. Nifedipine capsules, which had been widely used in this setting for nearly

20 years, are now to be used "with great caution, if at all," according to a Food and Drug Administration advisory, because of their propensity to cause quick and excessive hypotension. Perhaps the most important aspect of the treatment of a hypertensive urgency is to arrange quick follow-up for the patient so that chronic, better management of BP can be ensured.

The "acute target organ damage" that should be searched for when the primary care physician is faced with a very high BP and concern about a hypertensive emergency falls into four separate categories. Various neurologic emergencies should be considered (see Table 19–9) and appropriate steps taken to distinguish among them because the treatment is different. Hypertensive encephalopathy (typically a diagnosis of exclusion) improves dramatically and quickly after BP is reduced acutely; the hypertension during a stroke in evolution is typically *not* treated with BP-lowering drug therapy unless the BP exceeds 180/110 mm Hg. Cardiac and vascular emergencies include acute myocardial infarction and myocardial ischemia, pulmonary edema and acute heart failure, and acute aortic dissection. The latter is the condition that has the lowest target blood pressure (<120/80 mm Hg) and the least time to achieve it (typical recommendation: 20 minutes). Renal damage is manifested as either acute hematuria or acute elevation in serum creatinine; access to medical records to ascertain previous creatinine levels is obviously helpful here. Catecholamine-related hypertensive emergencies include either pheochromocytoma, drug (usually clonidine) withdrawal, or a crisis secondary to monoamine oxidase inhibitors.

Preeclampsia is the term often used for full-blown pregnancy-induced hypertension, and it includes many other criteria besides elevated BP. Nonetheless, one of the most important early treatments of this disorder is an appropriate antihypertensive drug regimen, which makes delivery of the infant much less dangerous. The recommended drug for each type of emergency and the BP target most frequently cited are found in Table 19–9. For most hypertensive emergencies, reduction of mean arterial pressure by 10% in the first hour and another 10% to 15% during the next few hours is appropriate; exceptions are aortic dissection and pregnancy-related hypertension (or eclampsia). Nitroprusside is the drug most commonly used for the treatment of hypertensive emergencies, although fenoldopam has both theoretical and practical advantages for patients with renal impair-

TABLE 19–9

Types of Hypertensive Crises, with Suggested Drug Therapy and Blood Pressure Targets

Type of Crisis	Drug of Choice	BP Target
	Neurologic	
Hypertensive encephalopathy	Nitroprusside*	25% reduction in mean arterial pressure over 2–3 hr
Intracranial hemorrhage or acute stroke in evolution	Nitroprusside* (controversial)	0%–25% reduction in mean arterial pressure over 6–12 hr (controversial)
Acute head injury/trauma	Nitroprusside*	0%–25% reduction in mean arterial pressure over 2–3 hr (controversial)
Subarachnoid hemorrhage	Nimodipine	Up to 25% reduction in mean arterial pressure in previously hypertensive patients, 130–160 mm Hg systolic in normotensive patients
	Cardiac	
Ischemia/infarction	Nitroglycerin or nicardipine	Reduction in ischemia
Heart failure	Nitroprusside* or nitroglycerin	Improvement in failure (typically 10%–15% decrease in BP)
Aortic dissection	Beta-blocker + nitroprusside*	120 mm Hg systolic in 30 min (if possible)
	Renal	
Hematuria or acute renal impairment	Fenoldopam	0%–25% reduction in mean arterial pressure over 1–12 hr
	Catecholamine Excess States	
Pheochromocytoma	Phentolamine	To control paroxysms
Drug withdrawal	Drug withdrawn	Typically only 1 dose necessary
	Pregnancy Related	
Eclampsia	$MgSO_4$, methyldopa, hydralazine	Typically <90 mm Hg diastolic, but often lower

*Some physicians prefer an intravenous infusion of either fenoldopam or nicardipine, neither of which has potentially toxic metabolites, over nitroprusside. Recent studies have also shown improvement in renal function during therapy with the former as compared with nitroprusside.

Updated from Elliott WJ, Black HR: Hypertensive crises. In Parrillo JE, Bone RC (eds): Critical Care Medicine: Principles of Diagnosis and Management. Philadelphia, Mosby–Year Book, 1995, pp 565–576.

ment and shares (with nicardipine) a lack of potentially toxic metabolites (cyanide, thiocyanate) associated with high doses or long infusions of nitroprusside.

Organizing for Successful Management

The goal of hypertension management is to prevent the morbidity and mortality associated with it and to do so in the "least intrusive" manner (physiologically and fiscally). Because hypertension is not a disease, but a condition that increases cardiovascular and renal risk, its long-term control is a continuing challenge. A protocol for a successful hypertension management visit is shown in Box 19–7. For many years it was thought that most patients with hypertension have no noticeable symptoms. Recent studies involving antihypertensive drugs without appreciable side effects have shown a significant decrease in headache when hypertensive patients are successfully treated. The quality of life in treated hypertensives was greatest in the group that achieved the lowest BP in both HOT and TOMHS, which suggests that there *may* be subtle symptoms attributable to elevated BP that improve when BP is lowered. It is nonetheless often difficult to convince a person with hypertension that taking a pill or changing one's lifestyle will result in tangible benefit, especially in the short term. It is also unfortunately true that treating hypertension (even successfully) does not reduce cardiovascular risk to the level of a normotensive person. This greater risk provides strong impetus for initiating lifestyle modifications early, even before the levels of BP that we call hypertension are present.

It is not surprising, therefore, that it is difficult in the long term to motivate patients to sustain their lifestyle modifications and adhere to the prescribed medications. National survey data indicate that only 27% of America's hypertensive population maintain their BP lower than 140/90 mm Hg; other parts of the world have even worse results. Many official reports have discussed and stressed efforts to improve adherence to medication. Economically, nonadherence is a very important issue inasmuch as about 10% of the money spent on hypertension is said to be wasted by people not taking their physician's advice and not taking their pills. This nonadherence results in unnecessary hospitalization, preventable strokes and myocardial infarctions, and a large portion of the admissions to nursing homes (where drug taking can be more carefully and efficiently supervised).

Education of the patient (and family) is the cornerstone of improving adherence; patients with educational or cognitive deficits are unlikely to follow instructions for very long. Some clinics have improved their hypertension control rates after a health educator was added to the hypertension treatment team. Behavioral suggestions are often useful: integrating pill taking into activities of daily living (e.g., taking pills when caring for teeth) or using a pill organizer (typically to organize pills according to days of the week that they are to be consumed). Increasing social support appears to be a beneficial strategy, especially for older individuals. The family member or caretaker can remind the patient of the need to take pills and keep office visits, as well as actually measure BP with a home device.

The primary physician has many opportunities to improve medication adherence. Probably the simplest method of assessing adherence to pill taking is to routinely ask about it. Medications that are taken once daily, without regard to food intake, and that are well tolerated appear to lead to better long-term adherence. Avoiding large, bad-tasting, or hard-to-swallow pills is important for many patients. Sensitivity of the physician to the patient's out-of-pocket expenses for medication is also important: many patients prefer fixed-dose combination pills because this strategy reduces their pharmacy copayment.

Missing appointments for follow-up care and monitoring of hypertension treatment has been associated with poorer outcomes, but several routine procedures can help minimize missed appointments. Reminders (either by telephone or by mail) have been shown to increase return visit rates. Scheduling a specific time and date with a known health care provider at the end of the office visit is more successful than "calling in for a future appointment." Decreasing waiting times, having convenient office hours, and having solicitous, caring office staff are also helpful.

Several characteristics of physicians have an impact on patient adherence to medications and their willingness to keep appointments. The Medical Outcomes

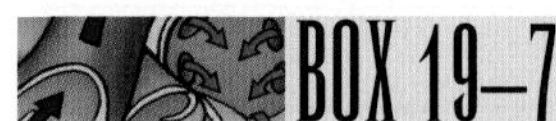
BOX 19–7

Protocol for a Successful Hypertension Management Visit

- Telephone or mailed reminder of the upcoming appointment date, time, and location (the day before the appointment)
- Greeting of the patient on arrival by helpful, friendly office staff
- Minimal time in the waiting room before being escorted to the examination/consulting room
- BP measurement (at least 3 readings) using proper technique after at least 5 minutes of quiet rest
- Discussion of adherence to lifestyle modifications
- Inventory of medications (if any) most accurately done by cataloging pill bottles)
- Interim history taking: adverse events (e.g., hospitalizations, emergency department visits, consultant visits), side effects (of drug therapy), home BP readings (if any), adherence assessment
- Brief, targeted physical examination
- Discussion of laboratory studies (already performed or needed)
- Discussion of BP measurement results and progress toward the BP goal (achieved or not)
- Prescription writing
- Opportunity for the patient's and family's questions to be addressed/answered
- Scheduling time and date for the next appointment

Study showed that physicians who are willing to involve the patient (when appropriate) in medical decision making are more successful in controlling BP. Physicians who are perceived as having effective communication skills, who encourage questions from the patient and appropriate family members, and who provide feedback about the patient's progress also achieved better results.

Most health care systems have accepted the treatment of hypertension as a worthwhile endeavor, one that is actually cost saving in high-risk patients and relatively cost-effective in others (vs. many other common medical interventions). Recent efforts by some health care systems to reduce health care costs by restricting pharmacy benefits, limiting the range and doses of drugs on an accepted formulary, and reducing accessibility of health care services have generally been ineffective in the long term. System-wide effort (often called "disease management programs") to encourage acceptance of generic drugs, increase the threshold for beginning antihypertensive drug therapy in low-risk patients, use one drug to treat both hypertension and a concomitant medical condition, and encourage adherence to medication taking has been more successful. The workload of the health care provider involved in these efforts can be increased by some of these procedures, but it is sometimes offset by case managers and other allied health professionals who perform some of these important tasks.

Hypertension control is an important public health goal that requires long-term commitment from the patient, the physician, and the health care system. When all work together toward a common goal, the recent progress in demonstrating the benefits of hypertension therapy in clinical trials can be easily and effectively translated to the primary care practice of medicine. Such commitment will eventually reduce the burden of disease and adverse cardiovascular and renal outcomes that were formerly associated with untreated elevated BP.

Evidence-Based Summary

- Screening for hypertension by measuring BP in asymptomatic individuals is recommended,[27] primarily because effective, relatively inexpensive drug treatments are available to prevent expensive and devastating stroke, heart attack, and other cardiovascular and renal events.[1]
- No direct evidence has shown that dietary interventions or exercise prevents cardiovascular events. A systematic review (18 trials, 2611 patients) of dietary advice to reduce weight has indicated that a reduction in weight of 3% to 9% correlates with about a 3-mm Hg reduction in systolic and diastolic BP[28]; weight loss is the most effective lifestyle modification to lower BP.[29] A systematic review (58 trials, 2161 patients) has indicated that salt restriction (by 118 mmol/24 hr) lowers BP by 3.9/1.9 mm Hg ($P < .001$ for both); weight loss and sodium restriction combined lowered BP more than either alone in several clinical trials.
- Systematic reviews of drug therapy for hypertension have shown that initial treatment with diuretics or beta-blockers (18 trials, 48,220 patients),[30] ACE inhibitors (4 trials, 12,124 patients),[21] or calcium antagonists (2 trials, 5520 patients)[21] is more effective in preventing cardiovascular events than placebo or no treatment is.
- A systematic review of 10 trials in 16,164 elderly hypertensive patients has shown more benefit with an initial diuretic than an initial beta-blocker.[31] One clinical trial concluded that an initial alpha-blocker was less effective than a diuretic in preventing heart failure (an important, but small component of a prespecified secondary endpoint).[19] Whether calcium antagonists are significantly less effective than other antihypertensive therapies initially is controversial[20, 21]; more primary data are expected in the next 2 years.
- A systematic overview of three trials consisting of 20,408 patients has indicated that the risk of stroke, coronary heart disease, and major cardiovascular events was reduced by 20%, 19%, and 15%, respectively, in the group receiving more intensive treatment.[21] These benefits were more obvious in high-risk patients (e.g., diabetics).

References

1. The Sixth Report of the Joint National Committee on prevention, detection, evaluation, and treatment of high blood pressure. Arch Intern Med 1997;157:2413–2446.
2. The World Health Organization/International Society of Hypertension Guidelines for the Management of Hypertension. J Hypertens 1999;17:151–185.
3. Burt VL, Whelton PK, Roccella EJ, et al: Prevalence of hypertension in the U.S. adult population: Results from the Third National Health and Nutritional Examination Survey, 1988–91. Hypertension 1995;25:305–313.
4. Elliott WJ, Black HR: Rationale and benefits of classification schemes for hypertension. Curr Opin Cardiol 1997;12:368–374.
5. Black HR, Yi J-Y: A new classification for hypertension, based on relative and absolute risk, with implications for treatment and reimbursement. Hypertension 1996;26:719–724.

6. Frohlich ED, Grim C, Labarthe DR, et al: Recommendations for human blood pressure determination by sphygmomanometers: Report of a Special Task Force Appointed by the Steering Committee, American Heart Association. Hypertension 1988;11:210A–222A.
7. Pickering T: Recommendations for the use of home (self) and ambulatory blood pressure monitoring. American Society of Hypertension Ad Hoc Panel. Am J Hypertens 1996;9:1–11.
8. Ogden LG, He J, Lydick E, Whelton PK: Long-term absolute benefit of lowering blood pressure in hypertensive patients according to the JNC VI risk stratification. Hypertension 2000;34:539–543.
9. Gueyffier F, Bulpitt C, Boissel JP, et al: Antihypertensive drugs in very old people: A subgroup meta-analysis of randomised clinical trials. INDANA Group. Lancet 1999; 353:793–796.
10. Sacks FM, Svetkey LP, Vollmer WM, et al: Effects on blood pressure of reduced dietary sodium and the Dietary Approaches to Stop Hypertension (DASH) diet. N Engl J Med 2001;344:3–9.
11. Clinical Guidelines on the Identification, Evaluation, and Treatment of Overweight and Obesity in Adults: The Evidence Report. Washington, DC, U.S. Government Printing Office, National Institutes of Health, 1998.
12. Safian RD, Textor SC: Medical progress: Renal-artery stenosis. N Engl J Med 2001;344:431–442.
13. Krijnen P, van Jaarsveld BC, Steyerberg EW, et al: A clinical prediction rule for renal artery stenosis. Ann Intern Med 1998;129:738–740.
14. Pacak K, Linehan WM, Eisenhofer G, et al: Recent advances in genetics, diagnosis, localization, and treatment of pheochromocytoma. Ann Intern Med 2001;134: 315–329.
15. Witteles RM, Kaplan EL, Roizen MF: Sensitivity of diagnostic and localization tests for pheochromocytoma in clinical practice. Arch Intern Med 2000;160:2521–2524.
16. Ganguly A: Primary aldosteronism. N Engl J Med 1998;339: 1828–1834.
17. Stewart PM: Mineralocorticoid hypertension. Lancet 1999; 353:1341–1347.
18. Neaton JD, Grimm RH Jr, Prineas RJ, et al: Treatment of Mild Hypertension Study: Final results. JAMA 1993;270: 713–724.
19. The ALLHAT Collaborative Research Group: Major cardiovascular events in hypertensive patients randomized to doxazosin vs. chlorthalidone: The Antihypertensive and Lipid-Lowering Treatment to Prevent Heart Attack Trial (ALLHAT). JAMA 2000;283:1967–1975.
20. Pahor M, Psaty BM, Alderman MH, et al: Health outcomes associated with calcium antagonists compared with other first-line antihypertensive therapies: A meta-analysis of randomised controlled trials. Lancet 2000;356:1949–1951.
21. Blood Pressure Lowering Treatment Trialists' Collaborative: Effects of ACE-inhibitors, calcium antagonists, and other blood-pressure–lowering drugs: Results of prospectively designed overviews of randomised trials. Lancet 2000;356:1955–1964.
22. The Heart Outcomes Prevention Evaluation Study Investigators: Effects of an angiotensin-converting enzyme inhibitor, ramipril, on death from cardiovascular causes, myocardial infarction, and stroke in high-risk patients. N Engl J Med 2000;342:145–153.
23. Hansson L, Zanchetti A, Julius S, et al, on behalf of the HOT Study Group: Effects of intensive blood pressure lowering and low-dose aspirin in patients with hypertension: Principal results of the Hypertension Optimal Treatment (HOT) randomised trial. Lancet 1998;351:1755–1762.
24. Turner R, Holman R, Stratton I, et al, for the United Kingdom Prospective Diabetes Study Group: Tight blood pressure control and risk of macrovascular and microvascular complications in type 2 diabetes: UKPDS 38. BMJ 1998;317:707–713.
25. Report of the National High Blood Pressure Education Program Working Group on High Blood Pressure in Pregnancy. Am J Obstet Gynecol 2000;183(Suppl):1–22.
26. Setaro JF, Black HR: Refractory hypertension. N Engl J Med 1992;327:543–547.
27. Littenberg B: A practice guideline revisited: Screening for hypertension. Ann Intern Med 1995;122:937–939.
28. Mulrow CD, Chiquette E, Angel L, et al: Dieting to Reduce Body Weight for Controlling Hypertension in Adults (Cochrane Review). Oxford, England, Update Software, 2001.
29. Trials of Hypertension Prevention Collaborative Research Group: The effects of nonpharmacologic interventions on blood pressure of persons with high normal levels: Results of the Trials of Hypertension Prevention, phase I. JAMA 1992;267:1213–1220.
30. Psaty BM, L SN, Siscovick DS, et al: Health outcomes associated with antihypertensive therapies used as first-line agents: A systematic review and meta-analysis. JAMA 1997;277:739–745.
31. Messerli FH, Grossman E, Goldboourt U: Are beta-blockers efficacious as first-line therapy for hypertension in the elderly: A systematic review. JAMA 1998;279:1903–1907.

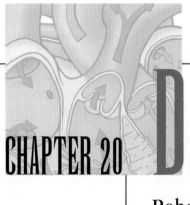

CHAPTER 20 Dietary Fat and Lipid Disorders

Robert H. Knopp

Approximately half of all deaths in the United States are caused by arteriosclerotic cardiovascular disease.[1] Although most deaths are due to coronary artery disease (CAD), a major fraction is also caused by arteriosclerotic disease of the peripheral vessels (see Chapter 37), especially ischemic cerebrovascular disease. Even though men have higher age-adjusted coronary mortality rates, women are as likely or even slightly more likely to die of arteriosclerotic disease because of their greater longevity.

Hyperlipidemia is one of the major causes of atherosclerosis (Fig. 20–1). In the U.S. population, total cholesterol levels rise with age until a plateau at about age 55, which is due in part to the premature death of persons with very elevated levels (Fig. 20–2). By comparison, the population average for the protective high-density lipoprotein (HDL) cholesterol levels are consistently higher in women than men but fluctuate by only a small amount with age (Fig. 20–3). The 3-hydroxy-3-methylglutaryl coenzyme A (HMG-CoA) reductase inhibitors, now called *statins*, can reduce the incidence of CAD and events by approximately one third in persons with hypercholesterolemia. However, many patients who are eligible for lipid-lowering therapy are not treated at all, and many who are treated do not reach appropriate therapeutic goals.[2,3] This chapter presents a commonsense view of the mechanisms of atherosclerosis, describes the interplay of the various lipoprotein fractions in the pathogenesis of atherosclerosis, and outlines therapeutic approaches to lipoprotein disorders that are commonly associated with arteriosclerotic vascular disease.

DEFINITIONS OF LIPID DISORDERS

All lipoprotein fractions play a role in atherogenesis (Fig. 20–4). Two major lipoproteins, low-density lipoprotein (LDL) and very low density lipoprotein (VLDL), promote atherosclerosis, whereas HDL cholesterol inhibits the process.

Exogenous and Endogenous Lipoprotein Pathways

The *exogenous lipoprotein pathway* begins with absorption of fatty acids and cholesterol from the intestine in the form of triglyceride-rich chylomicrons. These alimentary particles are very large, do not penetrate the arterial wall, and are not considered to be atherogenic. Major elevations in chylomicrons (e.g., triglyceride levels >2000 mg/dL) can cause pancreatitis when the chylomicrons infiltrate into the acini of the pancreas and induce a violent inflammatory response. Cutaneous evidence of infiltration can be seen in the form of white, nonexpressible papules, which are called eruptive

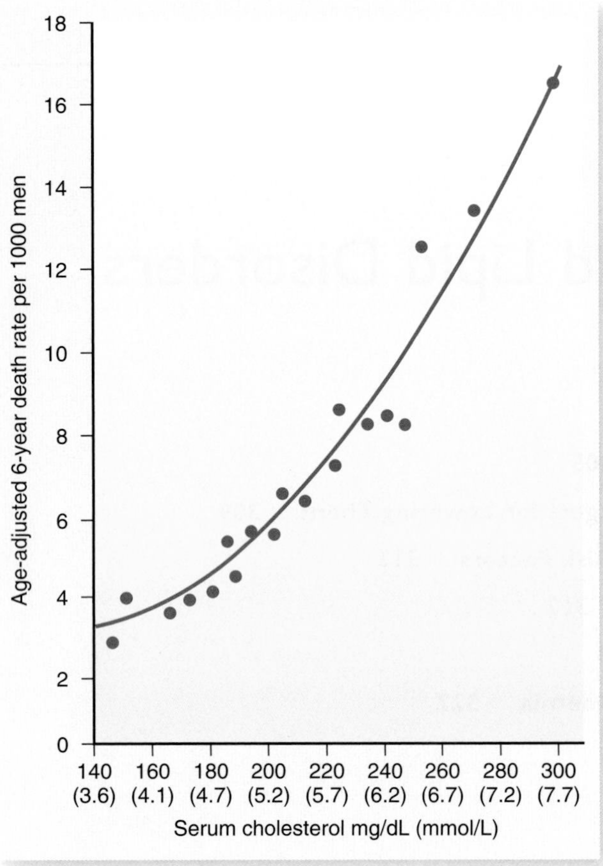

FIGURE 20–1. Relationship of serum cholesterol to coronary heart disease death in 356,222 men aged 35 to 57 years during an average follow-up of 6 years. Each point represents the median value for 5% of the population. Key points: (1) The risk increases steadily, particularly above 200 mg/dL (5.2 mmol/L), and (2) the magnitude of the increased risk is large—fourfold in the top 10% in comparison to the bottom 10%. (Data from Stamler J, Wentworth D, Neaton JD: Is the relationship between serum cholesterol and risk of premature death from coronary heart disease continuous and graded? Findings in 356,222 primary screenees of the Multiple Risk Factor Intervention Trial [MRFIT]. JAMA 1986;256:2823–2828; redrawn from Schaefer EJ: Overview of the Diagnosis and Treatment of Lipid Disorders. Cambridge, MA, Genzyme, 1995, p 11.)

xanthomas and are typically seen over shoulders, back, abdomen, buttocks, arms, and thighs. The three most common causes of severe hyperchylomicronemia with triglyceride levels above 2000 mg/dL are poorly controlled diabetes, excessive alcohol ingestion, and oral estrogen therapy superimposed on existing hyperlipidemia. Thus, most patients with lipid-induced pancreatitis are also prone to atherosclerosis.

Triglyceride is removed from chylomicrons by the enzyme lipoprotein lipase, which is tethered to the capillary endothelium. After triglyceride is removed, the resulting remnant lipoprotein is smaller and more cholesterol rich, and it has the potential for entering the arterial wall and initiating atherosclerosis. Levels of these remnant particles may be exaggerated postprandially if fasting lipid levels are elevated. Thus, a major goal of treatment is to reduce steady-state fasting lipoprotein levels and thereby reduce the accumulation of postprandial remnant particles. The postprandial rise in chylomicron remnants may also be reduced by a diet low in fat and cholesterol.

The *endogenous lipoprotein pathway* begins with secretion of triglyceride-rich particles from the liver in the form of VLDL (see Fig. 20–4). The enzyme lipoprotein lipase also removes triglyceride from VLDL to yield a VLDL remnant that is analogous to the chylomicron remnant. The VLDL remnant in turn is taken up in part by the liver but is also converted via further removal of triglyceride by a hepatic triglyceride lipase (hepatic lipase) to form LDL. Overproduction of lipoprotein from the liver can lead to elevations in VLDL, VLDL remnants, or LDL (or any combination of these lipoproteins), depending on the relative efficiency of removal of each lipoprotein: VLDL by lipoprotein lipase, the VLDL remnant by recognition of apoprotein E on its surface, conversion of VLDL to LDL by hepatic lipase, and removal of LDL by the LDL receptor.

HDL is generated when free cholesterol and phospholipid are taken from peripheral cells by apoprotein A-I; the process is mediated by a cell surface protein, ABC-AI. The free cholesterol transferred to the surface of HDL is esterified by the enzyme lecithin cholesterol acyltransferase (LCAT) and enters the neutral lipid core, the "baggage compartment" of the lipoprotein particle. This cholesterol ester is then either recycled to LDL by cholesterol ester transfer protein (CETP) or is delivered to the liver by hepatic lipase and the SRB-1 receptor (see Fig. 20–4).

Classification of Specific Lipid Disorders

The etiologic classification of lipid abnormalities (Table 20–1; see also Fig. 20–4) provides a rationale and approach to treatment. This schema also underscores the principle that all lipoprotein fractions are involved in atherogenesis and are amenable to treatment.

Familial Hypercholesterolemia. Familial hypercholesterolemia is associated with a reduction in activity of the LDL receptor, usually as a result of a polygenic, heterozygous or homozygous deficiency of the LDL receptor gene. LDL levels are generally about twice normal in the heterozygous state and four times normal in the homozygous state. Most of these patients have tendinous xanthomas (Fig. 20–5) or tuberous xanthomas (Fig. 20–6), a few have orbital xanthelasma, and most have a family history of early-onset CAD.

Rarely, marked LDL elevations are caused by a genetic defect in its associated apoprotein B so that LDL is not well recognized by the LDL receptor. This condition is known as apoprotein B–defective hypercholesterolemia. When hypercholesterolemia and premature CAD are found on both sides of the family, a polygenic basis is inferred.

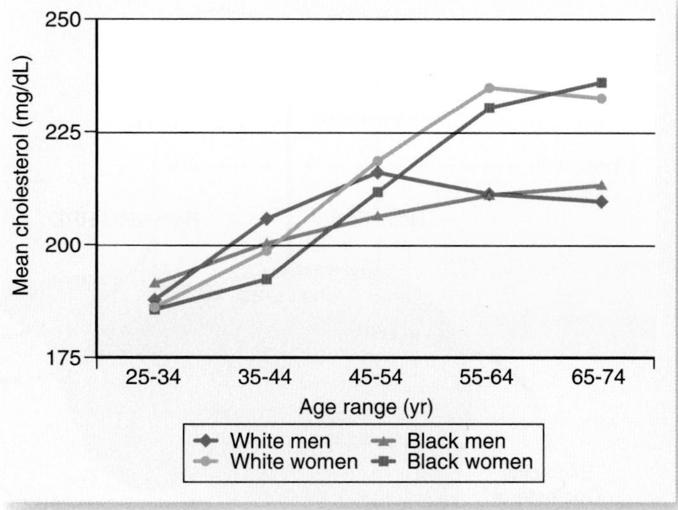

FIGURE 20–2. Mean total cholesterol (TC) values by age for white and black men and women. Data from the National Health and Nutrition Survey III, Phase 2, 1991 to 1994. (From Pignone MP, Phillips CJ, Atkins D, et al: Screening and treating adults for lipid disorders. Am J Prev Med 2001;20[3 Suppl]:77–89.)

Although these diagnostic distinctions are of scientific interest, all types of hypercholesterolemia require aggressive management. The first goal should be to upregulate the LDL receptor with a statin. However, if the condition is severe, combined drug therapy may be necessary to reach the target LDL level (see later) and correct any associated abnormalities in triglycerides and HDL.

Combined Hyperlipidemia. Overproduction of lipids occurs in a genetically heterogeneous disorder termed *combined hyperlipidemia*, which is called *familial combined hyperlipidemia* when it runs in families. The complicated physiology of the endogenous lipoprotein pathway explains why combined hyperlipidemia is not always manifested in the combined form but, instead, can occur as simple hypertriglyceridemia (e.g., excess VLDL), simple hypercholesterolemia (e.g., excess LDL), combined elevations in triglyceride and cholesterol (e.g., excess VLDL and LDL), or remnant removal disease in different family members or even in the same person at different times. From a therapeutic standpoint, combination drug treatment, usually involving a statin, niacin, or a fibrate (or any combination of these agents), is recommended for the best management of combined hyperlipidemia (see Table 20–1).

Familial Hypertriglyceridemia. An occasional patient with isolated familial hypertriglyceridemia, which is characterized by large buoyant VLDL and low total cholesterol and LDL levels, may not be at increased risk for CAD. A negative family history and the absence of physical signs are additional clues that these patients, unlike the great majority of hypertriglyceridemic persons, are not prone to atherosclerosis. These persons may not need to be treated, unless their triglyceride levels are at risk of rising into the pancreatitis range.

Low-HDL Disorders. The low-HDL syndromes *(hypoalphalipoproteinemia)* can be caused by a deficiency of apoprotein A-I production; by ABC-A1 deficiency, which leads to failure of apoprotein A-I to dock on the peripheral cell surface; by deficient cholesterol

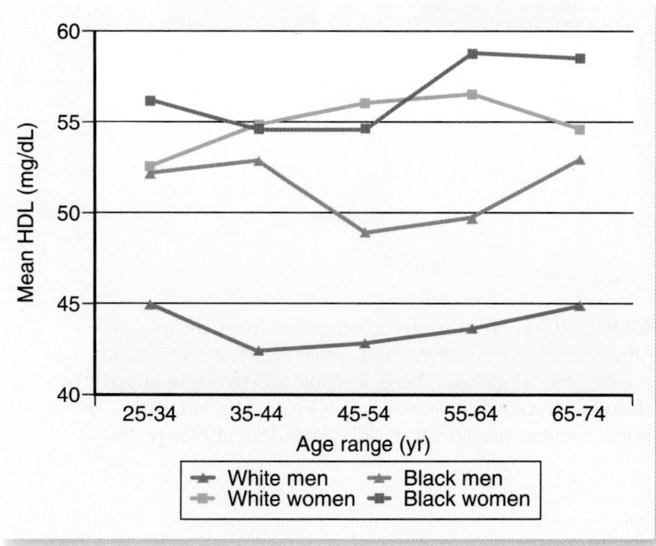

FIGURE 20–3. Mean high-density lipoprotein (HDL) cholesterol values by race and gender. Data from the National Health and Nutrition Survey III, Phase 2, 1991 to 1994. (From Pignone MP, Phillips CJ, Atkins D, et al: Screening and treating adults for lipid disorders. Am J Prev Med 2001;20[3 Suppl]:77–89.)

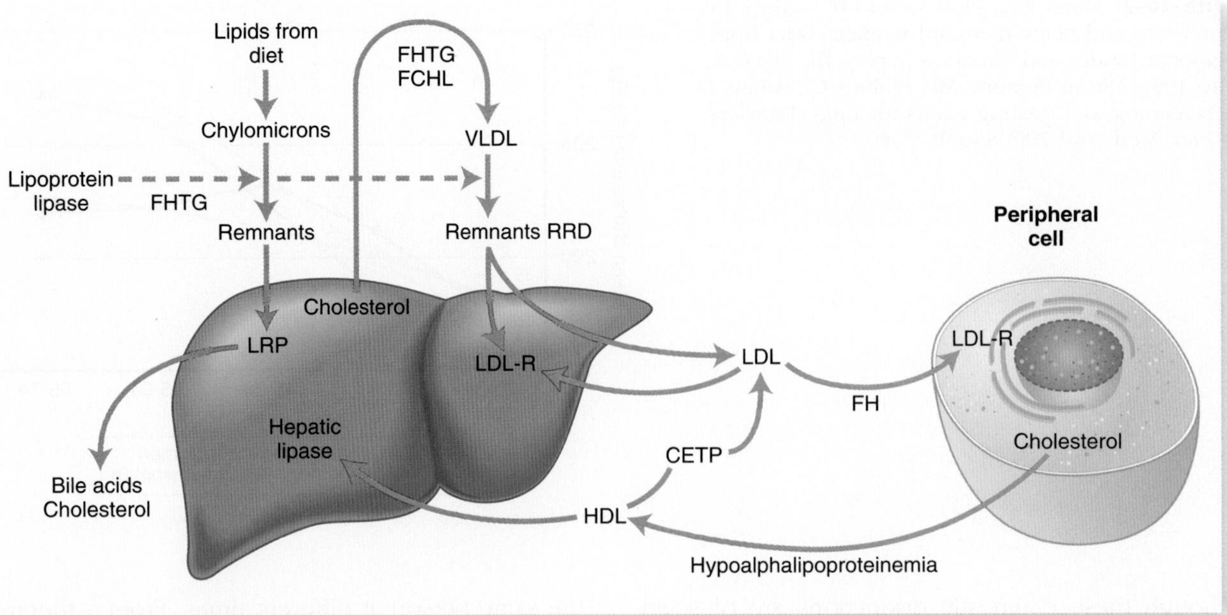

FIGURE 20–4. Pathways of lipid transport. Cholesterol is absorbed from the intestine and transported to the liver by chylomicron remnants, which are taken up by the low-density lipoprotein (LDL) receptor–related protein (LRP). Hepatic cholesterol enters the circulation as very low density lipoprotein (VLDL) and is metabolized to remnant lipoproteins after lipoprotein lipase removes triglyceride. The remnant lipoproteins are removed by LDL receptors (LDL-R) or further metabolized to LDL and then removed by these receptors. Cholesterol is transported from peripheral cells to the liver by high-density lipoprotein (HDL). Cholesterol is recycled to LDL and VLDL by cholesterol ester transport protein (CETP) or is taken up in the liver by hepatic lipase. Cholesterol is excreted in bile. The points in the process that are affected by the five primary lipoprotein disorders—familial hypertriglyceridemia (FHTG), familial combined hyperlipidemia (FCHL), remnant removal disease (RRD, also known as familial dysbetalipoproteinemia), familial hypercholesterolemia (FH), and hypoalphalipoproteinemia—are shown. The effects of drug therapy can also be understood from these pathways. Statins decrease the synthesis of cholesterol and secretion of VLDL and increase the activity of LDL receptors. Bile acid–binding resins increase the secretion of bile acids. Nicotinic acid decreases the secretion of VLDL and the formation of LDL and increases the formation of HDL. Fibrates decrease the secretion of VLDL and increase the activity of lipoprotein lipase, thereby increasing the removal of triglycerides. (Redrawn from Knopp RH: Drug treatment of lipid disorders. N Engl J Med 1999;341:498–511.)

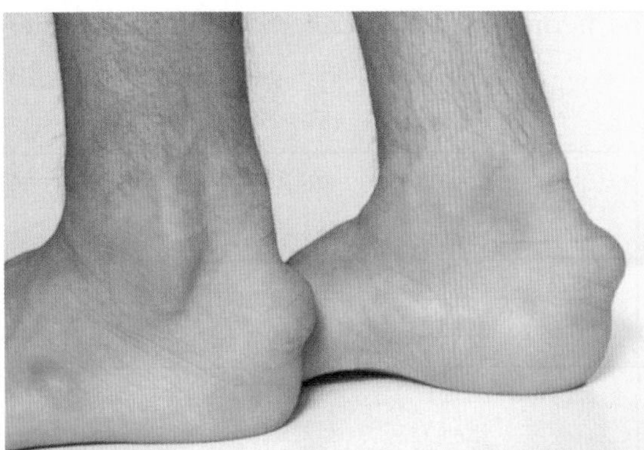

FIGURE 20–5. Tendinous xanthomas from diffuse infiltration of the tendons with cholesterol occur mainly on the extensor tendons. These lesions are strongly suggestive of familial hypercholesterolemia. (From Mir MA: Atlas of Clinical Diagnosis. London, WB Saunders, 1995, p 252.)

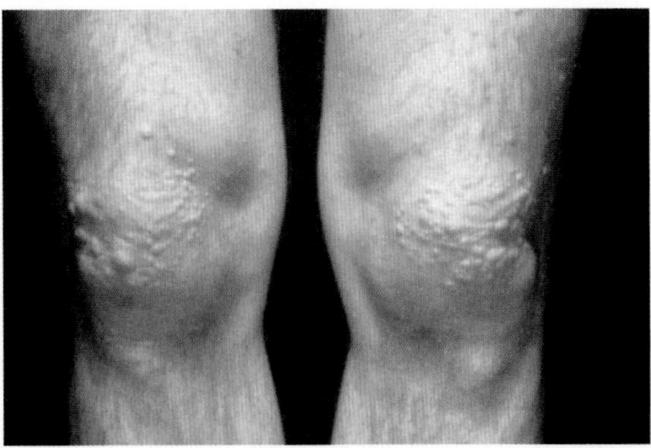

FIGURE 20–6. Tuberous xanthomas are yellowish nodules of varying size and occur on the elbows, buttocks, and knees. (From Mir MA: Atlas of Clinical Diagnosis. London, WB Saunders, 1995, p 252.)

TABLE 20–1

Primary Lipoprotein Disorders Amenable to Treatment by Diet and Drugs

Disorder	Mechanisms	Complications	Treatment*
Familial or polygenic hypercholesterolemia	Diminished LDL receptor activity Defective apolipoprotein B that is poorly recognized by the LDL receptor	CAD; occasionally PVD, stroke	Diet Statin Bile acid–binding resin Nicotinic acid Fibrate if statin intolerance
Familial combined hyperlipidemia†	Increased hepatic secretion of apolipoprotein B–rich VLDL and conversion to LDL	CAD, PVD, stroke	Diet and weight loss Statin Nicotinic acid Fibrate‡
Familial hypertriglyceridemia§	Decreased serum triglyceride removal resulting from decreased LPL activity Increased hepatic secretion of triglyceride-rich VLDL	Pancreatitis at triglyceride concentrations >2000 mg/dL; variable risk of CAD	Diet and weight loss Fibrate‡ Nicotinic acid n-3 fatty acids Oxandrolone
Remnant removal disease (familial dysbetalipoproteinemia)	Increased secretion of VLDL Impaired removal of remnant lipoproteins resulting from homozygosity ($\varepsilon_2/\varepsilon_2$) or heterozygosity ($\varepsilon_2/\varepsilon_3$ or $\varepsilon_2/\varepsilon_4$) for apolipoprotein E ε_2	PVD, CAD, stroke	Diet, weight loss Fibrate‡ Nicotinic acid Statin
Familial hypoalphalipoproteinemia (low-HDL syndrome)§	Diminished apolipoprotein A-I formation, increased removal, increased CETP or hepatic lipase activity	CAD, PVD (may be associated with hypertriglyceridemia)	Exercise and weight loss Nicotinic acid Fibrate‡ Statin

*Treatments may be given alone or in combination; the primary treatment is listed first, followed by other treatments in decreasing order of importance.

†Diabetes mellitus can greatly exacerbate the condition. The hyperlipidemia of diabetes is mechanistically closest to familial combined hyperlipidemia.

‡Combined treatment with a fibrate and a statin can increase the risk of myopathy.

§This disorder is characterized by low concentrations of HDL cholesterol.

CAD, coronary artery disease; CETP, cholesterol ester transfer protein; HDL, high-density lipoprotein; LPL, lipoprotein lipase; PVD, peripheral vascular disease; VLDL, very low density lipoprotein.

Reprinted, by permission, from Knopp RH: Drug treatment of lipid disorders. N Engl J Med 1999;341:498–511.

esterification, which prevents the accumulation of cholesterol in the HDL core; by high hepatic lipase levels, which enhance HDL cholesterol delivery to the liver; by increased cholesterol ester transfer to LDL; or by excessive plasma triglyceride levels, which prevent transfer of VLDL surface remnants (such as free cholesterol, phospholipid, and apoproteins) to HDL. The multiple etiologies of the low-HDL disorders defy any clinically useful diagnostic distinctions. A rule of thumb, however, is that the low-HDL disorders are usually associated with hypertriglyceridemia and if the hypertriglyceridemia is treated, the HDL level will rise. One exception to this rule is when apoprotein A-I levels are reduced, indicating the presence of a primary abnormality in the generation of HDL.

SCREENING FOR LIPID LEVELS AND TARGETS FOR LOWERING THEM

Screening

The National Cholesterol Education Program (NCEP) recommends screening all adults 20 years or older with a lipoprotein profile (total cholesterol, LDL cholesterol, HDL cholesterol, and triglyceride levels) every 5 years.[4] By comparison, the U.S. Preventive Services Task Force has taken a more conservative approach[5] (Box 20–1).

The advantages of earlier screening include the ability to detect familial lipid abnormalities and the opportunity to use levels above age-adjusted averages to encourage early lifestyle modifications. Screening is preferably performed in the fasting state, but total cholesterol and HDL levels are helpful even in nonfasting individuals. In persons with a family history of early CAD, measurement of additional lipid risk factors, such as elevated lipoprotein(a) (Lp[a]), homocysteine, or remnant levels (see later), can help justify more aggressive treatment of elevated lipid levels (Box 20–2).

A low LDL cholesterol level is less than 100 mg/dL, and a high HDL cholesterol level is greater than 60 mg/dL (Box 20–3). A high triglyceride level is more controversial; the current NCEP guidelines suggest a triglyceride goal of less than 200 mg/dL, but some authorities believe that an ideal fasting plasma triglyceride level is probably less than 150 mg/dL or even approaching 100 mg/dL.[6] When triglyceride levels are over 200 mg/dL, the small, dense, oxidizable LDL particles that are associated with an increased risk of CAD are almost always present. These particles are almost completely absent when the triglyceride level is less than 100 mg/dL.

BOX 20–1

USPSTF Recommendation for Screening Asymptomatic Adults for Lipid Disorders

1. In men 35 years and older and women 45 years and older, routine screening for lipid disorders is recommended. Treatment of abnormal lipids is recommended in people who are at increased risk for CAD. Grade A evidence
2. In younger adults (men aged 20 to 35 and women aged 20 to 45 years), screening for lipid disorders is recommended if they have other risk factors for CAD, including
   - Diabetes
   - A family history of cardiovascular disease before 50 years of age in male relatives or 60 years in female relatives
   - A family history suggestive of familial hyperlipidemia
   - Multiple CAD risk factors (e.g., tobacco use, hypertension).

   The USPSTF makes no recommendation for or against routine screening for lipid disorders in younger adults (men aged 20 to 35 years or women aged 20 to 45 years) in the absence of known risk factors for CAD.* Grade B evidence
3. Screening for lipid disorders should include measurement of total cholesterol and high-density lipoprotein cholesterol, which can be done on nonfasting or fasting samples
4. The USPSTF concludes that the evidence is insufficient to recommend for or against triglyceride measurement as part of routine screening for lipid disorders†
5. The USPSTF makes no recommendations about an upper age limit at which screening should be stopped
6. All patients, regardless of lipid levels, should be offered counseling about the benefits of a diet low in saturated fat and high in fruits and vegetables, regular physical activity, avoidance of tobacco use, and maintenance of a healthy weight
7. Drug treatment decisions should take into account
   - Overall risk of heart disease rather than lipid levels alone
   - Costs
   - Patients' preferences

*Author's note: Screening is appropriate in women considering oral contraceptives, especially if they are older than 35 years or beginning postmenopausal hormone replacement therapy.

†Author's note: Consideration of oral estrogen therapy or oral retinoids requires measurement of triglycerides.

CAD, coronary artery disease; USPSTF, U.S. Preventive Services Task Force.

Adapted from Screening adults for lipid disorders: Recommendations and rationale of the U.S. Preventive Services Task Force. Am J Prev Med 2001;20:73–76.

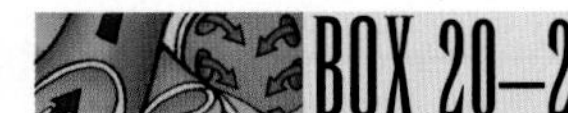

What Lipid Levels to Obtain in Screening and Follow-up

EVERYONE

Total cholesterol
LDL cholesterol
HDL cholesterol
Triglyceride

SPECIAL SITUATIONS

Lipoprotein analysis by ultracentrifugation: For direct LDL and VLDL cholesterol measurements when both total cholesterol and triglyceride levels are high and the fasting triglyceride level is >400 mg/dL

Lipoprotein(a): In patients with a family history or clinical evidence of premature vascular disease

Homocysteine: In patients with a family history or clinical evidence of premature vascular disease

Apoprotein A-I: When the triglyceride level is elevated and the HDL cholesterol level is low to determine whether the HDL reduction is primary (low A-I) or likely to respond to triglyceride lowering (A-I is normal)

Apoprotein B: When the triglyceride level is elevated and CAD risk is uncertain (high if apo-B is elevated, low if apo-B is low)

CAD, coronary artery disease; HDL, high-density lipoprotein; LDL, low-density lipoprotein; VLDL, very low density lipoprotein.

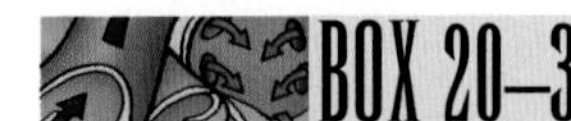

Classification of LDL, Total, and HDL Cholesterol (mg/dL)

LDL cholesterol	
<100	Optimal
100–129	Near or above optimal
130–159	Borderline high
160–189	High
≥190	Very high
Total cholesterol	
<200	Desirable
200–239	Borderline high
≥240	High
HDL cholesterol	
<40	Low
≥60	High
Triglyceride	
<150	Normal
150–200	Borderline high
200–499	High
≥500	Very high

HDL, high-density lipoprotein; LDL, low-density lipoprotein.

Adapted from Executive Summary of the Third Report of the National Cholesterol Education Program (NCEP) Expert Panel on detection, evaluation, and treatment of high blood cholesterol in adults (Adult Treatment Panel III). JAMA 2001;285:2486–2497.

Treatment

The NCEP recommends treating individual lipoprotein elevations to achieve specific targets. This approach has been most fully developed for LDL cholesterol, in which the targets are less than 160 mg/dL for persons with zero or one risk factor, less than 130 mg/dL for persons with two or more risk factors, and 100 mg/dL for patients with cardiovascular disease, diabetes, or a Framingham risk score of less than 20% in 10 years. The Framingham risk score can be used to refine LDL targets in persons with two or more risk factors. Less than 10% risk in 10 years is considered low risk, 10% to 20% is considered moderate risk, and more than 20% is considered a CHD risk equivalent[4,7] (Fig. 20–7; see also Fig. 18–1).

A minimum goal for HDL cholesterol is above 45 mg/dL in men and 55 mg/dL in women, especially persons at high risk or patients with CAD. Statins, niacin, and fibrates usually raise the HDL level. One hour of aerobic exercise per week (see Chapter 22) typically raises HDL levels by about 1 mg/dL. Moderate

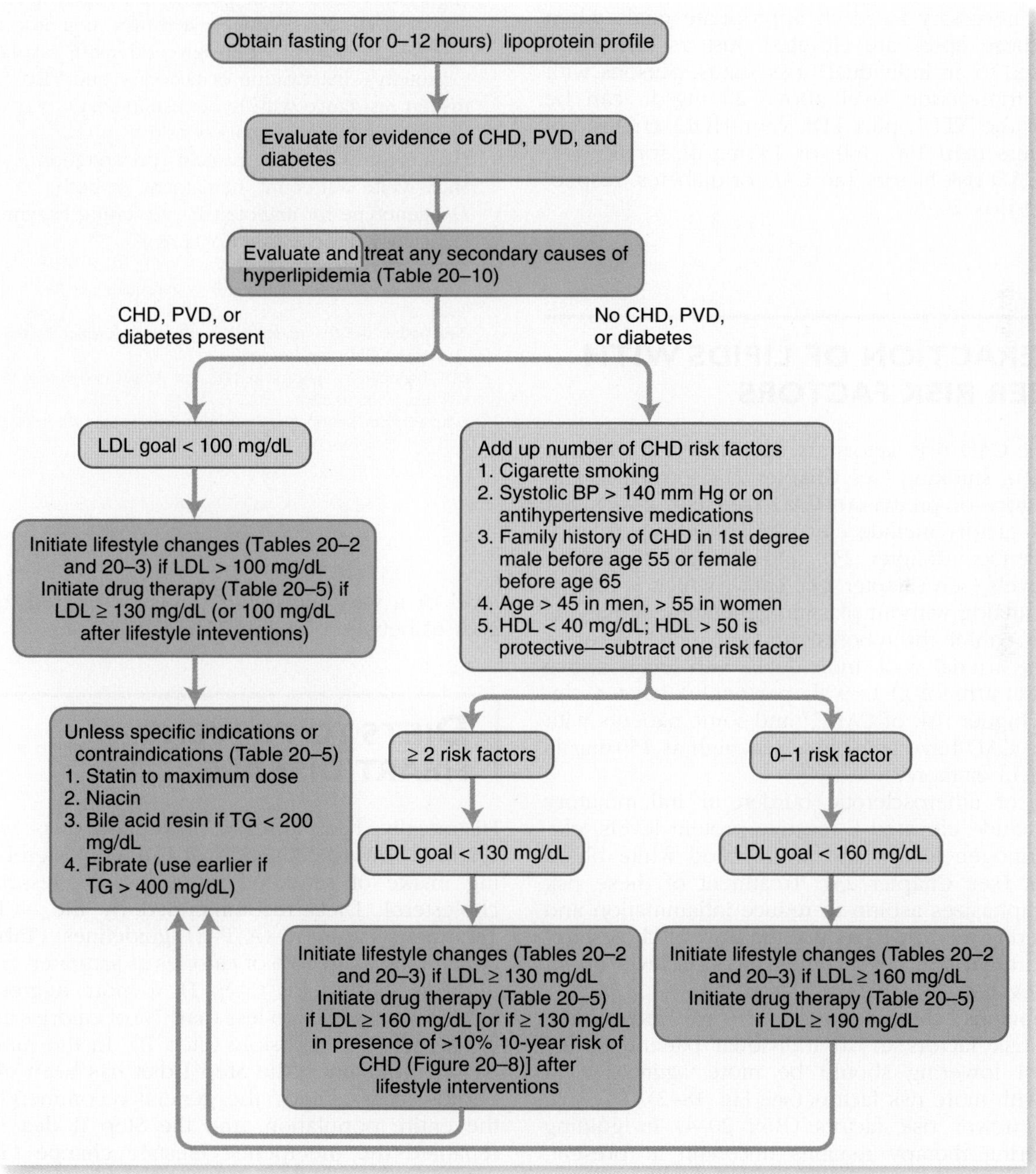

FIGURE 20–7. Approach to lipid screening and treatment. BP, blood pressure; CHD, coronary heart disease; HDL, high-density lipoprotein; LDL, low-density lipoprotein; PVD, peripheral vascular disease; TG, triglycerides. (Based on recommendations of the Executive Summary of the Third Report of the National Cholesterol Education Program [NCEP] Expert Panel on detection, evaluation, and treatment of high blood cholesterol in adults [Adult Treatment Panel III]. JAMA 2001;285:2486–2497.)

alcohol intake can also raise HDL levels (see Chapter 23). In the presence of CAD, however, it may not be possible to raise the HDL level to the ideal target. When an ideal HDL level cannot be reached, the only alternative is to be more aggressive with LDL lowering, an approach that is recommended whenever a patient has multiple risk factors that cannot be controlled or reversed.

In individuals with an LDL-to-HDL ratio of 5 or greater, a plasma triglyceride level above 200 mg/dL is associated with CAD.[8] High triglyceride levels also appear to be more important in women than men. In patients with CAD, combined lipid-lowering therapy with a triglyceride-lowering agent and an LDL-lowering agent are necessary to reach appropriate goals when both of these lipids are elevated. Just as LDL goals are adjusted to an individual's risk status, persons with a fasting triglyceride level above 200 mg/dL can be treated to the VLDL plus LDL (non-HDL) cholesterol goals of less than 190, 160, or 130 mg/dL for 0, 1, 2, or more CAD risk factors and CAD or diabetes, respectively (see Box 20–6).

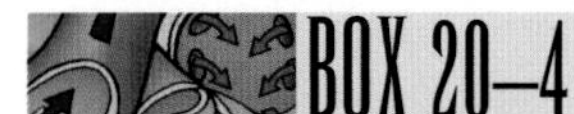
BOX 20–4

Other Risk Factors for Cardiovascular Disease*

Serum Lp(a) concentration 20 mg/dL (frequency distribution, 75th percentile) or 40 mg/dL (90th percentile)
Serum homocystine concentration >10 μmol/L (≥50th percentile)
Small, dense LDL particles
Ratio of serum VLDL cholesterol to triglycerides >0.3 (90th percentile) or >0.25 (75th percentile)
High concentrations of plasma fibrinogen, factor VIII, factor VII, plasminogen activator inhibitor type 1 (associated with hypertriglyceridemia); resistance to protein C inactivation of factors V and VIII
Insulin resistance with hyperinsulinemia
Visceral (intra-abdominal) obesity
High serum C-reactive protein concentration
High white cell count, hematocrit, or both
DD genotype for angiotensin-converting enzyme
Deficiency of antioxidant vitamins

To convert values for cholesterol to millimoles per liter, multiply by 0.026.
*See Figure 20–7 for "traditional" risk factors identified by the National Cholesterol Education Program.
HDL, high-density lipoprotein; LDL, low-density lipoprotein; VLDL, very low density lipoprotein.
Adapted from Knopp RH: Drug treatment of lipid disorders N Engl J Med 1999;341:498–511.

INTERACTION OF LIPIDS WITH OTHER RISK FACTORS

The classic CAD risk factors are age, hypertension (see Chapter 19), smoking (see Chapter 21), low HDL, and family history of premature CAD (see Fig. 20–7), but other risk factors include elevated Lp(a), hyperhomocystinemia (see Chapter 23), and elevated C-reactive protein levels (see Chapter 23). Lp(a), which is a plasminogen analog without plasmin-generating activity, is believed to inhibit thrombolysis and enhance LDL retention in the arterial wall. Individuals with levels above 40 mg/dL (140 nmol/L) (≈90th percentile) have a significantly higher risk of CAD,[8,9] and some patients with premature CAD have Lp(a) levels as high as 150 mg/dL (560 nmol/L) or more.

Indices of atherosclerotic burden or inflammatory activity include elevated C-reactive protein levels, elevated fibrinogen levels, and an elevated white blood cell count (see Chapter 23). Treatment of these risk factors emphasizes aspirin to reduce inflammation and lipid-lowering therapy to reduce the flow of cholesterol into the arterial wall, even when the LDL level is not greatly elevated.

The obvious clinical importance of determining all CAD risk factors in an individual patient is that cholesterol lowering should be more aggressive in patients with more risk factors (see Fig. 18–2). The role of other, newer risk factors (Box 20–4) in guiding lipid-lowering therapy remains uncertain at present. Nevertheless, in the presence of a markedly elevated homocysteine level despite folic acid supplementation (see Chapter 23), an elevated C-reactive protein level, or a markedly elevated Lp(a) level, more aggressive lipid lowering is logical. For example, some experts recommend that patients who have CAD, multiple risk factors, and either an elevated C-reactive protein level or a very high Lp(a) level be treated to an LDL goal of between 50 and 75 mg/dL.

DIETS TO PREVENT HEART DISEASE

Historically, heart disease prevention diets have been oriented toward reduction of LDL cholesterol by limiting intake of saturated fat and, to a lesser degree, cholesterol. Diets recommended by the NCEP Adult Treatment Panel II (ATP-II) guidelines (Table 20–2) contain less than 10% of calories as saturated fat, including *trans*-fatty acids (Step I); a more aggressive diet limits saturated fats to less than 7% of calories and *trans*-fats as much as possible (Step II). In the more recent ATP-III guidelines, the Step I diet has been eliminated because it is already the general recommendation for the entire population, and the Step II diet has been renamed the therapeutic lifestyle change (TLC) diet and modified to allow 25% to 35% of calories as fat. A consequence of extreme fat restriction below 25% of calories as fat is that substitution of carbohydrates for fats can cause hypertriglyceridemia, a reduction in HDL cholesterol, and possible endogenous generation of saturated fat, which prevents LDL from falling further.[10,11] For example, hypercholesterolemic women who follow

TABLE 20–2

Diets Recommended by the National Cholesterol Education Program

Nutrient	Step I Diet*	Step II Diet	ATP-III TLC Diet
Total fat:	<30% of calories	<30% of calories	25% to 35% of calories
Saturated fatty acids	<10% of calories	<7% of calories	<7% of calories
Polyunsaturated fatty acids	≤10% of calories	≤10% of calories	Up to 10% of calories
Monosaturated fatty acids	10% to 15% of calories	10% to 15% of calories	Up to 20% of calories
Carbohydrate	50% to 60% of calories	50% to 60% of calories	50% to 60% of calories
Protein	10% to 20% of calories	10% to 20% of calories	About 15% of calories
Cholesterol	<300 mg daily	<200 mg daily	<200 mg daily
Total calories	To desirable body weight	To desirable body weight	To desirable body weight

*In the ATP-III guidelines of the NCEP,[4] the Step I diet is no longer considered therapeutic for hyperlipidemia but is recommended for the general population, with the exception that a fat intake of 25% to 35% of the total calories is now recommended (with the higher percentage favored for patients with metabolic syndrome).

ATP, Adult Treatment Panel; TLC, therapeutic lifestyle diet.

Adapted from National Cholesterol Education Program: Summary of the second report of the National Cholesterol Education Program (NCEP) Expert Panel on Detection, Evaluation, and Treatment of High Blood Cholesterol in Adults (Adult Treatment Panel II). JAMA 1993;269:3015–3023; and reference 4.

the NCEP Step II diet have a reduction in HDL cholesterol that is sustained for as long as the diet is continued.[12] For these reasons, the ATP-III TLC diet allows 25% to 35% of calories as fat, and the American Heart Association has expanded its dietary guidelines rather than focusing only on fat restriction (Table 20–3). These recommendations emphasize the intake of fruits and vegetables, reduction of salt intake, maintenance of normal body weight, and intake of monounsaturated and polyunsaturated fat.[13] Similar flexibility is recommended for diabetic patients.

Although margarine may lower LDL cholesterol levels in comparison to butter, solid (stick) margarine and other hydrogenated solid fats, including those contained in crispy baked goods, contain *trans*-fatty acids, which are associated with an increased risk of CAD when compared with the *cis*-fatty acids present in soft (tub) margarine.[14] A Mediterranean diet, which includes a marked reduction in saturated fats, with most fats coming from plant sources such as olive oil and omega-3 fatty acids (fish oils), has been associated with a 50% or greater reduction in cardiac death, myocardial infarction, and all-cause mortality in CAD patients.[15] Increased consumption of omega-3 fatty acids, as found in fish, improves outcomes in patients with CAD and may be especially useful for reducing the risk of sudden arrhythmic death.[16] Strict adherence to a vegetarian diet with marked weight loss can lower LDL cholesterol by 35% to 40% and probably retards or even reverses the progression of angiographic CAD.

A heart disease prevention diet should include multiple elements, many of which do not deal directly with LDL cholesterol levels (Table 20–4). Although not all the elements are conclusively proved, the combination of effects has the potential to halve the incidence of CAD and, in aggregate, is potentially beneficial even if LDL cholesterol decreases little or not at all.

TABLE 20–3

Latest Dietary Recommendations from the American Heart Association

	Servings
Vegetables	3–5
Fruits	2–4
Carbohydrate	6 or more, complex and preferably whole grain
Protein	2 fish servings/wk Lean meat, fish, dry beans, eggs, nuts: 2–3 servings/day
Dairy (low fat)	2–3 servings
Fat	<30% if attempting to lose weight
Alcohol	≤2 drinks/day (men) ≤1 drink/day (women)
Salt	<6 g/day (2.3 g Na) (4.8 g Na = no added salt)

From Krauss RM, Eckel RH, Howard B, et al: AHA Dietary Guidelines: Revision 2000: A statement for healthcare professionals from the Nutrition Committee of the American Heart Association. Circulation 2000;102:2284–2299. By permission of the American Heart Association, Inc.

LIPID-LOWERING MEDICATIONS

Four main types of medication are available to treat lipid disorders: statins, nicotinic acid, fibric acid derivatives, and bile acid sequestrants, each with its own set of benefits (Table 20–5) and side effects (Table 20–6). Each type of medication, except nicotinic acid, significantly reduced the incidence of CAD in randomized trials (Table 20–7).

The Statin Drugs

The statin class of lipid-lowering medications has revolutionized the management of hyperlipidemia. Five statins are now available in the United States,[1] and several other statins are under development. One statin, cerivastatin, was withdrawn from the market because of its myotoxic side effects.

TABLE 20–4

Benefits of a Moderate Low Fat Diet on Cardiovascular Disease Risk Factors

Risk Factors	Intervention	Estimated Benefit for Reducing CAD
Cholesterol	Low SFA diet	~20%
	Low cholesterol intake	
	Fiber (soluble)	
	↑ Omega-3 fatty acids	
	Weight loss	
Syndrome X	Glucose ↓	20%
	Insulin ↓	
	Blood pressure ↓	
	Abdominal obesity ↓	
Homocysteine	Vitamins B_1, B_6, B_{12}, ↓ methionine	
Oxidative stress	Flavonoids	?
	Phytoestrogen	?
Triglyceride	Omega-3 fatty acids	~20%
HDL-C	Weight loss/exercise	~20%
	Alcohol/exercise	~20%
Blood pressure	↓ Salt, ↓ excessive alcohol	~10%
Nitric oxide	↓ Animal, ↑ plant protein	?
		Total ~70%

*It is not known whether lowering homocysteine levels prevents heart disease.

HDL-C, high-density lipoprotein cholesterol; SFA, saturated fatty acids.

Modified from Current concepts in dietary therapy for dyslipidemia. In Gotto AM Jr (ed): New York, Lawrence DellaCorte, 2001, pp 1–8.

TABLE 20–5

Drugs Affecting Lipoprotein Metabolism

Drug Class, Agents, and Daily Doses	Lipid/Lipoprotein Effects	Contraindications	Clinical Trial Results
HMG-CoA reductase inhibitors (statins)*	LDL ↓ 18%–55% HDL ↑ 5%–15% TG ↓ 7%–30%	Absolute: active or chronic liver disease Relative: concomitant use of certain drugs[†]	Reduced major coronary events, CHD deaths, need for coronary procedures, stroke, and total mortality
Bile acid sequestrants[‡]	LDL ↓ 15%–30% HDL ↑ 3%–5% TG, no change or increase	Absolute: dysbetalipoproteinemia, TG >400 mg/dL Relative: TG >200 mg/dL	Reduced major coronary events and CHD deaths
Nicotinic acid[§]	LDL ↓ 5%–25% HDL ↑ 15%–35% TG ↓ 20%–50%	Absolute: chronic liver disease, severe gout Relative: diabetes, hyperuricemia, peptic ulcer disease	Reduced major coronary events and possibly total mortality
Fibric acids[‖]	LDL ↓ 5%–20% (may be increased in patients with high TG) HDL ↑ 10%–20% TG ↓ 20%–90%	Absolute: severe renal disease, severe hepatic disease	Reduced major coronary events
Cholesterol absorption[¶]	LDL ↓ 18%	None	None

*Lovastatin (20 to 80 mg), pravastatin (20 to 80 mg), simvastatin (20 to 80 mg), fluvastatin (20 to 80 mg), atorvastatin (10 to 80 mg), rosuvastation (5 to 40 mg) (pending FDA approval).

†Cyclosporine, macrolide antibiotics, azole antifungal agents, and cytochrome P-450 inhibitors. Fibrates and niacin should be used with appropriate caution.

‡Cholestyramine (4 to 16 g), colestipol (5 to 20 g), and colesevelam (2.6 to 3.8 g).

§Immediate-release (crystalline) nicotinic acid (0.5 to 3 g), extended-release nicotinic acid (Niaspan) (0.5 to 2 g), and sustained-release nicotinic acid (0.5 to 2 g).

‖Gemfibrozil (600 mg twice daily), fenofibrate (200 or 160 mg once daily, depending on the form [generic versus trade, respectively]), and bezafibrate (400 mg; Canada only).

¶Ezetimibe, 10 mg once per day (pending FDA approval).

Adapted from Executive Summary of the Third Report of the National Cholesterol Education Program (NCEP) Expert Panel on detection, evaluation, and treatment of high blood cholesterol in adults (Adult Treatment Panel III). JAMA 2001;285:2486–2497.

CHD, coronary heart disease; FDA, Food and Drug Administration; HMG-CoA, 3-hydroxy-3-methylglutaryl coenzyme A; HDL, high-density lipoprotein; LDL, low-density lipoprotein; TG, triglycerides; ↓, decrease; ↑, increase.

TABLE 20–6

Side Effects of Lipid-Lowering Drugs

Drug and Site or Type of Effect	Effect
	Statins
Skin	Rash
Nervous system	Loss of concentration, sleep disturbance, headache, peripheral neuropathy
Liver	Hepatitis, loss of appetite, weight loss, and increases in serum aminotransferases to 2 to 3 times the upper limit of the normal range
Gastrointestinal tract	Abdominal pain, nausea, diarrhea
Muscles	Muscle pain or weakness, myositis (usually with serum creatine kinase >1000 U/L), rhabdomyolysis with renal failure
Immune system	Lupus-like syndrome (lovastatin, simvastatin, fluvastatin)
Protein binding	Diminished binding of warfarin (lovastatin, simvastatin, fluvastatin)
	Bile Acid–Binding Resins*
Gastrointestinal tract	Abdominal fullness, nausea, gas, constipation, hemorrhoids, anal fissure, activation of diverticulitis (cholestyramine, colestipol)
Liver	Mild serum aminotransferase elevations, which can be exacerbated by concomitant treatment with a statin
Metabolic system	Increases in serum triglycerides of approximately 10% (greater increases in patients with hypertriglyceridemia)
Electrolytes	Hyperchloremic acidosis in children and patients with renal failure (cholestyramine)
Drug interactions	Binding of warfarin, digoxin, thiazide diuretics, thyroxine, statins
	Nicotinic Acid
Skin	Flushing, dry skin, pruritus, ichthyosis, acanthosis nigricans
Eyes	Conjunctivitis; cystoid macular edema and retinal detachment (high dose)
Respiratory tract	Nasal stuffiness
Heart	Supraventricular tachyarrhythmias
Gastrointestinal tract	Heartburn, loose bowel movements or diarrhea
Liver	Mild increase in serum aminotransferases, hepatitis with nausea and fatigue
Muscles	Myositis
Metabolic system	Hyperglycemia (incidence, approximately 5%, higher in patients with diabetes), 10% increase in serum uric acid
	Fibrates
Skin	Rash
Gastrointestinal tract	Stomach upset, abdominal pain (mainly gemfibrozil), cholesterol-saturated bile, increase in incidence of gallstones from 1% to 2%
Genitourinary tract	Erectile dysfunction (mainly clofibrate)
Muscles	Myositis with impaired renal function (clofibrate > gemfibrozil > fenofibrate)
Plasma proteins	Interference with binding of warfarin necessitates a reduction in the dose of warfarin by approximately 30%
Liver	Increased serum aminotransferases

*Much less with colesevelam than the other resins.

Modified from Knopp RH: Drug treatment of lipid disorders. N Engl J Med 1999;341:498–511.

By inhibiting HMG-CoA reductase, primarily in the liver, the statins downregulate hepatic cholesterol synthesis and upregulate the LDL receptor. The result is enhanced uptake of LDL from the blood stream, as well as reduced cholesterol synthesis and reduced secretion of VLDL and LDL into the circulation. Statins are now the first-choice medication to lower LDL cholesterol. By reducing VLDL secretion, statins are also an important adjunct in the management of hypertriglyceridemia.

Side effects of statins occur in about 1% to 3% of patients, with muscle aches being the most common symptomatic complaint. Some well-informed patients confuse other musculoskeletal symptoms with true statin side effects. In other cases, the complaint may be real despite normal muscle enzyme levels, including creatine kinase (CK) and aspartate aminotransferase (AST) levels. When CK elevations are found, especially if they are 5 to 10 times the upper limit of normal, statins should generally be discontinued or reduced, even in the absence of symptoms, and alternative medications tried as needed. The mechanisms underlying CK elevations with statins and the interaction of statins with

TABLE 20–7

Primary Prevention Trials of Drug Therapy

Study Details	LRC*	Helsinki†	WOSCOPS‡	AFCAPS§
Year	1984	1987	1995	1998
Duration (yr)	7.4	5	4.9	5.2
Intervention (dose)	Cholestyramine (24 g qd)	Gemfibrozil (600 mg bid)	Pravastatin (40 mg qd)	Lovastatin (20–40 mg qd)
Inclusion	Men with TC >265 mg/dL and LDL >190 mg/dL	Healthy Finnish men (civil service or industrial employees); non-HDL cholesterol >200 mg/dL	Men with "elevated LDL cholesterol"	Men and women with average TC and below-average HDL
Number of subjects, intervention/control	1906/1900	2051/2030	3302/3293	3304/3301
Mean age (yr)	48	47	55	58
Male (%)	100	100	100	85
White (%)	95.5	~100	~100	89
Mean pre-Rx TC (mg/dL)	291.5	288.9	272	221
Mean pre-Rx LDL (mg/dL)	215.5	NR	192	150
Mean pre-Rx HDL (mg/dL)	45	47	44	Men, 36 Women, 40
Main outcome	Nonfatal MI, CHD death	Nonfatal MI, CHD death	Nonfatal MI, CHD death	Nonfatal MI, CHD death, unstable angina
Cumulative event rate‖	8.1/9.8	2.73/4.14	5.5/7.9	3.4/5.45
RRR (CI)	19 (3–32)	34 (8–53)	31 (17–43)	37 (21–50)

*Lipid Research Clinics Program: The Lipid Research Clinics Coronary Primary Prevention Trial Results. II. The relationship of reduction in incidence of coronary heart disease to cholesterol lowering. JAMA 1984;251:365–374.

†Frick MH, Elo O, Haapa K, et al: Helsinki Heart Study: Primary-prevention trial with gemfibrozil in middle-aged men with dyslipidemia. N Engl J Med 1987;317:1237–1245.

‡Shepherd J, Cobbe SM, Ford I, et al: Prevention of coronary heart disease with pravastatin in men with hypercholesterolemia. N Engl J Med 1995;333:1301–1307.

§Downs JR, Clearfield M, Weis S, et al: Primary prevention of acute coronary events with lovastatin in men and women with average cholesterol levels: Results of AFCAPS/Tex CAPS. JAMA 1998;279:1615–1622.

‖Event rates are cumulative incidences in percentages for the entire study period: intervention/control.

AFCAPS, Air Force Coronary Atherosclerosis Prevention Study; CHD, coronary heart disease; CI, confidence interval; HDL, high-density lipoprotein; LDL, low-density lipoprotein; MI, myocardial infarction; NR, not reported, RRR, relative risk reduction; Rx, treatment; TC, total cholesterol.

intrinsic disorders of muscle fatty acid oxidation are unknown. Minor asymptomatic rises in aminotransferase levels are found in up to 50% of individuals, but true hepatotoxicity, which is associated with fatigue, loss of appetite, and a moderate rise in aminotransferase levels, is rare. Minor increases in aminotransferase levels do not require a change in therapy if they are less than twice the upper limit of normal and are not associated with any constitutional symptoms. Current testing recommendations vary with the statin, but in general, the AST level should be measured when lipid levels are measured. AST is the preferred enzyme to monitor, in part because it is also found in muscle, so elevations can be an early sign of hepatitis or myotoxic effects. Other side effects occasionally seen with statins include gastrointestinal upset, particularly if taken without food, drug rash, and rarely, difficulty with sleep or concentration.

Because of the differences among the statins, each has advantages and disadvantages in certain types of patients (Table 20–8). *Lovastatin,* which is soon to become generic and should be taken with meals, can lower LDL by 40% at its maximal dose of 80 mg/day. Lovastatin is particularly associated with myotoxicity when used in combination with erythromycin, protease inhibitors, azole antifungals, and cyclosporine, all of which interfere with its hepatic metabolism by the cytochrome P-450 3A4 (CYP3A4) pathway (Table 20–9). Thus, lovastatin should not be given with drugs that are metabolized by the CYP3A4 pathway. Lovastatin is also associated with myositis in up to 5% of persons taking gemfibrozil, especially those with impaired renal function or smaller body mass. By comparison, the combination of a timed-release formulation of niacin with lovastatin does not appear to increase the risk of myotoxicity. Many physicians discontinue any statin use during hospitalization because of the possibility of unknown drug interactions.

Pravastatin differs from lovastatin in that a methyl group substitutes for a hydroxyl group. This minor structural change makes pravastatin more water soluble and hence less likely to affect the central nervous system. The occasional symptoms of sleeplessness, bad dreams, and poor daytime attentiveness that may be seen with lovastatin may be avoided with pravastatin. However, the most important difference is that

TABLE 20–8

Characteristics of Statins

Characteristic	Lovastatin	Pravastatin	Simvastatin	Atorvastatin	Fluvastatin	Rosuvastatin*
Maximal dose (mg/day)	80	80	80	80	80	40
Maximal (%) serum LDL cholesterol reduction produced	40	34	47	60	24	62
Serum LDL cholesterol reduction (%) produced by a 40-mg dose	34	34	41	50	24	57
Serum trigylceride reduction (%) produced by a 40-mg dose	16	24	18	29	10	28
Serum HDL cholesterol increase (%) produced by a 40-mg dose	8.6	12	12	6	8	10
Plasma half-life (hr)	2	1–2	1–2	14	1.2	~15
Effect of food on drug absorption	Increased	Decreased	None	None	Negligible	Negligible
Optimal time of administration	With meals	Bedtime	Evening	Evening	Bedtime	Evening
Penetration of central nervous system	Yes	No	Yes	No	No	No
Renal excretion of absorbed dose (%)	10	20	13	2	<6	10
Mechanism of hepatic metabolism	Cytochrome P-450 3A4	Sulfation	Cytochrome P-450 3A4	Cytochrome P-450 3A4	Cytochrome P-450 2C9	Noncytochrome pathway

*Olsson AG, Pears J, McKellar J, et al: Effect of rosuvastatin on low-density lipoprotein cholesterol in patients with hypercholesterolemia. Am J Cardiol 2001;88:504–508.

LDL, low-density lipoprotein; HDL, high-density lipoprotein.

Adapted from Knopp RH: Drug treatment of lipid disorders. N Engl J Med 1999;341:498–511.

pravastatin is metabolized by sulfation and possibly other mechanisms, and hence it can be used with care in combination with drugs that are metabolized by the CYP3A4 system. Thus, pravastatin is more widely used in patients taking protease inhibitors, cyclosporine, or azole antifungals, and it appears to be more compatible with gemfibrozil.[17] Pravastatin at a maximal dose of 80 mg yields an LDL-lowering effect nearly equal to that of lovastatin. In contrast to lovastatin, pravastatin should be taken on an empty stomach, ideally at bedtime. *Simvastatin* has a slightly greater lipid-lowering effect than lovastatin or pravastatin does, with maximal LDL lowering of 47% at an 80-mg dose.

Fluvastatin results in a 24% reduction in LDL at 40 mg/day and a 27% reduction at 80 mg/day. More recently, an 80-mg dose of fluvastatin in a timed-release form achieved a 38% reduction.[18] Fluvastatin might be an alternative to pravastatin because it is metabolized by the CYP2C9 pathway rather than the CYP3A4 pathway. However, experience is less with fluvastatin in combination with CYP3A4-metabolized drugs than with pravastatin (see Table 20–8).

TABLE 20–9

Drugs and Substances That Interfere with the Metabolism of Statins

Mechanism of Action	Effect	Drug or Substance
Inhibits cytochrome P-450 3A4	Raises serum drug concentrations	Clarithromycin, erythromycin, troleandomycin, cyclosporine, tacrolimus, delavirdine mesylate, ritonavir, lopinavir, saquinavir, fluconazole, itraconazole, ketoconazole, fluoxetine, grapefruit juice, mibefradil, nefazodone, verapamil, amiodarone
Induces cytochrome P-450 3A4	Lowers serum drug concentrations	Barbiturates, carbamazepine, griseofulvin, nafcillin, phenytoin, primidone, rifabutin, rifampin, troglitazone
Inhibits cytochrome P-450 2C9	May raise serum fluvastatin concentrations	Amiodarone, cimetidine, ranitidine, omeprazole, trimethoprim-sulfamethoxazole, fluoxetine, fluvoxamine, isoniazid, itraconazole, ketoconazole, metronidazole, sulfinpyrazone, ticlopidine, zafirlukast
Induces cytochrome P-450 2C9	May lower serum fluvastatin concentrations	Barbiturates, carbamazepine, phenytoin, primidone, rifampin

Adapted from Knopp RH: Drug treatment of lipid disorders. N Engl J Med 1999;341:498–511.

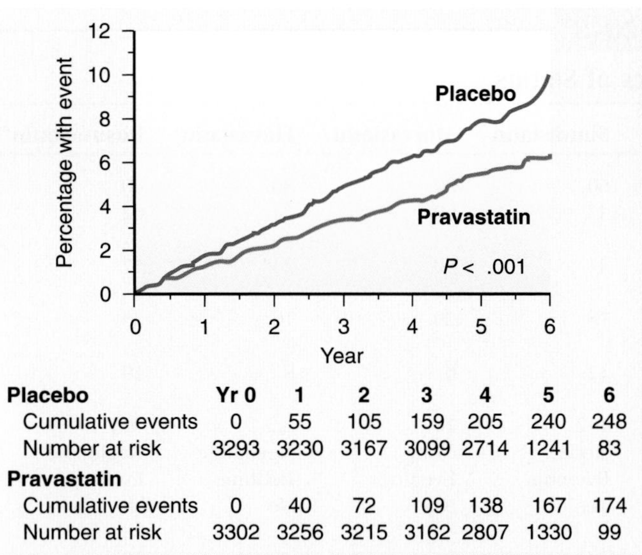

Placebo	**Yr 0**	**1**	**2**	**3**	**4**	**5**	**6**
Cumulative events	0	55	105	159	205	240	248
Number at risk	3293	3230	3167	3099	2714	1241	83
Pravastatin							
Cumulative events	0	40	72	109	138	167	174
Number at risk	3302	3256	3215	3162	2807	1330	99

FIGURE 20–8. Kaplan-Meier analysis of the time to a definite nonfatal myocardial infarction or death from coronary heart disease according to treatment group in a trial of pravastatin compared with placebo. (Redrawn from Shepherd J, Cobbe SM, Ford I, et al: Prevention of coronary heart disease with pravastatin in men with hypercholesterolemia. N Engl J Med 1995;333:1301–1307.)

Atorvastatin achieves the greatest LDL effect, with a maximal LDL reduction of 50% to 55% at 80 mg daily. Even at high doses, atorvastatin has been well tolerated in combination with other agents, including cyclosporine, tacrolimus, and the fibric acid derivatives, particularly fenofibrate. Atorvastatin-induced hepatotoxicity, which can be seen at the higher doses of the approved range, is manifested by elevated aminotransferase and alkaline phosphatase levels; occasionally, the bilirubin level will rise without overt hepatitis. The basis for this different pattern of hepatotoxicity with atorvastatin is unknown but may be related to its longer half-life, which is approximately 14 hours versus 1 to 3 hours for the other statins. Because of this longer half-life, atorvastatin can be given anytime during the day.

Another synthetic statin, rosuvastatin, is currently in development; it can yield a 60% to 65% decrease in LDL cholesterol at 80 mg/day. Rosuvastatin has a long half-life like atorvastatin, but it is hydrophilic like pravastatin. Its utility in combination with other lipid-lowering drugs is yet to be explored. Like pravastatin, it is metabolized by a non-cytochrome pathway.

In numerous trials of primary prevention (Fig. 20–8) and secondary prevention (Fig. 20–9) using lovastatin, pravastatin, or simvastatin, the effects of statins on lipoprotein levels yield a risk reduction benefit pre-

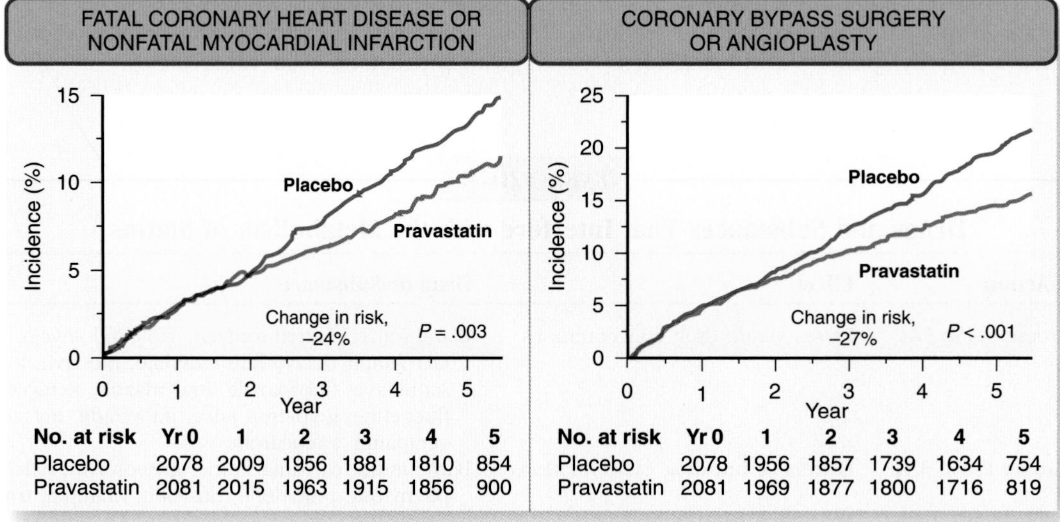

No. at risk	**Yr 0**	**1**	**2**	**3**	**4**	**5**
Placebo	2078	2009	1956	1881	1810	854
Pravastatin	2081	2015	1963	1915	1856	900

No. at risk	**Yr 0**	**1**	**2**	**3**	**4**	**5**
Placebo	2078	1956	1857	1739	1634	754
Pravastatin	2081	1969	1877	1800	1716	819

FIGURE 20–9. Kaplan-Meier estimates of the incidence of coronary events in the pravastatin and placebo groups. The *left* panel shows data for the primary endpoint—fatal coronary heart disease or nonfatal myocardial infarction. The *right* panel shows data for coronary bypass surgery or angioplasty. Changes in risk are those attributable to pravastatin. *P* values and changes in risk are based on Cox proportional hazards analysis. (Redrawn from Sacks FM, Pfeffer MA, Moye LA, et al, for the Cholesterol and Recurrent Events Trial Investigators: The effect of pravastatin on coronary events after myocardial infarction in patients with average cholesterol levels. N Engl J Med 1996;335:1001–1009.)

dicted by the Framingham equations[4,19] (see Fig. 20–1). Atorvastatin at 80 mg/day prevents recurrent events beginning 4 weeks after an acute coronary syndrome, and fluvastatin, pravastatin, and lovastatin have been shown to cause regression of CAD.[20] Statin therapy also improves immune tolerance to heart and renal transplants (pravastatin), diminishes fibrinogen levels, reduces blood viscosity, and activates endothelial nitric oxide synthase. In in vitro systems, some of these effects are independent of cholesterol lowering, but in vivo, most of the benefit seems to be due to the reduction in LDL and its penetration into the arterial wall, with a resultant reduction in inflammation and oxidative stress. The association of statin use with less osteoporosis may be a "healthy user" effect, although animal studies suggest a direct effect.

Even though statins are the preferred medications for the management of pure hypercholesterolemia, they are also highly appropriate for the management of combined hyperlipidemia with triglyceride-lowering drugs. Moreover, statins can be used with bile acid–binding resins to increase LDL lowering (Fig. 20–10). When statins are used concomitantly with niacin, fibrates, or both to treat combined triglyceride and HDL abnormalities, patients must be observed carefully for evidence of myotoxicity.

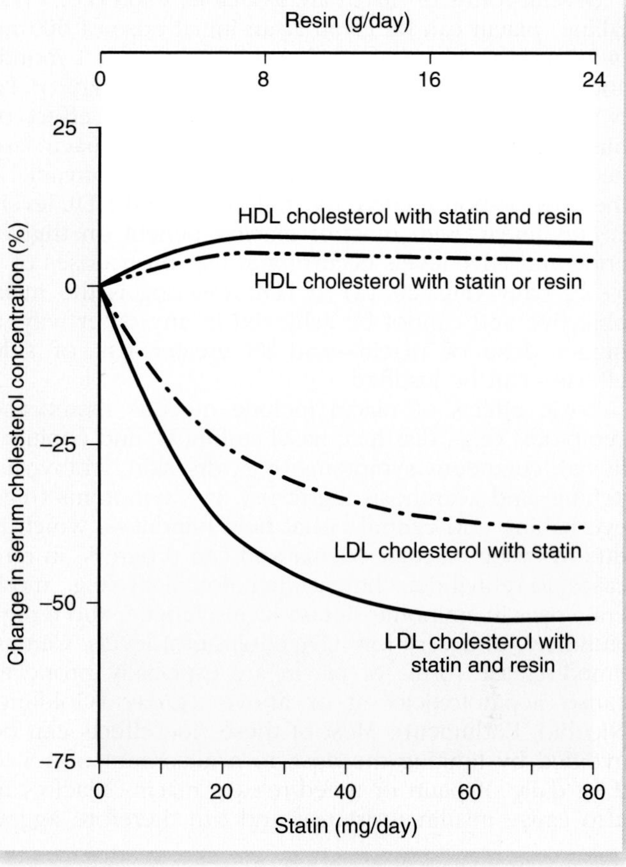

FIGURE 20–10. Effects of treatment with a statin and a bile acid–binding resin, alone or in combination, on serum high-density lipoprotein (HDL) and low-density lipoprotein (LDL) cholesterol concentrations. The effects of both drugs decline exponentially with increasing doses. Resin denotes bile acid–binding resin given as cholestyramine. (Adapted from Knopp RH: Drug treatment of lipid disorders. N Engl J Med 1999;341:498–511.)

Nicotinic Acid

Nicotinic acid, or niacin, was the first of the cholesterol-lowering drugs to be demonstrated to be effective in preventing CAD events and total mortality.[21] It lowers LDL by 15% to 20%, raises HDL by as much as 30%, and lowers plasma triglycerides and Lp(a) by as much as 30%. Niacin inhibits the mobilization of fatty acids from peripheral tissues (Fig. 20–11), with a resultant decrease in the formation of VLDL and LDL and an increase in HDL levels.[1]

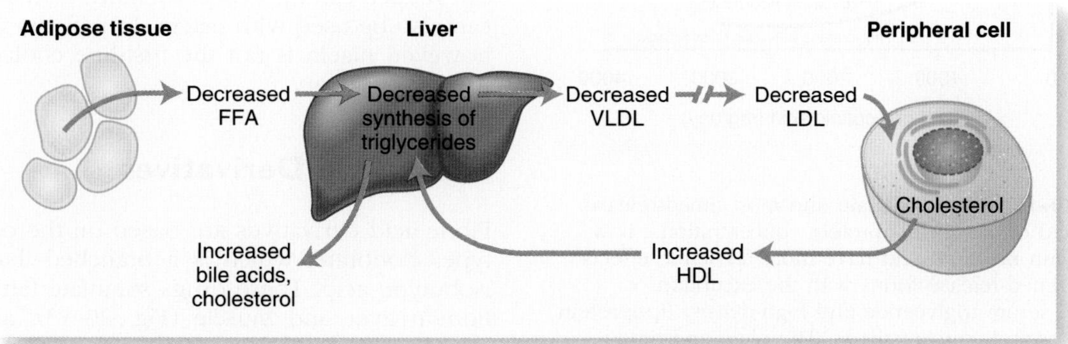

FIGURE 20–11. Mechanisms of action of nicotinic acid. Nicotinic acid inhibits the mobilization of free fatty acids (FFA) from peripheral adipose tissue to the liver. As a consequence of this decrease or an additional hepatic effect, the synthesis plus secretion of very low density lipoprotein (VLDL) is reduced, and formation of low-density lipoprotein (LDL) is also decreased. Nicotinic acid can also increase serum high-density lipoprotein (HDL) cholesterol concentrations by up to 30%; the mechanism responsible for this effect is unknown. (Redrawn from Knopp RH: Drug treatment of lipid disorders. N Engl J Med 1999;341:498–511.)

Several forms of niacin are available. Plain (i.e., crystalline) niacin can be given at an initial dose of 500 mg twice a day with meals and no hot liquids for 1 month and then increased to 500 mg three times a day or 1 g twice a day with meals. The LDL-lowering effect of niacin is linear, so relatively high doses of niacin are needed to achieve a substantial LDL benefit. Conversely, the dose-response curve for triglyceride and HDL levels is curvilinear, with most of niacin's benefit on triglyceride and HDL levels occurring at the lower doses of 1 to 2 g daily (Fig. 20–12). If LDL lowering is the main objective and cannot be achieved in any other way, a higher dose of niacin—and its greater risk of side effects—can be justified.

Toxic effects of niacin include mucous membrane symptoms (e.g., diarrhea, nasal stuffiness, and conjunctivitis), cutaneous symptoms (e.g., dry skin, ichthyosis, itching, and acanthosis nigricans), eye symptoms (e.g., eye itching and central visual field blindness, which is due to cystic macular edema and can progress, in rare cases, to retinal detachment), hepatotoxicity (e.g., moderate rises in aminotransferase levels, fatigue, and rarely, jaundice), and very low LDL cholesterol levels. Certain timed-release forms of niacin are especially prone to cause hepatotoxicity at or above 2 g/day (Goldline, Nicobid, Enduracin). Most of these side effects can be avoided by limiting the dose to a maximum of 1.5 to 2.5 g daily of plain or timed-release niacin. Niacin can also cause insulin resistance and can therefore aggravate or even precipitate diabetes. In established diabetes, the hyperglycemic effect of niacin can usually be managed with adjustment of diabetic medications.

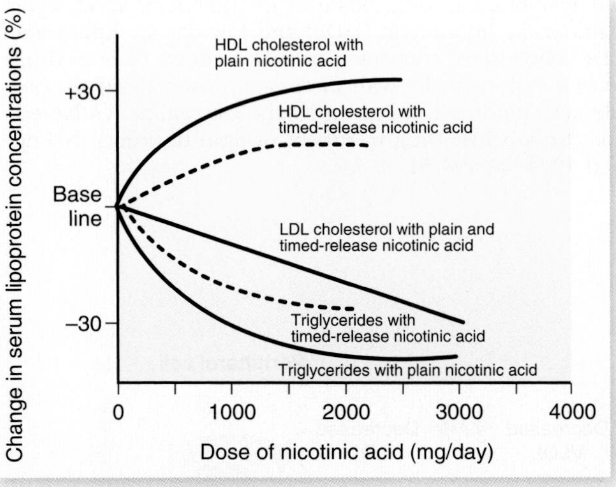

FIGURE 20–12. Effects of plain and most timed-release nicotinic acid on serum lipoprotein concentrations. Low doses of plain nicotinic acid have more favorable effects than most timed-release forms with the exception of Niaspan on serum triglyceride and high-density lipoprotein (HDL) cholesterol concentrations. The plain and timed-release forms have similar effects at any given dose on serum low-density lipoprotein (LDL) cholesterol concentrations. Most of the positive effects on serum triglyceride and HDL cholesterol concentrations occur with lower doses of nicotinic acid. (Redrawn from Knopp RH: Drug treatment of lipid disorders. N Engl J Med 1999;341:498–511.)

Unmodified niacin causes cutaneous flushing symptoms in 90% of persons. These symptoms are characterized by skin redness and warmth in the thorax and face occurring about 30 minutes after taking niacin and disappearing after about an hour. Flushing, which is the principal deterrent to using the drug, can be ameliorated by taking niacin with food, by avoiding the concurrent ingestion of hot liquids (such as hot coffee, tea, or soup), and by taking aspirin, 325 mg, 30 minutes before the niacin. In general, these measures will reduce the severity of flushing by about 50%, so the symptoms can be tolerated for the 3 to 4 days required for natural tachyphylaxis to develop to the prostaglandin-mediated flush. Thereafter, patients typically recognize only a tingle now and then after taking their niacin.

Unfortunately, approximately 10% to 30% of patients will not adapt to niacin flushing. These patients are candidates for the timed-release forms of niacin, one of the two best forms being Niaspan, an intermediate-release niacin taken at bedtime with an 8- to 12-hour duration of action. This approach inhibits the nocturnal rise in free fatty acids. Slo-Niacin, which is taken in the conventional manner with meals, is a reasonably well tolerated and efficacious alternative. The very long-acting niacins have a greater risk of toxicity, especially when more than 2 g is taken daily. Therefore, the general advice with all timed-release forms of niacin, including Niaspan and Slo-Niacin, is not to exceed a maximal dose of 2 or 2.5 g daily.

Niacin alone has been shown to reduce cardiovascular disease and all-cause mortality in a large secondary prevention trial.[21] It is especially useful in combined hyperlipidemia, in which virtually all lipoprotein species are disordered. Often, however, niacin is not sufficient when given alone and is best combined with a statin or a bile acid–binding resin. The combination of niacin and a resin can produce a 70% to 80% reduction in recurrent coronary events, as well as a reduction in the angiographic progression of CAD.[22,23] Statin plus niacin can reduce clinical events by more than 90%.[24] Fibrates can also be used with niacin. In patients with diabetes, however, niacin is not the first-line choice but can be used if necessary.[25]

Fibric Acid Derivatives

Fibric acid derivatives are based on the original prototype, clofibrate, which is a branched-chain analog of isobutyric acid. These drugs stimulate fatty acid oxidation in liver and muscle (Fig. 20–13), and they also increase lipoprotein lipase activity, increase apoprotein A-I synthesis, and downregulate apoprotein C-III levels. With enhanced fatty acid oxidation, re-esterification of free fatty acid to triglyceride in the liver is diminished, and secretion of VLDL is reduced. Similarly, enhanced fatty acid oxidation in muscle is associated with enhanced uptake of triglycerides. Thus, the fibrates

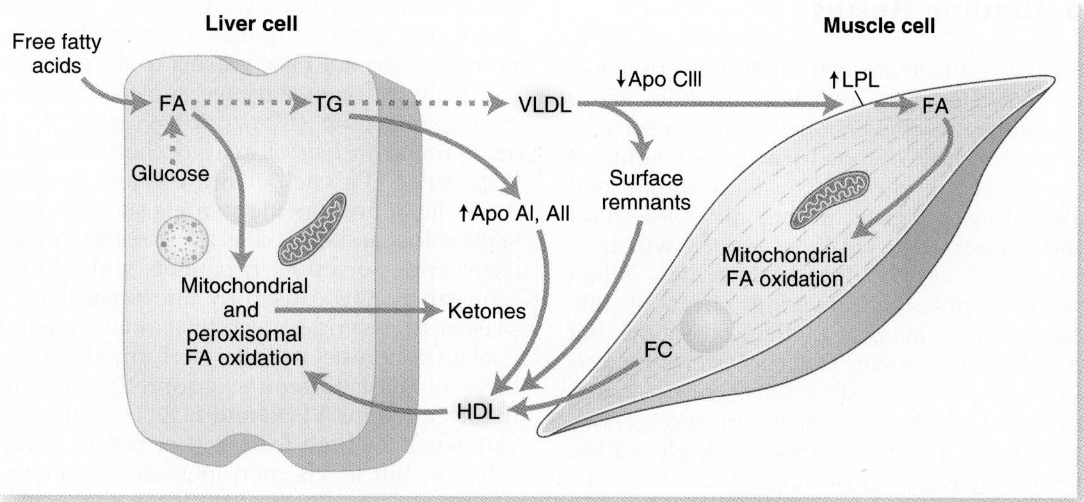

FIGURE 20–13. Metabolic effects of fibrates. *Bold lines* indicate increased transport, and *dashed lines*, diminished transport. Fibrates enhance the oxidation of fatty acids (FA) in liver and muscle and reduce the rate of lipogenesis in the liver, thereby reducing hepatic secretion of very low density lipoprotein (VLDL) triglycerides (TG). The increased uptake of triglyceride-derived fatty acids in muscle cells results from an increase in lipoprotein lipase (LPL) activity in adjacent capillaries and a decrease in the apolipoprotein C-III (Apo CIII) concentration, transcriptionally mediated by peroxisome proliferator–activated receptor alpha (PPARα). The enhanced catabolism of VLDL generates surface remnants, which are transferred to and increase high-density lipoprotein (HDL) levels. HDL concentrations are further augmented by an increase in transcription of apolipoprotein A-I (Apo AI). Other effects of fibrates include an increase in the size of LDL particles, increased removal of LDL, and a reduction in the levels of plasminogen activator inhibitor type 1. (Redrawn from Knopp RH: Drug treatment of lipid disorders. N Engl J Med 1999;341:498–511.)

decrease triglyceride levels both by diminishing production and by enhancing removal.

Typically, when triglyceride levels are elevated, LDL levels are low, and when plasma triglyceride levels are lowered (with a fibrate, niacin, weight loss, or fish oil), LDL levels rise, sometimes to surprisingly high levels. This LDL increase is not a toxic effect of the treatment but rather an unmasking of the persisting lipoprotein overproduction, which is now manifested in the LDL fraction because the metabolism of triglyceride-rich VLDL to LDL is no longer impaired. This effect usually occurs in persons with combined hyperlipidemia, and the combination of a statin with a fibrate can control the LDL level. If for some reason a statin cannot be used or is not tolerated, alternatives include niacin or an inhibitor of bile acid or cholesterol absorption.

Two fibrates are currently available in the United States: gemfibrozil and fenofibrate. Gemfibrozil can cause myotoxicity, especially when used with lovastatin, and erectile dysfunction. It is also associated with upper gastrointestinal intolerance, typically pain, in 10% to 15% of cases, particularly when taken as directed before meals. Fenofibrate seems to be free of most of these side effects, including myotoxicity; its primary toxic effect is skin rash, but hepatotoxicity occasionally occurs.

All fibrates increase biliary cholesterol concentrations and have the potential to precipitate gallstones, but this absolute increase in risk is small, from a baseline incidence of 1% to a frequency of about 2%. For this reason, fibrates are contraindicated in persons with gallstone disease. Of special importance is that all fibrates displace warfarin from albumin-binding sites. In general, the warfarin dose should be reduced by approximately 30%, but the international normalized ratio (INR) needs to be monitored carefully, especially at the beginning of therapy or with any change in dose.

Five major heart disease prevention studies have been performed with fibric acid derivatives. Two studies of clofibrate in the 1970s showed no benefit or a reduction in CAD that was partly offset by a significant increase in medical complications, including gallstones and biliary tract cancer. Subsequent large randomized trials showed a significant reduction in CAD events with gemfibrozil[26–28] and diminished progression of angiographic CAD in diabetic subjects with fenofibrate.[29]

A primary indication for fibric acid therapy is a triglyceride elevation to more than 1000 mg/dL, a range that can induce pancreatitis. Remnant removal disease (see Table 20–1) is another primary indication. Low HDL cholesterol is also somewhat amenable to fibrate therapy, but niacin is a better choice. Most frequently, fibric acid derivatives are used in combination with other agents, particularly statins, in the management of combined hyperlipidemia, especially when niacin fails or is not tolerated. To minimize the risk of myositis, a recommended approach is to add a statin at a low dose to the fibrate regimen and then increase the statin dose gradually. Fenofibrate appears to be the preferred fibrate in this setting. At each visit, the patient should be asked specifically about musculoskeletal symptoms, and a CK level should be drawn until clinical stability is ensured.

Bile Acid–Binding Resins

Bile acid–binding resins lower LDL cholesterol by interrupting the enterohepatic circulation of bile acids, thereby stimulating the conversion of cholesterol into bile acids by the enzyme 7-alpha-hydroxylase. Some of the cholesterol-lowering effect of resins is diminished by a compensatory increase in hepatic cholesterol synthesis and subsequent VLDL secretion, which is clinically manifested as a rise in triglycerides. When given alone, the cholesterol-lowering effect of bile acid–binding resins is inferior to that of statins but nevertheless sufficient to lower LDL cholesterol by 12% to 24% and reduce primary CAD events.[30] Concomitant use of a statin can block the increase in endogenous cholesterol synthesis, prevent the rise in triglycerides, and enhance the cholesterol-lowering effect of resins.

Cholestyramine and colestipol are composed of polar side chains on a synthetic carbon backbone that exchanges chloride for bile acids. Thus, hyperchloremia can be induced in susceptible individuals with impaired renal function. Constipation develops in about a third of patients, and a similar number of patients complain of abdominal fullness and gas. Nearly everyone complains about a gritty taste.

For these reasons, cholestyramine and colestipol are now used infrequently except in the most difficult patients. A newer resin, colesevelam, usually administered as three 0.625-mg tablets twice a day, can reduce LDL cholesterol levels by approximately 20% while increasing the prevalence of constipation from only 7% in a placebo group to 11% at a full dose of 3.8 g of colesevelam daily.[31] Colesevelam is therefore a valuable adjunctive therapy for severe hypercholesterolemia and in individuals who cannot tolerate statins.

Other Lipid-Lowering Therapies

Soluble fiber can lower LDL cholesterol modestly, by 5% to 10%, whether used as Metamucil, oat bran, guar gum, pectin, or fruit and vegetable fiber. All these agents, however, increase intestinal gas. Nonabsorbable plant sterols, such as sitosterol or sitostanol in the form of tub margarine (Benecol and TakeControl) taken as 2 to 3 tbsp daily, can competitively inhibit the gastrointestinal absorption of dietary and biliary cholesterol; they lower LDL cholesterol by as much as 12% to 15%.[32] Some patients will resist this treatment because it is more expensive than ordinary margarine, but its effect can sometimes be the equivalent of doubling the dose of a statin, which typically lowers LDL cholesterol by another 6% to 8%.

In postmenopausal women, oral estrogens or selective estrogen receptor modulators such as tamoxifen or raloxifene can lower LDL cholesterol by approximately 10% and raise HDL cholesterol modestly. Whether these interventions can reduce CAD is uncertain, in light of the adverse CAD effects of postmenopausal estrogen/progestin therapy (see Chapters 15 and 23). Estrogens increase triglyceride levels substantially when given orally to women with elevated baseline levels, but not when given by patch. Conversely, tamoxifen and raloxifene do not raise plasma triglyceride levels except in highly estrogen-sensitive subjects. The concentrated eicosapentaenoic (EPA)/docosahexaenoic (DHA) fatty acids found in fish oil may be helpful at doses of 4 to 9 capsules (1 g each) daily containing 67% EPA/DHA. Anabolic or androgenic steroids such as oxandrolone or stanozolol can be used as a last resort to reduce hepatic triglyceride secretion in patients with chronic or recurrent pancreatitis caused by uncontrollable elevations in plasma triglycerides despite standard medications.

LDL apheresis can be performed on a weekly or biweekly basis to remove apoprotein B, which contains the lipoproteins VLDL and LDL, from the blood stream. LDL levels will fall from 250 or 300 to 50 mg/dL within 3 hours, but levels then increase exponentially over a period of 1 to 2 weeks to a level only somewhat lower than the level at the initiation of pheresis therapy. This procedure can be lifesaving in unusual patients who have severe familial hypercholesterolemia and are unable take lipid-lowering medications or are nonresponsive or poorly responsive to drug treatment.

New Agents Affecting Intestinal Fat Absorption

Ezetimibe is the first pharmacologic inhibitor of intestinal absorption[33] both from the diet and via enterohepatic reabsorption. Its mechanism is currently unknown, but it lowers LDL cholesterol concentrations by approximately 18% at a maximal dose of 10 mg daily and is very well tolerated. Ezetimibe can also be used with statins to achieve the same additional 18% decrease in LDL cholesterol levels. Inhibitors of the intestinal bile acid transporter are also being studied in clinical trials.

A PRACTICAL APPROACH TO HYPERLIPIDEMIA

Goals of Therapy

Every person who has an LDL cholesterol level above their NCEP goal should be evaluated to be sure that they do not have a secondary cause of dyslipidemia such as diabetes, hypothyroidism, liver disease, or chronic renal failure (Table 20–10). Drugs that can increase LDL or decrease HDL (e.g., progestins, anabolic steroids, and corticosteroids) or that increase triglycerides (e.g., oral estrogens, beta-blockers, and alcohol) should be discontinued, if possible.

All individuals who still have an LDL cholesterol level above the NCEP goal should then be treated, beginning with lifestyle interventions (see Tables 20–2 and 20–3) and progressing to medications as needed to reach their goals (see Fig. 20–7). Simple administration of a statin at an initial dose may or may not be sufficient to attain the NCEP goal, and statin therapy is sometimes insuffi-

TABLE 20–10

Secondary Causes of Lipid Disorders

Increased LDL Cholesterol	Increased Triglyceride	Decreased HDL Cholesterol
Hypothyroidism	Obesity	Hypertriglyceridemia
Diabetes mellitus	Diabetes mellitus	Obesity
Obesity	Lack of exercise	Diabetes mellitus
Nephrotic syndrome	Alcohol intake	Cigarette smoking
Obstructive liver disease	Renal insufficiency	Lack of exercise
Progestins	Estrogens	Beta-blockers
Anabolic steroids	Beta-blockers	Progestins
High-dose thiazides	High-dose thiazides	Anabolic steroids

HDL, high-density lipoprotein; LDL, low-density lipoprotein.

Adapted from Schaefer EJ: Overview of the Diagnosis and Treatment of Lipid Disorders. Cambridge, MA, Genzyme, 1995, p 17.

cient at the maximal dose. Single-drug therapy typically reduces the incidence of CAD events by only 25% to 35%. Combinations of niacin, fibrates, and resins may be necessary to reach the desired lipid goals, which will result in further reductions in CAD. Even an LDL level of 100 mg/dL may not be sufficiently low for individuals with other untreatable risk factor such as a very elevated Lp(a), and one study has shown benefits from statins in patients with CAD and an intitial LDL cholesterol level below 100 mg/dL.[34] In patients who do not respond to prescribed therapies, attention should be paid to methods to improve adherence to both diet and drugs (Box 20–5).

Even in the face of a normal LDL level, the presence of a markedly elevated plasma triglyceride level or a low HDL level raises the risk for CAD. Approaches to an elevated triglyceride level emphasize aggressive treatment of LDL elevations, physical activity, weight loss, and medications if necessary (Box 20–6). In fact, the most common lipid abnormality seen in patients with CAD is combined (mixed) hyperlipidemia with an above average LDL cholesterol, a low HDL level, and an elevated triglyceride level. These patients often require the addition of niacin or a fibrate to a statin to normalize all three lipid levels. The recent ATP-III revision of the NCEP guidelines considers this situation by advising treatment of non-HDL cholesterol (i.e., LDL and VLDL cholesterol) to goals of less than 190 mg/dL for persons with zero or one CAD risk factor, less than 160 mg/dL for persons with two or more CAD risk

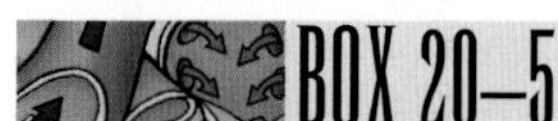

BOX 20–5

Interventions to Improve Adherence

FOCUS ON THE PATIENT

- Simplify medication regimens
- Provide explicit patient instruction and use good counseling techniques to teach the patient how to follow the prescribed treatment
- Encourage the use of prompts to help patients remember treatment regimens
- Use systems to reinforce adherence and maintain contact with the patient
- Encourage the support of family and friends
- Reinforce and reward adherence
- Increase visits for patients unable to achieve treatment goals
- Increase convenience and access to care
- Involve patients in their care through self-monitoring

FOCUS ON THE PHYSICIAN AND MEDICAL OFFICE

- Teach physicians to implement lipid treatment guidelines
- Use reminders to prompt physicians to attend to lipid management
- Identify a patient advocate in the office to help deliver or prompt care
- Use patients to prompt preventive care
- Develop a standardized treatment plan to structure care
- Use feedback from past performance to foster change in future care
- Remind patients of appointments and follow up on missed appointments

FOCUS ON THE HEALTH DELIVERY SYSTEM

- Provide lipid management through a lipid clinic
- Utilize case management by nurses
- Deploy telemedicine
- Utilize the collaborative care of pharmacists
- Execute critical care pathways in hospitals

Reproduced from Executive Summary of the Third Report of the National Cholesterol Education Program (NCEP) Expert Panel on detection, evaluation, and treatment of high blood cholesterol in adults (Adult Treatment Panel III). JAMA 2001;285:2486–2497.

factors, and less than 130 mg/dL for persons with CAD or diabetes (see Box 20–6).[4]

Randomized trials using statins have demonstrated the benefit of cholesterol-lowering therapy in a wide spectrum of patients (Fig. 20–14). Analyses of the cost-effectiveness of lipid-lowering therapy demonstrate that cholesterol reduction is associated with favorable cost-effectiveness ratios when used for *secondary prevention* in persons with existing CAD (Table 20–11), and it may actually save cost as well as years of life in high-risk patients. For *primary prevention* in persons without CAD, the cost-effectiveness of beneficial therapies to reduce LDL cholesterol depends on the individual's underlying risk of CAD: higher risk patients receive more absolute benefit for the same cost. Cost-effectiveness depends not only on the degree of elevation in LDL cholesterol itself but also on the presence of other CAD risk factors, including age and gender; cost-effectiveness ratios are similar in patients with diabetes and those with known CAD.[35] In general, dietary interventions are cost-effective across a wide range of assumptions.[36] The use of medications is critically dependent on the cost of the medications, with most recent analyses suggesting that costs per year of life saved with the use of nongeneric statins for primary prevention in patients without diabetes are consistently higher than, for example, the cost of a year of renal dialysis.[36] These findings emphasize why diet and lifestyle changes should be the first intervention and why physicians should strive to use lower cost medications whenever possible.

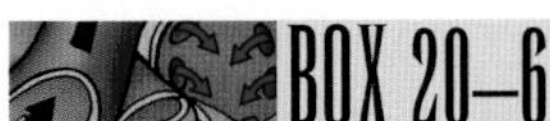
BOX 20–6

Treatment of Elevated Triglycerides (≥150 mg/dL)

1. Primary aim of therapy is to reach the LDL goal:
   - Intensify weight management
   - Increase physical activity
2. If triglycerides ≥500 mg/dL, lower triglycerides to prevent pancreatitis:
   - Very low fat diet (≤15% of calories from fat)
   - Weight management and physical activity
   - Fibrate or nicotinic acid
   - When triglycerides <500 mg/dL, turn to LDL-lowering therapy
3. If triglycerides ≥200 mg/dL after the LDL goal is reached, set secondary goal for non-HDL cholesterol (total cholesterol − HDL) 30 mg/dL higher than LDL goal:
   - <130 if CAD, peripheral vascular disease, or diabetes
   - <160 if ≥2 CAD risk factors
   - <190 if 0 or 1 CAD risk factors
4. If triglycerides 200–400 mg/dL after the LDL goal is reached, consider adding a drug if needed to reach the non–HDL cholesterol goal:
   - Intensify therapy with a statin, or
   - Add nicotinic acid or fibrate to further lower VLDL

CAD, coronary artery disease; HDL, high-density lipoprotein; LDL, low-density lipoprotein; VLDL, very low density lipoprotein.
Adapted from National Cholesterol Education Program: ATP III Guidelines At-A-Glance Quick Desk Reference. Bethesda, MD, National Institutes of Health, National Heart, Lung, and Blood Institute, 2001.

Illustrative Case Examples

Heterozygous Familial Hypercholesterolemia. A 58-year-old woman experienced the onset of angina at 33 years of age, a time when she smoked and used high-dose oral contraceptives. She underwent coronary artery bypass graft surgery shortly thereafter, with a repeat operation 11 years later. Her brother died of myocardial infarction at a young age. Her LDL cholesterol was 350 mg/dL, her HDL was 55 mg/dL, and her triglyceride level was 130 mg/dL. Now, with 80 mg/day of atorvastatin, 4 g daily of plain niacin in divided doses, and 3.8 g of colesevelam in two divided doses, her LDL level is 127 mg/dL, her HDL is 75 mg/dL, and her triglyceride level is 80 mg/dL. She had an unchanged angiogram at age 60 years. This case illustrates how very high doses of several drugs can be combined to treat severe hypercholesterolemia to a reasonable, even if not ideal level with good clinical results.

Combined Hyperlipidemia (Commonly Familial). A 58-year-old woman smoker had her first myocardial infarction at the age of 55 after an early menopause

TABLE 20–11

Cost-Effectiveness of Secondary Prevention with Simvastatin

	Cost-Effectiveness				
Group	***Age 35–44 yr***	***Age 45–54 yr***	***Age 55–64 yr***	***Age 65–74 yr***	***Age 75–84 yr***
Men	4,500*	1,800	3,900	6,700	9,900
Women	40,000	8,100	8,400	9,500	11,000

*Values are dollars per quality-adjusted life-year.

Reproduced with permission from Prosser LA, Stinnett AA, Goldman PA, et al: Cost-effectiveness of cholesterol-lowering therapies according to selected patient characteristics. Ann Intern Med 2000;132:769–779.

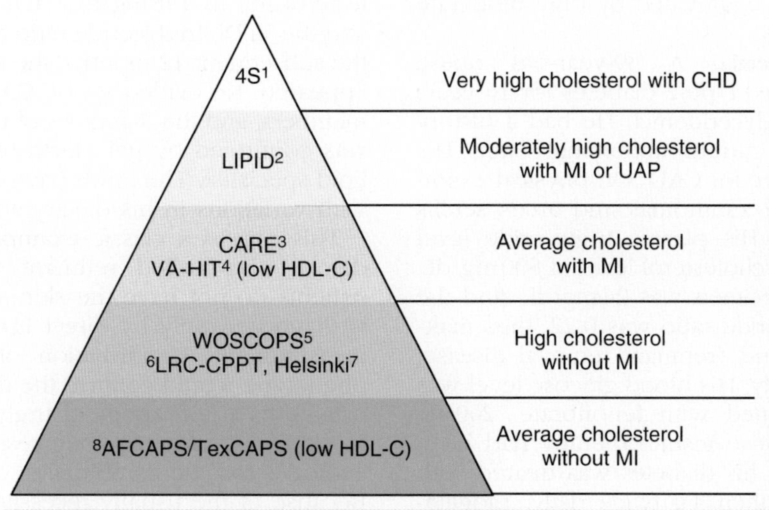

FIGURE 20–14. Large-scale clinical trials have supported the lipid hypothesis. The pyramid reflects relative applicability to the overall population, with the greatest number of individuals at the base and the fewest represented at the apex. CHD, coronary heart disease; HDL-C, high-density lipoprotein cholesterol; MI, myocardial infarction; UAP, unstable angina pectoris. [1]4S = Scandinavian Simvastatin Survival Study Group: Randomised trial of cholesterol lowering in 4444 patients with coronary heart disease: The Scandinavian Simvastatin Survival Study. Lancet 1994;344:1383–1389; [2]LIPID = The Long-Term Intervention with Pravastatin in Ischaemic Disease Study Group: Prevention of cardiovascular events and death with pravastatin in patients with coronary heart disease and a broad range of initial cholesterol levels. N Engl J Med 1998;339:1349–1357; [3]CARE = Sacks FM, Pfeffer MA, Moyte LA, et al, for the Cholesterol and Recurrent Events Trial Investigators: The effect of pravastatin on coronary events after myocardial infarction in patients with average cholesterol levels. N Engl J Med 1996:335;1001–1009; [4]VA-HIT = Rubins HB, Robins SJ, Collins D, et al, for the Veteran's Affairs High-Density Lipoprotein Cholesterol Intervention Trial Study Group: Gemfibrozil for the secondary prevention of coronary heart disease in men with low levels of high-density lipoprotein cholesterol. N Engl J Med 1999:341:410–418; [5]WOSCOPS = Caro J, Klittich W, McGuire A, et al: The West of Scotland Coronary Prevention Study: Economic benefit analysis of primary prevention with pravastatin. BMJ 1997;315:1577–1582; [6]LRC-CPPT = Lipid Research Clinics Program: The Lipid Research Clinics Coronary Primary Prevention Trial Results. II. The relationship of reduction in incidence of coronary heart disease to cholesterol lowering. JAMA 1984;251:365–374; [7]Helsinki = Frick MH, Elo O, Haapa K, et al: Helsinki Heart Study: Primary-prevention trial with gemfibrozil in middle-aged men with dyslipidemia. N Engl J Med 1987;317:1237–1245; [8]AFCAPS/TexCAPS = Downs JR, Clearfield M, Weis S, et al: The Air Force/Texas Coronary Atherosclerosis Prevention Study: Primary prevention of acute coronary events with lovastatin in men and women with average cholesterol level: Results of AFCAPS/TexCAPS. JAMA 1998;279:1615–1622. (From Gotto AM Jr, Farmer JA: Lipid-lowering trials. In Braunwald E, Zipes DP, Libby P [eds]: Heart Disease: A Textbook of Cardiovascular Medicine, 6th ed. Philadelphia, WB Saunders, 2001, p 1084.)

without hormone replacement. She has a history of CAD on both sides of her family, with varied lipid elevations. Laboratory studies revealed an LDL of 176 mg/dL, an HDL of 37 mg/dL, and a triglyceride level of 215 mg/dL. Lp(a), determined as a guide to the intensity of therapy, was 35 (about the 85th percentile). She was centrally obese, thus suggesting the metabolic syndrome. Her fasting blood glucose level was 110 mg/dL. The target LDL for this individual is less than 100 mg/dL, and this goal was reached with statin therapy alone. However, the triglyceride level remained at about 200 mg/dL, and her HDL level was only 37 mg/dL. Plain niacin was attempted, starting at 500 mg orally twice daily with meals. She avoided hot liquids and took an aspirin before the niacin, but she still had intolerable flushing and skin irritation with every dose for a week. As a result, an intermediate timed-release form of niacin was chosen. With this regimen, LDL fell to 75 mg/dL, HDL cholesterol was 45 mg/dL, and the triglyceride level was 130 mg/dL. This case illustrates conventional combination drug treatment of a nondiabetic person with combined hyperlipidemia. An LDL cholesterol level of 75 mg/dL or even lower is justifiable in a patient with CAD and an elevated Lp(a).

Benign Hypertriglyceridemia. A 60-year-old man who is 10 to 15 lb overweight has plasma triglyceride levels of 200 to 300 mg/dL, a cholesterol level of 178 mg/dL, an LDL of 78 mg/dL, and an HDL of 30 mg/dL. His apoprotein B level is 110 mg/dL (an average value), with an apoprotein A-I value of 135 (an average male value), thus indicating that the low HDL cholesterol level is due to the hypertriglyceridemia and can be corrected by lowering the triglyceride level. His fasting glucose is 96 mg/dL. He has no family history of CAD, and his physical examination is normal, including blood pressure. He has two to three alcoholic drinks per night. He was asked to abstain from alcohol for 1 week before his next visit, and his triglyceride level fell to 125 mg/dL, with an LDL of 110 mg/dL and HDL of 40 mg/dL. This patient was then instructed to follow a Step I diet, to exercise, and to limit his alcohol to one drink per night. Six weeks later he had repeat testing to confirm that his lipids remained normal. This example demonstrates the occasional case of benign hypertriglyceridemia with no apparent CAD risk, here aggravated by only moderate alcohol intake.

Severe Hypertriglyceridemia. A 39-year-old obese man had poorly controlled type 2 diabetes for 15 years associated with hypertriglyceridemia. He had a history of pancreatitis but no current abdominal pain. His family history was positive for CAD. On physical examination, he had eruptive xanthomas and arcus senilis without vascular bruits. His plasma triglyceride level was 15,000 mg/dL with a cholesterol level of 800 mg/dL. LDL in a centrifuged specimen was 24 mg/dL, and the VLDL cholesterol-triglyceride ratio was 0.22, thus making type III hyperlipidemia (remnant removal disease; see the next case) unlikely. His blood glucose level was 560 mg/dL. He was treated with fenofibrate, 200 mg daily (a full dose). Because insulin therapy had been unsuccessful in the past, his diabetes was treated with metformin, 500 mg and then 1 g twice daily, pioglitazone, 30 mg/day, and glibenclamide, 10 mg daily. One month later, the triglyceride level had fallen to 1500 mg/dL, the cholesterol level had fallen to 300 mg/dL, the LDL level was now up to 209 mg/dL, the blood glucose level had fallen to 175 mg/dL, and the patient's energy was much improved.

This case illustrates several points. First, diabetes is almost always associated with severe hypertriglyceridemia. Second, in obese type 2 diabetic patients, diabetes can usually be managed initially with a combination of oral agents. Third, this patient presumably has combined hyperlipidemia, and the elevation in LDL was unmasked by an improvement in the metabolism of VLDL to LDL. The next intervention is to reduce the LDL concentration, probably with a low-dose statin. Nicotinic acid is a second choice because of its potential to raise the blood glucose level in someone not taking insulin. Fish oil is another attractive option. Exercise and weight loss are also important adjunctive therapies, but they are not generally sufficient by themselves to manage severe hypertriglyceridemia.

Remnant Removal Disease (Also Known as Type III Hyperlipidemia). A 39-year-old overweight man had a cholesterol level of 835 mg/dL, a plasma triglyceride level of 1500 mg/dL, yellow streaks in his palmar creases bilaterally, and tuberous xanthomas over his elbows and knees. A full lipoprotein assay (ultracentrifuged or direct LDL method) was performed to differentiate type III hyperlipidemia from combined hyperlipidemia. The analysis showed an LDL cholesterol level of 45 mg/dL, VLDL cholesterol of 750 mg/dL, HDL of 25 mg/dL, a VLDL-triglyceride ratio of 0.40 (normal range, 0.10 to 0.30), an apoprotein B level of 300 mg/dL (upper limit, 140), an apoprotein A-I level of 136 mg/dL (average), and an Lp(a) level of 0.3 mg/dL (very low, the average is 10). He was treated with gemfibrozil, 600 mg twice a day, diet, and weight loss. His triglyceride level fell to 325 mg/dL, the cholesterol level declined to 200 mg/dL, and the HDL level increased to 45 mg/dL. The palmar xanthomas disappeared within 2 weeks, and the tuberous xanthomas decreased but did not disappear. For this reason and because of the persistent elevation in triglyceride level, pravastatin, 10 mg, was added to the regimen; the triglyceride level fell to 150 mg/dL, cholesterol fell to 145 mg/dL, HDL increased to 50 mg/dL, and the VLDL-triglyceride ratio normalized to 0.20. Over the subsequent 12 months, the tuberous xanthomas disappeared. No evidence of CAD was noted in his family members, and the diagnosis of remnant removal disease was confirmed by gel electrophoresis performed by a lipid specialist. The lipids have since waxed and waned with variations in his dietary adherence.

This case is a classic example of type III hyperlipidemia, also called remnant removal disease. Most patients do not have the skin signs, and the condition is diagnosed only by direct LDL and VLDL cholesterol measurement. Confirmation of an apoprotein E2/E2 phenotype would confirm the diagnosis. These patients usually have elevations of triglycerides and cholesterol to similar levels, and they respond very well to diet, exercise, and the combination of a fibrate with a statin. Because of the usually recessive nature of inheritance, these patients usually have little or no family history of CAD, but they are very susceptible to peripheral vascular disease. In the absence of the skin or laboratory features just described, treatment is similar to that for combined hyperlipidemia.

Primary Low HDL (Hyperalphalipoproteinemia). A 59-year-old man was referred for a cholesterol level of 220 mg/dL, LDL of 130 mg/dL, HDL of 30 mg/dL, and a triglyceride level of 320 mg/dL. His Lp(a) was 8 mg/dL. He has a distant family history of CAD. The apoprotein A-I level, which was measured to see whether he had a deficiency of HDL particles in addition to a low HDL cholesterol level, was 90 (low). When he was given a fibric acid, his LDL rose to 140 mg/dL, the triglyceride level fell to 120 mg/dL, and HDL remained at 30 mg/dL. His physical examination showed a right carotid bruit and an aortic ejection murmur; carotid ultrasound revealed 15% to 49% narrowings bilaterally. The addition of a low-dose statin reduced the LDL level to 70 mg/dL, but the HDL level remained in the 20- to 30-mg/dL range. Niacin was begun and increased gradually to 1500 mg/day, and the HDL cholesterol level increased to 35 mg/dL.

This case illustrates how a primary reduction in HDL is manifested as a low apoprotein A-I level and does not correct with triglyceride-lowering therapy. The best therapeutic approach is aggressive lowering of the LDL level. The addition of niacin may further lower LDL and triglyceride levels, but it does not generally raise HDL further. A typical, aggressive LDL cholesterol goal would be 50 to 75 mg/dL.

Estrogen-Induced Hypertriglyceridemia. A 54-year-old woman was given oral estrogen for menopausal symptoms and prevention of osteoporosis. Her uterus had been removed several years earlier for fibroids and dysfunctional bleeding. Her father died of a myocardial infarction at age 65. Hemorrhagic pancreatitis developed with a triglyceride level of 12,600 mg/dL and required months of hospitalization. With fibric acid therapy and 10 mg/day of a statin, her triglyceride level was 360 mg/dL; LDL cholesterol, 75 mg/dL; and HDL cholesterol, 35 mg/dL. After much deliberation, she began treatment with 0.1 mg of a patch estrogen for her menopausal symptoms, and her lipids remained in a similar range. Her glucose level also remained normal.

This case illustrates the serious consequences of oral estrogen treatment in a woman with underlying hypertriglyceridemia, and it also shows that such women can often be safely treated with patch estrogen. The severe hypertriglyceridemia is due to the fact that the "first pass" of oral estrogen through the liver increases triglyceride secretion.

Evidence-Based Summary

- Low HDL cholesterol is a risk factor for CAD, and high HDL cholesterol levels are protective. Currently, most therapies focus on reducing LDL cholesterol, with the recognition that some medications (e.g., niacin and, to a lesser degree, statins and fibrates) also raise HDL cholesterol levels. Nevertheless, interventions that raise HDL levels reduce CAD risks. By comparison, dietary interventions that focus on reduction of total and saturated fat commonly reduce HDL cholesterol levels; diets that substitute unsaturated fatty acids may provide benefits by offsetting this reduction in HDL cholesterol levels.
- The reduction in CAD associated with a reduction in LDL cholesterol levels closely parallels the curve describing the relationship between the LDL cholesterol level and CAD risk. Reductions in LDL cholesterol yield the predicted benefit regardless of whether they are achieved by diet or medications.
- Diets that decrease the intake of saturated fat, including *trans*-fatty acids, can lower the primary incidence of CAD and the risk of recurrent events in persons with existing CAD, with a benefit that is worth the cost.
- Reductions in LDL cholesterol levels with medications are associated with a reduced incidence of new-onset CAD and recurrent events in persons with CAD. These benefits extend to primary prevention in the setting of U.S. "average" LDL cholesterol levels and secondary prevention to reduce levels to below 100 mg/dL.
- The risk of CAD and hence the benefits of reducing LDL cholesterol levels are greater in patients with more CAD risk factors. As a result, the cost-effectiveness of lipid-lowering therapy depends on the patient's overall risk, as well as the LDL cholesterol lowering itself.
- Cholesterol-lowering medications in persons with existing CAD reap benefits at very reasonable costs, and in some cases they may save costs as well as lives. Primary prevention with medications is substantially more expensive, but the costs are likely to decline as the cost of medications declines. Niacin, because of its lower cost, is more cost-effective than statins, but it is oftentimes not as well tolerated. The choice of medications in specific patients must be individualized, and physicians should strive to use the most cost-effective regimens.
- Markedly elevated triglyceride levels are a risk factor for CAD, as well as for pancreatitis. Goals for reduction in triglyceride levels are guided by the ATP-III goals for non-HDL cholesterol, especially in patients with elevated LDL cholesterol levels. It is appropriate to address elevated triglyceride levels with weight loss, exercise, avoidance of alcohol and other agents that exacerbate hypertriglyceridemia, and, in high-risk situations, administration of triglyceride-lowering medications.

References

1. Knopp RH: Drug treatment of lipid disorders. N Engl J Med 1999;341:498–511.
2. Pearson TA, Laurora I, Chu H, Kafonek S: The Lipid Treatment Assessment Project (L-TAP): A multicenter survey to evaluate the percentages of dyslipidemic patients receiving lipid-lowering therapy and achieving low-density lipoprotein cholesterol goals. Arch Intern Med 2000; 160:459–467.
3. Yarzebski J, Spencer F, Goldberg RJ, et al: Temporal trends (1986–1997) in cholesterol level assessment and management practices in patients with acute myocardial infarction. Arch Intern Med 2001;161:1521–1528.
4. Executive Summary of the Third Report of the National Cholesterol Education Program (NCEP) Expert Panel on detection, evaluation, and treatment of high blood cholesterol in adults (Adult Treatment Panel III). JAMA 2001;285:2486–2497.
5. Pignone MP, Phillips CJ, Atkins D, et al: Screening and treating adults for lipid disorders. Am J Prev Med 2001; 20:77–89.
6. Miller M, Seidler A, Moalemi A, Pearson TA: Normal triglyceride levels and coronary artery disease events: The Baltimore Coronary Observational Long-Term Study. J Am Coll Cardiol 1998;31:1252–1257.
7. National Cholesterol Education Program: ATP III Guidelines At-A-Glance Quick Desk Reference. Bethesda, MD, National Institutes of Health, National Heart, Lung, and Blood Institute, 2001.
8. Assmann G, Schulte H, von Eckardstein A: Hypertriglyceridemia and elevated lipoprotein(a) are risk factors for major coronary events in middle-aged men. Am J Cardiol 1996;77:1179–1184.
9. Danesh J, Collins R, Peto R: Lipoprotein(a) and coronary heart disease: Meta-analysis of prospective studies. Circulation 2000;102:1082–1085.
10. Knopp RH, Walden CE, Retzlaff BM, et al: Long-term cholesterol-lowering effects of 4 fat-restricted diets in hypercholesterolemic and combined hyperlipidemic men. The Dietary Alternatives Study. JAMA 1997;278:1509–1515.
11. Knopp RH, Retzlaff B, Walden C, et al: One-year effects of increasingly fat-restricted, carbohydrate-enriched diets

on lipoprotein levels in free-living subjects. Proc Soc Exp Biol Med 2000;225:191–199.

12. Walden CE, Retzlaff BM, Buck BL, et al: Differential effect of National Cholesterol Education Program (NCEP) Step II diet on HDL cholesterol, its subfractions, and apoprotein A-I levels in hypercholesterolemic women and men after 1 year: The beFIT Study. Arterioscler Thromb Vasc Biol 2000;20:1580–1587.
13. Krauss RM, Eckel RH, Howard B, et al: AHA Dietary Guidelines: Revision 2000: A statement for healthcare professionals from the Nutrition Committee of the American Heart Association. Circulation 2000;102:2284–2299.
14. Oomen CM, Ocké MC, Feskens EJM, et al: Association between trans fatty acid intake and 10-year risk of coronary heart disease in the Zutphen Elderly Study: A prospective population-based study. Lancet 2001;357: 746–751.
15. De Lorgeril M, Salen P, Martin J-L, et al: Mediterranean diet, traditional risk factors, and the rate of cardiovascular complications after myocardial infarction: Final report of the Lyon Diet Heart Study. Circulation 1999;99:779–785.
16. Harper CR, Jacobson TA: The fats of life: The role of omega-3 fatty acids in the prevention of coronary heart disease. Arch Intern Med 2001;161:2185–2192.
17. Piscitelli SC, Gallicano KD: Interactions among drugs for HIV and opportunistic infections. N Engl J Med 2001;344: 984–996.
18. Ballantyne CM, Pazzucconi F, Pinto X, et al: Efficacy and tolerability of fluvastatin extended-release delivery system: A pooled analysis. Clin Ther 2001;23:177–192.
19. LaRosa JC, He J, Supputuri S: Effect of statins on risk of coronary disease: A meta-analysis of randomized controlled trials. JAMA 1999;282:2340–2346.
20. Schwartz GG, Olsson AG, Ezekowitz MD, et al: Effects of atorvastatin on early recurrent ischemic events in acute coronary syndromes: The MIRACL study: A randomized controlled trial. JAMA 2001;285:1711–1718.
21. Canner PL, Berge KG, Wenger NK, et al: Fifteen year mortality in Coronary Drug Project patients: Long-term benefit with niacin. J Am Coll Cardiol 1986;8:1245–1255.
22. Brown G, Albers JJ, Fisher LD, et al: Regression of coronary artery disease as a result of intensive lipid-lowering therapy in men with high levels of apolipoprotein B. N Engl J Med 1990;323:1289–1298.
23. Blankenhorn DH, Nessim SA, Johnson RL, et al: Beneficial effects of combined colestipol-niacin therapy on coronary atherosclerosis and coronary venous bypass grafts. JAMA 1987;257:3233–3240.
24. Zhao XQ, Brown BG, Chait A, et al: Simvastatin and niacin, antioxidant vitamins, or the combination for the prevention of coronary disease. N Engl J Med 2001;345: 1583–1592.
25. Elam MB, Hunninghake DB, Davis KB, et al: Effect of niacin on lipid and lipoprotein levels and glycemic control in patients with diabetes and peripheral arterial disease. The ADMIT Study: A randomized trial. JAMA 2000;284: 1263–1270.
26. Frick MH, Elo O, Haapa K, et al: Helsinki Heart Study: Primary-prevention trial with gemfibrozil in middle-aged men with dyslipidemia. N Engl J Med 1987;317:1237–1245.
27. Rubins HB, Robins SJ, Collins D, et al: Gemfibrozil for the secondary prevention of coronary heart disease in men with low levels of high-density lipoprotein cholesterol. Veterans Affairs High-Density Lipoprotein Cholesterol Intervention Trial Study Group. N Engl J Med 1999; 341:410–418.
28. Robins SJ, Collins D, Wittes JT, et al: Relation of gemfibrozil treatment and lipid levels with major coronary events: VA-HIT: A randomized controlled trial. JAMA 2001;285:1585–1591.
29. Diabetes Atherosclerosis Intervention Study Investigators: Effect of fenofibrate on progression of coronary-artery disease in type 2 diabetes: The Diabetes Atherosclerosis Intervention Study, a randomised study. Lancet 2001;357: 905–910.
30. Lipid Research Clinics Program: The Lipid Research Clinics Coronary Primary Prevention Trial Results. II. The relationship of reduction in incidence of coronary heart disease to cholesterol lowering. JAMA 1984;251:365–374.
31. Davidson MH, Dillon MA, Gordon B, et al: Colesevelam hydrochloride (CholestaGel): A new, potent bile acid sequestrant associated with a low incidence of gastrointestinal side effects. Arch Intern Med 1999;159:1893–1900.
32. Cater N: Historical and scientific basis for the development of plant stanol ester foods as cholesterol-lowering agents. Eur Heart J 1999;1(Suppl):36–44.
33. Dujovne CA, Bays H, Davidson MH, et al: Reduction of LDL cholesterol in patients with primary hypercholesterolemia by SCH 48461: Results of a multicenter dose-ranging study. J Clin Pharmacol 2001;41:70–78.
34. Heart Protection Collaborative Group: HRC/BHF heart protection study of cholesterol lowering with simvastatin in 20,536 high risk individuals. Lancet 2002;360:7–22.
35. Grover SA, Coupal L, Zowall H, Doras M: Cost-effectiveness of treating hyperlipidemia in the presence of diabetes. Who should be treated? Circulation 2000;102: 722–727.
36. Prosser LA, Stinnett AA, Goldman PA, et al: Cost-effectiveness of cholesterol-lowering therapies according to selected patient characteristics. Ann Intern Med 2000; 132:769–779.

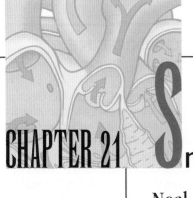

Smoking and Smoking Cessation

Neal L. Benowitz

EPIDEMIOLOGY AND ADVERSE EFFECTS

In the United States, approximately 25% of adults smoke cigarettes. Other forms of tobacco use in the United States include pipes and cigars (approximately 9% of men) and smokeless tobacco (snuff and chewing tobacco, 5.5% of men and 1% of women).

Tobacco smoke is an aerosol of droplets (particulates) containing water, tar, nicotine, and other alkaloids. It also contains several thousand different chemicals, many of which may contribute to human disease. With respect to cardiovascular disease, the chemicals of main concern have been oxidant gases, carbon monoxide, and nicotine.

Cigarette smoking is responsible for more than 400,000 premature deaths in the United States yearly, one third of which are deaths from cardiovascular disease. A lifelong smoker has a one in two chance of dying prematurely of a complication of smoking. Cigar and pipe smoking have been associated with an increased risk of coronary heart disease, whereas in most studies smokeless tobacco has not.

Cigarette smoking accounts for about 20% of cardiovascular deaths in the United States. Risk is increased for coronary heart disease, sudden death, cerebrovascular disease, and peripheral vascular disease, including aortic aneurysm. Cigarette smoking accelerates atherosclerosis and promotes acute ischemic events. The mechanisms of the effects of cigarette smoking are believed to include the following:

1. Endothelial dysfunction due to a reduced release of nitric oxide and the resulting impairment in vasodilatation
2. Development of an atherogenic lipid profile (smokers have, on average, higher low-density lipoprotein [LDL] cholesterol levels, more oxidized LDL, and lower high-density lipoprotein cholesterol levels than nonsmokers do)
3. Enhanced coagulability
4. Relative hypoxemia because of the effects of carbon monoxide
5. Hemodynamic stress because nicotine increases the heart rate and transiently increases blood pressure
6. Arrhythmogenesis, presumed to be related to catecholamine release, aggravation of myocardial ischemia, or both[1]

Carbon monoxide reduces the capacity of hemoglobin to carry oxygen and impairs the release of oxygen from hemoglobin to body tissues, both of which combine to result in a state of relative hypoxemia. In compensation for the reduced oxygen-carrying capacity, polycythemia often develops in smokers, with hematocrit values commonly reaching 50% or higher. This polycythemia, along with the increased fibrinogen levels found in cigarette smokers, increases blood viscosity, which adds to the risk of thrombotic events. Cigarette smoking also induces a chronic inflammatory state, as evidenced by increased blood levels of C-reactive protein. This chronic inflammation is thought to contribute to atherogenesis.

Cigarette smoking acts synergistically with other cardiac risk factors to increase the risk of ischemic heart disease. Although the risk of cardiovascular disease is roughly proportional to cigarette consumption, the risk persists even at levels as low as one to two cigarettes per day. Cigarette smoking reduces exercise tolerance in patients with angina pectoris and intermittent claudication. In patients who smoke, vasospastic angina is more common, and the response to vasodilator medications is impaired. In patients with coronary heart disease, the number of episodes and the total duration of ischemic episodes, as assessed by ambulatory electrocardiographic (ECG) monitoring, are substantially increased by cigarette smoking. The increase in the relative risk of coronary heart disease because of cigarette smoking is greatest in young adults, who would have a relatively low risk in the absence of cigarette smoking. Women who use oral contraceptives and smoke cigarettes have a synergistically increased risk of both myocardial infarction (MI) and stroke. Cigarette smoking is not a risk factor for hypertension per se, but it does increase the risk of complications, including the development of nephrosclerosis and progression to malignant hypertension.

After acute MI, the risk of recurrent MI is higher and survival is reduced by 50% over the next 12 years in persistent smokers as compared with quitters. After thrombolysis, the reocclusion rate is fourfold higher in smokers who continue than in those who quit. The risk of reocclusion of a coronary artery after angioplasty or occlusion of a bypass graft is increased in smokers. Smoking cessation reduces the excess risk of MI by 50% within 2 years of quitting. For persons who have quit for 10 to 14 years, their general cardiovascular risk declines to that of people who have never smoked.

Recently, cigarette smoking has been implicated as a contributor to morbidity and mortality in patients with left ventricular dysfunction,[2] with about a 40% increase in all-cause mortality, hospitalization, and MI in cigarette smokers. By comparison, risks in ex-smokers with left ventricular dysfunction appear to be similar to those who never smoked. In patients with heart failure, the magnitude of the reduction in mortality attributable to smoking cessation (30%) is at least comparable to the reduction in mortality associated with angiotensin-converting enzyme inhibitors, beta-blockers, or spironolactone (see Chapter 28).

Chewing tobacco and snuff deliver as much nicotine to the circulation as cigarette smoking does, and they are also a source of considerable sodium because of the addition of sodium bicarbonate as a buffer to facilitate nicotine absorption through the buccal mucosa. Smokeless tobacco does not, however, expose smokers to combustion gases. Smokeless tobacco can aggravate hypertension as a result of the sympathomimetic effects of nicotine, the effects of glycyrrhizinic acid (a potent mineralocorticoid found in licorice that is used to flavor some smokeless tobacco), and the increased sodium intake. The sodium load can also aggravate heart failure (see Chapter 28) and other edematous states (see Chapter 8).

ADDICTION TO NICOTINE AND SMOKING

Tobacco dependence has features of a chronic disease in that most users persist for many years and frequently cycle through episodes of cessation and relapse before they finally quit. Tobacco use is motivated primarily by the desire for nicotine. Drug addiction is defined as compulsive use of a psychoactive substance, the consequences of which are detrimental to the individual or society. Compulsive use is illustrated by the fact that 70% of smokers want to quit and 46% try to quit each year. Unfortunately, because of addiction, only 3% successfully quit each year.

Understanding addiction is useful in providing effective smoking cessation therapy.[3] Nicotine is absorbed rapidly from tobacco smoke into the pulmonary circulation; it then moves quickly to the brain, where it acts on nicotinic cholinergic receptors to produce its gratifying effects, which occur within 10 to 15 seconds after a puff. Smokeless tobacco is absorbed more slowly and results in less intense acute pharmacologic effects. With long-term use of tobacco, physical dependence develops and is associated with an increased number of nicotinic cholinergic receptors in the brain. When tobacco is unavailable, even for only a few hours, withdrawal symptoms often occur, including anxiety, irritability, difficulty concentrating, restlessness, hunger, craving for tobacco, disturbed sleep, and in some people, depression.

Addiction to tobacco is multifactorial, including a desire for the direct pharmacologic actions of nicotine, relief of withdrawal symptoms, and learned associations. Smokers report a variety of reasons for smoking, including pleasure, arousal, enhanced vigilance, improved performance, relief of anxiety or depression, reduced hunger, and control of body weight. Environmental cues—such as a meal, a cup of coffee, talking on the phone, an alcoholic beverage, or friends who smoke—often trigger an urge to smoke.

Smoking and depression are strongly linked in that smokers are more likely to have a history of major depression than nonsmokers are. Smokers with a history of depression are also likely to be more highly dependent on nicotine and have a lower likelihood of quitting. When they do quit, depression is more apt to be a prominent withdrawal symptom.

MANAGEMENT

Treatment of tobacco dependence should be viewed as a combination of behavioral modification and pharmacologic support. Evidence-based guidelines for the treatment of tobacco emphasize the identification of all tobacco users in a physician's practice and ascertaining each patient's intent with respect to quitting smoking[4,5] (Fig. 21–1). Identification of tobacco use is facilitated by the implementation of an office-based system so that

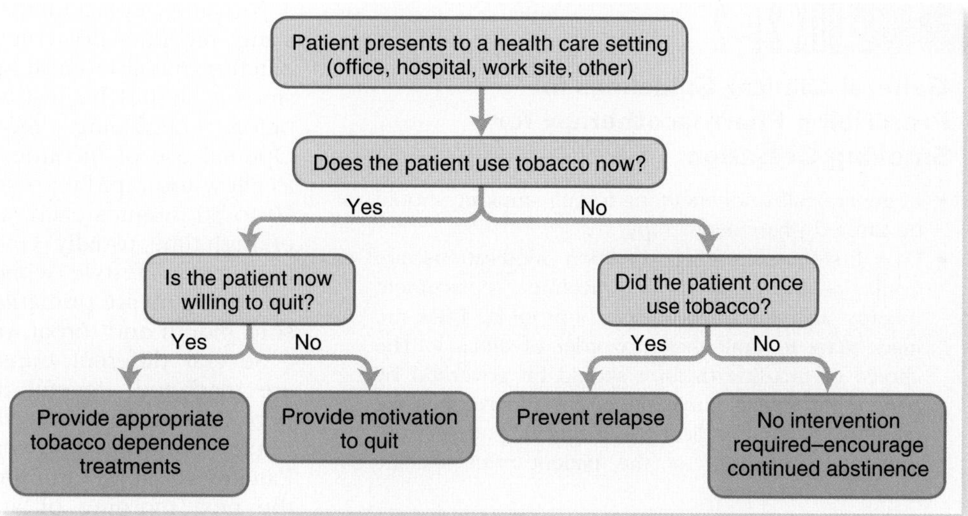

FIGURE 21–1. Algorithm for treating tobacco use.

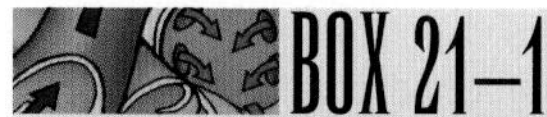

BOX 21–1

Brief Strategies to Help Patients Willing to Quit Tobacco Use—The "Five A's"

STRATEGIES FOR IMPLEMENTATION	ACTION
Ask—Systematically identify all tobacco users at every visit.	Implement an office-wide system that ensures that for every patient at every clinic visit, tobacco use status is queried and documented.
Advise—Strongly urge all tobacco users to quit.	In a clear, strong, and personalized manner, urge every tobacco user to quit.
Assess—Determine the patient's willingness to make an attempt at quitting.	Ask all tobacco users if they are willing to make an attempt at quitting at this time (e.g., within the next 30 days).
Assist—Aid the patient in quitting.	Help the patient with a plan for quitting. Provide practical counseling (problem-solving/skills training). Provide intratreatment social support. Help the patient obtain extratreatment social support. Recommend the use of approved pharmacotherapy except in special circumstances.
Arrange—Schedule follow-up contact.	Schedule follow-up contact, either in person or via telephone.

Adapted from A clinical practice guideline for treating tobacco use and dependence: A U.S. Public Health Service Report.[4]

patients are regularly queried about tobacco use at every visit. Tobacco use should be treated as a vital sign by using tobacco status stickers on patients' charts, electronic medical records, or computer reminder systems. The practice of routinely recording a patient's tobacco use status increases the odds ratio for quitting by twofold.

Brief strategies to help a patient quit (the "five A's"—Box 21–1), which can be implemented in as little as 3 minutes, increase cessation rates significantly. In a meta-analysis of 31 trials, brief physician advice increased quit rates by 70%.[5] Intensive behavioral treatment of tobacco dependence produces higher success rates than brief advice does and is cost-effective. However, these intensive programs are less widely available and may be less acceptable to patients than brief interventions. Nevertheless, clinicians with training in intensive smoking cessation therapy should be identified as a referral source for smokers who are interested.

A recent Public Health Service guideline recommends that all smokers trying to quit should be offered pharmacotherapy[4] (Box 21–2). In brief, two types of medications have been approved by the U.S. Food and Drug Administration (FDA) for smoking cessation—bupropion, which was originally marketed as an antidepressant drug, and nicotine (Table 21–1). Bupropion (approved only in sustained-release form) and nicotine (approved in various delivery forms) work primarily to relieve withdrawal symptoms and, to some extent, to reduce craving. Other drugs such as nortriptyline and clonidine have been shown in clinical trials to be effective in aiding smoking cessation but have not been approved by the FDA for this purpose. These

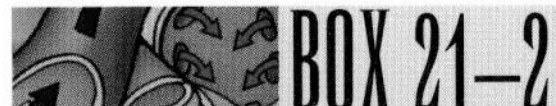
BOX 21–2

General Clinical Guidelines for Prescribing Pharmacotherapy for Smoking Cessation

- In general, all smokers trying to quit smoking should be offered pharmacotherapy.
- Five first-line smoking cessation medications are available—four types of nicotine replacement therapy and sustained-release bupropion. Data are inadequate to rank these in order of efficacy. The choice of first-line therapy should be governed by patient preference, familiarity of the clinician with the medication, contraindications in specific patients, and previous experience of the patient with specific pharmacotherapies.
- Second-line therapies include clonidine and nortriptyline. These drugs should be reserved for individuals with contraindications or failure of response to first-line medications.
- Several pharmacotherapies may delay, but not prevent weight gain after smoking cessation. It is recommended that patients start or increase physical activity, but strict dieting is discouraged because it appears to increase the likelihood of relapse to smoking. Patients should be reassured that weight gain after quitting is self-limited and poses much less of a risk to health than smoking does.
- Transdermal nicotine (patches) and nicotine gum appear to be safe for patients with chronic cardiovascular disease. Other medications are probably much safer than smoking in the presence of medical disease, but need further evaluation.
- In smokers with prolonged withdrawal symptoms or in an individual who is unable not to smoke in the absence of medication, long-term therapy with nicotine replacement medication or bupropion appears to be safe and reasonable.
- Research suggests that combining bupropion with nicotine patches or combining nicotine patches with ad libitum use of nicotine gum or nicotine nasal spray increases abstinence rates, compared with the rates produced by a single form of therapy.

Adapted from A clinical practice guideline for treating tobacco use and dependence: A U.S. Public Health Service Report.[4]

drugs tend to have greater side effects and are therefore viewed as second-line agents.

All of the pharmacologic treatments have been demonstrated in clinical trials to increase quitting rates, on average twofold, when compared with placebo treatment.[4,5] The absolute magnitude of the quit rates, which range from 3% to 15% in various studies, depend on the level of behavioral therapy and the characteristics of the smokers. Thus, pharmacotherapy combined with intensive behavioral therapy can result in quit rates as high as 30%.

Nicotine replacement medications include 2- and 4-mg nicotine polacrilex gum, transdermal nicotine patches, nicotine nasal spray, and nicotine inhalers. A smoker should be instructed to quit smoking entirely before beginning nicotine replacement therapy. Optimal use of nicotine gum includes instructions not to chew too rapidly, to chew 8 to 10 pieces per day for 20 to 30 minutes each, and to use the gum for a long enough time, usually 3 months or longer, for the smoker to learn a lifestyle without cigarettes. Side effects of nicotine gum are primarily local and include jaw fatigue, sore mouth and throat, upset stomach, and hiccups.

Several different transdermal nicotine preparations are marketed—several deliver 21 mg over a 24-hour period, and one delivers 15 mg over a period of 16 hours. Most have lower dose patches for tapering. Patches are applied in the morning and removed either the next morning or at bedtime, depending on the patch. Patches intended for 24-hour use can also be removed at bedtime if the patient is experiencing insomnia or disturbing dreams. Full-dose patches are recommended for most smokers for the first 1 to 3 months, followed by one to two tapering doses for 2 to 4 weeks each. Nicotine nasal spray, one spray into each nostril, delivers about 0.5 mg of nicotine systemically and can be used every 30 to 60 minutes. Local irritation of the nose commonly produces burning, sneezing, and watery eyes during initial treatment, but tolerance to these effects develops in 1 to 2 days. The nicotine inhaler actually delivers nicotine to the throat and upper airway, from which it is absorbed similar to nicotine from chewing gum. The inhaler is marketed as a cigarette-like plastic device and can be used ad libitum.

Bupropion is administered at 150 to 300 mg/day for 7 days before stopping smoking and then at 300 mg/day for the next 6 to 12 weeks.[6,7] Bupropion can also be used in combination with a nicotine patch. In excessive doses, bupropion can cause seizures, and it should not be used in individuals with a history of seizures or eating disorders (bulimia or anorexia). On average, nicotine medications or bupropion treatment doubles the cessation rates achieved with placebo treatment, and absolute rates of smoking cessation have increased from 12% (placebo) to 24% (active medication) in clinical trials.

Treating Tobacco Dependence in Patients with Cardiovascular Disease

For patients who have cardiovascular disease, smoking cessation is an imperative. The risks of smoking and, conversely, the benefits to be gained by quitting smoking are much greater in patients with cardiovascular disease than in those without such disease. However, physicians and patients have feared that nicotine may aggravate myocardial ischemia or peripheral vascular disease. Fortunately, postmarketing surveillance by the FDA found no evidence that nicotine patches increase the risk of MI.

TABLE 21–1

Suggestions for the Clinical Use of Pharmacotherapies for Smoking Cessation

Pharmacotherapy	Precautions/ Contraindications	Adverse Effects	Dosage	Duration	Availability	Cost Per Day
			First-line			
Sustained-release bupropion hydrochloride	History of seizure History of eating disorders	Insomnia Dry mouth	150 mg every morning for 3 days, then 150 mg twice daily (begin treatment 1–2 wk before quitting)	7–12 wk maintenance, up to 6 mo	Prescription only	$3.33
Nicotine gum	Temporomandibular joint disorder	Mouth soreness Dyspepsia	1–24 cigarettes/day: 2-mg gum (up to 24 pieces/day) ≥25 cigarettes/day: 4-mg gum (up to 24 pieces/day)	Up to 12 wk	OTC only	$6.25 for 10 2-mg pieces $6.87 for 10 4-mg pieces
Nicotine inhaler		Local irritation of mouth and throat	6–16 cartridges/day	Up to 6 mo	Prescription only	$10.94 for 10 cartridges
Nicotine nasal spray	Chronic nasal disorders, including rhinitis, polyps, and sinusitis	Nasal irritation Throat burning	8–40 doses/day	3–6 mo	Prescription only	$5.40 for 12 doses
Nicotine patch	Skin diseases such as atopic or eczematous dermatitis	Local skin reaction Insomnia	21 mg/24 hr 14 mg/24 hr 7 mg/24 hr 15 mg/16 hr	4 wk 2 wk 2 wk 8 wk	Prescription and OTC	$4.22 $4.51
			Second-line			
Clonidine	Rebound hypertension	Dry mouth Drowsiness Dizziness Sedation	0.15–0.75 mg/day	3–10 wk	Prescription only (oral formulation) Prescription only (patch)	$0.24 for 0.2 mg $3.50
Nortriptyline	Risk of arrhythmias	Sedation Dry mouth	75–100 mg/day	12 wk	Prescription only	$0.74 for 75 mg

OTC, over the counter.

Adapted from The Tobacco Use and Dependence Clinical Practice Guideline Panel, Staff, and Consortium Representatives: A clinical practice guideline for treating tobacco use and dependence. A US Public Health Service Report. JAMA 2000;283:3244–3254.

Several clinical studies have confirmed the relative safety of nicotine patches in patients with cardiovascular disease. In one study of 36 male smokers with severe coronary disease awaiting bypass surgery, sequential treatment with 21- and 14-mg nicotine patches significantly reduced the size of exercise-induced perfusion defects on quantitative thallium 201 single-photon emission computed tomography, even though most patients continued to smoke, albeit fewer cigarettes per day.[8] Despite increased plasma nicotine levels with the 14- and 21-mg patches versus smoking alone, no patient had a significant increase in myocardial ischemia while using the patches. The progressive reduction in the size of exercise-induced perfusion defects with higher nicotine doses was most closely related to the reduction in blood carboxyhemoglobin concentration, which decreased as a consequence of smoking fewer cigarettes. This study suggests that carbon monoxide or some other component of tobacco smoke rather than nicotine is most important in limiting myocardial nutrient supply in patients with coronary heart disease.

Two randomized trials and one case-control study have found transdermal nicotine to be safe in patients with cardiovascular disease. In a 5-week, placebo-controlled trial of 14 to 21 mg of transdermal nicotine per day in 156 patients with stable coronary artery disease, quit rates were low, so there was much concomitant smoking and patch use in each group.[9] The frequency of angina declined in the nicotine and placebo groups, with no difference between treatments. Ambulatory ECG monitoring revealed no differences in arrhythmias or ST segment changes in nicotine-treated versus placebo-treated patients. In a large Veterans Affairs cooperative study, 584 smokers with cardiovascular disease were treated with a 10-week course of either transdermal nicotine (beginning with 21 mg/day and tapering to 7 mg/day) or placebo.[10] Many participants continued to smoke during the study. The incidence of the primary outcome of death, MI, cardiac arrest, hospitalization for increased severity of angina, arrhythmias, or heart failure was similar in both groups. Most recently, a case-control study found no evidence of any increased risk of MI with the use of nicotine patches.[11]

Some pharmacologic considerations are useful in understanding the relative safety of nicotine in cardiovascular disease.[1] In general, nicotine medications deliver less nicotine than cigarette smoking does. The nicotine from cigarette smoke is absorbed rapidly into the lungs, from which it quickly reaches the arterial circulation and the heart, where it acts at high concentrations. Nicotine levels from slow-release drug delivery forms such as patches and gum result in much lower arterial concentrations and, therefore, less intense acute cardiovascular effects. Furthermore, substantial tolerance develops over time to many of the cardiovascular effects of nicotine. Thus, the cardiovascular effects of nicotine in doses as high as 66 mg transdermally (three patches) concomitant with cigarette smoking are no greater than the effects of cigarette smoking without nicotine patches.[12] Finally, cigarette smoking delivers not only nicotine but also other known cardiovascular toxins, such as carbon monoxide and oxidant gases. Cigarette smoking induces a hypercoagulable state, most likely related to the effects of oxidant gases, whereas nicotine alone does not.

The bottom line is that nicotine replacement therapy is much less hazardous than cigarette smoking. For individuals who need nicotine replacement therapy to stop smoking, the benefits far outweigh the risks, even in patients with severe cardiovascular disease and even if some smoking continues after the nicotine is started.

Less research has been conducted on the cardiovascular safety of bupropion in patients with cardiovascular disease. Bupropion is a sympathomimetic drug that can increase blood pressure and the heart rate in some patients. As a result, sufficient hypertension to require that bupropion be discontinued develops in some patients with cardiovascular disease.

Based on clinical evidence, it seems most reasonable to use nicotine replacement therapy as first-line therapy in patients with cardiovascular disease. If nicotine replacement fails or is not tolerated, bupropion, with careful monitoring of blood pressure, is an effective second choice.

Hospitalized Cardiovascular Patients

Hospitalized patients with cardiovascular disease are usually concerned about their health in the context of an acute illness, so the benefits of smoking cessation are likely to be perceived as more personal. As a result, hospitalized patients tend to be more highly motivated to quit smoking. In the United States, hospitals are smoke free, so smokers are, at least temporarily, in a smoke-free environment. Clinical trials of smoking cessation targeted to hospitalized smokers indicate a significant benefit in comparison to usual care.[13,14] Smoking cessation treatment can be provided by physicians, nurses, or smoking cessation counselors. Patients should be offered the option of pharmacotherapy, either while they are in the hospital or at discharge.

The timing of medications to promote smoking cessation in patients with acute cardiovascular events warrants careful consideration. Pharmacotherapy has generally been avoided in patients with recent MI, unstable or refractory angina, or life-threatening arrhythmias. However, cigarette smoking is far worse than nicotine for such patients. If patients are able to stop smoking only with nicotine medication, nicotine should be prescribed, regardless of the acuity of the cardiovascular condition. If the patient is having difficulty quitting smoking in the hospital, nicotine can be prescribed at that time. If the patient is able to abstain from smoking for several days in the hospital and then chooses to begin nicotine therapy at discharge or shortly thereafter, it is best to start such therapy at lower doses because some of the tolerance to nicotine will have been lost while the patient was not smoking in the hospital.

Cost-Effectiveness

A number of analyses confirm that smoking cessation therapy is effective and cost-effective. Assuming that brief physician counseling result in a quit rate of just 4.5%, the average cost per year of life saved has been estimated to be about $400 to $600 for men and about $750 to $950 for women, depending on age.[15] Incremental costs for adding a full course of nicotine patch therapy have ranged from $1800 to $2000 per year of life saved for men and $3000 to $4000 per year of life saved for women. Another analysis based on the cost of a specialized smoking clinic that offered both inpatient and outpatient smoking cessation treatments estimated an average cost of about $7000 per year of life saved.[16]

In the presence of cardiovascular disease, smoking cessation interventions are even more cost-effective because the benefit is greater. One analysis of the cost-effectiveness of a smoking cessation program after MI found that a nurse-managed program cost about $220 per year of life saved.[17] These costs per year of life saved, for individuals both with and without cardiovascular disease, are considerably lower than the cost per year of life saved for most accepted medical interventions, so smoking cessation treatment, with or without medication, is one of the most effective uses of health care resources.[18, 19]

Evidence-Based Summary

Brief Physician Advice

Brief physician advice to stop smoking has been examined in a systematic review of 31 trials involving 26,000 smokers in primary care, hospital wards, and outpatient clinics.[5] Brief advice significantly increased the odds of quitting by about 70%.

Intensive Counseling

Intensive counseling enhanced quit rates above those of brief counseling.[5] A systematic review of nine studies found that the odds of quitting significantly increased by 55% with intensive counseling versus brief advice or usual care.

Nicotine Replacement Medication

A systematic review of 90 clinical trials of nicotine chewing gum, transdermal patches, nasal spray, inhalers, sublingual tablets, and lozenges (the latter two of which are not yet available in the United States) found that the odds of quitting significantly increased by about 70% when compared with placebo.[5] For specific nicotine formulations, the data are as follows: nicotine gum, 48 trials involving 16,706 subjects, odds ratio of 1.63 (95% confidence interval [CI], 1.49 to 1.79); nicotine patches, 31 trials involving 15,777 subjects, odds ratio of 1.75 (CI, 1.57 to 1.94); nicotine nasal spray, 4 trials involving 887 subjects, odds ratio of 2.27 (CI, 1.61 to 3.20); and nicotine inhaler, 4 trials involving 976 subjects, odds ratio of 2.08 (CI, 1.43 to 3.04).

The available data indicate that the efficacy of different forms of nicotine replacement therapy is similar, so product selection should be guided by the preference of the patient and by the presence of medical contraindications. The few trials of a combination of nicotine products (e.g., nicotine patch plus gum or nasal spray) usually find incremental benefit when compared with a single preparation alone.

Bupropion

A systematic review of data from two large published trials and two small unpublished trials of bupropion plus behavioral counseling found that the odds of quitting increased significantly by nearly threefold.[5] One clinical trial found a greater cessation rate with a combination of bupropion and transdermal nicotine than with either agent alone.

Other Smoking Cessation Medications

Nortriptyline was found in two studies to increase the odds of quitting by nearly fourfold.[5] A systematic review of six clinical trials of clonidine found nearly a twofold increase in the odds of quitting, but the incidence of side effects was high, including sedation and orthostatic hypotension. Neither nortriptyline nor clonidine is approved for smoking cessation in the United States.

References

1. Benowitz NL, Gourlay SG: Cardiovascular toxicity of nicotine: Implications for nicotine replacement therapy. J Am Coll Cardiol 1997;29:1422–1431.
2. Suskin N, Sheth T, Negassa A, Yusuf S: Relationship of current and past smoking to mortality and morbidity in patients with left ventricular dysfunction. J Am Coll Cardiol 2001;37:1677–1682.
3. Benowitz NL: Nicotine addiction. Prim Care 1999;26:611–631.
4. The Tobacco Use and Dependence Clinical Practice Guideline Panel, Staff, and Consortium Representatives: A clinical practice guideline for treating tobacco use and

dependence. A US Public Health Service Report. JAMA 2000;283:3244–3254.

5. Lancaster T, Stead L, Silagy C, Sowden A: Effectiveness of interventions to help people stop smoking: Findings from the Cochrane Library. BMJ 2000;321:355–358.
6. Tashkin DP, Kanner R, Bailey W, et al: Smoking cessation in patients with chronic obstructive pulmonary disease: A double-blind, placebo-controlled, randomised trial. Lancet 2001;357:1571–1575.
7. Jorenby DE, Leischow SJ, Nides MA, et al: A controlled trial of sustained-release bupropion, a nicotine patch, or both for smoking cessation. N Engl J Med 1999;340:685–691.
8. Mahmarian JJ, Moye LA, Nasser GA, et al: Nicotine patch therapy in smoking cessation reduces the extent of exercise-induced myocardial ischemia. J Am Coll Cardiol 1997;30:125–130.
9. Transdermal Nicotine Study Group: Transdermal nicotine for smoking cessation. JAMA 1991;266:3133–3138.
10. Joseph AM, Norman SM, Ferry LH, et al: The safety of transdermal nicotine as an aid to smoking cessation in patients with cardiac disease. N Engl J Med 1996;335: 1792–1798.
11. Kimmel SE, Berlin JA, Miles C, et al: Risk of acute first myocardial infarction and use of nicotine patches in a general population. J Am Coll Cardiol 2001;37:1297–1302.
12. Zevin S, Jacob P 3d, Benowitz NL: Dose-related cardiovascular and endocrine effects of transdermal nicotine. Clin Pharmacol Ther 1998;64:87–95.
13. Rigotti NA, Arnsten JH, McKool KM, et al: Efficacy of a smoking cessation program for hospital patients. Arch Intern Med 1997;157:2653–2660.
14. Simon JA, Solkowitz SN, Carmody TP, Browner WS: Smoking cessation after surgery. A randomized trial. Arch Intern Med 1997;157:1371–1376.
15. Wasley MA, McNagny SE, Phillips VL, Ahluwalia JS: The cost-effectiveness of the nicotine transdermal patch for smoking cessation. Prev Med 1997;26:264–270.
16. Croghan IT, Offord KP, Evans RW, et al: Cost-effectiveness of treating nicotine dependence: The Mayo Clinic experience. Mayo Clin Proc 1997;72:917–924.
17. Krumholz HM, Cohen BJ, Tsevat J, et al: Cost-effectiveness of a smoking cessation program after myocardial infarction. J Am Coll Cardiol 1993;22:1697–1702.
18. Rigotti N: Treatment of tobacco use and dependence. N Engl J Med 2002;346:506–512.
19. Karnath B: Smoking cessation. Am J Med 2002;112:399–405.

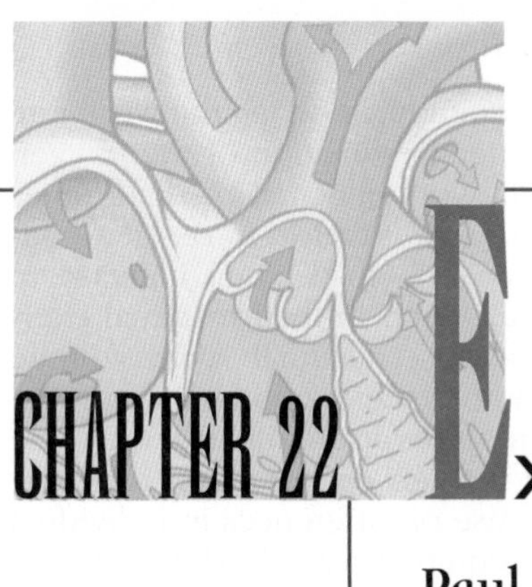

CHAPTER 22 Exercise and Heart Disease

Paul D. Thompson

The considerable benefits of vigorous physical activity and exercise are underestimated by most physicians, but overestimated by a few physicians and the general public. The human organism is extremely adaptable, and the somatic adaptations to chronic physical activity are one of the best manifestations of this plasticity. Regular physical exercise can increase muscle size and strength, bone density, maximal exercise and endurance capacity, cardiac dimensions and stroke volume, plasma volume, insulin sensitivity, high-density lipoprotein (HDL) cholesterol, and the skeletal muscle content of mitochondria and oxidative enzymes. A discussion of these adaptations is beyond the scope of this chapter, which will instead focus on what clinicians should understand (Box 22–1) to provide practical advice to their healthy patients and those with cardiac disease.[1]

EXERCISE PHYSIOLOGY AND THE PHYSIOLOGIC RESPONSE TO EXERCISE

Exercise requires an increase in oxygen uptake to meet the demands of exercising muscle. Oxygen uptake at any level of exercise is related to the cardiovascular system's ability to deliver oxygen and the exercising muscles' ability to consume it. The cardiovascular system's ability to deliver oxygen is dependent on cardiac output and the oxygen content of arterial blood.

The resting heart rate is determined by the parasympathetic nervous system and vagal tone. With the initiation of exercise, vagal tone is reduced and the heart rate increases. At approximately 50% of maximal exercise capacity, vagal influence is completely removed, and additional increases in heart rate are mediated by the sympathetic nervous system and circulating catecholamines. The maximal heart rate is generally estimated as age in years subtracted from 220 (220 – age), but the 95% confidence limits around this estimate are nearly ±40 beats per minute. The only accurate way to determine an individual's maximal heart rate is to perform a maximal exercise test, but patients who cannot reach their estimated maximal heart rate should be reassured that this "shortcoming" may be nothing more than normal individual variation.

Cardiac stroke volume and the arterial-venous oxygen difference ($PaO_2 - PvO_2$) increase acutely with exercise. $PaO_2 - PvO_2$ also widens during exercise for three reasons. First, exercising muscle extracts more oxygen than at rest, thereby reducing the oxygen content of the venous effluent from the muscular bed. Second, as cardiac output is redistributed from nonexercising tissue, such as the splanchnic bed, to the exercising musculature, more blood goes to active tissues that extract more oxygen. For example, approximately 25% of the resting cardiac output goes to the kidneys, but

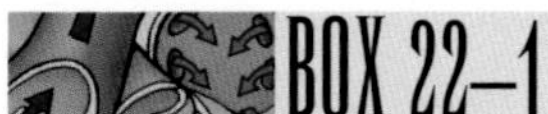

Definition of Terms and Concepts

Physical activity—any body movement required in daily living or as part of an exercise program

Exercise—physical activity undertaken for potential health benefits or to improve exercise capacity, although the terms *physical activity* and *exercise* can be used interchangeably

Exercise capacity—general exercise ability or the ability to perform a specified task

Physical fitness—overall exercise ability

Exercise training—a program of exercise designed to increase exercise capacity

Endurance exercise or *aerobic exercise*—repetitive motions against low-resistance: activities such as running, walking, cycling, and swimming

Strength exercise—repetitive muscle contractions against resistance; can be divided into

- *Isotonic* exercises such as weight lifting, where a fixed weight is moved through a range of motion
- *Isometric* exercise, in which the contraction is performed against any movable object

Resistance exercise training or *strength training*—an exercise program involving strength exercises and designed to increase skeletal muscle strength and size

Maximal exercise capacity—the highest amount of physical work that an individual can perform during an exercise test

Maximal oxygen uptake or *$\dot{V}O_2max$*—the greatest amount of oxygen that can be extracted from inspired air during an incremental exercise test and the physiologic measurement of maximal exercise capacity

Submaximal exercise—any exercise performed at a workload below maximal capacity

Endurance exercise capacity—an individual's ability to sustain either an aerobic or a strength exercise over time

One metabolic equivalent or *1 MET*—the amount of oxygen consumed at rest while seated, or approximately 3.5 mL/kg/min. METS are used to estimate endurance exercise workload

these small organs do not appreciably deplete the blood's oxygen content. Third, the arterial hemoglobin concentration increases during exercise because plasma volume is lost into the exercising muscle; this acute hemoconcentration explains the muscle swelling that occurs during exercise, a principle used by bodybuilders to maximize their muscles' size during competition.

Individuals differ in their exercise mechanical efficiency, and the most efficient exerciser consumes less oxygen during an exercise task. Despite this variation, a specific exercise task generally requires approximately the same oxygen uptake even when performed by different individuals. Consequently, knowing the work rate of exercise permits a general estimation of the oxygen required. The external work rate also determines cardiac output, and a 1-L/min increase in oxygen consumption should produce a 5- to 6-L/min increase in cardiac output. Individuals differ in their maximal exercise capacity primarily because maximal stroke volume and maximal cardiac output vary among individuals. The same physical task requires approximately the same absolute work rate and oxygen consumption in different individuals but, because of differences in individual exercise capacity, may require markedly different percentages of maximal exercise capacity (i.e., different relative work rates).

Identical external work rates can produce markedly different myocardial demand. Myocardial oxygen demand increases with increasing heart rate and systolic blood pressure; the product of heart rate multiplied by systolic blood pressure, which is termed the "rate-pressure product," is used clinically to estimate the myocardial oxygen demand of exertion. Both heart rate and systolic blood pressure increase linearly with an individual's relative work rate rather than with the absolute work rate. Consequently, identical external work rates can produce markedly different myocardial oxygen demands, depending on the individual's maximal exercise capacity. The implication of this observation is that a physical task requires less myocardial oxygen supply for a fit individual with high maximal exercise capacity than the same task requires for a less fit individual.

Maximal exercise capacity is determined by both cardiac and peripheral factors. Exercise performance is diminished by reductions in maximum heart rate and stroke volume from occult heart disease, a decrease in hemoglobin concentration from anemia, an inability to oxygenate red blood cells because of pulmonary disease, failure to shunt blood to exercising muscle, or muscle disease. Conversely, enhanced aerobic exercise capacity is almost always associated with superior cardiac performance and enhanced stroke volume. Superior exercise capacity is a marker of improved survival, probably because the heart has sufficient capacity to accept additional insult without the development of heart failure or other complications.

Strength training increases skeletal muscle size and strength, with little effect on maximal oxygen consumption and cardiac dimensions, whereas endurance exercise training increases maximal oxygen consumption and cardiac dimensions, with little effect on skeletal muscle size and strength. Aerobic activity reduces the risk of cardiovascular disease, but the role of strength training is uncertain.

The average increase in maximal oxygen consumption in healthy subjects after 3 to 12 months of training is approximately 20%.[2] Because exercise-induced increases in heart rate and systolic blood pressure are determined by the percent maximal capacity required and not by the absolute exercise workload itself, the same external workload or exercise task after training elicits smaller increments in heart rate and blood pressure.

PHYSICAL ACTIVITY FOR THE PREVENTION OF CORONARY HEART DISEASE

Essentially every study has shown that habitual physical activity reduces the incidence of coronary heart disease (CHD), regardless of whether physical activity is measured by type of employment, questionnaire, or performance on an exercise test. In a meta-analysis of published studies, being sedentary was associated with approximately twice the CHD risk as being active.[2] However, none of these studies are randomized trials, and individuals who choose physical activity may be innately different from sedentary individuals in other ways that explain their reduced risk. However, epidemiologic data remain the best evidence unless and until exercise is tested rigorously in a controlled trial.

More recent studies have addressed the issue of how much physical activity is required to reduce one's risk for CHD and whether there is a continuous relationship whereby more exercise is better or whether a threshold exists beyond which more exercise is no longer beneficial. Among 12,516 men in the Harvard Alumni Health Study, total physical activities requiring more than 6 metabolic equivalents (METs, see Table 25–1) were strongly associated with reduced cardiac events, whereas moderate (4 to 6 METs) and light (<4 METs) activity had no significant effect.[3] When compared with men who expended less than 500 kcal/wk, men expending 500 to 1000 kcal/wk experienced a 10% reduction, and men expending 1000 to 2000, 2000 to 3000, and over 3000 kcal/wk all had a similar 20% reduction. In women, 1 to 1.5 hours per week of walking is associated with lower CHD rates, independent of the pace of the walking.[4] These data suggest that benefit is gained from low levels of recreational activity, with a threshold effect at moderate levels of exertion, and that the accumulated energy expenditure is perhaps the most important factor.[5] As a result of this and other studies, the Centers for Disease Control and Prevention and the American College of Sports Medicine suggest that adults should perform 30 minutes of moderately intense physical activity on most and preferably all days of the week.[6]

The mechanism by which physical activity reduces CHD risk is not known. Regular exercise increases vagal tone and decreases the heart rate, changes associated with a decreased risk of malignant ventricular arrhythmia and sudden death.[7] Regular exercise may also directly increase coronary artery size, promote collateral vessel development, and improve coronary artery vasomotion.[8] Some of its benefits are also mediated by its effects on known CHD risk factors.

EXERCISE AS ADJUNCTIVE THERAPY FOR SELECTED RISK FACTORS

Exercise improves certain CHD risk factors, including triglycerides, HDL cholesterol, blood pressure, insulin insensitivity, and body weight. Some of the effects of exercise on such CHD risk factors as triglycerides, blood pressure, and insulin insensitivity do not require prolonged exercise training but occur acutely after a single exercise session and persist for several hours. However, exercise alone is rarely adequate therapy, except for mild abnormalities. In most patients, physical activity is best used as adjunctive therapy.

Blood Lipids (see Chapter 20)

Three to 6 months of exercise training reduces triglycerides, increases HDL cholesterol, and decreases low-density lipoprotein (LDL) cholesterol, but the average changes are small. A meta-analysis of 95 exercise training studies showed that the average change in HDL cholesterol was only +1.7 mg/dL[9] if subjects' body weight remained stable and +2.4 mg/dL if subjects lost weight. Triglycerides decreased 14 mg/dL in subjects who did not lose body weight and 21 mg/dL in subjects who lost weight; the changes in LDL cholesterol were −3 mg/dL and −11 mg/dL, respectively. By comparison, endurance athletes have HDL cholesterol concentrations 10 to 20 mg/dL higher than sedentary subjects and triglyceride levels 20 to 50 mg/dL lower.[10] Acute exercise in hypertriglyceridemic individuals can lower triglyceride levels by as much as 30% within hours, and walking at 30% of maximal exercise capacity for 2 hours decreases the appearance of postprandial triglycerides.[11] Consequently, an exercise regimen should be emphasized in patients with hypertriglyceridemia.

Blood Pressure (see Chapter 19)

Exercise training has a favorable, but modest antihypertensive effect that averages about a 5% reduction in systolic blood pressure and a 2% reduction in diastolic blood pressure[12]; the effect may be greater in hypertensive patients. Exercise also acutely reduces systolic blood pressure, an effect that can persist for up to 12 to 16 hours. As a result, some individuals with borderline or mild hypertension can normalize their blood pressure with daily or twice-daily exercise sessions. In most patients, however, exercise alone is unlikely to correct hypertension.

Blood Glucose and Insulin Sensitivity (see Chapter 23)

Habitual physical activity reduces the incidence of diabetes, and exercise training can improve insulin sensitivity and glucose control.[13,14] It is likely that the effect is greatest when vigorous exercise over a prolonged period of training is accompanied by weight loss. Patients with or at risk for type 2 diabetes should engage in an exercise program.

Body Weight (see Chapter 23)

The widespread availability of high caloric foods and the absence of physical activity explain why obesity is becoming an increasingly important problem in developed countries. Physical activity is an important part of weight reduction strategies and is commonly required for maintenance of lower body weight.

CARDIOVASCULAR RISKS OF EXERCISE IN APPARENTLY HEALTHY SUBJECTS

Although habitual physical activity reduces the incidence of CHD, vigorous exercise acutely increases the risk of myocardial infarction[15] (MI) and sudden cardiac death.[16]

TABLE 22–1

Cardiac Causes of Death in High-School and College Athletes ($N = 100$)

Cause of Death	Men	Women
Hypertrophic cardiomyopathy*	50	1
Probable hypertrophic cardiomyopathy	5	0
Coronary artery anomalies†	11	2
Myocarditis	7	—
Aortic stenosis	6	—
Cardiomyopathy	6	—
Atherosclerotic coronary disease	2	1
Aortic rupture	2	—
Subaortic stenosis	2	—
Coronary aneurysm	—	1
Mitral prolapse	1	—
Right ventricular dysplasia	—	1
Cerebral arteriovenous malformation	—	1
Subarachnoid hemorrhage	—	1

*Three also had coronary anomalies; one had Wolff-Parkinson-White syndrome.

†Includes anomalous left coronary artery (LCA) from the right sinus of Valsalva ($n = 4$), intramural left anterior descending (LAD) artery ($n = 4$), anomalous LCA from the pulmonary artery ($n = 2$), anomalous right coronary artery (RCA) from the left sinus ($n = 2$), hypoplastic RCA ($n = 2$), and ostial ridge of the LCA ($n = 2$). Three subjects with coronary anomalies also had hypertrophic cardiomyopathy and are tabulated with that group.

From Thompson PD: The cardiovascular risks of exercise. In Thompson PD (ed): Exercise and Sports Cardiology. New York, McGraw-Hill, 2000, pp 127–145.

Risk of Exertion for Children and Young Adults

Congenital and inherited cardiac abnormalities (see Chapter 34) and acquired myocarditis (see Chapter 29) are the predominant causes of exercise-related cardiac events in young individuals, usually defined as younger than 30 to 40 years (Table 22–1). Atherosclerotic disease is a rare cause of cardiac events in these subjects. The most common inherited cause of exercise deaths in young subjects in the United States is hypertrophic cardiomyopathy (see Chapter 29), but other congenital abnormalities such as coronary artery anomalies (see Chapter 34) and right ventricular dysplasia (see Chapter 30) are also frequently implicated.

The incidence of sudden death in young active subjects is low because of the low prevalence of these underlying abnormalities. Among high-school and college athletes, about one death occurs per year for every 133,000 males and 769,000 females within 1 hour of practice or competition.[17]

The rarity of exercise-related cardiac events in young subjects limits the value of any routine screening procedures. The American Heart Association currently recommends a personal and family history and physical examination before participation in high-school sports, as well as a repeat examination every 4 years by someone qualified to perform a cardiovascular examination and knowledgeable about the risks of exercise[18] (Box 22–2). For athletes with known cardiovascular disease, recommendations on eligibility for participation in competitive events are summarized in Table 22–2.[19]

BOX 22–2

Components of the Cardiovascular Preparticipation Screening

Questions should be asked about
- Exertional chest discomfort, syncope, dyspnea, and fatigue
- Individual history of cardiac murmurs, hypertension, or cardiac disease
- Family history of sudden death or conditions associated with sudden death

The physical examination should include
- Brachial artery blood pressure measurement
- Precordial auscultation with the athlete supine and standing
- Simultaneous palpation of radial and femoral pulses to exclude coarctation
- Inspection for stigmata of Marfan's syndrome

Adapted from Maron BJ, Thompson PD, Puffer JC, et al: Cardiovascular preparticipation screening of competitive athletes. A statement for health professionals from the Sudden Death Committee (clinical cardiology) and Congenital Cardiac Defects Committee (cardiovascular disease in the young), American Heart Association. Circulation 1996;94:850–856.

TABLE 22–2

Recommendations for Eligibility for Competition in Athletes with Several Common Cardiac Conditions*

Condition	Recommendation
Aortic stenosis	
Mild	No limitations
Moderate	Low-intensity† sports only, unless ETT demonstrates safety of moderate‡ activity
Severe	No competitive sports
Mitral valve prolapse	
No history of syncope, SVT, or VT; no family history of sudden death; no more than mild MR; no previous embolic events	No limitations
Any of the above	Low-intensity† sports only
Coronary artery disease§	
Normal resting EF, normal ETT, no known coronary stenoses >50% that have not been bypassed or dilated by angioplasty	Low-intensity† sports only unless ETT demonstrates safety of moderate‡ activity
Do not meet above criteria	Low-intensity† sports only; no competitive sports if exercise intolerance or exercise-induced arrhythmias

*These recommendations are for competitive athletes; more liberal recommendations may be appropriate for recreational activities in nonathletes.

†For example, bowling, golf.

‡For example, baseball, softball, table tennis, doubles tennis, volleyball.

§Even at the recommended level of exercise, these patients are at increased risk.

EF, ejection fraction; ETT, exercise tolerance test; MR, mitral regurgitation; SVT, supraventricular tachycardia; VT, ventricular tachycardia.

Adapted from the 26th Bethesda Conference: Recommendations for determining eligibility for competition in athletes with cardiovascular abnormalities. J Am Coll Cardiol 1994;24:845–899, *which includes full details for a wide range of cardiac conditions.*

Nevertheless, some advocate more extensive routine screening of competitive athletes. In an Italian study, 33,735 athletes were screened by electrocardiography and an exercise step test, with more formal exercise testing and echocardiography at the discretion of the examining physician. A total of 3016 were referred for echocardiography.[20] As a result, 621 athletes were denied permission to participate, with about 60% of the denials being due to cardiac issues, including 22 athletes with hypertrophic cardiomyopathy. Over an average of 8 years of follow-up, only 4 disqualified athletes died, and all of the 22 athletes with hypertrophic cardiomyopathy survived. Another 49 athletes who were not disqualified also died, for an annual death rate of 1 death per every 62,500 athletes. The authors compared the frequency of hypertrophic cardiomyopathy as a cause of death in the United States with their experience and concluded that the low rate of death caused by hypertrophic cardiomyopathy in their athletes was a result of the screening program. However, the prevalence of hypertrophic cardiomyopathy in the Italian athletes was only 0.06%, well below the 0.2% prevalence reported for young Americans,[21] and only four excluded athletes died. Finally, the annual death rate of 1 per 62,500 in these athletes is similar to, if not higher than, the rate reported for U.S. athletes subjected to a less formal evaluation program.[17] Based on such data, the current, less extensive screening recommendations of the American College of Cardiology appear appropriate.[18]

Probably as important as the screening of athletes, however, is the evaluation of exercise-related symptoms in children and young adults. Many victims of exercise-related sudden death had previous symptoms, such as syncope or chest discomfort, that were ignored or inadequately evaluated before the fatal event. Physicians should carefully evaluate symptoms in young subjects and refer questionable cases for further assessment by a cardiologist.

Finally, coaches and others who supervise athletic training and competition should be required to know the basics of cardiopulmonary resuscitation and have a basic plan for dealing with emergencies (see Chapter 24) so that young subjects with exercise-related events can be promptly managed. The role of external automatic defibrillators is not yet defined, but these instruments will probably have an increasing role as their cost decreases and their availability increases.

Risk of Exertion for Adults

Atherosclerotic CHD is the cause of most exercise-related cardiac events in adults, including exercise-related MI and sudden cardiac death. Adults may die during exertion as the result of a cerebrovascular accident, aortic stenosis, hypertrophic cardiomyopathy, or an intramyocardial coronary artery, but these conditions are rare in comparison to CHD events.

The pathologic precedent of exercise-related MI and sudden death in previously healthy adults is usually atherosclerotic plaque disruption followed by acute coronary thrombosis (see Chapter 27). Several mechanisms may lead to exercise-induced plaque disruption and thrombosis (Box 22–3), including arterial injury or thrombosis in a damaged arterial segment.[22] In patients with previous MI, death can also be due to ventricular fibrillation originating from areas of myocardial scarring in the absence of new plaque rupture.

The incidence of exercise-related sudden cardiac death is much greater in adults than younger subjects because of the higher prevalence of occult atherosclerotic CHD in adults. Nevertheless, exercise complications are still rare, with an estimated incidence of sudden death during exertion of only 1 death per year for every 15,000 individuals.[16] Although the absolute incidence of sudden cardiac death during exercise is low, the relative incidence during exercise is increased 5-fold in the habitually most active and more

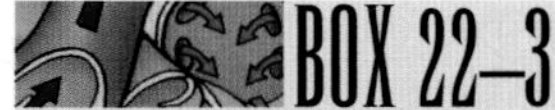

Exercise-Related Factors That Probably Contribute to Acute Coronary Events

Exercise-related factors initiating or exacerbating plaque rupture
- Increased heart rate
- Increased systolic blood pressure and sheer forces
- Increased coronary artery movement and twisting
- Exercise-induced coronary artery spasm
- Increased leukocyte-to-leukocyte adherence
- Increased circulating elastase

Exercise-related factors accelerating thrombus formation
- Deepening of plaque fissures by factors affecting plaque rupture
- Increased platelet aggregation (especially in unfit subjects)
- Increased platelet P-selectin
- Exercise-induced coronary spasm

than 50-fold in the habitually least active individuals in comparison to the incidence when sedentary.[23]

Cardiac events during exercise are more common in persons who exercise less frequently.[15,23] Less information is available for women than men, probably because of the delayed development of CHD in women, lower rates of vigorous physical activity in older individuals, and the overall lower incidence of sudden cardiac death in women.

Multiple studies have also demonstrated that vigorous exercise increases the risk of MI 2.1- to 10-fold.[15] Similar to the experience with sudden cardiac death, the exercise-related risk of MI is greatest for those who exercise rarely. The incidence of exercise-related MI is about seven times higher than the incidence of exercise-related sudden cardiac death, so the estimated annual incidence of MI during exercise is about 1 for every 2500 exercising men.[24]

Attempts to reduce the incidence of exercise-related cardiac events in adults have emphasized preparticipation exercise stress testing. For example, the American College of Sports Medicine[25] recommends exercise testing before initiation of a vigorous exercise program in men older than 40 and women older than 50 years, persons with more than one coronary disease risk factor, and persons with known CHD. Unfortunately, among ostensibly healthy asymptomatic individuals, a positive exercise stress test is a much better predictor of the development of angina pectoris than it is a predictor of MI or sudden cardiac death. For example, in a study of 916 Indiana state troopers monitored for a mean of 12.7 years, only 1 of 63 men with a positive electrocardiogram (ECG) response to exercise experienced an acute MI and 1 other experienced a sudden cardiac death,[26] whereas 25 MIs and 7 sudden cardiac deaths occurred in those with normal exercise ECGs. These findings are consistent with the current belief that hemodynamically significant coronary lesions are often tolerated until the appearance of angina, whereas acute MI and sudden cardiac death are frequently produced by plaque rupture and acute thrombosis in vessels without previous significant stenosis (see Chapters 25 and 27).

As a result, the *Guidelines for Exercise Testing*[27] issued by the American College of Cardiology and the American Heart Association considered the use of screening exercise tests before vigorous exercise activity to be not well established by evidence or opinion. Despite this tepid endorsement, many physicians continue to recommend such testing for their adult patients, possibly out of concern for legal liability.

Ultimate prevention of exercise-related CHD events, however, is possibly best accomplished by preventing the progression of CHD, stabilizing existing lesions with aggressive treatment, and identifying individuals in whom new symptoms have developed. Aggressive risk factor treatment (see Chapter 25) can stabilize coronary plaque and reduce acute cardiac events. Consequently, physically active individuals should receive aggressive risk factor treatment and not be allowed to believe that their exercise program is sufficient protection against CHD. It is also critically important that adults know the nature of prodromal cardiac symptoms and their need for prompt medical evaluation. Many victims of exercise-related sudden cardiac death previously experienced new symptoms, which they ignored. Physicians should ensure that their patients know to report not only new "chest pain" but also new exercise-related discomfort, tightness, or heartburn because such symptoms are often the initial symptom of CHD (see Chapters 6 and 25). Formal exercise testing in the setting of such symptoms is then extremely valuable in evaluating the symptoms (see Chapters 4 and 25).

EXERCISE IN PATIENTS WITH HEART DISEASE

Because exercise capacity is directly related to maximal cardiac stroke volume, exercise performance in patients with heart disease depends on the nature of the cardiac lesion, its severity, and its effect on the myocardium. Patients with cardiomyopathy (see Chapter 29) have reduced exercise capacity, in part because of the myocardium's inability to increase stroke volume during exercise. Differences in right ventricular function and habitual physical activity also contribute to variations in exercise capacity in patients with similar cardiac ejection fractions.

The effect of valvular disease on exercise performance also varies according to the valve involved, the nature of the lesion, and its severity (see Chapter 32). Mitral and aortic stenoses limit stroke volume and reduce exercise capacity. Mitral regurgitation also reduces exercise capacity because more time is spent in systole when regurgitation occurs. In contrast, aortic regurgitation occurs during diastole; time in diastole is reduced by tachycardia, so exercise capacity is often well preserved, even in those with substantial aortic insufficiency, if ventricular performance has not yet been reduced by the chronic volume overload.

In contrast, patients with CHD who have not sustained much myocardial damage may have normal exercise capacity. Patients with angina pectoris are not limited by stroke volume, but rather by exercise-induced chest discomfort. Classic angina pectoris occurs at a highly reproducible internal workload or rate-pressure product (see Chapter 25). This anginal threshold corresponds to the point at which myocardial oxygen demand cannot be adequately supplied by coronary flow because of fixed obstruction or abnormal coronary artery vasomotion. Exercise produces arterial dilatation in normal coronary arteries but can induce vasoconstriction in atherosclerotic coronary segments. Vasomotion may also explain the variability in angina by the time of day. Some patients experience "walk-through" angina during the beginning of exercise but can then perform the same or more demanding physical tasks without discomfort (see Chapter 25).

Response to Exercise Training in Patients with Heart Disease

Exercise training increases exercise capacity in patients with heart disease, but the magnitude of the increase in maximal oxygen consumption varies with the severity of the disease and the amount of myocardial injury. Patients with severely injured myocardium may be able to do nothing more than augment oxygen extraction and can therefore achieve only a very limited increase in exercise capacity with exercise training.

Patients with angina pectoris provide the clearest example of the physiologic adaptations that occur in patients with CHD. The increase in stroke volume with exercise training means that the same absolute external workload, which determines cardiac output, can be performed at a lower heart rate. The lower heart rate requires less myocardial oxygen supply and coronary blood flow. Consequently, a task that produced angina before exercise training can be performed after exercise training with no angina or with a delayed onset of angina.

In many studies of exercise training for patients with angina pectoris, angina continues to occur at the same rate-pressure product even though exercise capacity at the onset of angina is higher after training.[28] This finding implies no change in coronary blood supply. In some studies, however, the rate-pressure product at the onset of angina was higher after even brief exercise training, thus suggesting that exercise training can reduce exercise-induced coronary artery vasoconstriction.

The ability of exercise training to improve exercise capacity and reduce the frequency of angina makes exercise an effective adjunctive therapy for angina patients who are not candidates for angioplasty or coronary artery bypass procedures. In one study, among 18 patients with coronary disease whose exercise performance was limited by angina, only 7 continued to be limited by angina after just 12 weeks of an exercise training program.[29]

Assessment of only maximal effort capacity may underestimate many of the benefits of exercise on daily activities because few real-life tasks require maximal effort. Exercise training also has dramatic effects on submaximal working capacity in CHD patients. In one study, for example, time to exhaustion, as measured by treadmill walking at a workload requiring 80% of the individual's pretraining maximal oxygen consumption, increased 37% after 3 months of exercise training, whereas maximal oxygen consumption increased by only 16%.[30]

Does Therapeutic Exercise Improve Survival in CHD Patients?

No randomized studies have sufficient sample size to examine whether physical activity reduces subsequent cardiac events in patients with CHD. In a meta-analysis of 22 randomized trials of cardiac rehabilitation in over 4500 post-MI patients, those assigned to rehabilitation had a 20% to 26% reduction in mortality over the next 3 years, which was statistically significant during years 2 and 3.[31] However, 15 of the trials included other interventions, and the reduction in mortality in the 7 exercise-only studies, though of similar magnitude to what was found in all 22 studies, was not statistically significant. In a community-based observational study of men with established CHD, light to moderate physical activity was associated with lower all-cause mortality.[32] Whether therapeutic exercise would produce as pronounced a reduction in mortality in patients who now receive beta-adrenergic receptor blocking agents, angiotensin-converting enzyme inhibitors, lipid-lowering agents, antiplatelet agents, and modern reperfusion and revascularization procedures is unknown.

Exercise for Specific Types of Heart Disease

Heart Failure (see Chapter 28). Patients with heart failure have typically been prohibited from participating in exercise training programs, but recent studies suggest that some of the exercise intolerance in heart failure patients is produced by deconditioning. Multiple small studies have demonstrated increased exercise performance in heart failure patients after an exercise program, and large-scale trials to examine the effect of exercise training on morbidity and mortality are planned.

Claudication (see Chapter 37). Some of the most impressive increases in maximal exercise capacity from exercise training occur in patients with intermittent claudication. Summary data from 21 studies using exercise training as therapy for claudication showed that the average walking distance increased by 179%, or 225 m, to the onset of pain and 122%, or 397 m, to maximal pain.[33] Improvement was greatest in studies that trained subjects to the point of maximal tolerated pain, that continued for more than 6 months, and that used walking as the mode of training. These results are better than those reported for most surgical interventions and for all pharmacologic therapies.

Risk of Exercise in Individuals with CHD

Some of the risk of exercise in cardiac patients is probably related to exercise-induced ischemia, but aggressive medical and interventional therapy has reduced the prevalence of residual ischemia in most cardiac rehabilitation patients. One study[34] reported only one cardiac arrest for every 112,000 hours of exercise rehabilitation, one MI for every 294,000 hours, and one death for every 784,000 hours. It should be emphasized that this risk was for cardiac rehabilitation programs where prompt resuscitation was possible, so the incidence of one cardiac arrest for every 112,000 hours should be used to estimate the risk of death for cardiac patients participating in unsupervised exercise programs.

Risk of Exercise Stress Testing

The risk of exercise stress testing (see Chapter 4) varies with the prevalence of disease in the population being tested. The complication rate from seven reports in the usual clinical settings over the last 30 years suggests that approximately 1 MI, 2 episodes of ventricular fibrillation or major arrhythmia, 0.3 deaths, and fewer than 3 hospitalizations occur for every 10,000 exercise tests, or approximately 6 major complications per 10,000 exercise tests[35] (Table 22–3).

HOW TO INCORPORATE THERAPEUTIC EXERCISE INTO CLINICAL PRACTICE

Exercise has much to offer, not only in preventing and treating cardiovascular disease but also in preventing osteoporosis, treating depression, and delaying frailty. However, exercise is rarely recommended by most physicians, possibly because physicians do not feel comfortable making specific recommendations and because the composition of an "exercise prescription" appears complex,[36] and behavioral counseling to increase exercise is not routinely successful in changing patient behavior.[37] A physician's comfort level for routinely recommending exercise and success in changing patients' behavior can be increased by following several simple guidelines (Fig. 22–1).

Questions about a patient's usual physical activity and exercise habits should be a routine part of the review of systems. This approach signals the patient that exercise is important and provides a baseline for subsequent recommendations.

Recommendations for exercise should be based on the patient and on the physician's goal for the exercise program (Table 22–4). For general CHD prevention, the physician should recommend that patients perform 30 minutes of moderately intense physical activity on most and preferably all days of the week.[5] Brisk walking is an excellent option because it is simple and readily available. Patients who need to lose weight should be encouraged to exercise for longer periods because total energy consumption, not the intensity of exertion, is the key issue. Patients using exercise as a hygienic treatment of mild hypertension should be encouraged to exercise twice daily to obtain the acute exercise effect, which may persist for up to 13 hours.

TABLE 22–3

Cardiac Complications of Exercise Testing

Year	Site	# Tests	MI	VF	Death	Hospitalized	Comment
1971	73 U.S. Centers	170,000	NA	NA	1	3	34% of tests were symptom limited; 50% of deaths in 8 hr, 50% over the next 4 days
1977	15 Seattle facilities	10,700	NA	4.67	0	NR	
1977	Hospital	12,000	0	0	0	0	
1979	20 Swedish centers	50,000	0.8	0.8	6.4	5.2	
1980	1375 U.S. centers	518,448	3.58	4.78	0.5	NR	"VF" includes other arrhythmias requiring treatment
1989	Cooper Clinic	71,914	0.56	0.29	0	NR	Only 4% of men and 2% of women had CAD
1995	Geisinger Cardiology Service	20,133	1.42	1.77	0	NR	25% were inpatient tests supervised by non-MDs
Rates per 10,000 tests			**1.06**	**2.05**	**0.27**	**2.73**	

CAD, coronary artery disease; MI, myocardial infarction; NA, not available; NR, not recorded; VF, ventricular fibrillation.

Adapted with permission from Thompson PD: The cardiovascular risks of exercise. In Thompson PD (ed): Exercise and Sports Cardiology. New York, McGraw-Hill, 2000, pp 127–145.

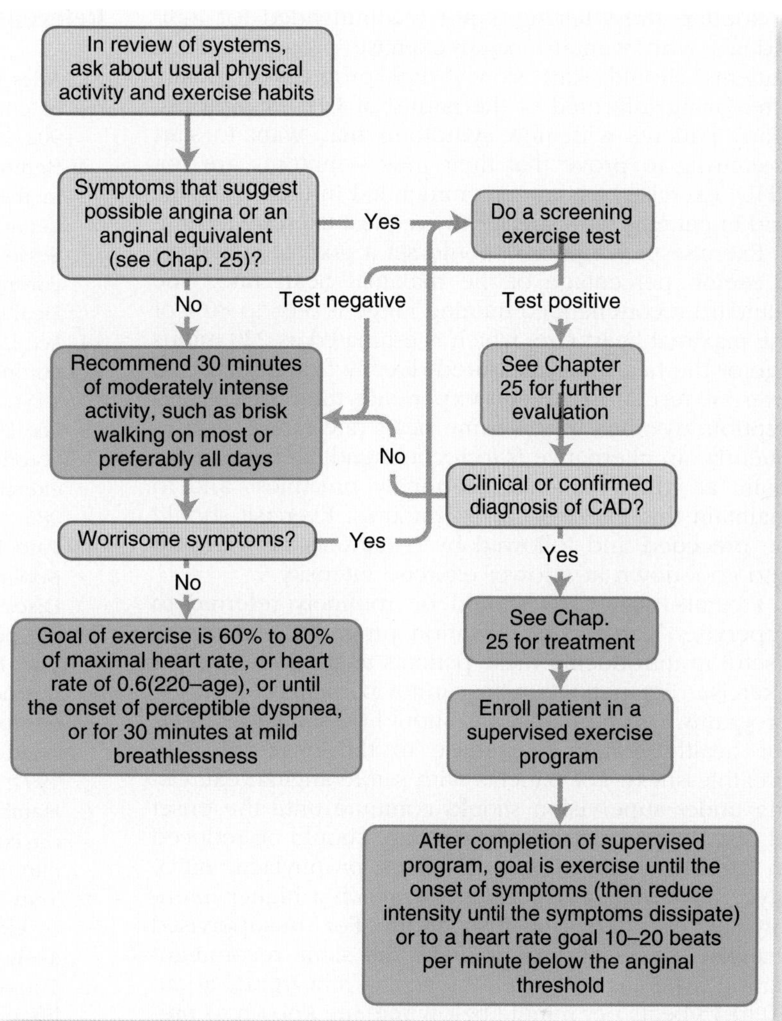

FIGURE 22–1. Guidelines for providing an exercise prescription in persons without known heart disease. CAD, coronary artery disease.

TABLE 22–4

Exercise Prescription According to Patient Characteristics

Characteristic	Training Regimen	Intensity	Type of Exercise	Frequency of Sessions (No./wk)	Duration of Each Session (min)
Age <65 yr, not overweight	High-intensity aerobic	75%–85% of maximal heart rate	Walking, jogging, cycling, rowing	3 or 4	30–45 (continuous or interval)
Age ≥65 yr	Low-intensity aerobic and resistance	65%–75% of maximal heart rate	Walking, cycling, rowing	3 or 4	30 (may be intermittent)
Overweight	Aerobic—high caloric expenditure	65%–80% of maximal heart rate	Walking	5 or 6	45–60
Age >65 yr and disabled, engaged in physical work, or overweight	Resistance	50%–75% of single-repetition maximal heart lift	Weight machine and dumbbells, with focus on upper part of legs, shoulders, and arms	2 or 3	10–20 (10 repetitions of each of 5 to 7 exercises)

Reprinted, by permission, from Ades PA: Cardiac rehabilitation and secondary prevention of coronary heart disease. N Engl J Med 2001;345:892–902.

Routine stress testing is not recommended for individuals who want to begin exercise programs. Such patients should start slowly and progress gradually after being informed of the nature of CHD symptoms. Many patients with new symptoms may want to start exercising to prove that their new symptoms are not CHD; exercise tests are recommended in these patients and in patients who specifically request exercise testing.

Exercise prescriptions should set a goal of achieving a certain percentage of the maximal heart rate. The standard recommended training range is 60% to 80% of the maximal heart rate, which is estimated as 220 minus age or the heart rate measured directly from a maximal exercise test. Most patients experience the onset of perceptible dyspnea in this same heart rate range. Consequently, an alternative is to recommend exercise to the point at which patients feel mildly breathless and to maintain this intensity for 30 minutes. Exercise should be preceded and followed by 5 minutes of warm-up and cool-down at a lower exercise intensity.

Patients with CHD should be routinely referred to supervised cardiac rehabilitation programs, which are useful in introducing these patients to the principles of exercise. For patients who cannot participate in these programs, recommendations should be similar to those for healthy patients—exercise to the onset of mild breathlessness. For patients with stable angina, exercising under supervision should continue until the onset of discomfort, and then the exercise should be reduced in intensity until the pain dissipates; prophylactic nitroglycerin permits CHD patients to reach a higher intensity of effort before discomfort. For unsupervised exercise, some physicians make the same recommendation, whereas others use the goal of a heart rate about 10 to 15 beats per minute below the rate known to precipitate angina. Similarly, patients with claudication should be encouraged to exercise to the onset of discomfort because this approach has been shown to yield the greatest improvements in effort tolerance.

Evidence-Based Summary

- The evidence is conclusive that exercise reduces such cardiac risk factors as hypertriglyceridemia, elevated blood glucose levels, hypertension, and body weight.
- Exercise training also improves exercise capacity in healthy subjects and in patients with CHD, heart failure, and claudication.
- Strong epidemiologic evidence suggests that exercise prevents the development of CHD, but randomized trials are not available to confirm this belief. Good evidence suggests that exercise training reduces mortality in post-MI patients, but this evidence is based on a meta-analysis of multiple trials of cardiac rehabilitation programs, most of which provided other risk factor interventions in addition to exercise training.

References

1. Ades PA: Cardiac rehabilitation and secondary prevention of coronary heart disease. N Engl J Med 2001;345:892–902.
2. Berlin JA, Colditz GA: A meta-analysis of physical activity in the prevention of coronary heart disease. Am J Epidemiol 1990;132:612–628.
3. Sesso HD, Paffenbarger RS, Lee IM: Physical activity and coronary heart disease in men: The Harvard Alumni Health Study. Circulation 2000;102:975–980.
4. Lee IM, Rexrode KM, Cook NR, et al: Physical activity and coronary heart disease in women. JAMA 2001;285:1447–1454.
5. Lee IM, Sesso HD, Paffenbarger RS: Physical activity and coronary heart disease risk in men: Does the duration of exercise episodes predict risk? Circulation 2000;102:981–986.
6. Pate RR, Pratt M, Blair SN, et al: Physical activity and public health. A recommendation from the Centers for Disease Control and Prevention and the American College of Sports Medicine. JAMA 1995;273:402–407.
7. Liao D, Cai J, Rosamond WD, et al: Cardiac autonomic function and incident coronary heart disease: A population-based case-cohort study. The ARIC Study. Atherosclerosis Risk in Communities Study. Am J Epidemiol 1997;145:696–706.
8. Hambrecht R, Wolf A, Gielen S, et al: Effect of exercise on coronary endothelial function in patients with coronary artery disease. N Engl J Med 2000;342:454–460.
9. Tran ZV, Weltman A, Glass GV, Mood DP: The effects of exercise on blood lipids and lipoproteins: A meta-analysis of studies. Med Sci Sports Exerc 1983;15:393–402.
10. Thompson PD, Cullinane EM, Sady SP, et al: High density lipoprotein metabolism in endurance athletes and sedentary men. Circulation 1991;84:140–152.
11. Aldred HE, Perry IC, Hardman AE: The effect of a single bout of brisk walking on postprandial lipemia in normolipidemic young adults. Metabolism 1994;43:836–841.
12. Thompson PD, Crouse SF, Goodpaster B, et al: The acute versus the chronic response to exercise. Med Sci Sports Exerc 2001;33(6 Suppl):438–445.
13. Tuomilehto J, Lindstrom J, Eriksson JG, et al: Prevention of type 2 diabetes mellitus by changes in lifestyle among subjects with impaired glucose tolerance. N Engl J Med 2001;344:1343–1350.
14. Boulé NG, Haddad E, Kenny GP, et al: Effects of exercise on glycemic control and body mass in type 2 diabetes mellitus: A meta-analysis of controlled clinical trials. JAMA 2001;286:1218–1227.
15. Giri S, Thompson PD, Kiernan FJ, et al: Clinical and angiographic characteristics of exertion-related acute myocardial infarction. JAMA 1999;282:1731–1736.
16. Thompson PD, Funk EJ, Carleton RA, Sturner W: Incidence of death during jogging in Rhode Island from 1975 through 1980. JAMA 1982;247:2535–2538.
17. Van Camp SP, Bloor CM, Mueller FO, et al: Nontraumatic sports death in high school and college athletes. Med Sci Sports Exerc 1995;27:641–647.
18. Maron BJ, Thompson PD, Puffer JC, et al: Cardiovascular preparticipation screening of competitive athletes. A statement for health professionals from the Sudden Death

Committee (clinical cardiology) and Congenital Cardiac Defects Committee (cardiovascular disease in the young), American Heart Association. Circulation 1996;94:850–856.

19. 26th Bethesda Conference: Recommendations for determining eligibility for competition in athletes with cardiovascular abnormalities. J Am Coll Cardiol 1994;24:845–899.
20. Corrado D, Basso C, Schiavon M, Thiene G: Screening for hypertrophic cardiomyopathy in young athletes. N Engl J Med 1998;339:364–369.
21. Maron BJ, Gardin JM, Flack JM, et al: Prevalence of hypertrophic cardiomyopathy in a general population of young adults. Echocardiographic analysis of 4111 subjects in the CARDIA study. Circulation 1995;92:785–789.
22. Li N, Wallen H, Hjemdahl P: Evidence of prothrombotic effects of exercise and limited protection by aspirin. Circulation 1999;100:1374–1379.
23. Siscovick DS, Weiss NS, Fletcher RH, Lasky T: The incidence of primary cardiac arrest during vigorous exercise. N Engl J Med 1984;311:874–877.
24. Thompson PD: The relative risk of myocardial infarction during exercise. In Fletcher G (ed): Cardiovascular Response to Exercise. Mount Kisco, NY, Futura, 1994, pp 291–300.
25. ACSM's Guidelines for Exercise Testing and Prescription, 6th ed. Philadelphia, Lippincott Williams & Wilkins, 2000.
26. McHenry PL, O'Donnell J, Morris SN, Jordan JJ: The abnormal exercise electrocardiogram in apparently healthy men: A predictor of angina pectoris as an initial coronary event during long-term follow-up. Circulation 1984;70:547–551.
27. Fletcher GF, Balady GJ, Amsterdam EA, et al: Exercise standards for testing and training. Circulation 2001;104:1694–1740.
28. Thompson PD, Cullinane E, Lazarus B, Carleton RA: Effect of exercise training on the untrained limb exercise performance of men with angina pectoris. Am J Cardiol 1981;48:844–850.
29. Ades PA, Grunvald MH, Weiss RM, Hanson JS: Usefulness of myocardial ischemia as predictor of training effect in cardiac rehabilitation after acute myocardial infarction or coronary artery bypass grafting. Am J Cardiol 1989;63:1032–1036.
30. Ades PA, Waldmann ML, Poehlman ET, et al: Exercise conditioning in older coronary patients: Submaximal lactate response and endurance capacity. Circulation 1993;88:572–577.
31. O'Connor GT, Buring JE, Yusuf S, et al: An overview of randomized trials of rehabilitation with exercise after myocardial infarction. Circulation 1989;80:234–244.
32. Wannamethee SG, Shaper AG, Walker M: Physical activity and mortality in older men with diagnosed coronary heart disease. Circulation 2000;102:1358–1363.
33. Gardner AW, Poehlman ET: Exercise rehabilitation programs for the treatment of claudication pain. A meta-analysis. JAMA 1995;274:975–980.
34. Van Camp SP, Peterson RA: Cardiovascular complications of outpatient cardiac rehabilitation programs. JAMA 1986;256:1160–1163.
35. Thompson PD: The cardiovascular risks of exercise. In Thompson PD (ed): Exercise and Sports Cardiology. New York, McGraw-Hill, 2000, pp 127–145.
36. Glasgow RE, Eakin EG, Fisher EB, et al: Physician advice and support for physical activity. Results from a national survey. Am J Prev Med 2001;21:189–196.
37. Eden KB, Orleans CT, Mulrow CD, et al: Does counseling by clinicians improve physical activity? Ann Intern Med 2002;137:208–215.

CHAPTER 23

Other Risk Factors for Coronary Heart Disease: Diet, Lifestyle, Psychological Disorders, and Estrogen Deficiency/Hormone Replacement Therapy

Frank B. Hu and JoAnn E. Manson

Coronary heart disease (CHD) remains the leading cause of mortality in the United States. and other industrialized countries. Because dietary and lifestyle change is a highly cost-effective means to lower CHD risk, it is critical to identify important nutritional and other modifiable risk factors for CHD. Several major lifestyle risk factors, such as cigarette smoking, obesity, and physical inactivity, have long been recognized. In more recent years, there have been important advances in our understanding of the role of specific dietary factors in the prevention of CHD, owing in part to several large prospective cohort studies of diet and chronic disease. In this chapter, we summarize current evidence regarding dietary and other lifestyle risk factors for CHD.

DIETARY FACTORS

Dietary Fat and Cholesterol

Major Types of Fat

Dietary fat intake is widely believed to play a role in the development of CHD. This belief is largely based on ecological studies relating dietary intake of saturated fat to rates of CHD in different countries. In the Seven Countries study, intake of saturated fat as a percentage of calories had a strong correlation with coronary death rates across 16 defined populations in seven countries ($r = 0.84$).[1] Interestingly, the correlation between the percentage of energy from total fat and CHD incidence was only modest (r = 0.39). Indeed, the regions with the highest CHD rate (Finland) and the lowest rate (Crete) had the same amount of total fat intake, at about 40% of energy, which was the highest among the 16 populations.

Randomized clinical trials would be ideal for testing dietary hypotheses. In most situations, however, dietary trials have been difficult to conduct because of practical considerations, including ethical issues and potential lack of compliance in the long term. Prospective cohort studies, in which diet is assessed before disease occurs, are generally considered the strongest nonrandomized design because they are less susceptible to biases that arise from the retrospective reporting of diet. Numerous prospective studies have examined the relationship between dietary fat intake and risk of CHD. The most detailed analyses of dietary fat and CHD were based on 14-year follow-up of 80,082 women from the Nurses' Health Study.[2] In this study, total amount of fat as compared with equivalent energy from carbohydrates was *not* significantly related to CHD risk. However, higher intakes of saturated and trans fats were associated with increased risk, whereas higher intakes of mono- and polyunsaturated fats *were* associated with *decreased* risk. Interestingly, on a gram-for-gram basis, the adverse effects of trans fat were much greater than those of saturated fat. When polyunsaturated and trans fats were examined in combination, risk was the lowest among those who had the lowest intake of trans unsaturated fat and the highest intake of polyunsaturated fat (e.g., those who consumed unhydrogenated soybean or corn oil instead of hard margarine) (relative risk [RR], 0.31; 95% confidence interval [CI], 0.11 to 0.88; $P = .01$) (Fig. 23–1). It was estimated that replacement of 5% of energy from saturated fat by unsaturated fats would reduce risk of CHD by 42% (23 to 56, $P < .001$), and replacement of 2% of energy from trans fat by unhydrogenated unsaturated fats would reduce risk 53% (34 to 67, $P < .001$). In contrast, replacement of 5% energy from saturated fat with carbohydrates was associated with a nonsignificant 14% decrease in CHD risk. These findings suggest that replacing saturated and trans fats with unhydrogenated mono- and polyunsaturated fats is more effective in preventing CHD than in reducing overall fat intake.

These results are consistent with those from metabolic studies of different types of fat on serum cholesterol (Table 23–1). It is well established that exchanging saturated fat for carbohydrate increases LDL as well as HDL cholesterol, whereas exchanging mono- and polyunsaturated fat for carbohydrate lowers LDL cholesterol and triglycerides and raises HDL cholesterol.[3] These findings are also consistent with dietary intervention trials showing benefits of high polyunsaturated fat diets in lowering CHD incidence or mortality. The major source of polyunsaturated fat is corn and soybean oils. The major non-animal sources of monounsaturated fat include olive and canola oils, nuts, and avocados. Both canola oil and nuts are also important sources of polyunsaturated fat.

Trans Fatty Acids

Trans fatty acids are formed when vegetable oils undergo the partial hydrogenation process to produce margarines and shortenings. This process makes vegetable oils more saturated and results in a solid state at room temperature. This process is also used to increase

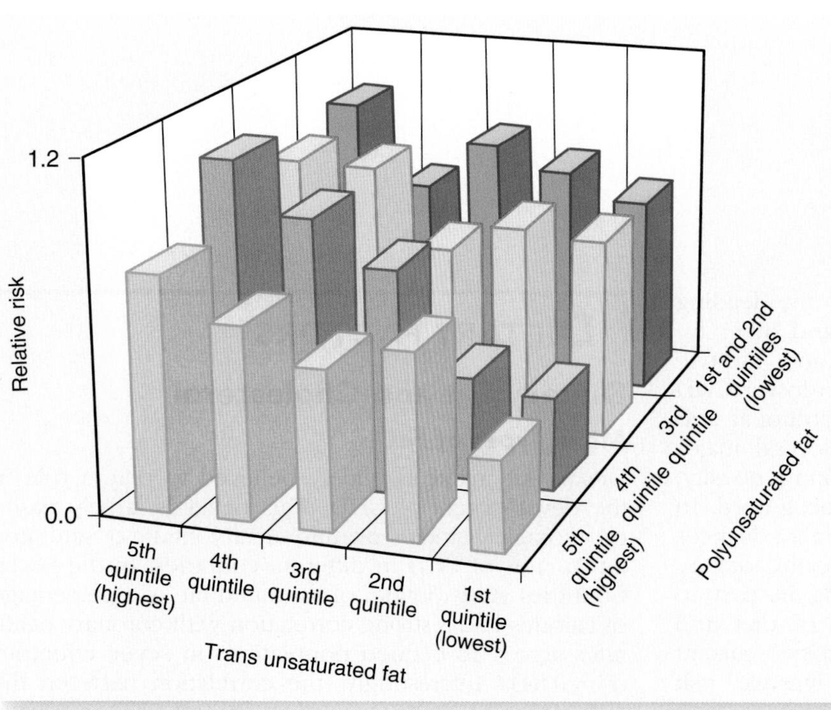

FIGURE 23–1. Multivariate relative risk of coronary heart disease according to dietary intake of trans unsaturated and polyunsaturated fats. The first and second quintiles for polyunsaturated-fat intake were combined to provide a sufficient number of women in each of the categories. The relative risks have been adjusted for age, time interval, body-mass index, cigarette smoking, menopausal status, parental history of premature myocardial infarction, use of multivitamins, use of vitamin E supplements, alcohol consumption, history of hypertension, aspirin use, physical activity, percentage of energy obtained from protein, saturated fat and monounsaturated fat, dietary cholesterol, and total energy intake. The reference group for all comparisons was the women with the highest intake of trans unsaturated fat and the lowest intake of polyunsaturated fat. (Redrawn from Hu FB, Stampfer MJ, Manson JE, et al: Dietary fat intake and risk of coronary heart disease in women. N Engl J Med 1997;337:1491–1499.)

TABLE 23–1

Types of Dietary Fat

Type of Fat	Main Sources	State at Room Temperature	Effect on Cholesterol Compared with Carbohydrates
Monounsaturated	Olives and olive oil, canola oil, peanut oil; cashews, almonds, peanuts, and most other nuts; peanut butter avocados	Liquid	Lowers LDL; raises HDL
Polyunsaturated	Corn, soybean, safflower and cottonseed oils; fish	Liquid	Lowers LDL; raises HDL
Saturated	Whole milk, butter, cheese, and ice cream; red meat; chocolate; coconuts, coconut milk, and coconut oil	Solid	Raises both LDL and HDL
Trans	Most margarines; vegetable shortening; partially hydrogenated vegetable oil; deep-fried chips: many fast foods; most commercially baked goods	Solid or semi-solid	Raises LDL*

*Compared with monounsaturated or polyunsaturated fat, trans fat increases LDL, decreases HDL, and increases triglycerides.

From Willett WC: Eat, Drink, and Be Healthy: The Harvard Medical School Guide to Healthy Eating. New York, Simon & Schuster, 2001.

shelf life of the products by destroying essential fatty acids, such as linolenic acid and linoleic acid, which tend to oxidize and become rancid, particularly when exposed to the high temperatures used for commercial deep-fat frying.

The major sources of trans fatty acids in the United States are stick margarines, vegetable shortenings, commercially baked products, and deep fried fast food.

Metabolic studies have consistently indicated adverse effects of trans fat intake on blood lipids and other cardiovascular risk factors. In particular, trans fatty acids raise LDL cholesterol levels and lower HDL cholesterol relative to natural *cis*-unsaturated fatty acids.[4] As such, the increase in the ratio of total to HDL cholesterol for trans fat is approximately double that for the same amount of saturated fat. In addition, trans fat increases lipoprotein(a) levels and plasma triglyceride levels, both of which have been associated with elevated risk of CHD.

Cholesterol and Eggs

Dietary cholesterol raises LDL cholesterol levels and causes atherosclerosis in numerous animal models. In controlled metabolic studies conducted in humans, dietary cholesterol raises levels of total and LDL cholesterol in blood, but the effects are relatively small compared with saturated and trans fatty acids, and individuals vary widely in their response to dietary cholesterol on plasma levels. Several epidemiologic studies have found a modest positive association between dietary cholesterol and risk of CHD. However, there is little direct evidence linking higher egg consumption, a major source of cholesterol, and increased risk of CHD. In a detailed study of 117,933 men and women, moderate egg consumption (up to 1 egg/day) had no overall impact on incidence of CHD or stroke. The null association of egg consumption with risk of CHD observed in this study may be somewhat surprising, considering the widespread belief that eggs are a major cause of heart disease. One egg contains about 20 mg cholesterol, but also appreciable amounts of protein, unsaturated fats, folate, B vitamins, and minerals. It is conceivable that the small adverse effect caused by cholesterol is counterbalanced by potential beneficial effects of other nutrients. These findings indicate that among healthy men and women, moderate egg consumption can be part of a nutritious and balanced diet.

N-3 Fatty Acids

There are two major classes of n-3 polyunsaturated fatty acids. Long-chain n-3 fatty acids such as eicosapentaenoic acid (20:5n-3; EPA) and docosahexaenoic acid (22:6n-3; DHA) are found in high concentrations in fish and fish oil. Alpha-linolenic acid (18:3n-3; ALA) is a shorter-chain n-3 fatty acid, which can be metabolized to longer-chain polyunsaturated n-3 fatty acids (i.e., EPA and DHA) through the desaturation-chain elongation pathway. The major sources of ALA in the diet are vegetable oils (especially soybean and canola oil), walnuts, and green leafy vegetables. Flaxseed has a higher amount of ALA, but it is not commonly consumed in the United States.

Several, but not all, prospective cohort studies have found an inverse association between fish consumption and risk of cardiovascular mortality in largely healthy populations. Fish and marine n-3 fatty acids may be particularly beneficial for preventing fatal CHD, especially sudden cardiac death. The diet and reinfarction trial (DART) showed that subjects who increased their fish intake to two servings per week, had a 29% reduction in total mortality after 2 years. The GISSI-Prevenzione trial showed that daily supplementation with marine n-3 fatty acids resulted in a 10% to 15% reduction in the main endpoints (death, nonfatal MI, and stroke).[6] Most of the reduction was attributable to the decrease in cardiovascular death, especially sudden cardiac death.

These two trials provide support for the therapeutic role of fish and fish oil in the treatment of MI patients.

There is growing evidence that a higher intake of ALA is also protective against CHD.

Several prospective cohort studies have found an inverse association between ALA intake and risk of CHD. In the Nurses' Health Study, the risk of fatal CHD was 50% lower among women in the highest quintile of ALA intake as compared with those in the lowest quintile. There was also an approximately 50% lower incidence of fatal CHD among women who consumed oil and vinegar salad dressing (a main source of ALA) 5 to 6 times or more per week compared to those who seldom consumed this salad dressing, even after taking into account salad intake.

The Lyon Diet Heart Study tested the effects of a "Mediterranean" diet enriched with ALA compared to a standard low fat diet among postmyocardial infarction patients.[5] The intervention diet included more bread, fruits, vegetables, fish, and poultry and less red meat and butter. After a mean follow-up of 27 months, coronary events were reduced by 73% and total mortality reduced by 70% in the treatment group.

There are several potential mechanisms by which n-3 fatty acids may reduce the risk of CHD. Animal studies have established that fish oil feeding effectively reduces the incidence and duration of cardiac arrhythmias. Significant reductions in the incidence of ventricular fibrillation and cardiac mortality were also observed in rats fed ALA-rich diets. In addition, ALA and its metabolite, EPA, can decrease generation of thromboxane A2, a pro-aggregatory vasoconstrictor, through their inhibitory action on the conversion of linoleic acid to arachidonic acid.

Carbohydrates

Glycemic Index and Glycemic Load

Traditionally, carbohydrates have been classified into simple or complex based on chemical structures. Most dietary recommendations have emphasized the use of complex carbohydrates or starches and avoidance of simple carbohydrates or sugars. This was based on the belief that simple sugars would be digested and absorbed more quickly, which would induce a more rapid postprandial glucose response. It is now recognized that many starchy foods such as baked potatoes and white bread produce even higher glycemic responses than simple sugars. That different carbohydrate-containing foods lead to different glycemic responses has led to the development of the concept of glycemic index (GI). GI is a ranking of foods based on the extent that blood glucose rises (the area under the curve for blood glucose levels) after ingesting a test food as compared to a standard weight (50 g) of reference carbohydrate (glucose or white bread). The GI depends largely on the rate of digestion and rapidity of absorption of carbohydrate. Typically, foods with a low degree of starch gelatinization (more compact granules), such as spaghetti and oatmeal and a high level of viscous soluble fiber such as barley, oats, and rye have a slower rate of digestion and lower GI values. The physical form of the food is another important determinant of GI. Whole grain products with intact bran and germ typically have lower GI values. In contrast, refined carbohydrate-containing foods such as white bread tend to have higher GI values because grinding or milling of cereals removes most of the bran and much of the germ and reduces the particle size, allowing for more rapid attack by digestive enzymes.

The overall blood glucose response is determined not only by the GI value of a food, but also by the amount of carbohydrate in the food. Thus, the concept of glycemic load (GL) (i.e., the product of the GI value of a food and its carbohydrate content) has been developed to represent both the quality and quantity of the carbohydrates consumed (Table 23–2). Using white bread as the reference, each unit of dietary GL represents the equivalent glycemic effect of 1 g of carbohydrate from white bread. The GL concept is highly advantageous because it represents a diet's overall ability to raise the blood glucose level. Several epidemiologic studies have found that GL, especially combined with low intake of cereal fiber, significantly elevated long-term risk of type 2 diabetes. High GL has also been associated with increased risk of CHD. The increased risk was more pronounced among overweight and obese women, suggesting that the adverse effects of a high GL diet are aggravated by underlying insulin resistance.

Fiber

Dietary fiber includes the cell walls of plants and other indigestable components of plants. Soluble fibers (pectins, gums, mucilages, and psyllium) lowers total and LDL cholesterol through increased bile acid excretion and decreased hepatic synthesis of cholesterol and fatty acids. However, based on a meta-analysis of 67 controlled trials, the magnitude of cholesterol-lowering effects of soluble fiber is only modest. For example, ingesting 3 g of soluble fiber from oats (3 servings of oatmeal) decreases cholesterol by only 2%. Thus, the cholesterol-lowering effects of fiber cannot explain the substantial reduction in risk of CHD associated with higher fiber consumption observed in numerous epidemiologic studies (discussed subsequently). Fiber may have many other benefits, however, including improving glycemic control and reducing hyperinsulinemia. A study has also suggested that low fiber consumption predicted higher fasting insulin levels and greater weight gain independent of dietary total and saturated fat intake.

Numerous prospective cohort studies have examined the relationship between fiber intake and risk of CHD and virtually all have found an inverse association. In the Nurses' Health Study, for each 10-g increase in total fiber intake, there was a 20% reduction in CHD risk. The strongest association was found for cereal fiber, as opposed to fruit and vegetable fiber. While research efforts should continue to investigate the biological effects of different types and sources of fiber, from a public health point of view, an increase in total dietary fiber, both soluble and insoluble and from different food

TABLE 23–2

Glycemic Index (GI) and Glycemic Load (GL) of Selected Common Foods

Food item	GI* (white bread = 100)	Serving size†	Grams of carbohydrates per serving	GL/ serving‡
White rice, low-amylose	125	1 cup	53	67
Baked potato	121	1	51	61
Corn flakes breakfast cereal	119	1 cup	24	29
Jelly beans	114	1 oz	26	30
Doughnut	108	1	23	25
Waffle	108	2	31	66
French fries	107	4 oz	35	37
Graham cookies	105	2	11	23
Honey	104	1 tbsp	17	18
Bagel	102	1	38	39
Watermelon	102	1 slice	17	17
Carrots	101	1/2 cup	8	8
White bread	101	1 slice	12	12
Wheat bread	98	1 slice	12	12
Sucrose	92	1 tsp	4	4
Raisins	91	1 oz	22	20
Ice cream	87	1/2 cup	16	14
White rice, high-amylose	84	1 cup	45	37
Orange juice	81	6 oz	20	16
Cake	80	1 piece	36	29
Brown rice	78	1 cup	45	35
Popcorn	78	1 cup	6	5
Sweet corn	78	1/2 cup	16	12
Sweet potato	77	1	25	19
Banana	75	1	27	20
Baked beans	68	1/2 cup	27	18
Parboiled rice	67	1 cup	43	29
Grapes	61	1/2 cup	14	9
Orange	61	1	16	10
All-bran breakfast cereal	60	1/2 cup	23	14
Apple juice	58	6 oz	22	13
Spaghetti	58	1 cup	40	23
Apple	51	1	21	11
Chickpeas	47	1 cup	45	21
Lentils	40	1 cup	40	16
Whole milk	38	1 cup	12	5
Kidney beans	38	1 cup	39	15
Grapefruit	36	0.5	10	2
Fructose	33	2 tbsp	31	10
Cherries	31	1 cup	24	7
Peanuts	20	1 oz	5	1

*The means of GI values were taken from Foster-Powell and Miller.

†The serving sizes and grams of carbohydrate/serving are from USDA.

‡GL is the product of the GI value of a food and its carbohydrate content per serving. Each unit of dietary GL represents the equivalent glycemic effect of 1 g of carbohydrate from white bread.

From Hu FB, van Dam RM, Liu S: Diet and risk of type 2 diabetes: The role of types of fat and carbohydrates. Diabetologia 2001;44:805–817.

sources (especially whole grains, fruits, vegetables, legumes, and nuts), should be encouraged.

Whole Grains

Whole grain products such as whole wheat breads, brown rice, oats, and barley tend to produce slower glycemic and insulinemic responses than highly processed refined grains. Whole grains are also rich in fiber, antioxidant vitamins, magnesium, and phytochemicals. Milling removes most of the bran and much of the germ. The resulting refined grain products have lost substantial amounts of dietary fiber, vitamins, minerals, essential fatty acids, and phytochemicals and contain more starch. Because of the loss of the outer bran layer and pulverization of the endosperm, refined grains are digested and absorbed more rapidly than whole grain products and thus tend to cause more rapid and larger increases in levels of blood glucose and insulin than do whole-grain products.[7]

Epidemiologic studies have consistently found an inverse association between whole grain consumption and risk of diabetes and CHD. In the Nurses' Health Study, a 25% lower risk of CHD (nonfatal MI and CHD death) was observed among women who ate nearly three servings of whole grains a day compared with those who ate less than one serving per week. In the United States, cereal grains are generally highly processed before they are used; only 2% of the 150 pounds of wheat flour consumed per capita in 1997 was whole wheat flour, and the average American gets less than one serving of whole grains a day. Thus, there is a great potential to reduce risk of type 2 diabetes and CHD by increasing consumption of whole grain products.

Antioxidants and Folate

Theoretically, vitamin E and other antioxidants can lower risk of CHD by blocking the oxidative modification of LDL-C, which appears to be an important step in the uptake of cholesterol into the arterial wall. A body of epidemiologic evidence has linked intake of vitamin E, especially supplements, and reduced risk of CHD. However, results from randomized clinical trials (such as the Alpha-Tocopherol, Beta-Carotene Cancer Prevention study, GISSI-Prevenzione Trial,[6] and the HOPE [Heart Outcomes Prevention Evaluation] study) have been largely negative. On the one hand, several clinical trials have ruled out any beneficial effects of supplementation with high doses of beta-carotene on cardiovascular events. On the other hand, large prospective cohort studies continue to supply strong evidence that high intakes of carotenoid-rich foods, such as fruits and vegetables, lower the risk of cardiovascular disease. In the analysis of the Nurses' Health Study, each one-serving-per-day increase in intake of fruits or vegetables was associated with a 4% lower risk for CHD and a 6% lower risk for ischemic stroke. The discrepancy between observational studies and supplementation trials raises the question whether the antioxidants coming from supplements, in high doses and not part of a balanced mix of antioxidants, function in the same way as those from diet.

Adequate folic acid is critical for preventing neural tube defects in newborns. Emerging evidence suggests that folate is beneficial in preventing cardiovascular disease, as well, because folic acid and other B vitamins are the primary determinants of plasma homocysteine concentrations, a recognized independent risk factor for CHD. In 1998, the recommended dietary allowance (RDA) for folic acid was raised to 400 micrograms per day, more than doubling the previous RDA set in 1989. A multivitamin supplement typically contains 400 μg of folic acid. Beginning in 1997, flour has been fortified with folate, adding about 100 μg per day of folate to the average American's diet. Most cold breakfast cereals are also fortified to provide 100 μg of folate per day. Other good dietary sources of folate include orange juice, spinach, and lentils.

Several epidemiological studies have found an inverse association between folate intake and risk of CVD. The Nurses' Health Study found a relative risk for CHD of 0.69 (95% CI, 0.55 to 0.87) for women in the highest quintile of folate intake (median 696 μg/d) compared to those in the lowest quintile of folate intake(median 158 μg/d). Of interest was that the inverse association between folic acid intake and CHD was strongest in women who had more than one alcoholic drink per day (RR = 0.27, 95% CI, 0.13 to 0.58). Several ongoing clinical trials are examining the effect of folate on CHD incidence, with results expected by 2005.

Plant Sterols

Plant sterols occur naturally in fruits, vegetables, vegetable oils, nuts, and grains. Over 40 plant sterols (phytosterols) have been described. The most abundant sterols are sitosterol, campesterol, and stigmasterol. Because these sterols are structurally similar to dietary cholesterol, except for methyl groups in the side chain, they inhibit cholesterol absorption in human intestines. Plant sterols have been known to lower blood cholesterol since the 1950s. Recently, a series of randomized trials conducted in the United States and Europe have confirmed the cholesterol-lowering effects of polyunsaturated fat magarines containing either sterol or stanol (saturated sterols). On average, adding 2 g of plant sterol or stanol to the diet reduces LDL cholesterol by 0.54 mmol/L in people aged 50 to 59 years, 0.43 mmol/L in those aged 40 to 49 years, and 0.33 mmol/L in those aged 30 to 39 years. Commercial products containing plant sterols or stanols (such as Benecol and Take Control) are widely available. One major concern is that plant sterols modestly lower blood concentrations of carotenoids and some fat soluble vitamins. Therefore, the long-term effects of these products need to be monitored.

Alcohol

Numerous epidemiologic studies have documented an inverse association between alcohol consumption and risk of CHD, in both men and women. In general, consumption of one or two drinks per day has corresponded to a reduction in risk of approximately 20% to 40%. Light-to-moderate alcohol consumption has also been associated with a lower risk of stroke. A point of controversy lies in whether one type of alcoholic drink confers more benefit than another. Several ecological studies have suggested that wine is more strongly associated with CHD risk reduction than are beer or liquors. In addition, clinical studies have found that polyphenols in red wine or purple grape juice reduce LDL oxidation and improve endothelial function. Most epidemiologic studies indicate that wine, beer, and liquor confer similar benefits on coronary risk, suggesting that the benefit of alcoholic drinks comes from alcohol per se rather than other components of each type of drink. A meta-analysis of 42 published controlled studies estimated that the HDL-raising effect of 30 g daily of alcohol accounted for 17% reduction in CHD risk and the reduction in fibrinogen accounted for 13% reduction in risk. These benefits were slightly negated by elevated triglyceride levels associated with alcohol consumption. Overall, changes in lipids and fibrinogens caused by an intake of 30 g of alcohol a day would predict a 25% reduction in CHD risk.

Despite convincing evidence for a beneficial effect of moderate alcohol consumption on CHD, public health recommendations regarding alcohol use are a matter of controversy. A major concern with any recommendation of alcohol use is the potential problem with heavy use and abuse, especially among young people. Alcohol consumption, even in moderate amounts, may increase risk of breast cancer in women. Thus, most experts recommend that if adults choose to drink alcoholic beverages, they should consume them only in moderation (no more than one drink (10 g) per day for women and no more than two drinks (20 g) per day for men).

CIGARETTE SMOKING

Cigarette smoking is a well-established cause of CHD, the leading cause of death in the United States. Between 1990 and 1994, an average of 430,700 Americans died each year of smoking-related illness; the largest proportion of these deaths being caused by cardiovascular disease. Smoking may confer even greater risk of CHD in women than in men. In the Nurses' Health Study, the number of cigarettes smoked per day was positively associated with the risk of fatal CHD (relative risk = 5.5 for greater than or equal to 25 cigarettes or more per day) and nonfatal MI (relative risk = 5.8). Even smoking 1 to 4 or 5 to 14 cigarettes per day was associated with a twofold to threefold increase in the risk of fatal CHD or nonfatal MI. Overall, cigarette smoking accounted for approximately half of these events in the cohort. Cumulative evidence indicates that regular exposure to passive smoking at home or work increases the risk of CHD among nonsmokers.[8] In the Nurses' Health Study, compared with women not exposed to passive smoking, the relative risks of total CHD—adjusted for a broad range of cardiovascular risk factors—were 1.58 (95% CI, 0.93 to 2.68) among those reporting occasional exposure and 1.91 (95% CI, 1.11 to 3.28) among women reporting regular exposure to passive smoking at home or work. In addition, there is increasing evidence that use of cigars and pipe tobacco is also associated with increased risk of CHD.

Smoking cessation substantially reduces risk of CHD. It has been estimated that stopping smoking eliminates one third of the excess risk of CHD within 2 years of cessation,[9] and the risk returns to the level of those who never smoked after 10 to 14 years of cessation. Similar benefits were observed for total mortality. Therefore, people who stop smoking will experience an immediate benefit as well as a further longer-term decline in the excess risk of CHD and total mortality.

OBESITY

Excessive body weight, even at average levels for the U.S. population, elevates cardiovascular risk factors and CHD incidence and mortality.[10] In the Nurses' Health Study, for increasing levels of current BMI (less than 21, 21 to less than 23, 23 to less than 25, 25 to less than 29, and greater than or equal to 29), the relative risks of nonfatal myocardial infarction and fatal coronary heart disease combined, as adjusted for age and cigarette smoking, were 1.0, 1.3, 1.3, 1.8, and 3.3 respectively (*P* for trend <.0001). In addition, weight gains during adulthood are associated with significantly increased risks of CHD and many other chronic diseases (Fig. 23–2). For example, as compared with women and men who maintained their weight within 2 kg (4 lb) of their weight at 18 to 20 years of age, those who gained 5.0 to 9.9 kg (11 to 22 lb) had 1.5 to 3-fold increased risks of CHD, hypertension, cholelithiasis, and type 2 diabetes. Abdominal adiposity, reflected by a higher ratio of waist to hip circumferences, predicts increased risk of CHD and type 2 diabetes, independent of BMI. A waist-to-hip ratio of >0.95 (or waist circumference ≥102 cm (40 inches)) in men and >0.80 (or waist circumference ≥88 cm (35 inches)) in women can be considered central obesity.

Because excess body fat is an important cause of CHD, weight control would be one of the most effective ways to reduce CHD risk (Fig. 23–3). Metabolic clinical trials indicate that a moderate weight loss (5% to 10% of initial body weight) leads to improvements in blood pressure, lipid levels, and glucose tolerance. Current strategies have not been very successful on a population basis, and the prevalence of obesity continues to increase. The public generally does not recognize the connection between overweight/obesity and diabetes or CHD. Clearly, more educational efforts are needed to increase the public's awareness about the health hazards of being overweight.

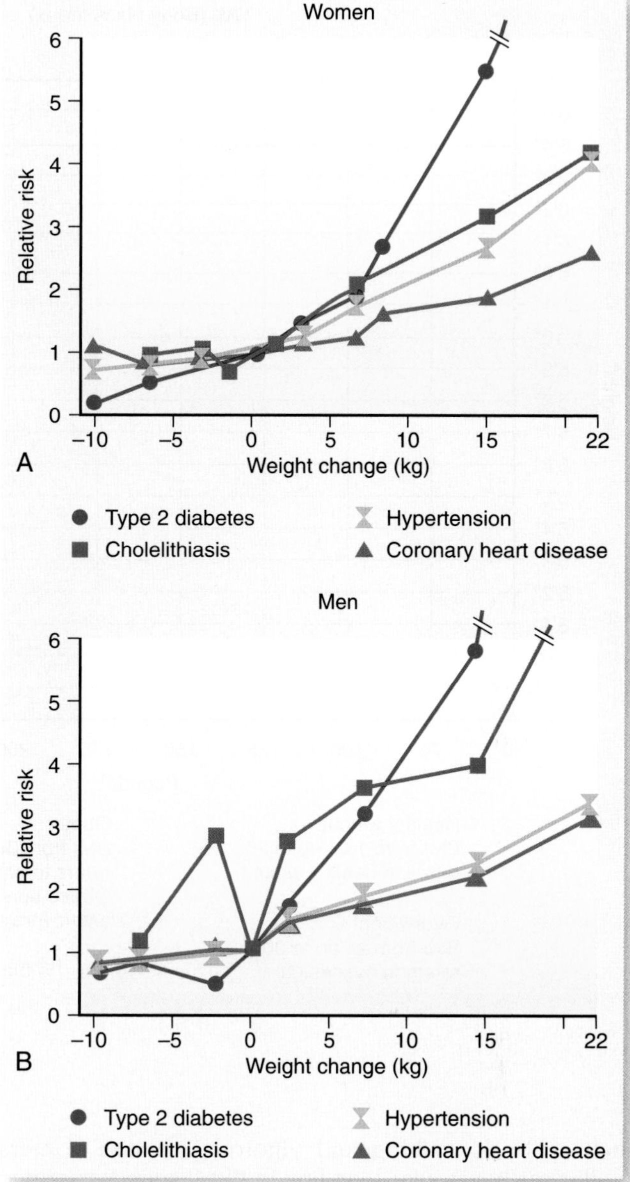

FIGURE 23–2. Relation between the change in weight and the relative risk of type 2 diabetes, hypertension, coronary heart disease, and cholelithiasis. Panel A shows these relations for change of weight from age 18 years among women in the Nurses' Health Study, initially age 30 to 55 years, who were followed for up to 18 years. Panel B shows the same relations for change of weight from age 20 years among men in the Health Professionals Follow-up Study, initially age 40 to 65 years, who were followed for up to 10 years. (Redrawn from Willett WC, Dietz WH, Colditz GA: Guidelines for healthy weight. N Engl J Med 1999;341:427–434.)

PHYSICAL ACTIVITY

More than 40 epidemiologic studies have addressed the relationship between exercise and CHD and most of the studies have found an inverse association between increasing total and vigorous activity and risk of CHD.[11] These studies indicate a 30% to 50% risk reduction in both men and women who engaged in regular physical activity, as compared with sedentary participants.

Increasing evidence also indicates that equivalent energy expenditure from moderate-intensity activity

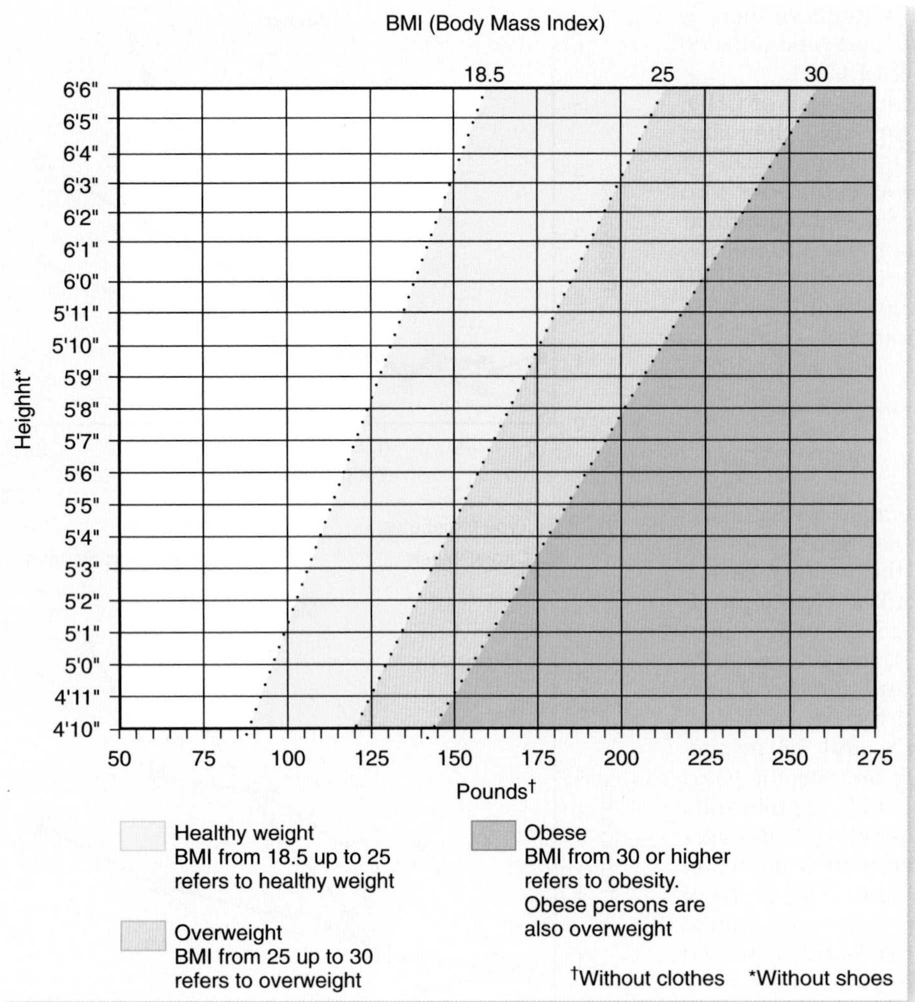

FIGURE 23–3. Chart for determination of body mass index (BMI). BMI measures weight in relation to height. The ranges shown are for adults. They are not exact ranges of healthy and unhealthy weights. They show that health risk increases, however, at higher levels of overweight and obesity. Even within the healthy BMI range, weight gains can carry health risks for adults. Directions for patient: Find your weight on the bottom of the graph. Go straight up from that point until you reach the line matching your height. Then look to find your BMI. (Redrawn from the Report of the Dietary Guidelines Advisory Committee on the Dietary Guidelines for Americans, 5th ed. Washington, DC, Center for Nutrition Policy and Promotion, 2000, p 3.)

such as brisk walking and vigorous exercise confers similar cardiovascular benefits. In the Insulin Resistance Atherosclerosis Study, both vigorous and nonvigorous activity were significantly associated with insulin sensitivity among 1467 men and women age 40 to 69 years. Among diabetic patients, daily walking combined with dietary therapy not only reduced body weight but also improved insulin sensitivity. Studies have shown that equivalent expenditures of energy in moderate or vigorous exercise led to similar reductions in adipose mass and had similar benefits on cardiorespiratory fitness and cardiovascular risk factors including blood pressure and lipids. In the Nurses' Health Study, there was a strong, graded, inverse relationship between energy expenditure in either walking or vigorous activity and the incidence of coronary disease. Among women who either walked briskly at least 3 hours per week or exercised vigorously for 1.5 hours per week, the risk was reduced by 30% to 40%. Similar benefits were observed for ischemic stroke and type 2 diabetes. These findings lend support to current federal guidelines that endorse moderate-intensity exercise, which is safe, achievable, and feasible for the majority of the population. Although vigorous exercise should not be discouraged for those who choose a higher intensity of activity, these results indicate that enormous public health benefits would accrue from the adoption of regular moderate-intensity exercise by those who are currently sedentary.

It is important to choose activities that one enjoys and can perform regularly (Box 23–1).

PSYCHOLOGICAL DISORDERS

It has been long suspected that psychosocial factors play a role in the development of CHD, although conclusive evidence regarding specific factors is still lacking. Cumulative evidence has implicated several psychosocial factors including anger, hostility, stress, lack of social support, and depression.[11] Clearly, these factors tend to be interrelated and it is difficult to tease out their independent effects.

In animal models, anger elicited increased coronary vascular resistance and ST-segment changes. Several epidemiological studies have suggested that high levels

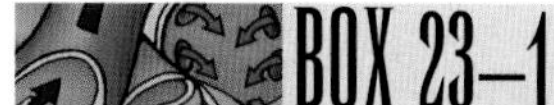

BOX 23–1

Examples of Physical Activities for Adults

For at least 30 minutes most days of the week, preferably daily, do any one of the activities listed below—or combine activities. Look for additional opportunities among other activities that you enjoy.

As part of your routine activities:

- Walk, wheel, or bike ride more, drive less.
- Walk up stairs instead of taking an elevator.
- Get off the bus a few stops early and walk or wheel the remaining distance.
- Mow the lawn with a push mower.
- Rake leaves.
- Garden.
- Push a stroller.
- Clean the house.
- Do exercises or pedal a stationary bike while watching television.
- Play actively with children.
- Take a brisk 10-minute walk or wheel in the morning, at lunch, and after dinner.

As part of your exercise or recreational routine:

- Walk, wheel, or jog.
- Bicycle or use an arm pedal bicycle.
- Swim or do water aerobics.
- Play racket or wheelchair sports.
- Golf (pull cart or carry clubs).
- Canoe.
- Cross-country ski.
- Play basketball.
- Dance.
- Take part in an exercise program at work, home, school, or gym.

From Report of the Dietary Guidelines Advisory Committee on the Dietary Guidelines for Americans, 5th ed. Washington, DC, 2001, p. 3.

of anger may increase the risk of CHD. In the Normative Aging Study of 1305 men, compared with men reporting the lowest levels of anger, the multivariate-adjusted relative risks among men reporting the highest levels of anger were 3.15 (95% confidence interval [CI]: 0.94 to 10.5) for total CHD (nonfatal MI plus fatal CHD) and 2.66 (95% CI: 1.26 to 5.61) for combined incident CHD events including angina pectoris (*P* for trend, .008).

Lack of social support has also been associated with CHD mortality. In the Health Professionals' Follow-up Study, compared with men with the highest level of social networks, socially isolated men (not married, fewer than six friends or relatives, no membership in church or community groups) were at increased risk for cardiovascular disease mortality (age-adjusted relative risk, 1.90; 95% CI: 1.07 to 3.37) and deaths from accidents and suicides (age-adjusted relative risk 2.22; 95% CI: 0.76 to 6.47). Socially isolated men were also at increased risk of stroke incidence (relative risk, 2.21; 95% CI: 1.12 to 4.35), but not incidence of nonfatal myocardial infarction. Lack of social support may also increase risk of recurrent myocardial infarction and cardiac mortality in persons with existing heart disease.

Increasing evidence supports a positive association between symptomatic depression and CHD risk. In the Normative Aging Study, men in the highest level of depression versus those in the lowest level of depression had multivariate-adjusted relative risks of incident CHD (total CHD and angina) of 1.46 (95% CI: 0.83 to 2.57), 2.07 (95% CI: 1.13 to 3.81), and 1.73 (95% CI: 0.97 to 3.10) for the three different depression scales. There were significant dose-response relations between level of depression measured by the MMPI-2 DEP scale and incidence of both angina pectoris (*p* value for trend, .039) and CHD (*p* value for trend, .016).

Despite substantial evidence from observational studies linking psychosocial factors and CHD, few studies have investigated whether behavioral intervention programs or treatment of depression reduces CHD incidence or mortality. In the Lifestyle Heart Study, Ornish and colleagues assigned 28 MI patients to an intervention group with low-fat, strict vegetarian diet, exercise, stress management, and yoga and 20 patients to a usual care group.[12] At year five, coronary atherosclerosis regressed in the experimental group but progressed in the control group, and significantly more "cardiac events" (MI, percutaneous transluminal coronary angioplasty, coronary artery bypass graft, cardiac hospitalization, deaths) occurred in the control group. Because multiple components were included in the intervention, it is unclear whether stress management had any independent effects.

MENOPAUSE AND POSTMENOPAUSAL HORMONE USE

The rate of CHD in women tends to increase abruptly after age 50, approximately the mean age at menopause, suggesting that estrogen deficiency may be a cause of CHD and postmenopausal hormone replacement therapy may reduce CHD risk. Moreover, several studies have suggested that an earlier age at menopause is associated with an increased risk of CHD, although this remains controversial. Numerous observational studies in the past three decades have, in aggregate, suggested that women who take estrogen have a risk of CHD that is 35% to 50% lower than the risk among women who do not take estrogen. Such an association is biologically plausible. Randomized trials have shown that estrogen therapy reduces plasma levels of LDL by 10% to 14% and increases plasma levels of HDL by 7% to 8%, changes known to be associated with a reduced risk of cardiovascular disease. Estrogen has also been shown to reduce levels of Lp(a) lipoprotein, inhibit oxidation of LDL, improve endothelial vascular function, and reverse postmenopausal increases in fibrinogen and plasminogen-activator inhibitor type 1—changes that should also reduce the risk of cardiovascular disease. At the same time, however, estrogen therapy may have potentially detrimental effects on cardiovascular biomarkers, such as increasing triglyceride levels; activating coagulation as a result of increases in factor VII, prothrombin fragments 1 and 2, and fibrinopeptide A; and increasing levels of C-reactive protein, a marker of inflammation associated with an increased risk of cardiovascular events.

The Women's Health Initiative (WHI), a randomized controlled primary prevention trial of estrogen/progestin (Prempro) among 16,608 postmenopausal women age 50 to 70 years in the United States, was stopped earlier than expected because of increased risk of breast cancer and because overall health risks clearly exceeded health benefits over an average follow-up of 5.2 years. In particular, estrogen plus progestin therapy increased breast cancer incidence by 26%, CHD incidence by 29%, stroke incidence by 41%, and incidence of pulmonary embolism by 111%, while the treatment decreased colorectal cancer by 37% and hip fracture by 34%. Although all-cause mortality was not affected by the treatment, overall health risks exceeded benefits from use of the regimen. These results provide strong evidence that combined estrogen plus progestin should *not* be initiated or continued for primary prevention of CHD (see Chapter 15 and Fig. 15–2).

Randomized trials of estrogen among women with preexisting CHD have not supported the role of hormone therapy in secondary prevention of CHD, either. The Heart and Estrogen/Progestin Replacement Study (HERS) randomized 2763 women with coronary disease to 0.625 mg of oral conjugated estrogen combined with 2.5 mg of continuous medroxyprogesterone acetate ($n = 1380$) or placebo ($n = 1383$). After 4.1 years, there was no overall protection against second coronary events for women assigned to treatment compared with those given placebo (RR = 0.99, 95% CI: 0.80 to 1.22). In the first year of the trial, the risk of major coronary disease events was 52% higher among treated women; in the second year, there was no relation between treatment and disease (RR = 1.00), and in the third year the relative risk was 0.87. By the fourth to fifth years of the trial, rates of coronary events were 33% lower in women assigned to hormone therapy. In the Estrogen Replacement and Atherosclerosis (ERA) study, a 3-year randomized clinical trial of atherosclerosis progression in women with heart disease, neither estrogen alone nor estrogen with progestin resulted in a decrease of plaque area, compared with placebo.

On the basis of the evidence from the WHI and the HERS, estrogen plus progestin therapy should *not* be initiated or continued for prevention of CHD or other chronic diseases in postmenopausal women. As discussed previously, a wide range of dietary and lifestyle approaches are available for the effective prevention of CHD.

Evidence-Based Summary

Compelling evidence indicates that CHD is heavily influenced by dietary and lifestyle factors. Whereas cigarette smoking, obesity, and physical inactivity have long been established as major causes of CHD, the role of specific dietary factors has not been clearly defined until more recently. Cumulative evidence from multiple lines of research indicates that types of fats and carbohydrates are probably more important than total amounts of fats and carbohydrates in determining risk of CHD. There can be some degree of flexibility in the amounts of fats and carbohydrates in a diet if healthy types of these nutrients are used to replaces unhealthy ones. The role of antioxidant vitamins, folate, and phytochemicals in the prevention of CHD is promising but not yet settled. Available evidence strongly suggests, however, that a dietary pattern rich in these nutrients, containing higher amounts of fruits, vegetables, whole grains, and nuts is likely to reduce risk of CHD.[14]

The combination of dietary and lifestyle factors is more powerful than a single factor alone.[15] In the Nurses' Health Study, women who did not smoke cigarettes, were not overweight, maintained a healthful diet (high in cereal fiber, fish, folate, polyunsaturated fat, and low in saturated and trans fat and glycemic load), exercised moderately or vigorously for half an hour a day, and consumed alcohol moderately (half a drink per day) had an incidence of coronary events that was more than 80% lower than that in the rest of the population (Table 23–3). Thus, when combined with pharmacologic treatment of hypertension and high lipid levels (if necessary), diet and lifestyle modification could prevent the majority of CHD events. Only about 3% of the Nurses' Health Study cohort met the criteria, however, for low risk defined by the guidelines, suggesting an even greater potential to prevent CHD in the general population by diet and lifestyle modification. Because unhealthy lifestyle factors such as smoking and psychosocial stress and disorders tend to cluster, it is important for physicians to consider the role of psychosocial variables in counseling their patients.

To promote healthy eating and lifestyle patterns, Willett has proposed a Healthy Eating Pyramid, a modified and improved version of the USDA Food Guide Pyramid.[14] In addition to nonsmoking, there are several other key dietary and behavioral changes emphasized by the Healthy Eating Pyramid:

1. Exercise daily.
2. Maintain body weight and, especially, prevent midlife weight gain.
3. Eat fewer bad fats (i.e., saturated and trans fats), replacing them with good fats (unhydrogenated unsaturated fats).
4. Eat fewer refined-grain carbohydrates and more whole-grain carbohydrates.
5. Abstain from cigarette smoking.
6. Eat plenty of vegetables and fruits.
7. Alcohol in moderation can be a healthy option unless contraindicated.
8. Take a multivitamin for nutritional "insurance."

The Healthy Eating Pyramid reflects the available evidence on diet and lifestyle described in this chapter (Fig. 23–4). These guidelines, if followed, have enormous potential to reduce risk of CHD.

TABLE 23–3

Risk of Coronary Events in Low-Risk Groups Defined According to Different Constellations of Modifiable Risk Factors for Coronary Disease among Current Nonsmokers in the Nurses' Health Study, 1980 to 1994*

Group	Percentage of Women in Group	No. of Coronary Heart Disease Events	Relative Risk (95% CI)†	Population Attributable Risk (95% CI)‡
Two low-risk factors§	16.4	62	0.68 (0.52–0.88)	28 (10–44)
Diet score in upper 2 quintiles				
Moderate to vigorous exercise ≥30 min/day				
Three low-risk factors¶	9.4	24	0.54 (0.36–0.82)	43 (17–62)
Diet score in upper 2 quintiles				
Moderate to vigorous exercise ≥30 min/day				
Body-mass index <25				
Four low-risk factors	4.0	5	0.25 (0.10–0.60)	74 (39–90)
Diet score in upper 2 quintiles				
Moderate to vigorous exercise ≥30 min/day				
Body-mass index <25				
Alcohol ≥5 g/day				

*CI denotes confidence interval.

†Relative risk was estimated from a multiple logistic-regression model and adjusted for age (in five-year categories), time periods (seven time periods), presence or absence of a parental history of myocardial infarction before the age of 60 years, menopausal status and use or nonuse of postmenopausal hormones, presence or absence of a history of hyper-tension, and presence or absence of a history of high cholesterol levels.

‡The population attributable risk is the percentage of coronary disease events in the population that are attributable to the nonadherence to the particular combination of lifestyle characteristics.

§The model was also adjusted for body-mass index and alcohol use.

¶The model was also adjusted for alcohol use.

From Stampfer MJ, Hu FB, Manson JE, et al: The primary prevention of coronary heart disease in women through diet and lifestyle. New Engl J Med 2000;343:16–22.

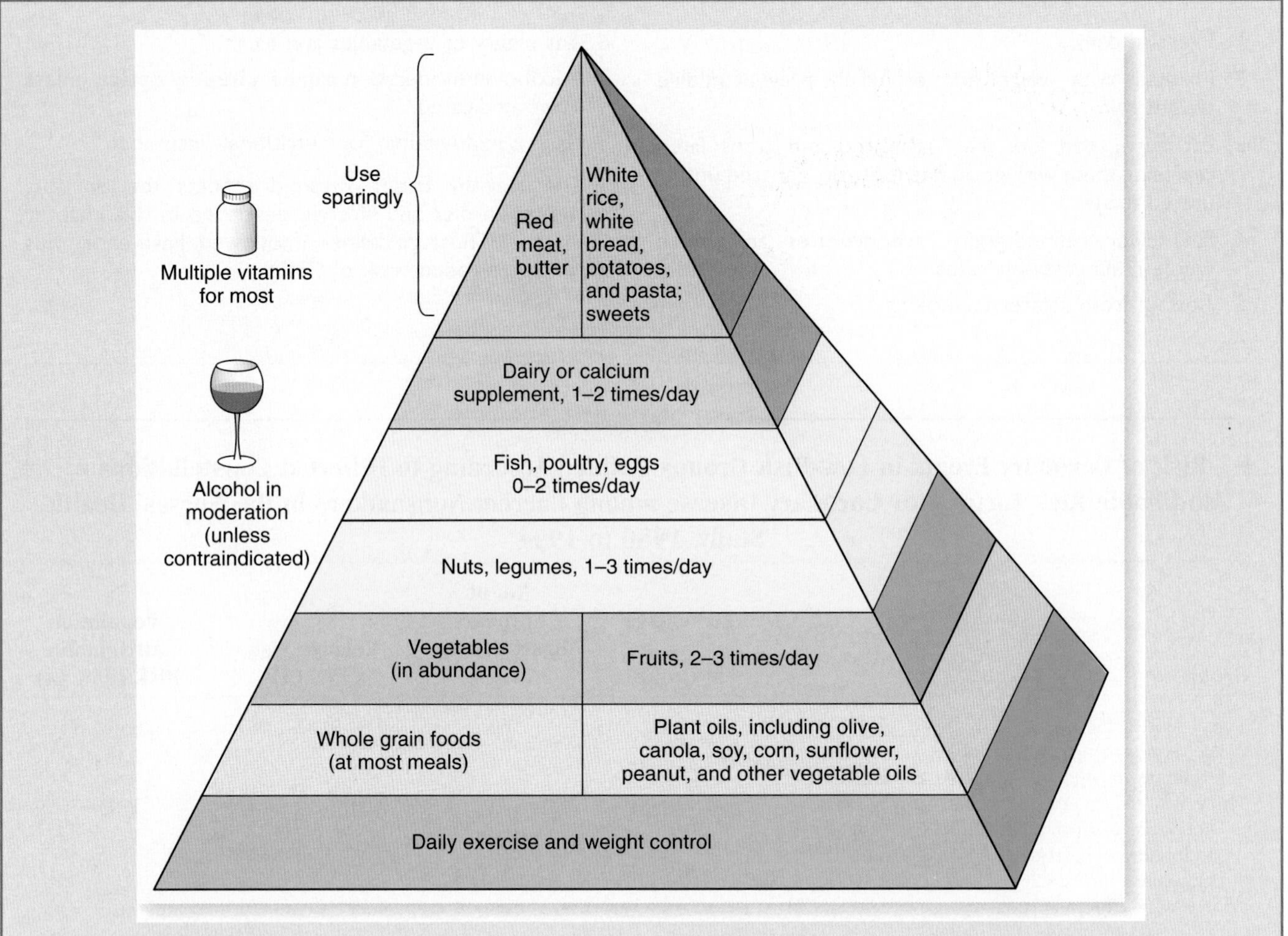

FIGURE 23–4. Healthy eating pyramid. (Redrawn from Willett WC: Eat, Drink, and Be Healthy: The Harvard Medical School Guide to Healthy Eating. New York, Simon & Schuster, 2001.)

References

1. Keys A: Seven countries: A multivariate analysis of death and coronary heart disease. Cambridge, MA, Harvard University Press, 1980.
2. Hu FB, Stampfer MJ, Manson JE, et al: Dietary fat intake and risk of coronary heart disease in women. N Engl J Med 1997;337:1491–1499.
3. Hu FB, Manson JE, Willett WC: Types of dietary fat and risk of coronary heart disease: A critical review. J Am Coll Nutr 2001;20:5–19.
4. Ascherio A, Katan MB, Zock PL, et al: Trans fatty acids and coronary heart disease. N Engl J Med 1999;340: 1994–1998.
5. de Lorgeril M, Renaud S, Mamelle N, et al: Mediterranean alpha-linolenic acid-rich diet in secondary prevention of coronary heart disease. Lancet 1994;343:1454–1459.
6. GISSI-Prevenzione Investigators. Dietary supplementation with n-3 polyunsaturated fatty acids and vitamin E after myocardial infarction: Results from the GISSI-Prevenzione trial. Lancet 1999;354:447–455.
7. Hu FB, van Dam RM, Liu S: Diet and risk of type 2 diabetes: The role of types of fat and carbohydrates. Diabetologia 2001;44:805–817.
8. Kawachi I, Colditz GA, Speizer FE, et al: A prospective study of passive smoking and coronary heart disease. Circulation 1997;95:2374–2379.
9. Kawachi I, Colditz GA, Stampfer MJ, et al: Smoking cessation and time course of decreased risks of coronary heart disease in middle-aged women. Arch Intern Med 1994;154:169–175.
10. Willett WC, Dietz WH, Colditz GA: Guidelines for healthy weight. N Engl J Med 1999;341:427–434.
11. Rozanski A, Blumenthal JA, Kaplan J: Impact of psychological factors on the pathogenesis of cardiovascular disease and implications for therapy. Circulation 1999;99: 2192–2217.
12. Ornish D, Scherwitz LW, Billings JH, et al: Intensive lifestyle changes for reversal of coronary heart disease. JAMA 1998;280:2001–2007.
13. Manson JE, Martin KA: Postmenopausal hormone replacement therapy. N Engl J Med 2001;345:34–40.
14. Willett WC: Eat, Drink, and Be Healthy: The Harvard Medical School Guide to Healthy Eating. New York, Simon & Schuster, 2001.
15. Stampfer MJ, Hu FB, Manson JE: The primary prevention of coronary heart disease in women through diet and lifestyle. N Engl J Med 2000;343:16–22.

PART 4

Recognition and Management of Patients with Specific Cardiac Problems

CHAPTER 24 Approach to Cardiovascular Emergencies

Robert A. Barish and Jerome F.X. Naradzay

The position of the primary care physician in the chain of survival has never been more important. Treating a cardiovascular emergency requires astute evaluation and immediate intervention. The primary care physician and patient must be prepared before mustering resources during the cardiovascular emergency. It is imperative that conversations between the patient and physician address advance directives, health care proxies, living wills, when to seek medical care, and when to go directly to an emergency department. This chapter presents information related to preparing for and treating cardiovascular emergencies.

PREPARING FOR AN EMERGENCY

Communication

The primary care physician must evaluate and treat an increasing number of patients with complex cardiovascular disease. The annual number of visits to physicians' offices is estimated to be more than 750 million.[1] It is clear that primary care physicians are challenged to evaluate more patients with cardiovascular disease outside acute care settings than ever before. Discharges for heart disease (e.g., ischemic heart disease, acute myocardial infarction, heart failure) in patients age 45 to 75 years and older have *increased* to more than 2 million per year, and the average length of stay in hospital for these illnesses has *decreased* to 4.5 days for patients age 45 to 64 years, to 4.8 days for those 65 to 74 years, and to 5.6 days for those 75 years and older.[1] These figures indicate that more patients with cardiac disease are coming to doctors' offices but spending less time in the hospital.

As a result of these changes, communication among the primary care physician, patient, and emergency physician has never been more important. The primary care physician must communicate with the emergency physician to avoid redundant testing and evaluation. It is up to the primary care physician to educate the patient about medical conditions, medications, and results of testing and evaluation, including guidance as to when to contact the primary care physician and when to go directly to the emergency department. To utilize hospital-based resources most appropriately, particularly during an emergency, the primary care physician must ensure hospital records are accurate and current. It is the primary care physician who will identify a high-risk patient, activate the emergency medical services (EMS) system, and transfer care to the emergency physician. Resources and time must be managed intelligently *before* an emergency arises.

Accessing Emergency Medical Services

Early access to the EMS system is essential for improving outcome for out-of-hospital cardiac arrests, strokes, and other cardiovascular emergencies. Automated defibrillation in out-of-hospital settings, such as airlines or even casinos, can markedly improve outcomes at an acceptable cost.[2] The chain of survival that started in the office must continue to the next link: the EMS provider. The primary care physician should notify the

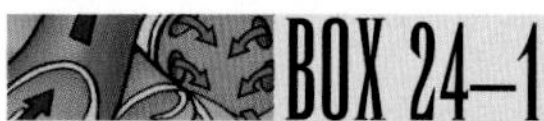

BOX 24–1

Types of EMS Providers*

EMS Level	Intervention
EMT-basic	Field stabilization of fractures; extrication techniques; oxygen administration; CPR
EMT-intermediate	Tracheal intubation, defibrillation, medications, intravenous access
EMT-paramedic	Intubation, intravenous medications, surgical airway, chest decompression, venous cutdown, transcutaneous pacing

*In addition to EMS personnel, first responders, such as police and fire department personnel, are required in many states to carry automatic external defibrillators.

CPR, cardiopulmonary resuscitation; EMS, emergency medical system; EMT, emergency medical technician.

medical dispatcher of the nature of the emergency, and together they should decide on the most appropriate level of prehospital response (Box 24–1).

The primary care physician should be familiar with resources available in local emergency departments and hospitals. Can the hospital initiate thrombolytic therapy for an acute ischemic stroke? Is echocardiography or intra-aortic balloon pump available on an emergency basis? Does the hospital provide primary angioplasty or thrombolysis for acute myocardial infarction? Can the hospital evaluate and treat acute aortic dissection?

Patient Education

Patients' decisions about where to seek medical care are influenced by many factors: financial concerns, marital harmony, "fear dimensions" of illness, socioeconomic status, experience with illness, residential instability, proximity to emergency departments, and accessibility of the primary care physician. Being cognizant of these, the primary care physician can help each patient better utilize health care resources.

A patient's decision to seek medical care will progress through phases influenced by self-assessment of the illness, consultation with supporters, and, finally, seeking formal medical evaluation. The two best predictors of where the patient seeks care are the patient's payment method and his or her problem-solving abilities. The primary care physician must attempt to influence the decision making process by being cognizant of factors that influence patients' decisions where to seek medical care and how to make educated decisions about their own illness. The primary care physician must focus on medical issues (e.g., compliance with treatment plans and severity of symptoms) and psychosocial issues (e.g., family and residential stability, fears of illness). Patients must be very well informed about their medical history, cardiac history, medications, surgical history, and the like. Primary care physicians should advocate the use of clinical information summaries (e.g., accurate medication lists, brief medical history) or electronic-chip health care medical smart cards. Precrisis education will focus on when to seek medical attention before symptoms progress to critical levels. Despite educational messages broadcast through various media, unnecessary delays in seeking treatment still exist when patients are having chest pain or symptoms consistent with a stroke.

It is imperative that primary care physicians educate each patient about symptoms germane to his or her medical history. For example, a patient with an abdominal aneurysm should know the warning signs of expansion or rupture. A patient with peripheral vascular disease should know how to distinguish between chronic claudication and occlusion. A handy summary or health care smart card can facilitate immediate care when the patient does seek medical attention.

A patient who contacts a primary care physician describing symptoms of a cardiovascular emergency should be encouraged to access EMS. The physician should notify the local emergency department of the impending arrival to reduce door-to-needle time and door-to–CT scan time. Hospitals, emergency departments, and primary care physicians' offices should work together to form a seamless, integrated patient care information system.

Advance Directives

Treating a cardiovascular emergency includes being prepared to address catastrophic events. Each patient must be well versed in the meaning and importance of a power of attorney for health care, living will, advance directive with instructions about end-of-life treatment (see Chapter 17), health care proxy and agents (including alternate agents), effective date and durability, and the agent's powers (Box 24–2). In addition to being ethically responsible, these discussions are required by the Patient Self-Determination Act, approved by Congress in 1991. This act requires health care providers to give information about advance directives to patients admitted to a health care facility and to document whether or not the individual has signed an advance directive.

Despite a federal law requiring hospitals, skilled nursing facilities, hospices, home health agencies, and health maintenance organizations (HMOs) serving persons covered by either Medicare or Medicaid to provide information about advance directives and explain legal choices in making decisions about medical care, disparity in making end-of-life decisions exists. Contributing to this disparity are misconceptions in patients' understanding of advance directives and the fact that less than half of patients are likely to discuss advance directives with their physicians. Physicians need to be aware of and understand end-of-life preferences among racial and ethnic groups.[3,4]

Explicit advance directives are essential and must replace nonspecific "do not resuscitate" orders. End-of-

BOX 24–2

An advance directive states, in writing, who can make decisions for the patient and what intervention is applicable when the patient cannot communicate owing to physical or mental illness. The Patient Self-Determination Act (PSDA) requires hospitals and nursing homes to tell patients about their right to refuse medical treatment.

Power of Attorney	The patient designates a **person**, called an agent, to make health care decisions for the patient in any situation in which the patient is unable to do so. Allows the agent to address a wide complexity of circumstances not covered in a living will. The agent must be intimately familiar with the patient.
Living Will	A **document** that allows patients to state in advance what types of medical treatment they do or do not desire if they develop a terminal illness. A living will can be as specific as needed but typically addresses a narrow range of conditions or predictions.

life and catastrophic illness directives can be customized to the patient's high-risk medical conditions. For example, if a patient has an abdominal aortic aneurysm, the directive can state: "I have an abdominal aortic aneurysm. I do not want resuscitation attempted if doctors diagnose aneurysm rupture."

Primary Care Physician's Office

The primary care physician's office should stock the supplies and medications necessary to stabilize a patient with a suspected cardiovascular emergency. Every physician's office should be equipped with basic equipment and medications needed for the initial treatment of cardiovascular emergencies (Box 24–3). Commercially available carts contain medications used during a cardiovascular emergency. Before the patient is transported to the emergency department, the primary care physician should contact the emergency physician. This communication can alert the emergency department staff and facilitate immediate management. In addition to this communication, sending prehospital electrocardiograms (ECGs), medication lists, and a medical history summary can reduce the time from evaluation to intervention.

BOX 24–3

Primary care office equipment and medications for evaluating and managing a cardiovascular emergency

Equipment

Supplemental oxygen and delivery systems: nasal cannula, bag-valve-mask, mouth-to-mask, intubation equipment
12-Lead electrocardiogram
Automatic external defibrillator
Transcutaneous pacemaker
Intravenous supplies
Medications needed to treat cardiac emergencies

Medications

Atropine sulfate injection 1 mg/10 mL
Diazepam injection, 10 mg/2 mL
Digoxin injection, 0.5 mg/2 mL
Diphenhydramine injection, 50 mg/mL
D-5-W, 500 mL
D-50-W, 50-mL syringe
Epinephrine 1:11,000 1-mL ampule
Epinephrine 1:10,000 syringe
Furosemide injection 20 mg/2 mL
Ipecac syrup, 1-oz bottle
Lidocaine HCl 2%, 100 mg/5 mL syringe
Nalbuphine ampules, 10 mg/mL
Naloxone injection ampule, 0.4 mg/mL
Nifedipine capsule, 10 mg
Nitrostat, 0.4-mg tablet (sublingual)
Prochlorperazine injection, 10 mg/2 mL
Propranolol injection, 1 mg/mL
Sodium bicarbonate 8.4%, 50 mEq/50 mL syringe
Solu-Cortef injection, 250-mg vial

TREATING THE PATIENT WITH A CARDIOVASCULAR EMERGENCY

The history and physical examination of the patient with symptoms of a suspected cardiovascular emergency are directed toward rapidly generating a differential diagnosis, with special emphasis on life-threatening conditions (Box 24–4). During a cardiovascular emergency, the benefits of the physician-patient relationship are most needed. The primary care physician can help the patient or emergency physician distinguish typical angina pectoris, headache, or common complaints from a true emergency. The primary care physician will know the results of a previous coronary angiogram, prior measurements of the diameter of an asymptomatic aortic aneurysm, or previous stroke deficits. Detailed medical information and knowledge of the patient's typical complaints contribute immensely to quick evaluation and treatment during emergency.

Consensus recommendations provide a directed approach, via algorithms, to manage potentially life-

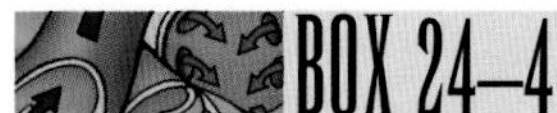

BOX 24–4

Cardiovascular Diagnosis Requiring Immediate Intervention

Acute myocardial infarction
Acute ischemic heart disease
Symptomatic dysrhythmia
Acute pulmonary edema or severe heart failure
Pericardial tamponade
Hypertensive crisis
  Pregnancy
  Aortic dissection
  Intracerebral event
  Renal failure
  Drug withdrawal
  Sympathomimetic use (e.g., cocaine, stimulants)
Pacemaker failure
Automatic implantable defibrillator discharge
Pulmonary embolism
Acute vascular occlusion
Acute stroke

threatening cardiovascular conditions. Resuscitation algorithms have been modified, taking into consideration equipment and medications likely to be available in a typical physician's office.[5] Actual office intervention will depend on equipment, medications, and staff available, but every physician's office should have an automatic external defibrillator, 12-lead ECG machine, and basic cardiopulmonary resuscitation (CPR) equipment. Universal treatment and EMS activation should be initiated early in the intervention of all cardiovascular emergencies.

The Adult Patient in Cardiac Arrest

For the adult patient in cardiac arrest, the primary care physician should initiate treatment delineated by the universal treatment algorithm (Fig. 24–1). The tenets of treatment include the following:

- Activate the EMS system.
- Prepare emergency equipment and medications.
- Record a 12-lead ECG or rhythm strip and immediately attempt to identify ventricular tachycardia (VT) or ventricular fibrillation (VF).
- Defibrillate if indicated.
- Assist breathing and circulation.
- Contact the emergency physician of impending transfer.

The primary care physician must identify and defibrillate VT or VF immediately.[6] Patients with acute coronary syndromes without decompensated dysrhythmia and acute stroke can be stabilized and prepared for transport. The emergency physician should be notified of the impending arrival of a cardiovascular emergency in order to prepare space, appropriate staff, and special equipment.

Life-Threatening Dysrhythmias

Life-threatening dysrhythmias can precede or occur at any time after the onset of other symptoms. These symptoms can range from nonspecific (weakness, shortness of breath, or chest pain) to castrophic collapse with cardiorespiratory arrest. The precipitating event for a malignant dysrhythmia can be as mundane as noncompliance with medication or as devastating as progression of an irreversible underlying disease. Lethal dysrhythmias can occur in the peri-infarct period, but they can also be the sequelae of an unrelated problem such as pulmonary disease, heart failure, aortic dissection, serum electrolyte abnormalities, or stroke. The primary care physician must immediately initiate treatment for VT and VF in the office but must not overlook co-morbid conditions that may require separate intervention (Figs. 24–1 through 24–8) (see Chapters 30 and 31). Amiodarone is preferable to lidocaine for shock-resistant ventricular fibrillation.[7]

Acute Myocardial Infarction

The keys to reducing myocardial tissue loss during an infarction are early diagnosis and rapid restoration of myocardial perfusion (see Chapter 27). Rapid diagnosis of an acute myocardial infarction depends simply on a heightened awareness that the patient's symptoms may have a cardiac source, checking an ECG, and obtaining appropriate serum markers of cardiac ischemia. The cornerstone of aborting or limiting an acute infarction (chemically or mechanically) is quick transfer to an emergency department, cardiac catheterization laboratory, or facility for cardiac bypass. Cardiac catheterization and rapid revascularization are indicated for patients at high risk for mortality, severe left ventricular function, or signs of shock (e.g., pulmonary congestion, tachycardia, hypotension).

For patients who complain of chest pain and who are suspected of having an acute cardiac ischemic event, the primary care physician can initiate oxygen therapy, nitroglycerin if the patient is not hypotensive, morphine for pain unresponsive to nitrates, and 160 to 325 mg aspirin (unless contraindications exist). A 12-lead ECG should be obtained and transmitted to the receiving hospital. Prehospital fibrinolytic therapy is recommended when a physician is present and the patient has diagnostic signs and 12-lead ECG demonstrating acute cardiac ischemia, or when out-of-hospital transport time is longer than 60 minutes.[5,8]

Ischemic Heart Disease

Patients with chest pain suggestive of cardiac ischemia (see Chapter 6) should undergo immediate assessment and intervention (Boxes 24–5 to 24–7). The physician

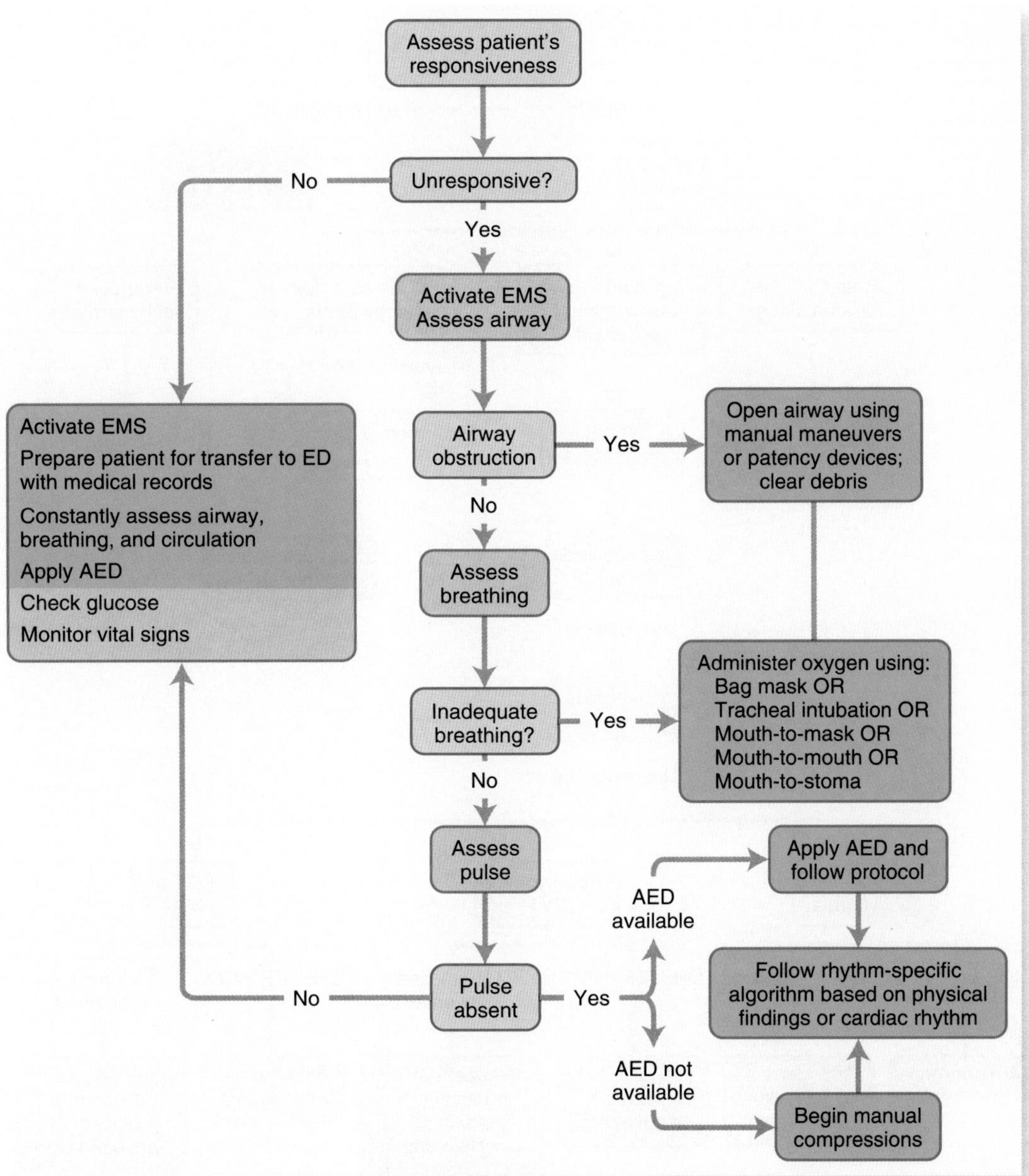

FIGURE 24–1. Universal algorithm for adult cardiovascular emergency. AED, automatic external defibrillator; EMS, emergency medical services.

BOX 24–5

Initial Assessment of Patients Complaining of Chest Pain

Measure vital signs
Measure oxygen saturation
Obtain IV access
Obtain 12-lead ECG
Brief history and examination
Obtain blood work for serum cardiac markers, electrolytes, and coagulation studies

From Guidelines 2000 for cardiopulmonary resuscitation and emergency cardiovascular care: International consensus on science. Circulation (Suppl) 102:I-1-I291, 2000.

BOX 24–6

Initial Intervention for Patients Complaining of Ischemic Cardiac Chest Pain

Oxygen at 4 L/min
Aspirin 160 to 325 mg
Nitroglycerin
Morphine IV (if pain not relieved with nitroglycerin)

Medication administration will be influenced by allergies or other contraindications. IV, intravenous.
From Guidelines 2000 for cardiopulmonary resuscitation and emergency cardiovascular care: International consensus on science. Circulation (Suppl) 102:I-1-I291, 2000.

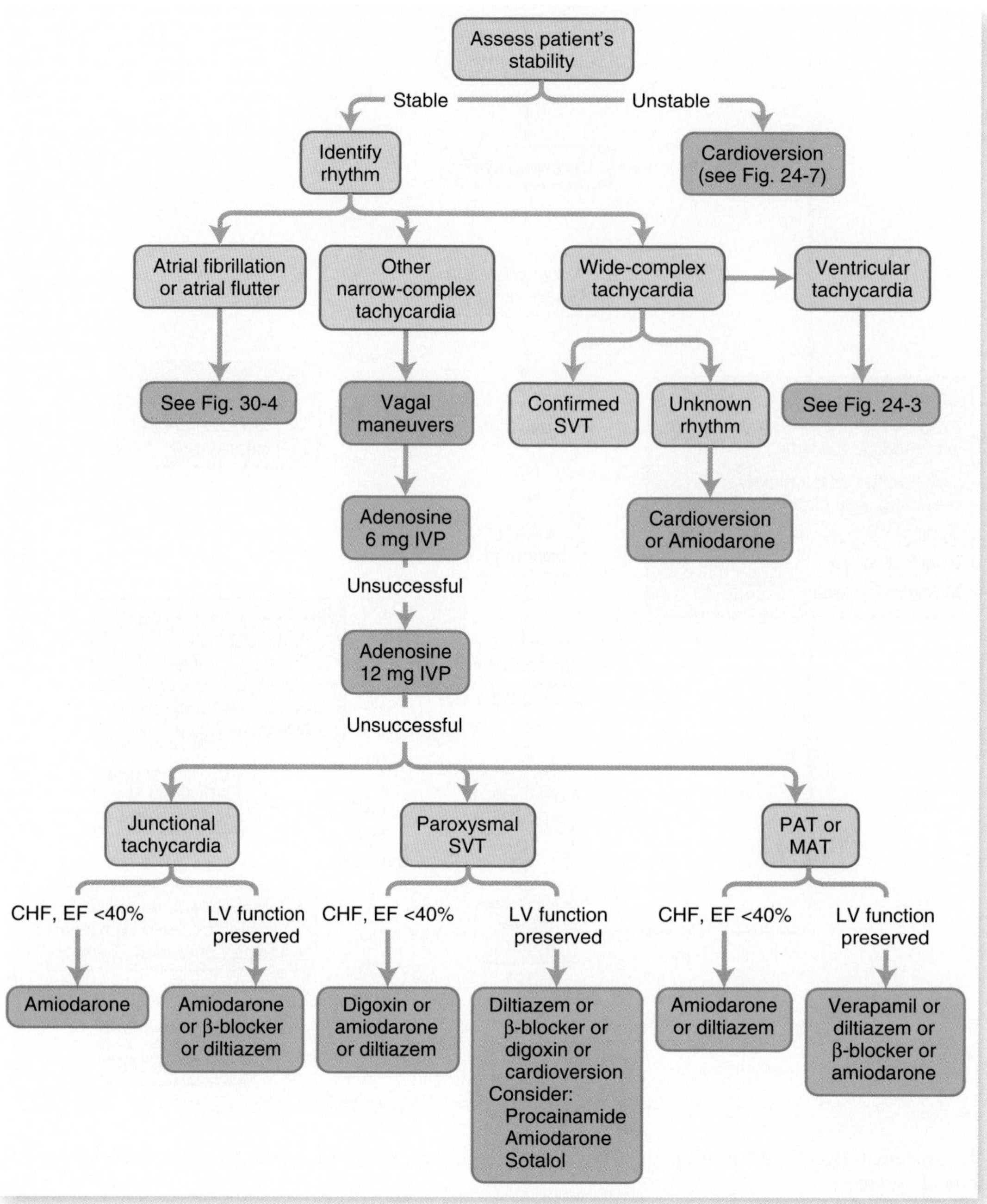

FIGURE 24–2. Tachycardia overview algorithm. CHF, congestive heart failure; EF, ejection fraction; IVP, intravenous push; MAT, multifocal atrial tachycardia; PAT, paroxysmal atrial tachycardia; SVT, supraventricular tachycardia. (Modified from Guidelines 2000 for cardiopulmonary resuscitation and emergency cardiovascular care: International consensus on science. Circulation [Suppl] 102:I1–I291, 2000.)

should immediately try to distinguish cardiac from noncardiac causes of the pain.

Hypertensive Crisis

The majority of patients with elevated blood pressure have essential hypertension with no underlying cause; the remaining patients have secondary hypertension with a potentially reversible cause (see Chapter 19). Elevated blood pressure must be evaluated carefully before initiating treatment (Box 24–8). A hypertensive emergency can be associated with a rapid deterioration of organ function due to inappropriately elevated blood pressure. The hypertensive condition may require immediate parenteral intervention (Table 24–1). Conversely, an elevated blood pressure may not require any intervention at all, and acutely lowering it may have a deleterious effect (e.g., acute cerebral ischemia). For less severe elevation of blood pressures (above 200 mm

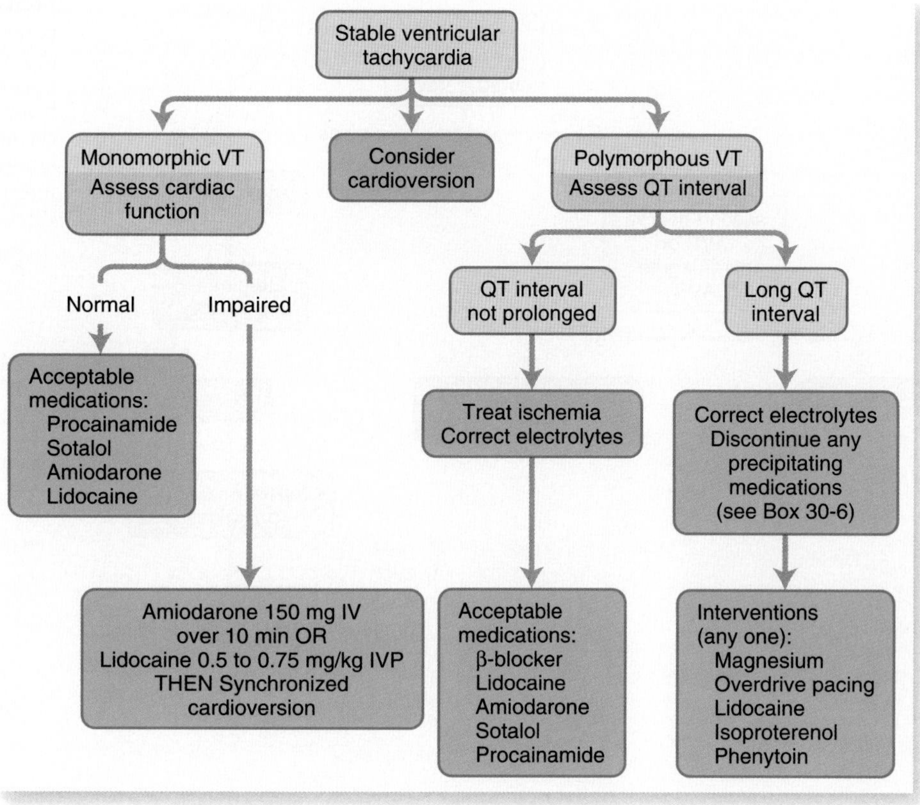

FIGURE 24–3. Stable ventricular tachycardia algorithm. VT, ventricular tachycardia. (Modified from Guidelines 2000 for cardiopulmonary resuscitation and emergency cardiovascular care: International consensus on science. Circulation [Suppl] 102:I1–I291, 2000.)

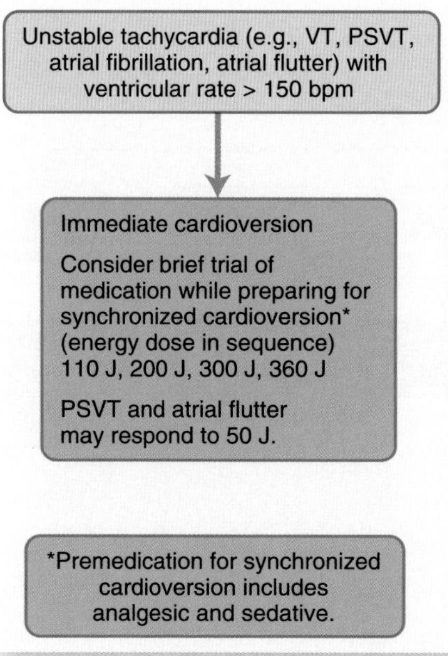

FIGURE 24–4. Unstable tachycardia algorithm. J, joules; PSVT, paroxysmal supraventricular tachycardia; VT, ventricular tachycardia. (Modified from Guidelines 2000 for cardiopulmonary resuscitation and emergency cardiovascular care: International consensus on science. Circulation [Suppl] 102:I1–I291, 2000.)

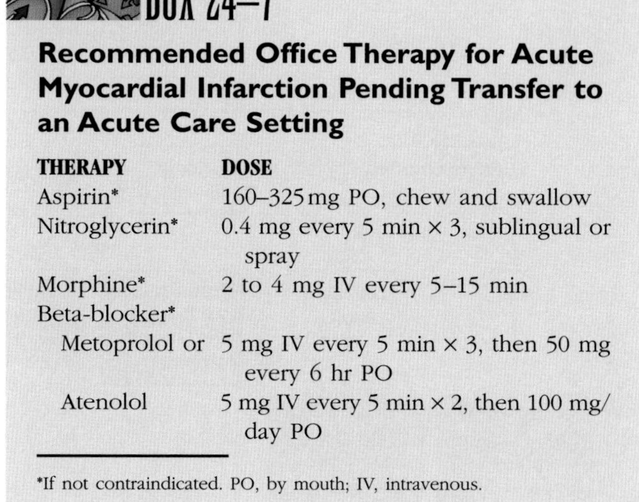

BOX 24–7

Recommended Office Therapy for Acute Myocardial Infarction Pending Transfer to an Acute Care Setting

THERAPY	DOSE
Aspirin*	160–325 mg PO, chew and swallow
Nitroglycerin*	0.4 mg every 5 min × 3, sublingual or spray
Morphine*	2 to 4 mg IV every 5–15 min
Beta-blocker*	
Metoprolol or	5 mg IV every 5 min × 3, then 50 mg every 6 hr PO
Atenolol	5 mg IV every 5 min × 2, then 100 mg/day PO

*If not contraindicated. PO, by mouth; IV, intravenous.

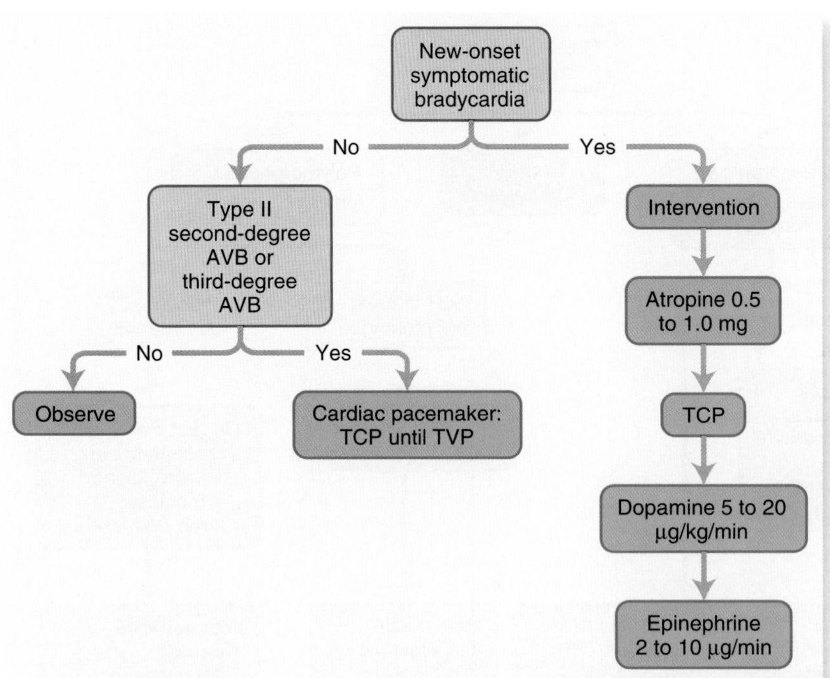

FIGURE 24–5. Emergent approach to the patient with bradycardia. AVB, atrioventricular block; TCP, transcutaneous pacer; TVP, transvenous pacer. (Modified from Guidelines 2000 for cardiopulmonary resuscitation and emergency cardiovascular care: International consensus on science. Circulation [Suppl] 102:I1–I291, 2000.)

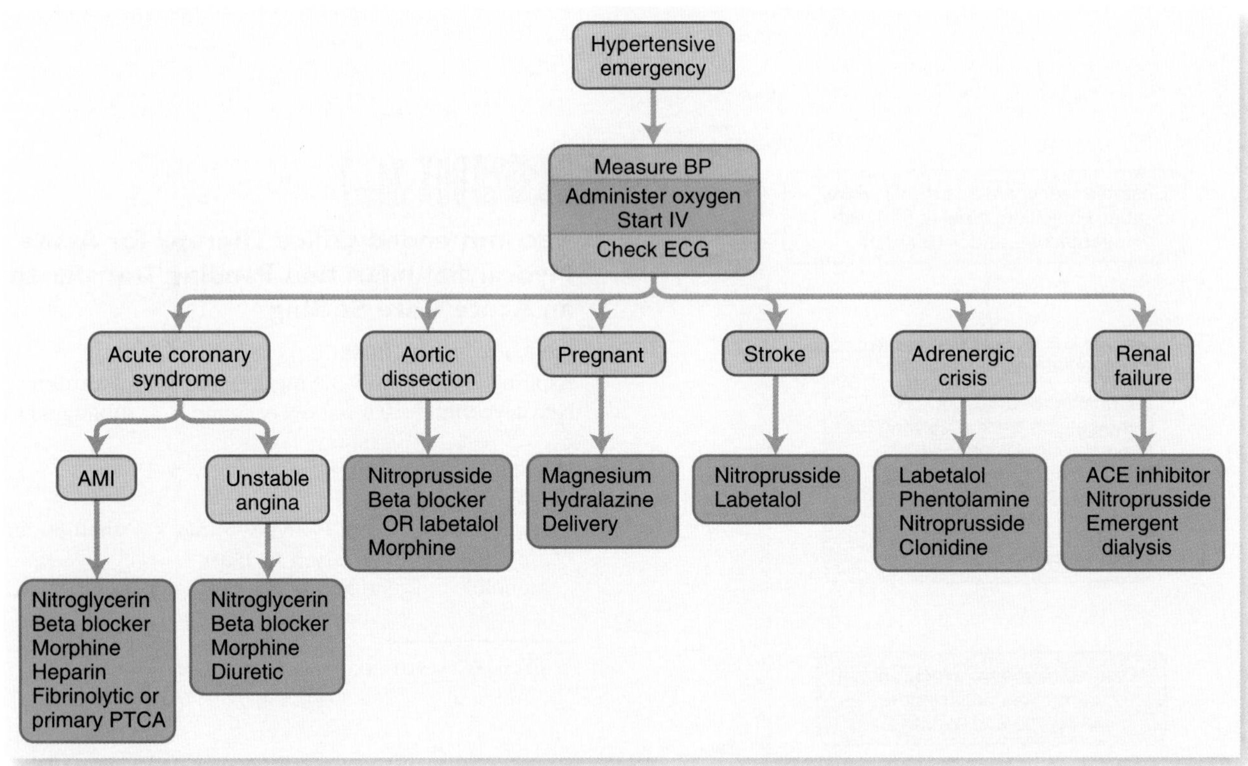

FIGURE 24–6. Emergency management of hypertension. Refer to text for doses and route of administration. Medications listed in the treatment boxes should be chosen after considering not only these common indications, but also their contraindications, as well as the patient's current medications, allergies, and conditions. Adrenergic crises include drug withdrawal, cocaine toxicity, and pheochromocytoma. ACE, angiotensin-converting enzyme; AMI, acute myocardial infarction; BP, blood pressure; ECG, electrocardiogram; IV, intravenous.

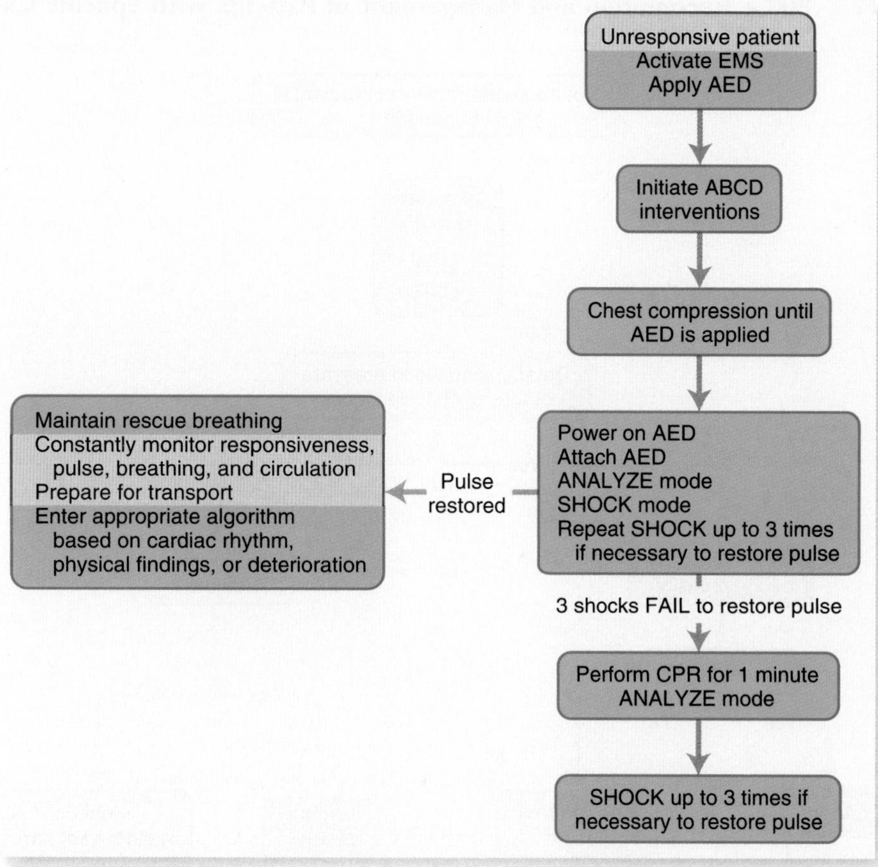

FIGURE 24–7. Automatic external defibrillator treatment algorithm. AED, automatic external defibrillator; CPR, cardiopulmonary resuscitation; EMS, emergency medical services. (Modified from Guidelines 2000 for cardiopulmonary resuscitation and emergency cardiovascular care: International consensus on science. Circulation [Suppl] 102:I1–I291, 2000.)

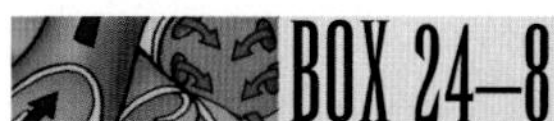

BOX 24–8

Evaluation of Patient with Hypertensive Crisis: Uncovering Reversible Causes and Evidence of End-Organ Injury

HISTORY

Onset and duration of hypertensive episode

Onset and duration of symptoms
- Pain symptoms: chest, neck, back, abdomen
- Neurologic symptoms
- Headache
- Altered mental status, speech, or vision
- Extremity weakness
- Seizure
- Medications
- Compliance history

Review of systems
- Coronary artery disease
- Aneurysm
- Stroke
- Pheochromocytoma
- Thyroid disease
- Renal disease
- Pregnancy
- Surgery

Social
- Cigarette smoking
- Cocaine or stimulant exposure
- Diet pills
- Stimulants

PHYSICAL EXAMINATION

Vital signs
- BP in each arm with appropriately sized cuff
- Repeat BP following a rest period
- Assess level of consciousness and distress

Head
- Artery palpation
- Intraocular pressure
- Funduscopic examination

Neck
- Jugular venous distention
- Carotid and vertebral auscultation for bruits
- Pain with movement

Respiratory
- Auscultatory findings of rales or wheezing

Cardiac
- S_3 gallop
- Aortic murmur

Extremities
- Comparative peripheral pulses
- Peripheral arterial flow and bruits
- Edema

Neurologic
- Complete system examination
- Visual field test by confrontation
- Language

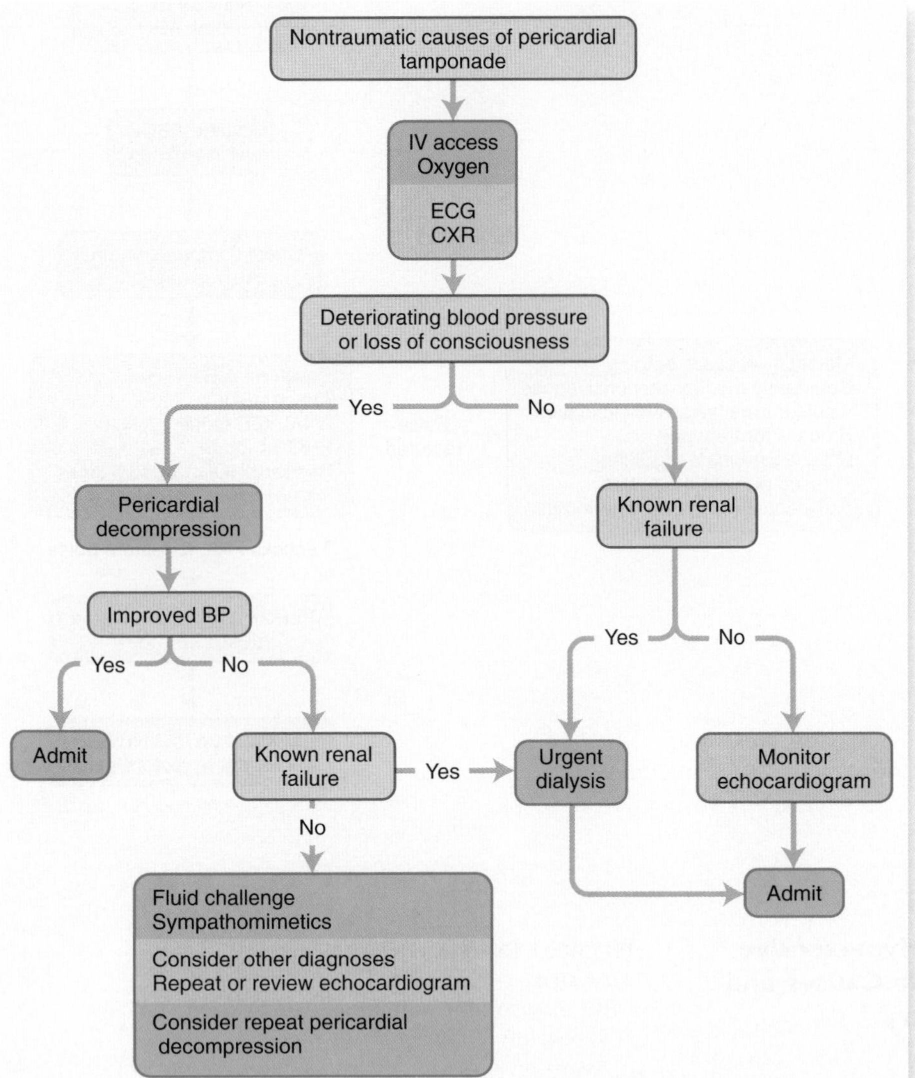

FIGURE 24–8. Emergency treatment of pericardial tamponade. BP, blood pressure; CXR, chest radiograph; ECG, electrocardiogram; IV, intravenous.

Hg systolic or 120 mm Hg diastolic) without evidence of end-organ abnormalities, oral medications can be used to lower the blood pressure (Table 24–2) and treat the underlying cause.

Acute Pulmonary Edema

Pulmonary edema can be associated with primary cardiac disease or noncardiac disease. Treatment must be started while the root cause is investigated (see Chapter 28). Common errors include not evaluating the patient for noncardiac causes of dyspnea or peripheral edema, attributing respiratory symptoms to chronic obstructive pulmonary disease, not identifying reversible causes of heart failure, failing to measure left ventricular function, and not properly evaluating the patient for myocardial ischemia. Rapid measurement of B-type natriuretic hormone levels can help identify heart failure as the cause of acute dyspnea.[9] In the majority of patients, acute heart failure is caused by a progression of underlying heart disease or myocardial ischemia.

Regardless of the cause, the symptoms of shortness of breath, labored respirations, and labored conversation must be treated (Box 24–9). The emphasis of treatment is on reducing fluid return to·the right heart by increasing venous capacitance and diuresis. The patient should be placed in the position of maximal comfort, preferably with the legs hanging over the side of the bed to increase venous dependency. Medications to treat acute pulmonary edema are listed in Table 24–3. Nesiritide, which is B-type natriuretic peptide, represents a new treatment approach that appears to be superior to dobutamine for acutely decompensated heart failure.[10]

Pericardial Emergencies

Disorders of the pericardium and pericardial space include pericarditis, constrictive pericarditis, and peri-

TABLE 24–1

Parenteral Treatment for Hypertensive Emergencies

Condition	Indications for Treatment	Treatment Options	Goal/Comments
Malignant/ accelerated hypertension	Persistent elevation of BP with evidence of end organ damage; DBP >140 mm Hg SBP >220 mm Hg, DBP 121–140 mm Hg, nonspecific symptoms: H/A, visual changes, nocturia, weakness, weight loss Retinopathy: flame hemorrhages, soft exudates, papilledema Proteinuria, hematuria, progressive azotemia, oliguria Progression to encephalopathy Hypokalemia DIC	IV nitroprusside, initial dose 0.1–5 μg/kg/min, titrate to effect every 5 min up to 10 μg/kg/min OR IV labetalol, 20–80 mg/min, additional bolus after 30 min as needed OR IV nicardipine, 5–15 mg/hr OR IV enalaprilat, 1.25 mg/6 hr	Lower BP over 1 hr; Contraindicated in pregnancy; cyanide toxicity with prolonged use; switch to a different drug when BP is controlled. Combined alpha and beta-blockade; contraindicated in beta-blocker–sensitive patients. Calcium antagonist; onset of action 5–15 min; allows smooth reduction in BP. ACE inhibitor; onset of action 15 min; best option if CHF or high renin states.
Aortic dissection	Clinical evidence, including symptoms of rupture, leak, or dissection	IV morphine 2 mg titrated to relieve pain and IV nitroprusside 0.2–0.5 μg/kg/min; OR IV esmolol 0.5 mg/kg over 1 min followed by 0.05 mg/kg/min for 4 min. Repeat up to 300 μg max; OR IV labetalol, 20–40 mg, doubling dose q 10 min	Reduce shear force by reducing peripheral resistance and ventricular contractility; goal is SBP <120 mm Hg.
Renal failure	Marked increase in BP, complications related to fluid overload such as acute CHF, IHD Acutely elevated creatinine	Emergent dialysis IV nitroprusside, 0.1–0.5 μg/kg/min	Treat CHF, IHD pending dialysis
Acute coronary syndrome	Chest pain, evidence of ischemia or infarction	0.3–0.4 mg SL, spray, or topical NTG OR IV nitroprusside, 0.2–0.5 μg/kg/min OR IV morphine 2 mg	Treat the underlying disease
Pulmonary edema	Respiratory distress, hypoxemia, IHD, pulmonary edema, complicating medical illness (i.e., AMI, CVA)	IV furosemide, 40–80 mg over 2 min OR IV bumetanide, 0.5–1.0 mg AND SL NTG 0.3 mg OR Transdermal NTG, 1–2 inches AND IV morphine 2 mg	Evaluate for precipitating event
Drug withdrawal; cocaine toxicity	Persistently elevated BP with evidence of end-organ damage	Start antihypertensive medication Benzodiazepine sedation	

AMI, acute myocardial infarction; CHF, congestive heart failure; CVA, cerebral vascular accident; DBP, diastolic blood pressure; DIC, disseminated intravascular coagulation; H/A, headache; IHD, ischemic heart disease; IV, intravenous; NTG, nitroglycerin; SBP, systolic blood pressure; SL, sublingual.

cardial tamponade (see Chapter 35). Pericardial disease can cause chest pain and can be difficult to distinguish from other causes of such pain (see Chapter 6).

Pericardial emergencies are caused by tamponade, which produces hypotension, tachycardia, pulsus paradoxus, elevated jugular venous pressure, and pulmonary vascular congestion. It may present with or progress to cardiovascular collapse. If time permits, an echocardiogram should be obtained to aid in diagnosis and intervention. Blood pressure can be supported with administration of intravenous fluid and the judicious use of inotropic agents. In the presence of cardiovascular collapse, however, emergent bedside pericardiocentesis may be lifesaving (Fig. 24–9).

TABLE 24–2

Oral Medications for Hypertensive Emergencies

Medication	Dose	Onset
Labetalol	200–400 mg	30 min–2 hr
Clonidine	0.1–0.2 mg	30–60 min
Captopril	25 mg	15–30 min
Nifedipine	10–20 mg	15–30 min

TABLE 24–3

Medications for Acute Pulmonary Edema

Medication	Dosage
Morphine sulfate	2–6 mg IV every 5–10 min
Diuretics	
Furosemide	40–100 mg IV
Bumetanide	1–2 mg IV
Torsemide	10–20 mg IV
Nitrates	
Nitroglycerin	0.4 mg SL 0.5–2 inches topical paste 10–500 mg/kg/min IV infusion
Nitroprusside	0.5–0.8 μg/kg/min IV infusion*
ACE inhibitor	
Enalaprilat	1.25 mg IV over several min
Digoxin	0.25–1 mg IV loading dose followed by 0.125–0.25 mg/day
Inotropic catecholamines†	
Dopamine	5–20 μg/kg/min IV infusion
Dobutamine	5–20 μg/kg/min IV infusion
Human B-type natriuretic peptide (nesiritide)	0.2 μg/kg bolus followed by a continuous infusion of 0.01 μg/kg per min
Phosphodiesterase inhibitors‡	
Amrinone	0.75 mg/kg IV loading over 2–3 min, followed by 5–15 μg/kg/min IV infusion*
Milrinone	50 μg/kg IV loading over 10 min, 375–750 ng/kg/min IV infusion*

Treatment should occur concurrently with search for underlying cause.
*Infusion titrated to improve clinical response.
†Pulmonary edema associated with hypotension.
‡Cardiogenic shock not responsive to standard therapy.
IV, intravenous; SL, sublingual; ACE, angiotensin-converting enzyme.

BOX 24–9

Signs Associated with Acute Pulmonary Edema

SIGNS

Diaphoresis
Tachypnea, labored conversation, and respiratory pattern
Hypertension*
Weak carotid pulse
Jugular venous distention
Rales
Wheezing
S_3, S_4
Hepatomegaly
Hepatojugular reflux
Ascites
Decreased peripheral perfusion: cool, clammy skin
Peripheral edema

LABORATORY FINDINGS

Abnormal ECG: dysrhythmia, low voltage QRS, inverted T waves, left atrial enlargement, left ventricular hypertrophy, myocardial ischemia, myocardial infarction
Abnormal arterial blood gas: hypoxemia, hypercapnia, mixed acidosis
Abnormal chest radiograph: alveolar consolidation, bilateral pulmonary infiltrates, cardiomegaly, pulmonary vascular redistribution, Kerley-A lines, Kerley-B lines

*Patients with cardiac ischemia or infarction can be hypotensive.
S_3, third heart sound; S_4, fourth heart sound; ECG, electrocardiogram.

Acute Vascular Occlusion

Sudden loss of a peripheral pulse combined with severe, steady pain and diminished or absent sensation and motor function of an extremity are cardinal signs of arterial insufficiency or frank occlusion (see Chapter 37). Patients who present within 6 hours of onset are considered to have an *acute* occlusion; their treatment differs from that of patients who present more than 6 hours after an occlusion (discussed later). In both groups of patients, pain should be treated aggressively, even though attempts to restore patency differ.

The differential diagnosis of acute arterial occlusion includes arterial embolic phenomena (thromboembolism and atheroembolism [microemboli]), arterial thrombosis, arterial inflammation (drug-induced, arterial vasculitis, and infectious arteritis), vasospasm, peripheral arteriovenous fistula, and arterial trauma (Table 24–4). The physical examination should assess skin temperature demarcation, pulse, sensory status, motor function, and tissue perfusion (e.g., appearance, ulcers, discoloration).

Evaluation is focused on diagnosing the cause and extent of vascular occlusion (Table 24–5). A vascular surgeon must be consulted immediately. Intravenous heparin can be initiated, but transient improvement does not obviate the need for rapid imaging, commonly with angiography. Pain management and treatment should begin without delay. To reduce tissue ischemia, initial treatment will include urine alkalization with sodium bicarbonate, forced intravenous saline hydration, and administration of a diuretic.

TABLE 24–4

Clinical Features of Acute Arterial Occlusion

Diagnosis	Cause and Source of Occlusion	Location of Occlusion	Treatment
Arterial embolism			
Thromboembolism	85% originate in the heart 60%–70% are caused by left ventricular thrombus, post–MI. Mitral stenosis Rheumatic valve disease Atrial fibrillation	Femoral and popliteal arteries	Fogarty catheter thrombectomy Heparinization Treat underlying rhythm
Atheroembolism	Microemboli composed of cholesterol, calcium, and platelets from proximal atherosclerotic plaques	Cortical vessels Lower extremity digits ("blue toe syndrome")	Treat underlying cause Local and conservative care Anticoagulation is contraindicated
Arterial thrombosis	In situ blood clot formation due to endothelial injury, altered arterial blood flow, acute vasculitis, trauma, severe atherosclerosis	Based on mechanism	Heparinization Direct arterial thrombolytic therapy Surgical thromboembolectomy/bypass
Inflammation			
Miscellaneous	Drugs, irradiation, trauma, infections, necrotizing (noninfectious)	Peripheral extremities	Reduce exposure to drug. Treat underlying infection. NSAIDs
Vasculitides	Possibly immune complex-mediated	Small vessels, retina, kidney, multiple organ dysfunction	Immunosuppression
Vasospasm	Mechanism unknown, possibly autonomic dysfunction	Distal small arteries	Vasodilator* Sympathectomy†
Trauma	In situ blood clot formation due to endothelial injury, altered arterial blood flow, acute vasculitis	Location of trauma	Thromboembolectomy/bypass

*Recommended agents: prazosin, nifedipine, reserpine, phenoxybenzamine, and pentoxifylline.

†Limited to Buerger's disease.

MI, myocardial infarction; NSAIDs, nonsteroidal anti-inflammatory drugs.

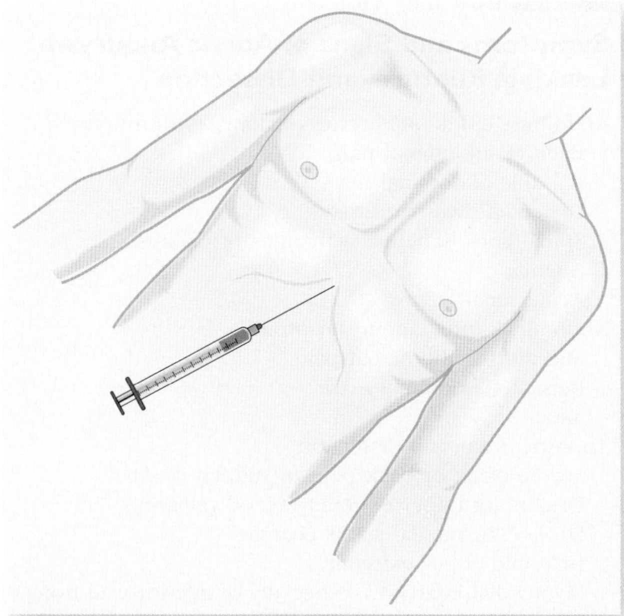

FIGURE 24–9. Subxiphoid approach for pericardiocentesis. With the patient's torso flexed 45 degrees, the physician inserts the needle under the xiphoid, directing it to the left of the sternum, while maintaining (approximately) a 45-degree angle between the needle and the skin surface. Constant aspiration of the plunger will produce a rapid return of blood when pericardial penetration has occurred.

TABLE 24–5

Differentiating Acute Arterial Embolus from Recent Thrombotic Occlusion

Character	Embolus	Thrombosis
Patient age	Not dependent on age	Older
Onset	Sudden	Gradual
Risk factor for embolus	Common	Uncommon
History of claudication	Uncommon	Common
Physical exam findings of vascular disease	Uncommon	Common
Skin temperature demarcation	Sharp	Poorly demarcated
Arteriogram	Minimal atherosclerosis, few collaterals	Diffuse atherosclerosis, well-developed collaterals
Ideal emergent treatment	Embolectomy	Heparinization Thromboembolectomy Bypass

Limb survival depends on restoring blood flow within 6 hours. When limb ischemia has been present for more than 6 hours, or reperfusion is restored following prolonged ischemia, metabolic acidosis can occur, leading to hyperkalemia, cardiac conduction disturbances, myoglobinuria, compromised renal function, or death.

Acute Pulmonary Embolism

There are an estimated 350,000 new cases of pulmonary embolism each year in the United States, including 100,000 new cases of fatal pulmonary embolism.[11] Pulmonary embolism can be difficult to diagnose because many of its signs and symptoms are not specific (see Chapter 38).

The primary care physician should have a heightened suspicion for pulmonary embolism in patients with unexplained dyspnea or chest pain. Rapid evaluation is required. Pending definitive diagnosis, oxygen, pain management, and basic interventions are required. In patients with a high clinical probability of acute pulmonary embolism (see Chapter 38), the primary care physician can initiate anticoagulation with heparin in the office even before a definitive diagnosis is established by scintigraphy or angiography. Heparin should be initiated with an intravenous bolus of 80 U/kg followed by an intravenous infusion of 18 U/kg/hr. Heparin therapy can be stopped later, with rapid restoration of natural clotting parameters, if pulmonary embolism is excluded. If the patient is diagnosed with pulmonary embolism, the physician can select anticoagulation with heparin, low-molecular-weight heparins, or unfractionated heparin.[9]

Abdominal and Thoracic Aortic Aneurysm

Abdominal aortic aneurysms generally expand asymptomatically, but patients also can present with pain, peripheral emboli from intra-aneurysmal clot, leaking, or frank rupture (Box 24–10) (see Chapter 36). In patients with rapidly expanding or leaking aneurysms, mild to severe pain is common in the midabdomen, flank, or lower back. Patients will complain of tenderness during palpation of a pulsatile abdominal mass. Lower extremity ischemia, spinal cord ischemia, or renal failure may develop rapidly. The signs of leak or rupture are dictated by the extent of hemorrhage. A leaking aneurysm may present with relative hypotension and a nagging backache, whereas rupture will present with profound hypotension and shock. The patient in shock with a suspected aneurysm rupture requires immediate surgical intervention. Patients with less catastrophic presentations require stabilization in a setting with the capability of managing sudden deterioration, performing diagnostic studies, and obtaining surgical consultation. The aneurysm's size, location, and luminal patency can be investigated with computed tomography, magnetic resonance imaging, ultrasonography, or aortography based on the patient's status. Painful expansion of a previously asymptomatic abdominal aortic aneurysm is commonly a sign of impending leak or rupture and should prompt immediate surgical consultation.

Thoracic aortic aneurysms are commonly caused by atherosclerosis, although Marfan's syndrome and other vasculitic processes can also be precursors (see Chapter 36). Thoracic aneurysms can present as expanding masses that place pressure on surrounding thoracic structures. Consequently, patients may develop hoarseness, cough, dysphagia, or the superior vena cava syndrome. A cardiothoracic surgeon should evaluate thoracic aneurysms for possible repair. Once a thoracic aneurysm begins to leak, or when it ruptures, cardiovascular collapse ensues rapidly and surgical treatment is unlikely to be beneficial.

Aortic Dissection

Aortic dissection may be caused by a tear in the aortic intima or by bleeding into the arterial wall media (Chapter 36). Patients commonly present with the sudden onset of severe chest pain or discomfort (see Box 24–10). Once aortic dissection is seriously considered, emergency cardiovascular surgery consultation is required. Initial management can be aimed at reducing blood pressure, unless the patient is already hypotensive. Nitroprusside and intravenous beta-adrenergic

BOX 24–10

Symptoms and Signs of Aortic Aneurysm Leaking, Rupture, and Dissection

Abdominal aortic aneurysm—leaking, but unruptured
- Back or abdominal pain
- Pulsatile abdominal mass
- Ischemic lower extremity
- Spinal cord ischemia with signs of paralysis
- Anemia
- Acute renal failure

Abdominal aortic aneurysm rupture
- Mid-diffuse abdominal pain
- Pulsatile abdominal mass
- Shock

Thoracic aneurysm dissection
- Severe chest or back pain of sudden onset
- Discordant upper extremity blood pressures
- Stroke/TIA/mental status change
- Ischemic upper extremity
- Myocardial infarction, especially of inferior wall from right coronary artery occlusion
- Acute aortic insufficiency from dissection into valve ring
- Pericardial tamponade from dissection leaking into pericardium

TIA, transient ischemic attack.

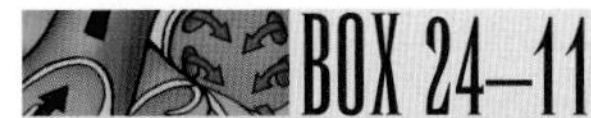

Treatment of Unstable Aortic Aneurysm

Large-bore IV access; avoid groin lines
IV nitroprusside 0.10 μg/kg/min to 10.0 μg/kg/min to achieve systolic pressure of about 110–120 mm Hg for abdominal aortic aneurysm and about 100 mm Hg for thoracic aortic dissection
IV beta-blockade
esmolol IV loading dose of 0.5 mg/kg over 1 min, followed by continuous infusion at a rate of 50 μg/kg/min for 3–5 min. Repeat bolus can be given and dose should be titrated up to achieve effect to a maximum infusion of 300 μg/kg/min; or propranolol 1 mg IV; or labetalol, 4 to 10 mg, titrated to achieve a heart rate of about 60 beats/min
Upright chest and abdominal flat plate radiograph
Crystalloid or colloid fluid resuscitation to treat hypotension
Radial artery (preferably right) cannulation for pressure monitoring
Contact surgical service
Type and cross-match 10 units of packed cells
Type and cross-match 4 units of fresh frozen plasma
Avoid hypothermia
Urethral catheter
Nasogastric tube

IV, intravenous.

antagonists are used to maintain relative hypotension and bradycardia.

Patients with proximal aortic dissection usually require emergency surgery. Uncomplicated distal dissections are commonly managed with medications; surgery is reserved for patients with persistent pain, extension of the dissection, or compromise of the arterial circulation to key organs (Box 24–11).

References

1. Cherry DK, Burt CW, Woodwell DA: National Ambulatory Care Survey: 1999 Summary. U.S. Department of Health and Human Services Publication No. 322, July 17, 2001. www.cdc.gov/nchs/about/major/ahcd/ahcd1.html. Accessed on October 11, 2000.
2. Groeneveld PW, Kwong JL, Liu Y, et al: Cost-effectiveness of automated external defibrillators on airlines. JAMA 2001;286:1482–1489.
3. Hopp FP, Duffy SA: Racial variations in end-of-life care. J Am Geriatr Soc 2000;48:658–663.
4. Mezey MD, Leitman R, Mitty EL, et al: Why hospital patients do and do not execute an advanced directive. Nurs Outlook 2000;48:165–171.
5. Guidelines 2000 for cardiopulmonary resuscitation and emergency cardiovascular care: International consensus on science. Circulation (Suppl) 2000;102:I1–I291.
6. Eisenberg MS, Mengert TJ. Cardiac resuscitation. N Engl J Med 2001;344:1304–1313.
7. Dorian P, Cass D, Schwartz B, et al: Amiodarone as compared with lidocaine for shock-resistant ventricular fibrillation. N Engl J Med 2002;346:884–890.
8. Morrow DA, Antman EA, Sayah A, et al: Evaluation of the time saved by prehospital initiation of reteplase for ST-elevation myocardial infarction. J Am Coll Cardiol 2002; 40:71–77.
9. Maisel AS, Krishnaswamy P, Nowak RM, et al: Rapid measurement of B-type natriuretic peptide in the emergency diagnosis of heart failure. N Engl J Med 2002;347: 161–167.
10. Silver MA, Horton DP, Ghali JK, Elkayam U: Effect of nesiritide versus dobutamine on short-term outcomes in the treatment of patients with acutely decompensated heart failure. J Am Coll Cardiol 2002:39:798–803.
11. Hull RD, Raskob GE, Brant RF, et al: Low-molecular-weight heparin vs heparin in the treatment of patients with pulmonary embolism. Arch Intern Med 2000;160: 2292.

CHAPTER 25 Recognition and Management of Patients with Stable Angina Pectoris

Kanu Chatterjee, C. Michael Gibson, and Lee Goldman

DEFINITION AND CLINICAL FEATURES

Angina pectoris is defined as chest discomfort or other related symptoms caused by myocardial ischemia. Angina is a *clinical diagnosis* that can be established only by a careful history (Box 25–1). Many investigations that are performed in clinical practice in patients with suspected or established angina document the presence or absence of myocardial ischemia or coronary artery disease (CAD), but not *angina*.

Angina pectoris is typically a "heaviness," "pressure," "squeezing," "suffocating," "grip-like" constriction or pain, but some patients have difficulty describing the discomfort or deny that their discomfort is truly pain (see Chapter 6). Angina is not generally sharp or stabbing, and it is not usually influenced by position or respiration.

The most frequent initial or primary location of angina is in the central portion of the chest and retrosternal area, but the left pectoral region, arms and hands, root of the neck, epigastrium, and even the right side of the chest may be initial sites. Occasionally, patients may complain of only interscapular or left infrascapular back pain. Discomfort that is located below the umbilicus or above the mandible is unlikely to be angina.

Anginal pain may be localized to one location, or it may radiate to one or both arms, the back, the epigastrium, the lower jaw, or any of the initial or primary locations. The duration of angina is variable, but it usually lasts 2 to 5 minutes. Very brief (<60 seconds) or prolonged (>30 minutes) discomfort occurs uncommonly in stable angina.

Angina is considered to be stable when it remains reasonably constant and predictable in terms of severity, initial features, character, precipitants, and response to therapy. Patients with progressively worsening angina (accelerated angina), one or more episodes of rest angina, angina after a recent myocardial infarction, or new-onset angina have *unstable* angina (see Chapter 26).

PATHOPHYSIOLOGY

Myocardial ischemia, whether silent or symptomatic, results from an imbalance between myocardial oxygen demand (consumption) and myocardial oxygen supply. Ventricular wall stress (which is determined by systolic

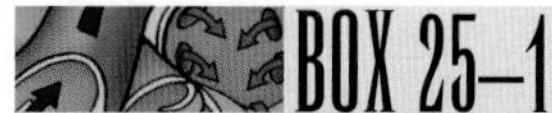

BOX 25–1

Clinical Features of Stable Angina Syndromes with Potential Mechanisms of Myocardial Ischemia

Angina of effort	Angina during predictable level of physical activity or during emotional stress (demand ischemia)
Walk-through angina	Angina at the onset of exercise, relieved during continued exercise (supply ischemia)
Vasospastic angina	Spontaneous angina at rest, usually not provoked by exercise (supply ischemia)
Nocturnal angina	Occurs soon after retiring, assuming recumbent position (demand ischemia)
	Occurs many hours after retiring (supply ischemia)
Postprandial angina	Angina during or soon after eating meals (supply and demand ischemia)
Syndrome X	Exertional angina (abnormal coronary vasodilatation during exercise) or vasoconstriction in response to certain stimuli in the presence of angiographically normal epicardial coronary arteries

blood pressure, ventricular volume, and wall thickness), heart rate, and myocardial contractility are the major determinants of myocardial consumption. Myocardial oxygen supply is determined primarily by coronary blood flow. Coronary blood flow is a function of myocardial perfusion pressure (aortic diastolic pressure) and the duration of diastole and is inversely proportional to coronary vascular resistance. Coronary vascular resistance, in turn, is determined by the severity of epicardial coronary artery stenoses, by changes in epicardial coronary artery tone, and by coronary arteriolar resistance; the latter is regulated by metabolic, neural, humoral, and autonomic activity. The mechanisms of myocardial ischemia in the various clinical subsets of stable angina are different. Angina may be predominantly due to an excessive increase in myocardial oxygen demand (e.g., exertional angina) or to a primary decrease in coronary blood flow (e.g., vasospastic or Prinzmetal's angina). When deciding on therapy to relieve myocardial ischemia, the mechanism should be considered in these clinical subsets.

DIAGNOSIS

History

Findings of Typical Effort Angina

Angina of effort, which is often termed *classic* angina, is characteristically induced by physical activity and is often precipitated more easily in cold weather or after eating. Some patients experience angina more frequently in the morning than during the remainder of the day despite less physical activity at this time. Exercising the upper extremities above the head precipitates angina more readily than exercising the lower extremities. Angina may also be triggered by emotional stress.

Relief of angina usually occurs within several minutes after cessation of exertion. Prompt relief within 2 to 3 minutes is also achieved with the use of sublingual nitroglycerin. Chest discomfort that is *instantaneously* relieved by nitroglycerin is unlikely to be angina pectoris.

In some patients, dyspnea, not chest discomfort, during activity is a manifestation of exercise-induced myocardial ischemia and is termed an *angina equivalent.* Both ischemic cardiac discomfort and cardiac dyspnea are worse during physical activity than at rest, and if patients are relieved of these symptoms during activity, it is unlikely that the symptoms are related to myocardial ischemia.

Severity

During the initial evaluation of patients with suspected or established angina, it is desirable to assess its severity as a guide to therapy. The New York Heart Association functional classification has largely been replaced by the Canadian Cardiovascular Society functional classifications or by classification systems based on activity levels that can be related to metabolic equivalents during treadmill exercise tests (see Chapter 4 and Table 25–1).

Risk Factors

During the initial evaluation of a patient with possible angina, the physician should determine whether risk factors for atherosclerotic CAD—including hyperlipidemia, diabetes mellitus, hypertension, cigarette smoking, obesity, and a family history of premature CAD—are present because these risk factors not only increase the likelihood that the patient has underlying coronary disease but also serve as potential targets for intervention. In women, menstrual status as well as hormone replacement therapy should be assessed because the risk of CAD rises in postmenopausal women (see Chapter 15). Inquiry should be made for a history of peripheral vascular disease or symptoms thereof, such as leg claudication and transient ischemic attacks, because the prevalence of CAD is substantially higher in patients with peripheral vascular disease, carotid artery disease, and thoracoabdominal aortic aneurysms.

Although CAD is by far the most frequent cause of angina, in the absence of atherosclerotic obstructive CAD, typical angina can be a symptom of hypertrophic

TABLE 25–1

Common Exercise Test Protocols

Protocol	Stage	Duration (min)	Grade (%)	Rate (mph)	Metabolic Equivalents at Completion	Functional Class
Modified Bruce protocol*	1	3	0	1.7	2.5	III
	2	3	10	1.7	5	II
	3	3	12	2.5	7	I
	4	3	14	3.4	10	I
	5	3	16	4.2	13	I
Naughton protocol†	0	2	0	2	2	III
	1	2	3.5	2	3	III
	2	2	7	2	4	III
	3	2	10.5	2	5	II
	4	2	14	2	6	II
	5	2	17.5	2	7	I

*Commonly used in ambulatory patients.

†Commonly used in patients with recent myocardial infarction, unstable angina, or other conditions that are expected to limit exercise.

cardiomyopathy, ischemic and nonischemic dilated cardiomyopathy, restrictive cardiomyopathy, and pulmonary hypertension. Clinical evaluation and appropriate investigations establish the diagnosis in such patients (see Chapters 6, 29, and 38).

Recognition of Other Clinical Subsets

Walk-Through Angina. In most patients with obstructive atherosclerotic CAD, the intensity of angina increases with continued physical activity. Some patients, however, have so-called walk-through angina. In this syndrome, the patient experiences angina at the beginning of physical activity (e.g., walking), but the angina then disappears despite continuation of the activity. The proposed mechanism for this phenomenon is thought to be an increase in coronary vascular tone and therefore a spontaneous reduction in coronary blood flow at the beginning of exercise, followed by reduced tone and better flow thereafter.

Mixed (Variable Threshold) Angina. The essential clinical feature of mixed angina is a substantial variation in the degree of physical activity that induces angina. These patients may likewise experience rest or nocturnal angina on certain occasions. Angina may also occur on exposure to cold, during emotional stress, or after meals. Dynamic vasoconstriction superimposed on fixed atherosclerotic coronary artery obstruction has been postulated as the mechanism for the variable exercise threshold.

Nocturnal Angina. In clinical practice, two types of nocturnal angina are encountered. Some patients experience angina within an hour or two after retiring. The mechanism of angina in this group of patients is likely to be an increase in venous return and hence increased intracardiac volume with a resulting increase in myocardial oxygen requirement. Other patients with nocturnal angina experience chest discomfort much later, in the early hours of the morning. In these patients, a primary reduction in coronary blood flow as a result of increased coronary vascular tone, perhaps related to different stages of sleep, has been postulated as the potential mechanism.

Postprandial Angina. Angina can occur after meals without any physical activity because of increased coronary vascular tone and a primary decrease in coronary blood flow. However, postprandial angina may occur only during physical activity after meals because of an associated increase in myocardial oxygen demand. Postprandial angina is almost always associated with significant atherosclerotic CAD.

Syndrome X. *Syndrome X* is defined as the presence of typical exertional anginal pain with angiographically normal coronary arteries. To establish the diagnosis, patients must have evidence of stress-induced myocardial ischemia by exercise electrocardiography, stress scintigraphy, or stress echocardiography in conjunction with anginal chest discomfort. Coronary angiography reveals normal or near-normal epicardial coronary arteries. Some of these patients have documented reductions in coronary vasodilator reserve, presumably caused by abnormalities in the coronary microcirculation. The syndrome may be more common in patients with hypertrophied myocardium of any cause. Although the symptoms of syndrome X do not respond well to medical management, the prognosis in terms of major coronary events appears to be benign.

Vasospastic Angina. Vasospastic (Prinzmetal's) angina occurs spontaneously at rest and may or may not be induced by exercise. The spasm is frequently noted in angiographically normal or near-normal coronary arteries, but it can also be at the site of a significant fixed stenosis. Vasospastic angina is often a cyclical phenomenon with paroxysms of severity.

Clinical Evaluation (Fig. 25–1)

The physical examination may be entirely normal in patients with stable angina. Cardiovascular examination

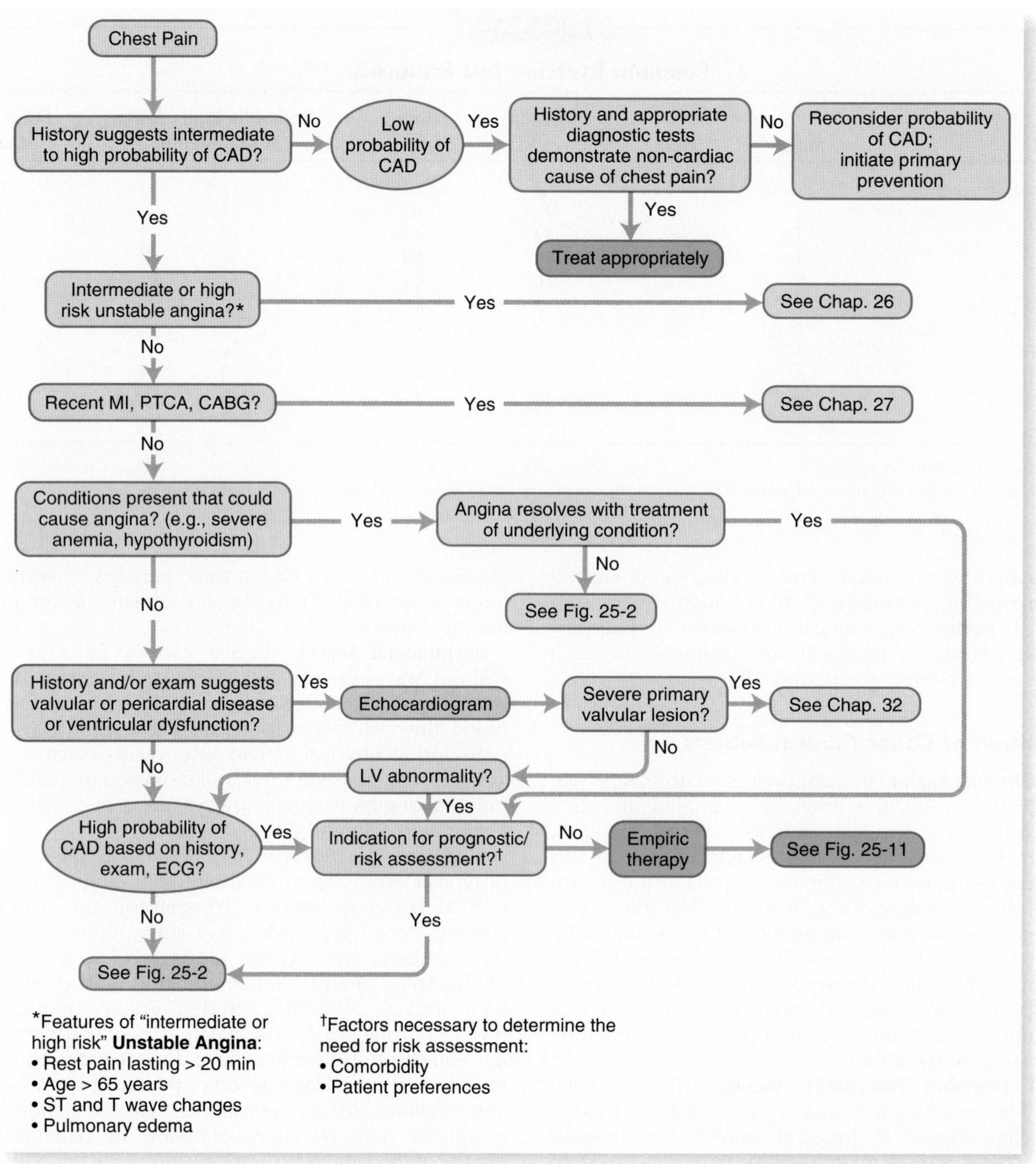

FIGURE 25–1. Clinical assessment of patients with chest pain suggestive of angina. CABG, coronary artery bypass graft surgery; CAD, coronary artery disease; ECG, electrocardiogram; LV, left ventricular; MI, myocardial infarction; PTCA, percutaneous transluminal coronary angioplasty. (Adapted from the American College of Cardiology/American Heart Association Task Force on Practice Guidelines: Management of Patients with Chronic Stable Angina. ACC/AHA/ACP-ASIM Pocket Guidelines. 2000, p 36.)

during ischemia, however, may reveal a transient third or fourth heart sound (or both sounds), a sustained outward (dyskinetic) systolic movement of the left ventricular apex, a murmur of mitral regurgitation, and paradoxical splitting of the second heart sound. The physical examination should also focus on detection of abnormal findings suggestive of left-sided and right-sided heart failure and other causes of angina, including aortic stenosis, cardiomyopathy, and pulmonary hypertension. The cardiovascular assessment should also include an examination of the peripheral pulses, funduscopic evaluation, and screening for risk factors for CAD, such as tendon xanthomas, xanthelasma, and corneal arcus, particularly in patients younger than 50

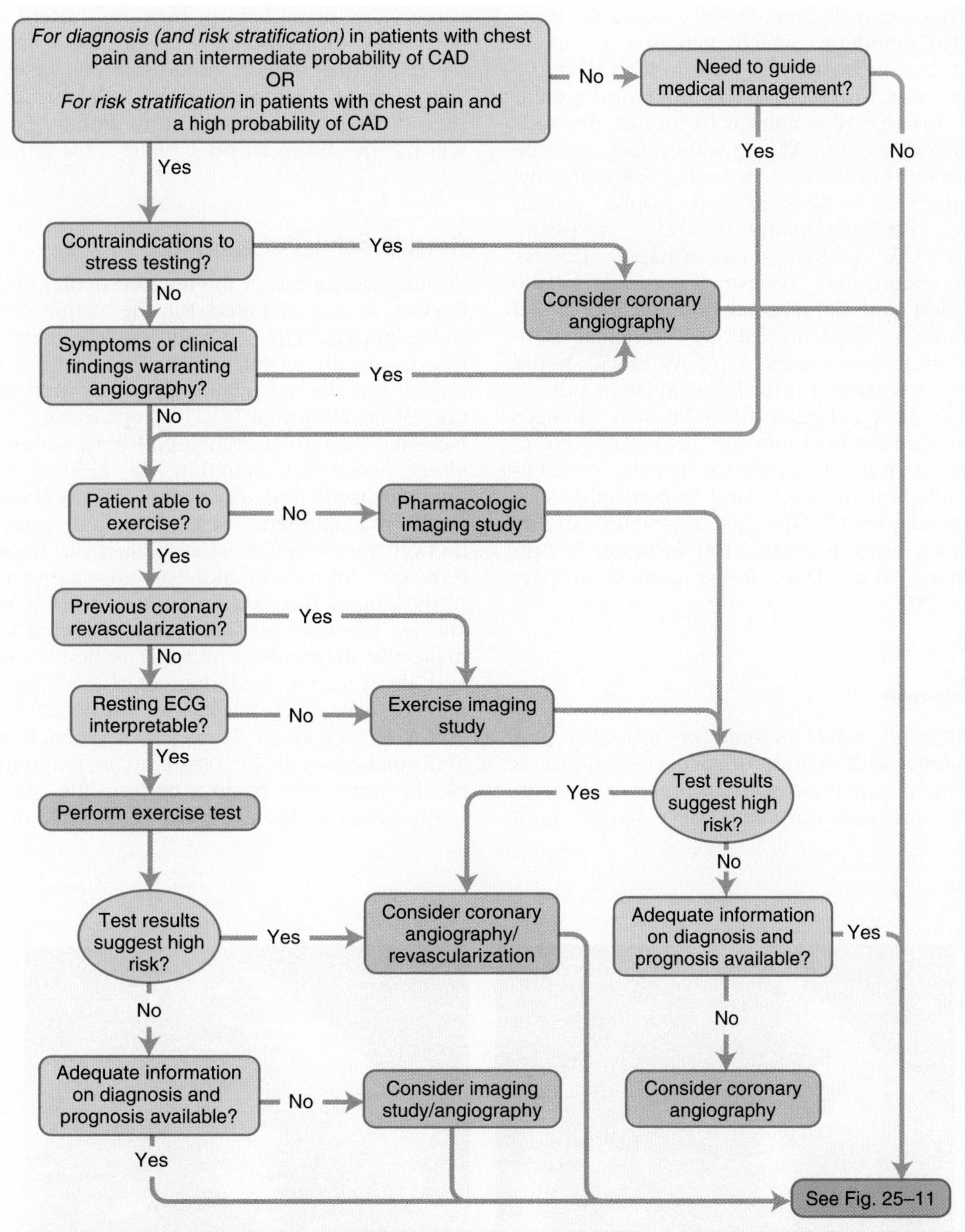

FIGURE 25–2. Approach to the use of stress testing and angiography for the evaluation of chronic stable angina. CAD, coronary artery disease; ECG, electrocardiogram. (Adapted from the American College of Cardiology/American Heart Association Task Force on Practice Guidelines: Management of Patients with Chronic Stable Angina. ACC/AHA/ACP-ASIM Pocket Guidelines. 2000, p 37.)

years. Palpation of peripheral arterial pulses, examination of the carotid arteries for bruits, and palpation of the abdomen for aneurysms are important because the presence of noncoronary atherosclerotic disease increases the likelihood of coronary disease. When palpation of the chest wall reproduces the chest pain, the pain is unlikely to be angina. The presence of a rub suggests pericardial or pleural disease.

Diagnostic Testing (Fig. 25–2)

Electrocardiography

The electrocardiogram (ECG) at rest is normal in approximately half of patients with chronic stable angina without a history of previous myocardial infarction. In the others, a variety of ECG findings may suggest ischemic heart disease. Q-waves suggest previous myocardial infarction, which increases the likelihood of CAD, but an isolated Q-wave in lead III and a Qs pattern in leads V_1 and V_2 are of equivocal significance in the absence of a clinical history of previous myocardial infarction or CAD. Q-waves may also be caused by other conditions, including hypertrophic cardiomyopathy, left ventricular hypertrophy, dilated nonischemic cardiomyopathy, and accessory atrioventricular (AV) pathways (see Chapter 12). ST segment depression and T-wave inversions in the resting ECG, left and right bundle branch block, left anterior hemiblock, atrial fibrillation, ventricular tachyarrhythmias, and various degrees of AV block should be considered indications for further evaluation but are not specific for CAD. For example, ST-T wave changes similar to myocardial ischemia are also observed in patients with intermittent ventricular pacing, intermittent left bundle branch block, and hypertrophic cardiomyopathy (Chapter 12). The new appearance of any of these ECG changes or pseudonormalization of preexisting changes on an ECG during pain is strongly suggestive of CAD.

Chest Radiograph

A chest radiograph, which should be routinely performed in patients with definite or suspected angina, is commonly normal in patients without previous myocardial infarction, previous coronary artery bypass graft surgery, or heart failure. Coronary artery calcification detected by fluoroscopy is associated with a high incidence of major-vessel atherosclerotic disease, but the sensitivity of fluoroscopy is low. Calcifications are best seen on ultrafast computed tomography (see later) and will not be observed on a plain chest radiograph.

Resting Echocardiography

Routine estimation of the left ventricular global ejection fraction is not required for the diagnosis of chronic stable angina. The left ventricular ejection fraction at rest is usually normal in patients who have chronic angina but do not have a previous myocardial infarction or an abnormal ECG, except in rare patients with ischemic dilated cardiomyopathy. In patients with previous myocardial infarction, the ejection fraction may be decreased, and the degree of decrease may help guide management. Segmental left ventricular wall motion abnormalities at rest (such as hypokinesis, or reduced wall motion; akinesis, absence of wall motion; or dyskinesis, the paradoxical motion of a wall segment and its failure to normally thicken during systole) help make the diagnosis of chronic ischemic heart disease, and the location and degree of wall motion abnormalities usually correlate with the location and extent of CAD (Fig. 25–3). However, segmental wall motion abnormalities may be observed in left bundle branch block, ventricular pacing, myocarditis, some forms of nonischemic cardiomyopathy (e.g., sarcoidosis, Chagas'

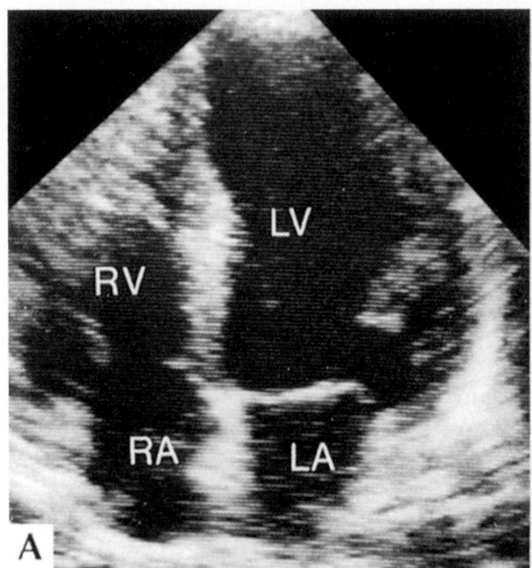

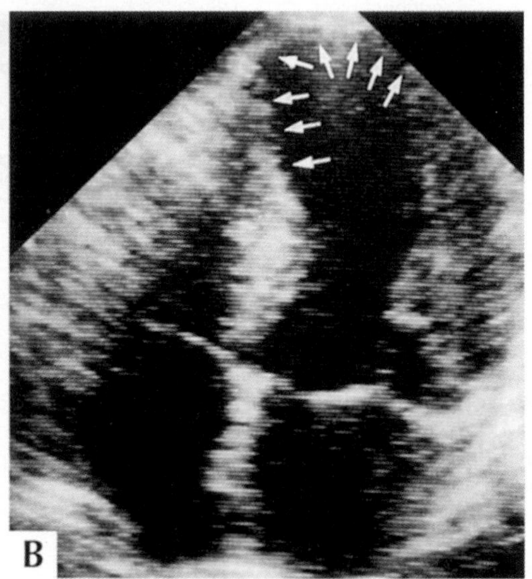

FIGURE 25–3. Wall motion abnormality is the hallmark of coronary artery disease on echocardiography. This abnormality is one of the earliest signs of myocardial ischemia or infarction. *A*, Two-dimensional echocardiographic apical four-chamber view at end-diastole. *B*, Two-dimensional echocardiographic apical four-chamber view at end-systole. The right ventricle (RV) and the septal and lateral walls at the base of the left ventricle (LV) demonstrate normal inward motion from diastole through systole; however, the distal septum and apex demonstrate akinesis (*arrows* in *B*). The wall motion abnormality demonstrated in this frame was caused by ischemia from a lesion in the mid-left anterior descending artery. LA, left atrium; RA, right atrium. (From Beller GA: Chronic ischemic heart disease. In Braunwald E [ed]: Essential Atlas of Heart Diseases, 2nd ed. New York, McGraw-Hill, 2001, p 85. Copyright © 2001 by McGraw-Hill, Inc. Used by permission of McGraw-Hill Book Company.)

heart disease), right ventricular volume overload, or previous cardiac surgery. Newer techniques such as tissue harmonic imaging and contrast echocardiography with intravenous injections of encapsulated gaseous microbubbles are currently experimental, but promising approaches for the diagnosis of ischemic heart disease. If an echocardiogram can be performed during ischemia, the presence of transient regional wall motion abnormalities and, occasionally, transient mitral regurgitation can be used to diagnose ischemic heart disease.

Ultrafast (Electron Beam) Computed Tomography

Although electron beam computed tomography (EBCT) is increasingly being used to detect coronary calcification as a means to screen for CAD, its sensitivity and specificity have varied widely, and its positive predictive value depends greatly on the types of patients in whom it is performed (see Chapter 4). Thus, routine use of EBCT for the diagnosis of CAD or for assessment of progression or regression of atherosclerosis is not currently recommended.[1,2]

Exercise Electrocardiography

The exercise ECG is more useful than the resting ECG for detecting myocardial ischemia and evaluating the cause of chest pain.[3,4] Down-sloping or horizontal ST segment depression or elevation (≥1 mm for ≥60 to 80 msec after the end of the QRS complex) is very suggestive of myocardial ischemia (see Chapter 4), particularly when these changes occur at a low workload during early stages of exercise, persist for more than 3 minutes after exercise, or are accompanied by chest discomfort that is compatible with angina (see Table 25–1; Fig. 25–4). Up-sloping ST segments are much less specific indicators of CAD.

An abnormal resting ECG associated with left ventricular hypertrophy, intraventricular conduction abnormalities, a preexcitation syndrome, electrolyte imbalance, or therapy with digitalis increases the probability that an exercise ECG will yield a false-positive result. In women, the lower previous probability of CAD is associated with more false-positive results on exercise ECG (see Chapters 4 and 15), but current consensus guidelines state that an exercise ECG in women is as sensitive as an exercise ECG in men for the initial evaluation of chest pain and diagnosis of CAD.[1] Similarly, exercise electrocardiography is routinely recommended in the elderly because of its relatively high sensitivity and low specificity despite occasional difficulties in performing the test (see Chapter 16). A fall in systolic pressure of 10 mm Hg or more during exercise or the appearance of a murmur of mitral regurgitation during exercise, along with other evidence of myocardial ischemia, increases the probability that an abnormal stress ECG is a true-positive test result that is indicative of significant CAD.

Treadmill exercise is generally preferable to bicycle exercise for detecting myocardial ischemia. In patients who cannot perform treadmill exercise, pharmacologic stress scintigraphy or echocardiography (see later) is

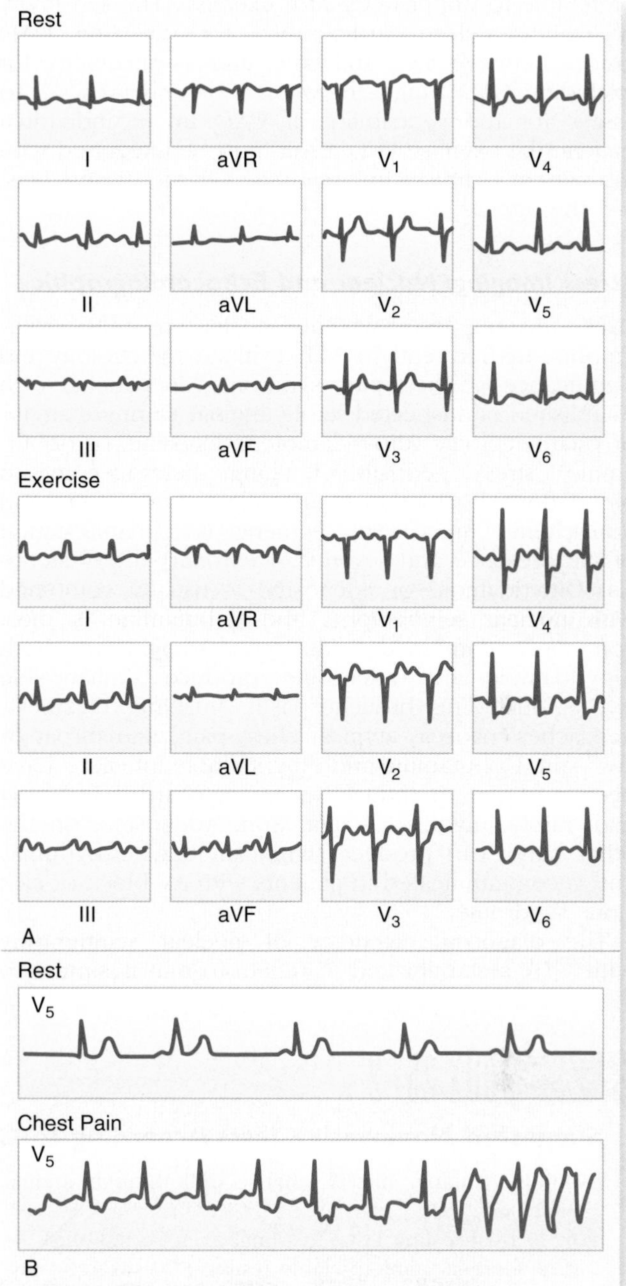

FIGURE 25–4. Diagnostic approaches for documenting myocardial ischemia in patients believed to have angina pectoris. *A*, Positive exercise test. Note the development of ST segment depression with exercise-associated angina. *B*, ST segment depression during ambulatory monitoring. Ambulatory (Holter) recordings in patients with angina and myocardial ischemia often demonstrate transient ST segment depression throughout the day. Most (>70%) such episodes are asymptomatic, but in patients with stable angina, symptomatic attacks are often recorded, as in this case. Note that the transient ischemic episode is accompanied by a brief burst of ventricular tachycardia. Patients who have positive electrocardiographic (ECG) exercise tests are far more likely to have demonstrable asymptomatic (or silent) ischemia on monitoring than are individuals with normal exercise tests. Episodes of angina can also occur without ECG abnormalities. (Redrawn from Abrams J: Medical therapy of stable angina pectoris. In Beller GA [vol ed]: Chronic Ischemic Heart Disease, vol 5. In Braunwald E [series ed]: Atlas of Heart Disease. Philadelphia, Current Medicine, 1995, p 7.5.)

preferable to upper body–arm exercise. The sensitivity of exercise electrocardiography for detecting CAD ranges between 45% and 68%, and its specificity for excluding CAD ranges between 77% and 90%.[1,3,4] To assess for the probability of CAD in an individual patient, the exercise ECG result must be integrated with the patient's clinical findings (see Chapter 2 and Figs. 2–5 through 2–7).

Stress Imaging: Nuclear and Echocardiographic

Stress imaging tests, whether nuclear or echocardiographic, are frequently used to evaluate the etiology and significance of chest pain syndromes in patients with established or suspected stable angina. During exercise or pharmacologic (dipyridamole, adenosine, or dobutamine) stress perfusion imaging, heterogeneity in blood flow distribution to the relatively ischemic and nonischemic myocardial segments is a manifestation of the presence and severity of coronary artery stenosis. Dipyridamole or adenosine is usually combined with nuclear scintigraphy, and dobutamine is most commonly combined with echocardiography. Both dipyridamole and adenosine produce similar side effects, including bronchospasm, flushing, dizziness, headaches, nausea, atypical chest pain, and throat or jaw pain. Dobutamine and dipyridamole infusions have been reported to induce severe myocardial ischemia and, rarely, myocardial infarction. Adenosine, on the other hand, can produce significant bradyarrhythmias and is contraindicated in patients with AV block or sick sinus syndrome.

The diagnostic accuracy of nuclear scintigraphy with ^{99m}Tc-sestamibi and ^{99m}Tc-tetrofosmin is similar to that of thallium 201, with a sensitivity and specificity of planar scintigraphy ranging between 83% and 90% and 88% and 90%, respectively.[1] Single-photon emission computed tomography is generally more sensitive than planar imaging for diagnosing CAD. Scintigraphy with dipyridamole also has high sensitivity, averaging about 90%, and acceptable specificity, averaging about 70%; the diagnostic performance of adenosine scintigraphy is similar to that of dipyridamole.

Myocardial perfusion imaging is recommended as the initial diagnostic test for patients with resting ECG abnormalities associated with a high rate of false-positive ECG results (see Figs. 4–2 and 25–2 and Box 25–2), such as the Wolff-Parkinson-White syndrome or 1 mm or more of ST depression at rest.[1,3,4] Pharmacologic stress is preferred in patients who are unable to exercise or who have an electronically paced ventricular rhythm or left bundle branch block. As with the exercise ECG, nuclear stress scintigraphy is less sensitive for the diagnosis of single-vessel CAD, particularly of the circumflex coronary artery.

Exercise or pharmacologic stress echocardiography compares changes in left ventricular segmental wall motion and thickening (Fig. 25–5) during peak stress versus at rest. A decrease in wall motion or thickening in one or more segments and compensatory hyperkinesis in complementary segments indicate myocardial ischemia. The average sensitivity of exercise and dobutamine stress echocardiography is approximately 86% and 82%, respectively, and the specificity is 88% and 83%, respectively; these values appear to be similar to those for stress nuclear myocardial perfusion imaging. Indications for exercise or dobutamine stress echocardiography as the initial diagnostic test in patients with

BOX 25–2

Suggested Noninvasive Tests According to Clinical Features of Patients with Stable Angina

Exertional angina, mixed angina, walk-through angina, postprandial angina with or without previous myocardial infarction

A. Normal resting ECG: treadmill exercise ECG test
B. Abnormal uninterpretable resting ECG: exercise myocardial perfusion scintigraphy (thallium 201 sestamibi)
C. Unsuitable for exercise, unable to exercise adequately: dipyridamole or adenosine myocardial perfusion scintigraphy, dobutamine stress echocardiography

Atypical chest pain with normal or borderline abnormal resting ECG or with nondiagnostic stress ECG, particularly in women: exercise myocardial perfusion scintigraphy

Vasospastic angina: ECG during chest pain, ST segment depressed during ambulatory ECG

Dilated ischemic cardiomyopathy with typical angina or for assessment of the extent of hibernating myocardium: assessment of regional and global ejection fraction by radionuclide ventriculography or two-dimensional echocardiography, radionuclide myocardial perfusion scintigraphy; in selected patients, flow and metabolic studies with positron emission tomography

Syndrome X: initially treadmill exercise stress ECG (after demonstration of presence of normal coronaries, coronary blood flow reserve can be assessed noninvasively by positron emission tomography)

Known severe aortic stenosis or severe hypertrophic cardiomyopathy with stable angina: exercise stress tests are contraindicated; dipyridamole or adenosine myocardial perfusion scintigraphy in selected patients

Mild aortic valvular disease or hypertrophic cardiomyopathy with typical exertional angina: treadmill myocardial perfusion scintigraphy under strict supervision or dipyridamole or adenosine myocardial perfusion scintigraphy

ECG, electrocardiogram.

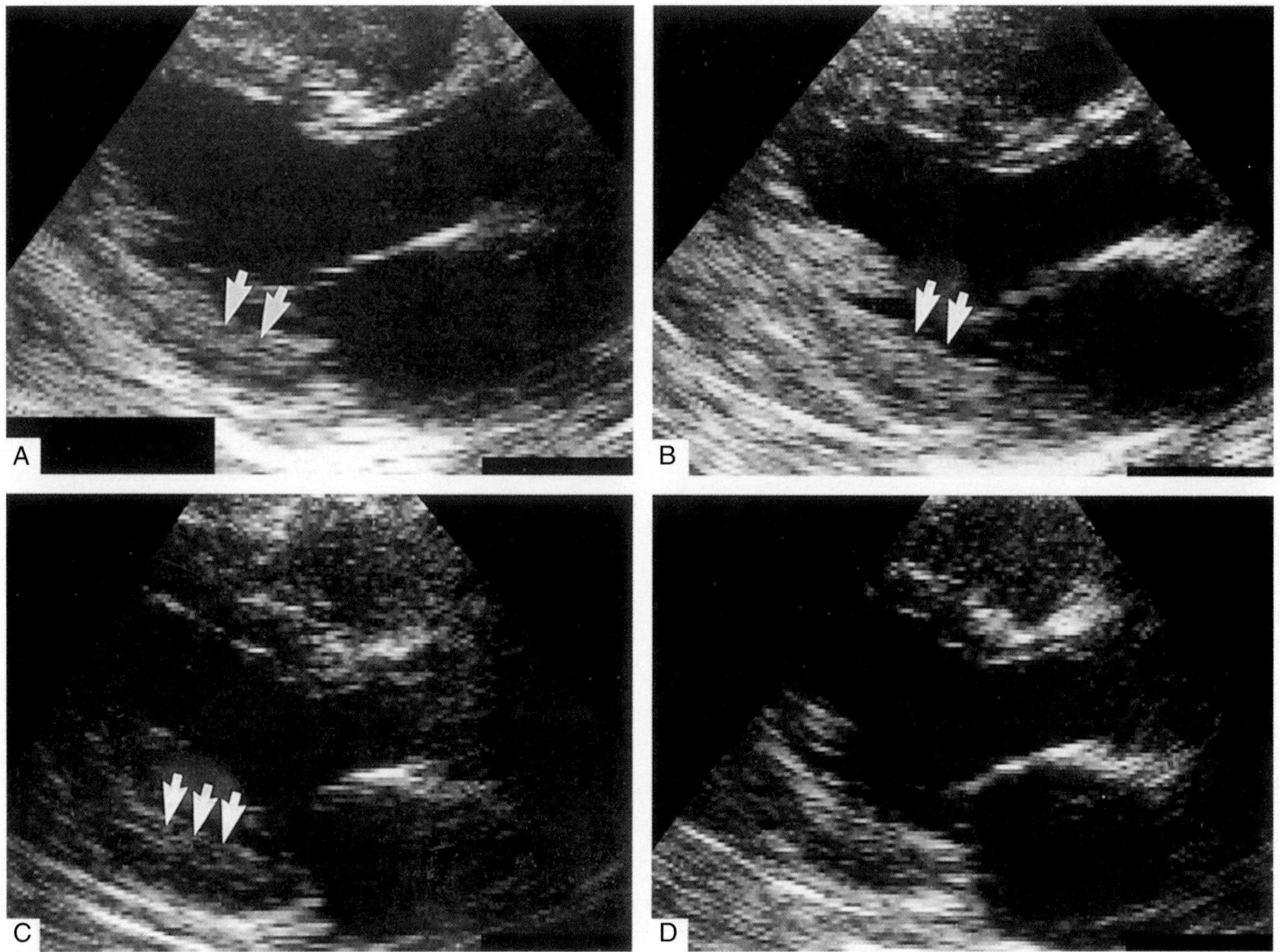

FIGURE 25–5. *A*, Stage I image of a patient at rest. Note the severe hypokinesis (*arrows*). *B*, Stage 2 image at low-dose dobutamine (5 μg/kg/min). Note the augmentation in wall motion of the previously hypokinetic zone (*arrows*). *C*, Stage 3 at peak dose (40 μg/kg/min). Note the akinesis (*arrows*). *D*, Stage 4 image at recovery. An initial improvement in inferoposterior wall motion was observed with low-dose dobutamine. The improvement deteriorates at high doses, however, thus suggesting that viable myocardium is still present in the infarct zone and is being supplied by a stenotic right coronary artery. Subsequent coronary angiography demonstrated 75% lesions in both the left circumflex and the posterior descending coronary arteries. (From Picard MH, Weyman AE: Echocardiography in chronic ischemic heart disease. In Beller GA [vol ed]: Chronic Ischemic Heart Disease, vol 5. In Braunwald E [series ed]: Atlas of Heart Diseases. Philadelphia, Current Medicine, 1995, p 4.13.)

chronic stable angina are similar to those for stress myocardial perfusion scintigraphy. Exercise nuclear imaging is less likely than an exercise ECG to give false-positive results in women, but nuclear imaging may yield false-positive results in patients with hypertrophic, dilated, and infiltrative cardiomyopathy. In patients with left bundle branch block, both exercise myocardial perfusion imaging and stress echocardiography have a high false-positive rate, so pharmacologic stress perfusion imaging is recommended.

Positron Emission Tomography

Positron emission tomography at rest and during pharmacologic stress (dipyridamole) can also assess regional coronary blood flow reserve, myocardial perfusion, and the presence and extent of hibernating myocardium. Rubidium 82 or ammonia (^{13}N) is used for assessment of myocardial perfusion, whereas labeled carbohydrates such as fludeoxyglucose F 18, lipids, and some amino acids can be used to assess myocardial metabolism and viable ischemic myocardium. With combined assessment of myocardial perfusion and metabolism, the sensitivity and specificity for the detection of CAD may approach 95%. However, positron emission tomography is a very expensive noninvasive test and is rarely used for the diagnosis of stable angina. Its added value is principally in difficult situations in which myocardial perfusion by traditional scintigraphy and assessment of left ventricular systolic function by echocardiography or radionuclide ventriculography do not reveal the extent of hibernating myocardium.[1]

Ambulatory ST Segment Monitoring

Many patients with CAD experience episodes of asymptomatic myocardial ischemia detectable by ST segment monitoring regardless of whether they have angina pectoris (Fig. 25–6). Patients with symptomatic angina also often have multiple additional episodes of asymptomatic ischemia, and the frequency and severity of these episodes correlate with prognosis. However, in clinical practice, ambulatory ST segment monitoring is seldom used for the diagnosis and management of stable angina. It is often useful, however, in the diagnosis and follow-up of patients with suspected vasospastic angina or in those with known asymptomatic coronary disease.

Selecting the Initial Test for Individual Patients

In patients with stable angina, mixed angina, walk-through angina, or postprandial angina with or without previous myocardial infarction, exercise electrocardiography is usually adequate to determine the presence and severity of myocardial ischemia, provided that the patient does not have changes on the resting ECG that will obscure the ischemia, such as a left bundle branch block or paced rhythm, and does not have a condition that predisposes to a false-positive test, such as a pre-excitation syndrome or digitalis use (see Fig. 25–2 and Box 25–2). The diagnosis of syndrome X is established by the presence of typical anginal discomfort accompanied by ischemic changes on exercise electrocardiography (or exercise stress scintigraphy), with subsequent demonstration of the absence of significant coronary artery obstruction by coronary arteriography.

In women with typical angina, exercise electrocardiography is also generally adequate. However, because of the higher incidence of false-positive results with stress electrocardiography in women, exercise perfusion scintigraphy and especially echocardiography are reasonable alternatives and should also be considered (see Chapter 15).

Exercise perfusion scintigraphy should be considered the test of choice when stress ECGs are uninterpretable, as in patients with bundle branch block, intraventricular conduction defects, left ventricular hypertrophy with baseline ST segment or T-wave abnormalities, preexcitation syndromes, or ST segment changes as a result of electrolyte imbalance or digitalis therapy. Stress perfusion scintigraphy is also more accurate than stress electrocardiography in determining the *extent* and *distribution* of ischemia.

Adenosine or dipyridamole perfusion scintigraphy and dobutamine echocardiography are the preferred noninvasive tests to assess for the presence and extent of myocardial ischemia in patients who are unable to exercise, and these tests are often recommended in patients with a blunted heart rate response because of

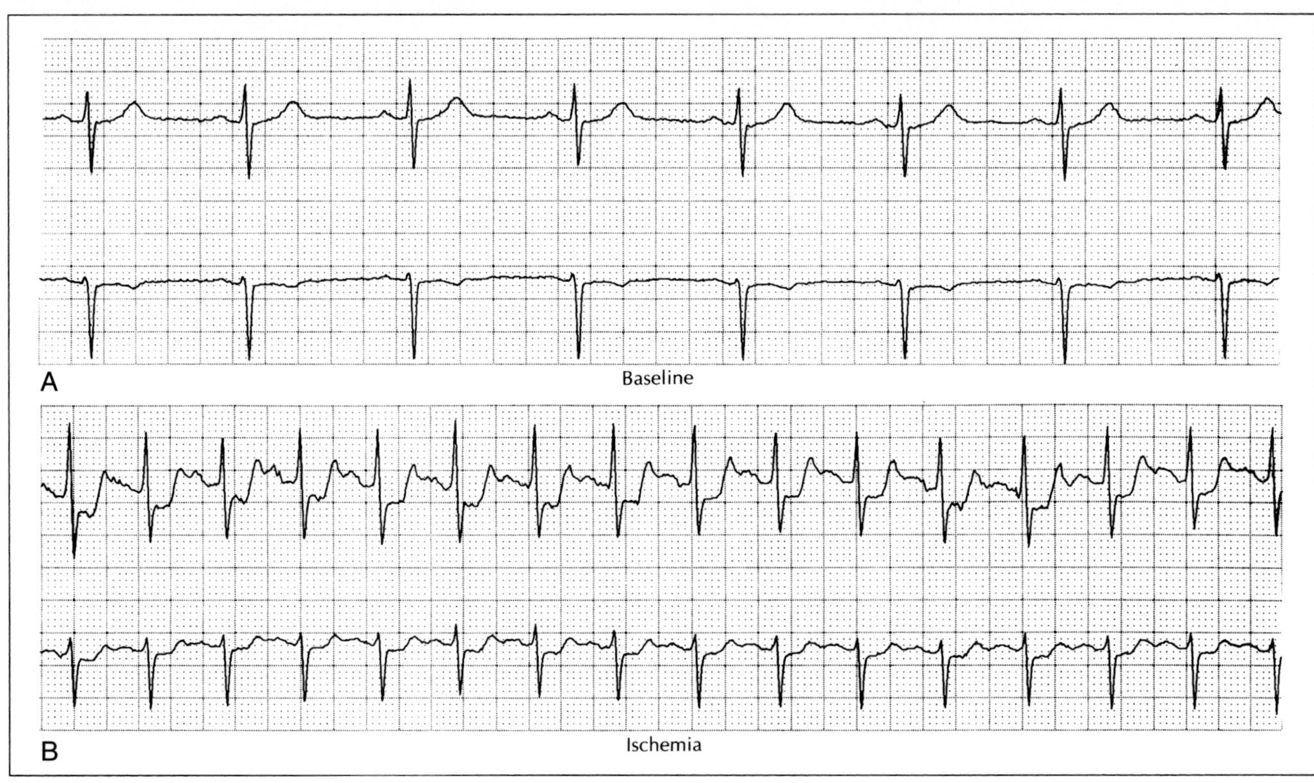

FIGURE 25–6. Detection of silent myocardial ischemia by ambulatory electrocardiographic monitoring. *A*, Baseline recording from an ambulatory electrocardiographic monitor. *B*, The same two leads showing 2 mm of ischemic-type ST segment depression while the patient, who had not experienced symptoms, was walking home. (From Bertolet BD, Pepine CJ: Silent myocardial ischemia. In Beller GA [vol ed]: Chronic Ischemic Heart Disease, vol 5. In Braunwald E [series ed]: Atlas of Heart Diseases. Philadelphia, Current Medicine, 1995, p 8.12.)

antianginal therapy. In patients with moderate or severe bronchospastic airway disease and poor exercise tolerance, dobutamine echocardiography is preferable to dipyridamole or adenosine scintigraphy.

In patients with suspected vasospastic (Prinzmetal's) angina, ST segment ambulatory monitoring is the best way to demonstrate spontaneous ST segment shifts with or without associated chest pain. This test may also be helpful in occasional patients who cannot perform treadmill exercise but have suspicious episodes of symptoms during specific activities or stress.

In patients with stable angina and documented previous myocardial infarction, assessment of left ventricular systolic function is desirable for selecting the appropriate therapy. In such patients, assessment for myocardial ischemia and ventricular function can be performed by the combination of a test for ischemia, such as exercise electrocardiography, and a test for left ventricular function, such as resting echocardiography, or by use of a single test such as resting and stress echocardiography.

Laboratory Tests

Hyperlipidemia and carbohydrate intolerance are established risk factors for CAD. Furthermore, correction of hyperlipidemia in patients with established CAD may reduce the incidence of death or nonfatal myocardial infarction (see Chapter 20). Thus, a fasting glucose level, as well as low-density lipoprotein (LDL) and high-density lipoprotein (HDL) cholesterol measurements, should be performed in all patients with suspected or documented ischemic heart disease (Box 25–3). Routine hematologic and thyroid function tests should also be performed to exclude significant anemia or abnormal thyroid function, which can be associated with worsening angina. Levels of triglycerides and lipoprotein(a) may also be risk factors for CAD, but the utility of measuring them is limited by the lack of data showing that treatment will alter risk.

Homocysteinemia has been found to be a risk factor for CAD, and folate, vitamin B_{12}, and vitamin B_6 can lower the homocysteine level (see Chapter 23). Although the therapeutic implications of lowering homocysteine levels have not been fully defined, homocysteine concentrations should be measured in patients with a strong family history of coronary disease, especially if it is not explained by traditional risk factors. Elevated fibrinogen and C-reactive protein levels[5] and increased platelet aggregability are also associated with a higher risk of coronary disease and adverse cardiac events. Other thrombogenic and hemostatic risk factors include plasminogen activator inhibitor-1 (PAI–1), factor VII, Von Willebrand factor, protein C, and antithrombin III. However, with the possible exception of C-reactive protein, these risk factors need not be routinely assessed in a patient with suspected or documented stable angina.

Coronary Arteriography

The principal indication for coronary angiography in patients with stable angina pectoris, with or without previous myocardial infarction, is for consideration of coronary revascularization (Box 25–4). Based on the results, a decision regarding medical treatment versus coronary revascularization can be made. However, even in the setting of presumed CAD ready for consideration of revascularization, 5% or more of patients may be unexpectedly found to not have significant CAD. On further testing, some patients will have syndrome X or previously undiagnosed structural heart disease, but others will have no obvious cardiac cause of their supposed anginal symptoms and will require evaluation for noncardiac causes of chest discomfort (see Chapter 6).

Diagnostic coronary arteriography is also indicated when patients have symptoms that are consistent with angina but noninvasive tests results are inconclusive or cannot be performed. Coronary arteriography is also recommended for diagnostic purposes in patients with known or possible angina pectoris who have survived

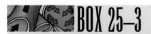

Other Laboratory Tests Suggested for Patients with Stable Angina

Low- and high-density lipoprotein cholesterol
Triglyceride level
Fasting glucose
Homocysteine level in patients with a strong family history, especially if not explained by other risk factors
Hematocrit
Test of thyroid function (thyroxine [T_4] level)
Consider C-reactive protein and lipoprotein(a) [Lp(a)] levels

BOX 25–4

Indications for Coronary Angiography

When revascularization surgery or angioplasty is contemplated because of symptoms or because stress ECG or thallium myocardial perfusion scintigraphy suggests high-risk coronary artery disease for which revascularization will improve the prognosis
Patients with atypical chest pain, when other diagnostic tests have failed to clarify the diagnosis
Suspected syndrome X
In patients with stable angina and valvular heart disease to delineate the coronary anatomy and to establish the mechanism of angina
In patients with known vasospastic angina to determine whether fixed coronary stenoses are present and in patients with suspected vasospastic angina to determine whether spasm can be provoked pharmacologically

ECG, electrocardiogram.

sudden cardiac death and in whom the results of noninvasive tests are inconclusive. When the diagnosis of vasospastic angina is strongly suspected but cannot be documented by noninvasive studies, coronary angiography with provocative testing (e.g., ergonovine) is indicated. Even when vasospastic angina can be diagnosed by noninvasive studies, coronary arteriography is indicated to determine whether fixed coronary artery stenoses are present in addition to the spasm. In patients who cannot undergo noninvasive testing because of disability, illness (e.g., severe chronic obstructive pulmonary disease), or morbid obesity, coronary angiography is indicated. In young symptomatic patients or in patients with suspected nonatherosclerotic CAD such as a coronary artery anomaly, Kawasaki's disease, coronary artery dissection, and radiation-induced coronary vasculopathy, coronary arteriography is indicated for diagnosis. In certain professionals (pilots, firefighters, police) with typical or atypical symptoms and inconclusive or highly suggestive evidence of myocardial ischemia by noninvasive testing, coronary angiography is indicated to establish the presence or absence of CAD. In patients with repeated admissions to the hospital for chest pain syndromes, coronary arteriography may be necessary to exclude CAD. Rarely, coronary arteriography is performed in patients with an overriding desire for a definitive diagnosis to relieve anxiety. In some diabetic patients, in whom symptoms may be difficult to analyze, coronary angiography may be required to establish the diagnosis and severity of CAD.

PROGNOSIS AND RISK STRATIFICATION

Extent of Coronary Disease and Degree of Left Ventricular Dysfunction

Approximately half of all patients with documented or suspected CAD are initially seen with stable angina pectoris. The average annual mortality rate associated with stable angina in patients with documented CAD ranges from 1% to 4%, but the prognosis varies widely, depending on several factors, especially the extent and severity of CAD and the state of left ventricular function (Fig. 25–7). Left main coronary artery stenosis with or without associated lesions of the other major coronary arteries carries a much worse prognosis, and the 4-year mortality in medically treated patients has been reported to be as high as 25%. The annual mortality rate in patients with one- and two-vessel disease is about 1.5%, but it is about 7% for those with three-vessel disease.

The severity of symptoms and exercise limitations also influence the prognosis (Fig. 25–8). The annual mortality rate of patients with three-vessel disease and good exercise capacity documented by exercise testing is about 4%, but it is approximately 10% in those with poor exercise capacity.

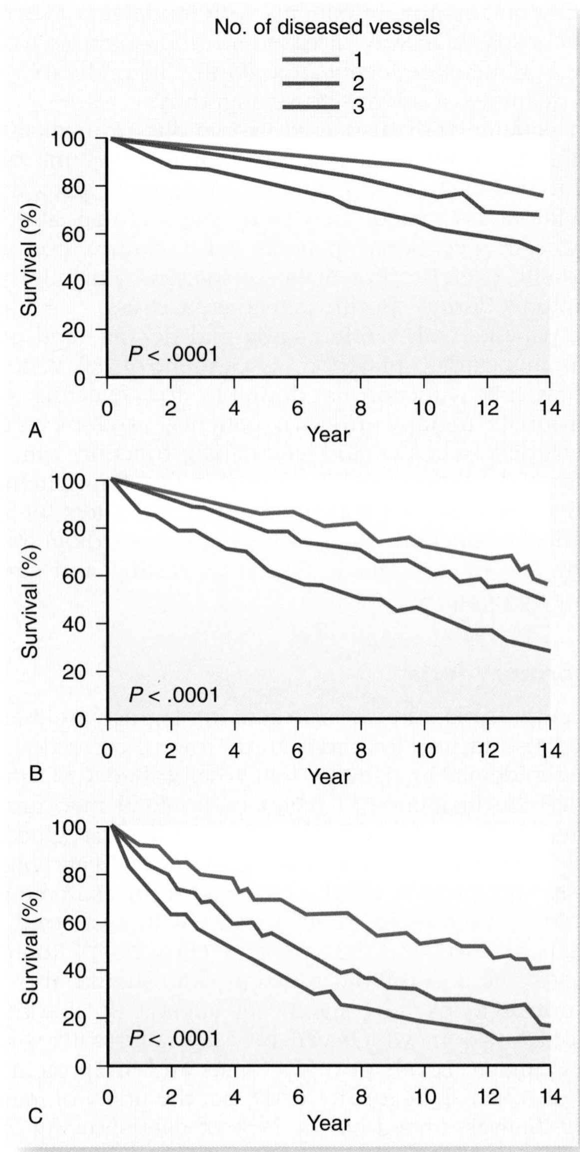

FIGURE 25–7. Graphs showing survival for medically treated Coronary Artery Surgery Study (CASS) patients. *A*, Patients with one-, two-, or three-vessel disease and ejection fractions of 50% to 100% by number of diseased vessels. *B*, Patients with one-, two-, or three-vessel disease and ejection fractions of 35% to 49% by number of diseased vessels. *C*, Patients with one-, two-, or three-vessel disease and ejection fractions of 0% to 34% by number of diseased vessels. (Redrawn from Emond M, Mock MB, Davis KB, et al: Long-term survival of medically treated patients in the Coronary Artery Surgery Study [CASS] Registry. Circulation 1994;90:2645. By permission of the American Heart Association, Inc.)

Impairment of left ventricular systolic function also adversely influences the long-term prognosis of patients with chronic stable angina. In patients with three-vessel CAD, the presence of an ejection fraction of less than 50% or evidence of clinical heart failure is associated with a mortality almost three times as high as the mortality in patients with normal ventricular function and a

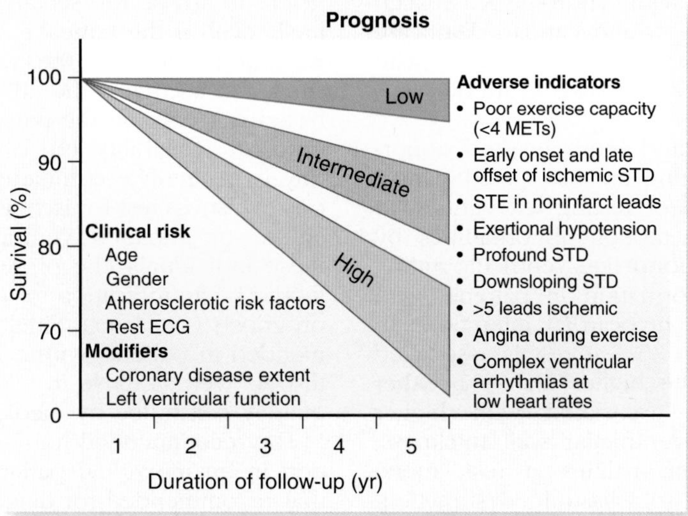

FIGURE 25–8. Actuarial survival curves of patients with normal or mildly impaired left ventricular function who have a low, intermediate, and high risk of mortality based on their exercise test results. Patients able to exercise to at least 7 metabolic equivalents (METs) with a normal exercise electrocardiogram (ECG) have an excellent 5-year prognosis for survival, even in the presence of obstructive coronary disease. The presence of several adverse indicators, such as poor exercise capacity and early onset and late offset of ischemic ST depression (STD) on the exercise ECG, place the patient in a high-risk group. Patients in the intermediate category, who have fewer adverse indicators than individuals in the higher risk group, fall into a subgroup for whom myocardial perfusion imaging can significantly enhance the prognostic information used to guide the decision for coronary angiography and revascularization. The survival curves shift downward for patients with moderate or severe left ventricular dysfunction. (From Beller GA: Chronic ischemic heart disease. In Braunwald E [ed]: Essential Atlas of Heart Diseases, 2nd ed. New York, McGraw-Hill, 2001, p 85. Copyright © 2001 by McGraw-Hill, Inc. Used by permission of McGraw-Hill Book Company; adapted from Chaitman BR: Exercise ECG testing. In Iskandrian AS [ed]: Myocardial Perfusion Imaging [Part I]: Diagnosis of Ischemic Heart Disease. New York, Cahners Healthcare Communications, 1993, pp 3–9.)

similar extent of CAD. The 5-year mortality rate may be as high as 90% in patients with three-vessel CAD, diffuse left ventricular systolic dysfunction, and an ejection fraction of less than 25%. Evidence of recent ulceration or rupture of unstable atherosclerotic plaques resulting in "acute" coronary syndromes is associated with a substantially increased short-term risk for cardiac death or nonfatal myocardial infarction.

Clinical Factors and Noninvasive Tests

In addition to coronary anatomy and left ventricular dysfunction, other clinical factors associated with a high risk of adverse outcomes include advancing age, the presence of risk factors for CAD (hypertension, diabetes, hyperlipidemia, smoking), peripheral vascular or arterial disease, and previous myocardial infarction (Box 25–5). In patients with chronic stable angina, the outcome is worse in patients with abnormal ECG findings, including evidence of one or more previous myocardial infarctions, left ventricular hypertrophy, persistent ST-T wave inversions, conduction abnormalities, atrial fibrillation, or ventricular arrhythmias. Chest radiographic findings of cardiomegaly, pulmonary venous congestion, left ventricular aneurysm, and left atrial enlargement indicate a higher risk for adverse cardiac events.

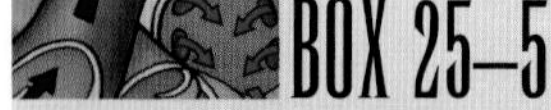

Indications for Coronary Angiography

CLINICAL MARKERS

Hypertension
Previous myocardial infarction
Diabetes
Hyperlipidemia
Smoking
Severe angina (class III or IV)
Peripheral vascular disease
ST segment depression on a resting ECG
Cardiomegaly on a chest radiograph

STRESS-INDUCED MARKERS

Failure to complete Bruce stage 1 or equivalent workload with >1 mm ST segment depression on a stress ECG; 2-mm or greater ST segment depression on a stress ECG irrespective of the level of exercise achieved; >10-mm Hg decrease in blood pressure or failure to increase blood pressure to >130 mm Hg
Left ventricular dysfunction with ST segment depression
Increased lung uptake in poststress thallium images
Multisegmental thallium 201 or technetium 99m sestamibi defects or multiple new echocardiographic wall motion abnormalities with or without associated depressed ventricular systolic function

The prognosis of patients with syndrome X is excellent, and myocardial infarction and cardiac death are extremely rare. The natural history of patients with atypical chest pain and normal coronary arteriograms appears to be benign.

Lower exercise capacity and more marked abnormalities on noninvasive testing are associated with a poorer prognosis. Detection of resting left ventricular global and segmental wall motion abnormalities by echocardiography or by radionuclide ventriculography can provide prognostic information in patients with stable angina and previous myocardial infarction; an ejection fraction of less than 35% at rest is associated with an annual mortality rate higher than 3%. Other echocardiographic findings associated with higher risk include increased left ventricular wall thickness, segmental wall motion abnormalities at rest, mitral regurgitation, and evidence of diastolic dysfunction. Echocardiographic detection of mobile and pedunculated left ventricular mural thrombi, which are usually observed in patients with previous anterior and apical infarctions, indicates an increased risk for thromboembolic complications, as well as other adverse cardiac events.

Approach to the Patient

The evaluation of a patient with known or suspected stable angina is designed to guide medical therapy and determine the potential indications for coronary revascularization.[1,2] Coronary revascularization is indicated to improve the quality or the duration of life, or both. Thus, it is used for the relief of symptoms that cannot be controlled to the satisfaction of the patient by medical therapy and in patients in whom the prognosis is likely to be improved. In making these decisions, the physician must consider not only the patient's clinical response to medical therapy but also the patient's overall medical condition, prognosis, and preferences.

As part of the initial evaluation of patients with established or suspected stable angina, the physician should assess the severity of myocardial ischemia, exercise capacity, and the status of left ventricular systolic function. Thus, every patient with stable angina who is able to exercise and in whom coronary revascularization is not excluded should have a noninvasive test of functional capacity and some test to evaluate the severity of ischemia and left ventricular function. The assessment must be sufficient to serve as a baseline functional evaluation and to determine whether the patient has disease that is severe enough that coronary revascularization will result in an improved prognosis, independent of relief of symptoms. For patients whose function is not at the level desired by the patient or physician, repeat functional assessment after medical management is helpful.

Noninvasive evaluation is especially important for identifying patients with reversible ischemia, and angiography should be recommended in these patients to determine whether the severity of the disease is sufficient to advise revascularization to improve the prognosis even if the patient's symptoms do not otherwise warrant it. Because the various tests are reasonably similar in accuracy, the choice among them should be based not only on the patient's characteristics but also on local availability and expertise. Coronary angiography is generally recommended in patients who have a positive stress test for ischemia and who also have heart failure or impaired ventricular function because, in these individuals, the presence of three-vessel disease would be an indication for revascularization to improve prognosis (see later). Similarly, angiography is recommended in patients with a high-risk noninvasive stress test, as well as those in whom symptoms are not adequately controlled by medical therapy.

The recommended noninvasive test for risk stratification in an individual patient is generally the same as that recommended for diagnosis[6] (see Box 25–2). If an exercise ECG is used, the Duke treadmill score can assess risk (see Table 4–2 and Fig. 4–5). In patients with a good score (+5 or higher), the annual mortality is only 0.25%; in patients with a very poor score (less than −10), it is 50%.

If stress imaging studies are performed, a normal stress perfusion scintiscan is associated with an annual rate of cardiac death and myocardial infarction of less than 1% even in the presence of known CAD. More extensive perfusion defects and the presence of lung uptake of thallium on stress images are associated with a poor prognosis (Figs. 25–9 and 25–10). Similarly, a negative stress echocardiogram indicates a 1% or lower mortality per year even in patients with known CAD. Progressively more severe global and segmental wall motion abnormalities during stress echocardiography correlate with future adverse cardiac events.

Coronary angiography is recommended for risk stratification in patients with a high probability of severe coronary artery disease (i.e., triple-vessel or left main CAD). Coronary angiography is also indicated in patients with refractory angina despite adequate medical therapy and in those who have survived sudden cardiac death. Coronary angiography for risk stratification is not indicated in patients with mild angina responding to medical therapy or in low-risk patients based on noninvasive testing.

MANAGEMENT (FIG. 25–11)

Antianginal and Anti-ischemic Therapy

Nitroglycerin and Nitrates

Nitroglycerin and other nitrates are endothelium-independent vasodilators that produce their beneficial effects both by decreasing myocardial oxygen requirements and by improving myocardial perfusion.[1] After entering the vessel wall, nitrates are converted to nitric oxide, which stimulates guanylate cyclase to produce cyclic guanosine monophosphate, the substance responsible for vasodilatation.

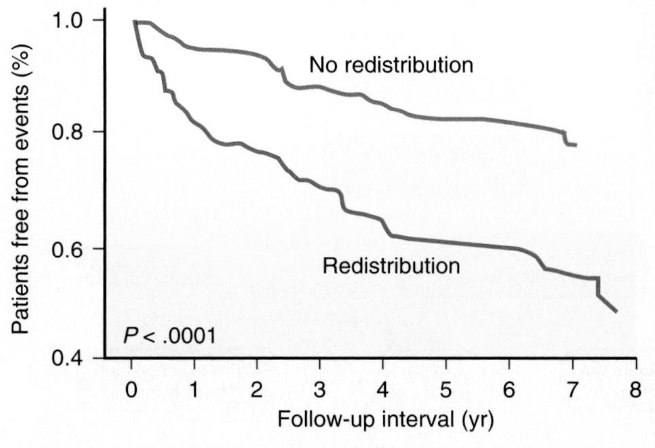

FIGURE 25–9. Event-free survival of patients with and without [201]T1 redistribution. Numerous investigators have shown that in addition to detection of coronary artery disease, important prognostic and functional information can be obtained from exercise and rest myocardial perfusion images. This illustration demonstrates the significant difference in event-free survival in patients who had angiographic coronary artery disease with and without evidence of [201]T1 redistribution. "Event-free" indicates freedom from death, nonfatal myocardial infarction, coronary bypass surgery, or angioplasty for 3 months or longer after completion of the study. The 5-year event-free survival rate was 82% for patients with no redistribution and 60% for patients with redistribution. (Redrawn from Wackers FJT: Stress radionuclide imaging for detecting and assessing prognosis of coronary artery disease. In Beller GA [vol ed]: Chronic Ischemic Heart Disease, vol 5. In Braunwald E [series ed]: Atlas of Heart Diseases. Philadelphia, Current Medicine, 1995, p 3.16.)

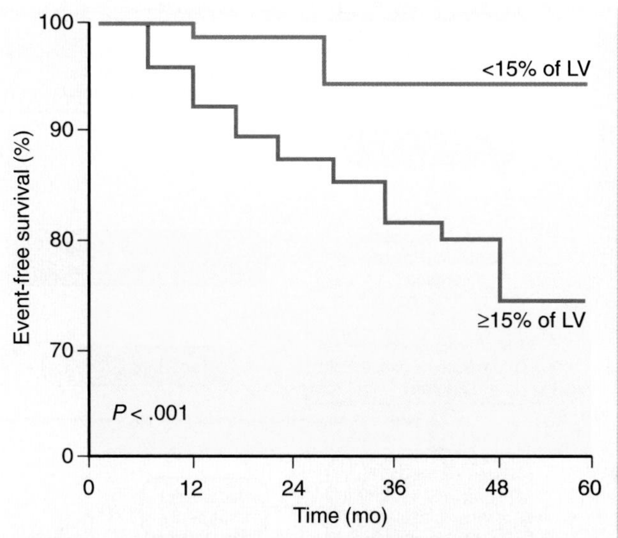

FIGURE 25–10. Correlation between event-free survival and the size of exercise-induced myocardial perfusion defects. A 2.5-year follow-up in 316 patients demonstrated a significant difference in event-free survival between the two groups. LV, left ventricle. (Redrawn from Wackers FJT: Stress radionuclide imaging for detecting and assessing prognosis of coronary artery disease. In Beller GA [vol ed]: Chronic Ischemic Heart Disease, vol 5. In Braunwald E [series ed]: Atlas of Heart Diseases. Philadelphia, Current Medicine, 1995, p 3.17.)

Nitrates dilate large epicardial coronary arteries and collateral vessels, relieve coronary vasospasm, and decrease the degree of coronary artery stenosis produced by an eccentric atherosclerotic plaque. Nitrates therefore have the potential to improve myocardial perfusion by coronary vasodilatation, by decreasing the degree of epicardial coronary artery stenosis, and by increasing collateral blood flow to the ischemic myocardium. Nitrates also decrease myocardial oxygen requirements by decreasing intracardiac volume as a result of reduced venous return secondary to peripheral venous dilatation and by reducing arterial pressure. These beneficial effects may be partly offset by a reflex increase in heart rate, which can be prevented by simultaneous beta-adrenergic blockade.

Nitrates are effective for the management of various clinical subsets of stable angina. In patients with exertional angina, nitrates improve exercise tolerance, the time to onset of angina, and ST segment depression during the treadmill exercise test. In patients with vasospastic angina, nitrates relax the smooth muscles of the epicardial coronary arteries and thereby relieve coronary artery spasm. In patients with mixed angina and postprandial angina, nitrates reduce myocardial oxygen demand and promote coronary vasodilatation. Nitroglycerin also exerts antithrombotic and antiplatelet effects in patients with stable angina.

A variety of nitrate preparations are currently available (Table 25–2). The onset of action of sublingual nitroglycerin tablets or nitroglycerin spray is within 1 to 3 minutes, thus making these drugs the preferred agents for acute relief of effort or rest angina. Nitroglycerin is also very useful for prophylaxis when taken several minutes before planned exertion. However, its short duration of action (20 to 30 minutes) makes it less practical for long-term prevention of ischemia in patients with stable angina.

For angina prophylaxis, long-acting nitrate preparations such as isosorbide dinitrate, mononitrates, transdermal nitroglycerin patches, and nitroglycerin paste are preferable. However, the major clinical problem with long-term continued nitrate therapy is nitrate tolerance. The most reliable method for prevention of nitrate tolerance is to ensure a nitrate-free period of approximately 10 hours, usually including the sleeping hours, in patients with effort angina. Isosorbide dinitrate should not be used more frequently than three times a day or a transdermal patch more often than every 12 hours.

The most common side effect of nitrate therapy is a throbbing headache, which tends to decrease with continued use. Although postural dizziness and weakness occur in some patients, frank syncope secondary to hypotension is relatively uncommon. Nitrates do not worsen glaucoma, once thought to be a contraindica-

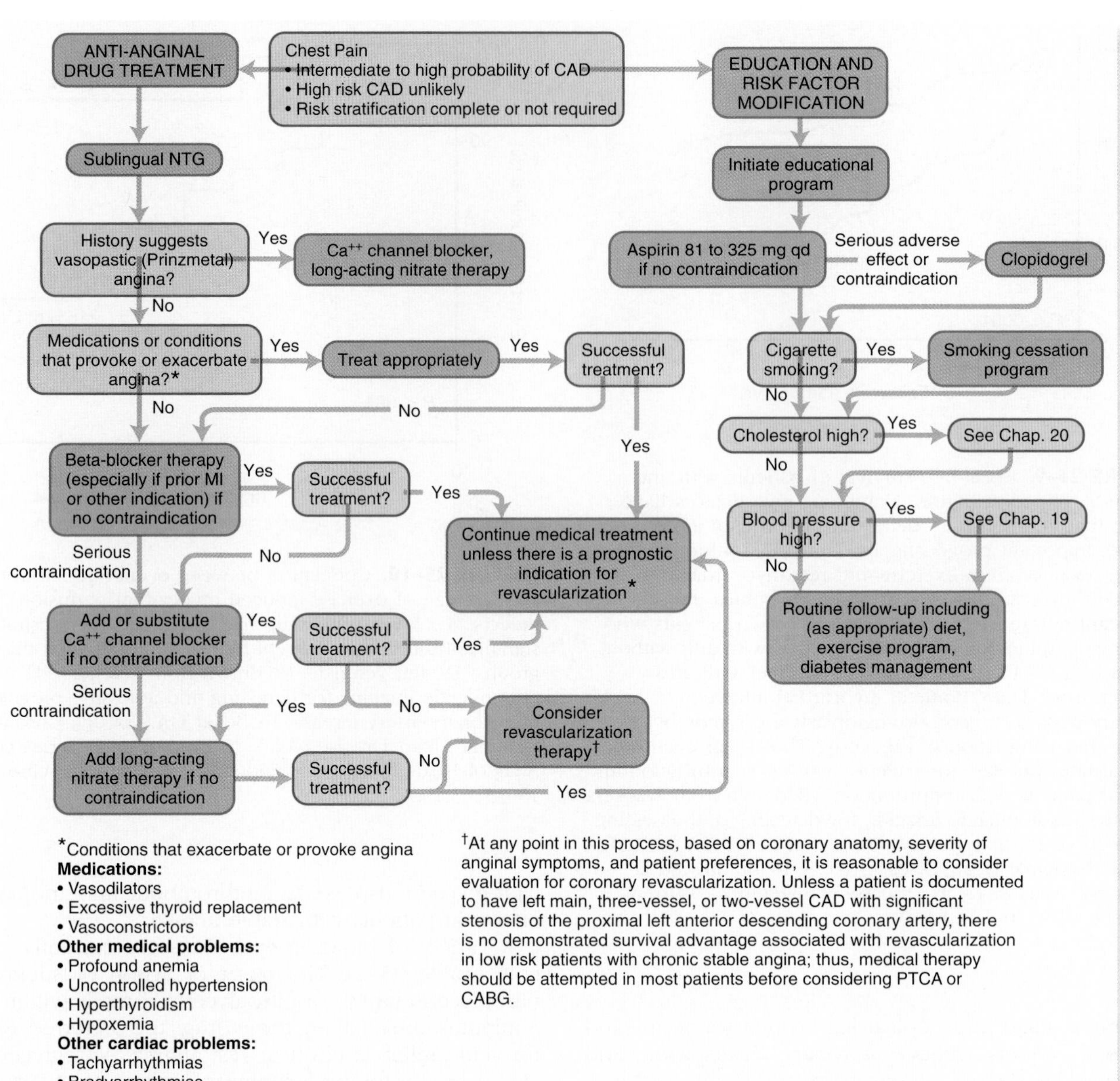

FIGURE 25–11. Treatment of stable angina. AS, aortic stenosis; CABG, coronary artery bypass graft surgery; CAD, coronary artery disease; NTG, nitroglycerin; MI, myocardial infarction; PTCA, percutaneous transluminal coronary angioplasty. (Adapted from American College of Cardiology/American Heart Association Task Force on Practice Guidelines. Management of Patients with Chronic Stable Angina. ACC/AHA/ACP-ASIM Pocket Guidelines. 2000, pp 38–39.)

tion to their use, and they can be used safely in the presence of increased intraocular pressure.

Beta-Adrenergic Blocking Agents

Beta-blocking drugs (Table 25–3) decrease the heart rate, blood pressure, and contractility and, as a result, reduce myocardial oxygen consumption. Slowing of the heart rate is associated with an increased left ventricular perfusion time. Exercise-induced increases in heart rate and blood pressure are also blunted. In patients with stable angina, beta-adrenergic blocking agents increase exercise duration and the time to onset of angina and ST segment depression, although the double product (heart rate multiplied by blood pressure) at which ischemia occurs remains unchanged.

Beta-blocking agents with $beta_1$-selectivity (such as metoprolol and atenolol) are preferable in patients with mild asthma, chronic obstructive pulmonary disease, insulin-dependent diabetes, or intermittent claudication. However, with increased doses of such agents, selectivity is lost, and both $beta_1$- and $beta_2$-receptors are blocked.

The major side effects of beta-blocker therapy include fatigue, impaired exercise tolerance, depression, insomnia, nightmares, sexual dysfunction, and worsening

TABLE 25–2

Nitroglycerin and Nitrates in Angina

Compound	Route	Dose	Duration of Effect
Nitroglycerin	Sublingual tablets	0.3–0.6 mg up to 1.5 mg	1½–7 min
	Spray	0.4 mg as needed	Similar to sublingual tablets
	Ointment	2% 6 × 6 in, 15 × 15 cm, 7.5–40 mg	Effect up to 7 hr
	Transdermal	0.2–0.8 mg/hr every 12 hr	8–12 hr during intermittent therapy
	Oral sustained release	2.5–13 mg	4–8 hr
	Buccal	1–3 mg 3 times daily	3–5 hr
	Intravenous	5–200 μg/min	Tolerance in 7–8 hr
Isosorbide dinitrate	Sublingual	2.5–15 mg	Up to 60 min
	Oral	5–80 mg 2–3 times daily	Up to 8 hr
	Spray	1.25 mg daily	2–3 min
	Chewable	5 mg	2–2½ hr
	Oral slow release	40 mg 1–2 times daily	Up to 8 hr
	Intravenous	1.25–5.0 mg/hr	Tolerance in 7–8 hr
	Ointment	100 mg/24 hr	Not effective
Isosorbide mononitrate	Oral	20 mg twice daily 60–240 mg once daily	12–24 hr

From Gibbons RJ, Chatterjee K, Daley J, et al: ACC/AHA/ACP-ASIM guidelines for the management of patients with chronic stable angina: A report of the American College of Cardiology/American Heart Association Task Force on Practice Guidelines. J Am Coll Cardiol 1999;33:2143. Reprinted with permission from the American College of Cardiology.

TABLE 25–3

Properties of Beta-Blockers in Clinical Use

Drugs	Selectivity	Partial Agonist Activity	Usual Dose for Angina
Propranolol	None	No	20–80 mg twice daily
Metoprolol	$Beta_1$	No	50–200 mg twice daily
Atenolol	$Beta_1$	No	50–200 mg/day
Nadolol	None	No	40–80 mg/day
Timolol	None	No	10 mg twice daily
Acebutolol	$Beta_1$	Yes	200–600 mg twice daily
Betaxolol	$Beta_1$	No	10–20 mg/day
Bisoprolol	$Beta_1$	No	10 mg/day
Esmolol	$Beta_1$	No	50–300 μg/kg/min
Labetalol*	None	Yes	200–600 mg twice daily
Pindolol	None	Yes	2.5–7.5 mg 3 times daily

*Labetalol is a combined alpha- and beta-blocker.

From Gibbons RJ, Chatterjee K, Daley J, et al: ACC/AHA/ACP-ASIM guidelines for the management of patients with chronic stable angina: A report of the American College of Cardiology/American Heart Association Task Force on Practice Guidelines. J Am Coll Cardiol 1999;33:2138. Reprinted with permission from the American College of Cardiology.

claudication and bronchospasm. Severe bradycardia, episodes of second- or third-degree heart block, unstable heart failure, and severe peripheral vascular disease are contraindications to the use of beta-blockers. Beta-blockers may increase the blood sugar level and impair insulin sensitivity, particularly when used concurrently with diuretics, and they may decrease the reaction to hypoglycemia in insulin-dependent diabetics. Beta-blockers increase triglyceride levels and reduce HDL cholesterol levels, but these changes are usually small and not of clinical significance except in occasional patients, in whom severe hypertriglyceridemia may develop.

The effective dose of any beta-blocking drug varies considerably from patient to patient. The resting heart rate should be reduced to between 45 and 60 beats per minute, and the heart rate during moderate exercise, such as climbing two flights of stairs at a normal pace, should be below 90 beats per minute. If beta-blockers induce symptomatic heart failure, the dose should be reduced or the drug should be temporarily discontinued while the heart failure is evaluated and treated (see Chapter 28). For maintenance treatment of stable angina, beta-blocking drugs with a relatively long half-life are preferable. Sudden withdrawal of beta-blocker therapy may result in worsening of angina and precipitation of acute ischemic episodes; it is preferable to taper these medications gradually over a period of 2 to 3 weeks.

Calcium Channel Blockers

All these agents reduce the transmembrane flux of calcium via the slow calcium channel. However, the dihydropyridines and nondihydropyridine types have different pharmacologic effects (Table 25–4).

The dihydropyridines, for example, nifedipine, exert a greater inhibitory effect on vascular smooth muscle than on the myocardium. Thus, the major therapeutic effect can be expected to be peripheral or coronary vasodilatation. These agents, however, also exert a negative inotropic effect and can therefore produce myocardial depression, which is less pronounced with amlodipine and nisoldipine. The peripheral vasodilata-

TABLE 25–4

Properties of Calcium Antagonists in Clinical Use

Drugs	Usual Dose	Duration	Side Effects
			Dihydropyridines
Nifedipine	*Immediate release*: 30–90 mg daily orally	Short	Hypotension, dizziness, flushing, nausea, constipation, edema
	Slow release: 30–180 mg orally		
Amlodipine	5–10 mg qd	Long	Headache, edema
Felodipine	5–10 mg qd	Long	Headache, edema
Isradipine	2.5–10 mg bid	Medium	Headache, fatigue
Nicardipine	20–40 mg tid	Short	Headache, dizziness, flushing, edema
Nisoldipine	20–40 mg qd	Short	Similar to nifedipine
Nitrendipine	20 mg qd or bid	Medium	Similar to nifedipine
			Miscellaneous
Bepridil	200–400 mg qd	Long	Arrhythmias, dizziness, nausea
Diltiazem	*Immediate release*: 30–80 mg 4 times daily	Short	Hypotension, dizziness, flushing, bradycardia, edema
	Slow release: 120–320 mg qd	Long	
Verapamil	*Immediate release*: 80–160 mg tid	Short	Hypotension, myocardial depression, heart failure, edema, bradycardia
	Slow release: 120–480 mg qd	Long	

From Gibbons RJ, Chatterjee K, Daley J, et al: ACC/AHA/ACP-ASIM guidelines for the management of patients with chronic stable angina: A report of the American College of Cardiology/American Heart Association Task Force on Practice Guidelines. J Am Coll Cardiol 1999;33:2141. Reprinted with permission from the American College of Cardiology.

tion caused by the dihydropyridines can also result in reflex adrenergic activation, tachycardia, and stimulation of the renin-angiotensin system. Intermittent adrenergic activation with short-acting dihydropyridines has been implicated as the mechanism for their potentially adverse cardiovascular effects.[1]

Nondihydropyridine calcium channel blockers such as verapamil and diltiazem slow the sinus node and may potentiate the bradycardia of beta-blockers. They are less potent peripheral vasodilators than the dihydropyridines and are less likely to cause hypotension, flushing, and dizziness.

Epicardial coronary artery spasm is effectively relieved and prevented by all calcium channel blockers, so these drugs are the agents of choice (along with nitrates) for the treatment of vasospastic angina. In patients with mixed, walk-through, postprandial, and late nocturnal angina, in which increased coronary vascular tone appears to contribute to the pathogenesis of the ischemia, the use of calcium channel blockers may be of benefit, particularly when nitrate therapy alone is inadequate.

In patients with stable exertional angina, calcium channel blockers improve exercise tolerance and the time to onset of angina and to ST segment depression during treadmill exercise tests as effectively as beta-blockers do. The mechanism of these beneficial effects is primarily decreased myocardial oxygen consumption. Calcium channel blockers and beta-adrenergic blocking drugs in combination can produce synergistic beneficial effects in stable angina.

Short-acting, immediate-release dihydropyridines such as nifedipine may increase the risk of myocardial infarction and mortality. Worsening congestive heart failure and increased mortality have also been observed with diltiazem in postinfarction patients with depressed left ventricular ejection fractions. However, second-generation vasoselective dihydropyridine calcium channel blockers such as amlodipine and felodipine are well tolerated by patients with left ventricular dysfunction and even overt clinical heart failure, and no increase in the risk of mortality has been described. Furthermore, vasoselective long-acting dihydropyridines (such as amlodipine) and extended-release nifedipine and slow-release verapamil and diltiazem have all been shown to reduce angina.

The general side effects of calcium channel blockers are constipation, peripheral edema, dizziness, and, occasionally, headache. With dihydropyridines, reflex tachycardia may produce palpitation. With diltiazem and verapamil, sinus bradycardia and AV block may occur. In choosing a particular calcium channel blocker in a given patient, the hemodynamic profile should be considered. Dihydropyridines are preferable in the presence of sinus bradycardia, sinus node dysfunction, or AV block, particularly when the blood pressure is not adequately controlled. Diltiazem or verapamil is preferable in patients with relative tachycardia.

Choices among Pharmacologic Agents for Angina

In patients with stable exertional angina, beta-blocker therapy is the preferred initial treatment (see Fig. 25–11). These agents reduce or prevent ischemia with a single daily dose, and their known long-term prognostic benefit after acute myocardial infarction (see Chapter 27) may also be generalizable to other patients with ischemic heart disease. In addition, all patients should be given nitroglycerin and instructions about its therapeutic and prophylactic use.

Calcium channel blockers are *not* the preferred initial therapy for the management of patients with stable exertional angina. In those with special circumstances or concomitant diseases, specific medications or combinations of medications are preferable. Calcium channel blockers are the preferred drug for vasospastic angina. For most patients, however, initial therapy should consist of the use of beta-adrenergic blocking agents, and nitrates should be added if the response to beta-blocker therapy is inadequate. Calcium channel blockers should be considered in patients who cannot tolerate beta-blockers or nitrates or who respond inadequately to these drugs. Extended-release nifedipine, second-generation vasoselective calcium channel blockers, and extended-release verapamil or diltiazem are the calcium blockers of choice.

BOX 25–6

Risk Reduction in Patients with Stable Angina

- Smoking cessation (see Chapter 21)
- Control of hypertension (see Chapter 19)
- Lipid management (see Chapter 20)
- Exercise prescription (see Chapter 22)
- Antiplatelet agents/anticoagulants
  - Aspirin: 75–325 mg daily
  - Clopidogrel: 75 mg daily if aspirin is not tolerated
  - Warfarin: international normalized ratio of 2.0–3.0 for postinfarction patients not able to take aspirin or clopidogrel
- Consider vitamin therapy for homocysteinemia (see Chapter 23)
- Angiotensin-converting enzyme inhibitors:
  - Postinfarction patients with or without depressed left ventricular function and with or without heart failure
  - High-risk patients, especially diabetics, without clinical heart failure
- Beta-blockers
  - Postinfarction patients
  - Continue in patients with depressed left ventricular ejection fractions (but reduce the dose if necessary)

Adapted from Gibbons RJ, Chatterjee K, Daley J, et al. ACC/AHA/ACP-ASIM guidelines for the management of patients with chronic stable angina: A report of the American College of Cardiology/American Heart Association Task Force on Practice Guidelines. J Am Coll Cardiol 1999;33:2143. Reprinted with permission from the American College of Cardiology.

Risk Factor Modification and Pharmacotherapy to Improve Prognosis (Box 25–6)

Smoking

Angina can be precipitated by the inhalation of tobacco smoke (tobacco angina). Smoking can also precipitate angina by causing a rise in the heart rate, as well as an increase in both systemic and coronary vascular resistance. Cigarette smoking promotes thrombosis, plaque instability, and arrhythmias. Of all the interventions to reduce coronary risk, none has more potential to improve life expectancy than smoking cessation (see Chapter 21). The beneficial effects of smoking cessation include a reduction in fibrinogen and carboxyhemoglobin, an improved lipid profile, decreased coronary vasoconstriction, and improved vascular endothelial function.

Hypertension

Control of hypertension is a critical goal in the management of angina pectoris (see Chapter 19). Treatment of hypertension will reduce myocardial oxygen demand and may reduce direct vascular endothelial injury.

Diet and Lipids

Control of hyperlipidemia is a critical part of the management of patients with stable angina from atherosclerotic CAD (see Chapter 20). A Mediterranean diet that is low in saturated fat and high in monounsaturated fat or fish can decrease cardiac mortality rates between 32% and 66%. In patients with documented CAD (i.e., in those with previous myocardial infarction, coronary artery bypass graft surgery [CABG], or percutaneous transluminal coronary angioplasty [PTCA] and in those with typical exertional angina) and with average or higher cholesterol levels, the use of 3-hydroxy-3-methylglutaryl coenzyme A (HMG CoA) reductase inhibitors (statins) decreases cardiovascular events and mortality by about 30% (see Chapter 20). Obesity is associated with an increased risk of CAD because of associated hypertension, glucose intolerance, and low HDL levels. Weight reduction, which is associated with improvements in many of these risk factors and also with a reduction in myocardial oxygen consumption, is highly desirable in patients with angina.[7] In low-risk patients, aggressive lipid lowering is better than revascularization for reducing future coronary events.[8]

Physical Inactivity and Exercise

Physical inactivity is a recognized risk factor for CAD (see Chapter 22). In patients with CAD, exercise training may increase exercise tolerance by improving physical conditioning.

Although moderate isotonic exercise should be encouraged, patients should be discouraged from performing very strenuous, vigorous exercise that can be expected to cause angina. Isotonic exercise such as walking is associated with peripheral vasodilatation and is preferable to isometric exercise such as weightlifting, which is associated with an increase in peripheral vasoconstriction. Patients should also be advised to avoid arm exercise, which is associated with a lower threshold for angina than is leg exercise. Patients should likewise be cautioned about exercising in cold or hot temperatures, which bring on angina more frequently than exercising at moderate temperatures.

Exercise programs should be guided by the results of exercise testing. It is desirable not to exceed 75% of the heart rate shown to induce ischemia as determined during the stress test. Exercise training is safe in patients with established CAD.

The mean maximal heart rate during sexual intercourse does not usually exceed 70% of the maximal predicted heart rate. Thus, if patients can achieve a heart rate of up to 120 beats per minute on an exercise tolerance test without angina, it is unlikely that sexual activity will precipitate symptoms. Patients should *not be* advised against sexual activity and, if necessary, should be encouraged to use nitrates prophylactically, unless they are also taking Viagra (sildenafil), which in combination with nitrates can precipitate severe hypotension.

Diabetes

Both type 1 (insulin-dependent) diabetes mellitus and type 2 (non–insulin-dependent) diabetes mellitus are risk factors for the development of cardiovascular disease. Adequate control of diabetes decreases microvascular complications and may also be useful for the primary and secondary prevention of CAD. In addition, because insulin resistance has been implicated in the genesis of atherosclerosis as a contributing factor in the pathogenesis of plaque instability, adequate control of diabetes appears to be highly desirable. Angiotensin-converting enzyme (ACE) inhibitor therapy appears to reduce the development of cardiovascular complications in diabetics, in whom aggressive control of hyperlipidemia is also advised.

Stress

Stress reduction programs, which commonly include exercise, meditation, and biofeedback training, may be of benefit in patients with stable angina. Treatment of depression and anxiety is also of benefit.

Hormone Replacement Therapy

Hormone replacement therapy in postmenopausal women can improve lipid profiles and measures of coronary vasodilatation (see Chapter 23). However, randomized trials of estrogen and progestin therapy in postmenopausal women with CAD have failed to show any decrease in adverse cardiac events despite these improved lipid profiles.[9] Hormone replacement therapy was actually associated with a higher incidence of CAD events in the first 2 years, as well as with more thromboembolic complications, gallbladder disease, and breast cancer. Thus, routine hormone replacement therapy is not recommended in postmenopausal women with coronary disease.

Vitamins and Antioxidants

Increased levels of homocysteine are associated with an increased risk for coronary, peripheral, and carotid artery disease. Deficiencies of vitamin B_6, vitamin B_{12}, and folate can cause hyperhomocysteinemia, and supplementation of these agents decreases homocysteine levels (see Chapter 23), although data to confirm the benefits of such therapy in decreasing the risk of adverse cardiac events are limited.[9]

Because oxidation of LDL cholesterol promotes and accelerates atherothrombosis, antioxidants (including vitamin C, vitamin E, and beta-carotene) have been evaluated as agents to decrease the risk of CAD. Prospective randomized clinical trials, however, have failed to demonstrate any beneficial effects of vitamin E or beta-carotene. The weight of evidence does not currently support the use of these three vitamins in the management of stable angina.

Alcohol

In epidemiologic studies, moderate alcohol consumption (approximately one to three drinks daily) has been associated with lower rates of cardiac events than has abstinence or higher consumption (see Chapter 23). Alcohol raises HDL cholesterol levels, but the precise mechanisms by which it is potentially beneficial are unknown. No prospective clinical trials have established the protective effects of alcohol, and the narrow purported therapeutic range makes it difficult to recommend alcohol as a beneficial intervention.

Antiplatelet and Antithrombotic Agents

Aspirin inhibits cyclooxygenase (COX) and the synthesis of platelet thromboxane A_2. In patients with stable angina, the use of aspirin is associated with about a 33% reduction in the risk of cardiac events. By comparison, the new selective COX-2 inhibitors may increase the risk of cardiac events. The recommended daily dose of aspirin is between 75 and 325 mg. Clopidogrel, a thienopyridine derivative, prevents adenosine diphosphate (ADP)-mediated activation of platelets by selectively and irreversibly inhibiting the binding of ADP to its platelet surface receptors. Clopidogrel appears to be slightly more effective but substantially more costly than aspirin in decreasing the combined risk of myocardial infarction, ischemic stroke, or vascular death in patients with CAD. Dipyridamole has antiplatelet effects, but when given orally, its vasodilatory effects enhance exercise-induced myocardial ischemia, so it should not be used as an antiplatelet agent in patients with angina.

Daily subcutaneous administration of low-molecular-weight heparin decreases fibrinogen levels and may be associated with improved exercise capacity in patients with stable angina. Long-term, low-intensity anticoagulation therapy reduces the risk of fatal and nonfatal myocardial infarction and coronary death in asymptomatic patients with risk factors for atherosclerosis. Current evidence suggests that long-term anticoagulation therapy is beneficial in some patients with stable angina, but whether used alone or in combination with aspirin, it appears to be no better than aspirin alone.

Angiotensin-Converting Enzyme Inhibition Therapy

Angiotensin inhibition has an antithrombotic effect, improves endothelial function, reduces ventricular remodeling, and may also stabilize atherosclerotic plaques. ACE inhibitors decrease total mortality, cardiovascular deaths, and strokes in patients with established CAD or at high risk for it even in the absence of heart failure or previous myocardial infarction.[11] ACE inhibitors are currently recommended in postinfarction patients with reduced systolic function and in patients with diabetes, but their indications may broaden in the future.

Approach to Patients with Possible Asymptomatic Ischemia

In some patients, angina may not be present, but asymptomatic (silent) ischemia may be suspected. Unlike patients with an angina equivalent such as exertional dyspnea, in whom the symptom can be used as a guide to therapy, patients with possible asymptomatic ischemia require a distinctive approach. In most cases, the asymptomatic ischemia is detected by a screening test (see Chapter 18) or by electrocardiographic monitoring during surgery or an unrelated illness.

Determining Whether a Positive Screening Test Is a True Positive or a False Positive

Because the prevalence of asymptomatic CAD varies by age, gender, and risk factors, interpretation of a positive screening test result varies among different types of patients. Assuming an overall prevalence of asymptomatic coronary disease of about 5% in the adult American population, an exercise ECG that shows 2 mm or more of ST depression (in the absence of underlying ST abnormalities, medications, or conditions known to cause false-positive results) or a clearly positive result on a myocardial perfusion scan increases the probability of coronary disease to about 50% (see Fig. 2–7). The combination of a strongly positive exercise ECG and a strongly positive myocardial perfusion scan raises the probability to about 90% and may be considered sufficient to make the clinical diagnosis of presumptive asymptomatic ischemia (Fig. 25–12). However, in asymptomatic men younger than 40 years and asymptomatic women younger than 50 years, in whom the prevalence of coronary disease is less than 5%, the combination of two positive test results predicts a probability of coronary disease of 80% or less. Similarly, when the results of the exercise ECG, myocardial perfusion scan, or exercise or stress echocardiogram are less indicative of ischemia—such as an exercise ECG showing less than 2 mm of ST segment depression at a high workload—the presence of asymptomatic myocardial ischemia is suggested but cannot be considered to be presumptive.

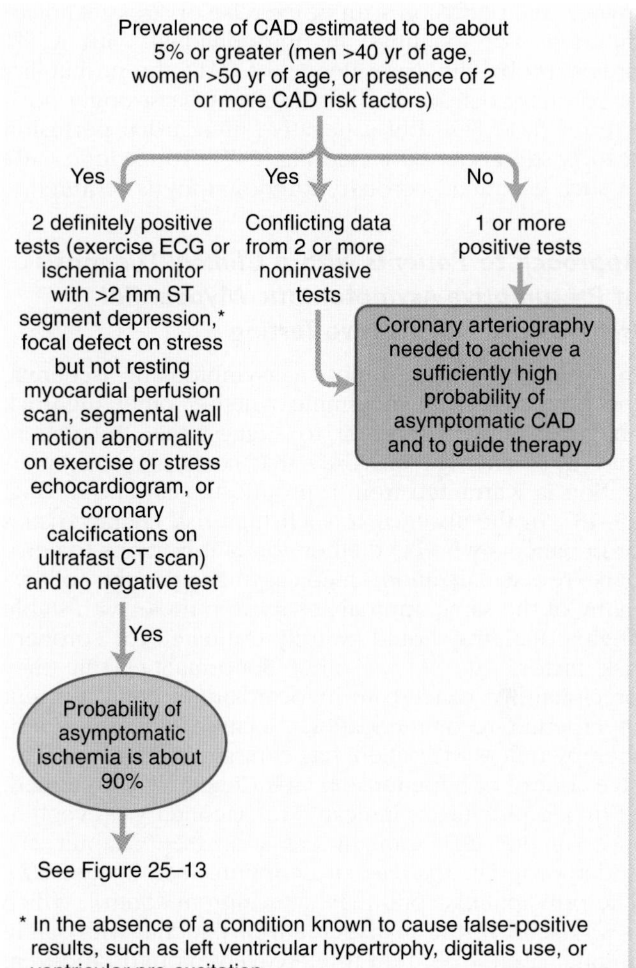

FIGURE 25–12. Making the clinical diagnosis of presumptive asymptomatic myocardial ischemia. CAD, coronary artery disease; CT, computed tomography; ECG, electrocardiogram.

In other situations with a lower pretest probability (prevalence) of coronary disease, coronary arteriography is required to make a definitive diagnosis. In addition, to determine whether the observed coronary artery stenosis is truly causing ischemia, correlation between the anatomic distribution of the coronary disease and the evidence for ischemia on noninvasive testing is helpful.

A strongly positive exercise ECG in an asymptomatic person cannot be neutralized by a negative result on a myocardial perfusion scan or exercise or stress echocardiogram. For example, in an individual with a 5% pretest probability (prevalence) of CAD, the probability of coronary disease in the presence of a strongly positive exercise ECG but a negative myocardial perfusion scan is still about 20% (see Fig. 2–7). To exclude CAD in such a patient, coronary arteriography is required.

Approach to Patients with a Clinical Diagnosis of Presumptive Asymptomatic Myocardial Ischemia by Noninvasive Testing

In patients with presumptive asymptomatic ischemia, the physician must determine whether other high-risk characteristics are present to suggest that the patient may have such severe CAD that coronary revascularization is warranted from a prognostic standpoint (Fig. 25–13). In the absence of such high-risk characteristics or in patients who have other contraindications to coronary revascularization, medical management follows many of the same approaches used in those with stable angina. Patients should be fully evaluated for coronary risk factors, as well as other abnormalities that may precipitate or exacerbate myocardial ischemia. Current therapeutic recommendations include routine aspirin therapy unless the patient has contraindications, aggressive control of hypertension (see Chapter 19), treatment of hyperlipidemia as indicated for secondary prevention (see Chapter 20), smoking cessation (see Chapter 21), and appropriate exercise prescriptions (see Chapter 22). The principal exception is that symptom control, which is so useful in the management of patients with stable angina, cannot be used to effectively monitor and treat patients with a clinical diagnosis of presumptive asymptomatic ischemia.

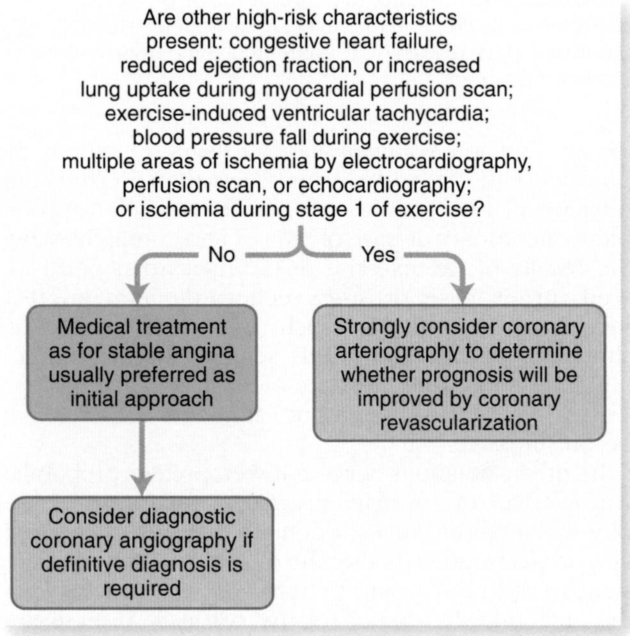

In patients with asymptomatic or minimally symptomatic ischemia, 100 mg/day of atenolol reduces the risk of subsequent symptomatic coronary events. Beta-blockers also aid in maintaining the blood pressure and heart rate below the individual's ischemia threshold as determined by formal exercise testing. Ambulatory electrocardiographic (Holter) monitoring should be used to adjust anti-ischemic therapy.

Although patients with totally asymptomatic ischemia may have a somewhat more favorable prognosis than symptomatic patients do, those with asymptomatic ischemia also appear to benefit from coronary revascularization if their anatomy is suitable (and would warrant revascularization if the ischemia were symptomatic). In such situations, revascularization can reduce ischemia, improve ischemia-free survival, and probably reduce coronary events. Thus, the approach to patients with diagnosed asymptomatic ischemia closely parallels that recommended for symptomatic patients with ischemia and anatomy of similar severity.

Are other high-risk characteristics present: congestive heart failure, reduced ejection fraction, or increased lung uptake during myocardial perfusion scan; exercise-induced ventricular tachycardia; blood pressure fall during exercise; multiple areas of ischemia by electrocardiography, perfusion scan, or echocardiography; or ischemia during stage 1 of exercise?

- No → Medical treatment as for stable angina usually preferred as initial approach → Consider diagnostic coronary angiography if definitive diagnosis is required
- Yes → Strongly consider coronary arteriography to determine whether prognosis will be improved by coronary revascularization

FIGURE 25–13. Approach to patients with a clinical diagnosis of presumptive asymptomatic myocardial ischemia by noninvasive testing.

Myocardial Revascularization

Two proven forms of myocardial revascularization have been developed for the treatment of chronic stable angina: catheter-based techniques (principally PTCA and coronary stenting, but also directional or rotational atherectomy) and CABG. Both of these therapies relieve angina and prevent subsequent adverse outcomes in patients with persistent class II or worse angina despite standard medical therapy.[12] Excimer laser angioplasty has no apparent benefit over these other, more standard catheter-based techniques.

Catheter-Based Revascularization

The principal indication for catheter-based revascularization is angina pectoris that fails to respond adequately to medical management in a patient with coronary artery lesions that are amenable to the procedure. The definition of an inadequate response to medical management is quite variable among patients and depends on the patient's lifestyle, occupation, and expectations. At one extreme are patients who are disabled by angina pectoris despite treatment with maximally tolerated doses of triple therapy (beta-adrenergic blockers, long-acting nitrates, and calcium antagonists) after lifestyle modifications that include achievement of optimal weight and cessation of smoking. At the other end of the spectrum are patients who consider medical therapy to have failed if control of angina pectoris requires doses of antianginal medications that cause side effects such as insomnia, fatigue, and sexual dysfunction. The usual candidate for a catheter-based intervention is somewhere between the extremes of this spectrum—that is, a patient who, although not totally disabled by angina, continues to experience angina regularly when engaging in activities of personal importance, such as recreational sports.

In randomized trials of medical therapy versus PTCA for patients with class II or III angina, PCI does not reduce the risk of death or nonfatal myocardial infarction,[8] but PTCA provides better relief of angina.[13] These results emphasize the need to tailor therapy to the individual patient.[14]

Ideal candidates for catheter-based revascularization have stable angina, are younger than 75 years and male, and have single-vessel, single-lesion CAD, without a history of diabetes. Lesions that are optimal for these procedures are short (<10 mm), concentric, discrete, and readily accessible. Catheter-based interventions are by no means excluded in patients without these features, but the risk of morbidity and mortality from the procedure is increased, particularly in patients with long (>20 mm), tortuous, irregular, angulated, calcified, severely stenotic (>90% stenosis) lesions and particularly when more than one such lesion is present in an artery. Overall, about 50% of patients with symptomatic CAD will be good candidates for PTCA (Fig. 25–14).

The major complication of PCI is abrupt closure, which is recognized angiographically before the patient leaves the laboratory and is usually accompanied by manifestations of acute ischemic chest pain and ECG changes. The incidence of abrupt closure of angioplasty followed by stenting is approximately 1%, and it occurs more commonly in patients older than 75 years; in women; in the presence of unstable angina, diabetes, and recent thrombolytic therapy; and with the angiographic features described previously. The mortality associated with catheter-based coronary revascularization in patients with stable angina is less than 1%, and it usually occurs after abrupt closure.[15] The frequency of this complication can be reduced by pretreatment with platelet glycoprotein IIb/IIIa receptor blockers.

Primary success of catheter-based interventions is generally defined as an absolute increase of 20% in luminal diameter and a final diameter obstruction of less than 50%. Such angiographic success can be anticipated in more than 90% of properly selected patients. Restenosis is usually defined as greater than 50% diameter stenosis and greater than 50% late loss of the acute luminal diameter. The incidence of this complication is approximately 30% to 40% after PTCA or atherectomy but appears to be reduced to about 20% after stenting. Drug-eluting stents are capable of reducing restenosis rates to less than 10%. Restenosis appears to occur more frequently in older patients, diabetics, and cigarette smokers and when lesions cause total coronary occlusion, involve the left anterior descending coronary artery, include thrombosis as well as plaque, or were complicated by severe dissection during the course of the procedure. Restenosis commonly occurs within 6 months after the procedure and is less frequent when the postprocedure lumen is larger. Recurrent severe angina occurs in approximately half the patients in whom angiographic restenosis develops, but it usually responds to repeat angioplasty (or stenting).

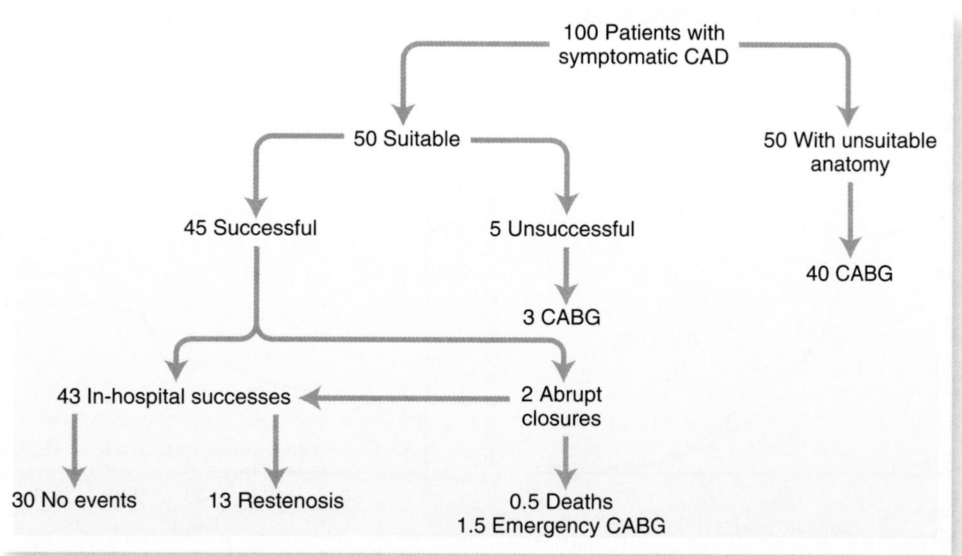

FIGURE 25–14. Limitations of balloon percutaneous transluminal coronary angioplasty (PTCA). Approximately 50% of patients who have symptomatic coronary artery disease (CAD) and are in need of revascularization are candidates for PTCA. The remaining patients are ineligible because of unfavorable coronary anatomy, which most commonly results from chronic total occlusion of more than 3 months in duration. Of suitable candidates, a small percentage have an unsuccessful procedure and subsequently require coronary artery bypass grafting (CABG). Abrupt vessel closure develops in a small proportion of patients who have a successful procedure, and restenosis necessitating a repeat procedure develops in 20% to 30% of patients. Thus, approximately 30% of all patients who need myocardial revascularization are successfully treated and free of complications after PTCA. (From Beller GA: Chronic ischemic heart disease. In Braunwald E [ed]: Essential Atlas of Heart Diseases, 2nd ed. New York, McGraw-Hill, 2001, p 100. Copyright © 2001 by McGraw-Hill, Inc. Used by permission of McGraw-Hill Book Company.)

The higher overall success rate of stenting—both at the time of the procedure (about 96% vs. 90% for balloon angioplasty) and at least 1 year after the procedure (Fig. 25–15)—appears to be worth the cost, especially if PTCA alone does not give an adequate angiographic result or if restenosis occurs.[16,17] Atherectomy results in a larger postprocedure coronary lumen than PTCA does and may be preferred over PTCA for certain types of coronary lesions, but it has been associated with no better and perhaps somewhat worse results than PTCA at 6 months in randomized studies of patients who are considered to be candidates for either procedure.

Coronary Artery Bypass Surgery

In this procedure, which is generally carried out after sternotomy and while on cardiopulmonary bypass, coronary obstructions (usually >70% narrowing of the luminal diameter) are bypassed with an internal mammary (arterial) or saphenous vein graft.[18] Arterial grafts have excellent long-term patency rates (90% at 10 years), whereas saphenous vein grafts show accelerated atherosclerosis, with approximately 50% patency at 10 years. Therefore, it is not surprising that internal mammary artery grafts are associated with a 27% reduction in 15-year mortality in comparison to saphenous vein grafts. When it is technically feasible, an arterial conduit, usually involving one or both internal mammary arteries, is recommended. For technical reasons, the left internal mammary artery is most conducive to a graft to the left anterior descending coronary artery, and the right internal mammary artery is most applicable to a graft to the right coronary artery. Patients who require more than two grafts generally receive a combination of arterial and venous grafts. Newer, minimally invasive CABG via a smaller thoracotomy incision or a thoracoscopic approach can potentially reduce the morbidity and hospital length of stay in eligible patients.

The operative mortality of CABG has stabilized at approximately 2%, with rates of 1% to 1.5% for uncomplicated patients with stable angina. The steady improvements in perioperative care have been offset by the progressively sicker patients who are referred for this procedure. With the widespread use of catheter-based interventions, an increasing fraction of those undergoing CABG are elderly patients who in the past would not have undergone such a procedure or who are poor candidates for any procedure because of advanced, serious, multivessel, multilesion disease. An increasing number of patients are undergoing repeat CABG because of atherosclerosis in venous bypass grafts, and these patients are likewise at higher risk.

Angina pectoris is relieved in more than 90% of patients who undergo CABG. Severe (class III or IV) angina occurs in 5% to 10% of patients at 3 years and increases gradually thereafter. Recurrence of angina is due to graft stenosis or progression of disease in nongrafted vessels. Therefore, it is essential for the revascularization to be as complete as possible.

Indications. CABG should be carried out to prolong life or improve its quality (Fig. 25–16). Prolongation of life has been demonstrated in patients with more than 50% luminal diameter obstruction of the left main coronary artery and in those with impaired left ventricular function (left ventricular ejection fraction <40%) and critical obstruction (>70% stenosis) in all

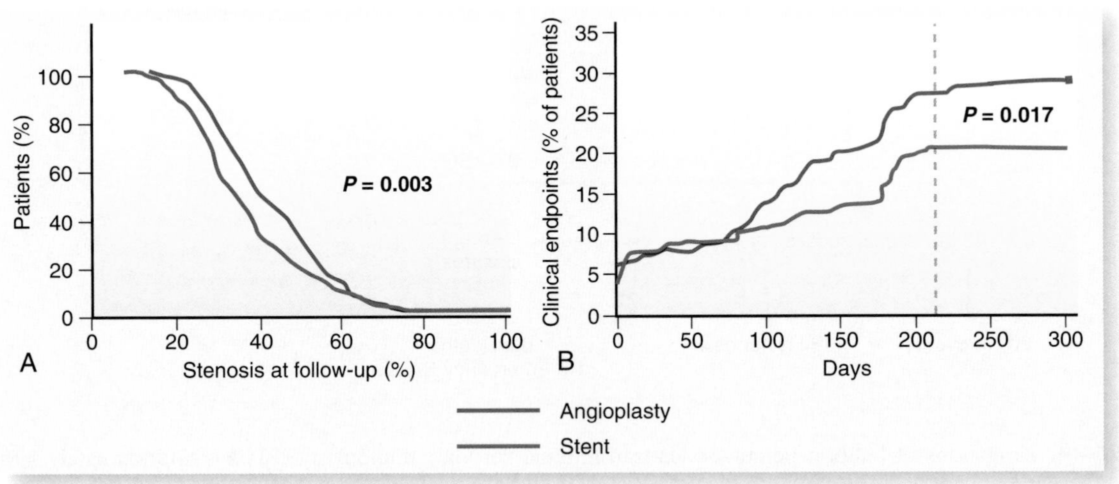

FIGURE 25–15. The Benestent Trial (Serruys PW, de Jaegere P, Kiemeneij F, et al: A comparison of balloon-expandable-stent implantation with balloon angioplasty in patients with coronary artery disease. N Engl J Med 1994;331:489–495) examined the cumulative frequency of the percent stenosis (*A*) and incidence of major clinical events (*B*) at follow-up for stent and balloon angioplasty treatment groups. Significant differences were found in both endpoints. The vertical *dashed line* in *panel B* indicates the end of the study. (From Beller GA: Chronic ischemic heart disease. In Braunwald E [ed]: Essential Atlas of Heart Diseases, 2nd ed. New York, McGraw-Hill, 2001, p 97. Copyright © 2001 by McGraw-Hill, Inc. Used by permission of McGraw-Hill Book Company.)

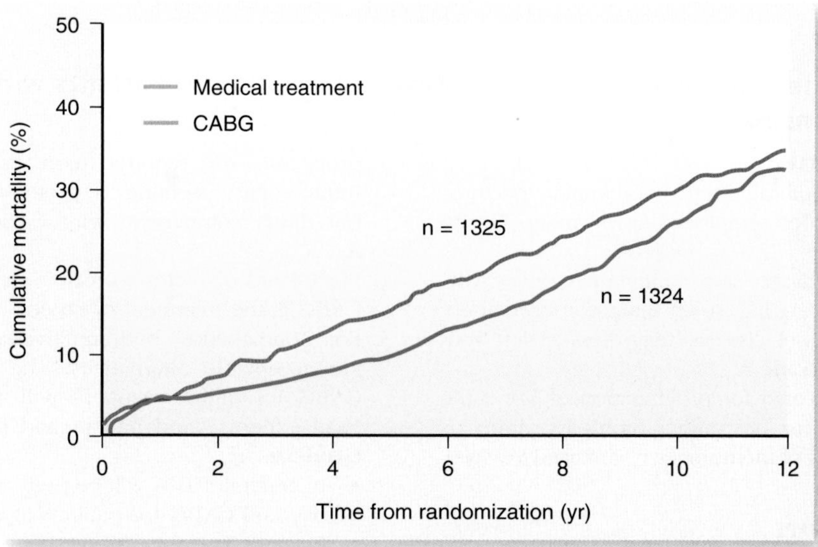

FIGURE 25–16. Overall survival after random allocation to medical treatment or coronary artery bypass graft surgery (CABG): pooled data from the major randomized trials. The advantage in favor of an initial strategy of CABG substantially widens for up to 5 to 7 years before again narrowing by 10 to 12 years. The survival advantage of CABG over medical therapy was proportional to the number of diseased coronary arteries (significant for three-vessel [relative risk {RR} = 0.58; $P < .001$] and left main coronary artery [RR = 0.32; $P = .004$] disease) and, in particular, to involvement of the left anterior descending (LAD) coronary artery (RR = 0.58, even if only one- or two-vessel disease). Relative benefits were similar regardless of left ventricular function (RR = 0.61 [normal]; RR = 0.59 [abnormal]). However, *absolute* benefit was greater in patients with an abnormal ejection fraction because the risk of death was twice as high in this group. (From Yusuf S, Zucker D, Peduzzi P, et al: Effect of coronary artery bypass graft surgery on survival: Overview of 10-year results from randomized trials by the Coronary Artery Bypass Graft Surgery Trialists Collaboration. Lancet 1994;344:563–570. © by The Lancet Ltd., 1994.)

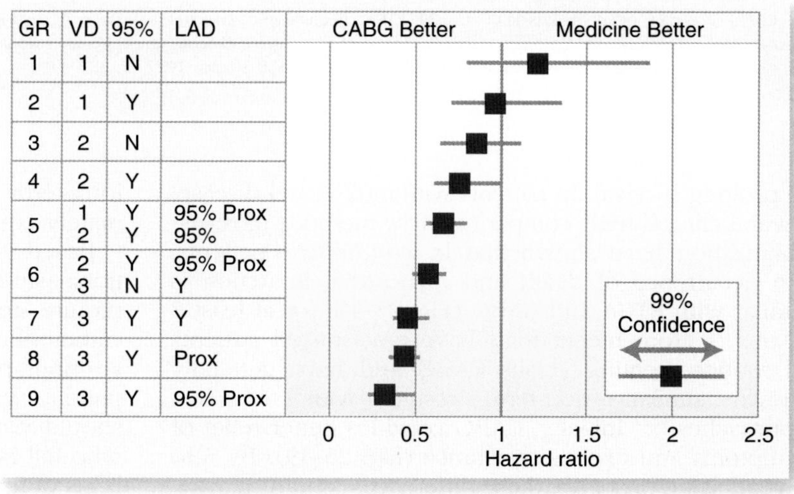

FIGURE 25–17. *A*, Adjusted hazard (mortality) ratios comparing coronary artery bypass grafting (CABG) and medical therapy for nine coronary anatomy severity groups (GR) according to the number of vessels diseased (VD), the presence or absence of 95% proximal stenosis (95%), and involvement of the left anterior descending coronary artery (LAD). (From Jones RH, Kesler K, Phillips HR III, et al: Long-term survival benefits of coronary artery bypass grafting and percutaneous transluminal angioplasty in patients with coronary artery disease. J Thorac Cardiovasc Surg 1996;111:1013.)

three major coronary arteries or in two arteries, one of which is the proximal left anterior descending artery (Fig. 25–17, Box 25–7). The presence of a high-risk result on a noninvasive test also increases the relative benefit of surgery. Patients with severe left ventricular dysfunction or failure obtain a survival benefit from CABG if the myocardium with impaired contractile function is viable, that is, is hibernating rather than necrotic.

The Choice between Catheter-Based Interventions and CABG

In patients with single-vessel disease who require revascularization for symptoms and who are determined to be suitable for *either* procedure by angiography, both percutaneous procedures and CABG provide substantial symptomatic benefit, but neither has been shown

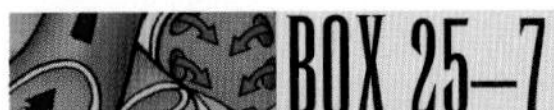
BOX 25–7

Current Recommendations for Myocardial Revascularization in Patients with Chronic Stable Angina

CABG VS. MEDICAL THERAPY

1. In patients with medically refractory angina pectoris, CABG is indicated for symptom improvement. **Grade A**.
2. In patients with medically stable angina pectoris, CABG is indicated to prolong life in left main coronary artery disease or three-vessel disease (regardless of left ventricular function). **Grade A**.
3. CABG may be indicated for prolongation of life if the proximal left anterior descending coronary artery is involved (regardless of the number of diseased vessels). **Grade A**.

PTCA VS. MEDICAL THERAPY

1. In patients with medically refractory angina pectoris, PTCA is indicated for symptom improvement. **Grade A**.
2. PTCA may be indicated in the presence of severe myocardial ischemia, regardless of symptoms. It is unclear whether PTCA improves survival in comparison to medical treatment in patients with one- or two-vessel disease. **Grade B**.
3. In the absence of symptoms or myocardial ischemia, PTCA is not indicated (merely for the presence of an anatomic stenosis). **Grade A**.

PTCA VS. CABG

1. For single-vessel disease, both PTCA and CABG provide excellent symptom relief, but repeat revascularization procedures are required more frequently after PTCA. Intracoronary stenting is preferred to regular PTCA, but direct comparison with CABG is limited. **Grade A**.
2. For treated diabetics with two- or three-vessel disease, CABG is the treatment of choice. **Grade A**.
3. For nondiabetics, both multivessel PTCA and CABG are acceptable alternatives. The choice of PTCA or CABG for initial treatment will depend primarily on local expertise and patient and physician preference. **Grade A**.
   - In general, PTCA will be preferred for patients at low risk and CABG for patients at high risk.
   - Large differences in mortality (40%–50%) are unlikely, but smaller, potentially important differences in mortality (20%–30%) cannot be excluded by the available data.
   - CABG is associated with more complete revascularization and superior early relief of angina, but these differences diminish after 3–5 years.
   - No significant differences in rates of myocardial infarction have been demonstrated.
   - Repeat revascularization procedures are required significantly more often after PTCA.
   - Initial cost, quality of life, and return to work are initially more favorable with PTCA than CABG, but these outcomes roughly equalize over 3–5 years.

CABG, coronary artery bypass graft surgery; PTCA, percutaneous transluminal coronary angioplasty. Adapted from Rihal CS, Gersh BJ, Yusuf S: Chronic coronary artery disease: Coronary artery bypass surgery vs. percutaneous transluminal coronary angioplasty vs. reduced therapy. In Yusuf S, Cairns JA, Camm AJ, et al (eds): Evidence-Based Cardiology. London, BMJ Books, 1999; pp 389–390.

to prolong survival. In patients with multivessel disease, several clinical trials comparing these methods of revascularization have shown that in *nondiabetic* patients, the occurrence of death and myocardial infarction is similar with PTCA and CABG (Fig. 25–18) for at least 8 years.[19,20] More recent trials have randomized patients to routine stenting versus CABG and have generally shown similar short-term results with the two approaches.[21,22] Initially, CABG provides better relief of symptoms and exercise tolerance (Fig. 25–19). By 3 to 5 years later, however, these differences tend to narrow because of repeated procedures in patients originally treated with PTCA and a decline in benefit from CABG, but overall, they are still slightly in favor of CABG.

Because of the high incidence of restenosis, the need for repeat revascularization is much higher in PTCA patients, approximately 50% at 5 years versus 5% to 10% after CABG. In diabetic patients with multivessel disease, survival is superior with CABG.[19]

Although the cost of catheter-based revascularization is lower than that of CABG initially, PTCA is associated with a greater need for repeat hospitalization, medical attention, and repeat revascularization. Therefore, the long-term costs of the two approaches are approximately equal.

Based on data from randomized trials and observational studies, patients with single-vessel disease who require revascularization are usually referred for a catheter-based intervention if they are deemed suitable arteriographically (Fig. 25–20). On the other hand, patients with left main CAD should undergo surgery, as should patients with three-vessel disease. In patients who fall between these two extremes and who, on the basis of findings on coronary arteriography, are suitable for both CABG and catheter-based interventions, either approach may be used with the following caveats: (1) surgical treatment is superior in diabetics with multivessel disease, and (2) CABG may be more desirable in nondiabetic patients who have two-vessel disease that involves the proximal left anterior descending coronary artery.

In practice, catheter-based revascularization is especially attractive in situations in which the risks associated with CABG are higher either in terms of overall mortality or in terms of neurologic side effects, each of which increases in the elderly, especially those older

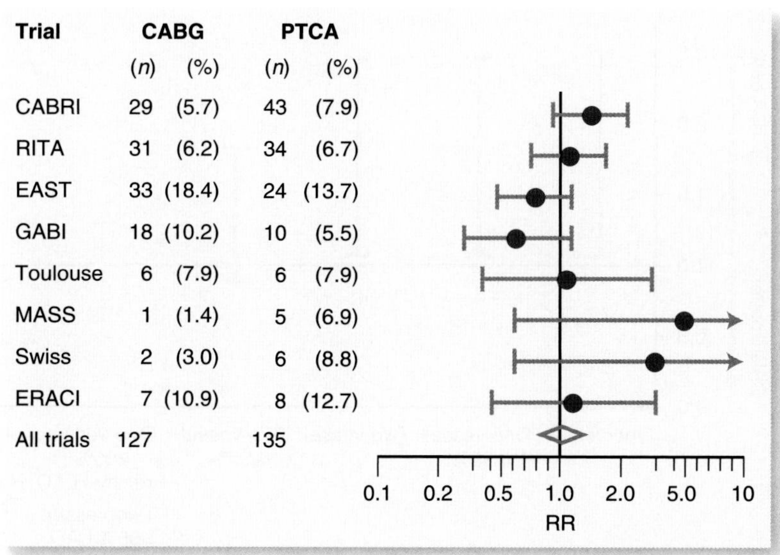

Trial CABG PTCA
(n) (%) (n) (%)
CABRI 29 (5.7) 43 (7.9)
RITA 31 (6.2) 34 (6.7)
EAST 33 (18.4) 24 (13.7)
GABI 18 (10.2) 10 (5.5)
Toulouse 6 (7.9) 6 (7.9)
MASS 1 (1.4) 5 (6.9)
Swiss 2 (3.0) 6 (8.8)
ERACI 7 (10.9) 8 (12.7)
All trials 127 135
0.1 0.2 0.5 1.0 2.0 5.0 10
RR

FIGURE 25–18. Cardiac death and myocardial infarction for the percutaneous transluminal coronary angioplasty (PTCA) group versus the coronary artery bypass grafting (CABG) group in the first year after randomization. CABRI, Coronary Angioplasty versus Bypass Revascularization Investigation; EAST, Emory Angioplasty versus Surgery Trial; ERACI, Argentine Randomized Trial of Percutaneous Transluminal Coronary Angioplasty versus Coronary Artery Bypass Surgery in Multivessel Disease; GABI, German Angioplasty Bypass Surgery Investigation; MASS, Medicine, Angioplasty, or Surgery Study; RITA, Randomized Interventional Treatment of Angina; RR, relative risk. (From Pocock SJ, Henderson RA, Richards AF, et al. Meta-analysis of randomised trials comparing coronary angioplasty with bypass surgery. Lancet 1995;346:1184–1189. © by The Lancet Ltd., 1995.)

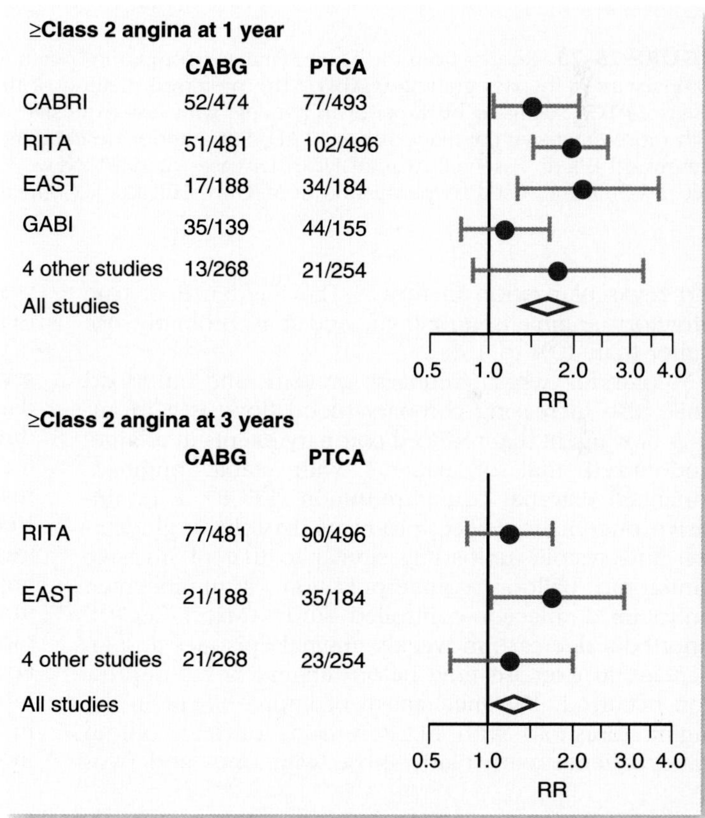

FIGURE 25–19. Prevalence of angina pectoris (at least class 2) 1 and 3 years after random allocation to transluminal coronary angioplasty (PTCA) or coronary artery bypass grafting (CABG). CABRI, Coronary Angioplasty versus Bypass Revascularization Investigation; EAST, Emory Angioplasty versus Surgery Trial; GABI, German Angioplasty Bypass Surgery Investigation; RITA, Randomized Interventional Treatment of Angina. (From Pocock SJ, Henderson RA, Richards AF, et al: Meta-analysis of randomised trials comparing coronary angioplasty with bypass surgery. Lancet 1995;346:1184–1189. © by The Lancet Ltd., 1995.)

than 75 years. In patients with life-limiting noncoronary diseases, the approach must be tempered by careful consideration of the patient's overall prognosis. In those who need an urgent noncardiac operation, a catheter-based approach, but not acute stenting, is generally preferable so that the patient can proceed to the noncardiac surgery without the morbidity of a thoracotomy (see Chapter 14).

In any case, the experience and skill of the operators available should be given strong consideration in the choice. The advantages and disadvantages of the two approaches should be explained to patients who fall into the middle groups, and the personal preferences of the patient and the family should be respected.

Refractory Angina

Refractory angina is diagnosed when an unacceptable frequency of angina, as perceived by the patient, continues despite adequate antianginal pharmacotherapy

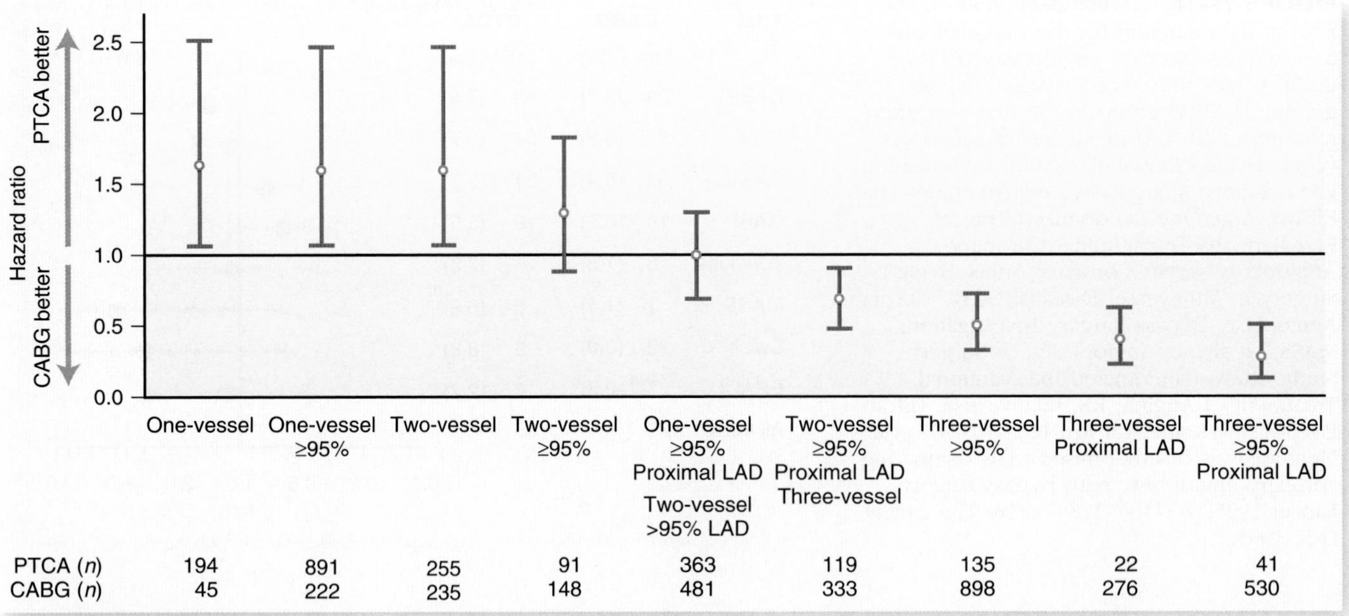

FIGURE 25–20. Results from the Duke database comparing percutaneous transluminal coronary angioplasty (PTCA) and coronary artery bypass grafting (CABG). The preferred method of therapy depends on the extent and severity of coronary disease. PTCA seems to be superior in patients with less extensive disease, whereas CABG is more advantageous for patients with more extensive coronary disease. LAD, left anterior descending. (From Beller GA: Chronic ischemic heart disease. In Braunwald E [ed]: Essential Atlas of Heart Diseases, 2nd ed. New York, McGraw-Hill, 2001, p 102. Copyright © 2001 by McGraw-Hill, Inc. Used by permission of McGraw-Hill Book Company.)

and revascularization therapy.[23] The incidence of true refractory angina is unknown, and it is probably not higher than 10% to 15%..

Nicorandil, which reduces preload and afterload while also increasing coronary blood flow, is a promising new agent that reduced coronary events in a large, randomized trial of patients with stable angina.[24] Enhanced external counterpulsation (EECP), a noninvasive pneumatic device, produces diastolic augmentation and systolic unloading similar to that of invasive intra-aortic balloon counterpulsation. A multicenter, randomized, placebo-controlled study (MUST-EECP)[25] reported a decrease in weekly anginal episodes and an increase in exercise time before angina or ST depression occurred. The mechanism of improvement in the angina threshold with EECP remains unclear, but in some patients, particularly those with one- and two-vessel CAD, myocardial perfusion improves in the ischemic segments.

Open heart or thoracoscopic transmyocardial laser revascularization (TMR) or percutaneous transmyocardial laser revascularization (PTMR) attempts to allow direct access of oxygenated blood from the left ventricular cavity to ischemic myocardium that cannot be revascularized by conventional methods. In a randomized clinical trial in which neither the patients nor the treating physicians were blinded, anginal class improved in TMR-treated patients in comparison to medically treated patients.[26] Despite a higher early mortality with TMR, it has been approved by the U.S. Food and Drug Administration for the treatment of refractory angina. In contrast, PTMR showed no benefit in a double-blind trial, and in one trial it increased mortality.

Evidence-Based Summary

The two principal goals of treatment are to (1) relieve angina and myocardial ischemia and (2) decrease the risks of adverse cardiac events—fatal and nonfatal myocardial infarction.

1. For maintenance treatment of angina and myocardial ischemia, beta-adrenergic blocking agents, calcium channel blocking agents, and long-acting nitrates appear to be equally effective. Combination therapy with two or all three of these classes of agents is frequently effective for better amelioration of anginal symptoms. Beta-blockers are the preferred monotherapy because of their known ability to prolong survival in patients who have survived a myocardial infarction (see Chapter 27) or who have heart failure (see Chapter 28).

2. Revascularization of ischemic myocardium either by catheter-based techniques or by CABG has a greater potential to relieve symptoms than medical therapy does; when revascularization is underused, subsequent outcomes are suboptimal.[27] Except in some specific anatomic subsets (e.g., patients with left main CAD, triple-vessel CAD, or double-vessel CAD that includes the proximal left anterior descending coronary artery), medical therapy for angina combined with therapy to decrease the risk of adverse cardiac events is associated with an equivalent or better short-term and long-term prognosis than mechanical revascularization is (see Box 25–7). For refractory angina, newer mechanical and pharmacologic interventions such as enhanced external counterpulsation, transmyocardial revascularization, and spinal cord stimulation may be of benefit in selected patients.
3. Proven therapies to decrease the risk of fatal and nonfatal myocardial infarction presently include antiplatelet agents, beta-adrenergic agents, lipid-lowering agents, and ACE inhibitors. Treatment with these medications should be considered irrespective of whether pharmacotherapy or catheter-based or surgical revascularization is used to relieve angina and myocardial ischemia.

References

1. Gibbons RJ, Chatterjee K, Daley J, et al: ACC/AHA/ACP-ASIM guidelines for the management of patients with chronic stable angina: A report of the American College of Cardiology/American Heart Association Task Force on Practice Guidelines. J Am Coll Cardiol 1999;33:2092–2197.
2. O'Rourke RA, Brundage BH, Froelicher VF, et al: American College of Cardiology/American Heart Association expert consensus document on electron-beam computed tomography for the diagnosis and prognosis of coronary artery disease. J Am Coll Cardiol 2000;36:326–340.
3. Gibbons RJ, Balady GJ, Beasley JW, et al: ACC/AHA guidelines for exercise testing: Executive summary. A report of the American College of Cardiology/American Heart Association Task Force on Practice Guidelines (Committee on Exercise Testing). Circulation 1997;96:345–354.
4. Lee TH, Boucher CA: Noninvasive tests in patients with stable coronary artery disease. N Engl J Med 2001;344:1840–1845.
5. Ridker PM, Rifai N, Clearfield M, et al: Measurement of C-reactive protein for the targeting of statin therapy in the primary prevention of acute coronary events. N Engl J Med 2001;344:1959–1965.
6. Williams SV, Fihn SD, Gibbons RJ: Guidelines for the management of patients with chronic stable angina: Diagnosis and risk stratification. Ann Intern Med 2001;135:530–547.
7. Kromhout D, Menotti A, Kesteloot H, Sans S: Prevention of coronary heart disease by diet and lifestyle. Circulation 2002;105:893–898.
8. Pitt B, Waters D, Brown WV, et al, for the Atorvastatin Versus Revascularization Treatment (AVERT) Investigators: Aggressive lipid-lowering therapy compared with angioplasty in stable coronary artery disease. N Engl J Med 1999;341:70–76.
9. Grady D, Herrington D, Bittner V: Cardiovascular disease outcomes during 6.8 years of hormone therapy. JAMA 2002;288:49–57.
10. Schnyder G, Roffi M, Pin R, et al: Decreased rate of coronary restenosis after lowering of plasma homocysteine levels. N Engl J Med 2001;345:1593–1600.
11. Heart Outcomes Prevention Evaluation Study Investigators: Effects of an angiotensin-converting enzyme inhibitor, ramipril, on cardiovascular events in high-risk patients. N Engl J Med 2000;342:145–153.
12. The TIME Investigators: Trial of invasive versus medical therapy in elderly patients with chronic symptomatic coronary-artery disease (TIME): A randomised trial. Lancet 2001;358:951–957.
13. Bucher HC, Hengstler P, Schindler C, Guyatt GH: Percutaneous transluminal coronary angioplasty versus medical treatment for non-acute coronary heart disease: Meta-analysis of randomised controlled trials. BMJ 2000;321:73–77.
14. Blumenthal RS, Cohn G, Schulman SP: Medical therapy versus coronary angioplasty in stable coronary artery disease: A critical review of the literature. J Am Coll Cardiol 2000;36:668–673.
15. Dove JT, Jacobs AK, Kennedy JW, et al: ACC/AHA guidelines for percutaneous coronary intervention (revision of the 1993 PTCA guidelines)—executive summary. A report of the American College of Cardiology/American Heart Association Task Force on practice guidelines (Committee to revise the 1993 guidelines for percutaneous transluminal coronary angioplasty). J Am Coll Cardiol 2001;37:2215–2238.
16. Kiemeneij F, Serruys PW, Macaya C: Continued benefit of coronary stenting versus balloon angioplasty: Five-year clinical follow-up of Benestent-I trial. J Am Coll Cardiol 2001;37:1598–1603.
17. Weaver WD, Reisman MA, Griffin JJ: Optimum percutaneous transluminal coronary angioplasty compared with routine stent strategy trial (OPUS-1): A randomised trial. Lancet 2000;355:2199–2203.
18. Cameron A, Davis KB, Green G, Schaff HV: Coronary bypass surgery with internal thoracic artery grafts: Effects on survival over a 15-year period. N Engl J Med 1996;34:216–219.
19. The BARI Investigators: Seven-year outcome in the bypass angioplasty revascularization investigation (BARI) by treatment and diabetic status. J Am Coll Cardiol 2000;35:1122–1129.
20. King SB, Kosinski AS, Guyton RA, et al: Eight-year mortality in the Emory angioplasty versus surgery trial (EAST). J Am Coll Cardiol 2000;35:1116–1121.
21. Serruys PW, Unger F, Sousa JE, et al: Comparison of coronary artery bypass surgery and stenting for the treatment

of multivessel disease. N Engl J Med 2001;344:1117–1124.

22. deFeyter PJ, Serruys PW, Unger F, et al: Bypass surgery versus stenting for the treatment of multivessel disease in patients with unstable angina compared with stable angina. Circulation 2002;105:2367–2372.
23. Kim MC, Kini A, Sharma SK: Refractory angina pectoris. J Am Coll Cardiol 2002;39:923–934.
24. The Impact of Nicorandil in Anqina Study Group: Effect of nicorandil on cornary events in patients with stable angina. Lancet 2002;359:1269–1275.
25. Arora RR, Crou JM, Jain D, et al: The multicenter study of enhanced external counterpulsation (MUST-EEOP); effect of EECP on exercise-induced myocardial ischemia and anginal episodes. J Am Coll Cardiol 1999;33:1833–1840.
26. Allen KB, Dowling RD, Fudge TL, et al: Comparison of transmyocardial revascularization with medical therapy in patients with refractory angina. N Engl J Med 1999;341:1029–1036.
27. Hemingway H, Crook AM, Feder G, et al: Underuse of coronary revascularization procedures in patients considered appropriate candidates for revascularization. N Engl J Med 2001;344:645–654.

CHAPTER 26 Recognition and Management of Patients with Unstable Angina and Non–ST Elevation Myocardial Infarction

Eugene Braunwald

CLINICAL MANIFESTATIONS

Clinical coronary artery disease includes a wide spectrum of conditions, ranging from acute ST elevation myocardial infarction (STEMI) at one end of the spectrum (see Chapter 27) to chronic stable angina (see Chapter 25) and asymptomatic ischemia at the other. Unstable angina (UA) and the closely related condition non–ST segment elevation (NSTEMI) are at the center of this spectrum and are referred to as UA/NSTEMI in this chapter.[1] This condition has features common to both STEMI and chronic stable angina. Unstable angina and acute myocardial infarction, both STEMI and NSTEMI comprise the acute coronary syndromes (ACS) (see Fig. 27–5). UA/NSTEMI are also referred to as *non–ST segment elevation ACS.*

Patients with UA/NSTEMI represent an increasing fraction of ACS patients. UA/NSTEMI is responsible for more than 1.4 million hospital admissions in the United States each year.[2] Approximately 60% of these admissions occur in patients older than 65 years, and almost half are women. Patients with this diagnosis are characterized by one or more of three features (Box 26–1): (1) angina of new onset (<2 months) that is severe (Canadian Classification III or IV) and brought on by minimal exertion; the new onset of chronic angina that is mild to moderate in severity (Canadian Classification I or II) is *not* considered to be UA; (2) increasing or crescendo angina—angina that is more severe, prolonged, or frequent—superimposed on a pattern of chronic stable angina; and (3) angina at rest. The distinction between NSTEMI and UA is based on the release in NSTEMI of biomarkers of myocardial necrosis (cardiac-specific troponin I or T or creatine-kinase [CK] MB).

Ischemic pain at rest also occurs in Prinzmetal's variant angina, but this condition is pathogenetically and clinically distinct from the UA secondary to coronary atherosclerosis and is discussed separately in this chapter.

Because UA is a heterogeneous condition, a classification based on five important features (Table 26–1) has been developed:[3, 4]

1. The severity of the clinical manifestations, ranging from new-onset or accelerated angina (the mildest) to acute angina at rest (the most severe)
2. The clinical circumstances that have precipitated UA, ranging from primary UA (i.e., without an extracardiac cause) (the mildest) to post AMI (the most serious)
3. The presence or absence of transient electrocardiographic changes during ischemic episodes
4. The release of biomarkers of necrosis
5. The intensity of anti-ischemic therapy at the time that the UA occurs.

TABLE 26–1

Braunwald Clinical Classification of Unstable Angina

Class	Definition	Death or Myocardial Infarction to 1 Year*, %
Severity		
Class I	New onset of severe angina or accelerated angina; no rest pain	7.3
Class II	Angina at rest within past month but not within preceding 48 hr (angina at rest, subacute)	10.3
Class III	Angina at rest within 48 hr (angina at rest, subacute)	10.8†
Clinical Circumstances		
A (secondary angina)	Develops in the presence of extracardiac condition that intensifies myocardial ischemia	14.1
B (primary angina)	Develops in the absence of extracardiac condition	8.5
C (postinfarction angina)	Develops within 2 weeks after acute myocardial infarction	18.5‡
Intensity of treatment	Patients with unstable angina may also be divided into three groups depending on whether unstable angina occurs (1) in the absence of treatment for chronic stable angina, (2) during treatment for chronic stable angina, or (3) despite maximal anti-ischemic drug therapy. The three groups may be designated subscripts 1, 2, or 3, respectively.	
Electrocardiographic changes	Patients with unstable angina may be further divided into those with or without transient ST-T wave changes during pain.	

*Data from TIMI III Registry: Cannon CP, McCabe CH, Stone PH, et al: Prospective validation of the Braunwald classification of unstable angina; Results from the Thrombolysis in Myocardial Ischemia (TIMI) III Registry (abstract). Circulation 1995;92(Suppl 1):1–19, Copyright 1995, American Heart Association.

†$p = .057$.

‡$p < .001$.

From Braunwald E: Unstable angina: A classification, Circulation 1989;80:410–414. Copyright 1989, American Heart Association.

BOX 26–1

Principal Presentations of Unstable Angina

Rest angina	Angina occurring at rest and within a week of presentation for medical care; usually lasts >20 min
New-onset angina	Angina of at least CCSC III severity with onset within 2 mo of initial presentation
Increasing angina	Previously diagnosed angina that is distinctly more frequent, longer in duration, or lower in threshold (i.e., increased by at least one CCSC within 2 mo of initial presentation to at least CCSC III severity)

From Archibald ND, Jones RH: Guidelines for treatment of unstable angina. *In* Califf, RM (vol. ed.): Acute Myocardial Infarction and Other Ischemic Syndromes. Braunwald E, (ser. ed.): Atlas of Heart Diseases. Vol. 8. Philadelphia Current Medicine, 1996.

CCSC, Canadian Cardiovascular Society Classification.

Both the incidence of adverse outcomes (death or MI) and the severity of obstructive disease found at coronary arteriography correlate with the higher classes of severity and clinical circumstances. Patients in class IIIC (post-MI patients with rest pain) who develop transient ST segment changes despite intensive anti-ischemic therapy have the worst prognosis, whereas those in class IB (patients without an extracardiac condition that leads to accelerated angina but who have no rest pain) who are not receiving anti-ischemic therapy, have no release of a biomarker of necrosis, and without electrocardiographic changes have the best outlook.

Pathophysiology

A large majority of patients with UA/NSTEMI have obstructive coronary artery disease, with the unstable state usually precipitated by an increase in coronary obstruction and, therefore, a reduction in oxygen supply.[5] The increase in obstruction may be caused by greater encroachment on the coronary lumen by the gradual enlargement of atherosclerotic plaques, but more commonly, one or more of three other processes are operative[1]:

1. Rupture or erosion of an atherosclerotic plaque causing exposure of the subendothelium and lipid core to platelets (Figs. 26–1 and 26–2), which adhere to the exposed tissue and become activated and bind to fibrinogen through glycoprotein IIa/IIb receptors.
2. An active thrombotic process caused by the coagulation cascade that is triggered by thrombin and that leads to fibrin formation. Thrombi are recognized as typical filling defects at coronary arteriography in almost half of patients with UA/NSTEMI (Fig. 26–3).

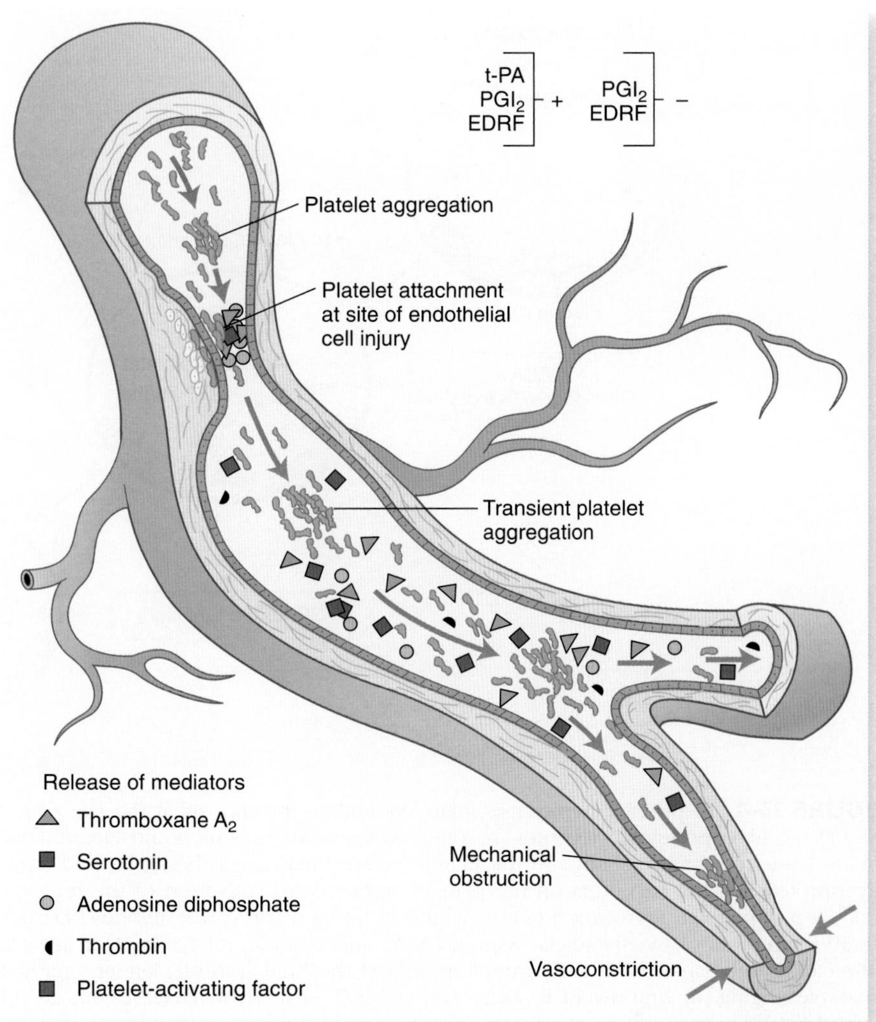

FIGURE 26–1. Schematic diagram suggesting probable mechanisms for the conversion from chronic coronary heart disease to acute coronary artery disease syndromes, including unstable angina. Endothelial injury, usually at sites of atherosclerotic plaques with plaque ulceration or fissuring, is associated with platelet adhesion and aggregation; and the release and activation of selected mediators—including thromboxane A_2, serotonin, platelet-activating factor, thrombin, or adenosine diphosphate—promotes platelet aggregation. Thromboxane A_2, serotonin, thrombin, and platelet-activating factor are vasoconstrictors at sites of endothelial injury. t-PA, tissue-type plasminogen activator; PGI_2, prostaglandin I_2; EDRF, endothelium-derived relaxing factor. (Redrawn from Willerson JT, Cohn JN [eds]: Cardiovascular Medicine, 2nd ed. New York, Churchill Livingstone, 2000, p 530.)

Thrombi have also been noted at coronary angioscopy in a large fraction of the remainder.

3. Coronary vasoconstriction caused by either an increase in neurogenically mediated coronary vascular tone or endothelial dysfunction that prevents the release of coronary vasodilators such as nitric oxide or prostacyclin, or both.

Because inhibition of platelet aggregation by aspirin and clopidogrel, interference with clot formation by heparin, and the administration of coronary vasodilators, such as nitrates and calcium antagonists, are all effective therapeutic measures in UA,[1, 5] it is likely that all three factors are involved in the majority of patients.

The culprit lesion in a coronary artery that is responsible for the development of UA/NSTEMI is usually a subtotal coronary occlusion that causes an imbalance between oxygen supply and demand, which in the case of NSTEMI is so severe that it causes myocardial necrosis. Alternatively, UA/NSTEMI may be caused by total coronary occlusion, but the presence of collateral vessels may prevent the development of infarction or limit the infarction to the subendocardium, and prevent the development of STEMI.

Clinical and Laboratory Findings

Like chronic stable angina, UA/NSTEMI occurs in both women and men, most often in the sixth to eighth decades of life, who have one or more of the major risk factors for coronary atherosclerosis (hypertension, hyperlipidemia, cigarette smoking, or diabetes mellitus). Clinical and laboratory features indicating the likelihood that symptoms result from an ACS secondary to coronary artery disease are shown in Table 26–2. In UA, the chest discomfort resembles that observed in chronic angina (see Chapters 6 and 25), but it is usually more severe and is more likely to be referred to as "pain." It is often described as squeezing, aching, or a feeling of tightness, dullness, or heaviness. Brief episodes of pain (several seconds), lancinating or darting pain, or pain that is continuous for more than 1 hour rarely occur in UA. The threshold of activity causing anginal discomfort is lower in UA than it is in stable angina, and sometimes angina occurs at rest or awakens the patient from sleep.[1] In UA, the episodes of pain occur with increased frequency, usually last longer (up to 30 minutes), and often occur at rest or at night; also, the pain generally radiates more widely. NSTEMI is usually characterized

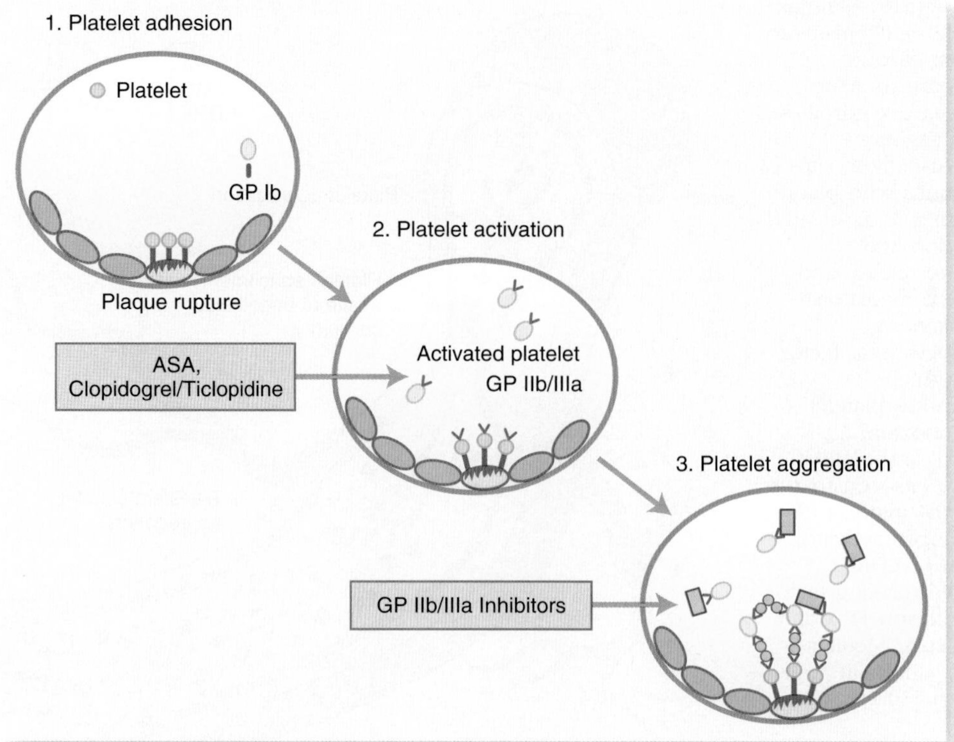

FIGURE 26–2. In primary hemostasis, platelets initiate thrombosis at the site of a ruptured plaque: platelet adhesion occurs via (1) the glycoprotein Ib receptor in conjunction with von Willebrand factor. This is followed by platelet activation (2), which leads to a shape change in the platelet, degranulation of the alpha and dense granules, and expression of glycoprotein IIb/IIIa receptors on the platelet surface with activation of the receptor, such that it can bind fibrinogen. The final step is platelet aggregation (3), in which fibrinogen (or von Willebrand factor) binds to the activated glycoprotein IIb/IIIa receptors of two platelets. Aspirin (ASA) and clopidogrel act to decrease platelet activation (see text for details), whereas the glycoprotein IIb/IIIa inhibitors inhibit the final step of platelet aggregation. (From Cannon CP, Braunwald E: Unstable angina. In Braunwald E, Zipes DP, Libby P [eds]: Heart Disease, 6th ed. Philadelphia, WB Saunders, 2001, pp 1232–1263.)

TABLE 26–2

Likelihood that Signs and Symptoms Represent an ACS Secondary to CAD

Feature	High Likelihood *Any of the following:*	Intermediate Likelihood *Absence of high-likelihood features and presence of any of the following:*	Low Likelihood *Absence of high- or intermediate-likelihood features but may have:*
History	Chest or left arm pain or discomfort as chief symptom reproducing prior documented angina Known history of CAD, including MI	Chest or left arm pain or discomfort as chief symptom Age >70 years Male sex Diabetes mellitus	Probable ischemic symptoms in absence of any of the intermediate likelihood characteristics Recent cocaine use
Examination	Transient MR, hypotension, diaphoresis, pulmonary edema, or rales	Extracardiac vascular disease	Chest discomfort reproduced by palpation
ECG	New, or presumably new, transient ST-segment deviation (≥0.05 mV) or T-wave inversion (≥0.2 mV) with symptoms	Fixed Q-waves Abnormal ST segments or T waves not documented to be new	T-wave flattening or inversion in leads with dominant R-waves Normal ECG
Cardiac markers	Elevated cardiac TnI, TnT, or CK-MB	Normal	Normal

CAD, Coronary artery disease; ECG, electrocardiogram; MR, mitral regurgitation.

From Braunwald E, et al: ACC/AHA guidelines for the management of patients with unstable angina and non–ST-segment elevation myocardial infarction. J Am Coll Cardiol 2000;36:970–1056.

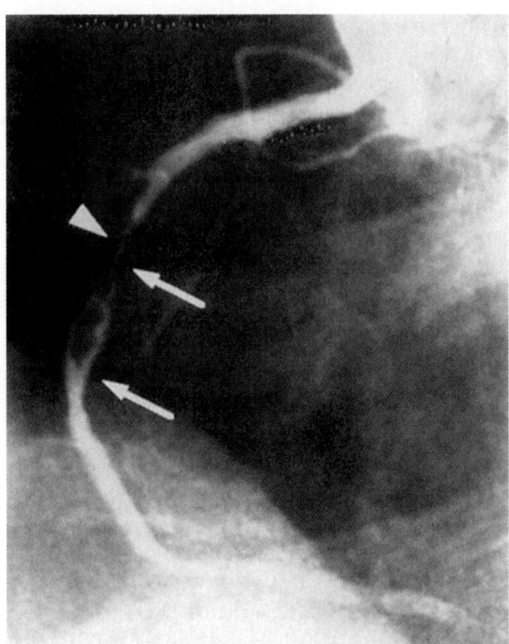

FIGURE 26–3. Intracoronary thrombus in unstable angina. This left anterior oblique right coronary arteriogram shows a severe stenosis in the mid-portion of the right coronary artery *(arrowhead),* followed by a large filling defect surrounded by contrast medium on all sides *(arrows).* (From Popma JJ, Bittl JA: Coronary angiography and intravascular ultrasonography. In Braunwald E, Zipes DP, Libby P [eds]: Heart Disease, 6th ed. Philadelphia, WB Saunders, 2001, p 410.)

by severe chest pain and can be distinguished from STEMI by the electrocardiogram. UA/NSTEMI, like STEMI, may be accompanied by dyspnea, presumably due to impaired function of a large segment of the left ventricle. Both UA and NSTEMI may present without chest pain but with pain in the arms, shoulder, or neck. In some patients, little or no pain is present, but instead dyspnea, nausea, and diaphoresis are the presenting symptoms.[5a]

Cocaine use, like Prinzmetal's angina, may cause UA secondary to coronary vasoconstriction. Cocaine users are usually younger than patients with UA secondary to atheroscerosis, often in their late teens or twenties. Cocaine use should be considered in young patients with UA.

Electrocardiogram

In the interval between episodes of ischemia, the electrocardiogram (ECG) may be normal, it may exhibit chronic nonspecific ST segment or T-wave changes, or it may show the Q-waves of a prior myocardial infarction. During ischemic pain, ST segment deviations or T-wave changes frequently occur and are usually transient; their persistence for more than 12 hours suggests that NSTEMI has occurred; this can be documented by the release of a biomarker. The diagnostic significance of ST segment and T-wave changes are greater if they are not present on a tracing before or subsequent to the pain. ST segment deviation is a marker of increased risk of an adverse clinical event (death or myocardial infarction).

Coronary Arteriography

When critical coronary artery obstruction is defined as more than 70% stenosis of the luminal diameter of one or more of the three major arteries and more than 50% of the left main coronary artery, three-vessel coronary artery disease is found in approximately 40% of patients with UA/NSTEMI, two-vessel disease in 20%, one-vessel disease in 15%,[1] left main coronary artery disease in 10%, and no critical obstruction in the remaining 15%. It has been postulated that vasoconstriction, most likely of the small coronary arteries and arterioles is responsible for ischemia in the approximately 15% of patients with UA/NSTEMI without obstructive epicardial coronary artery disease on coronary arteriography. The culprit lesions in UA/NSTEMI are often eccentric, with scalloped or overhanging edges, reflecting a disrupted atherosclerotic plaque or partially lysed thrombus (see Fig. 26–3).

Ventricular function, measured by contrast or radionuclide ventriculography or echocardiography, may be transiently impaired during and shortly after episodes of ischemia. Function may be permanently impaired in patients with previous MI.

Exercise Testing

After stabilization of symptoms, exercise testing can be carried out safely under a physician's observation and its results are of prognostic value. The prognosis is best in the approximately one third of patients with a normal exercise ECG or myocardial perfusion scintigram. In contrast, a "high-risk" exercise stress test or perfusion scintigram (see Chapters 6 and 25) defines a group of patients in whom subsequent fatal events, myocardial infarction, or failure of medical therapy is high. Patients with positive tests that are not deemed high risk have an intermediate prognosis.

Other Laboratory Tests

The release into the circulation of biochemical markers of myocardial cell injury, such as creatine kinase (CK) and its MB isoenzyme (CK-MB), troponin T, troponin I, and myoglobin, signifies the presence of cell injury and myocyte necrosis, and distinguishes NSTEMI from UA. Release of any of these biomarkers is associated with a higher risk of an adverse outcome.[6]

Natural History

The risk of death in UA/NSTEMI is intermediate between that of stable angina and STEMI. In one representative large clinical trial, the 30 day mortality rate was 3.5% and another 11.5% of patients developed MI or recurrent MI. After this period the event rate declined and became quite similar to that in patients with chronic stable angina.[7]

Management

In 2000, the American College of Cardiology and American Heart Association developed practice guidelines for the treatment of UA/NSTEMI.[2] An update has been published.[8]

Initial Therapy

Patients with symptoms suggesting UA should be referred immediately to the emergency department of a hospital or a specialized chest pain unit (Fig. 26–4). Ordinarily they should *not be* advised to go to a physician's office. The first step is to obtain a directed history, carry out a directed physical examination, and obtain a 12-lead ECG—if possible, while the patient is experiencing pain—to estimate the likelihood of the presence

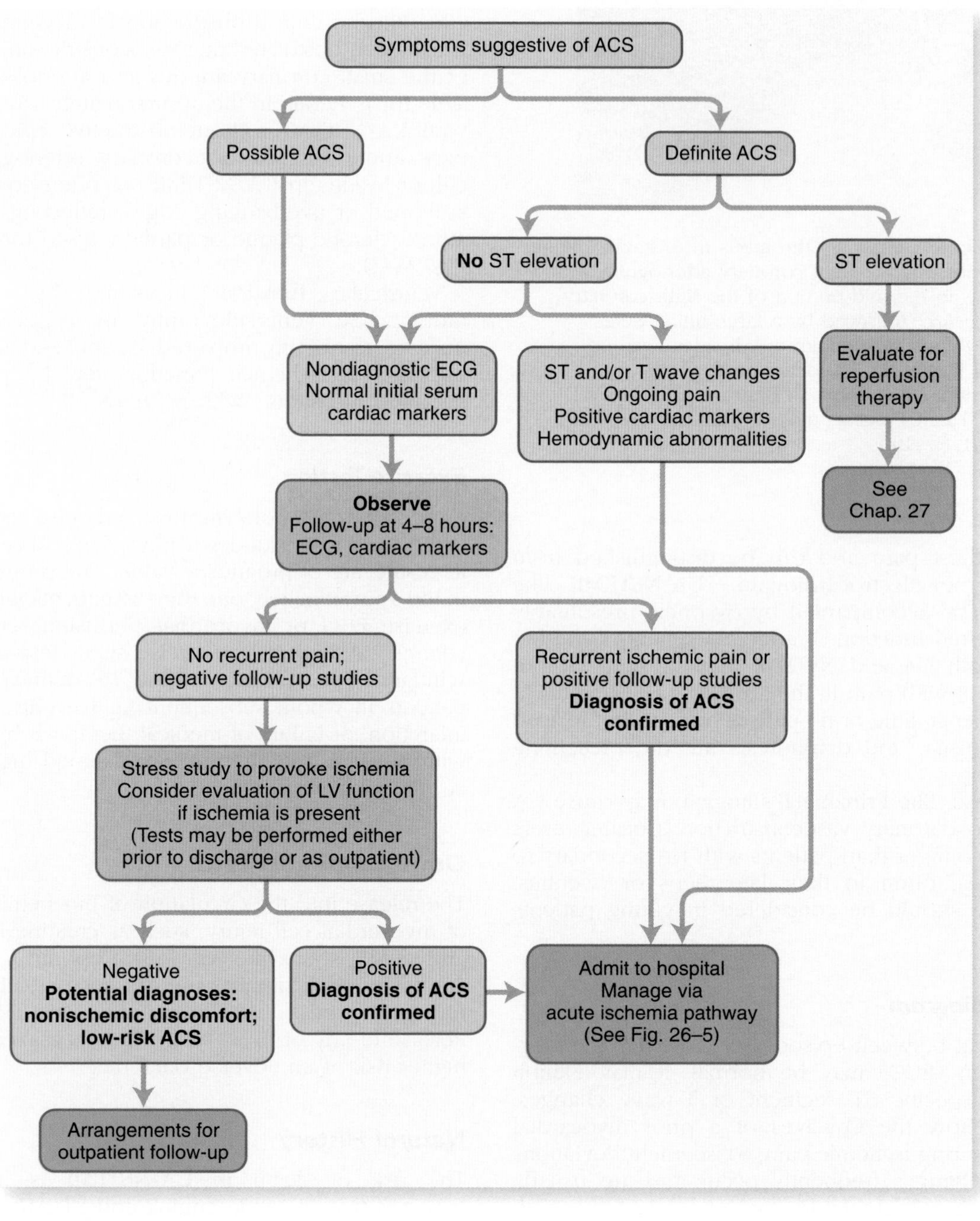

FIGURE 26–4. Algorithm for evaluation and management of patients suspected of having ACS. (Modified from Braunwald E, Antman EA, Beasley JW, et al: ACC/AHA guidelines for the management of patients with unstable angina and non–ST-segment elevation myocardial infarction. J Am Coll Cardiol 2000;36:970–1056.)

of significant coronary artery disease (Table 26–3). A history of prior myocardial infarction or definite angina, or the presence of ST segment deviations or marked T-wave changes during pain makes the likelihood of coronary artery disease high. A blood sample for biomarkers of cardiac injury should be obtained. The risk of death or nonfatal myocardial (re)infarction should then be determined (see Table 26–3). Advanced age (older than 75 years); prolonged, ongoing rest pain; the presence of left ventricular failure (third heart sound, rales, or transient mitral regurgitation); hemodynamic instability; and ventricular arrhythmia place the patient at high risk.

In patients at high or intermediate risk, therapy should be started wherever the patient is first encountered. Patients who have ongoing chest pain should be placed at bedrest and given supplemental oxygen. Unless there is a contraindication, they should be started on aspirin, clopidogrel, and heparin, as well as anti-ischemic therapy with beta-blockers and sublingual nitroglycerin (Tables 26–4 and 26–5). After initial treatment and stabilization in the emergency department, patients at high risk for adverse outcomes (see Table 26–3) should be transferred to an intensive care unit, whereas patients at intermediate risk may be placed in a regular bed with electrocardiographic monitoring. Patients at low risk may be managed as outpatients but should undergo detailed evaluation including a stress test within 72 hours.

Many aspects of the care of patients with UA/NSTEMI can be managed by primary care physicians. Cardiac consultation should be sought in high-risk patients, as well as in patients who fail to respond to therapy or who develop complications such as heart failure and those in whom coronary revascularization is considered.

Intensive Medical Treatment

All patients should be evaluated for noncoronary causes of UA, such as aortic valve disease or hypertrophic obstructive cardiomyopathy, as well as for extracardiac conditions, such as severe anemia, thyrotoxicosis, or infection, that may precipitate UA in a patient with chronic stable angina (i.e., secondary UA). Hematocrit, serum cholesterol (and fractions), and thyroxine levels should be measured routinely. Mild sedation or treatment with an anxiolytic drug is usually advisable. The aggressiveness of pharmacologic therapy depends on the severity of the ischemia and often requires multiple adjustments during hospitalization and after discharge.

TABLE 26–3

Short-Term Risk of Death or Nonfatal MI in Patients with UA*

Feature	High Risk *At least one of the following features must be present:*	Intermediate Risk *No high-risk feature but must have one of the following:*	Low Risk *No high- or intermediate-risk feature but may have any of the following features:*
History	Accelerating tempo of ischemic symptoms in preceding 48 hr	Prior MI, peripheral or cerebrovascular disease, or CABG, prior aspirin use	
Character of pain	Prolonged ongoing (>20 minutes) rest pain	Prolonged (>20 min) rest angina, now resolved, with moderate or high likelihood of CAD Rest angina (<20 min) or relieved with rest or sublingual NTG	New-onset CCSC III or IV angina in the past 2 weeks without prolonged (>20 min) rest pain but with moderate or high likelihood of CAD
Clinical findings	Pulmonary edema, most likely due to ischemia New or worsening MR murmur S_3 or new/worsening rales Hypotension, bradycardia, tachycardia Age >75 years	Age >70 years	
ECG	Angina at rest with transient ST-segment changes >0.05 mV Bundle-branch block, new or presumed new Sustained ventricular tachycardia	T-wave inversions >0.2 mV Pathological Q waves	Normal or unchanged ECG during an episode of chest discomfort
Cardiac markers	Markedly elevated (e.g., TnT or TnI > 0.1 ng/mL)	Slightly elevated (e.g., TnT >0.01 but <0.1 ng/mL)	Normal

*Estimation of the short-term risks of death and nonfatal cardiac ischemic events in UA is a complex multivariable problem that cannot be fully specified in a table such as this; therefore, this table is meant to offer general guidance and illustration rather than rigid algorithms.

CABG, coronary artery bypass graft; CAD, coronary artery disease; CCS, Canadian Cardiovascular Society Class; ECG, electrocardiogram; NTG, nitroglycerin; UA, unstable angina.

From Braunwald E, et al: ACC/AHA guidelines for the management of patients with unstable angina and non–ST-segment elevation myocardial infarction. J Am Coll Cardiol 2000;36:970–1056.

TABLE 26–4

Drugs Commonly Used in Intensive Medical Management of Patients with Unstable Angina

Drug Category	Clinical Condition	When to Avoid*	Dosage
Nitrates	Symptoms are not fully relieved with three sublingual nitroglycerin tablets and initiation of beta-blocker therapy	Hypotension	5–10 μg/min by continuous infusion Titrated up to 75–100 μg/min until relief of symptoms or limiting side effects (headache or hypotension with a systolic blood pressure <90 mm Hg or more than 30% below starting mean arterial pressure levels if significant hypertension is present) Topical, oral, or buccal nitrates are acceptable alternatives for patients without ongoing or refractory symptoms
Beta blockers[†]	Unstable angina	PR interval (ECG) >0.24 sec 2° or 3° atrioventricular block Heart rate <60 beats/min Blood pressure <90 mm Hg Shock Left ventricular failure with congestive heart failure Severe reactive airway disease	Metoprolol 5-mg increments by slow (over 1–2 min) IV administration Repeated every 5 min for a total initial dose of 15 mg Followed in 1–2 hr by 25–50 mg by mouth every 6 hr If a very conservative regimen is desired, initial doses can be reduced to 1–2 mg Propranolol 0.5–1.0 mg IV dose Followed in 1–2 hr by 40–80 mg by mouth every 6–8 hr Esmolol Starting maintenance dose of 0.1 $mg \cdot kg^{-1} \cdot min^{-1}$ IV Titration in increments of 0.05 $mg \cdot kg^{-1} \cdot min^{-1}$ every 10–15 min as tolerated by blood pressure until the desired therapeutic response has been obtained, limiting symptoms develop, or a dose of 0.20 $mg \cdot kg^{-1} \cdot min^{-1}$ is reached Optional loading dose of 0.5 mg/kg may be given by slow IV administration (2–5 min) for more rapid onset of action Atenolol 5-mg IV dose Followed 5 min later by a second dose 5-mg IV dose and then 50–100 mg orally every day initiated 1–2 hr after the IV dose
Calcium channel blockers	Patients whose symptoms are not relieved by adequate doses of nitrates and beta-blockers or in patients unable to tolerate adequate doses of one or both of these agents or in patients with variant angina	Pulmonary edema Evidence of left ventricular dysfunction	Dependent on specific agent
Morphine sulfate	Patients whose symptoms are not relieved after three serial sublingual nitroglycerin tablets or whose symptoms recur with adequate anti-ischemic therapy	Hypotension Respiratory depression Confusion Obtundation	2–5 mg IV dose May be repeated every 5–30 min as needed to relieve symptoms and maintain patient comfort

*Allergy or prior intolerance is a contraindication for all categories of drugs listed in this chart.

[†]Choice of the specific agent is not as important as ensuring that appropriate candidates receive this therapy. If there are concerns about patient intolerance owing to existing pulmonary disease, especially asthma, left ventricular dysfunction, or risk of hypotension or severe bradycardia, initial selection should favor a short-acting agent, such as propranolol or metoprolol or the ultra-short-acting agent esmolol. Mild wheezing or a history of chronic obstructive pulmonary disease should prompt a trial of a short-acting agent at a reduced dose (e.g., 2.5 mg IV metoprolol, 12.5 mg oral metoprolol, or 25 $\mu g \cdot kg^{-1} \cdot min^{-1}$ esmolol as initial doses) rather than complete avoidance of beta-blocker therapy.

Note: Some of the recommendations in this guide suggest the use of agents for purposes or in doses other than those specified by the U.S. Food and Drug Administration. Such recommendations are made after consideration of concerns regarding nonapproved indications. Where made such recommendations are based on more recent clinical trials or expert consensus.

IV, intravenous; aPTT, activated partial thromboplastin time; ECG, electrocardiogram; 2°, second-degree; 3°, third-degree.

From Braunwald E, Jones RH, Mark DB, et al: Diagnosing and managing unstable angina. Circulation 1994;90:613–622.

TABLE 26–5

Clinical Use of Antithrombotic Therapy

Drug	Dose
Oral Antiplatelet Therapy	
Aspirin	Initial dose of 162–325 mg nonenteric formulation followed by 75–160 mg/day of an enteric or a nonenteric formulation
Clopidogrel (Plavix)	75 mg/day; a loading dose of 4–8 tablets (300–600 mg) can be used when rapid onset of action is required
Ticlopidine (Ticlid)	250 mg twice daily; a loading dose of 500 mg can be used when rapid onset of inhibition is required; monitoring of platelet and white cell counts during treatment is required
Heparins	
Dalteparin (Fragmin)	120 IU/kg SC every 12 hr (maximum 10,000 IU twice daily)
Enoxaparin (Lovenox)	1 mg/kg SC every 12 hr; the first dose may be preceded by a 30-mg IV bolus
Heparin (UFH)	Bolus 60–70 U/kg (maximum 5000 U) IV followed by infusion of 12–15 U · kg^{-1} · h^{-1} (maximum 1000 U/h) titrated to a PTT 1.5–2.5 times control
Intravenous Antiplatelet Therapy	
Abciximab (ReoPro)	0.25 mg/kg bolus followed by infusion of 0.125 μg · kg^{-1} · min^{-1} (maximum 10 μg/min) for 12 to 24 hr
Eptifibatide (Integrilin)	180 μg/kg bolus followed by infusion of 2.0 μg · kg^{-1} · min^{-1} for 72 to 96 hr*
Tirofiban (Aggrastat)	0.4 μg · kg^{-1} · min^{-1} for 30 min followed by infusion of 0.1 μg · kg^{-1} · min^{-1} for 48 to 96 hr*

*Different dose regimens were tested in recent clinical trials before percutaneous interventions.

IV, intravenous; SC, subcutaneously; UFH, unfractionated heparin.

From Braunwald E, et al: ACC/AHA guidelines for the management of patients with unstable angina and non–ST-segment elevation myocardial infarction. J Am Coll Cardiol 2000;36:970–1056.

Nitrates

Nonhypotensive patients at high risk (see Table 26–3) and those whose symptoms that are not fully relieved with three 0.4 mg sublingual nitroglycerin tablets taken 5 minutes apart should receive intravenous nitroglycerin. This drug should be administered by continuous infusion commencing at a dose of 5 to 10 μg/min and titrated up by 10 μg/min every 5 to 10 minutes until relief of symptoms or limiting side effects occur. Once they have been symptom-free for 24 hours, patients on intravenous nitroglycerin should be switched to oral (e.g., isosorbide dinitrate SR, 40 mg qd or bid; isosorbide mononitrate SR, 60 mg to 240 mg qd) or transdermal (0.2 to 0.8 mg/hr q 12 hr) nitrate therapy.

Morphine Sulfate

When ischemic symptoms are not relieved by three serial sublingual nitroglycerin tablets or when symptoms recur despite adequate anti-ischemic therapy, in addition to intravenous nitroglycerin, morphine sulfate at a dose of 2 to 5 mg intravenously is recommended, unless contraindicated by hypotension or a history of intolerance. Morphine may be repeated every 5 to 10 minutes as needed to relieve symptoms and maintain patient comfort.

Beta-Adrenergic Blockers

Patients at high risk (see Table 26–3) and without contraindications (bradycardia, hypotension, left ventricular failure, atrioventricular block or reactive airway disease) should receive intravenous beta-blockers, for example, metoprolol in up to three 5-mg increments, atenolol, or esmolol (see Table 26–4). Intravenous treatment should be followed by oral beta-blockers (e.g., metoprolol, 50 to 200 mg twice daily). Intermediate- and low-risk patients do not require intravenous therapy and may be started on oral beta-blockers directly. Target heart rates of 50 to 60 beats per minute at rest are appropriate.

Calcium Antagonists

These drugs may be used to control ongoing or recurrent ischemic symptoms or hypertension in patients already on adequate doses of nitrates and beta-blockers, in those with contraindications or unable to tolerate adequate doses of one or both of these agents, and in those with Prinzmetal's angina (see later). Calcium antagonists should be avoided in patients with pulmonary edema or evidence of left ventricular dysfunction. Short-acting nifedipine should *not* be used in the absence of concurrent beta blockade. Diltiazem, immediate release 30 to 80 mg qid, or Verapamil (SR, 120 to 140 mg qd) is recommended.

Antiplatelet Agents

The combination of aspirin and clopidogrel is useful both acutely and chronically in patients with unstable angina (Fig. 26–5).[1, 2, 8, 9] The initial dose of aspirin should be 160 mg or 324 mg; subsequently, the dose should be 80 to 324 mg/day. Clopidogrel should be given as a loading dose of 300 mg initially followed by 75 mg/day. Patients at high risk and those in whom a percutaneous coronary intervention (PCI) is planned should receive an intravenous platelet glycoprotein IIb/IIIa receptor blocker (see Fig. 26–2).[2]

Heparin

Heparin (unfractionated [UFH], or low molecular weight [LMWH] is indicated in patients at high or intermediate risk of an adverse outcome and should be begun immediately and continued for 2 to 5 days or until coronary revascularization is performed.[2, 5] The initial dose of UFH is 60 to 70 (maximum, 5000) units/kg/min by intra-

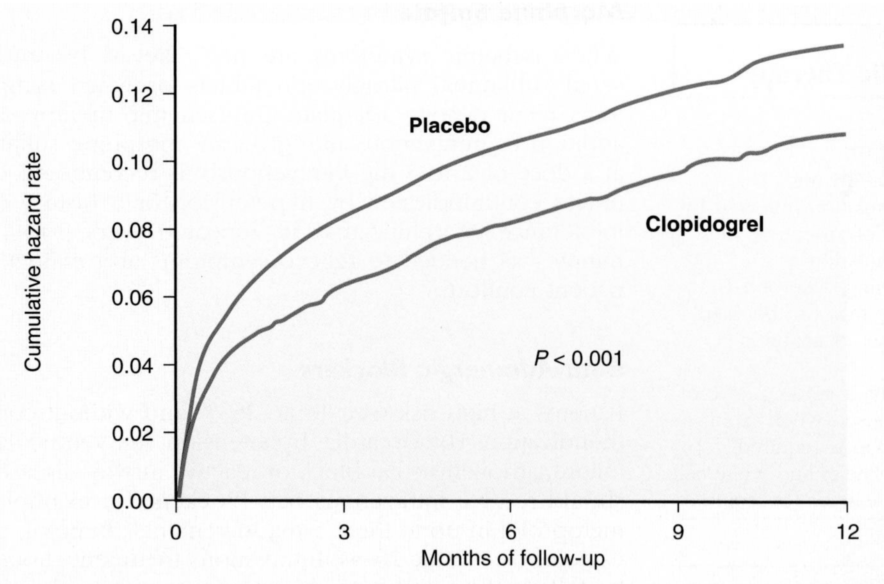

FIGURE 26–5. Cumulative hazard rates for the first primary outcome (death from cardiovascular causes, nonfatal myocardial infarction, or stroke) during the 12 months of the study. The results demonstrate the sustained effect of clopidogrel. (From The Clopidogrel in Unstable Angina to Prevent Recurrent Events (CURE) trial: Effects of clopidogrel in addition to aspirin in patients with acute coronary syndromes without ST-segment elevation. N Engl J Med 2001;345:494–502.)

venous bolus followed by an infusion of 12 to 15 (max 1000) units/kg/min, maintaining the activated partial thromboplastin time (aPTT) at 1.5 to 2.5 times control (see Table 26–5). When a therapeutic level has been achieved, the aPTT should be remeasured every 24 hours. Some studies suggest that LMWH (e.g., enoxaparin 30 mg IV bolus followed by 1 mg/kg subcutaneously bid) may be superior to unfractionated heparin.[10] Certainly, LMWH is more convenient than UFH to administer because it does not require monitoring and dose adjustments. Hemoglobin or hematocrit and platelet count should be measured daily while the patient is on heparin.

Fibrinolysis

Even though thrombosis plays a significant role in the pathogenesis of unstable angina, well-controlled studies have shown no benefit from fibrinolytic therapy.[2]

Cardiac Catheterization

If chest discomfort with objective evidence of ischemia persists for more than 1 hour after the commencement of aggressive medical therapy, or if the patient experiences pulmonary edema or hemodynamic instability, *emergency* cardiac catheterization and coronary arteriography should be strongly considered. Patients with continued ischemia despite therapy, especially those who are hypotensive, can benefit from stabilization by means of intra-aortic balloon counterpulsation as a bridge to cardiac catheterization or surgery, or both. Intra-aortic balloon counterpulsation may also be used to stabilize patients who require interhospital transfer. Early cardiac catheterization should also be considered in other patients with UA/NSTEMI who are at high risk, with ST segment deviations or a positive biomarker. This strategy may require transfer of the patient to a hospital with a cardiac catheterization laboratory.

Two randomized clinical trials, the FRISC II[11] and TACTICS-TIMI 18[12] trials have compared an *early invasive* strategy and an *early conservative* strategy in patients with UA/NSTEMI. In the early invasive strategy, cardiac catheterization was performed routinely and was followed by myocardial revascularization, which was carried out based on the anatomic findings. In the early conservative strategy, cardiac catheterization was performed only in patients who had persistent or recurrent pain or ischemia, or both, congestive heart failure, malignant ventricular arrhythmia, or a clearly positive, high-risk noninvasive study (see Chapter 25). Both trials demonstrated the superiority of the invasive approach, especially in patients at high risk (Fig. 26–6), and this approach is recommended for these patients. Cardiac catheterization and coronary arteriography are ordinarily *not* indicated, however, in patients with extensive comorbidities that contraindicate revascularization, as well as in those who do not wish to undergo this therapy.

Laboratory Testing

CK-MB or troponin T or I, or both, should be measured every 6 to 8 hours for the first 24 hours after admission. Troponins are especially useful in patients presenting 24 to 72 hours after symptom onset if serial CK-MB levels are normal. Serum lipid levels should be obtained, unless the patient has had a recent determination. Follow-up ECGs should be recorded every 8 hours for 24 hours, then every 24 hours, and whenever the patient has recurrent symptoms or a change in clinical status, and before discharge.

Medical Management

When ischemia at rest in a high-risk patient has been brought under control by medical management for at

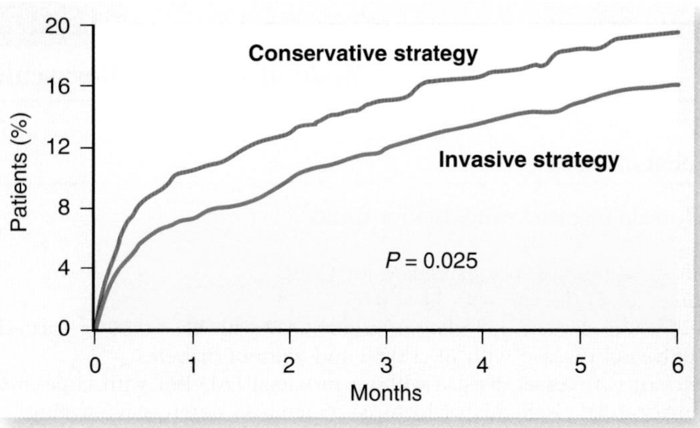

FIGURE 26–6. Cumulative incidence of the primary endpoint of death, nonfatal myocardial infarction, or rehospitalization for an acute coronary syndrome during the 6-month follow-up period. The rate of the primary endpoint was lower in the invasive-strategy group than in the conservative-strategy group (15.9% vs. 19.4%; odds ratio, 0.78; 95% confidence interval, 0.62 to 0.97; $P =$ .025). (From Cannon CP, Weintraub ES, Demopoulos LA, et al: Comparison of early invasive and conservative strategies in patients with unstable coronary syndromes treated with the glycoprotein IIb/IIIa inhibitor tirofiban. N Engl J Med 2001;344:1879–1887.)

least 24 hours, the patient may be transferred out of the intensive care or coronary care unit and placed on a maintenance medical regimen consisting of an oral long-acting nitrate (e.g., 10 to 60 mg isosorbide dinitrate PO, bid or tid), a beta-blocker, aspirin, clopidogrel, and heparin. During the following period of at least 24 hours, the patient should be observed closely in a monitored bed to identify ST segment or T-wave changes and arrhythmias. If ischemic episodes, left ventricular failure, serious tachyarrhythmias, or hypotension develops or recur on medical management, the patient should be returned to the intensive care unit or the cardiac catheterization laboratory or transferred to a hospital where such a facility is available.

Use and Timing of Noninvasive Tests

Exercise or pharmacologic stress testing should be performed before discharge in patients who have responded to medical therapy and have been free of angina at rest or minor exertion and of congestive heart failure for a minimum of 24 hours. It is also an integral part of the expeditious outpatient evaluation of low-risk patients with UA. The exercise treadmill test is a suitable mode of stress testing in patients with a normal resting ECG who are not taking digoxin. Patients with widespread or marked resting ST segment depression (≥1 mm), ST segment changes secondary to digoxin, left ventricular hypertrophy, left bundle branch block, intraventricular conduction defect, or ventricular preexcitation should be tested using myocardial perfusion scintigraphy. In patients unable to exercise owing to physical limitations, a pharmacologic stress should be used in combination with myocardial perfusion scintigraphy or echocardiography. Left ventricular function should be assessed. Left ventriculography may be carried out at the time of cardiac catheterization; alternatively, two-dimensional echocardiography or radionuclide ventriculography may be employed.

Myocardial Revascularization

The choice between the two modes of revascularization—surgery or PCI—depends largely on the coronary anatomy, as described in Chapter 25. The majority of patients can be managed by PCI, usually involving one or more coronary stents with the administration of an inhibitor of platelet glycoprotein IIb/IIIa receptors (Table 26–6).

Patients with multiple, diffuse lesions, those with left main coronary artery disease, three-vessel coronary artery disease, and significantly impaired left ventricular function (or a combination) are generally more suitable for coronary artery bypass grafting. The immediate risk of PCI and other catheter-based interventions in patients with unstable angina may be reduced by the prior administration of a platelet glycoprotein IIb/IIIa inhibitor (Fig. 26–7).

Discharge from Hospital and Postdischarge Care

Patients may be discharged after recovery from revascularization or, in those who do not undergo revascularization, 24 to 48 hours after ischemia has been controlled and noninvasive testing has been completed. Aspirin (80 to 324 mg/day) should be continued for an indefinite period, regardless of whether revascularization has been carried out. Clopidogrel (75 mg/day) should be continued for one year. Prior to hospital discharge, secondary prevention measures should be started—treating hypertension and hyperlipidemia, and embarking on an exercise program. There is now substantial evidence that patients at high- or intermediate risk should be started and continued on an angiotensin-converting enzyme inhibitor. Patients with an LDL cholesterol >100 mg/dL should be started on dietary treatment and a statin to reach this target at or prior to hospital discharge. Diabetes mellitus should be treated aggressively and a vigorous smoking cessation program should be undertaken. An effort to achieve ideal body weight and a graduated exercise program should be started. If chronic stable angina persists after hospital discharge, patients should be continued on a beta-blocker and long-acting nitrate, supplemented by sublingual nitroglycerin as needed.

TABLE 26–6

Mode of Coronary Revascularization for UA/NSTEMI

Extent of Disease	Treatment	Class/Level of Evidence
Left main disease,* candidate for CABG	CABG	I/A
	PCI	III/C
Left main disease, not candidate for CABG	PCI	IIb/C
Three-vessel disease with EF < 0.05	CABG	I/A
Multivessel disease including proximal LAD with EF < 0.50 or treated diabetes	CABG or PCI	I/A, IIb/B
Multivessel disease with EF > 0.50 and without diabetes	PCI	I/A
One- or two-vessel disease without proximal LAD but with large areas of myocardial ischemia or high-risk criteria on noninvasive testing	CABG or PCI	I/B
One-vessel disease with proximal LAD	CABG or PCI	IIa/B†
One- or two-vessel disease without proximal LAD with small area of ischemia or no ischemia on noninvasive testing	CABG or PCI	III/C†
Insignificant coronary stenosis	CABG or PCI	III/C

*≤50% diameter stenosis.

†Class/level of evidence I/A if severe angina persists despite medical therapy.

CABG, coronary artery bypass graft; EF, ejection fraction; LAD, left artery disease; PCI, percutaneous coronary intervention.

From Braunwald E, et al: ACC/AHA guidelines for the management of patients with unstable angina and non–ST-segment elevation myocardial infarction. J Am Coll Cardiol 2000;36:970–1056.

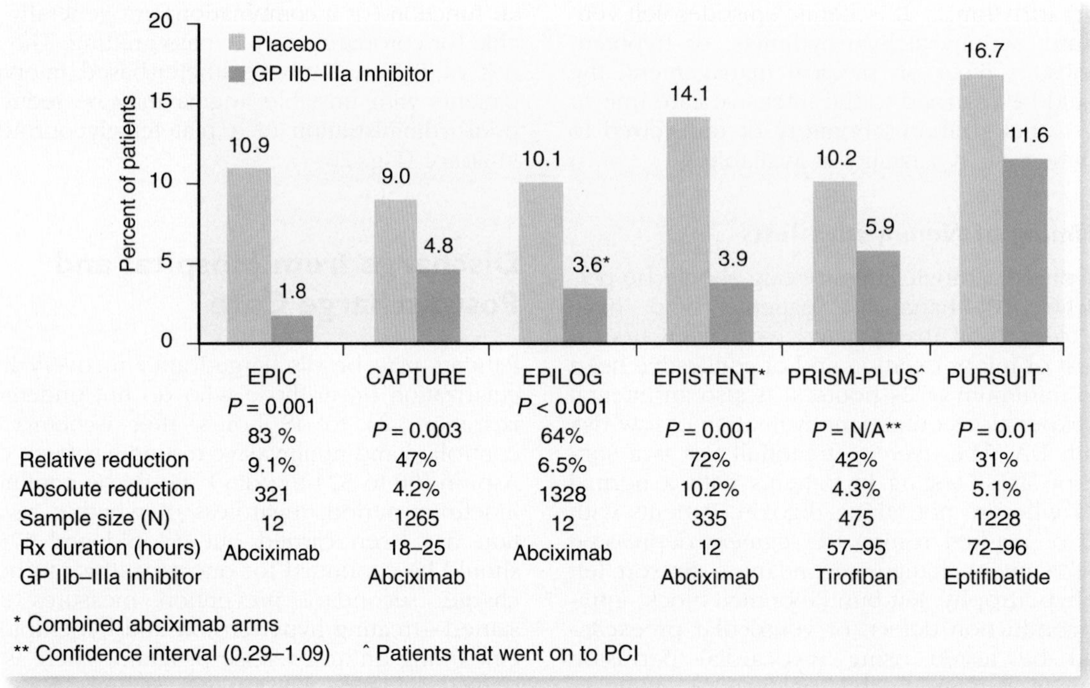

FIGURE 26–7. Death and MI at 30 days after PCI in patients with ACS: GP IIb/IIIa trials. (From Braunwald E, Antman EA, Beasley JW, et al: ACC/AHA guidelines for the management of patients with unstable angina and non–ST-segment elevation myocardial infarction. J Am Coll Cardiol 2000;36:970–1056.)

High-risk patients should be seen as outpatients in follow-up 1 to 2 weeks after discharge and lower-risk patients at 2 to 6 weeks. Patients should be advised to contact their primary care physician if symptoms recur or become more severe.

Initial Outpatient Management

Initial management on an outpatient basis is advisable in patients with UA considered to be at low risk of adverse events at the time of the initial evaluation (see

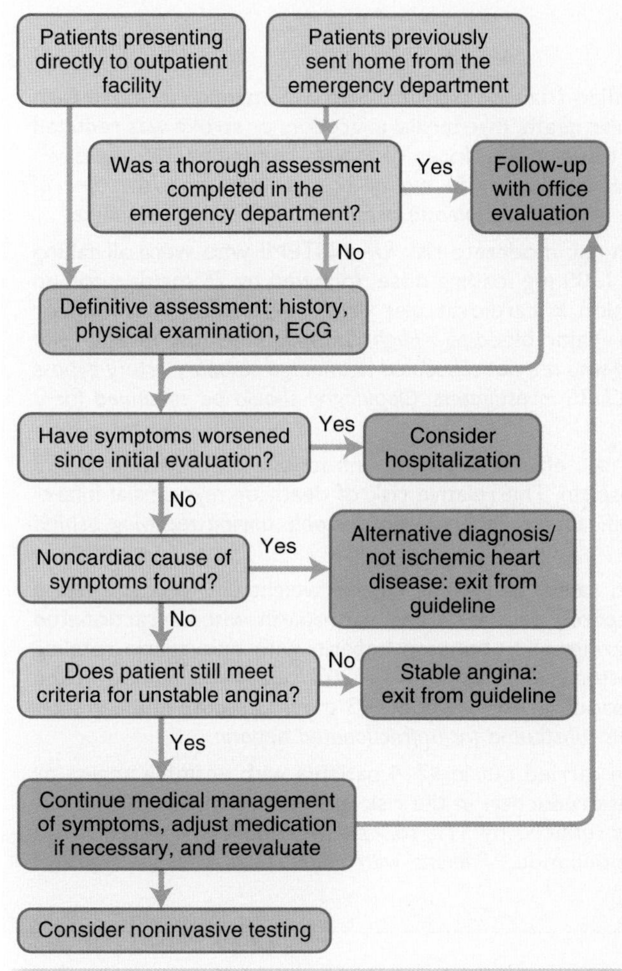

FIGURE 26–8. Algorithm for outpatient management of unstable angina. ECG, electrocardiogram. (From Archibald ND, Jones RH: Guidelines for treatment of unstable angina. In Califf RM, vol. ed: Acute Myocardial Infarction and Other Ischemic Syndromes. Braunwald E, series ed: Atlas of Heart Diseases, vol. 8. Philadelphia, Current Medicine, 1996.)

Fig. 26–8; see also Table 26–3 and Fig. 26–4). Workup should include a search for noncardiac factors that may have caused or precipitated UA or lack of compliance with a regimen previously designed for chronic stable angina. If the patient's symptoms are well controlled on the medical regimen, noninvasive stress testing and risk stratification may be undertaken on an outpatient basis.

Prinzmetal's Variant Angina

This uncommon form of angina also causes ischemic pain at rest. Its pathogenesis differs from the usual form of UA in that it is caused by severe focal spasm of one of the epicardial coronary arteries.[14]

Patients with Prinzmetal's angina are usually in their 40s or 50s, generally one or two decades younger than those with UA caused by coronary atherosclerosis. They often do not exhibit coronary risk factors, except for cigarette smoking. Prinzmetal's angina has been reported to occur in association with migraine, Raynaud's phenomenon, and aspirin-induced asthma. It may be precipitated by alcohol withdrawal, emotional distress, and the administration of 5-fluorouracil and cyclophosphamide. The attacks of pain occur most frequently in the early morning hours, may awaken the patient from sleep, are usually quite severe, and may be accompanied by tachyarrhythmias that can cause syncope. In contrast to the UA caused by coronary atherosclerosis, exercise capacity may be normal (unless the patient has coexistent atherosclerotic coronary artery disease [see later]). Again, in contrast to UA, the progression from exercise-induced angina to rest pain is rarely observed in Prinzmetal's angina.

The principal feature on laboratory investigation that distinguishes Prinzmetal's angina from UA is the ST segment *elevation* during ischemia in the former and the ST segment *depression* in the latter. ST segment elevation may be asymptomatic and detected on continuous (Holter) ECG monitoring. With prolonged, marked ST segment elevation, myocardial infarction can occur and transient intraventricular and atrioventricular conduction disturbances and ventricular tachyarrhythmias may develop.

Approximately one half of patients with Prinzmetal's angina also have a fixed obstructive lesion in a proximal coronary artery. The site of spasm is usually within 1 cm of the fixed obstruction. The diagnosis of Prinzmetal's angina can be confirmed in the catheterization laboratory by observing localized coronary spasm or inducing it with gradually escalating doses of intravenous ergonovine or the intracoronary injection of acetylcholine or by hyperventilation.

Management

Episodes of Prinzmetal's angina respond to nitrates, given sublingually or intravenously. Oral calcium antagonists are usually effective in preventing recurrence,[14] but these may have to be given at doses higher than those usually employed in the management of chronic stable angina or UA. The episodes of rest pain do not respond to, and cannot be prevented by, beta-blockade. Surgical or catheter-based revascularization is indicated in patients with Prinzmetal's angina who have a severe, discrete *fixed* obstruction and severe exercise-induced angina that does not respond adequately to medical therapy.

Prinzmetal's angina is often cyclical, with an acute, active phase characterized by frequent episodes of rest pain and followed by periods of inactivity. Patients who develop tachyarrhythmias during episodes of ischemia are at high risk of sudden death and require intensive therapy with calcium antagonists and nitrates. Patients who are maintained under active treatment with calcium antagonists and nitrates have an excellent prognosis with a 5-year survival rate of more than 90%.

Evidence-Based Summary

1. A systematic review of multiple randomized placebo-controlled trials of aspirin (75 to 325 mg/day) in more than 4000 patients with UA showed that the absolute risk of vascular death, myocardial infarction, or stroke was reduced by 5%, the relative risk by 35%. No additional benefit was observed in doses of aspirin exceeding 325 mg/day.[15] *Patients with unstable angina who are not allergic to aspirin should receive 75 mg to 325 mg daily from the time of diagnosis for an indefinite period. Patients who are allergic to or who cannot tolerate aspirin should receive clopidogrel.*
2. In one large trial, the CURE trial, 12,562 patients with high- or moderate-risk UA/NSTEMI who were all taking aspirin (75 to 325 mg/day) were randomized to clopidogrel (300 mg loading dose, followed by 75 mg/day) for up to 1 year. There was a 2.2% absolute (20% relative) reduction in cardiovascular death, myocardial infarction or stroke. There was a 1% absolute (37% relative) increase in major bleeding.[9] *High and moderate risk patients with UA/NSTEMI who are not at increased risk for major bleeding and who are not scheduled to undergo coronary artery bypass grafting should receive clopidogrel in the regimen used by the CURE investigators. Clopidogrel should be continued for 3 months and preferably for 1 year.*
3. A meta-analysis of six randomized controlled trials studied the effects of adding unfractionated heparin to 1353 patients with unstable angina, all of whom were receiving aspirin. The relative risk of death or myocardial infarction was reduced by 37%, reaching nominal statistical significance.[16] *Patients with unstable angina receiving aspirin should receive heparin for at least 48 hours.*
4. The totality of evidence regarding the relative efficacy and safety of low molecular weight and unfractionated heparin is not clear. Two large randomized trials that compared dalteparin and nadroparin with unfractionated heparin showed no significant difference.[2] Two trials comparing unfractionated heparin with enoxaparin totaling 7081 patients favored enoxaparin. A meta-analysis of the latter two trials shows a 20% relative reduction in the rate of death, MI, or urgent revascularization for all time periods to and including 43 days.[10] *Because of the greater convenience and strongly suggestive evidence, enoxaparin may be substituted for unfractionated heparin.*
5. Six randomized trials adding a GP IIb/IIIa inhibitor have been carried out in 4714 patients with unstable angina or non–ST segment elevation myocardial infarction. The absolute reduction in the risk of death or myocardial infarction ranged from 4.2% to 10.2%, while the relative risk was reduced by 31% to 72%. Benefit was observed with all three GP IIb/IIIa inhibitors—abciximab, tirofiban and eptifibatide.[2] *Patients with UA/NSTEMI who undergo PCI should receive a GPIIb/IIIa blocker.*

References

1. Cannon CP, Braunwald E: Unstable angina. In Braunwald E, Zipes DP, Libby P (eds): Heart Disease, 6th ed. Philadelphia: WB Saunders, 2001, pp 1232–1263.
2. Braunwald E, Antman EM, Beasley JW, et al: ACC/AHA guidelines for the management of patients with unstable angina and non–ST-segment elevation myocardial infarction. J Am Coll Cardiol 2000;36:970–1056.
3. Braunwald E: Unstable angina: A classification. Circulation 1989;80:410.
4. Hamm CW, Braunwald E: A classification of unstable angina revisited. Circulation 2000;102:118–122.
5. Theroux P, Fuster V: Acute coronary syndromes: Unstable angina and non–Q-wave myocardial infarction. Circulation 1998;97:1195–1206.

5a. Canto JG, Fincher C, Kiefer CI, et al: Atypical presentations among Medicare beneficiaries with unstable angina pectoris. Am J Cardiol 2002;90:248–253.

6. Antman EM, Tanasijevic MJ, Thompson B, et al: Cardiac-specific troponin I levels to predict the risk of mortality in patients with acute coronary syndromes. N Engl J Med 1996;335:1342–1349.
7. The PURSUIT trial investigators: Inhibition of platelet glycoprotein IIb/IIIa with eptifibatide in patients with acute coronary syndromes. The PURSUIT trial investigators: Platelet glycoprotein IIb/IIIa in unstable angina: Receptor suppression using Integrilin therapy. N Engl J Med 1998; 339:436–443.
8. Braunwald E, Antman EM, Beasley JW, et al: ACC/AHA 2002 guideline update for the management of patients with UA/NSTEMI. J Am Coll Cardiol 2002;40:1366.
9. Yusuf S, Zhao F, Mehta SR, et al: Effects of clopidogrel in addition to aspirin in patients with acute coronary syndromes without ST-segment elevation. N Engl J Med 2001; 345:494–502.
10. Antman EM, Cohen M, Radley D, et al: Assessment of the treatment effect of enoxaparin for unstable angina/non–Q-wave myocardial infarction: TIMI 11B ESSENCE Meta-analysis. Circulation 1999;100:1602–1608.
11. Wallentin L, Lagerqvist B, Husted S, et al: Outcome at one year after an invasive compared with a non-invasive strategy in unstable coronary artery disease: The FRISC II invasive randomized trial. Lancet 2000;356:9–16.
12. Cannon CP, Weintraub ES, Demopoulos LA, et al: Comparison of early invasive and conservative strategies in patients with unstable coronary syndromes treated with the glycoprotein IIb/IIIa inhibitor tirofiban. N Engl J Med 2001;344:1879–1887.
13. Gersh BJ, Braunwald E, Bonow RO: Chronic coronary artery disease. In Braunwald E, Zipes DP, Libby P (eds):

Heart Disease, 6th ed. Philadelphia, WB Saunders, 2001, pp 1272–1353.

14. Morikami Y, Yasue H: Efficacy of slow-release nifedipine on myocardial ischemic episodes in variant angina pectoris. Am J Cardiol 1991;68:580.
15. Antiplatelet Trialists' Collaboration. Collaborative overview of randomized trials of antiplatelet therapy I: prevention of death, myocardial infarction, and stroke by prolonged antiplatelet therapy in various categories of people. Br Med J 1994;308:81–106.
16. Eikelboom JW, Anand SS, Malmberg K, et al: Unfractionated heparin and low molecular weight heparin in acute coronary syndrome without ST elevation: A meta analysis. Lancet 2000;355:1936–1942.

CHAPTER 27

Recognition and Management of Patients with Acute Myocardial Infarction

Eugene Braunwald

Acute myocardial infarction (AMI) occurs in approximately 900,000 persons in the United States each year, and it is fatal in about one fourth of these cases.[1] Approximately half of these fatalities occur within 1 hour of the onset of symptoms and before the patient reaches the hospital; these fatalities account for a large percentage of all sudden cardiac deaths.

PATHOLOGY

On pathologic examination, AMI may be divided into full-thickness (i.e., transmural infarction) or subendocardial (i.e., nontransmural infarction).[2] The former occurs most commonly consequent to a platelet-fibrin thrombus on a ruptured plaque that had not been critically stenotic before the acute event, did not cause ischemia, and therefore did not lead to the formation of extensive protective collateral vessels. Nontransmural infarctions usually occur in the presence of severely narrowed coronary arteries that do not become totally occluded, become occluded only transiently, or become occluded for longer periods in the presence of abundant protective collaterals.

Pathogenesis

In almost all instances, AMI is a complication of coronary atherosclerosis. Atherosclerotic plaques can be classified in terms of severity (i.e., percentage diameter stenosis) and susceptibility to rupture or fissure. Unstable (i.e., "vulnerable") coronary atherosclerotic plaques (Fig. 27–1) are usually characterized by a relatively large lipid core that is separated from the circulating blood by a thin fibrous cap. Endothelial injury, which may be precipitated by stimuli such as flow shear stress, hypertension, hyperlipidemia, or their combination, may cause plaque fissuring or rupture (Fig. 27–2), exposing the thrombogenic core of collagen and lipids. In addition, activated macrophages in the atheroma destabilize the plaque by (1) secreting metalloproteinase enzymes, which degrade the interstitial matrix and contribute to plaque rupture, and (2) elaborating cytokines that inhibit vascular smooth muscle from forming plaque-

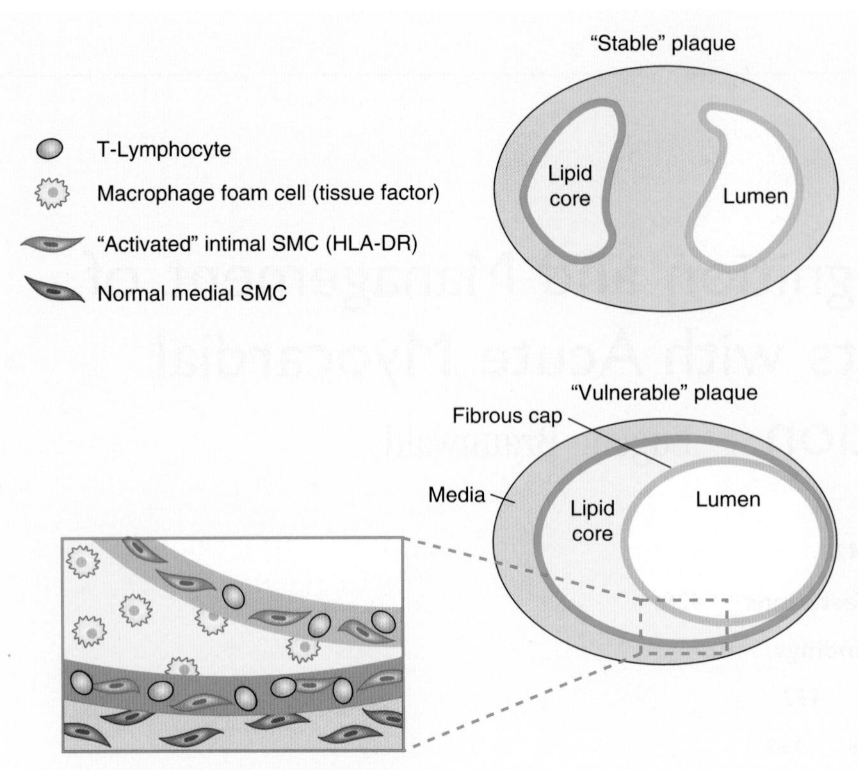

FIGURE 27–1. Comparison of the characteristics of "vulnerable" and "stable" plaques. Vulnerable plaques grow outward initially. The vulnerable plaque typically has a substantial lipid core and a thin fibrous cap separating the thrombogenic macrophages bearing tissue factor from the blood. At sites of lesion disruption, smooth muscle cells (SMCs) are often activated, as detected by their expression of the transplantation antigen human leukocyte antigen-DR (HLA-DR). In contrast, the stable plaque has a relatively thick fibrous cap protecting the lipid core from contact with the blood. Clinical data suggest that stable plaques more often show luminal narrowing detectable by angiography than do vulnerable plaques. (Redrawn from Libby P: Molecular bases of the acute coronary syndromes. Circulation 1995;91:2844.)

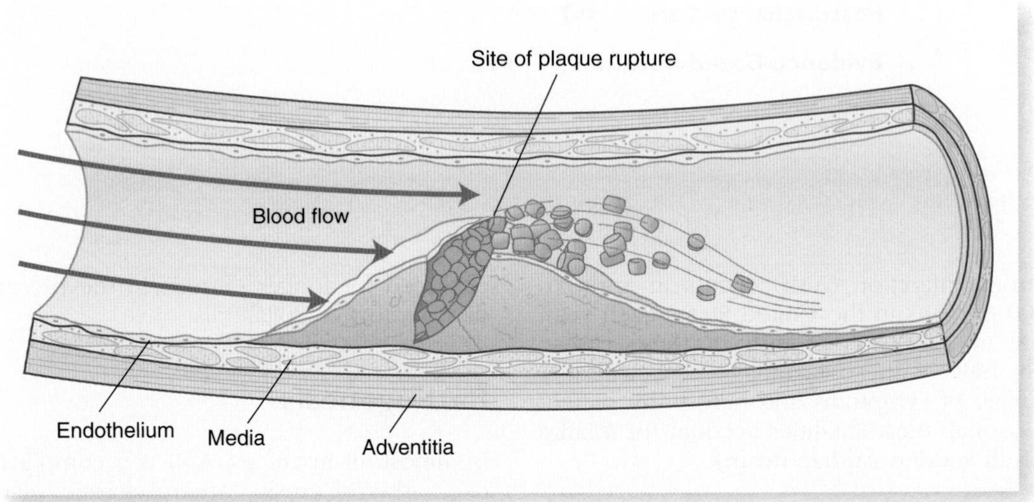

FIGURE 27–2. Diagram of arterial thrombus responsible for acute myocardial infarction (MI). Platelet adhesion and aggregation occur at the site of plaque rupture ("white thrombus"). Activated platelets exert procoagulant effects and the soluble coagulation cascade is activated. Fibrin strands and erythrocytes predominate within the lumen of the vessel and downstream in the "body" and "tail" of the thrombus. (Redrawn from Califf RM: Acute myocardial infarction and other acute ischemic syndromes. In Braunwald E [ed]: Essential Atlas of Heart Diseases, 2nd ed. Philadelphia, Current Medicine, 2001, p 61.)

stabilizing collagen. Exposure of the thrombogenic core causes platelet aggregation and the formation of a fibrin clot, resulting in total or subtotal arterial obstruction. Platelet aggregation also causes coronary vasoconstriction, which contributes to luminal narrowing.

In stable plaques the core is covered by a relatively thick fibrous cap separating it from contact with the blood (see Fig. 27–1), making the plaques unlikely to rupture. As stable plaques grow, they may produce very severe luminal narrowing and this condition is typically responsible for progressive exertional angina. Gradual progression may lead to total occlusion, which may cause infarction. In many such cases, however, the presence of collateral vessels, developed over months and years of plaque growth, prevents infarction despite complete occlusion.

In the absence of adequate collateral vessels, acute coronary obstruction causes severe transmural myocardial ischemia, electrocardiographic ST segment elevation and, if the latter is sustained for more than 20 to 30 minutes, infarction occurs (ST segment elevation myocardial infarction [STEMI]). Non-ST segment elevation myocardial infarction (NSTEMI) is most commonly caused by the development of a nonocclusive thrombus on a vulnerable plaque or by lysis (pharmacologically induced or spontaneous) of an occlusive thrombus. NSTEMI may also occur when—in the presence of a severely stenotic, flow-limiting atherosclerotic lesion—blood flow is further reduced by the development of hypotension, as may occur during surgery or severe infection. Alternatively, NSTEMI can be caused by an increase in myocardial oxygen requirements, produced by tachycardia or fever, or both, in the presence of stable, severe coronary obstruction. Rarely, severe persistent coronary vasospasm, as occurs in Prinzmetal's angina or cocaine abuse, may cause severe persistent ischemia and ultimately MI (see Chapter 26).

A number of pathologic processes other than atherosclerosis may also cause MI.[2] These include coronary emboli, congenital malformations of the coronary vessels, and a variety of inflammatory abnormalities of the coronary arteries (Box 27–1).

Pathophysiology

Severe ischemia or necrosis acutely impairs myocardial contraction and relaxation. If the mass of acutely

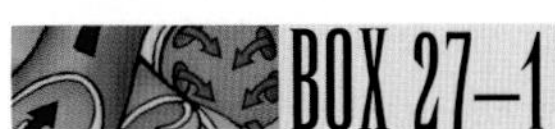

BOX 27–1

Conditions Other than Coronary Atherosclerosis That May Cause Acute Myocardial Infarction

Coronary emboli	Causes include aortic or mitral valve lesions, left atrial or ventricular thrombi, prosthetic valves, fat emboli, intracardiac neoplasms, infective endocarditis, and paradoxical emboli
Thrombotic coronary artery disease	May occur with oral contraceptive use, sickle cell anemia and other hemoglobinopathies, polycythemia vera, thrombocytosis, thrombotic thrombocytopenic purpura, disseminated intravascular coagulation, antithrombin III deficiency and other hypercoagulable states, macroglobulinemia and other hyperviscosity states, multiple myeloma, leukemia, malaria, and fibrinolytic system shutdown secondary to impaired plasminogen activation or excessive inhibition
Coronary vasculitis	Seen with Takayasu's disease, Kawasaki's disease, polyarteritis nodosa, lupus erythematosus, scleroderma, rheumatoid arthritis, and immune-mediated vascular degeneration in cardiac allografts
Coronary vasospasm	May be associated with variant angina, nitrate withdrawal, cocaine or amphetamine abuse, and angina with "normal" coronary arteries
Infiltrative and degenerative coronary vascular disease	May result from amyloidosis, connective tissue disorders such as pseudoxanthoma elasticum, lipid storage disorders and mucopolysaccharidoses, homocystinuria, diabetes mellitus, collagen vascular disease, muscular dystrophies, and Friedreich's ataxia
Coronary ostial occlusion	Associated with aortic dissection, luetic aortitis, aortic stenosis, and ankylosing spondylitis syndromes
Congenital coronary anomalies	Including Bland-White-Garland syndrome of anomalous origin of the left coronary artery from the pulmonary artery, left coronary artery origin from the anterior sinus of Valsalva, coronary arteriovenous fistula or aneurysms, and myocardial bridging with secondary vascular degeneration
Trauma	Associated with and responsible for coronary dissection, laceration, or thrombosis (with endothelial cell injury secondary to trauma such as angioplasty); radiation; and cardiac contusion
Augmented myocardial oxygen requirements exceeding oxygen delivery	Encountered with aortic stenosis, aortic insufficiency, hypertension with severe left ventricular hypertrophy, pheochromocytoma, thyrotoxicosis, methemoglobinemia, carbon monoxide poisoning, shock, and hyperviscosity syndromes

From Sobel BE: Acute myocardial infarction. In Bennett JC, Plum F (eds): Cecil Textbook of Medicine, 20th ed. Philadelphia, WB Saunders, 1996, p 302.

ischemic or necrotic myocardium is relatively small—less than 15% to 20% of the left ventricle—global ventricular function is usually maintained by increased contractile activity of the nonischemic myocardium. However, if the affected myocardium constitutes a larger fraction of the left ventricle—more than 20% to 25%—global ventricular function becomes depressed, and this may lead to impaired ventricular emptying and acute congestive heart failure.[2] When infarction is massive and involves more than approximately 35% of the left ventricle, pulmonary edema and/or cardiogenic shock owing to left ventricular pump failure may develop. In the case of transmural infarction, especially involving the anterior wall or apex, infarct expansion, a process consisting of dilatation and thinning of the area of infarction caused by a slippage between the muscle bundles, is common. This may lead to dyskinesia, that is, paradoxical systolic expansion, of the affected wall. Such areas of abnormal wall motion further increase the burden placed on the remaining viable myocardium and the likelihood of acute heart failure.

CLINICAL MANIFESTATIONS

History

A precipitating factor such as severe emotional stress, unusually vigorous exercise, or a serious illness is present in about half of patients developing MI. An approximately equal fraction of patients with AMI describe prodromal symptoms such as intermittent periods of rest pain not present previously or increasing intensity or frequency of preexistent angina. A higher frequency of onset of AMI occurs in the early morning hours, shortly after awakening, than at other times.

Chest Pain. (See also Chapter 6.) The majority of patients who are experiencing an AMI complain of prolonged (>30 min) chest pain characterized as "oppressive," "crushing," "constricting," "choking," or "viselike," and that is sometimes described with a clenched fist held against the sternum. Typically, the pain is retrosternal in location and spreads to the anterior chest, more commonly the left side; it often radiates down the arms, especially the ulnar aspect of the left arm, to the shoulders, upper extremities, jaw, neck, interscapular regions, and epigastrium. The pain is similar to that of angina pectoris but is more severe. Nausea, vomiting, and epigastric pain are common symptoms and may result in confusion with gastrointestinal disturbances such as esophagitis, gastritis, peptic ulcer, or acute cholecystitis. Indeed, patients with AMI may refer to their distress as "acute indigestion" or "heartburn." In some patients, only a dull ache or numbness is noted. In others, perhaps as many as one third of patients, especially elderly patients or those with diabetes, AMI may be painless and is discovered only by an incidental electrocardiogram (ECG). Approximately one half of these painless infarcts are not accompanied by any symptoms that the patient can recall, whereas in the others the history of an episode characterized by dyspnea, lightheadedness, a confused state, gastrointestinal upset, or chest pain not sufficiently intense to induce the patient to seek medical attention can be elicited. In a small fraction of patients, syncope is the presenting or an early complaint. Nervousness and apprehension, sometimes described as a feeling of impending doom, are also frequently mentioned.

Physical Examination

Patients experiencing an AMI often appear restless, anxious, and in obvious distress and sit up in bed clutching the chest. Pallor of the skin and perspiration may be prominent. Indeed, severe chest pain accompanied by diaphoresis points to the diagnosis of AMI. Large infarctions may cause pulmonary edema, with frothy pink sputum and a feeling of suffocation. Massive infarction causing cardiogenic shock (discussed later) results in cool and clammy skin, facial pallor, and cyanosis of the lips and nail beds. Although a variety of arrhythmias may occur in MI, mild sinus tachycardia at a rate of 100 to 110 beats per minute with frequent ventricular premature beats is the most common rhythm observed. Large infarctions usually lower both systolic and diastolic pressures by 10 to 20 mm Hg. Therefore, previously hypertensive patients often become normotensive, and previously normotensive persons may exhibit borderline hypotension, with systolic pressures between 90 and 110 mm Hg. A narrow pulse pressure (<30 mm Hg) reflects a depressed stroke volume in patients with more extensive infarctions. Patients with massive infarction and cardiogenic shock have, by definition, systolic pressures persistently below 80 mm Hg. Hypotension secondary to left ventricular dysfunction or pump failure is generally associated with sinus tachycardia and should be distinguished from the hypotension accompanied by bradycardia due to activation of vagal receptors and resultant excess parasympathetic stimulation; excess parasympathetic stimulation is seen most commonly in patients with inferior wall MI. Low-grade fever (to 38°C) develops within 24 hours of the onset of a large infarction.

The jugular venous pulse is normal except in patients with severe left ventricular or right ventricular failure, or both, in whom it is elevated, with prominent A- or V-waves (see Chapter 3). The carotid pulse is usually normal in contour, but it may be reduced in volume, suggesting a reduced stroke volume. Patients with heart failure may present with moist rales over more than one third of the lung fields, which do not clear on coughing. In patients with right ventricular infarction and resultant acute right ventricular failure, a positive hepatojugular reflux can often be elicited and accompanies hypotension.

The coronary atherosclerosis responsible for AMI may be associated with peripheral vascular disease and diminished or absent popliteal, dorsalis pedis, and posterior tibial pulses and an ankle/brachial artery index less than 0.8. Funduscopic examination may show the findings characteristic of hypertension or diabetes (see Chapter 3).

Cardiovascular Examination

AMI often acutely reduces stroke volume. As a consequence, precordial movements are reduced or even imperceptible on inspection and palpation and the peripheral pulses are weak. In patients with large transmural infarctions, the only precordial pulsations may be presystolic instead of systolic. An outward movement in early diastole, synchronous with the third heart sound (S_3), is sometimes palpable.

Auscultation. The heart sounds are usually normal in patients with small infarcts, but in patients with large infarcts the first heart sound (S_1) may be soft or indistinct and the pulmonary component of the second heart sound (S_2) accentuated. Severe left ventricular failure or left bundle branch block may cause paradoxical splitting of S_2 (see Chapter 3). An S_3, most easily audible at the apex, reflects left ventricular dysfunction. A fourth heart sound (S_4), best heard between the left sternal border and the apex, is a common finding in AMI and is of little prognostic significance. New, soft (grade 1 to 2/6) systolic murmurs are frequently audible at the apex and may be caused by mitral regurgitation secondary to papillary muscle dysfunction. A new, loud (grade ≥3/6) systolic murmur, accompanied by a thrill at or medial to the apex, suggests mitral regurgitation secondary to rupture of the head of a papillary muscle or a ventricular septal defect caused by perforation of the ventricular septum (discussed later). Pericardial friction rubs are heard along the left sternal border in approximately 15% of patients with AMI. They are usually evanescent and occur most commonly on the second or third day.

LABORATORY FINDINGS

Serum Markers

With myocyte death, intracellular macromolecules pass through the damaged cell membrane and the appearance of these substances in the blood stream signifies the presence of infarction.[3] The pattern of rise is helpful diagnostically, with the MB isoenzyme of creatine kinase (CK-MB) beginning to rise above normal levels approximately 4 to 6 hours after the onset of symptoms, reaching a peak in approximately 24 hours and returning to baseline within 3 or 4 days, unless reinfarction occurs. Although CK-MB has been the most widely used serum marker for confirming the diagnosis of AMI, its clinical value is limited by its lack of appearance during the first few hours of infarction and by its lack of total specificity, that is, its release with marked skeletal muscle damage.

Cardiac-specific troponin T (cTnT) and I (cTnI) are absent in extracardiac tissue, and their presence in the serum at any detectable concentration is highly specific for myocardial necrosis. The kinetics of the *initial* release of the cardiac-specific troponins are similar to those of CK and CK-MB, beginning to rise at 4 to 6 hours after the onset of infarction and reaching a peak at approximately 24 hours. Because they are components of the structural apparatus of myocytes, however, the troponins are released continuously for as long as 10 to 14 days from deteriorating cells, allowing the late diagnosis of infarction.[2] The release of cTnT and cTnI is enhanced by reperfusion of the infarction, whether it is induced therapeutically or occurs spontaneously, causing an earlier and higher peak value in serum. The assays for the troponins are becoming widely available and are replacing CK-MB. Hand-held devices that can provide a semiquantitative bedside measure of the troponins at the point of care, generally in the emergency department, are proving to be increasingly valuable in the rapid recognition of myocardial necrosis.

Myoglobin is a relatively small molecule that is rapidly excreted into the urine, and therefore, its duration of elevation after infarction is usually less than 24 hours, unlike CK-MB and the troponins, which remain elevated for longer periods. Although myoglobin is a very sensitive marker of muscle necrosis, it is nonspecific because it is a constituent of skeletal muscle and may be released from this tissue with even slight damage. Absence of an elevation of myoglobin between 3 and 12 hours following symptom development is useful, however, in excluding infarction.

An electrocardiogram should be obtained and CK-MB, cTnT, or cTnI should be measured at the time of presentation and again 6 to 8 hours later in patients with suspected infarction. Because values of serum CK-MB, cTnT, and cTnI usually remain normal during the first 4 hours after the onset of infarction, patients with a history consistent with possible AMI should not be discharged from the emergency department without several hours of observation. In patients with a low (<5%) clinical suspicion of AMI and no recurrent symptoms, the absence of new ischemic ECG changes or elevations of serum markers during a 6- to 12-hour observation period is adequate to exclude AMI with about a 99% certainty. In patients with a more classic history or with ECG changes suggestive of ischemia on presentation, 24 hours of negative serial ECGs and enzymes (every 6 to 8 hr) is required to reach a similar level of certainty.

Unless patients have other conditions requiring intensive care, this "rule out MI" care can be provided in a chest pain evaluation unit or stepdown unit (see Chapter 6).

Electrocardiography

Often, the first ECG sign of acute transmural ischemia is the development of transient, giant, so-called hyperacute, T-waves overlying the affected myocardium (Fig. 27–3). ST segment elevation is also observed in leads overlying the ischemia when the latter involves the epicardium (Fig. 27–4), whereas ST segment depression

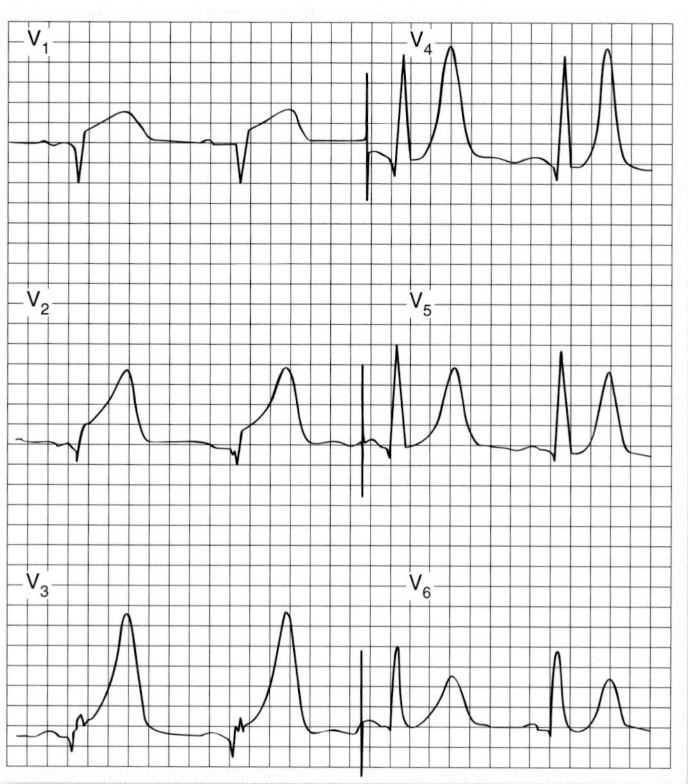

FIGURE 27–3. Hyperacute phase of anteroseptal myocardial infarction (MI). Note the tall positive T-waves (V_2 to V_3) along with ST segment elevations and Q-waves (V_1 to V_3). (From Goldberger AL: Electrocardiography. In Braunwald E, et al [eds]: Harrison's Principles of Internal Medicine, 15th ed. New York, McGraw-Hill, 2001, p 1268.)

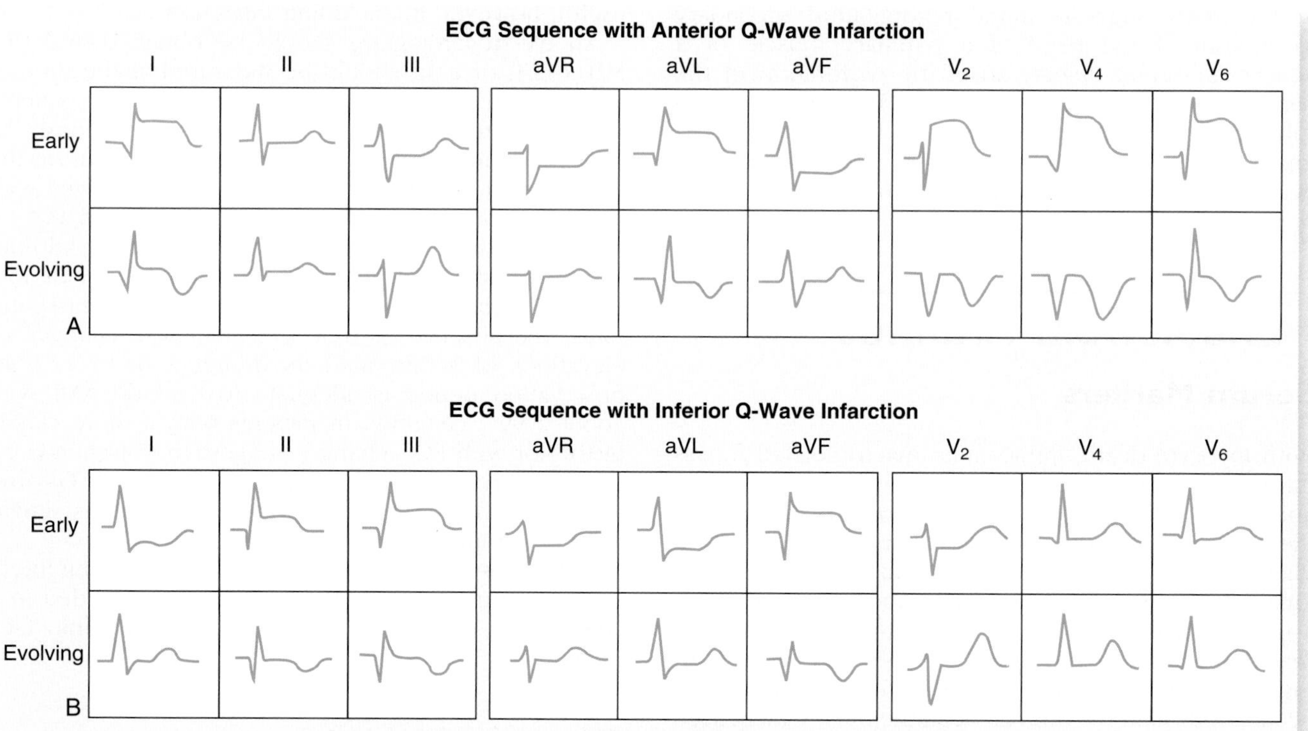

FIGURE 27–4. Sequence of depolarization and repolarization changes with acute anterior (*A*) and acute inferior (*B*) Q-wave infarctions. With anterior infarcts, ST elevation in leads I, aV_l (augmented voltage, unipolar left arm lead), and the precordial leads may be accompanied by reciprocal ST depressions in leads II, III, and aV_f (augmented voltage, unipolar left leg lead). Conversely, acute inferior (or posterior) infarcts may be associated with reciprocal ST depressions in leads V_1 to V_3. aV_r, augmented voltage, unipolar right arm lead. (*A* and *B*, Redrawn from Goldberger AL: Electrocardiography. In Braunwald E, et al [eds]: Harrison's Principles of Internal Medicine, 15th ed. New York, McGraw-Hill, 2001, p 1269; modified from Goldberger AL, Goldberger E [eds]: Clinical Electrocardiography: A Simplified Approach, 4th ed. St. Louis, Mosby–Year Book, 1990, pp 89–90, redrawn with permission of The McGraw-Hill Companies.)

occurs in the presence of subendocardial ischemia. Hyperacute T-wave changes and ST segment elevations are followed by T-wave inversions and sometimes by loss of the height of R-waves and the development of Q-waves, or both, in patients with STEMI. In patients who do not receive reperfusion therapy, ST segment elevations typically persist for 6 to 18 hours after the onset of chest pain, and as the ST segments become isoelectric, the T-waves become inverted and Q-waves develop in the same leads. In NSTEMI, T-wave inversion occurs early in the course of the infarction and may persist after the depressed ST segments have returned to isoelectricity and Q-waves usually do not develop.

For many years, infarcts with Q-waves were referred to as transmural infarcts, and non–Q-wave infarcts as *nontransmural infarcts*. Pathologic-ECG correlations do not support, however, such terminology and the preferred designations now are simply STEMI and NSTEMI (Fig. 27–5).

The infarction can be localized to the anterior septal region of the left ventricle if the aforementioned ECG changes occur in leads V_1 to V_3; to the apex of the left ventricle if they occur in leads V_4 to V_6; to the lateral wall with changes in leads V_5, V_6, and aV_l; and to the inferior wall with changes in leads II, III, and aV_f. Posterior wall infarction may cause reciprocal ST segment depression and paradoxical R-wave elevation in leads V_1 to V_4. Right ventricular infarction causes ST segment deviation and QS patterns in right-sided leads (V_1, V_{3R}, V_{4R}) and is usually accompanied by inferior wall infarction.[3]

In the minority of patients with AMI, the ECG is entirely normal or shows only minor ST segment and T-wave changes.

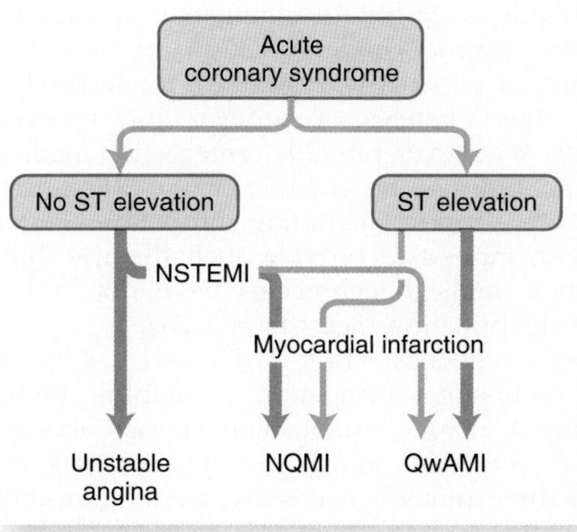

FIGURE 27–5. Nomenclature of ACSs. Patients with ischemic discomfort may present with or without ST-segment elevation on the ECG. The majority of patients with ST-segment elevation (*large arrows*) ultimately develop a Q-wave AMI (QwAMI), whereas a minority (*small arrows*) develop a non–Q-wave AMI (NQMI). Patients who present without ST segment elevation are experiencing either UA or an NSTEMI. The distinction between these two diagnoses is ultimately made based on the presence or absence of a cardiac marker detected in the blood. Most patients with NSTEMI do not evolve a Q-wave on the 12-lead ECG and are subsequently referred to as having sustained a non–Q-wave MI (NQMI); only a minority of NSTEMI patients develop a Q-wave and are later diagnosed as having Q-wave MI. Not shown is Prinzmetal's angina, which manifests with transient chest pain and ST-segment elevation but rarely MI. The spectrum of clinical conditions that range from upper segment to non–Q-wave AMI and Q-wave AMI is referred to as ACSs. (Adapted from Braunwald E, et al: ACC/AHA guidelines for the management of patients with unstable angina and non-ST segment elevation myocardial infarction. J Am Coll Cardiol 2000;36:970.)

Cardiac Imaging

Echocardiography (see Chapter 5 for further discussion)

The *two-dimensional echocardiogram* is useful in the evaluation of patients with acute chest pain. Typically, patients with AMI, especially transmural infarction, exhibit a regional wall motion disorder (akinesis or dyskinesis of the involved myocardium), which is readily recognized by transthoracic two-dimensional echocardiography. Echocardiography is particularly useful when the ECG is atypical or nondiagnostic, as when a conduction disturbance, particularly left bundle branch block, is present. It is useful in assessing left ventricular function and in the identification of right ventricular infarction and pericardial effusion, as well as left ventricular aneurysm and thrombus. This technique does not differentiate among old infarction, acute infarction, acute ischemia, or myocardial stunning (postischemic ventricular dysfunction).

Doppler echocardiography is helpful in the evaluation of patients with AMI and systolic heart murmurs, particularly in detecting and assessing the severity of tricuspid valvular regurgitation and in estimating right ventricular systolic pressure. It is especially useful in patients with cardiogenic shock or severe heart failure and new systolic murmurs, because it allows the detection of complications that may be surgically correctable (mitral regurgitation or ventricular septal defect), as well as ventricular aneurysm, pericardial effusion, and right ventricular infarction. Color Doppler echocardiography is also helpful in patients with a nondiagnostic ECG suspected of having an aortic dissection (see Chapter 36) in which it frequently demonstrates an intimal flap.

Nuclear Imaging

A variety of nuclear imaging techniques—radionuclide angiography, myocardial perfusion imaging, infarct avid scintigraphy, and positron emission tomography—show characteristic changes in AMI. The ease with which echocardiography can be performed compared with the necessity of moving a critically ill patient from the emergency department to a nuclear medicine department may limit the applicability of these other methods.

Differential Diagnosis

A typical history and ECG and release into the serum of a biomarker such as cTn or CK-MB are the three cornerstones to establishing the diagnosis of AMI. A joint committee of the European Society of Cardiology and the American College of Cardiology (ACC) has provided criteria for acute evolving or recent AMI as follows[4]:

1. Typical rise and gradual fall (troponin) or more rapid rise and fall (CK-MB) of biochemical markers of myocardial necrosis with at least one of the following: (a) ischemic symptoms, (b) development of pathologic Q-waves on the ECG, (c) ECG changes indicative of ischemia (ST segment elevation or depression), or (d) coronary artery intervention (e.g., coronary angioplasty) or
2. Pathologic findings of an acute MI

Although patients with unstable angina may have symptoms and ECG ST- and T-wave changes similar to those with AMI, they can subsequently be distinguished by the absence of development of new Q-waves and failure to release biomolecular markers into the serum (see Chapter 26).[5] Differentiation of AMI from acute pericarditis (see Chapter 35) may be challenging because the pain and ST segment elevations may be similar and serum markers sometimes rise slightly in pericarditis because of the associated epicardial injury. In pericarditis, the pain often persists for several days, ST segment elevations typically are more persistent and widespread than in AMI and occur in many (generally ≥6 of the 12) ECG leads, the ST segments often remain elevated for several days after the T-waves have become inverted, and Q-waves fail to develop.

MANAGEMENT

Prehospital Management (see Chapter 24)

The risk to life is highest during the first minutes after coronary occlusion and declines progressively in the hours, days, weeks, and years thereafter. Indeed, approximately half of all deaths associated with AMI occur during the first hour after its onset, and these are usually caused by ventricular fibrillation. Therefore, the overarching principle in the management of AMI is to shorten the time between the onset of symptoms and treatment to an absolute minimum. The three components of delay in the onset of treatment are (1) patient delay in seeking medical attention, (2) prehospital evaluation and transportation, and (3) evaluation and initiation of treatment in the hospital. Attention must be directed to reducing all three of these components.[2]

The general public and especially patients known to be at high risk of MI or reinfarction must be educated about the symptoms of AMI. They should be encouraged to seek urgent medical attention for chest discomfort, especially if it is accompanied by fatigue, dyspnea, or diaphoresis. It is useful for patients at especially high risk, such as those who have previously experienced an acute coronary syndrome (AMI or unstable angina), to have a copy of their resting ECG with them at all times to serve as a basis for possible future comparisons. Patients at high risk should be instructed to call emergency services through 911 with the onset of ischemic-type discomfort or to be taken directly to the nearest hospital that offers 24-hour emergency cardiac care. They should not be transported to the physician's office. While making arrangements for transportation, they should take one tablet of nitroglycerin sublingually, which may, if necessary and tolerated, be repeated twice at 5-minute intervals.

Care in the Ambulance. Patients who are recognized in the field by emergency medical services as having signs of pulmonary congestion, tachycardia, and systolic blood pressure less than 90 mmHg should, whenever possible, be transported to facilities in which cardiac catheterization and coronary revascularization can be carried out, so that the subsequent transfer to a hospital may be avoided.

It is highly desirable for emergency medical services to provide ventricular defibrillation, because it is lifesaving and if patients with AMI are immediately defibrillated, their chances of survival and recovery are excellent. Whenever possible, emergency medical personnel should also be capable of providing advanced cardiac life support, including intubation. Paramedics have been trained to provide such therapy, but basic emergency medical technicians have not and cannot provide defibrillation (see Chapter 24).

Use of a checklist (Box 27–2) and a 12-lead ECG during prehospital evaluation is helpful. Prehospital care should include establishing venous access, early relief of pain with morphine sulfate 5 mg every 5 minutes three times if necessary, the administration of nitroglycerin, and treatment of ventricular tachycardia with lidocaine (75 to 100 mg bolus followed by an infusion of 1 to 2 mg/min).

Prehospital Fibrinolysis. Because the earliest possible re-establishment of coronary reperfusion is of great importance, thrombolytic therapy should be begun as soon as possible in appropriate patients (discussed later). When treatment in the field allows initiation of thrombolytic therapy by more than 1 hour earlier than in the hospital, prehospital-initiated thrombolytic therapy can reduce relative mortality by 15% to 20% below that achieved by standard hospital-initiated treatment.[6] Prehospital fibrinolytic therapy may be especially useful in communities with transport delays of 90 minutes or longer. Prehospital fibrinolysis, however, requires very well trained and experienced emergency medical technicians in the ambulances as well as the capacity to transmit the ECG to the receiving hospital electronically. Without these elements, it is better to emphasize rapid transportation and shortening of the "door-to-needle" time once the patient reaches the emergency department.

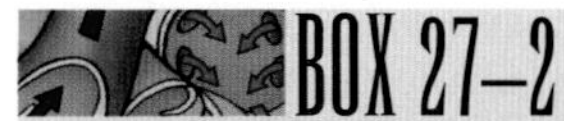BOX 27–2

Chest Pain Checklist for Use by EMT/Paramedic for Diagnosis of Acute Myocardial Infarction and Thrombolytic Therapy Screening

Check each finding below. If all (yes) boxes are checked and ECG indicates ST elevation or new BBB, reperfusion therapy with thrombolysis or primary PTCA may be indicated. Thrombolysis is generally not indicated unless all (no) boxes are checked and BP ≤180/110 mm Hg.

	Yes	*No*
Ongoing chest discomfort (≥20 min and <12 hr)	☐	__
Oriented, can cooperate	☐	__
Age > 35 yr (>40 yr if female)	☐	__
History of stroke or TIA	__	☐
Known bleeding disorder	__	☐
Active internal bleeding in past 2 wk	__	☐
Surgery or trauma in past 2 wk	__	☐
Terminal illness	__	☐
Jaundice, hepatitis, kidney failure	__	☐
Use of anticoagulants	__	☐

Systolic/diastolic BP
Right arm: __/__
Left arm: __/__

	Yes	*No*
ECG done	☐	__

*High-risk profile**	*Yes*	*No*
Heart rate ≥ 100 bpm	☐	__
BP ≤ 100 mm Hg	☐	__
Pulmonary edema (rales greater than halfway up)	☐	__
Shock	☐	__
Pain began	__	AM/PM
Arrival time	__	AM/PM
Begin transport	__	AM/PM
Hospital arrival	__	AM/PM

*Transport to hospital capable of angiography and revascularization if needed.

BBB, bundle branch block; BP, blood pressure, ECG, electrocardiogram; EMT, emergency medical technician; PTCA, percutaneous transluminal coronary angioplasty; TIA, transient ischemic attack.

Reprinted from Ryan, TJ, Anderson JL, Antman EM, et al: ACC/AHA guidelines for the management of patients with acute myocardial infarction. J Am Coll Cardiol 1996;28:1328–1428. Copyright 1996, with permission from the American College of Cardiology: adapted from the Seattle/King County EMS Medical Record.

Management in the Emergency Department (see Chapter 24)

If possible, initial evaluation should be completed within 10 minutes of arrival. The three principal goals of care in the emergency department are (1) stabilization, (2) triage, and (3) initiation of myocardial reperfusion. A clear plan for rapidly assessing the patient for reperfusion therapy is mandatory (Figs. 27–6 and 27–7). On arrival in the emergency department, patients with suspected AMI should immediately have a targeted cardiovascular history and physical examination and intravenous access should be established. A 12-lead ECG should be obtained, and the rhythm should be monitored continuously. Aspirin, at a dose of 160 or 325 mg, should be given to all patients with suspected AMI (regardless of whether thrombolytic therapy will be used and irrespective of the fibrinolytic agent) unless true aspirin allergy is present. If the first dose is chewed, a blood level is achieved more rapidly than if it is swallowed. Patients who have a true aspirin allergy may receive clopidogrel, 300 mg, instead.

Stabilization

Patients with acute chest pain thought to be caused by ischemia should receive one sublingual nitroglycerin tablet (0.3 or 0.4 mg), unless the initial systolic blood pressure is less than 90 mm Hg and the heart rate is less than 50 beats per minute or greater than 100 beats per minute. The nitroglycerin, which may be repeated twice at 5-minute intervals if the pain persists, also often improves hemodynamics in patients with AMI by dilating systemic and coronary arteries as well as systemic veins. Nitroglycerin should be avoided in patients suspected of having right ventricular infarction (see later) because of the potential for excessive reduction of preload. This drug often relieves ischemic pain in patients with unstable angina (see Chapter 26) or esophageal spasm, so that response to nitroglycerin should not be interpreted as a specific diagnostic intervention in the setting of acute chest pain.

Effective *analgesia* should be established with intravenous morphine (5 mg boluses given intravenously every 5 to 15 min) until severe pain has been relieved, unless it has been given in the ambulance. Respiratory depression secondary to morphine is unusual in patients with AMI and can be treated with naloxone (0.4 mg intravenously up to three times).

It is important to measure *blood* pressure repeatedly in patients receiving nitroglycerin and morphine, or both. If systolic arterial pressure declines below 100 mm Hg, and the patient does not have pulmonary congestion, the lower extremities should be elevated. If sinus bradycardia accompanies hypotension, atropine (0.5 to 1.0 mg intravenously repeated every 5 min to a total dose of 2.5 mg) is often helpful. Atropine is particularly effective in hypotensive patients after the administration of nitroglycerin, or with (1) sinus bradycardia or frequent premature contractions, (2) inferior infarction and atrioventricular (AV) block with narrow QRS complexes, (3) nausea and vomiting after the administration of morphine, and (4) type I second-degree AV block (see Chapter 31).

Oxygen saturation should be monitored with an oximeter in patients believed to have ongoing acute ischemic discomfort, and oxygen should be adminis-

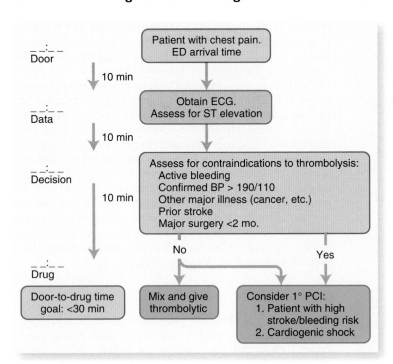

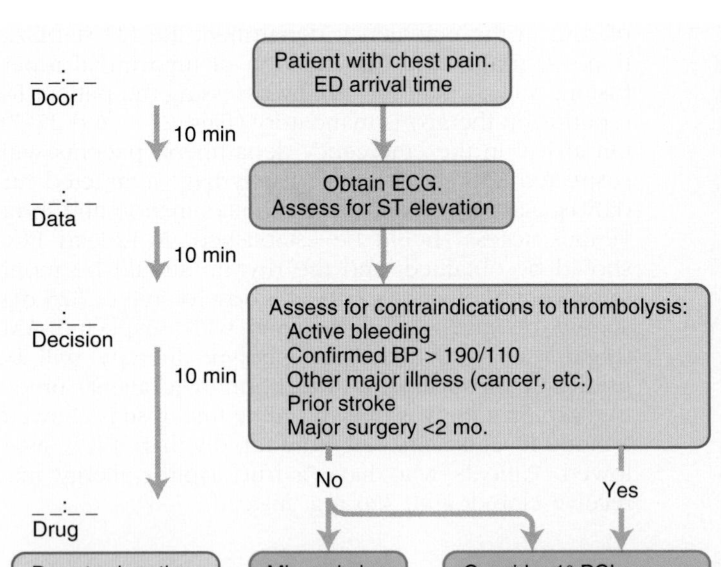

FIGURE 27–6. Thrombolysis critical pathways for acute myocardial infarction in the emergency department at Brigham and Women's Hospital. (From Cannon CP: Thrombolysis critical pathway. In Cannon CP, O'Gara PT [eds]: Critical Pathways in Cardiology. Philadelphia, Lippincott, Williams & Wilkins, 2001, pp 57–65. Adapted from Cannon CP, Antman EM, Walls R, et al: Time as an adjunctive agent to thrombolytic therapy. J Thromb Thrombolysis 1994;1:27–34, with permission.)

tered, usually by nasal prongs, in those with saturation under 90%. In patients in whom severe hypoxemia cannot be corrected by supplemental inspired oxygen, intubation and mechanical ventilation may be necessary.

Triage

After initial stabilization in the emergency department, patients should be triaged into three groups:

1. Patients with probable STEMI who require reperfusion therapy and have no contraindications (discussed later). If reperfusion is to be by means of fibrinolytic therapy, this should be initiated immediately in the emergency department before transfer to the coronary care unit (CCU). Alternatively, if reperfusion via percutaneous coronary intervention (PCI) is selected and the laboratory and team are available, the patient should be transferred immediately to the cardiac catheterization laboratory.
2. Patients with probable infarction who are not candidates for reperfusion therapy and who are not low-risk patients (see later) should be transferred to the CCU.
3. Patients considered to be at low risk may be admitted to a coronary observation (intermediate-care or stepdown) unit, which has the capability for continuous ECG monitoring and ventricular defibrillation. Low-risk patients include those who are stable with typical or atypical symptoms, but without ECG changes or with only minor ST–T-wave changes, as well as those who are pain-free, hemodynamically stable, and without co-morbid illness.

The ECG obtained in the ambulance or emergency department is at the center of the decision pathway for management because ST segment elevation in patients with typical clinical findings identifies those who may benefit from reperfusion therapy. Exceptions include patients in the very early phase of AMI, with hyperacute T-waves before the development of ST segment elevation (see Fig. 27–3), those with posterior infarction who have ST segment depression in leads V_1 through V_3, as well as those with presumably new left bundle branch block, all of whom may benefit from acute myocardial reperfusion. Some patients without ST segment elevations on presentation subsequently develop such elevation and thus become candidates for acute reperfusion therapy. Therefore, serial tracings should be obtained in patients with a history that suggests AMI and a nondiagnostic ECG.

Potential candidates for fibrinolytic therapy should be screened immediately for contraindications (Box 27–3). Approximately half of all patients with AMI do not qualify for thrombolysis because the admission ECG does not show ST segment elevations (or new left bundle branch block), because of contraindications to thrombolysis, or because they present more than 12 hours after the onset of symptoms. Efforts to shorten the time to presentation include education of patients at high risk of developing MI and their families.

Myocardial Reperfusion: Fibrinolytic Therapy

Because coronary thrombosis is the proximate cause of most cases of STEMI, it is not surprising that relief of the thrombotic obstruction—either by coronary fibrinolysis or a catheter-based intervention—is effective

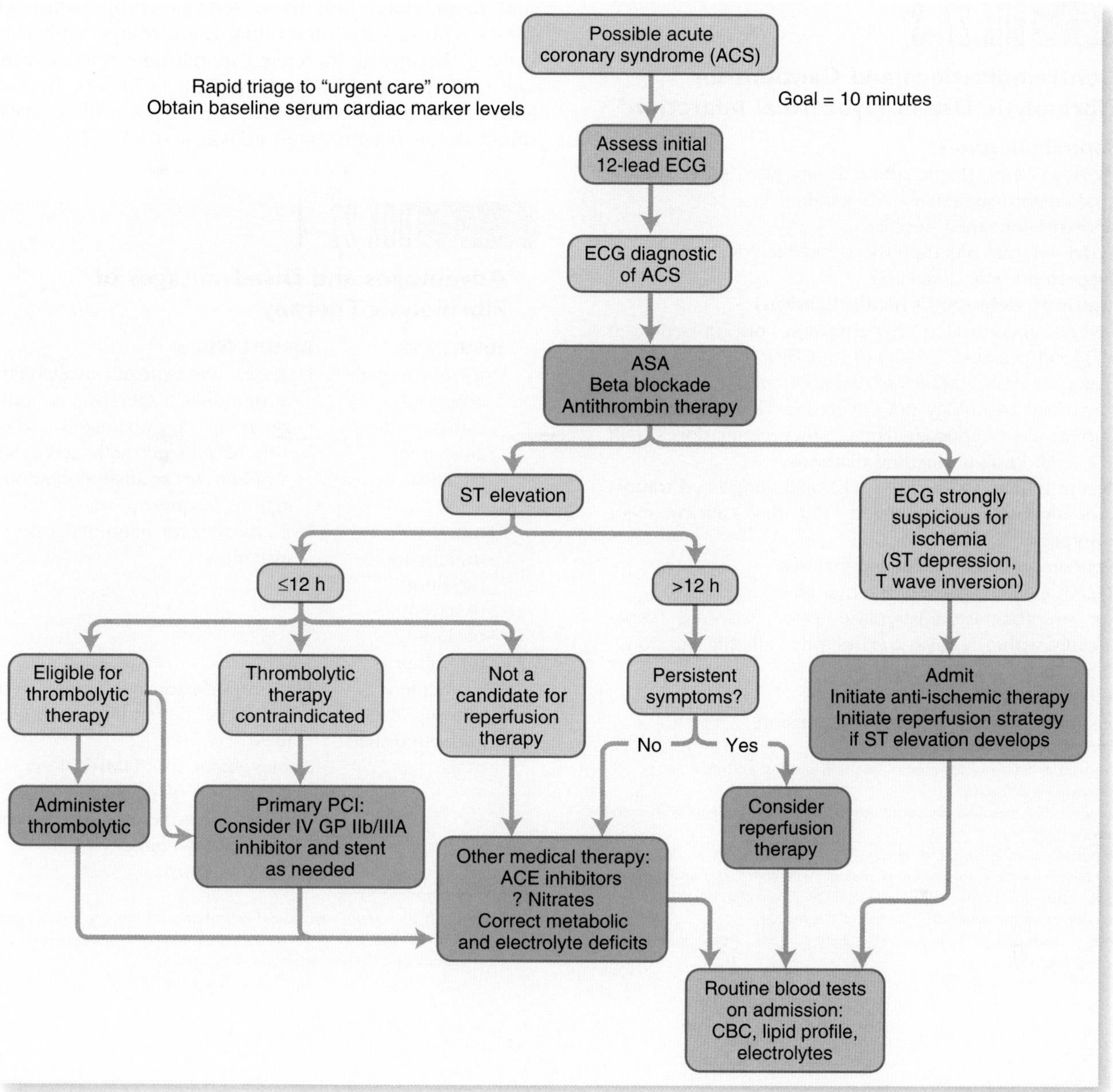

FIGURE 27–7. Algorithm for management of patients with suspected acute coronary syndrome (ACS) in emergency department. (Adapted from Antman EM, Braunwald E: Acute myocardial infarction. In Braunwald E [ed]: Heart Disease, 6th ed. Philadelphia, WB Saunders, 2001, p 1141.)

therapeutically if it is carried out before the infarct is completed. There is strong evidence that the beneficial effect of fibrinolytic therapy, expressed as the number of lives saved per thousand patients treated, is dependent on the time from symptom onset to initiation of therapy.[7] Although there is no definitive evidence of benefit in patients reperfused more than 12 to 24 hours after the onset of chest pain, reperfusion therapy may nonetheless still be considered in those who have ongoing ischemic pain and extensive, persistent ST segment elevation, even at this time. Because of the time dependency of the effectiveness of fibrinolytic therapy, the overall strategy must focus on reducing the "door-to-needle" time for the administration of fibrinolytic agents to 30 minutes or less and the "door-to-balloon" time in patients undergoing PCI (Fig. 27–8).

The benefit of fibrinolytic therapy has been demonstrated in both men and women and in patients with or without a history of previous MI; it is greater in patients with ST segment elevation in anterior as compared with inferior leads, as well as in patients with diabetes mellitus, hypotension, or tachycardia. The major complications are related to hemorrhage, with intracra-

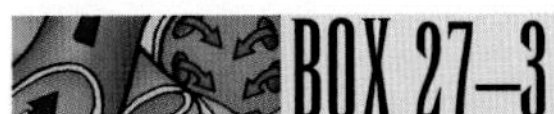

BOX 27–3

Contraindications and Cautions for Fibrinolytic Use in Myocardial Infarction*

Contraindications

Previous hemorrhagic stroke at any time; other strokes or cerebrovascular events within 1 yr
Known intracranial neoplasm
Active internal bleeding (does not include menses)
Suspected aortic dissection

Cautions/Relative Contraindications

Severe uncontrolled hypertension on presentation (blood pressure > 180/110 mm Hg)†
History of prior cerebrovascular accident or known intracerebral pathology not covered in Contraindications
Current use of anticoagulants in therapeutic doses (INR ≥ 2–3); known bleeding diathesis
Recent trauma (within 2–4 wk), including head trauma or traumatic or prolonged (>10 min) CPR or major surgery (<3 wk)
Noncompressible vascular punctures
Recent (within 2–4 wk) internal bleeding
For streptokinase/anistreplase: prior exposure (especially within 5 days–2 yr) or prior allergic reaction
Pregnancy
Active peptic ulcer
History of chronic severe hypertension

*Viewed as advisory for clinical decision making and may not be all-inclusive or definitive.

†Could be an absolute contraindication in low-risk patients with myocardial infarction.

Reprinted from Ryan TJ, Anderson JL, Antman EM, et al: ACC/AHA guidelines for the management of patients with acute myocardial infarction. J Am Coll Cardiol 1996;28:1328–1428. Copyright 1996, with permission from the American College of Cardiology.

INR, International Normalized Ratio; CPR, cardiopulmonary resuscitation.

nial hemorrhage the most serious complication (Box 27–4). The risk of intracranial hemorrhage with thrombolytic therapy is increased in patients with advanced age (>75 years), low body weight (<70 kg), hypertension (>180/100 mm Hg), and the use of a fibrin-specific direct tissue plasminogen activator (t-PA, r-PA, or TNK)

BOX 27–4

Advantages and Disadvantages of Fibrinolytic Therapy

ADVANTAGES	DISADVANTAGES
Does not require access to catheterization laboratory facilities	Despite widespread availability, thrombolytic therapy is only given in approximately 30%–40% of patients with acute MI; absolute or relative contraindications frequent
Treats the underlying problem of a central occluding thrombus	Not effective for hemodynamic instability
Documented efficacy in large, well-controlled trials	Early reperfusion rates range from 55%–80% depending on agent used
	Achievement of TIMI-3 flow in <50%–60% of patients
	Reliable assessment of reperfusion often not possible
	Residual stenosis

From Califf RM: Acute myocardial infarction and other acute ischemic syndromes. In Braunwald E (ed): Essential Atlas of Heart Diseases, 2nd ed. Philadelphia, Current Medicine, 2001, p 68.

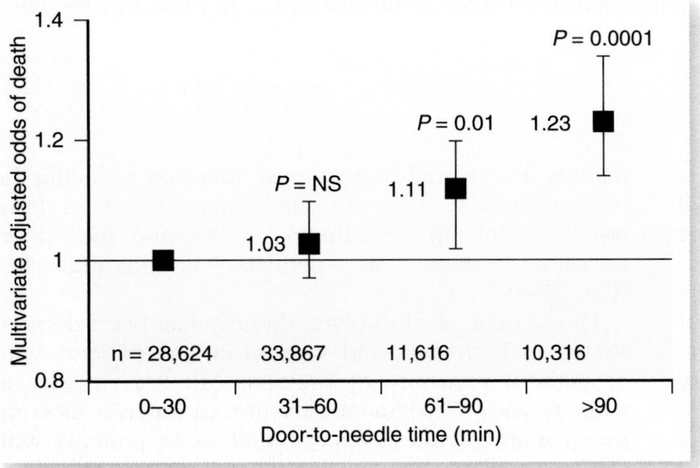

FIGURE 27–8. Relationship of door-to-drug time on multivariate (MV) adjusted mortality. (Reproduced from Cannon CP, Gibson CM, Lambrew ST, et al: Longer thrombolysis door-to-needle times are associated with increased mortality in acute myocardial infarction: An analysis of 85,589 patients in the National Registry of Myocardial Infarction. J Am Coll Cardiol 2000;35:376a, with permission.)

(as opposed to streptokinase). Although the relative benefit of thrombolysis appears to be reduced in patients 75 years or older, an effort to achieve myocardial reperfusion should still be made in such patients unless specific contraindications exist. These patients appear to be particularly benefited by primary PCI. Thrombolytic therapy is not advised in patients without ST segment elevation (except for the subgroup with posterior infarction with ST segment depression limited to leads V_1 and V_2).

Choice of Fibrinolytic Agent. There has been considerable debate concerning the choice of fibrinolytic agent.[2,8] Four such drugs, streptokinase, t-PA (Activase), r-PA (reteplase), and TNK t-PA (tenecteplase) have been approved and are now available. The first two have received the most intensive study. The advantage of t-PA over streptokinase is that it establishes earlier patency of the infarct-related artery, is associated with slightly better ventricular function, and in the large GUSTO (Global Utilization of Streptokinase and Tissue Plasminogen Activator for Occluded Coronary Arteries) I trial, it demonstrated a 1% lower absolute 30-day mortality (6.3% vs. 7.3%).[2] The usual front-loaded, accelerated regimen of t-PA is a 15-mg bolus, followed by 0.75 mg/kg over 30 minutes (maximum 50 mg), then 0.50 mg/kg over 60 minutes (maximum 35 mg). It requires cotherapy with heparin. The disadvantages of t-PA are a slightly greater risk of intracranial hemorrhage compared with streptokinase (0.6% vs. 0.3%). A 30-day mortality or nonfatal stroke composite clinical endpoint, however, which considered this serious complication, was shown in the GUSTO I trial to be slightly but statistically lower with t-PA (7.2%) than with streptokinase (8.1%). The other disadvantage of t-PA is its much greater cost than streptokinase.

The usual dose of streptokinase is 1.5 million units/100 mL given as a continuous infusion over 60 minutes. The major complications of this thrombolytic agent are fever, rash, hypotension, and very rarely, anaphylactic reaction. A disadvantage of streptokinase is that it may be ineffective in patients with antistreptococcal antibodies, which includes patients who have ever received the drug and those who have suffered a streptococcal infection during the preceding year.

The efficacy, risk of intracranial hemorrhage, and price of r-PA (reteplase) are similar to those of t-PA. It has, however, the advantage of simpler administration; two bolus injections of 10 million units are administered 30 minutes apart. TNK-tPA is a mutant of t-PA with reduced (slower) plasma clearance allowing for administration as a single bolus.[8] The approved dose is 0.53 mg/kg. The clinical outcomes from the use of t-PA, r-PA, and TNK-tPA are similar and these drugs may be considered to be interchangeable except that TNK-tPA can be administered as a single dose. This regimen maximizes convenience. Streptokinase may be acceptable in patients presenting more than 4 hours after the onset of chest pain, in those who are at lower risk of death (e.g., patients with inferior wall MI without hemodynamic disturbance), or in those whose risk of intracranial hemorrhage is high, that is, patients older than 75 years or with moderate hypertension (not severe enough to serve as an absolute contraindication) (see Box 27–3), or in situations in which cost considerations are dominant.

Irrespective of which agent is used, unnecessary venous or arterial interventions should be avoided in patients treated with thrombolysis.

Patients who receive the direct plasminogen activators (t-PA, rPA, or TNK-tPA) should receive intravenous heparin (60 U/kg bolus [maximum 4000 units]) followed by an infusion of 12 U/kg/hr maximum 1000 units/hr for approximately 48 hours. The activated partial thromboplastin time (aPTT) should initially be measured 3 hours after the start of fibrinolysis and then at least once every 24 hours, with adjustments to maintain an aPTT of 1.5 to 2.0 × control.[9] In patients who receive streptokinase, heparin should be added if there is a large anterior wall infarction, heart failure, or a mural thrombus visible on echocardiography. Heparin use is optional in other patients who receive streptokinase.

Emergency Catheter-Based Reperfusion (Percutaneous Coronary Intervention)

Primary PCI (primary angioplasty or stenting) is gaining increasing popularity as an effective means of achieving myocardial reperfusion in AMI.[10] The advantages of this approach are (1) achievement of reperfusion with a lower risk of hemorrhage, especially intracranial bleeding, than fibrinolytic therapy; (2) higher full-patency rates (approximately 90% compared with 60% for fibrinolytics); (3) more complete opening of the infarct-related artery, with less residual stenosis, lower reocclusion rates, less recurrent ischemia, and a lower likelihood of requiring coronary revascularization compared with fibrinolytic therapy; and (4) an elucidation of coronary anatomy that is often helpful in subsequent care (Box 27–5). Coronary stenting supported by platelet glycoprotein IIb/IIIa therapy is an attractive option.[11] The applicability of this strategy as a primary therapy for AMI is currently limited, however, to less than 20% of hospitals in the United States that have the skilled team and catheterization laboratory available around the clock and 7 days a week required for primary PCI.

The success of primary PCI is highly operator-dependent. In general, it should be limited to operators who perform more than 75 such procedures per year.[11] Patients with AMI who have failed PCI and have evidence of persistent ischemia or hemodynamic instability should be considered for urgent coronary bypass surgery. Therefore, primary PCI for AMI should, if possible, be limited to centers that have the capability for such procedures. Coronary bypass surgery is also recommended in patients with AMI who have persistent ischemia that is refractory to medical therapy and who are not candidates for fibrinolysis or catheter-based interventions. Under special circumstances, primary PCI may be carried out in hospitals without on site cardiac surgery departments (Box 27–6).

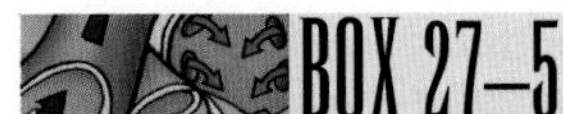

BOX 27–5

Advantages and Disadvantages of Direct Percutaneous Coronary Intervention

ADVANTAGES

Excellent reperfusion rates >90%
Achieves TIMI-3 flow in >90% patients
Rare contraindications (e.g., lack of arterial access, inability to receive heparin, unprotected left main coronary artery stenosis)
Can treat underlying residual stenosis as well as the thrombotic occlusion
Prompt identification of reperfusion
Identification of severity and extent of CAD facilitates triage and enhances therapeutic decision process, e.g., need for CABG in left main CAD patients
Effective for patients with hemodynamic instability
Facilitates diagnosis in patients with equivocal or indeterminant ECGs
Facilitates access for placement of hemodynamic support devices, e.g., IABP

DISADVANTAGES

Requires prompt, easy access to catheterization laboratory and trained personnel
Costs of maintenance of 24-hr laboratory facilities
Requires placement of large arterial sheaths
Limited controlled scientific data
Specific operator dependence

CABG, coronary artery bypass graft; CAD, coronary artery disease; IABP, intra-aortic balloon pump; TIMI-3 flow, normal perfusion.
From Califf RM: Acute myocardial infarction and other acute ischemic syndromes. In Braunwald E (ed): Essential Atlas of Heart Diseases, 2nd ed. Philadelphia, Current Medicine, 2001, p 67.

Even in hospitals with the available staff and facilities, valuable time may be lost between the patient's arrival in the emergency department and the opening of the occluded artery, thereby reducing the potential advantage of this approach. Even more time can be lost if patients are transferred from one hospital's emergency department to a second hospital that can perform the emergency intervention, and this strategy is usually not advisable. Registries of patients with AMI have shown a greater time delay between the onset of chest pain and reperfusion when primary angioplasty is performed than when thrombolytic therapy is administered.

When it is available without time delay ("door-to-balloon" time <1 hr), and when it can be performed by a skilled operator and trained team, emergency catheter-based reperfusion should be employed within 6 hours of the onset of symptoms in patients with STEMI who are in cardiogenic shock, are not eligible for fibrinolysis, and in those who are at relatively high risk of intracranial hemorrhage (age >75 years or hypertension, or both) as a consequence of thrombolysis. It can also be used as an alternative to thrombolysis in all candidates for this therapy.

Patients who have received fibrinolytic therapy should undergo coronary arteriography and, if the anatomic findings are appropriate, catheter-based revascularization if there is persistent chest pain and ST segment elevation 90 minutes after the onset of this therapy or if chest pain recurs and the ST segments become re-elevated.

Patients with AMI *without* ST segment elevations (NSTEMI) are not candidates for fibrinolytic therapy.[5] This important group of patients is discussed in Chapter 26. Other patients believed to have AMI who do not qualify for reperfusion therapy because of late arrival in the emergency department, nondiagnostic ECG changes, contraindications to fibrinolytic therapy without access to PCI, should receive aspirin, heparin, and intravenous beta-blockers, unless there are contraindications to these drugs.

Hospital Management

The CCU

The CCU should have a skilled, experienced staff and equipment for the monitoring of multiple ECG leads for cardiac rhythm and ST segment deviation, arterial oxygen saturation, and the invasive measurement of arterial pressure through an intra-arterial line and pulmonary artery pressure through a balloon flotation catheter. Equipment should also be available for defibrillation, standby percutaneous cardiac pacing, insertion of transvenous pacemakers, placement of an intra-aortic counterpulsation balloon, and noninvasive automatic monitoring of arterial pressure using a sphygmomanometric cuff.

General Measures

Analgesia with morphine, begun in the ambulance or emergency department, should be continued in the CCU as required. For the first 12 hours, patients should receive either nothing by mouth or a clear liquid diet and should be placed at bedrest (Box 27–7). Arterial

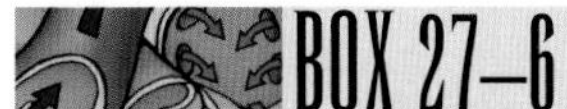
BOX 27–6

Operator, Institutional, and Angiographic Criteria for Primary PTCA Programs at Hospitals Without On-Site Cardiac Surgery

- The operators must be experienced interventionalists who regularly perform elective intervention.
- The nursing and technical CCL staff must be experienced in handling acutely ill patients and comfortable with interventional equipment. They must have acquired experience in dedicated interventional laboratories. They participate in a 24-hour, 7-day per week call schedule.
- The CCL itself must be well equipped, with optimal imaging systems, resuscitative equipment, and IABP support; it must be well stocked with a broad array of interventional equipment.
- The CCU nurses must be adept in the management of acutely ill cardiac patients, including invasive hemodynamic monitoring and IABP management.
- The hospital administration must fully support the program and enable the fulfillment of the above institutional requirements.
- Formalized written protocols must be in place for immediate and efficient transfer of patients to the nearest cardiac surgical facility.
- Primary PTCA must be performed routinely as the treatment of choice around the clock for a large proportion of patients with AMI, to ensure streamlined care paths and increased case volumes.
- Clinical and angiographic selection criteria for the performance of primary PTCA and for transfer for emergency CABG must be rigorous.
- An ongoing program of outcomes analysis and formalized periodic case review must exist.

AMI, acute myocardial infarction; CABG, coronary artery bypass graft; CCL, cardiac catheterization laboratory; CCU, cardiac care unit; IABP, intraaortic balloon pump; PTCA, percutaneous transluminal coronary angioplasty.

From McNamara NS, et al: In Cannon CP, O'Gara PT: Critical Pathways in Cardiology. Philadelphia; Lippincott, Williams and Wilkins, 2001; Adapted from Wharton TOP Jr, McNamara S, Fedele FA, et al: Primary angioplasty for the treatment of acute myocardial infarction: Experience at two community hospitals without cardiac surgery. J Am Coll Cardiol 1999;33:1257–1265.

oxygen saturation should be measured (usually with an oximeter), and hypoxemia should be corrected. Disturbances of acid-base balance or of electrolytes should be corrected, and in some instances, antianxiety agents (such as oral diazepam [2 to 10 mg] or oxazepam [15 to 30 mg] two to four times daily for 48 hours) may be helpful. Docusate sodium (200 mg daily) is useful as a stool softener. Patients who have no complications may use a bedside commode shortly after admission and should commence physical activity as shown in Box 27–8.

Patients with AMI can be discharged from the CCU after 24 hours if they are in Killip class I (Table 27–1) and if there are no complications (heart failure, hypotension, other hemodynamic instability, severe ventricular tachyarrhythmias, advanced AV block, large pericardial effusion, atrial fibrillation, persistent ischemic pain) or when they have been stable for 24 hours after successful treatment of a complication. After discharge from the CCU, patients should be followed in an intermediate CCU, where continuous monitoring of the ECG allows prompt, effective treatment of ventricular fibrillation and other serious arrhythmias.

The rate of progression from the CCU to the intermediate CCU, to a regular hospital floor, and to hospital discharge is governed by the patient's risk and clinical course. Patients without complications and not at high risk (discussed earlier) can generally be moved from the CCU to the intermediate CCU after 24 to 36 hours. If no complication supervenes during an additional 24 to 36 hours in the intermediate CCU, they can be moved to a regular hospital bed and discharged from the hospital by 4 to 6 days. Patients at higher risk may be moved from the CCU to the intermediate CCU after 2 or 3 days if their course has been stable. These patients may also benefit from longer observation (2 to 4 days) in the intermediate CCU and an equal time in a regular hospital bed. Unless complications occur or recur, even such higher-risk patients can generally be discharged by 8 to 10 days after admission.

Education. Efforts should be made to educate the patient about his or her illness while in the hospital. The nature of coronary artery disease, its risk factors, and the importance of diet, exercise, rehabilitation, smoking cessation, medication, and return to work and other life activities should be explained. This can be carried out by the primary care physician, nurses, and other health care professionals. Group instruction and videotaped programs may be useful, but these should be considered adjuncts and cannot take the place of one-on-one contact with a caregiver.

Complications

Hemodynamic Disturbances

Based on clinical examination, patients can be divided into four groups based on the Killip classification (see

BOX 27–7

Sample Admitting Orders

Condition	Serious
IV	NS or D_5W to keep vein open.
Vital signs	q ½ hr until stable, then q 4 hr and prn. Notify if HR < 60 or > 10: BP < 90 or > 150; RR < 8 or > 22. Pulse oximetry × 24 hr.
Activity	Bedrest with bedside commode and progress as tolerated after approximately 12 hr.
Diet	NPO until pain-free, then clear liquids. Progress to a heart-healthy diet (complex carbohydrates =50%–55% of kilocalories, monounsaturated and unsaturated fats ≤30% of kilocalories), including foods high in potassium (e.g., fruits, vegetables, whole grains, dairy products), magnesium (e.g., green leafy vegetables, whole grains, beans, seafood), and fiber (e.g., fresh fruits and vegetables, whole-grain breads, cereals).
Medications	Nasal O_2 2 L/min × 3 hr.
	Enteric-coated ASA daily (165 mg).
	Stool softener daily.
	Beta blockers?
	Consider need for analgesics, nitroglycerin, anxiolytics.

IV, intravenous; NS, normal saline solution; D_5W, 5% dextrose in water; prn, as required; HR, heart rate; BP, blood pressure; RR, respiratory rate; NPO, nothing by mouth; ASA, acetylsalicylic acid.

Reprinted from Ryan TJ, Anderson JL, Antman EM, et al: ACC/AHA guidelines for the management of patients with acute myocardial infarction. J Am Coll Cardiol 1996;28:1328–1428. Copyright 1996, with permission from the American College of Cardiology.

BOX 27–8

Activity Progression after Myocardial Infarction

GENERAL GUIDELINES

When progressing through the stages noted below, specific activities should be stopped for increasing shortness of breath or the patient's perception of fatigue or detection of an increase in the heart rate of >20–30 beats/min^{-1}. Vital signs should be monitored before and after progression from one stage to the next and also from one level to the next within each stage. Energy-conserving techniques should be emphasized and the use of prophylactic nitroglycerin should be reviewed with the patient.

STAGE I (DAYS 1–2)

Use a bedpan or commode. Feed self-prepared tray with arm and back support. Complete assistance with bathing. Passive ROM to all extremities. Active ankle motion (with footboard if available). Emphasis on relaxation and deep breathing.

Partially bathe upper body with back support. Bed to chair transfers for 1–2 hr per day. Active ROM to all extremities 5–10 times (sitting or supine).

STAGE II (DAYS 3–4)

Bathe, groom, self-dress sitting on bed or chair. Bed-to-chair transfers ad lib. Ambulate in room with gradual increase in duration and frequency.

May shower or stand at sink to bathe. May dress in own clothes. Supervised ambulation outside of room (100–600 ft several times per day) (33–200 m).

Partially bathe upper body with back support. Bed to chair 20–30 min daily. Active assisted to active ROM all extremities: 5–10 times (sitting or supine).

STAGE III (DAYS 5–7)

Ambulate 600 ft (200 m) 3 times per day. May shampoo hair (e.g., activity with arms over head).

Supervised stair walking.

Predischarge exercise tolerance test.

ROM, range of motion; ad lib., as desired.

From Antman EM: General hospital management. In Julian D, Braunwald E (eds): Management of Acute Myocardial Infarction. London, WB Saunders, 1994, p 34.

Table 27–1). Invasive monitoring, with a pulmonary artery flotation (Swan-Ganz) catheter and an intra-arterial line, is indicated in patients in class IV with a systolic pressure below 80 mm Hg and pulmonary rales, as well as in patients with pulmonary edema that is not corrected by intravenous furosemide (discussed later), and in patients with hypotension that is not readily corrected with fluid administration, leg raising, or atropine. Although there should be no hesitation to insert a pulmonary artery catheter in appropriate patients, this procedure should be carried out by an experienced operator. Complications of inserting a pulmonary artery catheter occur in approximately 4% of cases and include sepsis, pulmonary infarction, and very rarely, pulmonary artery rupture. Cardiac output should be measured in these patients with the indicator dilution technique with injection of the indicator (cool saline) into the right atrium and sampling (with a thermistor) in the pulmonary artery.

Hemodynamic assessment allows patients to be classified as shown in Table 27–1 and treated as shown in Table 27–2. Hypoperfusion is identified by a cardiac index below 2.2 L/min/m^2, whereas pulmonary congestion is reflected by a pulmonary capillary wedge pressure (PCWP) above 18 mm Hg. Treatment should be tailored to the hemodynamic abnormality. Patients who are hypotensive or have hypoperfusion but a PCWP below 18 mm Hg may be suffering from hypovolemia and should receive a bolus of 100 mL normal saline solution, followed by 50-mL increments every 5 minutes until the systolic arterial pressure reaches 110 mm Hg or

TABLE 27–1

Hemodynamic Classifications of Patients with Acute Myocardial Infarction

A. Based on Clinical Examination		**B. Based on Invasive Monitoring**	
Class	***Definition***	***Subset***	***Definition***
I	Rales and S_3 absent	I	Normal hemodynamics PCWP < 18, CI > 2.2
II	Rales over <50% of lung	II	Pulmonary congestion PCWP > 18, CI > 2.2
III	Rales over >50% of lung fields (pulmonary edema)	III	Peripheral hypoperfusion PCWP < 18, CI < 2.2
IV	Shock	IV	Pulmonary congestion and peripheral hypoperfusion PCWP > 18, CI < 1.8

S_3, third heart sound; PCWP, pulmonary capillary wedge pressure; CI, cardiac index.

A and *B*, from Antman EM, Braunwald E: Acute myocardial infarction. In Braunwald E, Zipes DP, Libby P (eds): Heart Disease, 6th ed. Philadelphia, WB Saunders, 2001, p. 1174; (A) modified from American Journal of Cardiology, Vol. 20, Killip TI, Kimball J: Treatment of myocardial infarction in a coronary care unit. A two-year experience with 250 patients, pp 457. Copyright 1967, with permission from Excerpta Medica Inc; and (B) data from Forrester J, Diamond G, Chatterjee K, et al: Medical therapy of acute myocardial infarction by the application of hemodynamic subsets. N Engl J Med 1976;295:1356.

TABLE 27–2

Choice of Pharmacologic Agents in Patients with Acute Myocardial Infarction Based on Hemodynamic Parameters

Drug Effect	**Furosemide**	**IV Nitrates**	**Dobutamine**	**Dopamine**	**ACE Inhibitors**
Preload	↓	↓	—	↑	↓
Afterload	—	Minimal ↓	Minimal ↓	↑	↓
Sinus tachycardia	No	Yes	Minimal	Yes	No, minimal
			Parameters		
Moderate heart failure, PCWP ≥20	Yes	Yes	Yes, if BP >70	Yes, if BP <70 and oliguria (on dobutamine)	Oral maintenance weaning nitroprusside
Severe heart failure, PCWP >24, cardiac index <2.5 L/min/m^2	Yes	Yes, if BP >95	Yes, if BP >70	Yes, if BP <70	Yes
Cardiogenic shock if BP <95 PCWP >18, cardiac index <2.5 L/min/m^2	CI	CI	Yes	Yes IABP	RCI
Right ventricular infarction, JVP ↑	CI	CI	Useful with titrated volume infusion	Relative CI ↑ PA pressure	CI

Key: Yes, useful; ↓, decrease; —, no change; ↑, increase.

ACE, angiotensin-converting enzymes; BP, systolic blood pressure (mm Hg); CI, contraindication; IABP, intra-aortic balloon pump; JVP, jugular venous pressure; PA, pulmonary artery; PCWP, pulmonary capillary wedge pressure; RCI, relative contraindication.

Modified from Khan MG: Complications of myocardial infarction and postinfarction care. In Khan MG (ed): Heart Disease: Diagnosis and Therapy. Baltimore, Williams & Wilkins, 1996, p. 66.

the PCWP exceeds 18 mm Hg. Patients with pulmonary congestion or rales involving more than one-third of the lung fields that do not clear on coughing, and with a systolic arterial pressure exceeding 100 mm Hg should receive a diuretic (e.g., furosemide, 20 to 40 mg intravenously repeated every 4 hr). Normotensive patients with pulmonary congestion despite diuretics should receive vasodilator therapy. The vasodilator of choice is intravenous nitroglycerin given in a dose of 5 μg/min, with the dose increased by 10 μg/min every 5 minutes to a maximum of 200 μg/min until the hemodynamics have been optimized or until the systolic arterial pressure has declined to 90 mm Hg. In patients with persistent heart failure, oral vasodilators, especially angiotensin-converting enzyme (ACE) inhibitors, should be used.

Cardiogenic Shock

This severe form of ventricular failure is characterized by markedly elevated ventricular filling pressure (PCWP >20 mm Hg), very low cardiac index (<1.8 L/min/m^2), persistent severe systemic hypotension (systolic arterial pressure <80 mm Hg), and evidence of organ hypoperfusion such as a clouded sensorium, cool extremities, oliguria, or metabolic acidosis (Fig. 27–9). Cardiogenic shock is most commonly caused by extensive damage to the left or right ventricular myocardium or by a mechanical defect (ventricular septal rupture or papillary muscle rupture) (Table 27–3 and Fig. 27–10). Cardiogenic shock occurs in approximately 10% of patients with AMI and usually is not present at the time of admission but develops during the course of hospitalization.

Management. In the patient with cardiogenic shock owing to left ventricular dysfunction but without a mechanical defect (ventricular septal defect or mitral regurgitation), continuous hemodynamic assessment is essential. Inotropic stimulation with a sympathomimetic agent is usually indicated. When systolic arterial pressure is very low (<70 mm Hg), norepinephrine 2 to 10 μg/kg/min is the drug of choice. In patients with moderate hypotension (systolic arterial pressure 70 to 90 mm Hg), dopamine (5 to 20 μg/kg/min) is used. When the systolic arterial pressure is higher (≥90 mm Hg), dobutamine (2 to 20 μg/kg/min) may be the optimal agent.

In patients in whom cardiogenic shock persists despite inotropic support as outlined previously, intra-aortic balloon counterpulsation, with insertion of the balloon percutaneously or via an arterial cutdown in the femoral artery, is indicated. The balloon is inflated during early diastole and deflated just before the onset of systole. This augments coronary blood flow and lowers the pressure against which the left ventricle ejects and results in a small (approximately 15%) increase in cardiac output and moderate (approximately 5 mm Hg) lowering of PCWP.

Despite the favorable hemodynamic effects of the combination of the administration of sympathomimetic amines and intra-aortic balloon counterpulsation, these therapies have only a minor beneficial effect on mortality. Therefore, after stabilization with inotropic agents and intra-aortic balloon counterpulsation, cardiac catheterization and coronary arteriography should be carried out unless myocardial revascularization is contraindicated or not feasible. Coronary revascularization—either via a catheter-based technique or by means of coronary bypass grafting—is performed whenever possible. The SHOCK trial randomized patients with shock to emergency revascularization or initial medical

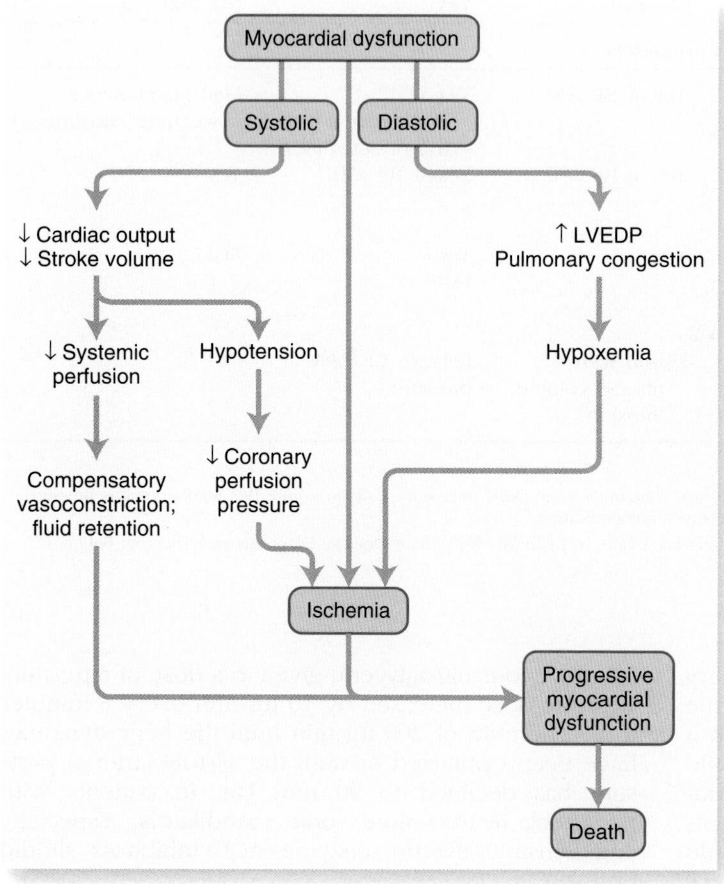

FIGURE 27–9. The vicious circle in cardiogenic shock. LVEDP, left ventricular end-diastolic pressure. (From Hollenberg SM, Kevinsky CJ, Parrillo JE: Cardiogenic shock. Ann Intern Med 1999;131:47–59.)

TABLE 27–3

Acute Myocardial Infarction—Mechanical Complications, Incidence, Timing, and Mortality

	% of Total Acute Infarcts	Incidence and Timing (%)	% of Total Rupture	% of Total In-Hospital Mortality	Type of Infarct
Cardiac rupture	3–10	Up to 40; day 1 Up to 50; days 2–3		8–17*	
Free wall	2–6*†	25; day 1 10; days 4–7	85	7–14	Lateral
Papillary muscle rupture	1	25; days 1–2 or 6–10 75; days 3–5	5	1	Commonly inferoposterior
Ventricular septal rupture	1–2	25; days 1–2 or 6–14 75; days 3–5	10	1–2	60% anterior 40% inferior
Severe mitral regurgitation	<2	days 1–5			
LV aneurysm	7–12	3 mo			90% anterior 10% inferior

*Am Heart J 1989;117:809.

†J Am Coll Cardiol 1991;68:961.

LV, left ventricular.

Modified from Khan MG: Complications of myocardial infarction and postinfarction care. In Khan MG (ed): Heart Disease: Diagnosis and Therapy. Baltimore, Williams & Wilkins, 1996, p. 83.

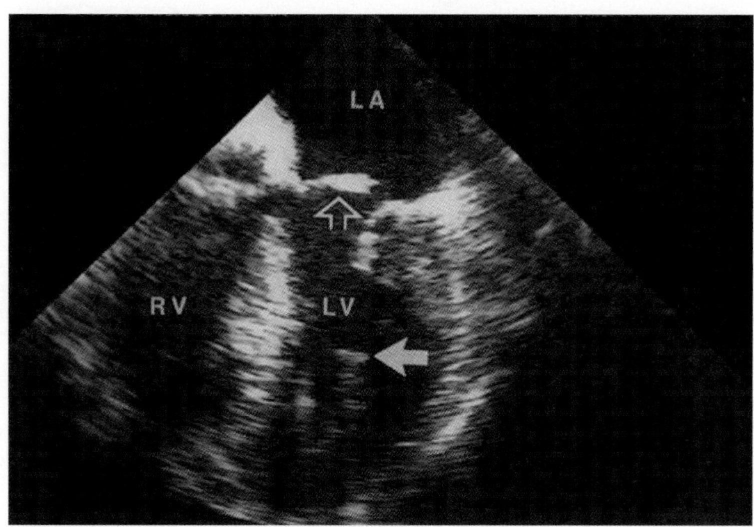

FIGURE 27–10. Transesophageal echocardiogram in the four-chamber view demonstrating a failed anterior leaflet of the mitral valve (*open arrow*) after acute MI and chordal rupture. The solid arrow indicates the base of the posterior papillary muscle. LA, left atrium; LV, left ventricle; RV, right ventricle. (Courtesy of Alan Mogtader, MD, St. Luke's–Roosevelt Hospital Center and Columbia University, New York. From Hochman JS, Palazzo A, Holmes DR, Jr: Cardiogenic shock complicating acute myocardial infarction. In Califf RM [volume ed]: Acute Myocardial Infarction and Other Acute Ischemic Syndromes. Braunwald E [series ed]: Atlas of Heart Diseases. Philadelphia, Current Medicine, 2001.)

stabilization.[13] Six-month mortality was 50% in the revascularization group compared to 63% in the medically treated group. Subgroups of patients in cardiogenic shock that showed particular benefit from early revascularization were those who were younger than 75 years, had a prior MI, and were treated less than 6 hours from onset of infarction.

A New Systolic Murmur

The presence of a new loud systolic heart murmur suggests the presence of a mechanical complication, an interventricular septal defect due to rupture of the ventricular septum,[16] or massive mitral regurgitation secondary to rupture of the head of a papillary muscle. These complications, which may accompany cardiogenic shock, can be recognized and differentiated by two-dimensional echocardiography with Doppler flow imaging (Fig. 27–11; see also Fig. 27–10). Alternatively, they may be recognized by means of a balloon flotation catheter, in which an oxygen stepup is observed as the catheter is advanced from the right atrium into the right ventricle in the presence of a ventricular septal defect, or a tall V-wave is observed in the PCWP in the presence of mitral regurgitation.

Management

If one of the previously mentioned mechanical defects is suspected, and after aggressive therapy has been agreed, on following discussion with the patient or

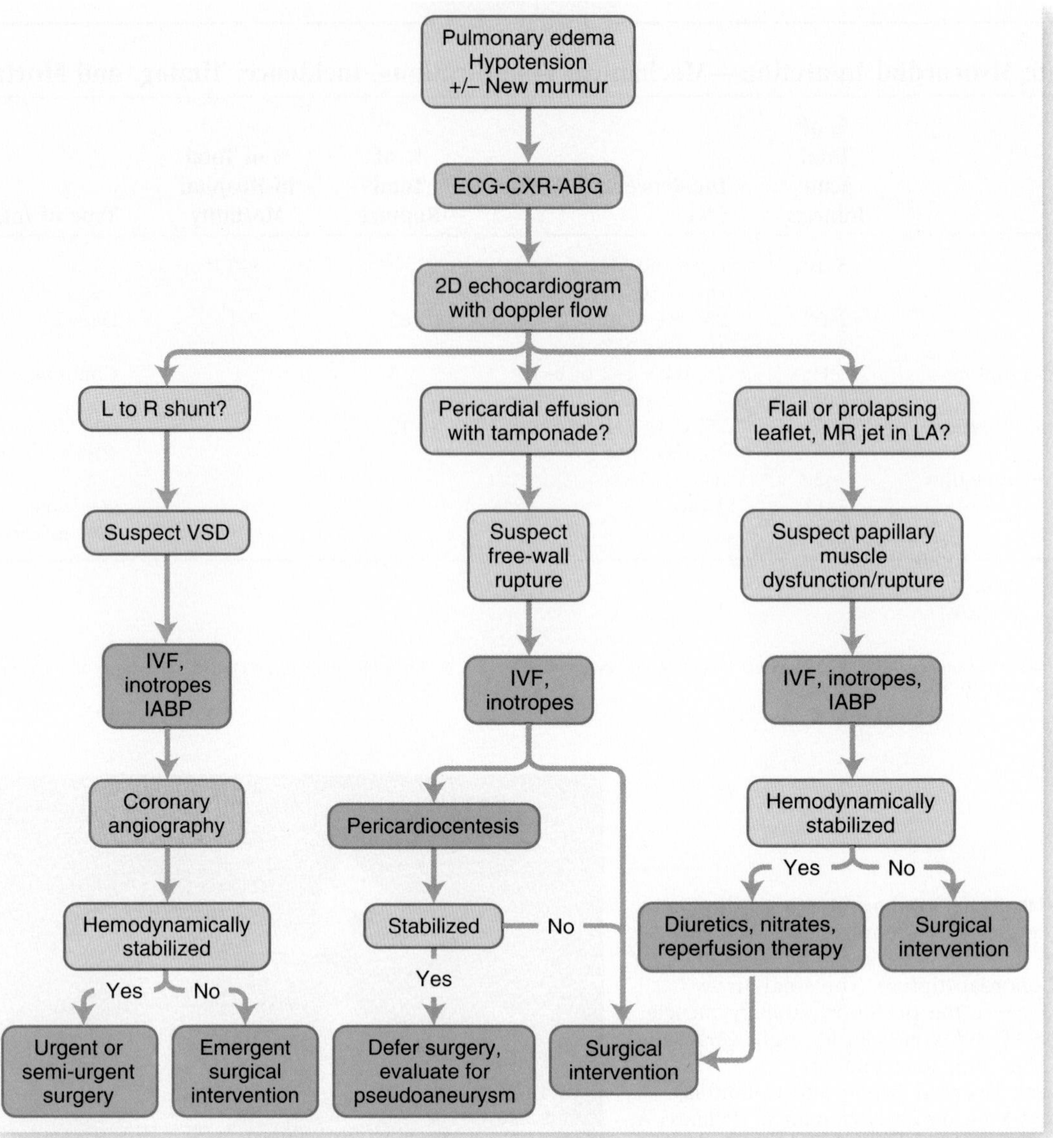

FIGURE 27–11. The management of patients with postinfarction mechanical complications is determined by the site of the involvement and the degree of hemodynamic compromise. (From Becker RC: Complicated myocardial infarction. In Cannon CP, O'Gara PT [eds]: Critical Pathways in Cardiology. Philadelphia, Lippincott, Williams & Wilkins, 2000, pp 107–130.)

relatives, the diagnosis should be confirmed by cardiac catheterization and coronary angiography. Intra-aortic balloon counterpulsation is often useful for stabilizing the patient before operation. Surgical correction of the defect (mitral valve repair or replacement) is commonly combined with coronary revascularization.

Right Ventricular Infarction

This usually is seen in patients with coexistent inferior left ventricular infarction and rarely (<5%) occurs in an isolated form.[3] Right ventricular infarction should be suspected in patients with inferior left ventricular infarction with unexplained, persistent hypotension, clear lung fields, and elevated jugular venous pressure (Box 27–9). Right atrial pressure is elevated, right ventricular pulse pressure is reduced, and PCWP is usually normal or only slightly raised. The ECG typically shows ST segment elevations in right precordial leads, especially V_{4R} (the right precordial lead in the V_4 position). The right atrial pressure pulse usually reveals a prominent Y descent, whereas the right ventricular pressure tracing shows an early diastolic drop and plateau, that is, a "square root sign" similar to that observed in constrictive pericarditis (see Chapter 35). Kussmaul's sign—an increase in jugular venous pressure with inspiration—in the presence of an inferior wall AMI, suggests right ventricular involvement. Echocardiography often reveals right ventricular dilatation. The reduction of

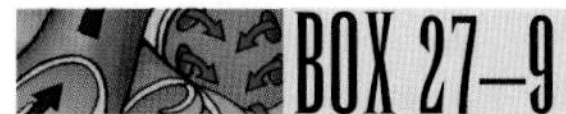
BOX 27–9

Potential Complications of Right Ventricular Infarction

Cardiogenic shock
High degree atrioventricular block
Atrial fibrillation or atrial flutter
Ventricular tachycardia or fibrillation
Ventricular septal rupture
Right ventricular thrombus with or without pulmonary embolism
Tricuspid regurgitation
Pericarditis
Right-to-left shunt via patent foramen ovale

From Becker RC: Complicated myocardial infarction. In Cannon CP, O'Gara PT: Critical Pathways in Cardiology. Philadelphia, Lippincott, Williams and Wilkins, 2001.

preload (hypovolemia, diuretic use, nitroglycerin) intensifies hypotension.

Treatment consists of the expansion of plasma volume with saline solution and, if this is insufficient, the addition of dobutamine. Pulmonary artery pressure monitoring is needed if the hypotension does not respond to fluids or if the patient develops signs suggestive of left ventricular failure. It is especially important to maintain AV synchrony in patients with right ventricular infarction, and AV sequential pacing is highly desirable in patients with heart block and hypotension.

Arrhythmias (see also Chapters 30 and 31)

The majority of patients with AMI develop one or more cardiac arrhythmias.[2] Many of these are transient and benign and do not require specific therapy. Others are more serious and life-threatening and require prompt treatment.

Tachyarrhythmias

Supraventricular Tachyarrhythmias. Sinus tachycardia is a common arrhythmia in AMI and is typically associated with increased sympathetic activity, persistent pain, hypotension, left ventricular failure, and anxiety. Treatment consists of correction of the underlying disorder and the use of beta-adrenergic blockers unless there is a contraindication to the use of these drugs (discussed later).

Atrial fibrillation occurs in approximately 15% of patients with AMI. It is seen most often during the first 24 hours, may be transient, and is more frequent in patients with left ventricular failure, with large anterior wall MIs, or with AV block, and in the elderly. In the absence of heart failure, a beta-adrenergic blocker (e.g., metoprolol 5 mg by intravenous bolus every 5 to 10 min for three doses followed by 25 or 50 mg orally every 6 hr) is often effective. In patients with atrial fibrillation and left ventricular failure in whom beta-blockers are contraindicated, and who are not receiving maintenance digitalis therapy, digoxin 0.4 mg intravenously followed 4 hours later by another 0.2 to 0.4 mg is useful. In patients with severe hemodynamic compromise or ongoing ischemia, electrocardioversion beginning with 50 joules, with the energy gradually increased if the first shock is not successful, is indicated. Amiodarone, 200 mg/day for 6 weeks, is useful for suppressing recurrence of atrial fibrillation. Patients with recurrent atrial fibrillation should receive oral anticoagulants to prevent thromboembolism.

Ventricular Premature Beats. These are detectable by monitoring in a large majority of patients with AMI. Even if these beats are frequent, that is, more than 5 per minute, are of multiform configuration, occur in bigeminal rhythm, or if they occur early ("R on T"), prophylactic suppression with antiarrhythmic agents such as lidocaine or procainamide is not necessary when patients are closely monitored.[15] Indeed, such prophylaxis may even be harmful. It is now considered best to treat such premature beats with intravenous beta-blockers and to screen for and correct electrolyte or acid-base disturbances, hypoxemia, or heart failure.

Accelerated Idioventricular Rhythm. A ventricular rhythm with a rate of 60 to 120 beats per minute (sometimes termed slow ventricular tachycardia) occurs during the first 2 days in 10% to 20% of patients with AMI. Accelerated idioventricular rhythm is especially common after successful reperfusion. Treatment with atropine or atrial pacing is indicated when the AV dissociation causes hemodynamic compromise.

Ventricular Tachycardia. This arrhythmia is classified as either nonsustained (<30 sec) or sustained (>30 sec) and as monomorphic or polymorphic. Sustained ventricular tachycardia, with a ventricular rate >150 beats per minute that causes hypotension or other hemodynamic compromise, requires immediate therapy with electric countershock. When the tachycardia is polymorphic, it should be treated with an unsynchronized discharge of 200 joules, whereas monomorphic ventricular tachycardia should be treated with a synchronized discharge of 100 joules. The energy should be increased in 50-joule increments if the patient does not respond to the first shock. When the ventricular rate is slower than 150 beats per minute and the ventricular tachycardia is well tolerated hemodynamically, the following pharmacologic regimens may be employed:

1. **Lidocaine:** A bolus of 1.0 to 1.5 mg/kg followed by supplemental bolus injections of 0.5 to 0.75 mg/kg every 5 to 10 minutes to a maximum of 3 mg/kg followed by a maintenance infusion of 20 to 50 μg/kg/min. The dose should be reduced in older patients (>70 years). Patients with heart failure and hepatic dysfunction should have slower infusion rates of 10 to 20 μg/kg/min.
2. **Procainamide:** A loading infusion of 12 to 30 mg/min should be followed by a maintenance infusion of 1 to 4 mg/min.

3. **Amiodarone:** 75 to 150 mg infused over 10 minutes followed by an infusion of 1.0 mg/min for 6 hours and then reduced to 0.5 mg/min.

Ventricular Fibrillation. Three major forms of ventricular fibrillation occur in patients with AMI. *Primary* ventricular fibrillation occurs early (<48 hr from the onset), suddenly, and unexpectedly in the absence of left ventricular failure. The incidence of this arrhythmia has declined strikingly during the past two decades. *Secondary* ventricular fibrillation usually also occurs early, but it is associated with (and secondary to) left ventricular failure and cardiogenic shock. *Late* ventricular fibrillation occurs more than 48 hours after MI and also frequently accompanies ventricular dysfunction. On the one hand, primary ventricular fibrillation, even when treated successfully, may increase mortality during the hospital course, but the postdischarge prognosis is not altered. On the other hand, both secondary and late ventricular fibrillation are associated with a worse prognosis because they are usually associated with extensive myocardial damage.

Ventricular fibrillation should be treated as rapidly as possible with an electric shock of 200 to 300 joules. If unsuccessful, 300 to 400 joules should be used. If ventricular fibrillation persists, epinephrine (5 to 10 mL/1–1:10,000 intracardiac or 1 mg intravenously) is indicated. Additional adjunctive treatment includes intravenous lidocaine (1.5 mg/kg), bretylium (5 to 10 mg/kg), or amiodarone (75 to 150 mg bolus), or a combination. After defibrillation, patients should re-ceive an intravenous beta-blocker (e.g., 5 mg metoprolol) repeated twice at 5-min intervals if tolerated, and infusion of an antiarrhythmic drug (lidocaine 2 mg/min, procainamide 1 to 4 mg/min, or amiodarone 1.0 mg/min for 6 hours followed by 0.5 mg/min) for 12 to 24 hours and then should be reassessed for the need for future therapy. Serum electrolytes should be measured; hypokalemia and hypomagnesemia should be treated as well.

Bradyarrhythmias

Sinus Bradycardia. This arrhythmia occurs early in the course of infarction in about one-third of patients, and is more common in patients with inferior or posterior than with anterior infarction. Beta-blockers should be held. Intravenous atropine should be administered if the heart rate is less than 50 beats per minute, or if the heart rate is between 50 and 60 beats per minute and the patient is hypotensive or exhibits frequent ventricular ectopic beats. Elevation of the legs may be helpful in hypotensive patients with bradycardia without pulmonary congestion. If the bradycardia persists despite atropine and the patient remains symptomatic or hypotensive, electric pacing is indicated.

First-Degree AV Block and Mobitz Type I Second-Degree AV Block. Each of these arrhythmias occurs in approximately 10% of patients with AMI and generally do not require treatment, except for the discontinuation of drugs which interfere with AV conduction (digitalis, beta-blockers, verapamil, diltiazem). Atropine is indicated in patients with Mobitz type I second-degree AV block and bradycardia (<50 beats/min) or hypotension.

Mobitz Type II Second-Degree Block and Third-Degree AV Block. When associated with anterior wall MI, these forms of heart block are usually characterized by wide QRS complexes. These patients are at high risk and should be treated with temporary transvenous pacing. AV sequential pacing should be employed when there is left ventricular failure. When these forms of block are associated with inferior infarction, they are usually accompanied by ventricular rates above 40 beats per minute and narrow QRS complexes and are secondary to an intranodal lesion. This latter form of block is usually transient and should be treated with atropine. If it fails to respond, temporary transvenous pacing should be employed.

Intraventricular Block. Block in a single division of the conduction system (left anterior divisional block, left posterior divisional block, or right bundle branch block) is associated with large infarcts and therefore with higher mortality. Patients with such blocks require careful observation for the development of more advanced forms of block but no specific therapy. Bifascicular block (right bundle branch block with either left anterior or posterior divisional block or left bundle branch block) is usually secondary to extensive myocardial necrosis and should be managed initially with the application of transcutaneous pacing electrodes in a standby mode that is activated if ventricular rate drops below a preset threshold. Although transcutaneous external temporary pacing is associated with discomfort, it can be employed for brief periods in patients at risk of developing high-degree AV block before a transvenous pacemaker is inserted.

Pacing (Table 27–4)

Temporary transvenous ventricular pacing is carried out by inserting a pacing catheter percutaneously through the jugular, subclavian, or femoral veins and advancing it to the right ventricular apex. AV dual-chamber pacing is required in some patients to achieve hemodynamic compensation and requires insertion of a second catheter into the right atrial appendage. In patients with persistent third-degree or Mobitz type II second-degree AV block, permanent pacing is indicated.

Recurrent Chest Pain

Recurrent ischemia and acute pericarditis are the most important causes of recurrent chest discomfort. The first task is to distinguish between these two causes.

Recurrent Ischemia or Reinfarction. This occurs in approximately 25% of patients and is the most important cause of recurrent pain during the first 18 hours of AMI. This diagnosis is aided by the development or

TABLE 27–4

Acute MI: Nonmedical Therapies

Modality	Indications	Comments
Pulmonary artery (Swan-Ganz) catheterization	Hypotension unresponsive to fluids Unexplained tachycardia, tachypnea, hypoxemia, or acidosis Suspicion of ventricular septal rupture or acute mitral regurgitation Refractory pulmonary edema	Swan-Ganz allows determination of wedge pressure, cardiac output, and systemic vascular resistance, which can be used to distinguish cause of hypotension Selected hemodynamic subsets: RV infarction: ↑ RA pressure, RA/PCW pressure ratio >0.9, ↓ CO Cardiogenic shock: ↓ BP, ↓ CO, ↑ PCW pressure, ↑ SVR Acute MR: ↑ PCW pressure (prominent V-wave may be seen); CO usually ↓ Acute VSD: ≥8% oxygen stepup from RA → RV and PA, CO calculations are falsely elevated (reflecting L → R shunting with ↑ pulmonary flow) Acute tamponade: ↓ BP, paradoxical pulse, RA ~ PCW pressure, ↓ CO; prominent X-descent may be seen on RA tracing. May need echo to distinguish from RV infarct Massive pulmonary embolism: ↓ BP, ↓ CO, ↑ PA pressure and PVR, normal PCW pressure
Temporary pacemaker Prophylactic	New LBBB Bifascicular block: RBBB with left anterior or left posterior fascicular block Alternating LBBB and RBBB	Prophylactic pacing (usually for 48–72 hr) is recommended to prevent hemodynamic collapse in the event that conduction delay progresses to 3° AV block Transcutaneous or transvenous leads are acceptable; transcutaneous leads are quickly placed and avoid bleeding complications if thrombolytics or anticoagulants have been given
Therapeutic	Asystole Mobitz II 2° AV block 3° AV block Bradycardia with hypotension	Transvenous lead is recommended; a transcutaneous lead may be needed until the transvenous lead is in place when hemodynamic or clinical instability is present Temporary pacing may not be required if bradycardia or 3° AV block occurs with inferior MI and resolves with atropine AV sequential pacing may be preferred over ventricular pacing in severe LV dysfunction/hypertrophy and RV infarction; optimization of AV synchrony ("atrial kick") may facilitate cardiac output

AV, atrioventricular; BP, blood pressure; CO, cardiac output; LBBB, left bundle branch block; L → R, left-to-right; LV, left ventricular; MI, myocardial infarction; MR, mitral regurgitation; PA, pulmonary artery; PCW, pulmonary capillary wedge; PVR, pulmonary vascular resistance; RA, right atrial; RBBB, right bundle branch block; RV, right ventricular; SVR, systemic vascular resistance; VSD, ventricular septal defect; 2°, second-degree; 3°, third-degree.

Modified from Grines CL: Myocardial infarction. *In* Freed M, Grines C (eds): Essentials of Cardiovascular Medicine. Birmingham, MI: Physicians' Press, 1994, pp. 112–113.

recurrence of ST segment and T-wave changes, usually in the same leads in which Q-waves appeared, and sometimes by re-elevation of CK-MB or other biochemical markers of myocardial necrosis.

Patients with recurrent ischemia should receive intravenous nitroglycerin and intravenous beta-blockers, heparin, and aspirin (if they are not already receiving these drugs). Unless there are obvious contraindications to revascularization, such as a serious co-morbid condition, they should undergo urgent coronary arteriography and, depending on the anatomic findings, PCI or surgical revascularization (Fig. 27–12).

Pericarditis (see Chapter 35). This complication is observed most frequently 24 hours to 6 weeks after STEMI and occurs in approximately 20% of patients. Although the discomfort may resemble post-MI angina, it frequently radiates to the trapezius ridge and the left shoulder and becomes worse during deep inspiration. It is often, but not uniformly, associated with a pericardial friction rub, concave upward ST segment elevation and PR segment depression, and a pericardial effusion that can be detected by two-dimensional transthoracic echocardiography. The treatment of choice is aspirin, up to 650 mg four times daily. Corticosteroids and nonsteroidal anti-inflammatory drugs should be avoided because these agents may interfere with myocardial healing. Patients with pericarditis who receive anticoagulants should be observed carefully for increasing pericardial effusion due to bleeding into the pericardial sac.

Cardiac Rupture

Rarely, recurrent pain may also be caused by cardiac rupture.[16] The risk factors for this catastrophic complication are infarcts that are first infarcts, anterior in loca-

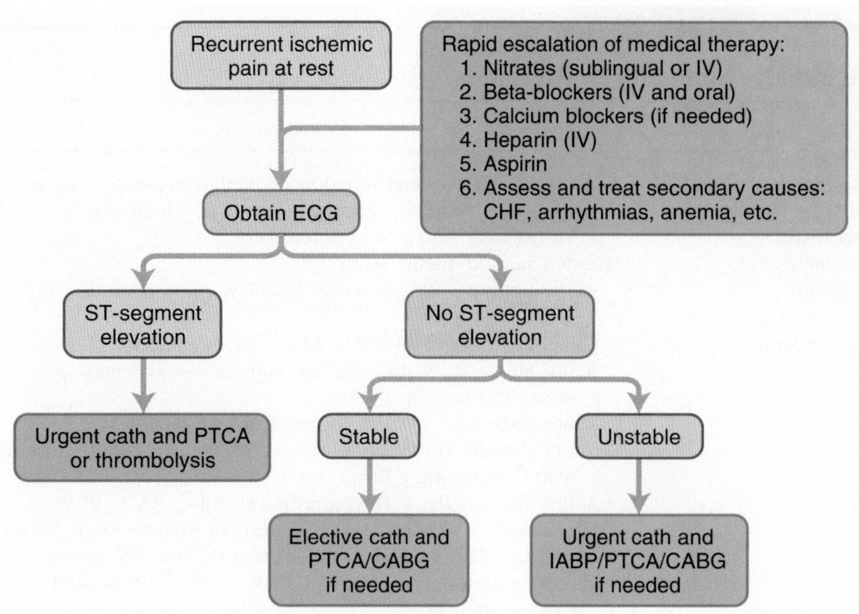

FIGURE 27–12. Treatment of recurent ischemic events. (From Cannon CP, Ganz LI, Stone PH: Complicated myocardial infarction. In Rippe JM, Irwin RS, Fink MP, Cerra FB [eds]: Intensive Care Medicine, 3rd ed. Boston, Little, Brown, 1995.)

tion, and occurring in older patients (>70 years), in women, and in patients with a history of hypertension. This event is associated with cardiac tamponade and requires immediate pericardiocentesis and emergency surgical repair (see Chapter 35).

PHARMACOTHERAPY

Beta-Adrenergic Blockers

These drugs diminish myocardial oxygen consumption by reducing heart rate, arterial blood pressure, and myocardial contractility. Several multicenter trials have shown the benefits of early treatment, that is, less than 4 hours after onset of pain, with intravenous beta-blockade followed by oral therapy. Patients who present later can be started on oral therapy that is usually continued for an indefinite period.

When given intravenously in the acute stage, beta-blocker therapy has been shown to reduce the rate of development of definite MI, infarct size, and the incidence of tachyarrhythmias, sudden death, and total mortality. When administered chronically, these drugs reduce the incidence of reinfarction, sudden death, and total mortality. Contraindications to beta-blockers are shown in Box 27–10. If complications such as heart failure, heart block, or bronchospasm develop, beta-blockers should be withdrawn or their dose decreased until complications resolve.

Two useful regimens are intravenous atenolol 5 to 10 mg followed by oral atenolol 100 mg daily, or metoprolol 15 mg intravenously in three divided doses, followed by 100 mg orally twice a day.

BOX 27–10

Contraindications to Acute Beta-Adrenergic Blockade

Heart rate less than 60 bpm
Systolic arterial pressure less than 100 mm Hg
Moderate or severe LV failure
Signs of peripheral hypoperfusion
PR interval greater than 0.24 sec
Second- or third-degree AV block
Severe chronic obstructive pulmonary disease
History of asthma
Severe peripheral vascular disease
Insulin-dependent diabetes mellitus

LV. left ventricular, AV, atrioventricular.
Reprinted from Ryan TJ, Anderson JL, Antman EM, et al: ACC/AHA Guidelines for the management of patients with acute myocardial infarction. J Am Coll Cardiol 1996; 28: pp 1328–1428. Copyright 1996, with permission from the American College of Cardiology.

ACE Inhibitors

By lowering ventricular afterload and preload, ACE inhibitors reduce the incidence of congestive heart failure, ventricular dilatation, and remodeling.[17] These drugs appear to be useful when begun as early as 1 day after infarction. When continued for several years, they improve clinical outcome in patients with left ventricular dysfunction and heart failure.

In the absence of contraindications (hypotension, known hypersensitivity, bilateral renal artery stenosis, and possible pregnancy), an oral ACE inhibitor should be given to all hemodynamically stable AMI patients with ST segment elevation. ACE inhibitor therapy should be begun within the first 24 hours, after reperfusion therapy has been completed and the blood pressure has stabilized. Left ventricular function should be evaluated before hospital discharge, and ACE inhibition should certainly be continued for an indefinite period in patients with hypertension, heart failure, prior infarction, evidence of a reduced ejection fraction (<40%), anterior infarction, or with large regional wall motion abnormalities. There is growing evidence that when well tolerated, these drugs should also be continued indefinitely even in patients without any of these findings. A number of regimens—such as lisinopril, 5 mg/day for 2 days and then 10 mg daily, or trandolapril, 2 mg/day for 2 days followed by 4 mg/day—may be employed.

Nitroglycerin

This drug exerts favorable pharmacologic actions by reducing right and left ventricular preload and afterload and causes coronary vasodilatation. It should be administered when the patient is first encountered. There is no clear-cut evidence that the routine administration of nitroglycerin is beneficial in patients with uncomplicated MI who receive reperfusion therapy. Intravenous nitroglycerin (5 to 10 μg/min, up to 150 μg/min as long as hemodynamic stability is maintained) is, however, the drug of choice with the recurrence of ischemia. It is also useful in nonhypotensive patients with left ventricular failure and may be used for 24 to 48 hours in patients with large Q-wave anterior wall MIs to reduce ventricular remodeling and dilatation. It may then be continued orally or topically for 4 to 6 days in these patients.

Calcium Antagonists

These drugs have not been shown to reduce mortality in AMI. Indeed, because it has been suggested that immediate-release nifedipine is associated with a dose-related increased risk of in-hospital mortality, this drug should not be used in patients with AMI. Verapamil (240 to 480 mg/day in divided doses or once daily with sustained release) or diltiazem (120 to 360 mg daily in three or four doses or once daily with sustained release) may be useful in controlling attacks of recurrent ischemia or atrial fibrillation in patients without heart failure or AV block. These agents are especially useful in patients who cannot tolerate or who have contraindications to beta-blockers.

POST-MI RISK STRATIFICATION

Risk stratification before hospital discharge is an important aspect of management and determines whether coronary angiography is indicated. The first step is to determine whether the clinical variables indicating a relatively high risk for future cardiac events are present (Fig. 27–13). Patients who have had recurrent ischemia at rest or with mild activity, who have had evidence of congestive heart failure, or who are known to have an ejection fraction below 40%, and in whom there are no contraindications for revascularization, should undergo cardiac catheterization and coronary arteriography. Revascularization should then be carried out if the coronary anatomy is suitable and there are no contraindications. Patients who have had an episode of ventricular fibrillation or sustained ventricular tachycardia more than 48 hours after AMI should be considered for electrophysiologic study and implantation of an automatic internal cardioverter defibrillator (AICD) (see Chapter 30). Coronary angiography is often performed routinely 1 to 2 days after admission in patients with non-ST segment elevation MI (NSTEMI) or unstable angina (see Chapter 26) who appear on clinical grounds to be candidates for coronary revascularization, and who are cared for in cardiac centers. Revascularization may then be carried out if the coronary anatomy is appropriate.

Patients without these clinical indicators of high risk should undergo an assessment of left ventricular function (echocardiogram or radionuclide angiogram and submaximal stress test) before hospital discharge. In patients who have an interpretable ECG and who can exercise, a submaximal exercise test (see Chapter 4) is suitable. If the test is negative, they may return for a symptom-limited exercise test at 3 to 6 weeks. If that too is negative, they can remain on medical therapy and risk factor reduction. Conversely, if the resting ejection fraction is under 40% or the stress test is markedly abnormal (≥2 mm ST segment depression, hypotension at peak exercise, or low working capacity) (see Chapter 4), and there are no obvious contraindications to revascularization, coronary angiography should be carried out.

In patients in whom the ECG is uninterpretable because of resting ST–T-wave abnormalities, digitalis therapy, or left bundle branch block, rest and exercise radionuclide myocardial perfusion scintigraphy (with thallium or sestamibi) or rest and exercise echocardiography should be performed. Patients who cannot exercise should undergo a pharmacologic stress imaging study such as adenosine or dipyridamole myocardial perfusion scintigraphy or echocardiography with dobutamine stress. A marked abnormality in any of these tests, or a resting ejection fraction below 40%, measured by echocardiography or a radionuclide technique, should be followed by coronary angiography.

Ambulatory ECG monitoring (Holter monitoring) for ischemia or arrhythmia was widely employed in the past, but it is not recommended for routine management. It may be useful in patients who have experienced symptomatic arrhythmias.

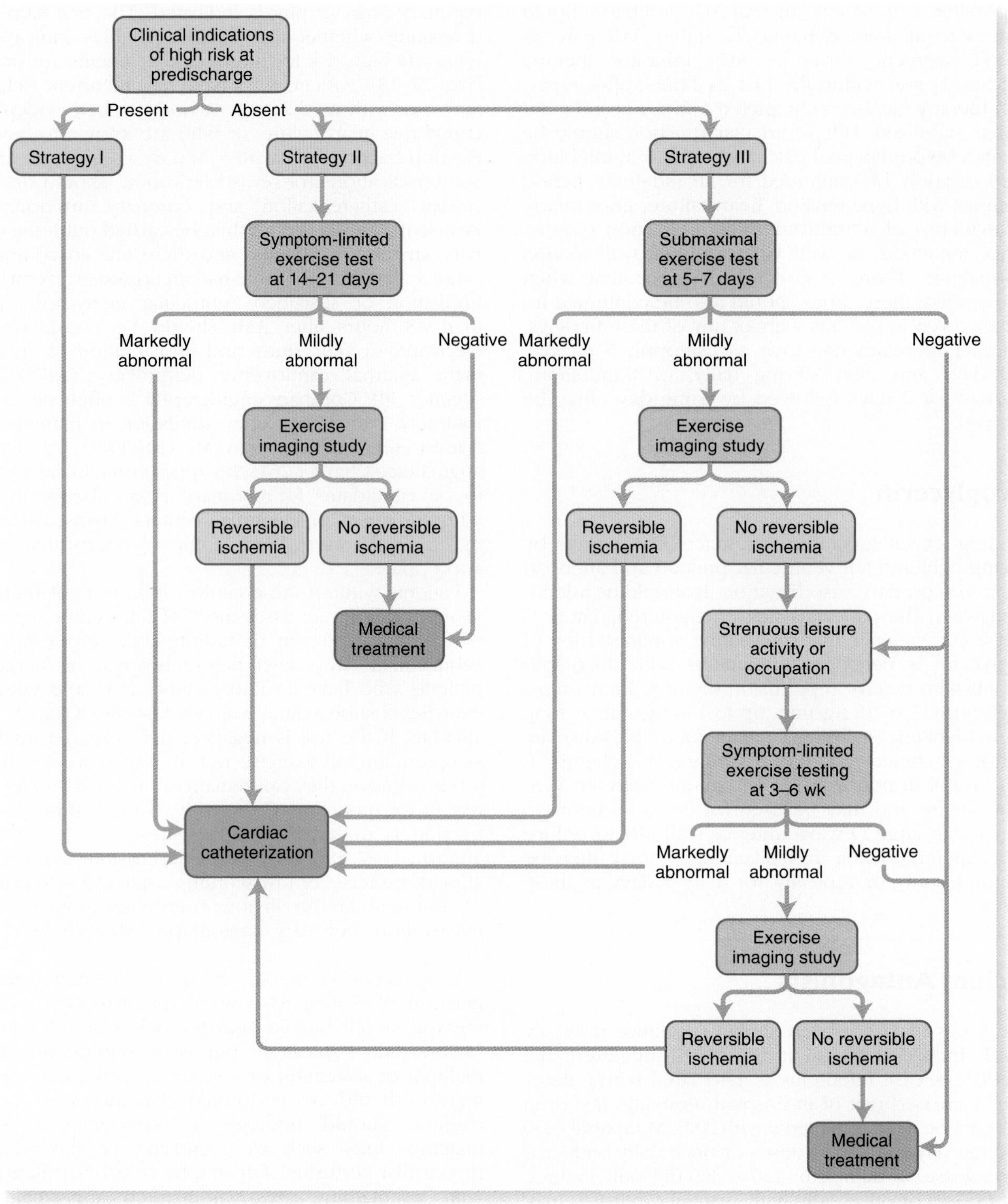

Clinical indications of high risk at predischarge

Present — Absent

Strategy I

Strategy II

Strategy III

Symptom-limited exercise test at 14–21 days

Submaximal exercise test at 5–7 days

Markedly abnormal

Mildly abnormal

Negative

Markedly abnormal

Mildly abnormal

Negative

Exercise imaging study

Exercise imaging study

Reversible ischemia

No reversible ischemia

Reversible ischemia

No reversible ischemia

Medical treatment

Strenuous leisure activity or occupation

Symptom-limited exercise testing at 3–6 wk

Cardiac catheterization

Markedly abnormal

Mildly abnormal

Negative

Exercise imaging study

Reversible ischemia

No reversible ischemia

Medical treatment

FIGURE 27–13. Management algorithm for risk stratification after acute myocardial infarction (MI). Patients with clinical indicators of high risk at hospital discharge (*left*), such as recurrent ischemia at rest or depressed left ventricular function, should be considered candidates for revascularization and referral to cardiac catheterization for ultimate triage to either angioplasty/coronary artery bypass graft surgery or medical therapy and risk factor reduction. Patients with life-threatening arrhythmias, such as sustained ventricular tachycardia or ventricular fibrillation should be considered for diagnostic cardiac catheterization, electrophysiology study, and management with implantation of a cardioverter-defibrillator either alone or in conjunction with amiodarone (strategy I). Patients without indicators of high risk at hospital discharge can be evaluated either with a symptom-limited exercise test at 14 to 21 days (strategy II) or a submaximal exercise test before discharge (strategy III). Patients with a negative exercise test or no evidence of reversible ischemia on an exercise imaging study can be managed with medical therapy and risk factor reduction. (From Ryan TJ, Antman EM, Brooks NH, et al: 1999 Update: ACC/AHA Guidelines for the Management of Patients with Acute Myocardial Infarction: Executive Summary and Recommendations. A Report of the American College of Cardiology/American Heart Association Task Force on Practice Guidelines [Committee on Management of Acute Myocardial Infarction]. Circulation 1999;100:1016–1030.)

Postdischarge Care

The primary care physician plays a critical role in postdischarge care and in the prevention of reinfarction. Perhaps most important is education regarding the nature of coronary artery disease and the risk factors for recurrent infarction. Lifestyle modifications are of paramount importance. These include smoking cessation. It should be emphasized to the patient that within 2 years of discontinuing smoking, the risk of a nonfatal recurrent MI falls to the level observed in patients who never smoked.

Cardiac Rehabilitation

This includes an organized program of exercise training and education about coronary risk factor modification, an American Heart Association Step I diet, smoking cessation, and weight optimization. These measures have been shown to improve the quality of life, reduce ischemic symptoms, and lower the incidence of subsequent coronary events. Because mortality is higher in patients after AMI without social support, every effort should be made to provide such support. This includes not only strengthening family ties but also encouraging participation in group activities and, whenever possible, return to work. Unless the patient is limited by symptoms of ischemia or heart failure, physical activity should be encouraged on hospital discharge. Physical conditioning programs should be undertaken; level walking, biking, and light calisthenics should be increased progressively. A negative, symptom-limited stress test at 3 to 6 weeks after discharge can be taken as a signal to increase physical activities to include swimming, rapid walking, and jogging. It is useful for the exercise to be undertaken as part of an organized rehabilitation program that includes instruction in diet, achievement of optimal weight, and smoking cessation. In patients with a mildly abnormal symptom-limited exercise test at 3 to 6 weeks, physical activity should be encouraged, but not to the level that will regularly provoke symptoms of ischemia.

Hypertension (see also Chapter 19)

It is imperative to treat post-MI hypertension. In view of the long-term benefits of ACE inhibitors and beta-blockers in these patients, this combination of antihypertensive drugs is preferred. A third agent, usually a diuretic, is added if hypertension persists despite treatment with the combination. The major long-term side effect of ACE inhibitors is cough, and if it develops, the dose may be reduced (e.g., lisinopril, 10 mg to 5 mg). The major side effects of long-term beta-adrenergic blockers are fatigue, depression, and sexual dysfunction.

Lipid-Lowering Therapy (see also Chapter 20)

A lipid profile should be obtained on all patients with MI. Because cholesterol levels may fall after 24 to 48 hours, it is important that these measurements be obtained on admission, otherwise a 6-week wait is necessary for the cholesterol to reach pre-MI levels. It is desirable to fractionate the cholesterol. The National Cholesterol Education Program has suggested that the target LDL be below 100 mg/dL.[18] Diet is a mandatory component of cholesterol lowering with the American Heart Association Step I diet. Three large randomized trials[18] have shown that the incidence of recurrent coronary events can be reduced with statin therapy in post-MI patients and these drugs are very helpful in achieving reductions of cholesterol. Patients with LDL at target levels (<100 mg/dL) with low HDL and/or elevated triglycerides should be considered for fibrate or niacin therapy. Compliance with diet and pharmacotherapy is enhanced if therapy is begun before hospital discharge.

Medical Therapy

The greatest mortality benefit from chronic beta-blockade is observed in patients with impaired ventricular function and ventricular arrhythmias. In the absence of contraindications (see Box 27–10), a beta-blocker and aspirin 160 or 325 mg/day[19] should also be continued indefinitely. Treatment with an ACE inhibitor for an indefinite period is strongly recommended in patients with evidence of congestive heart failure, an ejection fraction below 40%, or a large regional wall motion abnormality, and should be considered in all post-MI patients.

The widespread use of aspirin has greatly diminished the need for warfarin in the post-MI patient. At the present time, the latter is limited to secondary prevention of infarction in patients who are unable to take aspirin, to those with persistent or paroxysmal atrial fibrillation or a documented left ventricular thrombus, or to those with extensive wall motion abnormality.

Class I *antiarrhythmic drugs* should not be used routinely prophylactically in post-MI patients with frequent and complex ventricular ectopy. Patients with severe *symptomatic* ventricular tachyarrhythmias should be treated with beta-blockers, undergo screening for provokable ischemia, and be considered for specialized procedures such as implantation of antitachycardia devices or ablation of arrhythmogenic foci (see Chapter 30).

Evidence-Based Summary

1. A systematic review involving 18,773 patients with acute MI in placebo-controlled trials showed that aspirin was associated with absolute and relative reductions of 2.4% and 21%, respectively, for death of any cause, 1.2% and 5.5%, respectively, for nonfatal reinfarction, and 0.2% and 41%, respectively, for nonfatal stroke. All of these reductions were statistically significant.[19]

   In the absence of aspirin allergy, aspirin (160 mg or 326 mg) should be chewed or swallowed immediately and continued for several years.

2. In a systematic review involving 58,600 patients with MI or suspected MI in placebo-controlled trials, fibrinolytic therapy was associated with absolute and relative reductions of mortality in 30 days of 1.9% and 18%, respectively. Greatest absolute reduction occurred in patients with anterior infarcts (3.7%) versus inferior infarcts (0.8%).[20] The benefit was greater the earlier treatment was administered, with risk reduction falling by 0.16% with each hour that therapy was delayed.[21] The risk of hemorrhagic stroke averaged 0.51% with streptokinase, 0.72% with t-PA.[22] Independent predictors for intracranial hemorrhage were age older than 65 years, weight less than 70 kg, hypertension on admission, history of cerebral vascular disease, and use of t-PA.[23]

   In the absence of contraindications fibrinolytic therapy should be administered immediately to patients with ST elevation MI or bundle branch block.

3. In a systematic review of 54,234 patients enrolled into 82 randomized trials of beta-blockade in acute MI,[24] there was a relative reduction of 23% in mortality over 6 to 48 months. Older patients and those with large infarcts demonstrated the greatest benefit.

   In patients without contraindication to these agents (see Box 27–10) beta-blockers should be administered within hours of the development of acute MI and continued for several years.

4. In an overview involving 98,496 patients with acute MI randomized to an angiotensin converting enzyme (ACE) inhibitor or placebo, 30-day mortality was reduced by 0.5%, with absolute benefit greater in patients with Killip class II to III, tachycardia (>100 beats/min), and anterior infarction.[25]

   In the absence of contraindications, ACE inhibitor should be initiated within the first 24 hours in patients with acute MI.

5. In a systematic review of 2606 patients with acute MI enrolled into 10 randomized trials of percutaneous transluminal coronary angioplasty (PTCA) or fibrinolytic therapy, the absolute reduction of mortality with PTCA was 2.1% and there was a 42% relative reduction of death or reinfarction.

   Primary PTCA, when carried out promptly and by experienced operators, is at least as effective as, and possibly more effective than, fibrinolytic therapy in reducing death, reinfarction, and hemorrhagic stroke in acute MI.

References

1. American Heart Association: 2002 Heart and Stroke Statistical update. Dallas, American Heart Association, 2002.
2. Antman EM, Braunwald E: Acute myocardial infarction. In Braunwald E (ed): Heart Disease, 6th ed. Philadelphia, WB Saunders, 2001, pp 1114–1231.
3. Kinch JW, Ryan TJ: Right ventricular infarction. N Engl J Med 1994;30:1211.
4. The Joint European Society of Cardiology/American College of Cardiology Committee: Myocardial infarction redefined—a consensus document of the Joint European Society of Cardiology/American College of Cardiology Committee for the redefinition of myocardial infarction. J Am Coll Cardiol 2000;36:959.
5. Braunwald E, Antman EM, Beasley JW, et al: ACC/AHA guidelines update for the management of patients with unstable angina and non-ST segment elevation myocardial infarction. J Am Coll Cardiol 2002;40:1366.
6. Morrison LJ, Verbeejk PR, McDonald AC et al: Mortality and prehospital thrombolysis for acute myocardial infarction: A meta-analysis. JAMA 2000;283:2686.
7. Fibrinolytic Therapy Trialists' (FTT) Collaborative Group: Indications for fibrinolytic therapy in suspected acute myocardial infarction collaborative overview of early mortality and major morbidity results from all randomized trials of more than 1000 patients. Lancet 1994;343:311.
8. ASSENT-2 Investigators: Single-bolus tenecteplase compared with front-loaded alteplase in acute myocardial infarction: The ASSENT-2 double-blind randomized trial. Lancet 1999;354:716.
9. Menon V, Berkoqitz SD, Antman E, et al: New heparin dosing recommendations for patients with acute coronary syndromes. Am J Med 2001;110:641.
10. Grines CL, Browne KF, Marco J, et al: A comparison of immediate angioplasty with thrombolytic therapy for acute myocardial infarction. The Direct Angioplasty in Myocardial Infarction Study Group. N Engl J Med 1993;328:673.
11. Canto JG, Every NR, Magid DJ, et al: The volume of primary angioplasty procedures and survival after acute myocardial infarction. National Registry of Myocardial Infarction 2 Investigators. N Engl J Med 2000;342:1573.
12. Montalescot G, Barragan P, Wittenberg O, et al: for the ADMIRAL Investigators: Platelet glycoprotein IIb/IIIa inhibition with coronary stenting for acute myocardial infarction. N Engl J Med 2001;344:1895.
13. Hochman JS, Sleeper LA, Webb JG, et al: Early revascularization in acute myocardial infarction complicated by cardiogenic shock. Should we emergently revascularize

occluded coronaries for cardiogenic shock? N Engl J Med 1999;341:625.

14. Enshaw BS, Granger CB, Birnbaum Y, et al: Risk factors, angiographic patterns, and outcomes in patients with ventricular septal defect complicating acute myocardial infarction. Circulation 2000;101:27.
15. Sadowski ZP, Alexander JH, Skrabucha B, et al: Multicenter randomized trial and a systematic overview of lidocaine in acute myocardial infarction. Am Heart J 1999;137:792.
16. Slater J, Brown RJ, Antonelli TA, et al: Cardiogenic shock due to cardiac free-wall rupture or tamponade after acute myocardial infarction: A report from the SHOCK Trial Registry. J Am Coll Cardiol 2000;36(3 suppl A): 1117.
17. Latini R, Maggioni AP, Flather M, et al: ACE inhibitor use in patients with myocardial infarction: Summary of evidence from clinical trials. Circulation 1995;92:3132.
18. Expert Panel on Detection, Evaluation and Treatment of High Blood Cholesterol in Adults: Executive summary of the third report of the National Cholesterol Education Program (NCEP) expert panel on detection, evaluation, and treatment of high blood cholesterol in adults (adult treatment panel III). JAMA 2001;285:2486.
19. Antiplatelet Trialists Collaboration: Collaborative overview of randomized trials of antiplatelet therapy I: Prevention of death, myocardial infarction, and stroke by prolonged antiplatelet therapy in various categories of people. Br Med J 1994;308:81–106.
20. Collins R, Peto R, Baigent BM, Sleight DM: Aspirin, heparin and fibrinolytic therapy in suspected acute myocardial infarction. N Engl J Med 1997;336:847–860.
21. The GUSTO Investigators: An international randomized trial comparing four thrombolytic strategies for acute myocardial infarction. N Engl J Med 1993;329:673–682.
22. Berkowitz SD, Granger CB, Pieper KS, et al: Incidence and predictors of bleeding after contemporary thrombolytic therapy for myocardial infarction. Circulation 1997;95:2508–2516.
23. Freemantle N, Cleland J, Young P, et al: Beta-blockade after myocardial infarction: systematic review and meta regression analysis. Br Med J 1999;318:1730–1737.
24. ACE Inhibitor Myocardial Infarction Collaborative Group: Indications for ACE inhibitors in the early treatment of acute myocardial infarction: Systematic overview of individual data from 100,000 patients in randomized trials. Circulation 1998;97:2201–2212.
25. Weaver WD, Simes RJ, Betriu A, et al: Comparison of primary coronary angioplasty and intravenous thrombolytic therapy for acute myocardial infarction: A quantitative review. JAMA 1997;1278:2093–2098.

CHAPTER 28 Recognition and Management of Patients with Heart Failure

Lynne Warner Stevenson

Heart failure is commonly defined as a condition in which an abnormality in cardiac function is responsible for the inability of the heart to pump the quantity of blood required for ordinary activity from a normal filling pressure. Heart failure affects approximately 1% to 2% of the population. In most Western nations, heart failure accounts for 3% of the entire national health care budget, with 60% to 70% of that cost resulting from hospitalization. Now that medical therapies have been shown to improve survival and diminish the need for hospitalization in all stages of heart failure, identification and diligent treatment of these patients have become especially important.[1–3] The primary care physician is likely to continue to play a vital role in the recognition and routine ongoing care of many of these patients.

DIAGNOSIS AND ASSESSMENT

The first step is to identify a patient with heart failure (Table 28–1). Patients with a history of myocardial infarction, valvular heart disease, or severe hypertension merit particular vigilance for evidence of heart failure. The possibility of heart failure should be considered in any patient with reduced exercise tolerance, although many other causes may be responsible for this symptom. The symptoms and signs of elevated filling pressure at rest (e.g., orthopnea, edema, jugular venous distention) are more specific but generally occur later in the disease. Many patients with chronic pulmonary disease in whom the concomitant diagnosis of heart failure is missed receive months of bronchodilator therapy for presumed exacerbation of bronchoconstriction. Patients with abdominal pain secondary to congestive hepatomegaly caused by heart failure may undergo extensive gastrointestinal evaluation unless the signs of elevated right heart pressure are appreciated. These symptoms and signs of heart failure occur in both patients with low ejection fraction (systolic dysfunction) and those with preserved ejection fraction (diastolic dysfunction causing abnormalities in cardiac filling and relaxation) (see later).

A bedside assay for brain natriuretic peptide (BNP), which is secreted from the ventricles under stress, has been proposed as a sensitive assay to rule out cardiac disease as a cause of dyspnea of unknown etiology.[4] Sufficient experience has not yet accrued to determine the reliability of this assay outside investigational settings.

TABLE 28–1

Clinical Evidence Suggesting the Diagnosis of Heart Failure

Type of Evidence	Highly Suggestive	Less Specific
Symptoms	Orthopnea	Decreased exercise tolerance
	Paroxysmal nocturnal dyspnea	Nocturnal cough Discomfort when bending
Signs	Jugular venous distention S_3 gallop Displaced left ventricular impulse Rales Narrow pulse pressure Pulsatile hepatomegaly	Tachycardia Hypotension Ascites Peripheral edema
Chest radiograph	Cardiomegaly	Pleural effusion
Screening laboratory tests	Elevated natriuretic peptide level	
Response to diuretics	Decreased orthopnea Improved exercise tolerance Rapid weight loss >3 lb without dizziness	

S_3, third heart sound. Adapted from Kannel WB, Belander AJ: Epidemiology of heart failure. Am Heart J 1991;1221:951.

History

The cardinal symptoms and signs of heart failure generally reflect the hemodynamic abnormalities. They initially occur during heavy exertion, then during routine activity, and ultimately at rest (see Table 3–2). The severity of heart failure has traditionally been scored by the New York Heart Association (NYHA) classification and the Specific Activity (Goldman) scale (see Table 3–2). When heart failure progresses slowly to the symptomatic stage, the first symptom is often *exertional dyspnea* (see Chapter 7) or *fatigue*. At the initial evaluation and at each subsequent visit, the duration and frequency of activity responsible for these symptoms should be elicited. Specific questions could include the number of blocks that the patient can walk, tolerance for climbing stairs, and difficulty with routine chores such as making the bed and getting the mail. An inability to dress without stopping to rest usually signifies the presence of severe heart failure. Patients with severe limitation of exercise but no clinical evidence of cardiac disease require elicitation of a careful history to identify other causes of fatigue such as pulmonary disease or anemia.

Orthopnea is the symptom most sensitive to baseline elevation of left ventricular filling pressure.[5] Though usually described as dyspnea in the recumbent position, orthopnea may occasionally be manifested as nocturnal cough or severely disturbed sleep. The spouse may describe *Cheyne-Stokes* respirations (cyclical hyperventilation and hypoventilation or apnea) during the patient's sleep. *Paroxysmal nocturnal dyspnea* also reflects severely elevated left ventricular filling pressure that may be present chronically or episodically, such as during episodes of myocardial ischemia. Many patients with systemic venous congestion describe anorexia, early satiety, or abdominal discomfort. These gastrointestinal symptoms can occur even in the absence of edema or ascites but are often accompanied by hepatomegaly.

The history should also include questions related to the cause of the heart failure. For example, does the patient have a history of myocardial infarction or a heart murmur in childhood that could be indicative of congenital heart disease? Has early coronary artery disease, an enlarged heart, arrhythmias, or sudden death suggesting genetic abnormalities associated with either coronary artery disease or cardiomyopathy developed in family members? Patients with heart failure should also be questioned about symptoms suggestive of transient cerebral ischemic attacks or peripheral embolic events from intracardiac thrombi. In addition, any history of cardiac arrest, syncope or presyncope, unexplained dizziness, or sustained palpitations should raise concern regarding cardiac dysrhythmias, which in patients with heart failure generally warrant immediate evaluation by a specialist.

Physical Examination (Box 28–1)

The cardiovascular examination should include a careful assessment of vital signs. The arterial pulse should be examined for rhythm, intensity, and pulsus alternans, which often indicates severe left ventricular dysfunction. Postural vital signs should be measured in any patient complaining of dizziness or weakness when standing or walking and should be routinely monitored during adjustment of therapy with diuretics, angiotensin-converting enzyme (ACE) inhibitors, and

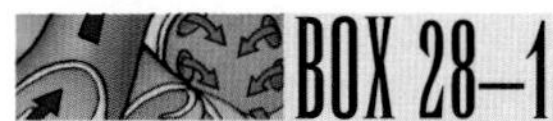
BOX 28–1

Physical Findings in Patients with Heart Failure

VITAL SIGNS
Pulse rate, rhythm, and quality
Determination of proportional pulse pressure
Blood pressure response to the Valsalva maneuver
Positional blood pressure
Respiratory rate, depth, and periodicity
Temperature

CARDIOVASCULAR SIGNS
Elevated jugular venous pressure
Abdominojugular neck vein reflex
Cardiomegaly on palpation/percussion
Chest wall pulsatile activity
Gallop rhythm on auscultation
Heart murmurs
Diminished S_1 or S_2
Prominent P_2
Friction rub
Peripheral pulses
Temperature of extremities

NEUROLOGIC SIGNS
Mental status abnormalities

PULMONARY SIGNS
Rales
Rhonchi
Friction rub
Wheezes
Dullness to percussion

ABDOMINAL SIGNS
Ascites
Hepatosplenomegaly
Pulsatile liver
Decreased bowel sounds
Ileus

SYSTEMIC SIGNS
Edema
Cachexia
Petechiae/ecchymoses
Rash
Arthritis

P_2, second pulmonic heart sound; S_1, first heart sound; S_2, second heart sound.
Adapted from Young JB: Assessment of Heart Failure. *In* Colucci WS (vol ed): Cardiac Function and Dysfunction. In Braunwald E (series ed): Atlas of Heart Failure, 2nd ed. Philadelphia, Current Medicine 1999, p 7.6.

beta-blockers. A decline of over 10 mm Hg in systolic blood pressure with standing rarely occurs in patients with heart failure unless they have hypovolemia, excessive vasodilator effect, or autonomic neuropathy such as may be seen in amyloidosis or in some elderly patients. In addition to auscultation of the lungs for rales, rhonchi, wheezes, or effusion, the respiratory rate and depth and any periodic respiratory pattern should be observed. Other components of the directed examination should focus on potential causes of the heart failure (systemic disease such as thyrotoxicosis or alcoholism), exacerbating factors such as infection, and indications of the severity of disease such as cachexia.

Clinical Assessment of the Resting Hemodynamic Profile

Based on both the history and physical examination, patients can rapidly be classified according to the presence or absence of congestion or compromised perfusion[6] (Fig. 28–1). Patients frequently have a profile of normal filling pressure and perfusion despite a depressed left ventricular ejection fraction. Ventricular filling pressure can be normal or elevated regardless of cardiac output, whereas cardiac output can be normal or depressed regardless of filling pressure. Many patients with a low ejection fraction can still maintain normal or near-normal stroke volume with ventricular dilatation, whereas some patients with a normal ejection fraction may have a low stroke volume if the ventricular cavity is small. Heart failure can be characterized by four clinical profiles:

- No congestion with adequate resting cardiac output
- Congestion with adequate resting cardiac output
- Congestion with inadequate cardiac output
- No congestion with inadequate cardiac output[6]

The last profile occurs predominantly in patients with heart failure who have received intensive diuretic therapy, but it may occasionally appear in patients with modest diuretic requirements.[7]

Elevated filling pressure in chronic heart failure is suggested by the presence of orthopnea (left ventricle) and jugular venous distention (right ventricle). Hepatic enlargement and pulsation confirm elevated right atrial pressure accompanied by tricuspid regurgitation. Rales (which may reflect alveolar edema) often develop in patients with new heart failure and an acute increase in pulmonary capillary wedge pressure to over 20 mm Hg. However, rales are often absent in patients with chronic heart failure despite left ventricular filling pressure that is chronically elevated to three times normal or even higher because the pulmonary lymphatic system can adapt chronically to increase alveolar fluid clearance 10- to 20-fold. Dyspnea and orthopnea, however, develop as a consequence of interstitial edema and the resultant decreased lung compliance, even in the absence of rales (see Chapter 7).

An inadequate cardiac output causing chronic hypoperfusion may not be apparent from the patient's general clinical appearance. However, cool extremities, altered mentation, and progressive deterioration in renal function, when present, suggest hypoperfusion at rest. Narrowing of the proportional pulse pressure ([systolic pressure—diastolic pressure]/systolic pressure) may be a helpful clue to severely reduced cardiac output.[5] A proportional pulse pressure below 25% suggests a

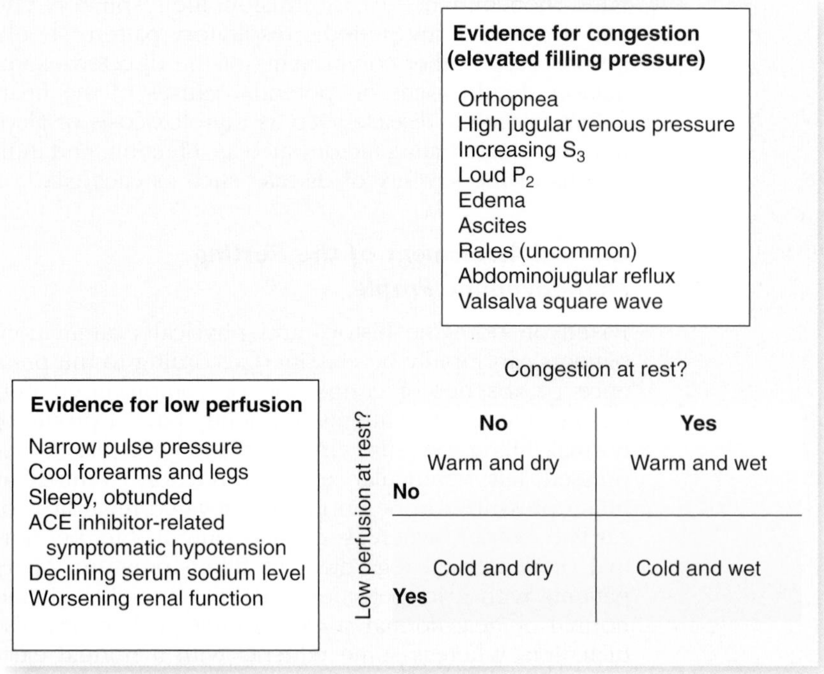

Evidence for congestion (elevated filling pressure)

Orthopnea
High jugular venous pressure
Increasing S_3
Loud P_2
Edema
Ascites
Rales (uncommon)
Abdominojugular reflux
Valsalva square wave

Evidence for low perfusion

Narrow pulse pressure
Cool forearms and legs
Sleepy, obtunded
ACE inhibitor-related symptomatic hypotension
Declining serum sodium level
Worsening renal function

Low perfusion at rest?	Congestion at rest? No	Congestion at rest? Yes
No	Warm and dry	Warm and wet
Yes	Cold and dry	Cold and wet

FIGURE 28–1. A 2 × 2 table of hemodynamic profiles for patients with heart failure. Most patients can be classified in a 2-minute bedside assessment according to the signs and symptoms shown. This classification helps guide initial therapy and the prognosis for patients with advanced heart failure.

cardiac index less than 2.2 L/min/m^2, which represents a critical level of decreased perfusion. In some older patients with low cardiac output, pulse pressure may be relatively preserved because of decreased vascular elasticity.

Laboratory Evaluation

The electrocardiogram (ECG) may provide clues to the cause and severity of heart failure. A completely normal ECG is rare in patients with symptomatic heart failure. Patients with left ventricular dilatation often exhibit an RV_6 greater than RV_5 and a tall R-wave (>11 mm) in aVL. Low voltage suggests chronic constrictive pericarditis, cardiac tamponade, severe chronic obstructive pulmonary disease, or cardiac amyloidosis. A myocardial infarct pattern with deep Q- or QS-waves suggests that ischemic heart disease is the cause of the heart failure. Poor R-wave progression in the precordial leads is common in both ischemic and nonischemic cardiomyopathy. Left bundle branch block or less specific intraventricular conduction delays can result from ischemic heart disease and also commonly occur in patients with nonischemic cardiomyopathy. The left ventricular voltage of hypertrophy and atrial abnormalities frequently occur in patients with the syndrome of heart failure and preserved ejection fraction. Sinus tachycardia (heart rate >100 beats/min) reflects the high sympathetic tone characteristic of cardiac decompensation and occurs more prominently in younger patients.

Echocardiography (see Chapter 5) provides considerable information without risk or discomfort and is a key test in the evaluation of patients with established or suspected heart failure.[1] The echocardiogram can be used to detect both systolic and diastolic dysfunction. Predominant systolic dysfunction is a more common cause of heart failure and is characterized by a low ejection fraction and dilated ventricle. However, almost half of cases of heart failure in elderly patients occur in the setting of a left ventricular ejection fraction greater than 40%, and ventricular hypertrophy and abnormalities in left ventricular relaxation and filling are frequently, but not always detectable in this population (see "Heart Failure in Special Patient Groups").[8]

A patient with newly diagnosed heart failure deserves specialized evaluation to determine the cause of the ventricular dysfunction and to guide further therapy directed toward decreasing progression of the disease and improving clinical status. Echocardiography often suggests potential causes of heart failure such as ischemic heart disease, primary valvular disease, or amyloidosis. Regional wall motion abnormalities on echocardiography can occasionally occur in nonischemic cardiomyopathy but strongly suggest coronary artery disease. Patients who have left ventricular dysfunction and symptoms suggestive of ischemia should undergo evaluation if their general condition renders them eligible for revascularization. Endomyocardial biopsy is not routinely indicated.

A chest radiograph may be the first image documenting the presence of cardiac disease, and it occasionally suggests the cause, as in left ventricular aneurysm, mitral stenosis, or congenital heart disease (see Chapter 13). Because the left ventricle often dilates in the anteroposterior direction, the cardiac silhouette may appear deceptively normal. Once heart failure is advanced, the enlarged right ventricle forms the left border of the cardiac silhouette. Enlargement of vessels to the upper lobes, fluid in the fissures, peribronchial cuffing, and pulmonary interstitial and alveolar edema are all indicative of pulmonary venous hypertension (Fig. 28–2). Measurement of thyroid-stimulating hormone, serum iron studies for hemochromatosis, and determination of the hematocrit may be helpful in the search for a cause (Table 28–2). Serologic testing for collagen vascular disease and human immunodeficiency virus is recommended in selected patients. Blood tests for electrolytes, renal and hepatic function, and coagulation studies can reflect the severity of the disease and are thus useful for management. Brain natriuretic peptide, the levels of which vary with alterations in intracardiac filling pressure, has been proposed as a marker of disease severity and response to therapy, but this application has not been adequately tested in general clinical settings.[4]

Potentially Reversible Factors

A careful search should be made for reversible or precipitating factors that could have caused or exacerbated the heart failure (Box 28–2). In many patients, symptomatic heart failure is precipitated by an acute disturbance that places an extra hemodynamic load on the heart, such as an infection or tachyarrhythmia. Perhaps the most frequent cause of reversible cardiac decompensation is nonadherence with the therapeutic regimen. An increase in dietary sodium intake or inappropriate discontinuation of medications can precipitate heart failure in patients with asymptomatic left ventricular dysfunction.

In patients with *ischemic heart disease* and new or worsening heart failure, the possibility of reversible ischemia causing myocardial hibernation should be considered.[1] Revascularization is often performed for angina or large areas of viable myocardium with impairment in blood flow at rest or low-level exercise. The benefit of revascularization is most clearly established when left ventricular dysfunction is accompanied by left main coronary artery disease or severe angina.

Although *hypertension* is now less common than previously as a cause of heart failure, it may be an important contributor, particularly in African Americans.[9] Even modest elevations in arterial pressure can further compromise a ventricle impaired by another process such as a previous myocardial infarction. Therefore, hypertension should be treated aggressively.

BOX 28–2

Potentially Reversible Factors in Heart Failure

- Nonadherence to the medical regimen
- Superimposed systemic infection
- Myocardial ischemia
- Primary valvular disease
- Tachycardias
- Hypertension
- Heavy alcohol consumption
- Cocaine, amphetamines, or excessive use of bronchodilators
- Anemia
- Hemochromatosis
- Thyroid disease (hyperthyroidism or hypothyroidism)
- Obesity
- Eating disorders (in particular consider hypocalcemia and hypophosphatemia)
- Pregnancy
- Medications exacerbating fluid retention
- Pulmonary embolism

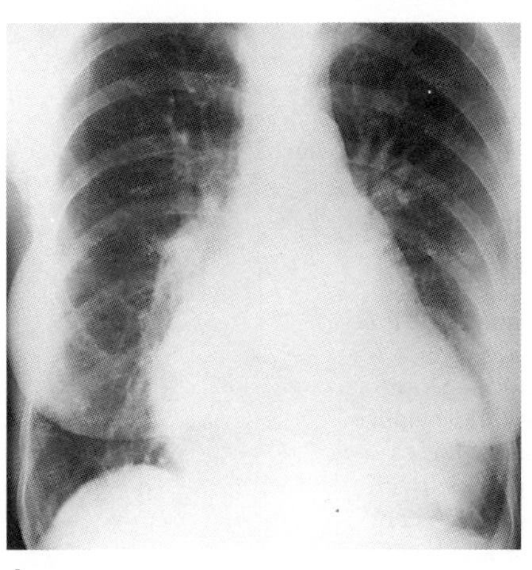

A

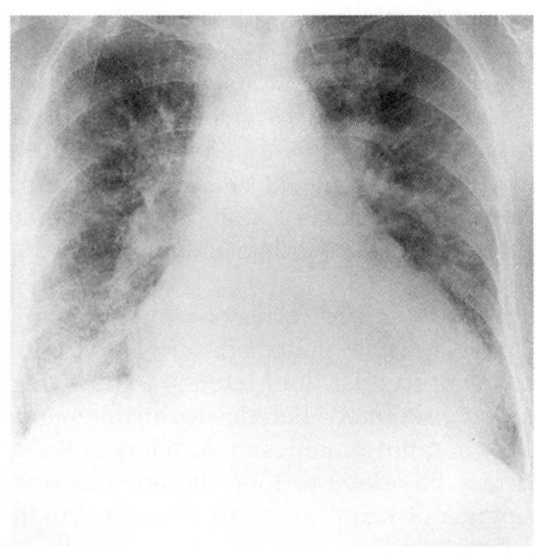

B

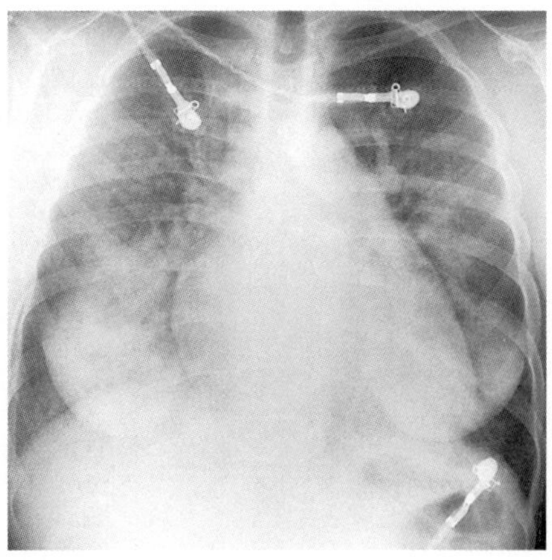

C

FIGURE 28–2. Cardiac radiograph in heart failure. *A,* Pulmonary blood flow redistribution showing enlargement of the upper lobe vessels with ischemic cardiomyopathy and elevated pulmonary pressure. *B,* Pulmonary interstitial edema. The vessels are indistinct and enlarged, and peribronchial cuffing is present. *C,* Pulmonary alveolar edema in a patient with clinical congestive heart failure. The central parahilar distribution of edema, termed *bat wing* edema, is typical of fluid overload from cardiovascular disease or other causes such as renal failure. (From Steiner RM, Levin DC: Radiology of the heart. In Braunwald E [ed]: Heart Disease, 5th ed. Philadelphia, WB Saunders, 1997, pp 204–239.)

TABLE 28–2

Selected Recommendations from Guidelines for Heart Failure

Topic	Recommendation	Strength of Evidence*
Initial evaluation	Patients with symptoms highly suggestive of heart failure should undergo echocardiography or radionuclide ventriculography to measure left ventricular function even if physical signs of heart failure are absent	C
Diagnostic testing	Practitioners should perform a chest radiograph; ECG; CBC; serum electrolytes, serum creatinine, serum albumin, and liver function tests; and urinalysis for all patients with suspected or clinically evident heart failure. A TSH level should also be checked in all patients with heart failure and no obvious cause and in patients who have atrial fibrillation or other signs or symptoms of thyroid disease Routine use of myocardial biopsy is not recommended, but it may be indicated in some cases to establish diagnoses with specific implications for subsequent therapy	C
Screening for arrhythmias	Screening evaluation for arrhythmias such as ambulatory ECG is not routinely warranted	A
Prevention in asymptomatic patients	Asymptomatic patients with moderately or severely reduced left ventricular systolic function (EF <35%–40%) should be treated with an ACE inhibitor	A
Activity recommendations	Regular exercise should be encouraged for all patients with stable NYHA class I–III heart failure	B
Diet	Dietary sodium should be limited to less than 4g, with more severe restriction to 2g daily in patients with persistent or recurrent fluid retention	C
ACE inhibitors	Patients with heart failure secondary to left ventricular systolic dysfunction should be given a trial of ACE inhibitors unless specific contraindications exist: (1) history of intolerance or adverse reactions to these agents, (2) serum potassium level >5.5 mEq/L that cannot be reduced, or (3) symptomatic hypotension. Patients with systolic blood pressure <90 mm Hg have a higher risk of complications and should be managed by a physician experienced in using ACE inhibitors in such patients Caution and close monitoring are also required for patients who have a serum creatinine level greater than 3.0 mg/dL or an estimated creatinine clearance of less than 30 mL/min	A
Angiotensin receptor blockers	Patients unable to tolerate ACE inhibitors because of disabling cough should be given a trial of angiotensin receptor antagonists. Patients unable to tolerate ACE inhibitors because of hypotension, hyperkalemia, or renal failure face similar risks from angiotensin receptor antagonists, which should not be prescribed for them	B
Beta-adrenergic blockers	Patients with stable heart failure should undergo initiation of therapy with a beta-adrenergic blocker unless specific contraindications exist: bradycardia with a heart rate lower than 60 beats/min, severe pulmonary disease with bronchospasm, systolic blood pressure <80 mm Hg, marked fluid retention, or recent need for intravenous therapy for heart failure decompensation. Beta-blockers should be initiated with low doses, patient education regarding potential side effects, and close supervision	A
Diuretics	Diuretics should be prescribed to restore and maintain as normal a fluid balance as possible. There is no indication for the use of diuretics for heart failure except to treat fluid retention and hypertension. Most patients who have required diuretics for maintenance of fluid balance will continue to require diuretics in addition to the other therapies	B
Spironolactone	Spironolactone may be added to loop diuretic therapy in patients with class IV symptoms of heart failure or class III symptoms after recent heart failure hospitalization. Specific contraindications are a current or recurrent history of hyperkalemia, serum creatinine level >2.0 mg/dL, and unstable renal function likely to deteriorate to a creatinine level >2.0 mg/dL. Potassium supplementation should be stopped or drastically reduced, with serum levels monitored closely during initiation and follow-up of spironolactone therapy	B

Topic	Recommendation	Strength of Evidence*
Digoxin	Digoxin is used routinely in patients with severe heart failure and added to the medical regimen of those with mild or moderate heart failure who remain symptomatic after optimal management with other medications	B
Hydralazine/isosorbide dinitrate	The combination of isosorbide dinitrate and hydralazine is an acceptable alternative in patients with contraindications or intolerance to ACE inhibitors and may be added as adjunctive therapy when symptoms persist despite aggressive therapy with ACE inhibitors and diuretics	B
Anticoagulation	Anticoagulation is not routinely recommended in the absence of atrial fibrillation, intracardiac thrombi, or previous embolic events	C

ACE, angiotensin-converting enzyme; CBC, complete blood count; ECG, electrocardiogram; EF, ejection fraction; NYHA, New York Heart Association; TSH, thyroid-stimulating hormone.

*Strength of evidence: A, good evidence of treatment from randomized trials; B, fair evidence; C, expert opinion.

Data from Hunt SA, Baker DW, Chin MH, et al: ACC/AHA guideline for the evaluation and management of chronic heart failure in the adult: Executive summary. A report of the American College of Cardiology/American Heart Association Task Force on Practice Guidelines (Committee to Revise the 1995 Guidelines for the Evaluation and Management of Heart Failure). J Am Coll Cardiol 2001;38:2101–2113.

Heavy alcohol consumption has been estimated to cause approximately 10% of all cases of dilated cardiomyopathy in adults and is probably underrecognized. Even two drinks daily may be sufficient to worsen heart failure in patients with left ventricular dysfunction of other cause. Illicit drug use may also contribute to cardiomyopathy. *Cocaine* may cause acute coronary syndromes but can also produce a chronic cardiomyopathy similar to that seen with pheochromocytoma.

Tachyarrhythmias can cause cardiomyopathy in otherwise normal hearts, but more frequently they aggravate left ventricular dysfunction of other cause. Atrial fibrillation, present in approximately 20% of patients with heart failure, is a major target for therapy because rates during exertion are often excessive. Conversion to sinus rhythm or at least aggressive rate control is often associated with marked clinical improvement.

Both *hyperthyroidism* and *hypothyroidism* may compromise cardiac function, and these conditions should therefore be considered, especially in patients receiving amiodarone because the iodine contained in this antiarrhythmic drug can cause these disorders. *Severe* obesity is the most common metabolic abnormality contributing to heart failure; weight loss often improves symptoms and sometimes the ejection fraction as well. Severe obesity may also be associated with sleep apnea, which can compromise cardiac function. *Pregnancy* may unmask previously asymptomatic heart disease, but it can also cause a cardiomyopathy (peripartum cardiomyopathy). *Anemia,* both acute and chronic, can precipitate decompensation in patients with previously stable left ventricular dysfunction.

Patients with heart failure are at risk for deep venous thrombosis and *pulmonary embolism* (see Chapter 38), which in turn can exacerbate heart failure and precipitate acute decompensation.

A variety of *drugs* may exacerbate heart failure. First-generation calcium antagonists have been associated with clinical deterioration and decreased survival in patients with heart failure. Usually prescribed for hypertension, angina, or control of the ventricular response in atrial fibrillation, these agents should be replaced by other therapies in most patients with cardiac decompensation. Antiarrhythmic agents that severely depress myocardial contractility, such as disopyramide and sotalol, may aggravate systolic heart failure. Beta-blockers are beneficial in many patients with heart failure (see later), but they may exacerbate heart failure when initiated rapidly or given in high doses or to patients with severe congestive symptoms. Nonsteroidal anti-inflammatory agents can cause fluid retention and deterioration in renal function and hence worsen the symptoms and signs of heart failure.

MANAGEMENT OF HEART FAILURE (FIG. 28–3)

The goals of therapy are to reduce the symptoms of heart failure, prevent or reverse progression of ventricular dysfunction, and prolong survival.[1] The relative importance of these goals varies with the presence and severity of the symptoms of heart failure. In the asymptomatic or mild stages of heart failure, emphasis is placed on arresting disease progression, whereas in later stages of decompensation, improving the quality as well as the length of life should be emphasized.[7] Exacerbating factors such as anemia or thyroid disease should be treated and monitored aggressively.

Asymptomatic Left Ventricular Dysfunction

An asymptomatic reduction in the left ventricular ejection fraction may be diagnosed by echocardiography or radionuclide angiography after cardiomegaly is found incidentally on a routine chest radiograph, during evaluation for a suspected arrhythmia or embolic event, or after referral for atypical chest pain. A history of myocardial infarction warrants screening to detect

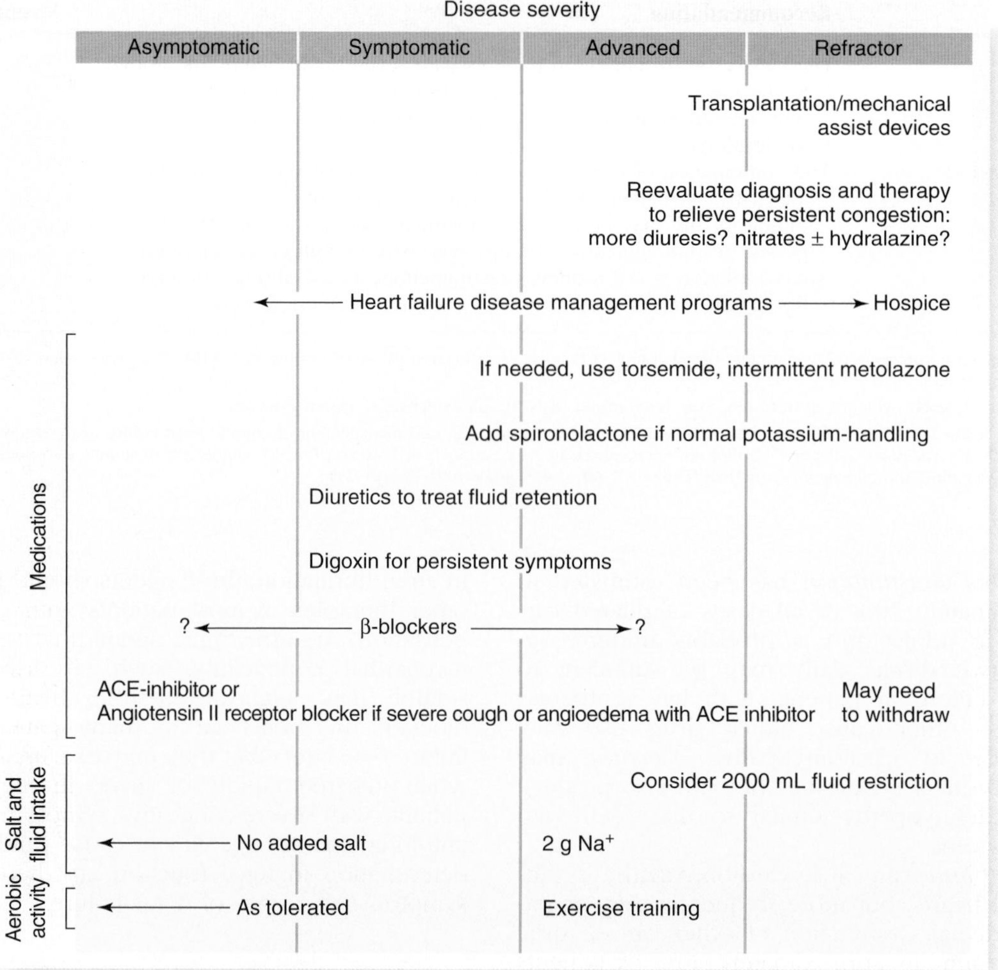

FIGURE 28–3. Step diagram demonstrating the addition of therapies in relation to the clinical severity of heart failure with a reduced left ventricular ejection fraction. Angiotensin-converting enzyme (ACE) inhibitors are prescribed at every level of disease severity. Angiotensin receptor blocking agents are a reasonable alternative for patients who cannot tolerate ACE inhibitors because of angioedema or severe cough. Beta-adrenergic blocking agents are prescribed for patients with mild to moderate symptoms of heart failure, but they are not initiated in patients with severe symptoms of heart failure unresponsive to stabilization with other therapies. Diuretics are prescribed to maintain fluid balance, with spironolactone added in patients with severely symptomatic disease when renal function and potassium handling are preserved. When severe symptoms persist, patients may benefit from the addition of nitrates with or without hydralazine. Transplantation and mechanical assist devices are relevant to only a very small population with advanced heart failure. Restriction of sodium and fluid intake is increasingly required as heart failure becomes more severe. Heart failure management programs are most cost-effective in patients at high risk for repeated heart failure hospitalization. (From Nohria A, Lewis E, Stevenson LW: Medical management of advanced heart failure. JAMA 2002;287:628–640.)

asymptomatic left ventricular dysfunction because such patients have been shown to benefit from intervention. ACE inhibitors are the only class of drugs that have clearly been demonstrated to benefit asymptomatic patients with left ventricular dysfunction.[10] Beta-blockers have been shown to improve outcomes in asymptomatic patients with depressed ventricular function after myocardial infarction, and their use is likely to extend to all stable patients with a left ventricular ejection fraction less than 40%.[11–13] It is critical that physicians provide appropriate therapy and monitoring for concomitant conditions to lower risk, administer lipid-lowering therapies for management of coronary artery disease and hypertension, and ensure careful control of diabetes to decrease progression to clinical heart failure.[1]

Symptomatic Heart Failure

The development of symptoms heralds a worsening prognosis for patients with left ventricular dysfunction. Therapy for symptomatic heart failure requires continual adjustment of medications and lifestyle to maximize clinical status, maintain freedom from congestion and postural hypotension, and establish optimal neurohormonal antagonism to improve the long-term outcome.

Relief of Congestion

After confirming the diagnosis and addressing potentially reversible factors, the approach to symptoms of heart failure requires assessment of the patient's hemodynamic profile as discussed previously (see Fig. 28–1). When symptoms or signs of excess circulating volume are observed, diuresis should be initiated with loop diuretics.[1] ACE inhibitors can be started but should not be titrated upward until fluid balance is re-established, except in patients with severe hypertension. As a general goal in patients with systolic heart failure, filling pressure should be reduced to the level at which orthopnea, edema, rales, and ascites are absent and jugular venous pressure is normal.[1] In patients with evidence of congestion without hypoperfusion (warm and wet, see Fig. 28–1), diuretic therapy is generally adequate to restore stability. Diuretic doses should be increased, with the addition of metolazone or another thiazide when necessary, until an adequate response is achieved.[7] When congestion is complicated by hypoperfusion, therapy to improve cardiac output with vasodilating or intravenous inotropic agents is often required to achieve adequate diuresis. In patients with heart failure and preserved ejection fraction,[8] optimal filling pressure may be higher than normal, but it is usually possible to achieve relief of symptomatic congestion at rest and during routine activity. Diuretic use may occasionally be discontinued when the underlying or exacerbating cause of heart failure resolves. In most cases, however, once needed, diuretic therapy should be continued in patients with chronic heart failure, but dosing regimens should be flexible to avoid recurrent fluid overload.[1,7]

Neurohormonal Antagonists—ACE Inhibitors and Beta-Blocking Agents

Symptoms of heart failure develop in some patients while already taking ACE inhibitors for previous hypertension or asymptomatic left ventricular dysfunction. In other patients, left ventricular dysfunction is not diagnosed until they have symptomatic heart failure. During acute decompensation, ACE inhibitors do not generally improve symptoms, but initiation is usually tolerated during diuresis unless it is accompanied by severe hypotension or renal dysfunction.

Beta-blockers are now recommended for all stable patients with heart failure secondary to systolic dysfunction, unless a specific contraindication is present (see later).[1] In contrast to ACE inhibitors, suppression of the adrenergic nervous system with beta-blockers more often causes acute clinical deterioration, particularly when patients have suspected congestion or hypoperfusion. Initiation of beta-blockers is not recommended in patients with decompensated heart failure; instead, they are deferred until re-establishment of good fluid balance and stable blood pressure.[1,13] Both ACE inhibitors and beta-blockers have been shown to improve symptoms over time, decrease left ventricular remodeling, decrease recurrent ischemic events, and prolong survival in patients with left ventricular dysfunction.

Maintenance of Perfusion

Systemic perfusion, which is a function of cardiac output, can usually be maintained even when the left ventricular ejection fraction is low. The "arithmetic of cardiac output" indicates that stroke volume can be preserved despite a low ejection fraction in the presence of ventricular dilatation. For example, in patients with chronic heart failure and a left ventricular ejection fraction one third of normal (20%), left ventricular end-diastolic volumes may exceed three times normal. Stroke volume is often normal or only marginally reduced, and a slight compensatory tachycardia may contribute to normal cardiac output at rest. However, as left ventricular dilatation progresses, functional mitral regurgitation often develops despite an anatomically normal mitral valve. This dynamic mitral regurgitation is very sensitive to changes in loading conditions and may cause a marked reduction in forward stroke volume. As heart failure progresses, similar factors operate on the right ventricle, with tricuspid regurgitation affecting right ventricular stroke volume. Systemic perfusion may also decline early when the ejection fraction falls acutely before compensatory dilatation has occurred; in addition, it may decline in diseases with a restrictive component that limits dilatation, such as radiation- or doxorubicin (Adriamycin)-induced cardiomyopathy.

Most patients with a low ejection fraction and impaired perfusion derive benefit from peripheral vasodilatation, which reduces both the load on the left ventricle and mitral regurgitation. When cardiac output is adequate to maintain perfusion, patients frequently tolerate systolic blood pressure that is lower than normal, as long as they do not have marked postural hypotension. Patients with severe heart failure may tolerate systolic pressure as low as 80 mm Hg with optimal medical therapy.[7] Older patients may be less able to tolerate such low blood pressure because of cerebrovascular disease, difficulty maintaining equilibrium while walking, and impaired autonomic postural responses. Patients with clinical evidence of poor perfusion at rest frequently have persistent limiting symptoms leading to referral for evaluation of advanced heart failure.[7]

Hospitalization for Heart Failure

Indications for hospital admission are summarized in Box 28–3. New heart failure symptoms of *rapid onset*, even if relatively mild, should be considered grounds for admission because deterioration can occur rapidly. Patients with substantial volume overload generally require admission to achieve safe and effective diuresis unless their fluid and electrolyte responses to high doses of diuretics have previously been well characterized and clinical evaluation can be repeated several

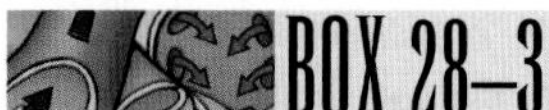

BOX 28–3

Indications for Hospital Admission in Patients with Heart Failure

Rapid onset of new symptoms of heart failure
New myocardial infarction or ischemia
Symptomatic arrhythmias
- Syncope or presyncope
- Cardiac arrest
- Multiple discharges from an implantable defibrillator
- Atrial fibrillation with exacerbated heart failure

Symptoms of cerebral ischemia or peripheral embolism events
Decompensation of chronic heart failure

NEED FOR IMMEDIATE HOSPITALIZATION

Pulmonary edema or respiratory distress in the sitting position
Arterial desaturation to <90% in the absence of a known cause of hypoxemia
Heart rate >120 beats/min (unless in chronic atrial fibrillation)
Systolic blood pressure <75 mm Hg
Decreased mentation attributed to hypoperfusion

NEED FOR URGENT HOSPITALIZATION

New evidence of simultaneous congestion and hypoperfusion
New development of severe hepatic distention, tense ascites, or anasarca
Decompensation in the presence of acutely worsening noncardiac conditions, such as pulmonary or renal disease or dysfunction

CONSIDER HOSPITALIZATION

Rapid fall in serum sodium to <130 mEq/L
Rising serum creatinine at least twofold to >2.5 mg/dL
Persistent symptoms of resting congestion despite repeated outpatient clinic visits

BOX 28–4

Expectations from Hospitalization for Heart Failure

Elucidation of the cause or exacerbating factors, if necessary
Plan of treatment for reversible conditions
Achievement of optimal fluid status and definition of "dry weight" or plan for achieving dry weight at home (often unsuccessful if not achieved before discharge)
Definition of optimal vasodilator doses and associated blood pressure limits
Institution of therapy for ischemia, if needed
Institution of therapy for arrhythmias, if needed
Adequate anticoagulation regimen, if indicated
Estimation of capacity for daily activity after discharge
Decision regarding home health care
Education of patient and family (see Box 28–6)
Provision of written information to the patient, including
- Wallet card indicating the diagnosis and medical regimen
- Written medication schedule
- Scheduled office evaluation in 5–10 days
- 24-hr phone number to reach medical staff familiar with the current regimen
- Instructions regarding indications for urgent call (see Box 28–5)

times weekly. Patients with evidence of fluid overload and hypoperfusion ("cold and wet") usually require multiple simultaneous adjustments in therapy that cannot be provided in an outpatient setting. Patients in whom worsening of congestion is accompanied by deteriorating renal function often need inpatient management, even if systemic perfusion otherwise appears to be well maintained.[7]

For patients admitted primarily for treatment of heart failure, the plan for hospitalization should include the components shown in Box 28–4. Routine use of intravenous inotropic infusions is discouraged because of the high incidence of arrhythmias and ischemic events and no sustained benefit.[7] However, when used, inotropic infusions should be discontinued at least 48 hours before discharge to determine the efficacy and tolerability of the planned oral regimen. Focus should be on re-establishment of fluid balance and redesign of the outpatient medical regimen to prevent readmission, which may be provided most effectively by a specialist or a team experienced in caring for such patients both in the hospital and during their transition after discharge (see later).

A major factor in achieving a successful outcome after discharge is the adequacy of patient education, including specific instructions about when to contact the medical care system (Box 28–5). These instructions should be provided in the hospital and reiterated after discharge. It is increasingly being recognized that after hospitalization for heart failure, patients should be monitored in a dedicated program of heart failure management, if available (see later), that can provide specialized physician, nurse, and in some cases, nutritionist support until the outpatient course becomes stable.[14]

Patient Education

Patient education about heart failure often emphasizes the necessary lifestyle restrictions imposed by this condition and reinforces the unfortunate concept of the "failure" of a vital organ. Rather than referring to the heart as "failing," it is more positive to refer to it as "handicapped" and to emphasize that handicaps require special provisions but can often be overcome. Too often, all the "don'ts" are covered first, and the "dos" are relegated to the last few minutes of the counseling

BOX 28–5

Specific Instructions to Patients Regarding When to Contact a Physician*

Weight gain ≥3 lb not responding to predesignated diuretic change
Uncertainty about how to increase diuretics
New swelling of the feet or abdomen
Worsening shortness of breath with mild exercise
Onset of inability to sleep flat in bed or awakening from sleep because of shortness of breath
Worsening cough
Persistent nausea/vomiting or inability to eat
Worsening dizziness or new spells of sudden dizziness not related to sudden changes in body position
Prolonged palpitations

If you, the patient, experience any sudden severe symptoms, you may need to call 911 or the equivalent emergency phone number to arrange a trip to the emergency room. (These sudden severe symptoms may include *but are not limited to* chest pain, severe shortness of breath, loss of consciousness not resulting from sudden standing, new cold or painful arm or foot, sudden new visual changes, or impairment in speech or strength in an extremity.)

**Note:* This is only a sample list and is not intended to include all potential problems for which a patient with heart failure should seek urgent medical advice.

BOX 28–6

Education of Patients and Family

GENERAL INFORMATION
Cause or probable cause of heart failure
Explanation of symptoms of heart failure
Patient as leader of the care team
Role of family members or other caregivers
Availability of a qualified local support group
Advisability of vaccinations against influenza

OUTLOOK WITH HEART FAILURE
Potential for good function and survival
Undulating disease course
Life expectancy
Advance directives
Family recognition of risk for sudden death

SELF-MONITORING
Heart failure diary
Daily measurement of weight
Home blood pressure monitoring, if appropriate
Surveillance for common symptoms
Instructions for when to contact the care team (see Box 28–5)

MEDICATIONS
Explanation and schedule of medications
Probable side effects and appropriate responses
Plan of diuretic adjustment for weight increase, with subsequent electrolyte management
Anticoagulation management, if necessary
Availability of less costly medications or financial assistance

DIET
Sodium restriction, label reading, and meal planning
Lipid restriction for patients with known vascular disease
General fluid limit (even if liberal)
Alcohol restriction or elimination

ACTIVITY
Recommendations for work, leisure activities
Regular aerobic activity
Sexual activity
Encouragement of midday rest period, if appropriate

session. Instead, the positive aspects of activity should be outlined prominently (Box 28–6).

Exercise/Activity

To avoid physical deconditioning, ambulatory patients with stable heart failure should be encouraged to participate in a regular program of specific, uninterrupted exercise at least 4 days a week (e.g., a walking program outdoors or in an enclosed mall during inclement weather). An exercise program can begin by asking the patient to walk at a comfortable pace for 10 minutes, with increases first in duration and then in speed. Stationary bicycles and home treadmills can be set at low workloads equivalent to walking. Heavy weightlifting and other significant isometric effort increase impedance to ventricular ejection and should *not* be part of the regimen. Daily activities such as housework and shopping are encouraged but are not equivalent to specific, uninterrupted exercise. An exercise prescription helps convince both the patient and family that the clinical condition is helped and not hurt by activity.

Many patients and families worry that the heart will be irreversibly damaged by prolonged activity during travel or family events. It may be helpful to reassure them that such activity is unlikely to injure the heart itself, although the patient may experience fatigue and need to compensate by decreasing activity the next day. Trials of exercise training in heart failure have consistently shown benefit.[14]

In general, patients without evidence of congestion at rest can safely participate in sexual activity. Dyspnea is less likely if pillows are used to elevate the chest and head. Some patients take 0.3 to 0.6 mg of sublingual nitroglycerin before sexual activity to reduce breathlessness.

In making recommendations regarding employment, heavy or sustained isometric work should be avoided, and patients should not routinely lift more than 20 lb. For patients working outside the home, extra rest on weekends is advisable, and it may sometimes be necessary to curtail professional, community, and family responsibilities to allow continued employment. Intermittent rest such as a scheduled nap or afternoon rest period each day is often helpful to prevent excessive fatigue. Recovery at home for several days is indicated after a bout of overt heart failure.

Sodium and Fluid Restriction

After having emphasized what patients *can* do, it is necessary to be very firm about restrictions on sodium and, in some cases, fluid intake.[6] For many patients, sodium restriction is perceived as a severe penalty, and considerable education and encouragement regarding other seasoning options are required. Patients with hypertension or early left ventricular dysfunction should be advised to avoid adding salt at meals and should limit their intake of salty foods such as potato chips, cheese, and canned soup. Once the daily furosemide requirement exceeds 80 mg, patients should limit their daily sodium intake to 2 g, which can be accomplished by emphasis on fresh foods and careful attention to labels on packaged food. If patients remain clinically stable for more than 3 months without any need for frequent adjustment of diuretics, they may *occasionally* indulge in pizza or "fast" food. However, they should be warned to watch their weight closely after such exceptions. Though not encouraged, such transgressions, when carefully managed in stabilized patients, may ultimately lead to better overall quality of life and adherence to therapy.

Even before heart failure becomes severe, patients should understand that their ability to excrete an excess fluid load is impaired. Patients with frequent exacerbations of heart failure may require lower doses of diuretics and fewer hospitalizations when limited to 2 qt of fluid intake daily. The fluid content of fruits should be estimated and included. Tighter restrictions may be necessary when the serum sodium concentration is below 125 mEq/L, which frequently requires in-hospital management. To make the most of a limited fluid allotment, patients should drink fluids other than water and may want to include ice, frozen juice, and frozen grapes as part of their daily fluid intake.

Other Dietary Restrictions

Alcohol consumption should be restricted in all patients with a reduced left ventricular ejection fraction because decrements in left ventricular function can be detected after the consumption of even one alcoholic beverage. Recommendations vary from complete abstinence to no more than one to two alcoholic beverages per week. Patients with alcoholic cardiomyopathy must abstain completely.

Most patients whose heart failure is associated with ischemic heart disease should be counseled about the need to reduce their intake of fat and cholesterol. An American Heart Association Step I diet is indicated in such patients, although during periods of acute decompensation and shortly thereafter, the risk from fat intake assumes a lower priority.

Adherence to the Medical Regimen

Considerable work has been done to determine the causes and correction of nonadherence to the medical regimen. The complexity and cost of the medication schedule are major factors, as are a lack of education and understanding about the disease and poor social and family support.[6] Simplification of the regimen may represent a positive tradeoff for some patients if adherence is improved over that with a regimen more parallel to those tested in large trials.

Predicting Survival

Patients with heart failure and their families seek and deserve to know the prognosis. However, even specialists in the field are repeatedly humbled by their inability to predict how long these patients will survive. Therefore, it is a disservice to cite a specific period of time during which patients and family unconsciously count down the days, at the end of which nothing happens. If it seems essential to provide a range, the cliché of "less than 6 months to live" should be avoided, and instead, the longest possible range in which the outcome could be positive should be offered—"Many patients like you are alive over a year later." At the same time, it is vital to inform families that a patient with serious heart disease can die suddenly at any time. Although the specter of sudden death is often frightening, it is important to inform patients and families at the outset that half of all deaths in patients with heart failure are sudden. This expectation may allow important conversations to take place in time and also prevent years of self-recrimination for a sudden death that occurred after traveling, arguing, or bringing in the groceries. It is important for patients to prepare and update advance directives regarding their preferences for life-sustaining therapies.[6,7]

Clinical status remains the strongest predictor of survival. In patients with NYHA class I or II heart failure, the average annual mortality is 5% to 10%, depending on the index event. Those in NYHA class III have an annual mortality of approximately 20%, whereas patients with persistent class IV symptoms have an annual mortality of 50% or greater. Even after the development of class IV symptoms, the potential for improvement is illustrated by the experience with ambulatory patients awaiting cardiac transplantation, up to one third of whom may improve sufficiently to leave the transplant list for a quality of life and 2-year survival that are equivalent to that attained after transplantation.

In patients with mild to moderate symptoms of heart failure, the left ventricular ejection fraction is a strong prognostic indicator, with a predicted 3-year mortality of almost 50% in patients with an ejection fraction less than 20% and a mortality of approximately 25% with an ejection fraction between 30% and 35%. Although the prognosis for patients with predominantly diastolic dysfunction has not been well defined, overall mortality appears to be lower in this group than in those with systolic dysfunction.[8,16]

The prognosis is better in patients in whom acute decompensation has been precipitated by a specific event, such as infection, than in those in whom it appears to be related to progression of the underlying illness. The potential for spontaneous improvement in left ventricular function should also be recognized, particularly in patients with heart failure symptoms of recent onset. Such improvement is most likely for patients without ischemic heart disease, in whom an unrecognized viral infection may have caused reversible dysfunction.

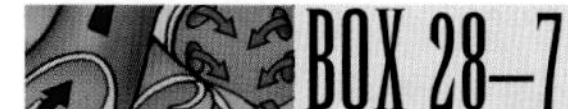
BOX 28–7

Clinic Flow Sheet for Chronic Heart Failure*

VITAL INFORMATION

Blood pressure (sitting, standing [after 3 min])
Heart rate (sitting, standing)
Clinic weight/home weight
Recent emergency department or hospital visits
Recent need for extra diuretics

CURRENT SYMPTOM STATUS

Routine activity level
Specific exercise
Limitation while dressing
Orthopnea/paroxysmal nocturnal dyspnea
Gastrointestinal symptoms
Angina
Palpitations/syncope
Symptoms of embolic events

CARDIOVASCULAR EXAMINATION (+ VITAL SIGNS ABOVE)

Jugular venous pressure
Peripheral edema
Ascites
Hepatomegaly
Lung sounds
Warmth of extremities
Change in S_3, S_4, or murmurs

SUMMARY

Fluid overload (yes/no)
Activity level (I–IV)
Compared with last visit (worse/same/better)
Clinically stable (yes/no)

*To be recorded at each encounter.
S_3, third heart sound; S_4, fourth heart sound.
Adapted from Grady KL, Dracup K, Kennedy G, et al: Team management of patients with heart failure. Circulation 2000;102:2443–2456.

Continuing Care

The most important aspect of continuing care in patients with heart failure is the ability to recognize early signs of clinical deterioration.[6] Symptoms of congestion and those suggestive of arrhythmias or embolic events should be sought. Syncope or other evidence of life-threatening arrhythmias in a patient with heart failure usually warrants hospital admission for specialized evaluation (see Box 28–4). Physicians who treat patients with chronic heart failure often find it helpful to maintain a specific flow sheet for both symptoms and signs (Box 28–7).

Interval Laboratory Evaluations

Electrolytes, creatinine, and blood urea nitrogen (BUN) should be measured within 24 to 48 hours of a major diuresis, after a major change in therapy, with the development of severe decompensation, and every 3 to 6 months in patients who are in stable, mild heart failure while receiving a constant target dose of an ACE inhibitor alone. Once major symptoms of heart failure have developed, serum sodium is a very sensitive indicator of the patient's overall state of compensation. A level below 134 mEq/L in a patient with major symptoms generally indicates that the heart failure is progressing and not likely to respond to simple adjustments in therapy. A serum sodium concentration of less than 125 mEq/L or a decline of 5 mEq/L to less than 130 mEq/L often warrants hospital admission. Magnesium levels should be determined initially and after major changes in the diuretic regimen.

A white blood cell count should be obtained before and after ACE inhibitor therapy is begun to check for the rare case of agranulocytosis. The hematocrit should be determined when a stable patient deteriorates. The ECG does not generally need to be repeated at every visit, except in patients receiving antiarrhythmic therapy (to check the QT interval) or when recent symptoms suggest ischemia or arrhythmias. Chest radiographs are not routinely necessary during follow-up but may be useful for identifying pneumonia or other pulmonary processes that may be causing exacerbations of dyspnea.

Once the clinical assessment and routine laboratory tests are completed, it is important to synthesize the information into an overall assessment of volume status and stability.[6] If changes in the medical regimen are required, they should be made gradually, if possible. For example, for postural hypotension in the absence of suspected hypovolemia, vasodilator doses can be decreased by 25%. For suspected volume depletion, the diuretic can be stopped for 1 or 2 days and restarted at doses that are 25% lower. Drugs for heart failure should rarely be discontinued abruptly except in the event of toxicity or allergy.

Indications for Referral

Specialized evaluation is often indicated at the time that heart failure is first diagnosed to facilitate identification or exclusion of contributing causes. Cardiac specialists can also work with primary care physicians in managing acute, severe decompensation and establishing a long-term treatment program. The latter may ordinarily be supervised by the primary care physician. When difficulty is anticipated or encountered with initiation of ACE inhibitors or beta-blockers, referral for specialized management may allow successful establishment of the regimen over a 3- to 6-month period, followed by return to primary care supervision. A declining serum sodium level or a progressive increase in creatinine indicates progression of disease that may warrant more aggressive intervention. The most common indication for referral is the appearance or persistence of symptoms limiting routine daily activities (class III or IV) despite attempted therapy with an ACE inhibitor, beta-blocker, digoxin, and diuretics, as discussed later.

COMMON MEDICATIONS FOR HEART FAILURE

ACE Inhibitors

Three agents have been shown to improve outcomes at all stages of heart failure when the left ventricular ejection fraction is less than 40%.[1] For a patient with a new diagnosis of heart failure and no volume overload, ACE inhibitors are the first agents administered. The usual starting doses in this setting are 5 mg/day of lisinopril, 2.5 mg of enalapril twice daily, or 12.5 mg of captopril three times daily. The latter, a short-acting agent, is sometimes used for initiation when hypotension and renal dysfunction are potential concerns. Approximately 5% to 10% of patients with mild to moderate heart failure cannot tolerate ACE inhibitors, most often because of cough. Currently, no good evidence is available to suggest that the frequency of cough varies with different agents. In many patients with heart failure treated with ACE inhibitors, cough is actually a sign of elevated left-sided filling pressure and diminishes with treatment of the heart failure. Of the remaining patients, some can tolerate moderate doses of these agents. ACE inhibitors may occasionally have to be discontinued because of hyperkalemia. Angioneurotic edema and agranulocytosis are rare complications of ACE inhibition.

Upward titration of oral ACE inhibitors should proceed, generally in the outpatient setting. Target doses (Table 28–3) should be sought and at times exceeded in patients with persistently elevated blood pressure. Randomized controlled trials suggest that any additional benefit from doses of an ACE inhibitor that are at "target" or higher (such as 40 mg lisinopril) as opposed to moderate (5 to 10 mg lisinopril) is minor. ACE inhibitors often improve renal function in patients with mild to moderate heart failure. In addition, they are recommended for decreasing progression of diabetic nephropathy. Serum creatinine frequently rises by a few tenths of a milligram during ACE inhibitor therapy, which is not a reason to discontinue treatment with these drugs. However, in severe heart failure, inhibition of the renin-angiotensin system may occasionally cause a progressive reduction in the glomerular filtration rate. Renal artery stenosis should be considered if renal function deteriorates markedly with ACE inhibitor therapy. When the serum creatinine level exceeds 2 mg/dL or the serum BUN level exceeds 50 mg/dL, ACE inhibitor therapy should be initiated or adjusted only by experienced physicians. Angioedema is a rare, but life-threatening side effect of ACE inhibitors that may appear long after drug initiation, and it precludes rechallenge with ACE inhibitors.

Symptomatic hypotension occurring repeatedly even with low doses of ACE inhibitors in a patient with persistent heart failure symptoms suggests marked neurohormonal activation characteristic of advanced disease, which should be evaluated by a specialist.[7] An inability to tolerate ACE inhibitors because of renal dysfunction or symptomatic hypotension may occur in up to 20% of patients with advanced heart failure.[7]

Angiotensin Receptor Blockers

ACE inhibitors do not completely block the renin-angiotensin system. By blocking the receptors, angiotensin receptor blockers (ARBs) act more distally and completely in the pathway. These antagonists do not increase bradykinin and prostaglandins, which may contribute to both the benefits and side effects seen with ACE inhibitors. The benefit of ACE inhibitors appears to exceed that of ARBs as single agents.[17] The use of ARBs with ACE inhibitors has been shown to cause a larger decrease in left ventricular dimensions and neurohormonal activation and a clinically small decrease in hospitalizations.[18] Too much neurohormonal antagonism may be deleterious, however, and concern has been raised that ARBs may worsen outcomes in patients already receiving both ACE inhibitors and beta-blockers.

ARBs are indicated for the treatment of left ventricular dysfunction when ACE inhibitors are not tolerated because of cough, angioedema, or rash. Because they have similar mechanisms of action, ARBs are not an alternative therapy when hypotension, hyperkalemia, or renal dysfunction prevents the use of ACE inhibitors. The combination of ACE inhibitors and ARBs can be very effective in the treatment of hypertension in patients with heart failure. ARBs are *not* currently recommended in patients already receiving both ACE inhibitors and beta-blocking agents.[18]

Beta-Adrenergic Receptor Antagonists (Beta-Blockers)

Beta-blockers have now been shown to benefit patients with mild to moderate symptoms of heart failure, as well

TABLE 28–3

Oral Medications Commonly Used in the Treatment of Heart Failure

Drug	Initial Dose (mg)	Target Dose (mg)	Recommended Maximal Dose (mg)
ACE inhibitors			
Captopril	6.25*–12.5 tid	50 tid	100 qid
Enalapril	2.5 bid	10 bid	20 bid
Lisinopril	5 qd	20 qd	40 qd
Quinapril	5 bid	20 bid	†
Ramipril	1 bid	5 bid	†
Nitrates			
Isosorbide dinitrate	10 tid	As needed with ACE inhibitors (40 mg tid with hydralazine)	80 tid
Mononitrates	Little experience in heart failure		
Nitrate patches	Generally considered to be less effective than isosorbide dinitrate		
Beta-receptor blockers			
Bisoprolol	1.25 qd		10 qd
Carvedilol	3.125 bid		25–50 bid
Metoprolol tartrate	6.25 bid		75 bid
Metoprolol CR/XL	12.5–25 qd		200 qd
Digoxin	0.125 qod–0.25 qd	No titration except to avoid toxicity	
Hydralazine	25 tid	75 qid	150 qid
Loop diuretics (often first-line diuretic)			
Furosemide	10–40 qd	As needed	240 bid
Bumetanide	0.5–1.0 qd	As needed	10 qd
Torsemide	20‡	As needed	200 mg daily
Thiazide diuretics (less commonly used than loop diuretics)			
Hydrochlorothiazide	25 qd	As needed	50 qd
Chlorthalidone	25 qd	As needed	50 qd
Thiazide-related diuretics			
Metolazone (usually given only in conjunction with a loop diuretic)	1.25–2.5 mg* ½ hr before loop diuretic dose	As needed, most effective with intermittent use	10 bid
Potassium-sparing diuretics			
Spironolactone	25 qd or qod	25 qod–bid	50 bid§
Amiloride	5 qd	As needed	20 qd§

*Given as a single test dose initially.

†Little experience with doses above the target doses in heart failure.

‡A dose of 20 mg assumes previous loop diuretic therapy with a decreasing response.

§These doses may lead to a high risk of life-threatening hyperkalemia in heart failure and are rarely used.

ACE, angiotensin-converting enzyme.

Adapted from Hunt SA, Baker DW, Chin MH, et al. ACC/AHA guidelines for the evaluation and management of chronic heart failure in the adult: Executive summary. A report of the American College of Cardiology/ American Heart Association Task Force on Practice Guidelines (Committee to Revise the 1995 Guidelines for the Evaluation and Management of Heart Failure). J Am Coll Cardiol 2001;38:2101–2113.

as patients after myocardial infarction.[3,11–13] It is likely that they will also be found to be beneficial in asymptomatic patients with nonischemic left ventricular dysfunction. Recent studies and subset analyses suggest that they are tolerated and also beneficial in a group of patients stabilized after recent severe symptoms of heart failure.[13] However, it should be noted that patients with significant volume overload or recent need for intravenous medication for heart failure were excluded from these studies. Other contraindications include resting bradycardia or advanced conduction system disease, severe bronchospasm, and symptomatic hypotension.

As inhibitors of the adrenergic nervous system that supports a failing circulation, beta-blockers can precipitate or aggravate heart failure, even when initiated at the recommended low starting dose of 12.5 mg of long-acting metoprolol (CR-XL) or 3.125 mg of carvedilol twice daily (see Table 28–3). Doses can be escalated at intervals of 1 to 2 weeks initially and then at 2 to 4 weeks, with the nighttime dose sometimes increased first. The measured benefit has been greatest when target doses have been reached, but beneficial effects have also been seen at low doses. Patients should be vigilant for signs of fluid retention and should understand that they may temporarily feel a mild decrease in energy for the first week after dose escalation. Hypotension and dizziness may be slightly greater with carvedilol than the other diuretics because of its concomitant peripheral vasodilatation. The benefit of improved left ventricular ejection fraction and decreased heart size may be seen as early as 3 months. Whereas some patients feel remarkably improved by this time, others improve more slowly. In some patients, beta-blockers cause a persistent fatigue that limits activity despite improved cardiac function. A small number of patients experience severe depression that may necessitate discontinuation of the beta-blocker.

Diuretics

Diuretics should be administered for control of congestion and fluid retention (see Fig. 28–3). Although thiazide diuretics are well tolerated and effective in mild heart failure, these agents are frequently inadequate for the chronic prevention of fluid retention in moderate or severe heart failure and have been associated with hyponatremia. Recurrent fluid retention often responds best to a loop diuretic such as furosemide at initial daily oral doses of 10 or 20 mg. Patients may start diuretic therapy on an outpatient basis. They should be instructed to weigh themselves daily and should be contacted by telephone within 3 days of initiating diuretic therapy to discuss the response and possible adjustment in dose. Patients should then return to see their physician within the next 3 to 7 days for further clinical assessment, including repeat determination of the serum potassium concentration.

During the initiation of diuretic therapy in ambulatory patients, weight loss should not exceed 2 lb daily. If no response to a given initial dose is seen, it should be increased by at least 50%. If no improvement is noted after two dose increases, hospitalization may be necessary to establish safe and effective diuresis. Intravenous administration of loop diuretics may be required to initiate diuresis in patients who are already receiving high doses of oral diuretics. Early experience with the oral loop diuretic torsemide indicates that its better absorption and earlier peak effect than furosemide may improve diuretic responsiveness without any need for intravenous administration in some cases.[7] Once optimal fluid balance has been restored, the maintenance dose of the diuretic is lower than that required to initiate diuresis. When the total daily dose of furosemide is less than 80 mg, once-daily diuretic dosing in the morning may decrease the inconvenience of nocturia.

Monitoring fluid status requires continued vigilance. The adjustment in diuretics for heart failure has been compared with the adjustment in insulin for diabetes; needs change from day to day, depending on many factors. Guided by daily weights, most ambulatory patients can become responsible for their own flexible diuretic regimens. They are generally instructed to double their loop diuretic (not thiazides or potassium-sparing diuretics) when a weight gain of 2 lb or more occurs. Once the baseline weight has been reestablished, the previous dose can be resumed. When daily doses of furosemide exceed 160 mg, evaluation of the entire regimen by a specialist may be helpful.[7]

Intermittent use of metolazone (2.5 or 5.0 mg) for weight gain refractory to doubling of the dose of furosemide frequently restores fluid balance and response to the loop diuretic. Because even a 2.5-mg dose of this diuretic in conjunction with furosemide can cause brisk diuresis, serious hypotension, electrolyte depletion, or a combination of these effects, the first dose of metolazone in patients already receiving a loop diuretic may be most safely administered in the hospital setting. Chronic, regular use of metolazone is rarely indicated because it loses much of its diuretic effect over time and causes electrolyte depletion.

Aldosterone Antagonists

At one time, aldosterone antagonists were used primarily as potassium-sparing agents in patients requiring high potassium replacement to prevent diuretic-induced hypokalemia. In addition to its effects on electrolyte excretion, aldosterone may have multiple other desirable effects on myocardial and vascular structure and function. Inhibition of aldosterone's effects with spironolactone in the Randomized Aldactone Evaluation Study (RALES) reduced mortality and decreased recurrent class IV symptoms or hospitalization in patients with severe heart failure.[19] These patients received large doses of loop diuretics, had serum creatinine concentrations less than 2.0 mg/dL, did not receive any routine potassium replacement, and underwent vigilant monitoring of electrolytes and renal function. Caution is necessary to avoid hyperkalemia when adding a potassium-sparing agent such as spironolactone to a regimen that includes ACE inhibitors, ARBs, or both agents, particularly when diabetes or preexisting renal disease may further compromise regulation of potassium.

Spironolactone and other potassium-sparing diuretics should be considered only in patients who have stable renal function and are receiving loop diuretics. The peak effect may not be evident for several days, during which time serum potassium levels need to be checked frequently. Even after a stable regimen has been established, hyperkalemia may occur,[20] particularly in the setting of volume depletion. Aldosterone antagonists should be discontinued during any interruption of loop diuretic therapy. Spironolactone has not been studied or recommended for treatment of mildly symptomatic heart failure or for treatment without loop diuretics. Gynecomastia occurs in about 10% of patients taking spironolactone.[19]

Electrolyte Replacement

Diuretic therapy causes urinary loss of both potassium and magnesium. ACE inhibitors reduce potassium excretion, but many patients with adequate renal function require potassium supplementation during daily therapy with loop diuretics such as furosemide despite ACE inhibitor therapy. Dietary supplementation is rarely adequate. Salt substitutes, most of which contain potassium, can improve compliance with sodium restriction but should be used in moderation because excessive consumption can cause hyperkalemia.

Serum potassium levels should generally be maintained between 3.8 and 4.5 mEq/L in patients with heart failure. *Hypokalemia* is a well-recognized complication of diuretic therapy that can aggravate arrhythmias and precipitate severe muscle cramps during rapid diuresis. Unless hypokalemia is very severe or life threatening, potassium should be replaced by oral administration. Patients who require loop diuretics often receive maintenance doses of 20 to 60 mEq of oral potassium daily, usually no more than 20 mEq at one time. The dangers of *hyperkalemia* are less well recognized but are equally important. A serum concentration of potassium greater than 6 mEq/L, particularly when the level has risen quickly, can depress myocardial contractility and cause arrhythmias resembling ventricular tachycardia. Aggressive repletion of potassium in the presence of ACE inhibitors and potassium-sparing diuretics has led to many episodes of life-threatening hyperkalemia, one of the causes of sudden death in heart failure. Hospitalized patients with heart failure are at greater risk for cardiac arrest from hyperkalemia than from hypokalemia.

Severe *hypomagnesemia* can also occur as a consequence of diuretic therapy and can precipitate or aggravate ventricular arrhythmias. Hypomagnesemia can exacerbate hypokalemia, and some patients require chronic supplementation of both minerals. Magnesium is generally replaced to levels of approximately 2 mg/dL, but chronic supplementation has not proved to be of benefit.

Vasodilators

Nitrates

The addition of a nitrate to ACE inhibitor therapy may improve exercise tolerance in patients with severe exertional dyspnea. The combination of hydralazine and nitrates is useful when ACE inhibitors are not tolerated. Nitrate therapy is generally introduced with isosorbide dinitrate at a dose of 10 mg three times daily, and the dose may be gradually increased to 40 mg three times daily. Although nitrate tolerance is a well-recognized problem, it is rarely clinically evident when oral nitrates are taken three times daily with a nitrate-free interval of at least 10 hours at night. The only common side effect of nitrates is headache, which frequently improves after 24 to 48 hours of therapy but may require acetaminophen. Sublingual nitroglycerin (0.3 to 0.6 mg) is very effective for rapid, temporary relief of pulmonary edema or congestion and may be used every few minutes on an emergency basis until more definitive therapy is available. In some patients, exertional dyspnea may be decreased by nitroglycerin or sublingual isosorbide dinitrate before embarking on strenuous activity.

Hydralazine

Hydralazine, by itself, is an arterial vasodilator only and does not reduce ventricular filling pressure to the same extent that nitrates and ACE inhibitors do. The combination of hydralazine and isosorbide dinitrate has been shown to decrease mortality as well as improve left ventricular ejection fraction and exercise capacity in patients with heart failure. However, this combination has been found to be less beneficial than ACE inhibition in mild to moderate heart failure. The major indications for hydralazine in combination with nitrates in heart failure are intolerance of ACE inhibitors and persistent heart failure symptoms or hypertension despite ACE inhibitors.

Calcium Antagonists

Even though calcium antagonists cause vasodilatation in heart failure, the overall benefit appears to be reduced by their negative inotropic effect and by the reflex activation of the sympathetic nervous system that they can induce. Although these drugs should not be used as vasodilators in systolic heart failure, they may be useful as antihypertensive agents or for control of the ventricular rate in atrial fibrillation in patients with heart failure and a preserved ejection fraction.

Digitalis

Cardiac glycosides are the oldest drugs still currently prescribed for heart failure. Although digitalis compounds improve contractility, their clinical benefit may result primarily from their effect on the autonomic nervous system. Digitalis is commonly used in patients with heart failure and atrial fibrillation to decrease the ventricular rate, but it is usually inadequate as a single agent in this regard. Digitalis is used in symptomatic patients with normal sinus rhythm and systolic heart failure to improve functional status and decrease hospitalization. The benefit is most apparent in patients with a low ejection fraction and severe symptoms. In patients with sinus rhythm, digitalis does not appear to improve survival.[21]

For treatment of heart failure, "loading" with high doses of digitalis is not necessary. In most patients with normal renal function, 0.125 or 0.25 mg of digoxin is the daily dose. Doses may need to be lower in the elderly or in patients with impaired renal function, in whom dosing may be reduced to alternate days. Doses of digoxin should generally be halved when initiating amiodarone, which increases serum digoxin levels.

Digoxin levels are generally checked only when toxicity is a concern, such as when renal function declines or after the institution of drugs that can reduce digoxin clearance, such as amiodarone, quinidine, and verapamil. Serum levels of 0.8 to 1.2 ng/dL may be optimal. Serum levels above 1.5 ng/dL are generally thought to be excessive, whereas levels below 0.5 ng/dL are considered ineffective. Signs of digitalis toxicity include nausea, confusion, visual disturbances, ventricular or junctional tachyarrhythmias, and atrioventricular block. When toxicity is suspected, an ECG should be obtained and the serum potassium level determined.

Nonsteroidal Anti-inflammatory Agents

These drugs inhibit prostaglandin activity, which helps preserve renal function and fluid excretion in patients with heart failure. Exacerbation of heart failure in patients with advanced disease may result from even one or two doses. Because these agents are available without prescription, patients may forget to mention their use. Musculoskeletal pain should instead be treated with acetaminophen or aspirin when possible. For attacks of gout in patients with impaired renal function and heart failure, first-line therapy may instead be colchicine or steroid therapy in severe cases.

TREATMENT OF RELATED CONDITIONS

Arrhythmias

Prevention of Sudden Arrhythmic Death

Up to half of all deaths in patients with chronic heart failure are sudden. Although ventricular tachycardia and fibrillation can cause sudden death in heart failure patients, multiple other causes are possible and include myocardial infarction, pulmonary or systemic emboli, hyperkalemia, and primary bradyarrhythmias. Cardiac arrest and syncope in heart failure merit careful evaluation for treatable causes, including ventricular tachyarrhythmias.

The approach to using internal cardioverter-defibrillators (ICDs) is evolving rapidly because of information from randomized controlled trials (see Chapter 30). The most widely accepted indication is a history of sustained ventricular tachycardia or ventricular fibrillation. ICDs have also been shown to improve survival in patients with a history of coronary artery disease with spontaneous sustained or nonsustained ventricular tachycardia and an electrophysiologic study that is positive for inducible ventricular tachycardia.[22] More recently, ICD implantation has prolonged life in patients with severely depressed ventricular function with previous myocardial infarction (left ventricular ejection fraction ≥0.30) without specific makers of arrhythmia risk.[22a]

All major trials of ICDs have largely addressed outpatient populations and have excluded patients with class IV symptoms of heart failure. Although successful resuscitation is common in patients who have class IV symptoms, the benefit for overall survival is not established. Patients in whom hemodynamic compensation cannot be maintained and in whom the 1-year survival from a hemodynamic standpoint is anticipated to be less than 1 year may not be appropriate candidates for ICDs.

ICDs provide highly effective therapy to prevent death from ventricular tachyarrhythmias. They are also, however, associated with a significant rate of inappropriate shocks related to incorrect sensing of atrial arrhythmias, other artifacts, and damaged or defective leads. Such shocks can at times provoke anxiety and impair emotional and social functioning.

Atrial Fibrillation

The prevalence of atrial fibrillation increases with the severity of heart failure, and it occurs in up to 30% in patients with severe symptoms. Because tachycardia can cause or exacerbate heart failure, control of the ventricular rate is critical. Digoxin is rarely adequate to control the ventricular rate with activity, which usually requires beta-adrenergic blocking agents or amiodarone. Although some patients clearly feel better in sinus rhythm, no trial evidence has shown the superiority of sinus rhythm over a controlled ventricular rate and anticoagulation in patients with chronic atrial fibrillation. Amiodarone is usually the preferred drug for treatment of atrial fibrillation in heart failure. Dofetilide helps maintain sinus rhythm and has not been shown to increase mortality in this group, but worsening renal function decreases drug excretion and thereby increases the risk of the life-threatening rhythm *torsades de pointes*. Type I antiarrhythmic agents such as quinidine and procainamide may help maintain sinus rhythm but increase the risk of sudden death and worsening heart failure and are therefore contraindicated. When sinus rhythm cannot be maintained and the ventricular response cannot be controlled pharmacologically, ablation of the atrioventricular node with pacemaker placement may be indicated.

Bradyarrhythmias

A significant proportion of instances of syncope and sudden death in heart failure may result from bradyarrhythmias. Patients should have a pacemaker implanted for symptomatic bradycardia and consideration of whether an implantable defibrillator is warranted because the current ICDs all include backup bradycardia pacing. When pacemaker dependence is anticipated, patients with heart failure in whom atrioventricular synchrony can be maintained may best be supported with dual-chamber devices.

Biventricular Pacing

The prevalence of prolonged intraventricular conduction evident from a wide QRS complex on the ECG increases with worsening heart failure. The resulting ventricular dyssynchrony may further impair left ventricular contraction and increase secondary mitral regurgitation. Simultaneous pacing of the right and left ventricles can improve contractility and exercise capacity in some patients with class III symptoms of heart failure.[23] Biventricular pacing can be considered when the QRS duration exceeds 150 msec and persistent heart failure symptoms limit daily activity despite optimization of other therapies.

Amiodarone

Amiodarone is the safest and most effective agent for preventing atrial and ventricular arrhythmias in heart failure. Even patients with severe heart failure generally tolerate oral amiodarone without an exacerbation of heart failure symptoms, but they may require lower loading doses than those used in patients without heart failure. However, because amiodarone reduces the clearance of digoxin and warfarin, the doses of these agents must be reduced. Major side effects of amiodarone include pulmonary toxicity, liver dysfunction, hyperthyroidism, hypothyroidism, and neuropathy. Initiation and adjustment of this drug should be supervised by a physician with extensive experience in treating heart failure.

Prevention of Embolic Events

The annual incidence of systemic and pulmonary embolism in patients with chronic heart failure is 2% to 5%. By comparison, the risk of severe bleeding complications from anticoagulation in the general population is 0.8% to 2.5% yearly, but this risk may be higher in patients whose warfarin requirements are unpredictably reduced by intermittent hepatic congestion. Therefore, anticoagulation is not *routinely* recommended in the current guidelines for the treatment of heart failure, although this issue remains controversial.[1] However, anticoagulation is indicated in heart failure patients with additional specific risks for embolic events, such as atrial fibrillation, a history of pulmonary or arterial embolic events, and mobile intracardiac thrombi or marked apical dyskinesis visualized on echocardiography. The risk associated with chronic warfarin anticoagulation in patients with heart failure may be reduced by careful maintenance of the international normalized ratio (INR) at relatively low levels (2.0 to 2.5).

Controversy continues regarding whether the use of aspirin decreases the benefit of ACE inhibitors. Current recommendations consider aspirin acceptable when antiplatelet therapy is required for prevention of cardiac and cerebral ischemic events.[1] The newer agent clopidogrel has not been shown to adversely interact with ACE inhibitors, but it is more costly than aspirin.

Treatment of Sleep Disturbances

The frequency of nocturnal sleep disturbances may approach 30% as heart failure progresses. Some patients are prone to arterial desaturation during sleep, particularly with a Cheyne-Stokes breathing pattern or sleep apnea. For such patients, nocturnal oxygen therapy may improve sleep, daytime symptoms, and occasionally, cardiac function. Formal sleep studies should be considered when abnormal breathing patterns are observed by the clinician or stated to occur by the patient or spouse during sleep.

Supplemental Oxygen Therapy

Most patients with heart failure do not have arterial oxygen desaturation and do not benefit from chronic oxygen supplementation, which serves only to reinforce the image of debility. Patients with oxygen desaturation, particularly in the context of underlying lung disease, may benefit from oxygen therapy. Occasional patients with refractory fluid overload describe feeling less dyspneic with chronic oxygen supplementation, which may reflect a placebo effect or direct suppression of central dyspnea by increased dissolved oxygen.

ADVANCED HEART FAILURE

Patients who have persistent symptoms that limit daily activity (NYHA class III or IV symptoms) despite attempted therapy with an ACE inhibitor, beta-blocker, and diuretics as tolerated are considered to have advanced heart failure.[7] Such patients have frequently had a recent hospitalization for heart failure. Careful re-evaluation of hemodynamic status should be undertaken, particularly for evidence of fluid retention causing congestive symptoms. Relief of congestion is the primary goal of therapy for advanced heart failure.[1,7] Particularly when accompanied by evidence of low perfusion, patients may require therapy with an intravenous vasodilator or inotropic agent for restabilization. Hemodynamic monitoring is useful in some patients to identify baseline hemodynamic profiles and response to therapy.

The optimal blood pressure needed to reduce left ventricular workload while maintaining peripheral perfusion in patients with advanced heart failure may be lower than that usually tolerated, with systolic blood pressure commonly as low as 80 to 90 mm Hg. Up to 20% of patients with advanced heart failure may be unable to tolerate an ACE inhibitor because of symptomatic hypotension or progressive renal dysfunction. The balance between cardiac and renal compensation is particularly delicate in patients with advanced heart failure, who frequently have aggravated renal dysfunction before diuresis has been adequate to relieve the symptoms.

Moderately elevated levels of creatinine (>2.0 mg/dL) and BUN (>50 mg/dL) may have to be accepted to maintain relief from congestive symptoms. Continued increases in serum creatinine require close surveillance, but most patients achieve a stable level early after therapy has been intensified. Some show gradual improvement in renal function as their hemodynamic status stabilizes. In other patients, particularly those with intrinsic renovascular disease associated with atherosclerosis, hypertension, and diabetes, a compromise must be achieved between impaired renal function and the intensive diuresis and vasodilatation required to relieve cardiac symptoms. Such compromise usually requires the participation of a specialist.[7]

Management of heart failure includes frequently scheduled contact with these patients to identify and intervene for early signs of recurrent fluid retention. In selected, highly motivated patients, instruction in home blood pressure measurement may facilitate minor adjustments in medications. Once an effective regimen has been initiated, further changes must be made very carefully. Even for symptomatic hypotension attributed to excessive vasodilatation or diuresis, medication doses should in general be reduced rather than discontinued. Any change in vasodilator or diuretic medication requires re-evaluation within 3 days. A beta-blocker should be initiated only after evidence of clinical stability, but it may nonetheless need to be withdrawn with evidence of worsening heart failure.

Refractory Heart Failure

When patients continue to have heart failure symptoms at rest or with minimal exertion despite repeated trials of all standard therapies, their heart failure may be termed refractory.[1] It is estimated that 100,000 patients in the United States younger than 80 years have refractory heart failure for which cardiac replacement therapy might be considered. For the population older than 80 years, co-morbidities combined with the debility of heart failure generally preclude surgical intervention.

Cardiac Transplantation

This procedure provides a good quality of life and a 60% to 70% 5-year survival rate in carefully selected patients (Box 28–8). Unfortunately, this option is limited by the donor heart supply to fewer than 2500 patients yearly in the United States. Transplant recipients assume the burden of rejection, immunosuppression, and accelerated graft coronary artery disease.[24] More than half of recipients continue to be restricted in their activities, and less than half return to work. The primary care

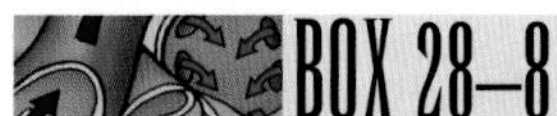

BOX 28–8

Selection Criteria for Cardiac Transplantation

ACCEPTED INDICATIONS

Peak Vo_2 ≤10 mL/kg/min with achievement of anaerobic metabolism

Severe ischemia consistently limiting routine activity and not amenable to bypass surgery or angioplasty

Recurrent symptomatic ventricular arrhythmias refractory to all accepted therapeutic modalities

PROBABLE INDICATIONS

Peak Vo_2 <14 mL/kg/min and major limitation in daily activities

Recurrent unstable ischemia not amenable to revascularization

Instability of fluid balance/renal function despite compliance with weight monitoring, flexible use of diuretic drugs, and salt restriction

INADEQUATE INDICATIONS

Ejection fraction ≤20%

History of previous functional class III or IV symptoms of heart failure

Previous ventricular arrhythmias

Peak Vo_2 >15 mL/kg/min without other indications

CONTINUING EVALUATION

Clinical assessment by heart failure/transplant team at least every 1–2 mo

Re-evaluation at 6-mo intervals to include assessment of clinical stability, pulmonary pressures, and measurement of peak oxygen consumption

CONTRAINDICATIONS

General

- Any noncardiac condition that would itself shorten life expectancy or increase the risk of death from rejection or from the complications of immunosuppression, particularly infection

Specific

- Physiologic advanced age (various programs)
- Active infection
- Active ulcer disease
- Recent pulmonary infarction
- Severe diabetes mellitus with end-organ damage
- Severe peripheral vascular disease
- *Pulmonary function (FEV_1, FVC) <60% or a history of chronic bronchitis
- *Creatinine clearance <40–50 mL/min
- *Bilirubin >2.5 mg/dL, transaminases >2 times normal
- *Pulmonary artery systolic pressure >60 mm Hg
- *Mean transpulmonary gradient >15 mm Hg
- Active substance abuse
- High risk of noncompliance

*May need to demonstrate reversibility after aggressive therapy to improve hemodynamic status.

FEV_1, forced expiratory volume in 1 second; FVC, forced vital capacity; Vo_2, volume of oxygen consumption.

Adapted from Mudge GH, Goldstein S, Addonizio LJ, et al: Cardiac transplantation: Recipient guidelines/prioritization. J Am Coll Cardiol 1993;22:21. Reprinted with permission from the American College of Cardiology.

physician should refer patients with advanced heart failure to heart failure/transplant centers for evaluation early in their disease if they are potentially eligible.

Mechanical Cardiac Support Devices

Ventricular support devices have been used as a "bridge" to transplantation in almost 25% of the patients currently undergoing transplantation. The major complications are infection, thrombosis, and device failure. A recent trial extended the potential application of an implantable left ventricular assist device to "destination" therapy for patients not eligible for transplantation.[25] However, the high cost and complication rate restrict the use of these devices at the present time.

End-of-Life Considerations

The number of patients with end-stage heart failure is increasing because of both success of earlier interventions and the aging of the population. The current drugs and ICDs have reduced the chance of sudden death during earlier stages of disease, thus leaving more patients to progress to refractory symptoms of fluid retention and low cardiac output.[7] As the prospect of hemodynamic collapse approaches, it is critical to review end-of-life choices with the patient and family.[26] Distinction should be made between intervention for a potentially reversible condition and intervention to postpone a welcome death that offers the only relief.

TABLE 28–4

Systolic versus Diastolic Dysfunction in Heart Failure

Parameters	Systolic	Diastolic
History		
Older age	+	+++
Coronary heart disease	++++	+
Hypertension	++	++++
Diabetes	+	+++
Valvular heart disease	++++	+
Flash pulmonary edema	+	+++
Paroxysmal dyspnea	++	+++
Physical examination		
Narrow pulse pressure	+++	–
Cardiomegaly	+++	+
Soft heart sounds	++++	+
S_3 gallop	+++	+
S_4 gallop	+	+++
Mitral regurgitation	+++	+
Edema	++	++
Jugular venous distention	+++	++
Chest radiogram		
Cardiomegaly	+++	+
Pulmonary congestion	+++	+++
Electrocardiogram		
Low voltage	+++	–
Left ventricular hypertrophy	++	++++
Left ventricular dilatation	+++	–
Q-waves	+++	+
Echocardiogram		
Low ejection fraction	++++	–
Left ventricular dilatation	+++	–
Atrial dilatation alone	+	+++
Left ventricular hypertrophy	++	++++
Mitral regurgitation	+++	++

S_3, third heart sound; S_4, fourth heart sound.

Adapted from Young JB: Assessment of heart failure. In Colucci WS (vol ed): Cardiac Function and Dysfunction. In Braunwald E (series ed): Atlas of Heart Failure, 2nd ed. Philadelphia, Current Medicine 1999, p 7.12.

HEART FAILURE IN SPECIAL GROUPS

Heart Failure and Preserved Ejection Fraction

Clinical Profile

Heart failure with "preserved" ejection fraction, usually defined as an ejection fraction over 40%, accounts for approximately 40% of all cases of heart failure in the United States, a proportion that increases with increasing age.[8,16] The different features in systolic and diastolic heart failure are summarized in Table 28–4. In systolic heart failure, the primary functional abnormality is impaired contractility, which is associated with a marked reduction in left ventricular ejection fraction, usually to less than 40% in symptomatic patients. When heart failure occurs with an ejection fraction of over 40%, impaired ventricular relaxation and compliance lead to elevation of ventricular end-diastolic pressure with little reduction in the ejection fraction. This condition is often termed "diastolic dysfunction," although some component of systolic dysfunction may also be present.[8] Diastolic dysfunction may be caused by reduced ventricular diastolic capacity, as occurs in hypertrophic, restrictive, or hypertensive cardiomyopathy, constrictive pericarditis, myocardial infiltration, or impaired ventricular relaxation. Heart failure related to diastolic dysfunction is most commonly identified in elderly patients with hypertension and diabetes, although these conditions can cause systolic dysfunction as well.

Because stroke volume is the product of ejection fraction and ventricular diastolic volume, any process that restricts myocardial dilatation leads to a lower stroke volume and cardiac output and thus more severe limitation in cardiac reserves. In the extreme example of hypertrophic cardiomyopathy, the left ventricular ejection fraction may be as high as 80%, but even 80% of a severely diminished left ventricular cavity volume can yield a low stroke volume. More commonly, stroke volume is normal at rest but fails to increase appropriately during exercise. This condition is often associated with avid fluid retention, particularly in patients who are also obese. "Flash" pulmonary edema occurs frequently and can sometimes be attributed to triggers such as an exacerbation of hypertension or a concomitant infection, but it often remains unexplained. Renal artery stenosis, which is associated with a high renin state causing myocardial hypertrophy and vasoconstriction, is an occasional cause of recurrent flash pulmonary edema.

Physical examination usually reveals a fourth heart sound (see Table 28–4). The symptoms and signs of elevated left- and right-sided filling pressure can be as severe as in systolic failure but are not often accompanied by evidence of hypoperfusion. The diagnosis is best confirmed by echocardiography, which may demonstrate abnormal ventricular filling patterns in the presence of relatively preserved systolic function and little, if any, ventricular dilatation.

Management

The tendency to retain fluid is often the most prominent feature on clinical assessment in patients with impaired diastolic function. These patients should be treated with diuretics until the symptoms and signs of fluid retention resolve or resolution is prevented by postural hypotension or an unacceptable reduction in renal function. Without specific trial data demonstrating the efficacy of therapies, most attention should be devoted to treating hypertension and elevated heart rates, which further compromise diastolic filling.[16] ACE inhibitors (or ARBs if ACE inhibitors are not tolerated) are the most reasonable first-line drugs for the hypertension. Beta-blockers help control both hypertension and heart rate. The atrial contribution to ventricular filling should be maintained whenever possible, even with repeated cardioversion in some patients. Digoxin is occasionally indicated to control the heart rate in atrial fibrillation, although beta-blockers, amiodarone, or verapamil may be more effective for this purpose. When sinus rhythm cannot be maintained and rate control cannot be achieved, atrioventricular node ablation with implantation of a pacemaker may be indicated. Beyond these efforts, calcium antagonists may improve diastolic function in some patients, but their benefits in the absence of hypertension have not been proved, and some concern exists regarding higher mortality.

The Elderly

Half of all patients with heart failure in the United States are older than 70 years, and nearly 1 in 10 persons older than 80 has heart failure. Predominant diastolic dysfunction as a cause of heart failure is increased in the elderly, but systolic heart failure with a low ejection fraction still accounts for approximately half of the cases.[16] Heart failure in these patients is frequently combined with diffuse coronary artery disease or aortic valve sclerosis. Vascular disease in the carotid arteries and lower extremities and noncardiac co-morbid conditions such as diabetes mellitus, pulmonary disease, and renal disease may complicate the diagnosis and management.

The options and intensity of therapy for heart failure are limited by the aging circulation. Whereas younger patients often tolerate systolic blood pressure as low as 80 mm Hg, patients older than 70 years should probably be maintained at a systolic pressure of at least 90 mm Hg; those with cerebrovascular disease may require a systolic pressure of 120 mm Hg or even higher. Because of altered autonomic regulation, the unacceptable postural hypotension resulting from vasodilator therapy may be a greater problem in the elderly, who are also more prone to progressive renal dysfunction during diuresis. However, in most elderly patients, by careful manipulation of therapeutic measures, an acceptable balance can be reached in which jugular venous pressure, creatinine, and BUN are all slightly elevated but stable.

Women account for only about 20% of the heart failure population younger than 70 years because coronary artery disease and dilated cardiomyopathy occur more commonly in men. In patients older than 70 years, women represent an increasing fraction of the heart failure population, a reflection of the higher incidence of heart failure with preserved ejection fraction in elderly women and their longer life expectancy.[16]

African Americans

Heart failure appears to occur at an earlier age and with greater severity in African Americans.[9] The prevalence of hypertension is consistently higher, and coronary disease is less often implicated as the etiology of heart failure. The worse prognosis for African Americans in multiple study populations persists after adjustment for socioeconomic factors that may limit adherence to medical therapy. Genetic polymorphisms in components of neurohormonal regulation may be found to explain some differences in response to hypertension and to ACE inhibitors and beta-blockers.

Evidence-Based Summary

ACE INHIBITORS

A systematic review of ACE inhibitors versus placebo involved 12,763 patients with heart failure or left ventricular failure enrolled in five randomized clinical trials.[2] Mortality was reduced from 29.1% in the placebo group to 23.4% in the ACE inhibitor group. Readmission for heart failure was also significantly reduced from 15.5% to 11.9%. These benefits were observed in all subgroups (age, sex, cause of heart failure, and NYHA class). No systematic differences between different ACE inhibitors were observed. Cough, hypotension, hyperkalemia, and renal dysfunction were the principal adverse effects.

BETA-BLOCKERS

In a systematic overview of 18 placebo-controlled randomized controlled trials of 3023 patients with NYHA class II or III heart failure, beta-blockers reduced mortality from 12% (placebo) to 8%.[3] Two more recent, large randomized controlled trials that enrolled 6538 class II to class IV patients reported that mortality was significantly reduced from 17.3% with placebo to 11.8% with bisoprolol ($P < .0001$)[11] and from 11% with placebo to 7.2% ($P = .0062$)[12] per patient year with metoprolol. A large trial demonstrated benefit in patients with recent class IV symptoms of heart failure after excluding those with clinical evidence of volume retention or therapy with intravenous inotropic agents.[13] No adverse effects were observed when doses were gradually escalated.

DIGOXIN

A systematic review of digoxin in seven randomized controlled trials of patients with heart failure and sinus rhythm found less clinical deterioration with digoxin but no effect on mortality.[27] One large randomized controlled trial compared digoxin with placebo in 6800 patients.[22] Mortality was similar (35.1% for placebo vs. 34.8% for digoxin—not significant). However, the number of patients requiring hospital admission for heart failure was reduced from 35% with placebo to 27% with digoxin ($P < .001$). This trial showed more apparent benefit in patients with a lower ejection fraction and more severe heart failure symptoms at baseline. Digoxin did not increase hospitalizations for ventricular tachyarrhythmia, supraventricular arrhythmia, or myocardial infarction. Patients previously stable with digoxin were more likely to have worsening symptoms when digoxin was replaced with placebo.

ANGIOTENSIN RECEPTOR BLOCKERS

In a trial of 3152 patients, an ARB was found to be slightly less effective than an ACE inhibitor for prevention of hospitalization.[17] In a trial of 5010 patients with class II to class III heart failure, the addition of an ARB had no impact on mortality, but it decreased hospitalizations for heart failure from 18% to 14% over a 4-year period, with the largest benefit observed in patients who were not taking an ACE inhibitor.[18] Some concern was raised about excess adverse events when an ARB was added in patients taking an ACE inhibitor and beta-blocker. Other large trials addressing the role of angiotensin receptor antagonists are ongoing.

ALDOSTERONE RECEPTOR ANTAGONISTS

One major randomized controlled trial has been conducted in 1663 patients with severe heart failure (NYHA class III and IV) and ejection fractions less than 35% who were receiving ACE inhibitors and diuretics; mortality was reduced from 46% in placebo recipients to 35% in spironolactone-treated patients ($P < .001$).[19] Gynecomastia occurred in 10% of the spironolactone-treated patients (1% in the placebo group). No excess of hyperkalemia was noted in this trial.

IMPLANTABLE CARDIAC DEFIBRILLATORS

A total of 1016 patients with left ventricular dysfunction (ejection fraction <40% but not in class IV) and serious ventricular arrhythmias (resuscitation from ventricular fibrillation, syncope, or sustained ventricular tachycardia) were randomized to ICD implantation or pharmacologic antiarrhythmic drug treatment. Three-year mortality was reduced from 36% (drug treatment) to 25% (ICD therapy) ($P < 0.02$).[28] In 196 patients with nonsustained ventricular tachycardia who had ventricular tachycardia inducible at electrophysiologic study, mortality was reduced from 39% to 16% with ICD therapy.[22] In 1232 stable patients with severely depressed left ventricular function >1 month after myocardial infarction without specific arrhythmia risk, ICD implantation reduced mortality from 19.8% to 14.2% ($p = 0.016$), a 31% relative risk reduction.[22a]

EXERCISE

Three randomized controlled trials of exercise training have shown benefit in patients with heart failure.[14] Exercise capacity, left ventricular function, survival, and rehospitalization were improved. Further study is needed because only 189 patients were included in the combined trials.

References

1. Hunt SA, Baker DW, Chin MH, et al: ACC/AHA guidelines for the evaluation and management of chronic heart failure in the adult: Executive summary. A report of the American College of Cardiology/American Heart Association Task Force on Practice Guidelines. J Am Coll Cardiol 2001;38:2101–2113.
2. Flather M, Yusuf S, Kober L, et al, for the ACE-Inhibitor Myocardial Infarction Collaborative Group: Long-term ACE-inhibitor therapy in patients with heart failure or left ventricular dysfunction: A systematic overview of data from individual patients. Lancet 2000;355:1575–1581.
3. Lechat P, Packer M, Chalon S, et al: Clinical effects of beta adrenergic blockade in chronic heart failure. A meta-analysis of double-blind, placebo controlled, randomized trials. Circulation 1998;98:1184–1191.
4. Dao Q, Krishnaswamy P, Kazanegra R, et al: Utility of B-type natriuretic peptide in the diagnosis of congestive

heart failure in an urgent-care setting. J Am Coll Cardiol 2001;37:379–385.

5. Stevenson LW, Perloff JK: The limited reliability of physical signs for estimating hemodynamics in chronic heart failure. JAMA 1989;261:884–888.
6. Grady KL, Dracup K, Kennedy G, et al: Team management of patients with heart failure: A statement for healthcare professionals from The Cardiovascular Nursing Council of the American Heart Association. Circulation 2000;102:2443–2456.
7. Nohria A, Lewis E, Stevenson LW: Medical management of advanced heart failure. JAMA 2002;287:1–12.
8. Zile MR, Gaasch WH, Carroll JD, et al: Heart failure with a normal ejection fraction: Is measurement of diastolic function necessary to make the diagnosis of diastolic heart failure? Circulation 2001;104:779–782.
9. Yancy CW: Heart failure in blacks: Etiologic and epidemiologic differences. Curr Cardiol Rep 2001;3:191–197.
10. Pfeffer MA, Braunwald E, Moye LA, et al: Effect of captopril on mortality and morbidity in patients with left ventricular dysfunction after myocardial infarction. Results of the survival and ventricular enlargement trial. The SAVE Investigators. N Engl J Med 1992;327:669–677.
11. The Cardiac Insufficiency Bisoprolol Study II (CIBIS-II): A randomised trial. Lancet 1999;353:9–13.
12. Effect of metoprolol CR/XL in chronic heart failure: Metoprolol CR/XL Randomised Intervention Trial in Congestive Heart Failure (MERIT-HF). Lancet 1999;353:2001–2007.
13. Packer M, Coats AJ, Fowler MB, et al: Effect of carvedilol on survival in severe chronic heart failure. N Engl J Med 2001;344:1651–1658.
14. McAlister FA, Lawson FM, Teo KK, Armstrong PW: A systematic review of randomized trials of disease management programs in heart failure. Am J Med 2001;110: 378–384.
15. Packer M, Gheorghiade M, Young JB, et al: Withdrawal of digoxin from patients with chronic heart failure treated with angiotensin-converting-enzyme inhibitors. RADIANCE Study. N Engl J Med 1993;329:1–7.
16. Dauterman KW, Massie BM, Gheorghiade M: Heart failure associated with preserved systolic function: A common and costly clinical entity. Am Heart J 1998;135(Suppl): 310–319.
17. Pitt B, Poole-Wilson PA, Segal R, et al: Effect of losartan compared with captopril on mortality in patients with symptomatic heart failure: Randomised trial—the Losartan Heart Failure Survival Study ELITE II. Lancet 2000;355: 1582–1587.
18. Cohn JN, Tognoni G: A randomized trial of the angiotensin-receptor blocker valsartan in chronic heart failure. N Engl J Med 2001;345:1667–1675.
19. Pitt B, Zannad F, Remme WJ, et al: The effect of spironolactone on morbidity and mortality in patients with severe heart failure. Randomized Aldactone Evaluation Study Investigators. N Engl J Med 1999;341:709–717.
20. Effectiveness of spironolactone added to an angiotensin-converting enzyme inhibitor and a loop diuretic for severe chronic congestive heart failure (the Randomized Aldactone Evaluation Study [RALES]). Am J Cardiol 1996;78: 902–907.
21. The Digitalis Investigation Group: The effect of digoxin on mortality and morbidity in patients with heart failure. N Engl J Med 1997;336:525–533.
22. Moss AJ, Hall WJ, Cannom DS, et al: Improved survival with an implanted defibrillator in patients with coronary disease at high risk for ventricular arrhythmia. Multicenter Automatic Defibrillator Implantation Trial Investigators. N Engl J Med 1996;335:1933–1940.

22a. Moss AJ, Zareba W, Hall WJ, et al: Prophylactic implantation of a defibrillator in patients with myocardial infarction and reduced ejection fraction. N Engl J Med 2002;346:877–883.

23. Cazeau S, Leclercq C, Lavergne T, et al: Effects of multisite biventricular pacing in patients with heart failure and intraventricular conduction delay. N Engl J Med 2001;344:873–880.
24. Mudge GH, Goldstein S, Addonizio GS, et al: Recipient guidelines/prioritization for cardiac transplantation: The 24th Bethesda Conference. Am J Cardiol 1993;22:21–31.
25. Rose EA, Gelijns AC, Moskowitz AJ, et al: Long-term mechanical left ventricular assistance for end-stage heart failure. N Engl J Med 2001;345:1435–1443.
26. Stevenson LW: Rites and responsibility for resuscitation in heart failure: Tread gently on the thin places. Circulation 1998;98:619–622.
27. Jaeschke R, Oxman AD, Guyatt GH: To what extent do congestive heart failure patients in sinus rhythm benefit from digoxin therapy? A systematic overview and meta-analysis. Am J Med 1990;88:279–286.
28. A comparison of antiarrhythmic-drug therapy with implantable defibrillators in patients resuscitated from near-fatal ventricular arrhythmias. The Antiarrhythmics versus Implantable Defibrillators (AVID) Investigators. N Engl J Med 1997;337:1576–1583.
29. Belardinelli R, Georgiou D, Cianci G, Purcaro A: Randomized, controlled trial of long-term moderate exercise training in chronic heart failure: Effects on functional capacity, quality of life, and clinical outcome. Circulation 1999;99:1173–1182.

CHAPTER 29

Recognition and Management of Patients with Cardiomyopathies

G. William Dec

The cardiomyopathies are a diverse group of cardiac disorders characterized by primary involvement of the ventricular myocardium. The myocardial dysfunction is not related to coronary atherosclerosis or to valvular, congenital, or hypertensive heart disease. The World Health Organization has recommended that the cardiomyopathies be classified by their anatomic appearance and abnormal physiology into dilated, hypertrophic, and restrictive types. Dilated cardiomyopathies are characterized by biventricular dilatation and impaired systolic function; hypertrophic cardiomyopathies by abnormal wall thickening, myocardial hypercontractility, and impaired diastolic function; and restrictive cardiomyopathies by an abnormally stiff myocardium with impaired ventricular relaxation but well-preserved contractile function[1] (Table 29–1).

DILATED CARDIOMYOPATHIES

Pathology

Cardiac enlargement is the hallmark of dilated cardiomyopathy. Dilatation of all four cardiac chambers is typical (Fig. 29–1), although the disease sometimes involves only one side of the heart. Even though the thickness of the ventricular wall may be mildly increased, the increase is insufficient to match the degree of ventricular dilatation. Histopathologically, evidence of varying degrees of myocyte degeneration, eccentric hypertrophy, and atrophy of the myofibrils is noted. Interstitial and replacement fibrosis may be extensive.

A wide variety of diseases may directly affect the myocardium and result in either permanent or transient systolic dysfunction. Dilated cardiomyopathy probably represents a common expression of myocardial damage that has resulted from one or more myocardial insults yet to be defined. All potentially reversible causes of dilated cardiomyopathy should be considered, particularly excessive alcohol consumption, toxins such as cocaine or drug hypersensitivity myocarditis, ischemic heart disease, and endocrine disorders (Box 29–1).

Alcoholic Cardiomyopathy

Excessive alcohol consumption is one of the most common identifiable causes of dilated cardiomyopathy.[1] Substantial evidence indicates that chronic alcohol use depresses cardiac function. The typical patient with alcoholic cardiomyopathy is a middle-aged man who has consumed at least 80 g of alcohol daily for at least a decade. Because alcohol use has increased in adolescents, it is no longer rare to see young adults with this disorder. Alcoholic liver disease is rare in such patients. The cardiac failure is reversible in most patients with recently diagnosed cardiomyopathy if total abstinence from alcohol is achieved.

TABLE 29–1

Hemodynamic and Morphometric Features of the Cardiomyopathies

Feature	Dilated	Hypertrophic	Restrictive
LV ejection fraction	<45%	65%–90%	50–70% <40% (late)
LV cavity size	Increased	Normal or decreased	Normal Increased (late)
Stroke volume	Markedly decreased	Normal or increased	Normal or increased
Volume-mass ratio	Increased	Decreased	Markedly decreased
Diastolic compliance	Normal to decreased	Markedly decreased	Markedly decreased
Other features	Mild/moderate MR/TR 15 common	Dynamic obstruction MR may be present	Often mimics constrictive pericarditis

LV, left ventricular; MR, mitral regurgitation; TR, tricuspid regurgitation.

Adapted from DeSanctis RW, Dec GW: The cardiomyopathies, Section 1, Subsection XIV. In Dale DC, Federman D (eds): Scientific American Medicine. New York, Scientific American, 1995.

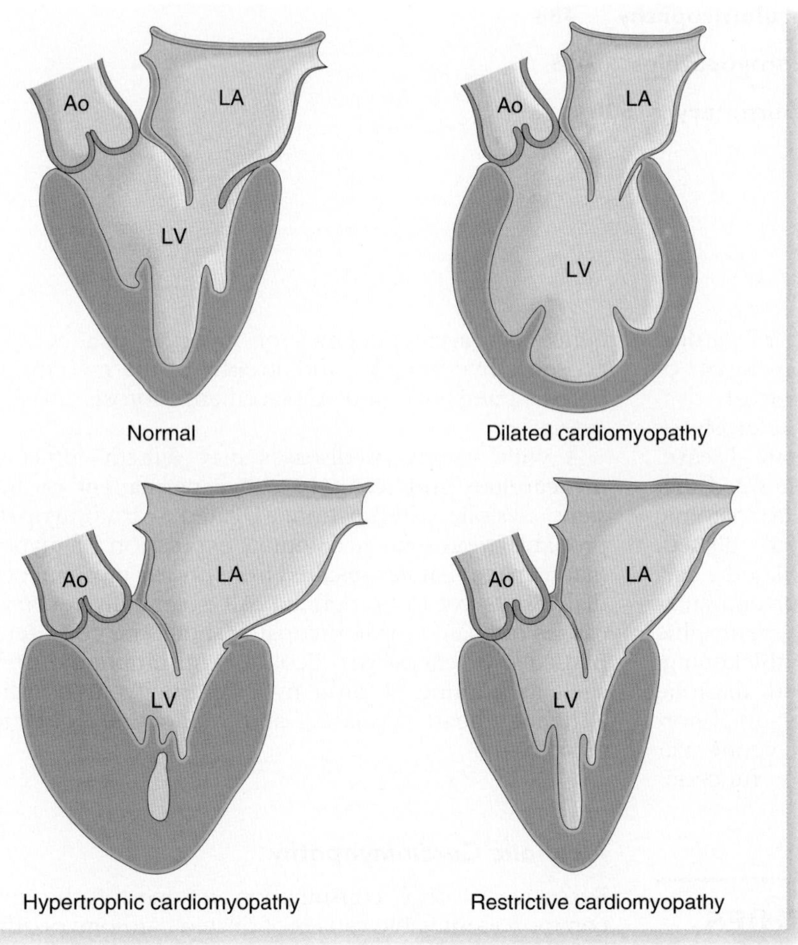

FIGURE 29–1. Schematic representation of the three morphometric types of cardiomyopathy—dilated, hypertrophic, and restrictive. Ao, aorta; LA, left atrium; LV, left ventricle. (Redrawn from Waller BF: Pathology of the cardiomyopathies. J Am Soc Echocardiogr 1988;1:4–19.)

Toxic Cardiomyopathy

Dilated cardiomyopathy can result from chronic exposure to drugs or toxins—the most common being cocaine or antineoplastic chemotherapeutic agents, especially the anthracycline drugs. *Anthracycline cardiotoxicity* is directly related to cumulative doses of the drug and increases dramatically in patients who receive more than 400 to 450 mg/m^2. Patients with preexisting left ventricular dysfunction or those who receive either concomitant mediastinal irradiation or other antineoplastic drugs such as dactinomycin, cyclophosphamide, mitomycin, or dacarbazine are at increased risk for anthracycline cardiotoxicity. Although congestive heart

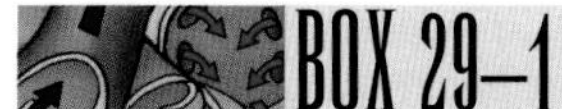

BOX 29–1

Causes of Potentially Reversible Dilated Cardiomyopathy

TOXINS
Ethanol
Cobalt
Antiretroviral agents (AZT, ddI, ddC)
Phenothiazines
Cocaine
Mercury

METABOLIC ABNORMALITIES
Nutritional (thiamine, selenium, carnitine, and taurine deficiencies)
Endocrinologic (hypothyroidism, acromegaly, thyrotoxicosis, pheochromocytoma)
Electrolyte disturbances (hypocalcemia, hypophosphatemia)
Hemochromatosis

INFLAMMATORY/INFECTIOUS/INFILTRATIVE
Infectious
- Viral (coxsackievirus, adenovirus, cytomegalovirus)
- Rickettsial (Rocky Mountain spotted fever, Q fever)
- Bacterial (diphtheria)
- Parasitic (toxoplasmosis, trichinosis)
- Spirochetal (leptospirosis, Lyme disease)

Inflammatory/infiltrative
- Collagen vascular disorders (sarcoidosis)
- Hypersensitivity myocarditis
- Hemochromatosis
- Peripartum

MISCELLANEOUS
Tachycardia induced
Idiopathic

AZT, zidovudine (azidothymidine); ddC, zalcitabine (dideoxycytidine); ddI, didanosine (dideoxyinosine).

failure may develop acutely during drug administration, a latent period of many months or even years is more commonly observed. Mortality can exceed 60% once overt heart failure has developed.

Human Immunodeficiency Virus Cardiomyopathy

Cardiomyopathy is also common in patients with acquired immunodeficiency syndrome (AIDS) (Box 29–2). Evidence of ventricular dysfunction has been reported in up to 20% of patients with AIDS and is usually associated with a reduced CD4 cell count.[2] Fluctuations in ejection fraction are not uncommon in such patients. Myocarditis is evident at autopsy in approximately 50% of patients who die of active human immunodeficiency virus (HIV) infection. Myocardial dysfunction in patients with AIDS may result from active intracellular HIV replication (HIV myocarditis) or opportunistic infections such as toxoplasmosis or

BOX 29–2

Cardiac Lesions in Patients with Acquired Immunodeficiency Syndrome

Myocarditis
Endocarditis
Pericarditis
Dilated cardiomyopathy
Kaposi's sarcoma
Malignant lymphoma
Arteriopathy
Myocardial infarction

From Glazier JJ: Specific heart muscle disease. In Abelmann WH (vol ed): Cardiomyopathies, Myocarditis and Pericardial Disease, vol 2. In Braunwald E (series ed): Atlas of Heart Disease. Philadelphia, Current Medicine, 1994, p 4.2.

cytomegalovirus affecting the heart. More importantly, reversible cardiac toxicity has been described for commonly used drugs such as zidovudine (also known as AZT [azidothymidine]) and interferon alfa, agents commonly used to treat HIV and its complications. As HIV-infected patients live longer, it can be anticipated that more of them will have cardiac involvement.

Peripartum Cardiomyopathy

This specific dilated cardiomyopathy usually develops during the last 6 weeks of pregnancy or the first 3 months after parturition. A minority of cases have been shown by endomyocardial biopsy to result from active myocarditis. Peripartum cardiomyopathy is more commonly observed in women with preeclampsia or multiple births. Although most cases resolve with restoration of normal ventricular function, approximately 20% of patients may be left with chronic left ventricular dysfunction or require transplantation for rapidly progressive disease. Subsequent pregnancies should be avoided if residual cardiomegaly or impaired contractile function persists. Recurrence is rare if ventricular function has normalized.

Inflammatory Heart Disease

Viral myocarditis is a frequent cause of acute dilated cardiomyopathy, particularly in children and adolescents. It has long been hypothesized that subclinical viral myocarditis can initiate an autoimmune reaction that culminates in the development of an unequivocal dilated cardiomyopathy. Although coxsackievirus and echoviruses frequently cause myopericarditis, these forms of myocarditis are usually mild and self-limited. Even though enteroviral RNA can be recovered from endomyocardial biopsy fragments in 25% to 50% of patients with dilated cardiomyopathy, biopsy evidence of both an inflammatory infiltrate and myocyte necrosis is required to establish a histologic diagnosis of acute myocarditis. When rigorous histologic criteria are used, only about 5% to 10% of patients with dilated cardiomyopathy have unequivocal evidence of myocarditis. The percentage is even lower when symptoms have been present for more than 1 year. Myocarditis should be considered in patients with acute biventricular dysfunction, unexplained life-threatening ventricular arrhythmias, or widespread T-wave inversions that occur during or immediately after an acute viral illness. The natural history of acute myocarditis is variable and ranges from early death from chronic dilated cardiomyopathy to complete recovery (Fig. 29–2).

Familial Cardiomyopathy

Cases of familial dilated cardiomyopathy are more frequent than had previously been recognized. Indeed, 20% of patients with idiopathic dilated cardiomyopathy have at least one first-degree relative with impaired ventricular function. Except for a family history, no clinical or histopathologic characteristics distinguish familial from nonfamilial forms of the disease. The mode of inheritance is generally autosomal dominant, but it can be genetically heterogenous, as indicated by reports of autosomal recessive, X-linked recessive, and mitochondrial inheritance. Specific mutations in cardiac cytoskeletal proteins (dystrophin, desmin, tafazzin, and lamin A/C) result in defects in transmission of contractile force.[3] Skeletal muscle dysfunction accompanies all but the lamin A/C mutations. Recently, mutations in sarcomere protein genes (beta-myosin heavy chain, troponin T, and actin) have been reported to produce dilated cardiomyopathy. Genotypic identification of specific mutations in patients with dilated cardiomyopathy may ultimately lead to the identification and treatment of asymptomatic carriers who are at risk for the development of symptomatic disease.

Idiopathic Dilated Cardiomyopathy

More than 75 specific heart muscle diseases can produce dilated cardiomyopathy.[1] However, in a sizable minority of cases, a cause is not evident despite extensive evaluation, and these patients are labeled as having idiopathic dilated cardiomyopathy. This condition probably represents a final common pathway of a variety of toxic, metabolic, and infectious processes that result in acute or ongoing myocardial damage. Although clinical findings of idiopathic dilated cardiomyopathy do not differ substantially from most secondary forms of dilated cardiomyopathy, the prognosis may vary by disease etiology[4] (Fig. 29–3).

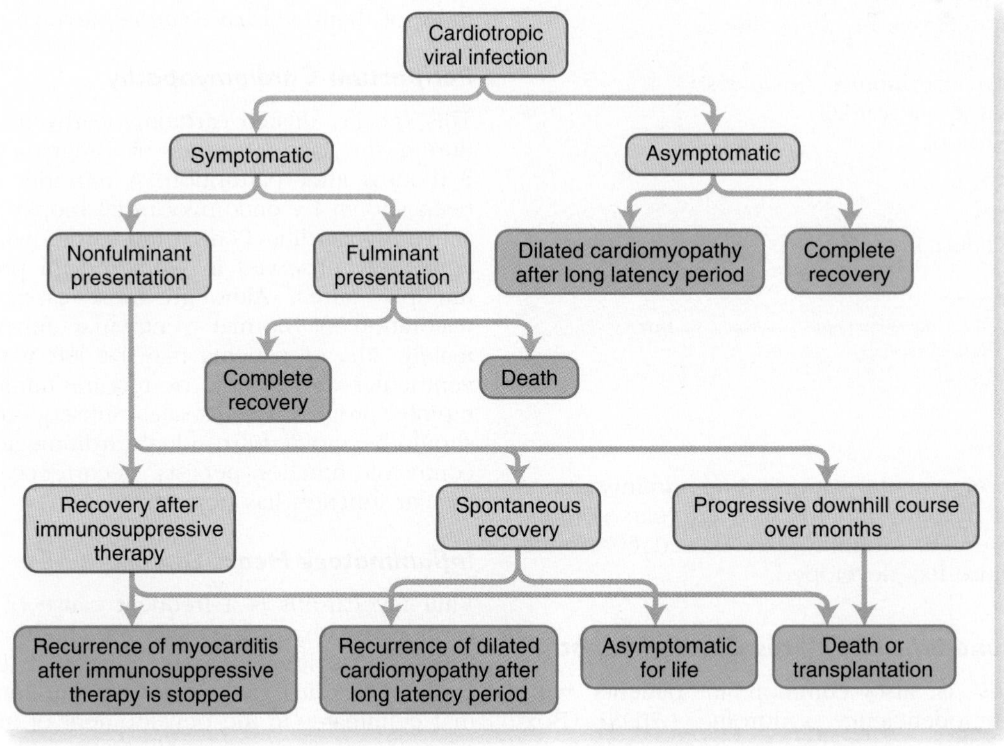

FIGURE 29–2. Natural history of human myocarditis. Most patients with mild symptoms of acute myocarditis are not seen by cardiologists, and most of these patients appear to recover fully. Of the patients with symptomatic heart disease typically seen by cardiologists, a small number have fulminant manifestations and either die in the acute stage or appear to recover completely. Of the remaining patients with myocarditis, a few have a progressive downhill course over a period of months to years that ends in death from heart failure or intractable arrhythmias. Some spontaneously recover and remain asymptomatic for life, whereas others have an asymptomatic period followed by the development of dilated cardiomyopathy. (Redrawn from Herskowitz A, Ansari AA: Myocarditis. In Abelmann WH [vol ed]: Cardiomyopathies, Myocarditis, and Pericardial Disease, vol 2. In Braunwald E [series ed]: Atlas of Heart Diseases. Philadelphia, Current Medicine, 1995, pp 9.1–9.24.)

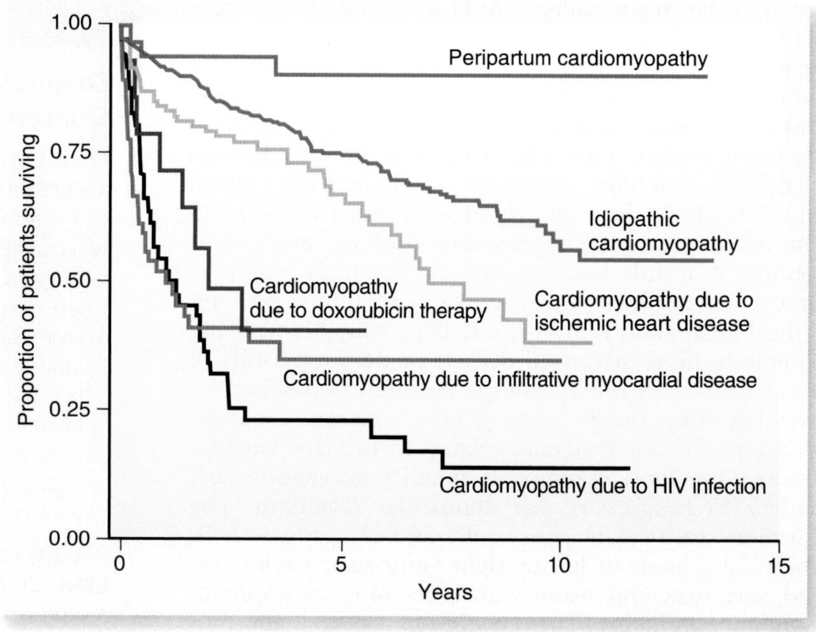

FIGURE 29–3. Influence of disease etiology on long-term survival in patients with dilated cardiomyopathy. (Redrawn, by permission, from Felker GM, Thompson RE, Hare JM, et al: Underlying causes and long-term survival in patients with initially unexplained cardiomyopathy. N Engl J Med 2000;342:1077–1084.)

Ischemic Cardiomyopathy

It is uncertain whether intermittent bouts of myocardial ischemia can produce dilated cardiomyopathy in patients with *normal* epicardial coronary vessels. Although abnormal microvascular reactivity, possibly caused by coronary vasospasm, could lead to myocardial necrosis and scarring, little direct evidence supports this theory. Small-vessel disease or microvascular dysfunction is more common in patients with dilated cardiomyopathy who have angina-like chest pain than in those with symptoms of congestive heart failure.

Recurrent or extensive myocardial infarction can lead to a cardiomyopathic picture consisting of ventricular dilatation, impaired contractility, and heart failure symptoms. Chronically ischemic but viable (so-called hibernating) myocardium can contribute to left ventricular dysfunction and ischemic cardiomyopathy. Not uncommonly, patients, particularly those with long-standing diabetes mellitus, may lack a history of angina pectoris or previous myocardial infarction despite extensive coronary artery disease, and such individuals may be clinically indistinguishable from those with idiopathic dilated cardiomyopathy. Given the high prevalence of ischemic heart disease, the possibility that impaired ventricular function may be improved through coronary revascularization should always be considered. The potential of coronary revascularization (through either coronary bypass surgery or angioplasty) is directly proportional to the extent of ischemic, but noninfarcted myocardium that can be adequately revascularized.

Clinical Manifestations

Patients with acute myocarditis generally have an acute manifestation characterized by sudden onset of heart failure, palpitations, pleuritic or angina-like chest pain, or even cardiogenic shock. The development and progression of symptoms are usually more gradual in patients with dilated cardiomyopathy. A minority of patients may have asymptomatic left ventricular dysfunction for months or years. The most common features are those related to left ventricular failure, particularly fatigue and dyspnea. Diminished cardiac output results in fatigue and generalized weakness. Exercise intolerance is also common and is related to both impaired cardiac output and reduced skeletal muscle performance. Right heart failure is often a late feature and is associated with a particularly poor prognosis. Exertional or rest dyspnea secondary to chronic pulmonary congestion is a frequent symptom. Acute pulmonary edema frequently occurs in acute myocarditis, but it is uncommon in chronic dilated cardiomyopathy. It often occurs in response to a precipitating event such as a respiratory infection or an alteration in cardiac rhythm.

Palpitations are common and reflect the occurrence of either atrial or ventricular ectopic beats. Syncope is a rare initial manifestation. Ischemic chest discomfort occurs in 25% to 50% of patients despite angiographically normal coronary arteries and is believed to be due to a reduction in dilator reserve of the coronary vasculature. Nonanginal chest pain secondary to pulmonary emboli or abdominal pain secondary to hepatic congestion is commonly observed in the late stages of disease.

Physical Findings

The physical findings reflect the underlying severity of the left ventricular dysfunction and range from subtle signs such as unexplained premature ventricular beats or cardiomegaly on chest films to overt, decompensated biventricular heart failure. Although pulmonary rales may be heard in patients with acute dilated cardiomyopathy, clear lung fields are most common. The jugular venous pulse is often elevated, and a prominent V-wave and brisk Y descent indicative of tricuspid regurgitation are often evident. Precordial palpation typically reveals a diffuse, laterally displaced, and heaving apical impulse; often, the right ventricle is palpable as well. The most prevalent auscultatory findings are gallop sounds. A fourth heart sound (S_4 or atrial) gallop is almost universally heard when sinus rhythm is present. A third heart sound (S_3 or ventricular) gallop is typically audible in more advanced disease or during periods of decompensation. An S_3 gallop can often be elicited by stressing the heart with gentle exercise. Systolic murmurs are not generally related to primary valvular disease; the most common is mitral regurgitation secondary to progressive left ventricular dilatation. The murmurs are usually pansystolic and of grade I–II/VI. They are related to left or right ventricular cavity size and may wax and wane with worsening or improvement in heart failure. The presence of a systolic murmur louder than grade II/VI should suggest the possibility of primary valvular disease.

Signs of right heart failure are initially present in less than 50% of patients, but they commonly develop as left ventricular dysfunction worsens and the patient enters a chronic phase of heart failure (see Chapter 28).

Diagnostic Evaluation

Noninvasive Studies

Patients with unexplained dilated cardiomyopathy (see Chapter 13) should undergo a diagnostic evaluation initially limited to studies necessary to determine the type of cardiac abnormality, uncover correctable causative factors, evaluate the prognosis, and guide treatment. The American College of Cardiology and American Heart Association Task Force on Heart Failure has issued guidelines on the diagnostic approach to patients with heart failure (and cardiomyopathy), as summarized in Box 29–3.[5] Any evaluation should begin with a careful search for reversible secondary causes of dilated cardiomyopathy. Screening blood studies should include serum phosphorus, calcium, creatinine, urea nitrogen, and serum iron (to rule out hemochromatosis).

The chest film may suggest sarcoid or demonstrate infiltrates indicating an eosinophilic syndrome. It typically reveals cardiomegaly, often with four-chamber enlargement. Pulmonary venous redistribution is a frequent finding, whereas interstitial or alveolar edema is uncommon.

The electrocardiogram (ECG) is usually abnormal but may initially show only nonspecific repolarization abnormalities, atrial or ventricular enlargement, or sinus tachycardia. A wide variety of arrhythmias (most importantly, atrial fibrillation or ventricular tachycardia) may occur as a result of patchy interstitial fibrosis. Conduction system abnormalities are noted in more than 80% of patients and may include first-degree atrioventricular (AV) block, left anterior hemiblock, nonspecific conduction delays, and most commonly, left bundle branch block. Interestingly, right bundle branch block is quite rare. Conduction abnormalities are more common in patients with long-standing disease, progress over time, and are markers of increasing interstitial fibrosis or myocyte hypertrophy. Left ventricular hypertrophy and poor R-wave progression are also frequent ECG findings. Localized QS-waves resembling the typical pattern

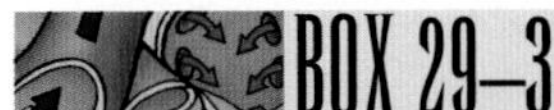

Diagnostic Evaluation of New-Onset Dilated Cardiomyopathy

CLASS I STUDIES (USUALLY INDICATED, ALWAYS ACCEPTABLE)

- CBC and urinalysis
- Electrolytes, renal function, glucose, phosphorus, calcium, albumin, TSH level
- Chest film, electrocardiogram
- Transthoracic Doppler echocardiogram
- Noninvasive stress testing in patients who lack angina but have a high probability of underlying ischemic heart disease, a known previous myocardial infarction, or extensive areas of hibernating myocardium (*Note:* Patients should be suitable candidates for revascularization if extensive ischemia is detected)

CLASS II STUDIES (ACCEPTABLE BUT OF UNCERTAIN EFFICACY: CONTROVERSIAL)

- Serum iron/ferritin
- Noninvasive stress testing in all patients with unexplained dilated cardiomyopathy
- Coronary angiography in all patients with unexplained dilated cardiomyopathy
- Endomyocardial biopsy in patients with
  - Cardiomyopathy of recent onset (generally <6 mo) and rapid deterioration in ventricular function
  - Clinically suspected myocarditis
  - Cardiomyopathy and a systemic disease known to involve the myocardium (e.g., sarcoidosis, hemochromatosis)

CLASS III STUDIES (GENERALLY NOT INDICATED)

- Routine 24-hr ambulatory ECG monitoring
- Serial echocardiography in clinically stable patients
- Routine right heart catheterization to guide medical therapy
- Endomyocardial biopsy in chronic dilated cardiomyopathy
- Cardiac catheterization in patients who are not candidates for revascularization, valve replacement, or cardiac transplantation

CBC, complete blood count; ECG, electrocardiogram; TSH, thyroid-stimulating hormone.

Adapted from American College of Cardiology/American Heart Association Task Force Report: Guidelines for the evaluation and management of heart failure. J Am Coll Cardiol 1995;26:1384–1385.

of myocardial infarction in the anterior leads may be noted when extensive left ventricular fibrosis is present, even without a discrete myocardial scar, or when present in multiple leads. QS-waves more often reflect previous myocardial infarction and, in patients with cardiomyopathy, are indicative of an ischemic origin.

Transthoracic Doppler echocardiography is the most useful initial noninvasive diagnostic procedure because it can rapidly assess systolic and diastolic function, chamber dimensions, and ventricular wall thickness and exclude clinically significant valvular heart disease. The left ventricular ejection fraction is usually less than 40%. Although global hypokinesis is often found, segmental wall motion abnormalities may occur in up to 60% of patients because of altered regional wall stress and thus cannot be reliably used to differentiate ischemic from nonischemic causes. Doppler interrogation often detects clinically inaudible mild to moderate mitral and tricuspid regurgitation. Myocardial contractile reserve, as indicated by a rise in the left ventricular ejection fraction during dobutamine echocardiography, appears to predict late spontaneous improvement in ventricular function and geometry over time.

Patients with a previous myocardial infarction and congestive heart failure, but without angina pectoris, are commonly evaluated with stress testing to detect ischemic or hibernating myocardium (see Chapter 25). Dobutamine stress echocardiography and positron emission tomographic imaging have the highest sensitivity and specificity for detecting viable myocardium. Quantitative stress thallium or technetium sestamibi scintigraphy may also provide clinically relevant information regarding myocardial viability.

Invasive Studies

Cardiac catheterization is not necessary in all patients with dilated cardiomyopathy and is not indicated for serial assessment. Right heart catheterization is most useful for tailoring medical therapy in patients with severe symptoms despite optimal treatment. Baseline hemodynamic assessment before the initiation of conventional medical therapy is seldom indicated. Coronary angiography is recommended in patients with symptomatic angina pectoris, significant areas of ischemic myocardium on noninvasive stress imaging, and unexplained cardiomyopathy and a high probability of coronary artery disease (e.g., those with multiple coronary risk factors, segmental left ventricular dysfunction on echocardiography, or QS-waves on ECG); the latter patients are potential candidates for coronary revascularization.

Right ventricular endomyocardial biopsy has generally been used to differentiate patients with myocarditis from those with idiopathic dilated cardiomyopathy. The low diagnostic yield (<10%) and lack of an effective treatment of myocarditis have limited its clinical relevance. Biopsy should be reserved for patients with rapidly progressive ventricular dysfunction and clinically suspected giant cell myocarditis (based on a preceding viral prodrome, associated pericarditis, or elevation of creatine kinase or troponin levels) or those in whom an active systemic disease and possible cardiac involvement (e.g., sarcoidosis, hemochromatosis, or Löffler's eosinophilic myocarditis) are suspected.

Differential Diagnosis

Dilated cardiomyopathy must be distinguished from valvular heart disease, coronary artery disease, and hypertensive heart disease. Features that aid in differentiating dilated cardiomyopathy with accompanying functional mitral regurgitation from that caused by primary mitral valve disease include the absence of a history of mitral valve prolapse, the absence of significant mitral valve calcification, the relative infrequency of atrial fibrillation, the severe depression of ventricular function, and the presence of left atrial enlargement that is proportional to the degree of left ventricular dilatation.

The clinical manifestations of end-stage aortic valve disease, either stenosis or regurgitation, may also resemble those of dilated cardiomyopathy. The murmur of severe aortic stenosis may be faint, but it is rarely absent. A severe elevation in left ventricular end-diastolic pressure may mask signs of aortic regurgitation and cause the diastolic murmur to disappear. Suspicion of aortic valve disease should be confirmed by noninvasive or invasive cardiac evaluation. Hypertensive heart disease is usually the result of severe, long-standing systolic and diastolic hypertension. Diastolic heart failure (see Chapter 28) rather than systolic contractile dysfunction is the more common finding in this disorder.

Natural History

Asymptomatic cardiomegaly, the first stage of dilated cardiomyopathy, may go undetected for months or years. Although the rate of progression from asymptomatic cardiomegaly to overt symptomatic disease is unknown, symptomatic patients generally have a poor prognosis. The most common complication of dilated cardiomyopathy is progressive heart failure, which is the cause of death in 75% of patients. Sudden cardiac death from ventricular arrhythmias or electromechanical dissociation is also frequent, especially in patients with episodes of ventricular tachycardia and severe left ventricular dysfunction. Evidence of systemic or pulmonary embolism, or both, may be found at autopsy in up to 50% of patients with chronic dilated cardiomyopathy. Emboli can also cause catastrophic complications, including embolic myocardial infarction, but they are an infrequent (<5%) cause of death.

The prognosis varies considerably, with some patients experiencing a fulminant course resulting in death or organ transplantation within weeks or months of initial evaluation. Conversely, many patients do remarkably well for years. Survival data from tertiary referral centers initially reported mortality rates of 25% to 30% at 1 year and approximately 50% at 5 years. The poor survival in early retrospective series may have reflected a substantial referral bias in that patients with more advanced disease or treatment failures are more likely to be referred to tertiary centers. More recent observations suggest substantially better survival, with an average 5-year mortality of 20% (see Fig. 29–3). This reduction in mortality probably reflects earlier disease detection, a shift to population-based studies, and better treatment. A minority of patients may have a remarkably long period of clinical stability. Spontaneous improvement in ventricular function (an increase in ejection fraction >10%) occurs in 20% to 40% of cases and occurs most frequently within 6 months of the initial examination. Improvement in ventricular function is independent of the initial ejection fraction but is more likely to occur in patients with acute, rather than chronic dilated cardiomyopathy. Active myocardial inflammation detected by biopsy or radionuclide imaging techniques and lesser degrees of myocardial damage as seen on endomyocardial biopsy specimens correlate weakly with the likelihood of spontaneous improvement in ventricular function.

The most reliable prognostic indicator is the severity of left ventricular dysfunction (Box 29–4). Although the relationship is certainly not linear, the lower the ejection fraction or the greater the degree of left ventricular enlargement, the poorer the long-term prognosis. Other morphologic features that are associated with a poor prognosis include lesser degrees of left ventricular hypertrophy, a more spherical ventricular cavity, and right ventricular dysfunction.

Clinical features that portend a more favorable prognosis include female gender, age younger than 55 years, and New York Heart Association class less than IV. Syncope, a persistent S_3, and right-sided heart failure on physical examination all predict a poor prognosis. Although elevated serum concentrations of norepinephrine, atrial and brain natriuretic factor, and renin have been shown to have prognostic value, they are seldom used in clinical practice. Cardiopulmonary exercise testing can provide important prognostic information and quantify a patient's extent of functional limitation. Maximal systemic oxygen uptake below 10 mL/kg/min predicts a 1-year mortality rate as high as 50% and is frequently used to identify patients in need of cardiac transplantation. Careful subjective assessment of daily functional capacity provides similar, albeit less quantitative prognostic information and is the preferred method for monitoring most patients, except those with advanced symptoms who are being considered for investigational therapies or transplantation.

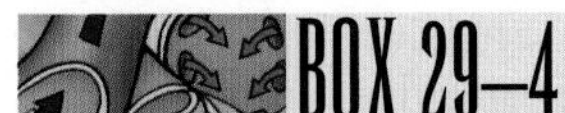
BOX 29–4

Predictors of Poor Outcome in Dilated Cardiomyopathy

CLINICAL FEATURES

NYHA class IV symptoms
Older age (>55 yr) at initial evaluation
Male gender
Ischemic cause
History of syncope
Persistent S_3 gallop
Right-sided heart failure signs
Inability to tolerate ACE inhibitors

HEMODYNAMIC AND VENTRICULOGRAPHIC FINDINGS

Left ventricular ejection fraction <20%
Right ventricular dysfunction
Pulmonary hypertension
Right atrial pressure >8 mm Hg
Pulmonary capillary wedge pressure >16–18 mm Hg
Cardiac index <2.2 U/min/m^2

NEUROHORMONAL ABNORMALITIES

Hyponatremia (serum sodium <137 mmol/L)
Enhanced sympathetic tone (elevated plasma norepinephrine or resting sinus tachycardia)
Increased plasma atrial or brain natriuretic factor, renin

FUNCTIONAL LIMITATIONS

Maximal oxygen uptake <12 mL/kg/min

ARRHYTHMIA PATTERN

History of previous cardiac arrest
Symptomatic or asymptomatic nonsustained runs of ventricular tachycardia
Second- or third-degree AV block

ACE, angiotensin-converting enzyme; AV, atrioventricular; NYHA, New York Heart Association; S_3, third heart sound.

Management

Medical Therapy

In addition to the general management of heart failure described in Chapter 28,[5] disease-specific therapies should also be considered. Abstinence from alcohol should be prescribed whenever alcoholic cardiomyopathy is suspected. Phlebotomy is useful in treating hemochromatosis, but it is most effective when instituted before the development of significant left ventricular dysfunction. Correction of metabolic or endocrinologic abnormalities such as hyperthyroidism, hypothyroidism, acromegaly, or pheochromocytoma typically results in restoration of normal ventricular function. Adequate rate control of rapid atrial fibrillation can also lead to resolution of the cardiomyopathy.

Anticoagulation. Patients with dilated cardiomyopathy have an increased risk for systemic or pulmonary embolism because of blood stasis in the hypocontractile ventricle. The risk is greatest in patients with severe left ventricular dysfunction, established or paroxysmal atrial fibrillation, a history of thromboembolism, or echocardiographic evidence of intracardiac thrombi. Controlled trials have not evaluated the efficacy of systemic anticoagulation for dilated cardiomyopathy patients in normal sinus rhythm. Chronic warfarin therapy for such patients should be reserved for those with a high risk of thromboembolism (severe heart failure, mural ventricular thrombus, history of systemic or pulmonary embolization, recent thrombophlebitis), and the international normalized ratio should be adjusted to achieve a value of 2 to 3.

Antiarrhythmic Therapy. A variety of ventricular arrhythmias, including nonsustained asymptomatic ventricular tachycardia, are present during 24-hour ambulatory monitoring in most patients with dilated cardiomyopathy. Sudden cardiac death accounts for 20% to 40% of the mortality in this population. Unfortunately, Holter monitoring, signal-averaged ECG, and even electrophysiologic testing have not proved useful for risk stratification of patients with dilated cardiomyopathy and asymptomatic nonsustained ventricular tachycardia. Antiarrhythmic drugs have not been shown to decrease mortality, and many of these drugs actually increase the risk through proarrhythmic actions. Thus, the empirical use of antiarrhythmic medications (other than beta-adrenergic blockers) in patients with asymptomatic dilated cardiomyopathy cannot be supported at this time.

However, patients with dilated cardiomyopathy and aborted sudden cardiac death, cardiac syncope, or symptomatic ventricular tachyarrhythmias do benefit from suppression of arrhythmia. Although many respond to empirical amiodarone, the low rates of long-term success, the high incidence of drug toxicity, and the increased proarrhythmic risk suggest that an implantable cardioverter-defibrillator, rather than chronic antiarrhythmic therapy, should now be considered the preferred treatment in such patients. Its effect on long-term survival in patients with advanced disease is less clear because many patients will be spared an arrhythmic death only to die of progressive heart failure within 2 to 3 years.

Surgical Therapy

Given the high prevalence of ischemic heart disease and its role as the principal cause of heart failure in North America, the possibility that ventricular function may be improved through coronary revascularization should always be considered in patients with symptomatic ischemic dilated cardiomyopathy.[6] Systolic dysfunction may reflect not only a fixed scar but also the partially reversible effects of intermittent or prolonged ischemia (i.e., hibernating myocardium) (see Chapter 25). For patients with ischemic cardiomyopathy but not angina pectoris, the potential benefit of coronary bypass surgery or multivessel angioplasty is directly proportional to the extent of ischemic, but noninfarcted myocardium that can be adequately revascularized. The presence of reversible ischemia can often be surmised from a history of angina pectoris or demonstration of ischemic ECG changes. A favorable surgical outcome is more likely if reversible defects in two or more myocardial regions can be demonstrated by thallium scintigraphy or positron emission tomography during exercise or pharmacologic stress testing. Accumulating evidence is indicating that surgical revascularization, even in the absence of angina pectoris, can improve symptoms of heart failure, exercise capacity, and long-term prognosis in carefully selected patients with extensive multivessel coronary artery disease and significantly impaired ventricular function. Patients most likely to benefit have three-vessel coronary artery disease, good distal vessels, a left ventricular ejection fraction exceeding 20%, mild or absent mitral regurgitation, and a left ventricular end-diastolic dimension less than 70 mm.

Mitral valve repair can provide symptomatic benefit for selected patients with severe (4+) mitral regurgitation and medically refractory heart failure symptoms. Cardiac transplantation is an effective treatment in dilated cardiomyopathy patients with advanced heart failure, but its use is limited to a small percentage of such patients because of an inadequate number of cardiac donors (see Chapter 28). Electrically driven, totally implantable left ventricular assist devices, particularly the Novacor and Heartmate models, may ultimately be a better long-term solution for severe, intractable heart failure.

Referral to Cardiologists

Most patients with dilated cardiomyopathy do not require referral to a cardiologist for subspecialty consultation. In general, patients who may benefit from specialized cardiovascular consultation include those who have failed conventional therapy and have progressive heart failure symptoms (Box 29–5). Patients with acute myocarditis, as well as those being considered for transplantation or enrollment in an investigational heart failure trial, should also be referred.

BOX 29–5

Dilated Cardiomyopathy: Indications for Cardiology Referral

Progressive left ventricular dilatation, deterioration in ejection fraction, or worsening symptoms despite medical therapy

Active myocarditis

Consideration of endomyocardial biopsy in patients with rapidly progressive cardiac symptoms associated with a systemic disease known to affect the myocardium

Syncope

Symptomatic or asymptomatic nonsustained ventricular tachycardia on ambulatory or in-hospital ECG monitoring

Patients with NYHA class III/IV heart failure symptoms who are being considered for cardiac transplantation or participation in a heart failure clinical trial

Consideration of coronary angiography or coronary revascularization in patients with known ischemic cardiomyopathy and anginal symptoms or a positive stress imaging study

ECG, electrocardiogram; NYHA, New York Heart Association.

Likewise, those who may require an invasive procedure, either endomyocardial biopsy or coronary angiography, should be considered for referral. Finally, patients with known or suspected ischemic cardiomyopathy and poor ventricular function who are being considered for revascularization should undergo cardiac evaluation.

HYPERTROPHIC CARDIOMYOPATHY

Hypertrophic cardiomyopathies are characterized by inappropriate myocardial hypertrophy, often predominantly involving the interventricular septum, and a hyperdynamic left ventricle.[7] The myocardial hypertrophy is disproportionate to the accompanying hemodynamic load. The most prominent pathophysiologic abnormality in hypertrophic cardiomyopathy is diastolic dysfunction related to abnormal left ventricular stiffness. A distinctive clinical feature of the disease in some patients with hypertrophic cardiomyopathy is a dynamic pressure gradient in the subaortic outflow region of the left ventricle (see Table 29–1).

Etiology

Although hypertrophic cardiomyopathy may appear to develop sporadically, this condition is usually genetic. A hereditary pattern is evident in the family history in more than 50% of patients, and it is transmitted as an autosomal dominant trait.[8] Genetic linkage techniques reveal that most familial cases are due to an abnormality on chromosome 14, which contains the gene responsible for encoding the beta heavy chain of cardiac myosin. However, a number of different genotypic abnormalities may be responsible for the development of cardiac hypertrophy, including abnormalities in troponin I and T, alpha-tropomyosin, and myosin-binding protein C.[8] Convincing evidence has now been presented that the specific genetic defect strongly predicts prognosis. Specific mutations associated with an increased risk of sudden death and a dramatic reduction in life expectancy have been identified. It is anticipated that in the near future, screening for genotypic abnormalities will be widely available and may permit more aggressive treatment of asymptomatic patients in the hope of preventing sudden cardiac death or altering disease progression.

Hypertrophic cardiomyopathy must be differentiated from hypertensive concentric left ventricular hypertrophy. A characteristic form of hypertensive cardiomyopathy has increasingly been recognized in elderly patients. Typical features include excessive concentric left ventricular hypertrophy disproportionate to the severity of the hypertension, vigorous systolic contractility, and impaired diastolic function. Women and African Americans are more commonly affected, and beta-blockers often improve symptomatic pulmonary congestion.

Pathology/Pathophysiology

The hallmark of hypertrophic cardiomyopathy is unexplained hypertrophy, predominantly of the left ventricle and usually with thickening of the interventricular septum that is often disproportionately greater than that of the ventricular free wall. In its severest forms, the left ventricular hypertrophy may reach such massive dimensions that the walls encroach on the left ventricular cavity, which becomes small, elongated, and slitlike.[7, 9] The left ventricular papillary muscles are greatly hypertrophied, and the anterior papillary muscle is displaced medially and anteriorly. Movement of the septal leaflet of the mitral valve may be restricted by the hypertrophied septum. The opposition of the anterior mitral leaflet to the hypertrophied septum often causes obstruction to left ventricular outflow (Fig. 29–4).

Unlike the ventricular hypertrophy observed in hypertension, in which myocytes enlarge uniformly and remain in an orderly pattern, the histopathology of hypertrophic cardiomyopathy is unusual, with myofibrils demonstrating an extensive pattern of disarray. Typically, they are enlarged, vary in size and shape, and show strikingly heterogeneous morphology. This disarray may in part explain the abnormal diastolic stiffness and arrhythmias that characterize hypertrophic cardiomyopathy.

Hypertrophic cardiomyopathy may occur in either an obstructive or a nonobstructive form, depending on the presence or absence of a dynamic subaortic outflow pressure gradient. Opposition of the anterior mitral leaflet and the hypertrophied septum results in dynamic outflow obstruction. Conditions that reduce left ventricular cavity size (e.g., reduced venous return) bring the mitral leaflet and septum into closer proximity and promote obstruction. Conditions that enlarge the left ventricle (e.g., increased venous return) separate them and reduce the obstruction. Interventions that increase myocardial contractility also increase outflow tract obstruction, whereas negative inotropic agents (such as beta-blockers and calcium channel blockers) have the opposite effect. In addition to the presence or absence of outflow obstruction, concomitant mitral regurgitation may also contribute to symptoms. Although the dynamic systolic outflow tract obstruction may create impressive murmurs and receives significant attention in most patients, the symptoms of hypertrophic cardiomyopathy are primarily related to the increased left ventricular stiffness, which produces elevated left ventricular filling pressure and dyspnea.

Clinical Manifestations

Most patients with hypertrophic cardiomyopathy are either asymptomatic or only mildly symptomatic and are identified during screening of relatives of a patient with the disease. The most common symptoms include dyspnea, exertional angina pectoris, palpitations, syncope, and near-syncope. The disease is most often identified in adults during their third or fourth decades

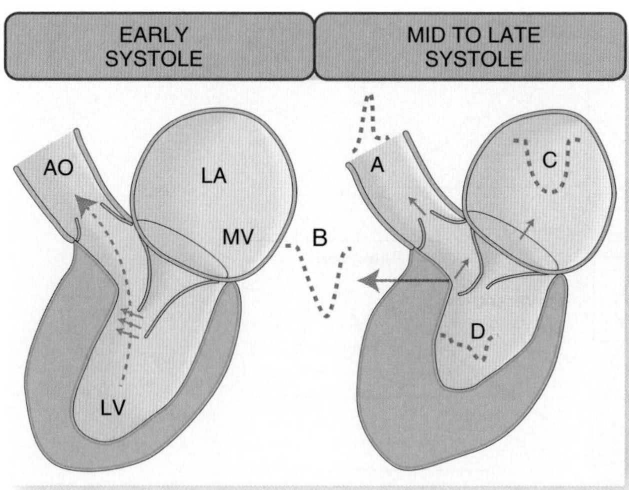

FIGURE 29–4. *Left,* Proposed mechanism of mitral valve leaflet (MV) systolic anterior motion (SAM) in early systole in patients with hypertrophic cardiomyopathy. Ventricular septal hypertrophy causes a narrowed outflow tract, as a result of which the ejection velocity is rapid and the path of ejection *(dashed line)* is closer to the MVs than normal. Such outflow results in Venturi forces (*three short oblique arrows* in the outflow tract) drawing the anterior or posterior MVs, or both, toward the septum. Subsequent MV-septal contact results in obstruction to left ventricular outflow and concomitant mitral regurgitation, as seen in the *right panel.* By mid systole, SAM-septal contact is well established and causes marked narrowing of the left ventricular outflow tract with obstruction to outflow. AO, aorta; LA, left atrium; LV, left ventricle. *Right,* Proximal to the level of SAM-septal contact, *converging lines* indicate acceleration of the jet just proximal to the obstruction and narrowing of the jet width. Distal to the obstruction, *arrows* and *diverging lines* indicate the high-velocity flow that emanates from the site of SAM-septal contact and is directed posterolaterally at a considerable angle from the normal path of aortic outflow. In late systole, although forward flow continues into the outflow tract and aorta, the volume of flow is much less than in early nonobstructed systole. Typical Doppler flow patterns are shown. A, integrated Doppler flow signal in the ascending aorta; B, high outflow tract velocity recorded by continuous-wave (CW) Doppler at the site of SAM-septal contact; C, presence of mitral regurgitation recorded by CW Doppler; D, late-systolic velocity peak that can be recorded in the apical region of the left ventricle. (Redrawn from Wigle ED: Hypertrophic cardiomyopathy: A 1987 viewpoint. Circulation 1987;75:312. By permission of the American Heart Association, Inc.)

of life. Unfortunately, the first clinical manifestation of disease may be sudden cardiac death. The extent of hypertrophy and the severity of symptoms bear a general relationship, but it is not absolute in that some patients have severe symptoms with only mild hypertrophy whereas others have marked hypertrophy and are virtually asymptomatic. The most common symptom is dyspnea, which is due to elevated left ventricular diastolic filling pressure secondary to impaired diastolic function. Angina pectoris occurs in 20% to 25% of symptomatic patients and may be due to the markedly increased oxygen requirement of the hypertrophied myocardium and the increased pressure resulting from outflow tract obstruction, from abnormalities in small intramyocardial arterioles, and from decreased myocardial blood flow as a result of elevated left ventricular diastolic filling pressure. Angina that is relieved by the patient assuming a recumbent position is a hallmark of hypertrophic disease but is rarely encountered. Myocardial infarction may occur in older patients in whom concomitant atherosclerotic coronary disease develops.

Syncope or near-syncope typically occurs during or shortly after completing physical exercise. Exertional syncope may result from excessive peripheral vasodilatation, inadequate cardiac output from either outflow tract obstruction or impaired diastolic filling, or cardiac arrhythmias. Peripheral vasodilatation is poorly tolerated in the obstructive form of hypertrophic cardiomyopathy because it worsens outflow tract obstruction. Syncope may also occur in the nonobstructive form of disease secondary to inadequate diastolic filling or arrhythmias ranging from atrial or ventricular tachycardias and asystole to complete heart block. Although these symptoms in children or adolescents identify patients at increased risk for sudden death, many adult patients may have a history of near-syncope or frank syncope dating back many years.

Atrial fibrillation is a late consequence of hypertrophic cardiomyopathy and is poorly tolerated because of loss of the presystolic atrial contribution to cardiac output and the rapid ventricular response rate, which impairs diastolic filling. Systemic embolism is a common complication of atrial fibrillation in hypertrophic cardiomyopathy, and long-term anticoagulation is necessary.

Physical Findings

Findings on physical examination depend on the presence or absence of left ventricular outflow tract obstruction, the severity of this obstruction, and the presence or absence of concomitant mitral regurgitation. In asymptomatic patients, examination typically reveals a left ventricular lift and a loud S_4 (Fig. 29–5). The initial carotid upstroke is very rapid and forceful. If obstruction to left ventricular outflow is present, a bisferiens character with a rapid initial upstroke followed by a second slower carotid impulse may be palpable (see Chapter 3). A single brisk upstroke may be converted to a double impulse if maneuvers that elicit outflow tract obstruction are undertaken.

Precordial palpation typically reveals a hyperdynamic systolic impulse and an apical impulse that is displaced laterally and inferiorly. A presystolic impulse generated by vigorous atrial contraction is often palpable.

Auscultation almost always reveals a prominent S_4 if normal sinus rhythm is maintained; an S_3 is less frequently encountered. Fluctuation in splitting of the second heart sound may be noted and depends on the

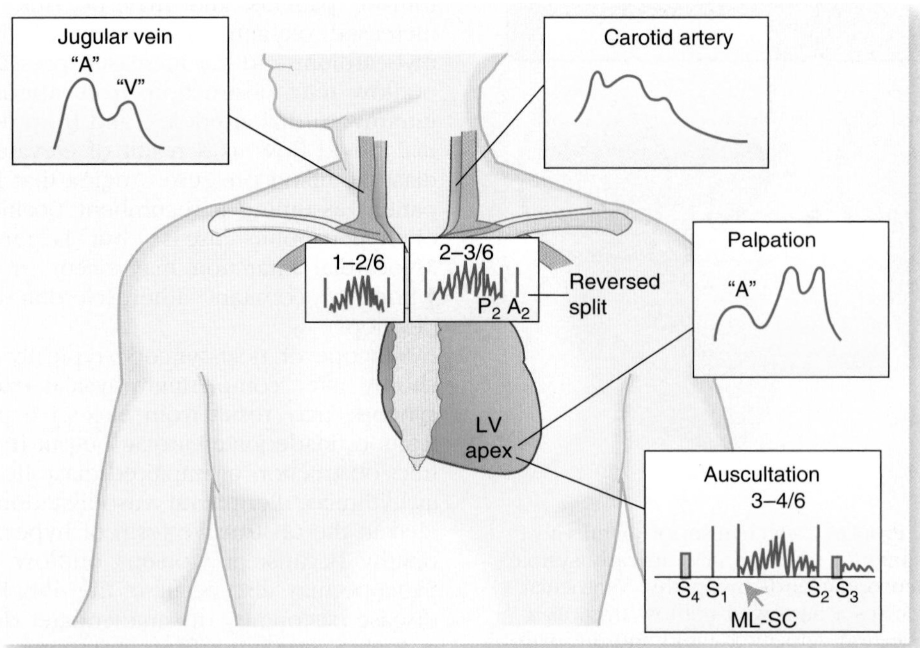

FIGURE 29–5. Physical examination in patients with subaortic obstructive hypertrophic cardiomyopathy (HCM). Seven physical signs in subaortic obstructive HCM are not found in nonobstructive HCM. On palpation, a spike-and-dome arterial pulse can often be felt in the carotid artery or in a peripheral pulse. On palpation of the left ventricular (LV) apex, one may find a triple apex beat caused by a palpable left atrial gallop and a double systolic impulse—one impulse comes before the onset of obstruction and the other after it. On auscultation, at or just medial to the LV apex is heard a late-onset, diamond-shaped systolic murmur of grade III to IV/VI in intensity. This murmur is produced by both the subaortic obstruction and the concomitant mitral regurgitation, which causes the murmur to radiate to both the left sternal border and the axilla. Because of the mitral regurgitation, a short diastolic inflow murmur is often heard after the third heart sound (S_3). Rarely, a mitral leaflet–septal contact (ML-SC) sound may be heard preceding the systolic murmur at the apex. If the fourth heart sound (S_4) is palpable, a double apex beat will be heard that is quite different in timing and significance from the double systolic apex beat that occurs in subaortic obstructive HCM. In nonobstructive HCM, there is either no apical systolic murmur or, at most, a grade 1 to 2/6 murmur of mitral regurgitation. In any type of HCM, a grade 1 to 3/6 systolic ejection murmur at or below the pulmonary area may be heard. This murmur may reflect obstruction to right ventricular (RV) outflow. Examination of the jugular venous pulse frequently reveals a prominent A-wave that rises on inspiration and reflects RV diastolic dysfunction. Rarely, this A-wave is accompanied by an RV S_4. A_2, aortic second sound; P_2, second pulmonic heart sound; S_1, first heart sound; S_2, second heart sound. (Redrawn from Wigle ED, Kitching AD, Rakowski H: Hypertrophic cardiomyopathy. In Abelmann WH: Cardiomyopathies, Myocarditis, and Pericardial Disease, vol 2. In Braunwald E [series ed]: Atlas of Heart Diseases. Philadelphia, Current Medicine, 1995, pp 2.1–2.22.)

degree of outflow tract obstruction at any instant. The murmurs of hypertrophic cardiomyopathy may be caused by outflow tract obstruction or mitral regurgitation or by both lesions. The systolic murmur characteristic of hypertrophic cardiomyopathy is harsh in character and has a crescendo-decrescendo pattern. It is most easily audible between the left sternal border and the cardiac apex and often radiates to the axilla. A holosystolic murmur, loudest at the cardiac apex, should suggest accompanying mitral regurgitation. The murmur of hypertrophic cardiomyopathy demonstrates marked variability during different maneuvers. The Valsalva maneuver or abrupt standing accentuates the outflow murmur by decreasing left ventricular chamber size, whereas squatting or isometric handgrip diminishes the murmur by increasing left ventricular cavity size. Bedside maneuvers to differentiate the murmur of hypertrophic disease from aortic stenosis or mitral regurgitation are summarized in Table 29–2.

Diagnostic Evaluation

Noninvasive Studies

The ECG typically shows left ventricular hypertrophy, nonspecific repolarization abnormalities or a strain pattern, and left atrial enlargement. Unexplained left ventricular hypertrophy or repolarization abnormalities may be the only sign of any abnormality in asymptomatic patients. Abnormal QS-waves mimicking a previous myocardial infarction, often evident in the anterolateral or inferior leads (creating a pseudoinfarct pattern), are due to the massive septal hypertrophy. Deeply inverted apical T-waves help identify patients with a variant of hypertrophic cardiomyopathy primarily involving the apex. ECG abnormalities often precede other clinical evidence of disease, and the diagnosis of hypertrophic cardiomyopathy should be considered in any young patient whose ECG suggests

TABLE 29–2

Bedside Maneuvers to Differentiate the Murmur of Obstructive Hypertrophic Cardiomyopathy from That of Valvular Heart Disease

	Response of Murmur		
Maneuver	**Hypertrophic Cardiomyopathy**	**Aortic Stenosis**	**Mitral Regurgitation**
Valsalva, hypervolemic tachycardia, standing *(decreased LV cavity)*	Increased	Decreased	Decreased
Squatting, passive leg elevation, isometric handgrip *(increased cavity size)*	Decreased	No change or slight increase	No change or slight increase

LV, left ventricular.

a previous silent myocardial infarction or unexplained left ventricular hypertrophy.

The chest film is not usually helpful. Varying degrees of left ventricular or left atrial enlargement may be evident.

Echocardiography is the most useful initial study for confirming the diagnosis of hypertrophic cardiomyopathy. The cardinal echocardiographic feature is unexplained left ventricular hypertrophy. Asymmetric hypertrophy of the interventricular septum with a septal-to-left ventricular free wall thickness greater than 1.3:1 is highly suggestive of the disease, though not pathognomonic (Fig. 29–6). Considerable variability in the degree and pattern of hypertrophy may be evident with concentric hypertrophy, asymmetric hypertrophy, apical hypertrophy, or a hypertrophied posterior free wall.

Echocardiography also reveals the presence and severity of left ventricular outflow tract obstruction and may document whether it is fixed or labile in nature. Systolic motion of the anterior (septal) mitral valve leaflet often accompanies hypertrophic cardiomyopathy when outflow tract obstruction exists (see Fig. 29–4). Although systolic anterior motion has rarely been described in other conditions, it is highly specific (97%) for obstructive hypertrophic cardiomyopathy. In addition to quantifying the degree of outflow tract obstruction, Doppler echocardiography is useful in assessing the severity of concomitant mitral regurgitation. Echocardiography is also extremely useful in monitoring disease progression, particularly in children and young adults with familial disease. Provocative measures such as the Valsalva maneuver and pharmacologic vasodilatation with amyl nitrite are useful adjuncts to resting echocardiographic interrogation because they produce or intensify obstruction.

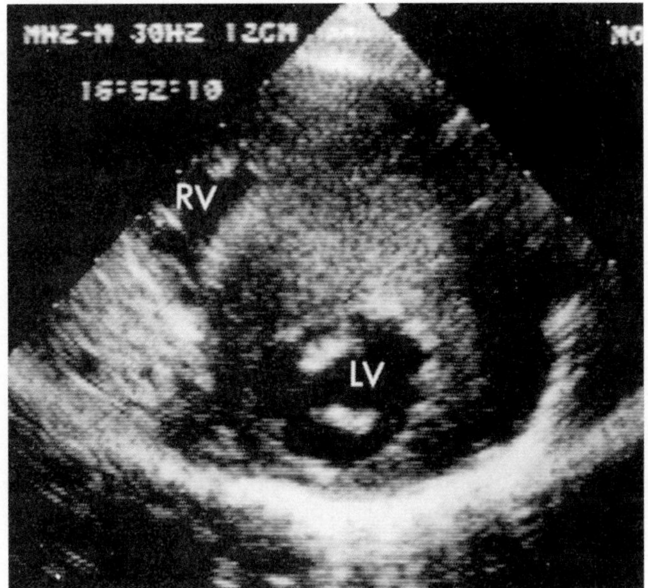

FIGURE 29–6. A short-axis echocardiographic image at the mitral valve level illustrates marked asymmetric ventricular hypertrophy. LV, left ventricle; RV, right ventricle. (From Levine RA: Echocardiographic assessment of the cardiomyopathies. In Weyman AE [ed]: Principles and Practice of Echocardiography, 2nd ed. Philadelphia, Lea & Febiger, 1994, p 784.)

Invasive Studies

Catheterization typically reveals elevated left ventricular end-diastolic filling pressure and a prominent A-wave. The gradient in the outflow tract of the left ventricle (Fig. 29–7), if present, may be fixed or labile and ranges over 150 mm Hg. Left ventriculography characteristically shows a small hyperdynamic chamber. The papillary muscles are thickened, mild mitral regurgitation is common, and the apex of the ventricle is often obliterated in systole. Cardiac catheterization is usually reserved for patients in whom the diagnosis remains uncertain despite echocardiography or for those in whom surgical or catheter-based intervention is being considered for relief of progressive symptoms. As the diagnostic accuracy of echocardiographic studies has increased, the need for invasive evaluation of hypertrophic cardiomyopathy has declined.

Electrophysiologic studies are indicated in high-risk patients, particularly those with a history of previous cardiac syncope, documented cardiac arrest, or symptomatic ventricular tachycardia. Its role in other subsets of patients, such as asymptomatic individuals

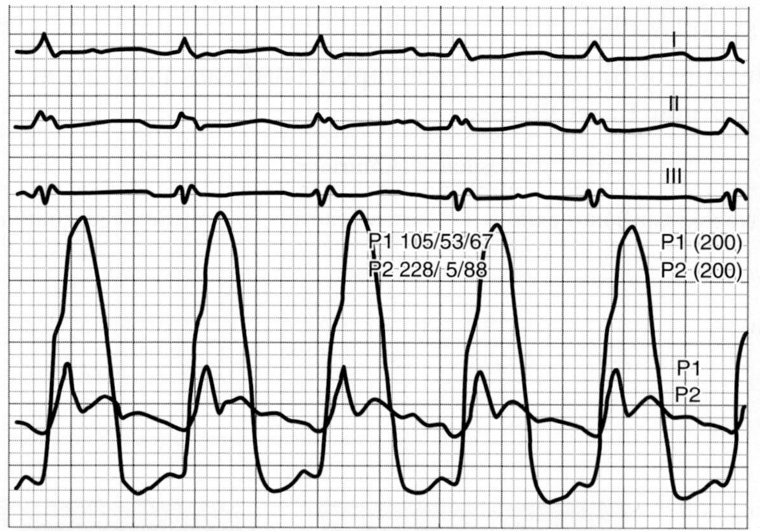

FIGURE 29–7. Simultaneous left ventricular and aortic pressure tracings in a patient with severe left ventricular outflow tract obstruction. In the left ventricular tracing is a prominent atrial contraction that contributes to the elevation in left ventricular end-diastolic pressure. The aortic pressure tracing waveform demonstrates a characteristic spike-and-dome rapid upstroke with a second peak that occurs in late systole before the incisura (providing the bisferiens feature of the carotid pulse on physical examination). The notch on the upstroke of the left ventricular pressure tracing coincides with the time of contact between the mitral valve and the septum as a result of systolic anterior motion of the mitral valve in this condition. (Redrawn from McKenna WJ, Elliot PM: Hypertrophic cardiomyopathy. In Topol E [ed]: Textbook of Cardiovascular Medicine, Philadelphia, Lippincott-Raven, 1998.)

with a family history of sudden cardiac death, remains unclear.

Differential Diagnosis

Hypertrophic cardiomyopathy may be confused with the left ventricular hypertrophy associated with chronic, severe untreated hypertension. A pattern of asymmetric septal hypertrophy will differentiate the two entities, as will the history of previous blood pressure readings. The concentric form of hypertrophic cardiomyopathy has many similarities to hypertensive hypertrophic disease of the elderly. The latter entity is typically seen in older women with a previous history of hypertension and diabetes mellitus. Occasionally, restrictive or infiltrative diseases such as amyloidosis may produce marked concentric hypertrophy. Hypertrophic cardiomyopathy is occasionally confused with valvular or subvalvular aortic stenosis, chronic mitral regurgitation, infundibular pulmonic stenosis, or a small ventricular septal defect. The brisk carotid upstrokes and the variable systolic murmur with maneuvers are useful in identifying hypertrophic cardiomyopathy.

Long-term athletic training may produce an increase in left ventricular end-diastolic cavity dimension, wall thickness, and contractility that is commonly referred to as "the athlete's heart." This condition is a physiologic form of hypertrophy in which left ventricular wall thickness is usually mildly increased, and overlap may exist between mild morphologic expression of hypertrophic cardiomyopathy and a more pronounced degree of physiologic hypertrophy such as that observed in rowers or weightlifters. Hypertrophic cardiomyopathy is more likely than physiologic hypertrophy when (1) hypertrophic cardiomyopathy is documented in a relative of the athlete, (2) evidence of impaired left ventricular filling is seen on transmural Doppler echocardiography, usually demonstrated as a diminished peak early-diastolic filling rate, (3) the left ventricular wall is thicker than 15 mm, and (4) the left ventricular cavity is smaller than 45 mm.[7,9]

Natural History

The clinical course of hypertrophic cardiomyopathy is highly variable, although the rate of progression is generally more rapid in children and adolescents (particularly during the teenage growth years). The extent of left ventricular hypertrophy usually remains stable over time in adults; however, hypertrophy may develop during adolescence despite an initial normal echocardiogram. Progression of hypertrophic cardiomyopathy to left ventricular dilatation and systolic dysfunction (i.e., the development of dilated cardiomyopathy) occurs in up to 10% of adult patients with long-standing symptomatic disease. The best predictor of long-term outcome appears to be the specific mutation responsible for the genetic defect. Death is most often sudden in hypertrophic cardiomyopathy and may occur in previously asymptomatic individuals or in those with a stable clinical course. The clinical features that best predict sudden death are a young age (<30 years) at diagnosis and a family history of hypertrophic cardiomyopathy with sudden death. A history of syncope is ominous in children but less so in adults. Ventricular tachycardia on ambulatory monitoring is also associated with increased risk, particularly in patients with a history of alterations in consciousness. Although the presence or severity of an outflow tract gradient does not correlate with the risk of sudden death, the extent of left ventricular hypertrophy does predict a risk for sudden death.[10]

In patients seen at major referral centers, annual mortality averages 5% to 6% for children and 3% for adults. However, community-based studies have indicated an annual mortality of only 1%.

Management

Medical Therapy

Management of patients with hypertrophic cardiomyopathy should be aimed at alleviating symptoms, preventing complications, and reducing the risk of sudden cardiac death[9] (Fig. 29–8). Whether asymptomatic or minimally symptomatic patients should be treated remains controversial. Some clinicians favor the use of beta-adrenergic blocking drugs or calcium channel blockers to delay progression of the disease or the occurrence of sudden death. Low-dose amiodarone has also been advocated for asymptomatic patients with runs of nonsustained ventricular tachycardia. None of these treatments can be currently recommended for asymptomatic patients because evidence of their efficacy is lacking.

Beta-blockers have traditionally been the mainstay of medical therapy for patients with mild to moderate symptoms. They provide effective relief of angina, dyspnea, and syncope and improve exercise capacity in a third to half of all patients. Although the level of ventricular ectopy often decreases, beta-adrenergic blockade has not been convincingly shown to decrease the risk of sudden death or, indeed, to alter survival in patients with hypertrophic cardiomyopathy.

Calcium channel blockers (particularly verapamil) are often useful in patients who fail to respond to beta-blockers, and they have been shown to improve symptoms in up to 60% of patients unresponsive to beta-blocker therapy. Although their negative inotropic properties usually lessen outflow obstruction, rarely, their peripheral vasodilating properties may actually increase obstruction and worsen symptoms. Verapamil has also been shown to prevent silent myocardial ischemia during exercise. The addition of a low-dose diuretic such as a thiazide may provide symptomatic improvement in patients with persistent dyspnea. For those who have refractory symptoms with a single agent, the combination of a beta-blocker and a calcium channel blocker may provide substantial clinical

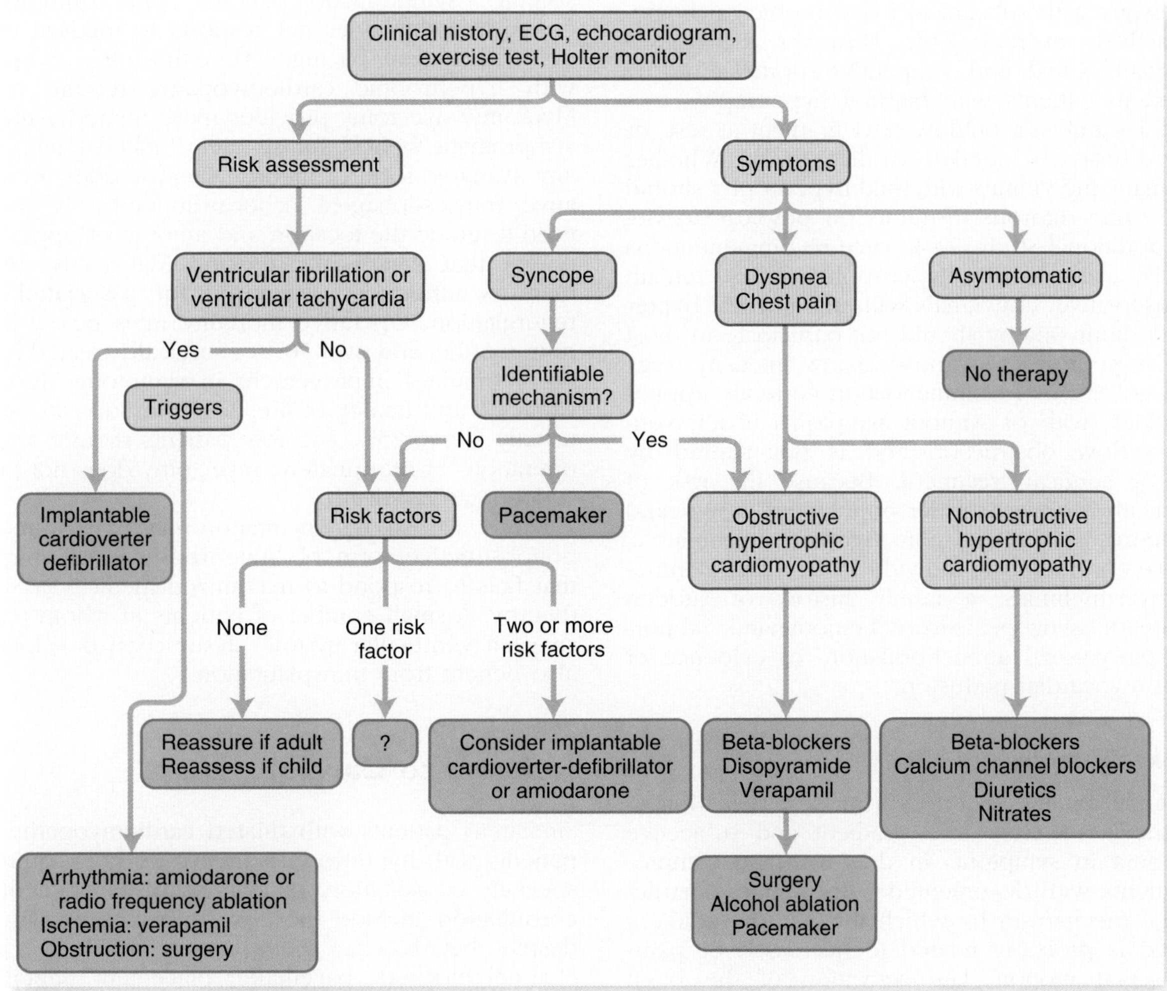

FIGURE 29–8. Algorithm for the management of patients with known hypertrophic cardiomyopathy. ECG, electrocardiogram. (Redrawn from Elliot PM, McKenna WJ: Hypertrophic cardiomyopathy. In Crawford MH, DiMarco JP [eds]: Cardiology. New York, Mosby, 2001, p 12.9.)

improvement. Disopyramide is a type I antiarrhythmic agent that possesses potent negative inotropic properties. It has been shown to reduce obstruction and to improve symptoms in patients with the obstructive form of disease. Dosages typically range from 150 to 200 mg orally four times daily. The drug has significant disadvantages, including anticholinergic effects and a decline in hemodynamic benefits over time.

Patients at high risk of sudden cardiac death should ordinarily receive an implantable cardioverter-defibrillator (ICD). These include patients who have been resuscitated from sudden cardiac death; who have had multiple episodes of syncope; or who have developed sustained ventricular tachycardia during electrophysiologic testing, nonsustained ventricular tachycardia on Holter monitoring, a flat or hypotensive response to exercise, or a ventricular wall thickness exceeding 30 mm. Amiodarone may be useful in patients with a history of sudden cardiac death or symptomatic ventricular arrhythmias. The decision to use antiarrhythmic drug suppression versus an implantable defibrillator must be individualized (see Chapter 30).

Exercise Prohibition. Strenuous exercise should be prohibited because it increases the risk of sudden death. Many persons with subclinical hypertrophic cardiomyopathy actively exercise daily. However, the risk of sudden death is real, and competitive sports should be prohibited in patients with marked hypertrophy, evidence of a significant outflow tract gradient at rest, or a family history of sudden cardiac death. Whether asymptomatic individuals with mild hypertrophy should have the same rigorous restraints on physical activity requires additional study. Task force recommendations on exercise in those with hypertrophic disease remain quite conservative. Individuals with unequivocal hypertrophic cardiomyopathy should not participate in most competitive sports except those of low intensity (e.g., bowling, golf). This recommendation currently applies to individuals with or without symptoms of left ventricular outflow obstruction and is not altered by medical or surgical treatment. Because the risk of sudden death is lower in older populations (>30 years) with hypertrophic disease, more vigorous athletic activity may be considered in individuals who lack ventricular tachyarrhythmias, a family history of sudden cardiac death, syncope, severe hemodynamic abnormalities, paroxysmal atrial fibrillation, or evidence of abnormal myocardial perfusion.

Pacemaker Therapy

AV sequential pacing produces a modest reduction in the ventricular outflow tract gradient and subjective improvement in symptoms in drug-resistant, symptomatic patients with documented outflow tract obstruction.[11] The mechanism by which the outflow gradient is reduced is probably related to decreased or paradoxical septal motion, late activation of the basal septum, or decreased left ventricular contractility. For AV sequential pacing to be successful in reducing outflow tract obstruction, there must be complete ventricular capture, which requires careful optimization of the AV delay. Patients older than 65 years appear most likely to benefit. Its effect on long-term prognosis is unknown. However, cardiac pacing is ineffective in treating the nonobstructive form of the disease.

Controlled Septal Infarction

Infusion of absolute ethanol into the proximal septal branches of the left anterior descending artery creates a small infarction of the upper ventricular septum and a dramatic reduction in outflow tract obstruction. Success rates in excess of 90% have been reported with echocardiographic guidance.[12] However, 10% to 15% of patients may require permanent pacing, and several deaths have been reported. The risk of late ventricular dilatation or life-threatening arrhythmias remains unknown. Hence, this procedure should be reserved for older patients or those with co-morbid conditions known to increase the risk of myectomy surgery.

Surgical Therapy

Surgical myotomy/myectomy is recommended for persistently symptomatic patients with outflow tract obstruction that does not respond to medical therapy or synchronized pacing.[13] Less than 10% of patients with hypertrophic cardiomyopathy require surgery. Myotomy/myectomy provides more hemodynamic and symptomatic benefit for severely limited patients than any available form of medical therapy does. Intraoperative transesophageal echocardiography is routinely used to guide the location and amount of upper septal muscle that is surgically resected. Mitral valve replacement is infrequently required for associated mitral regurgitation. Operative mortality rates below 5% are now routine, and over 70% of surgically treated patients report marked improvement in symptoms, functional capacity, and quality of life. Ten-year survival rates are usually above 85%, and few patients require a second operation.[13] Unfortunately, myectomy does not prevent sudden cardiac death.

Rarely, cardiac transplantation may be required for a nonobstructive form of hypertrophic cardiomyopathy that fails to respond to maximized medical or surgical therapy. A small number of patients in whom progressive left ventricular systolic dysfunction develops may also benefit from transplantation.

Referral to Cardiologists

Similar to patients with dilated cardiomyopathy, most patients with hypertrophic disease do not require subspecialty consultation. Patients who may benefit from consultation include those with persistent symptoms despite beta-blocker therapy and in whom calcium channel blockers, pacemaker placement, septal ablation, or myectomy is being considered (Box 29–6). Likewise, patients at high risk for sudden cardiac death require consultation. Finally, patients who fail medical or surgical treatment or those with progressive left ven-

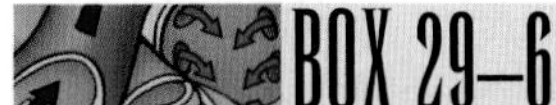

BOX 29–6

Hypertrophic Cardiomyopathy: Indications for Cardiology Referral

NYHA class III/IV angina or heart failure symptoms despite conventional therapy
Children/adolescents/young adults with asymptomatic hypertrophic disease and a family history of sudden death
Syncopal spells
Nonsustained ventricular tachycardia on ambulatory monitoring
Competitive athletes with a heart murmur or ECG evidence of substantial hypertrophy
Refractory heart failure or anginal symptoms leading to consideration of myectomy, dual-chamber pacing, or controlled septal infarction
Refractory symptoms or deterioration in left ventricular function leading to consideration of cardiac transplantation

ECG, electrocardiogram; NYHA, New York Heart Association.

tricular systolic dysfunction and who are in need of transplantation should undergo timely referral.

RESTRICTIVE CARDIOMYOPATHIES

Restrictive cardiomyopathies are the least commonly encountered form of heart muscle disease in Western countries. The hallmark of these disorders is abnormal diastolic function—the ventricular walls are excessively stiff and impair normal ventricular filling. Systolic function usually remains unimpaired until late in the disease. Varying degrees of myocardial fibrosis, hypertrophy, endocardial thickening, or secondary infiltration are usually responsible for the disorder. Although cardiac amyloidosis and idiopathic primary restrictive cardiomyopathy are the most commonly diagnosed causes, restrictive cardiomyopathy can result from a variety of other conditions (Box 29–7). Unlike dilated and hypertrophic disease, restrictive cardiomyopathy rarely has a familial component.

Pathophysiology

The ventricular myocardium is rigid and noncompliant, impedes ventricular diastolic filling, and produces elevations in cardiac filling pressure. Systemic and venous congestion and decreased stroke volume and cardiac output are the consequences of this abnormal diastolic filling. The clinical and hemodynamic picture of restrictive cardiomyopathy mimics that of constrictive pericarditis.

BOX 29–7

Causes of Restrictive Cardiomyopathy

MYOCARDIAL
Noninfiltrative
  Idiopathic
  Scleroderma
Infiltrative
  Amyloidosis
  Sarcoidosis
  Gaucher's disease
  Hurler's disease
Storage diseases
  Hemochromatosis
  Fabry's disease
  Glycogen storage diseases

ENDOMYOCARDIAL
Endomyocardial fibrosis
Hypereosinophilic syndrome
Carcinoid
Metastatic malignancies
Radiation injury
Anthracycline toxicity

From Wynne J, Braunwald E: Restrictive and infiltrative cardiomyopathies. In Braunwald E (ed): Heart Disease, 5th ed. Philadelphia, WB Saunders, 2001, p 1775.

Clinical Manifestations

Congestive heart failure is the most common clinical manifestation,[14] and exertional dyspnea is a prominent feature. Exercise intolerance is also frequently encountered because of an inability of the patient to increase cardiac output by tachycardia without further compromising diastolic ventricular filling. As in constrictive pericarditis, clinical evidence of right-sided heart failure without evidence of underlying pulmonary disease of sufficient severity to serve as an explanation is a frequent initial finding.

Physical Findings

Careful examination of the jugular venous pulse is essential for establishing the correct diagnosis. The elevated diastolic filling pressure results in chronic venous hypertension manifested as an increase in jugular venous pressure. An inspiratory increase in venous pressure (Kussmaul's sign) is commonly seen. The most prominent waveform is the Y descent. Precordial examination is generally unremarkable. The apex beat is usually in its normal position within the midclavicular line in the fifth left intercostal space. It is more likely to be palpable than in constrictive pericarditis, where the pericardium is usually quiet. An S_3 or S_4 (or both) is usually present. Mitral regurgitation and tricuspid regurgitation are frequently observed in restrictive cardiomyopathy, but they are quite uncommon in constrictive pericarditis. Hepatomegaly, ascites, and peripheral edema occur in more advanced cases.

Diagnostic Evaluation

Noninvasive Studies

The chest film often displays pulmonary congestion as a reflection of the elevated ventricular diastolic pressure. Cardiomegaly is either mild or absent, and pleural effusions are seen in advanced disease. Atrial enlargement is common when AV regurgitation has developed. The ECG is seldom normal but frequently demonstrates only nonspecific repolarization changes. The findings of low voltage, left axis deviation, and pseudomyocardial infarction should suggest an infiltrative process such as amyloidosis.[15]

Infiltrative diseases may be entirely confined to the heart or may be part of a more generalized systemic process. A complete blood count, erythrocyte sedimentation rate, serum protein electrophoresis, and renal and hepatic function studies should be undertaken. Additional blood studies (such as iron, iron binding, and ferritin) should be individualized.

Echocardiography confirms normal left and right ventricular size and systolic function and is useful for excluding hypertrophic cardiomyopathy or unsuspected valvular heart disease. Left ventricular wall mass is increased in patients with infiltrative diseases but may be normal in those with primary restrictive disease. The classic Doppler echocardiographic finding is rapid ventricular inflow and early cessation of flow in diastole. These filling characteristics result in a tall E-wave and a blunted A-wave (reflecting atrial inflow). However, the E-wave–to–A-wave ratio is load dependent and cannot reliably define the extent or severity of diastolic dysfunction. Echocardiographic findings are also often useful for differentiating restrictive cardiomyopathy from constrictive pericarditis. Patients with constriction have greater respiratory-dependent variations in left ventricular isovolumetric relaxation time and peak mitral valve velocity during early diastole. Echocardiography is not sufficiently accurate to quantify the degree of pericardial thickening or unequivocally establish a diagnosis of pericardial constriction.

Magnetic resonance imaging and computed tomography are quite useful for differentiating constrictive disease from restrictive cardiomyopathy. Both imaging techniques can accurately quantify the degree of pericardial thickening.

Invasive Studies

The characteristic hemodynamic feature of restrictive cardiomyopathy is a deep and rapid early decline in ventricular pressure at the onset of diastole, followed by a rapid rise to a plateau phase in early diastole (Fig. 29–9). This dip and plateau in pressure has been termed the "square root" sign and is evident in both atrial and ventricular pressure tracings. Right atrial pressure is elevated, and a prominent Y descent is noted. The X descent may also be rapid, and the combination may result in a characteristic M-waveform in the right atrial pressure tracing. Although both right- and left-sided filling pressure is elevated, patients with restrictive cardiomyopathy typically have left ventricular filling pressure that exceeds right ventricular filling pressure by more than 5 mm Hg. This difference may be further accentuated by exercise.

Right ventricular endomyocardial biopsy is often useful in differentiating primary restrictive disease from an infiltrative process or constrictive pericarditis. Because of sampling error, however, a normal biopsy does not completely exclude the possibility of restrictive disease.

Differential Diagnosis

Restrictive cardiomyopathies must always be differentiated from constrictive pericarditis, a distinction that is not always easily made on the basis of clinical or hemo-

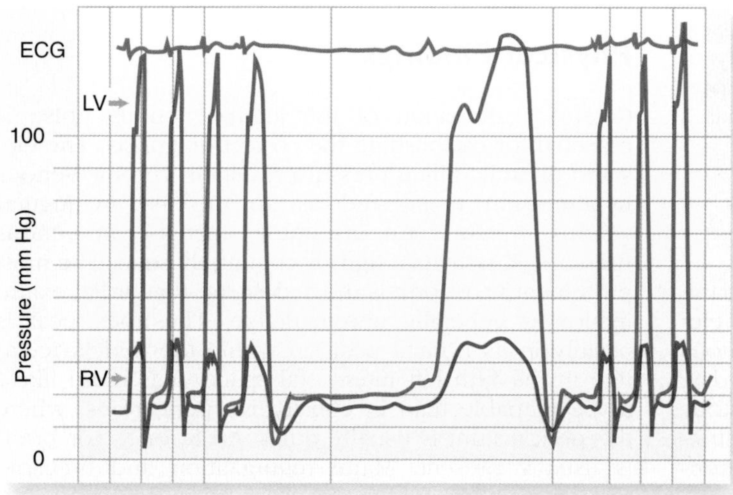

FIGURE 29–9. Right ventricular (RV) and left ventricular (LV) pressure tracings in a patient with idiopathic restrictive cardiomyopathy. A dip-and-plateau pattern is seen in both ventricles, and diastolic filling pressures are elevated. The plateaus occur at different pressures, approximately 16 mm Hg for the RV tracing and 20 mm Hg for the LV tracing. The diagnosis of restrictive disease was confirmed by thoracotomy. ECG, electrocardiogram. (Redrawn from Benotti JR, Grossman W, Cohn PF: The clinical profile of restrictive cardiomyopathy. Circulation 1980;61:1206. By permission of the American Heart Association.)

dynamic findings (Table 29–3). In general, constrictive pericardial disease involves both ventricles equally and produces a plateau of filling pressures. Thus, in constrictive pericarditis, the left ventricular end-diastolic, left atrial, pulmonary capillary wedge, right ventricular end-diastolic, and right atrial pressures are within 5 mm of one another and have similar configurations. Conversely, restrictive cardiomyopathies tend to cause greater impairment in left than right ventricular diastolic filling. Thus, left-sided filling pressures almost always exceed that on the right side by more than 5 mm Hg; in questionable cases, provocative testing with a fluid load may be helpful to see whether right- and left-sided pressures diverge, a finding in restrictive cardiomyopathy. Furthermore, pulmonary artery systolic pressure is often above 50 mm Hg—a pressure level that is distinctly uncommon in constrictive disease. Patterns of diastolic filling, as determined by Doppler echocardiography or radionuclide ventriculography, may also help distinguish the two entities (see earlier). Magnetic resonance imaging is usually an essential study to differentiate the two conditions. In some cases, endomyocardial biopsy or, very rarely, surgical thoracotomy may be necessary to differentiate surgically correctable constrictive pericarditis from restrictive cardiomyopathy.

Prognosis and Treatment

The prognosis in restrictive cardiomyopathy is one of symptomatic progression; less than 10% of patients survive more than 10 years after the onset of symptoms. Conventional treatment is directed toward relief of congestive symptoms. Diuretics are used to reduce peripheral edema and ascites and to decrease exertional dyspnea. Although angiotensin-converting enzyme (ACE) inhibitors and calcium channel blockers are often prescribed in an effort to improve diastolic filling, these agents must be used cautiously because of their peripheral vasodilating properties. No medical treatment has been shown to prolong survival. Corticosteroids and cytolytic agents may play a role in the treatment of specific causes of restrictive cardiomyopathy (see later).

Specific Causes of Restrictive Cardiomyopathy

Primary Restrictive Cardiomyopathy

Patients are considered to have a *primary* restrictive cardiomyopathy if they have a history of heart failure, normal left ventricular end-diastolic volume, elevation of ventricular filling pressure at catheterization, and the absence of an explainable cause for the diastolic dysfunction, such as an infiltrative process, coronary artery disease, coronary vasculitis, or hypertrophic cardiomyopathy. Endomyocardial biopsy typically shows varying degrees of myocyte hypertrophy and interstitial fibrosis and thus differentiates this disorder from hypertrophic disease. Restrictive hemodynamics and complete heart block may be present in this disorder despite the

TABLE 29–3

Differentiation of Restrictive Cardiomyopathy from Constrictive Pericardial Disease

Feature	Restrictive Cardiomyopathy	Constrictive Pericarditis
	Physical Examination	
Pulsus paradoxus	Uncommon	Uncommon
Palpable apical impulse	May be present	Absent
S_3 gallop	May be present	Absent
AV regurgitation murmur	Common	Rare
Pericardial knock	Absent	May be present
	Electrocardiogram	
Low voltage	Uncommon (exception: amyloidosis)	Commonly present
	Chest Film	
Cardiomegaly	Mild LV prominence	Absent
Pericardial calcification	Absent	Seen in 30%–50%
	Hemodynamics	
"Square root" sign		
LV diastolic pressure exceeds	Frequently evident	Almost always
RV diastolic pressure by 15 mm Hg during exercise, volume loading	Very common	Rare
Kussmaul's sign	Uncommon	Common (>80%)
	MRI	
Pericardial thickening	Absent	Virtually always evident

AV, atrioventricular; LV, left ventricular; MRI, magnetic resonance imaging; RV, right ventricular; S_3, third heart sound.

absence of significant fibrosis on biopsy.[14] Complete heart block, skeletal myopathy, and a dominant pattern of inheritance have been described in a rare familial form. Mean survival has been reported to be approximately 9 years after symptom onset and 5 years after the development of heart failure.

Hypereosinophilic Syndrome

Endomyocardial fibrosis is a common form of restrictive disease in equatorial Africa but is rarely encountered in nontropical countries. Marked hypereosinophilia (>1500 eosinophils/mm^3) of any cause can result in endomyocardial disease. The clinical diagnosis of idiopathic hypereosinophilic syndrome (so-called Löffler's endocarditis) is characterized by unexplained peripheral eosinophilia of greater than 6 months' duration and associated evidence of end-organ involvement. The heart is involved in more than 75% of patients. The central nervous system, kidneys, lungs, gastrointestinal tract, and skin are other common sites. Cardiac involvement is usually biventricular; endocardial fibrosis and thrombus formation are the characteristic pathologic lesions. Clinical features include weight loss, persistent fever, cough, skin rash, and heart failure. Although asymptomatic involvement may be present early in the disease, more than 50% of patients have symptoms of overt heart failure. AV valvular regurgitation is common because of the extensive fibrosis. Likewise, large mural thrombi are often evident on echocardiography, and systemic embolization is a frequent complication. The echocardiogram commonly demonstrates localized thickening of the posterobasal left ventricular free wall with marked limitation of motion of the posterior mitral leaflet. The left ventricular apex may be obliterated by thrombus, and varying degrees of mitral and tricuspid regurgitation are present on Doppler echocardiography.

Treatment. Therapy with corticosteroids and hydroxyurea may substantially improve survival. Medical therapy with diuretics, afterload-reducing agents, and warfarin anticoagulation can often control symptoms. Surgical treatment offers symptomatic improvement once the fibrotic stage of the disease has developed.

Cardiac Amyloidosis

Amyloidosis is a systemic disease caused by the extracellular deposition of insoluble amyloid protein fibrils within tissues.[15] Amyloid may be deposited in almost any organ, but clinically significant disease does not result unless extensive infiltration has occurred. Primary amyloidosis is caused by the production of an amyloid protein composed of portions of immunoglobulin light chain (so-called AL amyloid) by a monoclonal population of plasma cells, often as a consequence of multiple myeloma. Secondary amyloidosis is caused by the production of a nonimmunoglobulin protein (termed AA) and is found in a variety of chronic inflammatory diseases. Six different forms of familial amyloidosis are now recognized and result from abnormal production of prealbumin protein. Finally, senile amyloidosis is due to production of yet another prealbumin protein. It is becoming increasingly common as the average age of the population increases. Although clinically significant cardiac involvement is present in up to 50% of patients with primary amyloidosis, the heart is involved in less than 10% of cases of secondary amyloidosis. Likewise, familial amyloidosis is only occasionally associated with overt cardiac dysfunction and, then, only late in the course of the disease. Cardiac amyloidosis is more common in men than women, and it is rarely seen before the age of 30 years, even in the familial forms.

Pathologically, the walls of both ventricles are firm, rubbery, and noncompliant. Amyloid is visible between myocardial fibers. The intramural coronary arteries and veins frequently also contain amyloid deposits.

The most common manifestation of cardiac amyloid is that of right-sided heart failure from restrictive physiology. Paroxysmal dyspnea and orthopnea are usually absent early in the disease. Although systolic function is typically normal at initial evaluation, progressive deposition of amyloid frequently results in systolic dysfunction. The course of this disease is marked by relentless progression of heart failure. Orthostatic hypotension secondary to autonomic nervous system involvement is a well-recognized occurrence.

The ECG is frequently abnormal. The most characteristic feature is diffusely diminished QRS voltage, which is evident in approximately 50% of all patients. Left axis deviation, atrial fibrillation, pseudo–myocardial infarction patterns, and ventricular arrhythmias are frequently evident with more severe infiltration.

Echocardiography is extremely sensitive in detecting clinically significant cardiac amyloid. Typical findings include increased ventricular wall thickness, small size of the left ventricular cavity, and atrial dilatation. Thickened ventricular walls and a granular, sparkling texture are highly suggestive of amyloidosis (Fig. 29–10). The sparkling pattern results from amorphous amyloid deposition that replaces collagen fibers within the myocardium. Echocardiographic findings also predict the prognosis, with the poorest survival rates noted in patients with the greatest ventricular wall thickness.

Abdominal fat pad aspiration is the single most useful diagnostic technique because it combines ease of performance, sensitivity, and specificity (Table 29–4). Endomyocardial biopsy is useful for establishing the diagnosis of cardiac amyloidosis if the abdominal fat pad aspirate does not prove to be diagnostic.

Treatment. Treatment of cardiac amyloidosis is generally palliative and ineffective. Diuretics should be judiciously used to control symptoms of venous congestion. Digitalis and calcium channel blockers are relatively contraindicated because of their selective binding to amyloid fibers. Insertion of a permanent pacemaker is useful in patients with symptomatic conduction system disease or marked bradycardia. Several disease-specific treatment regimens have been studied, including prednisone, melphalan, and colchicine.[16] Colchicine may be partially effective in familial amyloidosis; combination therapy with prednisone and melphalan produces a modest improvement in survival for patients with AL

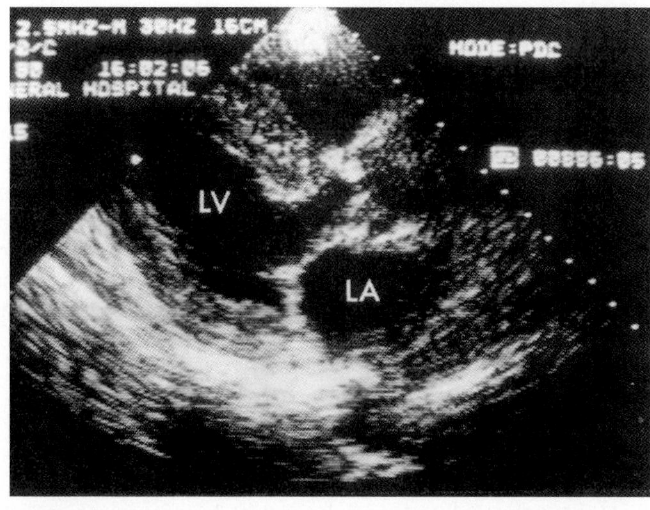

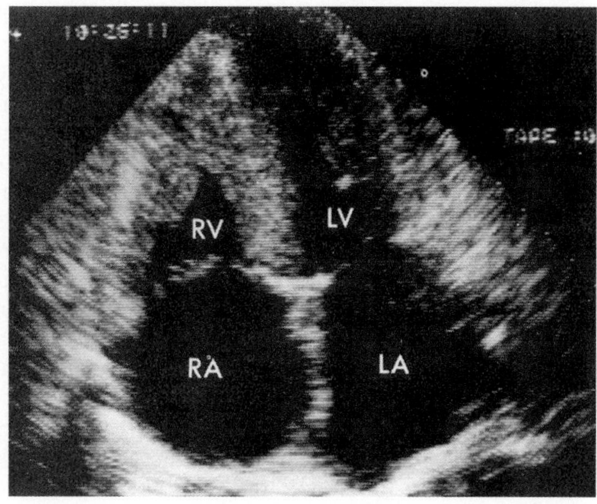

A B

FIGURE 29–10. *A,* Parasternal long-axis echocardiographic image showing a "sparkling" granular myocardial texture in the interventricular septum in a patient with biopsy-proved amyloidosis. LA, left atrium; LV, left ventricle. *B,* An apical four-chamber echocardiographic image demonstrates biventricular hypertrophy in a patient with biopsy-proved amyloidosis. (From Levine RA: Echocardiographic assessment of the cardiomyopathies. In Weyman AE [ed]: Principles and Practice of Echocardiography. 2nd ed. Philadelphia, Lea & Febiger, 1994, p 810.)

TABLE 29–4

Sensitivity of Noninvasive and Invasive Diagnostic Studies for Cardiac Amyloidosis

Diagnostic Test	Sensitivity (%)
Electrocardiography	
Low voltage	63–80
Q waves	60–93
Echocardiography	
Speckled appearance	45–87
Interatrial septal thickening	60
Tissue biopsy	
Abdominal fat pad aspiration	80
Rectal biopsy	70–85
Bone marrow biopsy	50–56
Skin biopsy	50–90
Endomyocardial biopsy	100
Radionuclide imaging	
^{99m}Tc-pyrophosphate scintigraphy	23

From Pereira NL, Dec GW: Restrictive and infiltrative cardiomyopathies. In Crawford H, DiMarco JP (eds): Cardiology, London, Mosby, 2001, pp 5–14.5

amyloid.[16] Results with other agents have been disappointing. Combined heart and bone marrow transplantation is being studied as treatment of primary amyloidosis.

Hemochromatosis

Hemochromatosis is characterized by excessive deposition of iron in a variety of tissues, including the heart, liver, testes, and pancreas. Cardiac involvement leads to a mixed dilated/restrictive cardiomyopathy with both systolic and diastolic dysfunction evident. The severity of the myocardial dysfunction is directly proportional to the quantity of iron deposited within the myocardium.

Hemochromatosis may occur as a familial or idiopathic disorder, in association with a defect in hemoglobin synthesis, in chronic liver disease, or as a result of excessive iron supplementation. Cardiac involvement is the initial manifestation in up to 15% of patients and may include either arrhythmias or heart failure. Whereas repolarization abnormalities and supraventricular arrhythmias are common, AV conduction defects and ventricular tachyarrhythmias are rarely noted. Echocardiographic abnormalities typically include increased ventricular wall thickness, enlarged cardiac chambers, and systolic dysfunction. Cardiac involvement is usually evident from the clinical, echocardiographic, and laboratory features. However, endomyocardial biopsy may occasionally be necessary to confirm the diagnosis.

Treatment. Treatment should consist of repeated phlebotomy, which is most effective if instituted before irreversible end-organ damage has developed. Chelation therapy with deferoxamine is most beneficial if begun early in the disease process, but it can provide clinical benefit even if symptomatic cardiomyopathy has developed. Combined heart-liver transplantation should be considered for selected patients with progressive heart failure in whom serious compromise has not yet developed in other end organs.

Cardiac Sarcoidosis

Sarcoidosis is a multisystem granulomatous disease that frequently involves the myocardium. Granulomatous involvement may occur in any region of the heart, but the left ventricular free wall and interventricular septum are the most common sites. Although clinical involvement is evident in only 5% of patients, cardiac involvement is present at autopsy in 20% to 30% of cases.

Cardiac infiltration by granulomas is associated with progressive fibrosis and leads to increased left ventricular stiffness. Impaired systolic contractile function may also occur as the disease progresses. Endomyocardial biopsy is positive in approximately 50% of patients, but a negative biopsy does not exclude the diagnosis because of the patchy nature of the disease. Myocardial sarcoidosis typically affects young or middle-aged adults of either gender and is usually associated with generalized sarcoidosis. The clinical spectrum includes ventricular arrhythmias, conduction system abnormalities, heart failure, and sudden cardiac death.[17] Syncope is a common manifestation and requires prompt evaluation. ECG abnormalities may include repolarization abnormalities, varying degrees of AV block, and QS-waves mimicking myocardial infarction. Myocardial imaging with thallium 201 or gallium 67 frequently demonstrates abnormal segmental uptake indicative of myocardial involvement.

The clinical course of the disease is highly variable, with a minority of patients having extensive myocardial involvement but few symptoms and others having rapid progression to death or transplantation. The most common cause of death is sudden cardiac death from ventricular tachyarrhythmias or high-grade AV block from direct involvement of the conduction system.

Treatment. Treatment of cardiac sarcoidosis remains unsatisfactory. Permanent pacing is useful when a high-grade AV block is present. Antiarrhythmic treatment or cardioverter-defibrillator implantation is frequently required for patients with recurrent ventricular tachyarrhythmia. Case reports have suggested that corticosteroids may halt disease progression or improve function, but controlled trials are lacking. Cardiac transplantation remains an option for individuals with progressive symptoms. Disease may recur in the cardiac allograft but is usually responsive to enhanced immunosuppression.

Referral to Cardiologists

Unlike the dilated and hypertrophic forms, restrictive cardiomyopathy is rare, and most patients should be referred to a cardiologist for consultation. The goals of such referral are to (1) differentiate primary restrictive disease from infiltrative causes, (2) differentiate restrictive cardiomyopathy from constrictive pericarditis, (3) develop the most appropriate treatment strategy, and (4) evaluate patients for disease-specific treatment protocols or transplantation.

Evidence-Based Summary

Dilated Cardiomyopathy

- A familial pattern is present in approximately 20% of patients with idiopathic dilated cardiomyopathy. Specific genotypic abnormalities have generally involved cytoskeletal support proteins rather than sarcomeric contractile elements.[3]
- Spontaneous improvement in ventricular function occurs in 20% to 40% of patients with idiopathic dilated cardiomyopathy. Individuals most likely to improve have a short duration of symptoms and mild ventricular dilatation and demonstrate contractile reserve on dobutamine stress echocardiography. The 5-year survival rate averages 75% to 80% in individuals who do not demonstrate echocardiographic improvement.[4]
- Echocardiography is the most useful initial noninvasive diagnostic procedure. Although global hypokinesis characterizes many cardiomyopathies, segmental wall motion abnormalities may be observed in 60% of individuals. Coronary angiography is indicated for patients with symptomatic angina pectoris, significant areas of ischemic myocardium on noninvasive testing, or unexplained left ventricular dysfunction and a high probability of coronary artery disease. Dobutamine stress echocardiography and positron emission tomographic imaging are best for assessing viable, but hibernating myocardium that may improve with revascularization.[5, 6]
- Pharmacologic therapy does not differ by etiology of the dilated cardiomyopathy. ACE inhibitors, beta-blockers, and diuretics remain the cornerstones of treatment. Chronic warfarin therapy should be reserved for patients at high risk for thromboembolism, particularly those with a documented mural ventricular thrombus, a previous history of embolization, or atrial fibrillation. Empirical use of antiarrhythmic agents has not been shown to decrease the risk of sudden death. An implantable cardioverter-defibrillator should be considered in patients with aborted sudden cardiac death, cardiac syncope, or symptomatic ventricular tachyarrhythmias.[5]

Hypertrophic Cardiomyopathy

- A familial pattern is evident in more than 50% of patients with hypertrophic cardiomyopathy. The disease is transmitted as an autosomal dominant trait. Genotypic studies have identified single-point mutations in sarcomeric contractile proteins. Although abnormalities of beta heavy chain myosin are most common, other abnormalities include mutations in troponin I and T, alpha-tropomyosin, and cardiac myosin-binding protein C.[8]
- The most common form of hypertrophic disease is unexplained concentric left ventricular hypertrophy. Dynamic outflow tract obstruction and mitral regurgitation are also frequent findings. Common symp-

toms include dyspnea (secondary to diastolic dysfunction), exertional angina pectoris, palpitations, syncope, and near-syncope.[7]

- Annual mortality averages 3% for adults at referral centers and less than 1% in community-based series. Specific genotypes strongly predict the prognosis. Clinical features that predict sudden death are young age at diagnosis, a family history of sudden death, syncope, extensive left ventricular hypertrophy, and documented ventricular tachycardia.[7, 9, 10]
- Echocardiography is the most useful tool for establishing the diagnosis. Marked variability in the pattern and extent of hypertrophy is evident. When suspected, echocardiography should be performed with provocative measures, such as the Valsalva maneuver or administration of amyl nitrate, to evaluate the presence and severity of left ventricular outflow tract obstruction.[9]
- Beta-blockers, often administered in high dose, remain the mainstay of medical therapy for patients with mild to moderate symptoms of angina or exertional dyspnea. Calcium channel blockers and negative inotropic agents such as disopyramide may be useful for patients who fail to respond to beta-blockade. Patients with refractory symptoms and marked subaortic obstruction should be considered for DDD pacing, controlled septal infarction, or surgical septal myectomy. An implantable cardioverter-defibrillator should be considered in patients at high risk for sudden death.[9, 11–13]

Restrictive Cardiomyopathies

- Cardiac amyloidosis and idiopathic primary restrictive cardiomyopathy are the most commonly diagnosed forms of restrictive heart disease. Restrictive cardiomyopathies must always be differentiated from pericardial constriction, a distinction that is not always possible from the clinical and hemodynamic findings. Magnetic resonance imaging is the diagnostic procedure of choice.
- Echocardiography is extremely sensitive in detecting cardiac amyloidosis. The occurrence of unexplained left ventricular hypertrophy and a granular "sparkling" appearance should suggest the diagnosis. Greater degrees of hypertrophy are associated with a poorer prognosis. An abdominal fat pad biopsy is most useful in defining the abnormal protein pattern (AL, AA, or prealbumin).[15]
- Treatment of restrictive cardiomyopathies is generally palliative and ineffective. Diuretics and nitrates should be administered to control venous congestion. Combination therapy with prednisone and melphalan may prolong survival by 6 to 12 months for primary amyloidosis.[16]

References

1. DeSanctis RW, Dec GW: The cardiomyopathies. In Dale D, Federman D (eds): Scientific American Medicine. New York, Scientific American, 2000, pp 1–28.
2. Rerkpattanapipat P, Wongpraparut N, Jacobs LE, Kotler MN: Cardiac manifestations of acquired immunodeficiency syndrome. Arch Intern Med 2000;160:602–608.
3. Fatkin D, MacRae C, Sasakit T, et al: Missense mutations in the rod domain of the lamin A/C gene as causes of dilated cardiomyopathy and conduction-system disease. N Engl J Med 1999;341:1715–1724.
4. Felker GM, Thompson RE, Hare JM, et al: Underlying causes and long-term survival in patients with initially unexplained cardiomyopathy. N Engl J Med 2000;342: 1077–1084.
5. American College of Cardiology/American Heart Association Task Force Report: Guidelines for the evaluation and management of chronic heart failure in the adult. Circulation 2001;104:2996–3007.
6. Bax JJ, Poldermans D, Elhendy A, et al: Improvement of left ventricular ejection fraction, heart failure symptoms and prognosis after revascularization in patients with chronic coronary artery disease and viable myocardium detected by dobutamine stress echocardiography. J Am Coll Cardiol 1999;34:163–169.
7. Wigle ED, Rakowski H, Kimball BP, Williams WG: Hypertrophic cardiomyopathy. Clinical spectrum and treatment. Circulation 1995;92:1680–1692.
8. Maron BJ, Moller JH, Seidman CE, et al: Impact of laboratory molecular diagnosis on contemporary diagnostic criteria for genetically transmitted cardiovascular diseases: Hypertrophic cardiomyopathy, long-QT syndrome, and Marfan syndrome. A statement for healthcare professionals from the Councils on Clinical Cardiology, Cardiovascular Disease in the Young, and Basic Science, American Heart Association. Circulation 1998;98:1460–1471.
9. Spirito P, Seidman CE, McKenna WJ, Maron BJ: The management of hypertrophic cardiomyopathy. N Engl J Med 1997;336:775–785.
10. Spirito P, Bellone P, Harris K, et al: Magnitude of left ventricular hypertrophy and risk of sudden death in hypertrophic cardiomyopathy. N Engl J Med 2000;342: 1778–1785.
11. Ommen SR, Nishimura RA, Squires RW, et al: Comparison of dual-chamber pacing versus septal myectomy for the treatment of patients with hypertrophic obstructive cardiomyopathy. A comparison of objective hemodynamic and exercise end points. J Am Coll Cardiol 1999;34: 191–196.
12. Lakkis NM, Nagueh SF, Kleiman NS, et al: Echocardiography-guided ethanol septal reduction for hypertrophic obstructive cardiomyopathy. Circulation 1998;98:1750–1755.
13. Robbins RC, Stinson EB: Long-term results of left ventricular myotomy and myectomy for obstructive hypertrophic cardiomyopathy. J Thorac Cardiovasc Surg 1996;111:586–594.

14. Ammash NM, Seward JB, Bailey KR, et al: Clinical profile and outcome of idiopathic restrictive cardiomyopathy. Circulation 2000;101:2490–2496.
15. Falk RH, Comenzo RL, Skinner M: The systemic amyloidoses. N Engl J Med 1997;337:898–909.
16. Kyle RA, Gertz MA, Greipp PR, et al: A trial of three regimens for primary amyloidosis: Colchicines alone, melphalan and prednisone, and prednisone and colchicines. N Engl J Med 1997;336:1202–1207.
17. Perreira N, Dec GW: Restrictive cardiomyopathies. In Crawford MH, DiMarco JP (eds): Cardiology. London, Mosby, 2000, pp 14.1–14.10.

CHAPTER 30

Recognition and Management of Patients with Tachyarrhythmias

Melvin M. Scheinman and Vineet Kaushik

In assessing patients with suspected or known tachyarrhythmias, the physician must determine the possible severity of the arrhythmia and any underlying cardiologic and noncardiologic conditions. This chapter reviews the common cardiac arrhythmias seen by primary care physicians, identifies the appropriate diagnostic procedures for different types of patients, and indicates when further specialized care is required.

OFFICE EVALUATION OF PATIENTS WITH A SUSTAINED ARRHYTHMIA

History

The office evaluation of a patient with a new sustained arrhythmia should be brief and directed toward specific questions that relate to proper diagnosis and therapy. Arrhythmias are often evanescent; hence, one of the most important initial maneuvers is to record the arrhythmia on a 12-lead electrocardiogram (ECG). While the ECG is being recorded, the physician must discern several key elements in the history. For example, was the arrhythmia preceded or was it accompanied by anginal chest pain? Does the patient have a previous history of structural heart disease? A new-onset sustained arrhythmia in a patient with established cardiac disease should suggest the presence of ventricular tachycardia (VT). In contrast, a history of abrupt-onset tachycardia in a younger, otherwise healthy individual would favor a diagnosis of supraventricular tachycardia (SVT).[1]

An accurate drug history may be of paramount importance. VT in younger patients should raise the possibility of cocaine use or tricyclic antidepressant overdose. The type and amount of drug therapy, particularly antiarrhythmic therapy, is extremely important. Has the patient been treated with digitalis preparations, quinidine-type drugs, or sotalol, and what is the time relationship of the new arrhythmia to starting the drug? It is also important to record the use of diuretic agents because severe electrolyte disorders, particularly hypokalemia, may exacerbate arrhythmias related to the use of antiarrhythmic drugs.

The clinician should assess for the presence of severe hypoxia or acid-base disturbances. Patients with severe lung disease will often have atrial fibrillation, multifocal atrial tachycardia, or frequent ventricular premature depolarizations. Other important noncardiac causes of cardiac arrhythmias include hyperthyroidism and pheochromocytoma; sinus tachycardia is common with both of these diagnoses. Atrial fibrillation is a frequent sequela of hyperthyroidism, whereas both SVT and VT may be associated with pheochromocytoma.

The Physical Examination

The physical examination is geared toward assessment of the nature of the arrhythmia, as well as its hemodynamic consequences. If the physical examination shows evidence of periodic large A-waves in the jugular venous pulse, as well as variation in the intensity of the first heart sound and in systolic blood pressure, the presence of atrioventricular (AV) dissociation and hence VT should be suspected. Findings on physical examination also guide the response to therapy. For example, signs (and symptoms) of cardiac failure or severe hypotension mandate emergency measures that should be initiated in the office (see Chapter 24 and later under "Treatment").

Interpretation of the Electrocardiogram

The 12-lead ECG is key to understanding the arrhythmia and its mechanism (see Chapter 12). The first analysis is directed toward differentiation of the arrhythmia into narrow-complex versus wide-complex tachycardia (Box 30–1). A QRS complex of 0.12 second or longer in any lead is diagnostic of a wide-complex tachycardia. Wide-complex tachycardias are further divided into those resulting from VT, from SVT with aberrant conduction (or bundle branch block), or from preexcited tachycardias. The latter are less common but may occur in patients with accessory pathways who have arrhythmias manifested as antegrade conduction over a bypass tract. If one discerns evidence of AV dissociation during wide-complex tachycardia, a diagnosis of VT is certain. Because only 20% of patients with VT show clear-cut evidence of AV dissociation, a stepwise approach can help distinguish VT from SVT with aberrancy (Fig. 30–1). It is important to remember that SVT with wide QRS complexes may be seen in patients with hyperkalemia, tricyclic overdose, or various antiarrhythmic agents (i.e., flecainide). In all series of patients with wide-complex tachycardia, VTs outnumber SVTs by about 3:1.

Distinction among narrow-complex tachyarrhythmias can usually be based on ECG criteria: the regularity of the rhythm (see Box 30–1) and the relationship of the P-wave to the QRS complex (Fig. 30–2). The physician must first distinguish sinus tachycardia from tachyarrhythmias. Sinus tachycardia is defined as a sinus rate above 100 beats per minute, and it rarely exceeds 180 beats per minute in an adult. It can often be distinguished from paroxysmal SVT (PSVT) by readily discernible P-waves that are upright in the inferior leads (leads II, III, and aVF), by its gradual onset and cessation, by its occasional gradual slowing in response to carotid sinus pressure, or by its variation in response to respiration or activity.

Sinus tachycardia may be precipitated by serious conditions such as hypovolemia, heart failure, infection, anemia, electrolyte abnormalities, and thyrotoxicosis. It may also be stimulated by adrenergic agents, coffee, tea, tobacco, alcohol, or vagolytic agents. Frequently, however, it is related to emotion or stress. The sinus tachycardia itself does not require any treatment, but it serves to call attention to associated medical problems.

In most adults, atrial fibrillation, atrial flutter, and SVTs cannot be conducted at rates exceeding about 160 to 180 beats per minute because of delay in the AV node. As patients become older, these maximal rates decline.

If conduction to the ventricle exceeds 160 to 180 beats per minute with a wide QRS complex, an accessory pathway should be suspected. Conversely, if patients have atrial fibrillation, atrial flutter, or other nonsinus rhythms with rates below 100 to 120 beats per minute in the absence of medications, intrinsic disease of the AV node should be suspected. Because an SVT itself may be a manifestation of sinus node dysfunction, these patients with slow AV conduction commonly have the so-called bradycardia-tachycardia syndrome (see Chapter 31). In patients with the bradycardia-tachycardia syndrome, it is often impossible to treat the tachyarrhythmia successfully with medications without simultaneously causing symptomatic bradycardia. The patient may require catheter ablation of the source of the SVT, the combination of ablation of the AV node and a pacemaker to guard against symptomatic bradycardia, or the combination of medications to prevent the tachyarrhythmia and a pacemaker.

BOX 30–1

Types of Tachycardia

- Wide-complex tachycardias: QRS ≥0.12 sec
  - Ventricular tachycardia (with or without detectable AV dissociation)
    - Monomorphic (each beat looks similar)
    - Polymorphous—beats vary, often with an oscillating pattern; torsades de pointes
  - Supraventricular tachycardia (with or without apparently conducted or retrograde P-waves)
    - With aberrant conduction in the His-Purkinje system in the ventricles
    - With antegrade conduction via an accessory pathway
- Narrow-complex tachycardias: QRS <0.12 sec
  - Irregularly irregular—atrial fibrillation (see Fig. 30–3)
  - Irregular
    - Multifocal atrial tachycardia
    - Any supraventricular rhythm with irregular AV conduction or superimposed premature beats
  - Regular
    - Sinus tachycardia
    - Atrial flutter (see Fig. 30–5)
    - Paroxysmal supraventricular tachycardia (see Fig. 30–2)
      - AV nodal reentry
      - Accessory pathway
    - Ectopic atrial tachycardia from an accelerated atrial focus (see Fig. 30–2)
    - Junctional ectopic tachycardia

AV, atrioventricular.

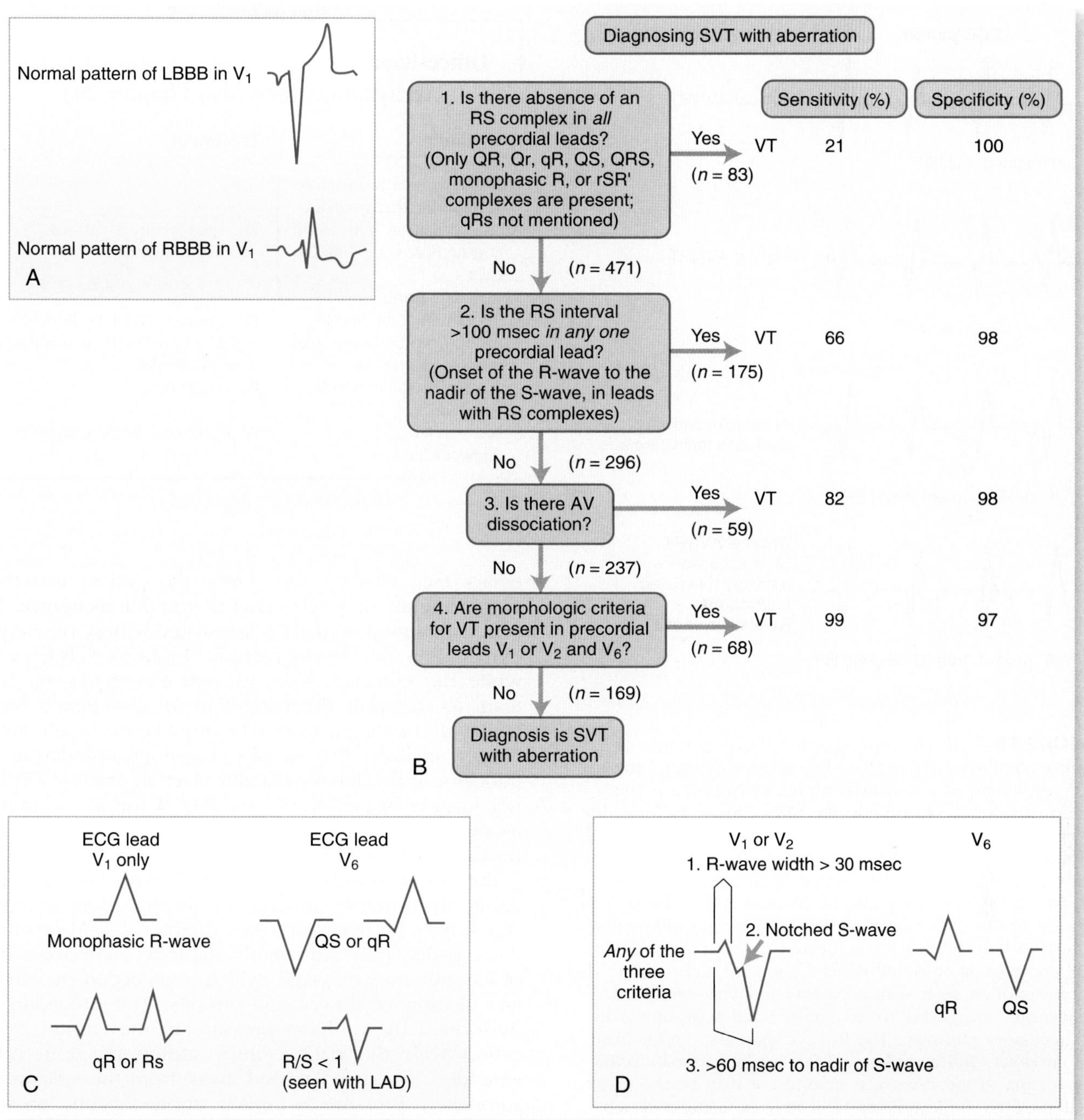

FIGURE 30–1. The 12-lead electrocardiogram (ECG) in the differential diagnosis of wide-complex tachycardia. Brugada and colleagues analyzed 384 cases of ventricular tachycardia (VT) and 170 cases of supraventricular tachycardia (SVT) with aberrancy, for a total of 554 patients with tachycardia (those taking antiarrhythmic medications were excluded). They then devised a systematic approach for diagnosing wide–QRS complex tachycardia with regular rhythm. *A*, The first step is to exclude sinus tachycardia or atrial tachycardia with a right (RBBB) or left (LBBB) bundle branch block, which can usually be done by finding P-waves: the ST segment and T-wave are always smooth unless distorted by a P-wave. However, missing this diagnosis should not affect the ability to diagnose VT or SVT, unless the patient is taking QRS-lengthening drugs. *B*, Steps in the diagnosis of SVT with aberration. A "Yes" answer at any point indicates that no further steps need be taken. When the answer is "No," proceed to the next step. The cumulative sensitivity with this method is 97% and the specificity is 99%. AV, atrioventricular. *C*, Morphologic criteria favoring the diagnosis of VT in the presence of RBBB-type QRS complexes (dominant positive in V_1). LAD, left axis deviation. *D*, Morphologic criteria used to diagnose VT in the presence of LBBB-type QRS complexes (dominant *negative* in V_1). (Adapted from Brugada P, Brugada J, Mont L, et al: A new approach to the differential diagnosis of a regular tachycardia with a wide QRS complex. Circulation 1991;83:1649. By permission of the American Heart Association, Inc.)

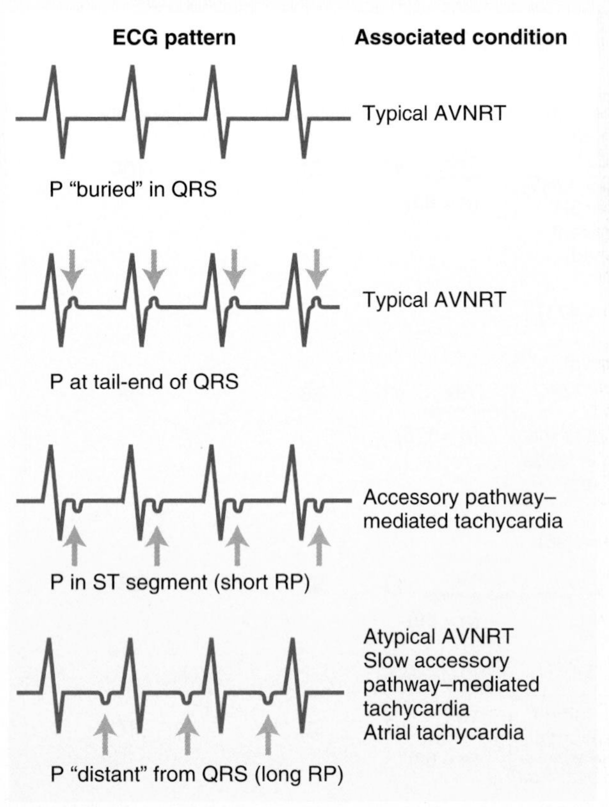

FIGURE 30–2. Electrocardiographic (ECG) patterns of narrow-complex tachycardias. The most important clue to the mechanism of a narrow-complex tachycardia is the relationship of the P-wave to the QRS complex. No visible P-wave often means that the P-wave is buried in the QRS complex, usually as a consequence of typical atrioventricular (AV) nodal reentry. With typical AV nodal reentry, the P-wave may also be located just at the start or the end of the QRS complex, thereby giving a qRs or Rsr' pattern. When the P-wave is located close to the previous QRS complex, it is identified as a short RP tachycardia. This pattern is often seen with accessory pathway–mediated tachycardia and is due to retrograde atrial activation over the accessory pathway. The P-wave may also be far from the previous QRS complex and is classified as a long RP tachycardia. If the P-wave is inverted, it may be the result of atypical AV node reentry, or it may be using a slowly conducting accessory pathway in the retrograde direction. AVNRT, atrioventricular nodal reentry tachycardia. If the P wave is upright with a long RP tachycardia, the rhythm may be either sinus tachycardia or atrial tachycardia. (Redrawn from Grogin HR: Supraventricular tachycardia. In Scheinman M [vol ed]: Arrhythmias: Electrophysiologic principles. In Braunwald E [series ed]: Atlas of Heart Diseases, vol 9. Philadelphia, Current Medicine, 1996, pp 5.1–5.17.)

Management

If patients are initially seen with hemodynamically unstable VT, ventricular flutter or fibrillation, or atrial fibrillation associated with a very rapid response as a result of accelerated conduction over an accessory pathway, immediate direct-current cardioversion is necessary (see Chapter 24). Once the patient is stable, arrangements must be made for expeditious transfer for hospital admission. If VT is associated with stable hemodynamics, a trial of drug therapy (Table 30–1) is in order while the clinician waits for the emergency medical team to transport the patient to an emergency room facility. If the diagnosis of VT cannot be excluded, initial therapy includes the use of intravenous amiodarone or lidocaine if the left ventricular ejection fraction (EF) is not known or is low (EF <40%).[2] If the EF is known to be preserved (EF >40%), intravenous lidocaine or procainamide may be used (Table 30–2).

TABLE 30–1

Office-Based Treatment of Sustained Cardiac Arrhythmias (See Also Chapter 24)

Arrhythmia	Treatment
Hemodynamically unstable ventricular trachycardia Atrial fibrillation with rapid conduction via a bypass tract Ventricular fibrillation	Emergency direct-current countershock
Hemodynamically stable monomorphic ventricular tachycardia	IV amiodarone or IV lidocaine; if LVEF >40%, IV procainamide or IV sotalol
Polymorphous ventricular tachycardia	IV magnesium
Supraventricular tachycardia	IV adenosine or IV verapamil

IV, intravenous; LVEF, left ventricular ejection fraction.

For patients with a regular SVT who are hemodynamically unstable, emergency direct-current countershock may be necessary (see Chapter 24). Most often, these patients are sufficiently stable to allow for a trial of carotid sinus massage, which is preceded by careful auscultation of the carotid arteries. The procedure is performed by applying pressure to the carotid bifurcation with the patient in a supine position, neck extended, and head turned away from the side being stimulated. Pressure is initially applied lightly on one side only, then more firmly for about 5 seconds in a massaging or rotating manner to stimulate carotid sinus baroreceptors and cause a reflex increase in vagal tone. Care must be taken to not massage atherosclerotic carotid arteries, from which some risk of embolization may ensue. Although massage of each side individually may be beneficial, simultaneous bilateral massage should never be performed.

Carotid sinus massage often causes a gradual slowing of sinus tachycardia, may increase the degree of AV block in patients with atrial flutter, may somewhat slow the rate of atrial fibrillation, and may cause sudden termination of a reentrant SVT. It can rarely terminate in VT.

As an alternative to carotid sinus massage, patients may use the Valsalva maneuver or may suddenly immerse their face in cold water. Application of pres-

TABLE 30–2

Common Antiarrhythmic Medications

Class	Drug	IV Loading Dose	Maintenance Dose	Major Side Effects	Excretion
1A	Quinidine sulfate	10 mg/kg	200–400 mg PO q6h	Diarrhea, thrombocytopenia, torsades de pointes, tinnitus, hypotension	Hepatic
	Quinidine gluconate	—	324–628 mg PO q8h	Same as above	Hepatic
	Procainamide	10–15 mg/kg	1000 mg PO q8h	Nausea, lupus syndrome, torsades de pointes	Renal/hepatic
1B	Lidocaine	1 mg/kg	1–4 mg/min IV	Seizures, respiratory arrest	Hepatic
1C	Flecainide	—	100–150 mg PO q12h	Headache, visual disturbances, ventricular tachycardia	Hepatic/renal
	Propafenone	—	150–300 mg q8h	Metallic taste, nausea, ventricular arrhythmias	Hepatic/renal
III	Amiodarone	5 mg/kg IV or 1.2 g/day × 10 days PO	200–400 mg/day	Thyroid, pulmonary fibrosis, corneal deposits, hepatic fibrosis, gray-blue skin discoloration	Lacrimal ducts/hepatic
	Sotalol	—	80–160 mg q12h	Bradycardia, bronchospasm, fatigue, increased heart failure, torsades de pointes	Renal
	Ibutilide	1 mg over 10-min period	—	Polymorphous VT, nausea	Hepatic/renal
	Dofetilide	—	Depends on GFR and QT interval	Polymorphous VT	Renal

GFR, glomerular filtration rate; IV, intravenously; PO, orally; VT, ventricular tachycardia.

sure to the eyeballs should not be tried because retinal detachment has been reported. Each of these maneuvers, which may be taught to the patient if proven to be successful under a physician's observation, is associated with an increase in vagal tone that may be adequate to terminate an SVT. However, patients with symptoms consisting of more than palpitations alone, such as those with dyspnea, dizziness, or chest pain, need further medical attention urgently if simple attempts are not rapidly successful.

If carotid massage is unsuccessful in a patient with a regular PSVT, intravenous adenosine or verapamil is remarkably effective (>95%) in terminating the episode. If the SVT is readily terminated and was not associated with evidence of acute myocardial ischemia or hemodynamic instability, hospitalization is not required, but the patient should be referred to a cardiac specialist for further treatment. A wide variety of effective pharmacologic and nonpharmacologic treatment modalities are currently available (Box 30–2), and early referral to a specialist is recommended to help choose the most appropriate therapy.

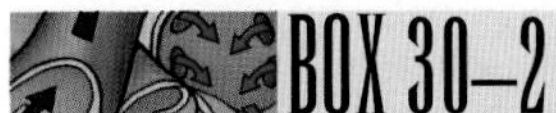
BOX 30–2

Rhythms for Which Catheter Ablation Is Performed

PROCEDURE OF CHOICE
Atrial flutter
Paroxysmal supraventricular tachycardia

CONSIDER IN SPECIAL OR REFRACTORY CASES
Atrial fibrillation
Some forms of ventricular tachycardia

DIAGNOSIS AND TREATMENT OF SPECIFIC TACHYARRHYTHMIAS

Atrial Fibrillation

Diagnosis

Atrial fibrillation, which is the most common sustained clinical arrhythmia, is diagnosed by obtaining a 12-lead ECG and finding an irregularly irregular ventricular rhythm without discrete P-waves (Fig. 30–3). The QRS complex is usually narrow because of its supraventricular origin, but it may be wide if aberrant conduction or a bundle branch block is present. Atrial fibrillation associated with the Wolff-Parkinson-White syndrome may occur at a very rapid rate and be life threatening. This arrhythmia is diagnosed by its very rapid irregular rate associated with wide preexcited QRS complexes, and it requires emergency treatment (see later).

Epidemiology. Approximately 4% of the population older than 60 years has sustained atrial fibrillation, with

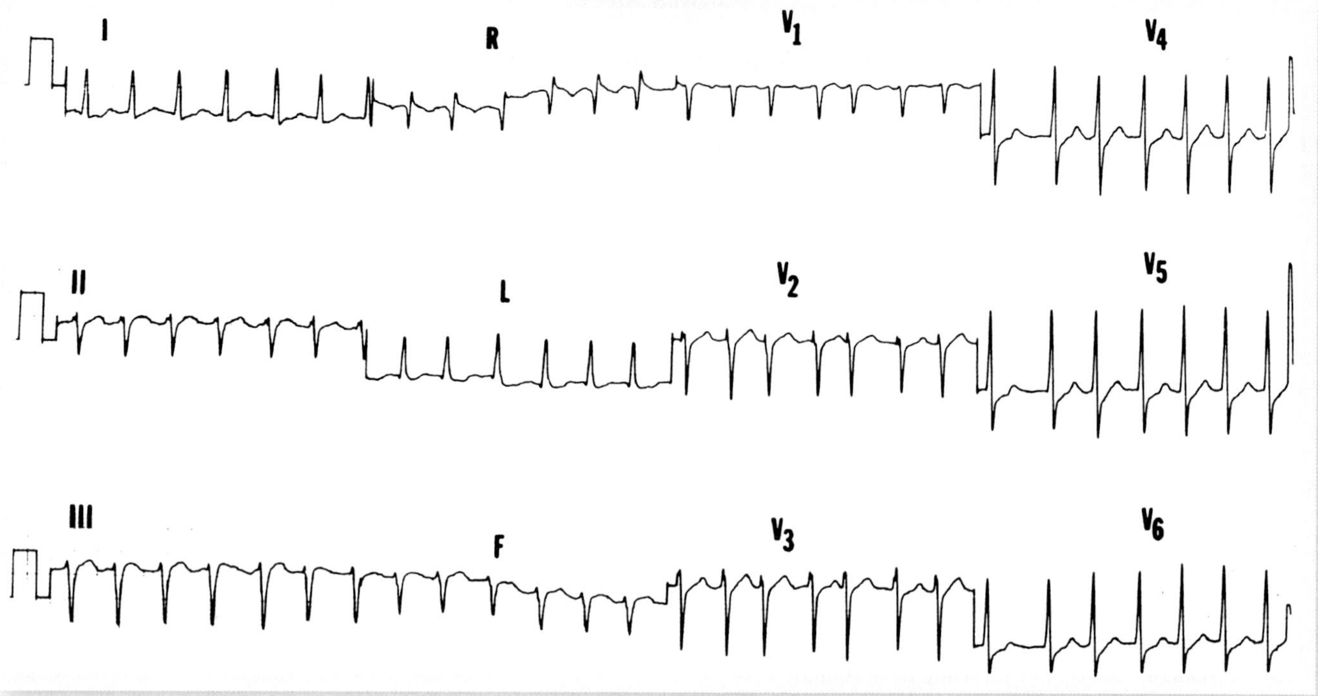

FIGURE 30–3. A 12-lead electrocardiogram showing atrial fibrillation with a rapid ventricular response. Note that the ventricular rate is irregularly irregular, and no discrete P-waves are recorded.

a particularly steep increase in prevalence after the seventh decade of life.[3] Other risk factors include heart failure, hypertensive cardiovascular disease, coronary artery disease, and valvular heart disease. Moreover, both sustained and paroxysmal atrial fibrillation have important implications for the development of a cerebrovascular accident (CVA) or the risk of death. It is estimated that 15% to 20% of CVAs in nonrheumatic patients are due to atrial fibrillation, and the incidence is even higher in those with rheumatic mitral valve disease.

Risk and Precipitating Factors. When called on to manage patients with new-onset atrial fibrillation, it is important to establish the precipitating factors because the type of associated condition determines the long-term prognosis (Box 30–3). In some patients, episodes of atrial fibrillation may be initiated by caffeine, alcohol, or marijuana. Atrial fibrillation may result from acute intercurrent ailments. For example, this arrhythmia may occur in patients with hyperthyroidism or lung disease or after either cardiac or pulmonary surgery, especially in older patients. Atrial fibrillation is also seen in patients with acute pulmonary embolism, myocarditis, or acute myocardial infarction, particularly when the latter is complicated by either occlusion of the right coronary artery or acute heart failure. When atrial fibrillation occurs in these settings, it almost always abates spontaneously if the patient recovers from the underlying problem. Hence, management usually involves the administration of drugs to control the heart rate, but chronic antiarrhythmic therapy is not generally needed.

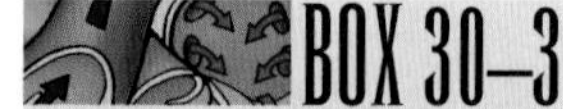

Precipitating Factors for Atrial Fibrillation

ASSOCIATED CARDIAC ABNORMALITIES

Hypertension, heart failure, coronary artery disease
Valvular heart disease (especially mitral or tricuspid)
Inflammatory/infiltrative disease (pericarditis, amyloid)
Congenital (e.g., atrial septal defect)
Metastatic cancer to the atrium or pericardium
Triggering arrhythmias (atrial flutter, paroxysmal supraventricular tachycardia)

OTHER PRECIPITANTS

Drugs or intoxicants (e.g., alcohol, carbon monoxide)
Postoperative, especially after cardiac or pulmonary surgery
Acute or chronic pulmonary disease
Enhanced vagal tone/enhanced sympathetic tone
Metabolic abnormalities, e.g., hypokalemia, hyperthyroidism, pheochromocytoma
Exertion related

LONE ATRIAL FIBRILLATION

Alternatively, atrial fibrillation may occur in association with structural cardiac disease. Important associated conditions include rheumatic mitral stenosis, hypertension, hypertrophic cardiomyopathy, and chronic heart failure. In contrast to patients with acute intercurrent ailments, those with structural heart disease may expect (even with antiarrhythmic therapy) many recurrences until chronic atrial fibrillation supervenes.

When atrial fibrillation is not associated with a precipitating cardiac or noncardiac diagnosis, patients are known as "lone fibrillators." The natural history of the atrial fibrillation in these patients is similar to that in patients with structural cardiac disease in that episodes of atrial fibrillation are likely to recur and, eventually, the arrhythmia becomes sustained.

Management (Fig. 30–4)

The objectives of therapy include (1) achieving rate control, (2) restoring sinus rhythm (when feasible), and (3) decreasing the risk of CVA.

Initial Evaluation. The initial evaluation of patients with new-onset atrial fibrillation includes a detailed history keying on possible precipitating factors, as well as the presence of organic cardiac disease. As such, the initial evaluation includes, at a minimum, a careful physical examination, 12-lead ECG, chest radiograph, echocardiogram, and tests of thyroid function. Further testing will depend on various aspects of the history or physical examination. For example, if atrial fibrillation is usually precipitated by exercise, an exercise treadmill test is appropriate. In a patient with frequent episodes of paroxysmal atrial fibrillation, a 24- to 48-hour Holter recording may discern whether the atrial fibrillation is triggered by another arrhythmia, such as when a premature atrial complex during a rapid paroxysmal atrial tachycardia causes the immediate onset of atrial fibrillation.

Rate Control. If the patient has atrial fibrillation and a rapid rate associated with severe heart failure or cardiogenic shock, emergency direct-current cardioversion is indicated. For patients with atrial fibrillation associated with a rapid rate but with stable hemodynamics, attempts to achieve acute rate control are indicated. Drugs to slow the rate of atrial fibrillation include digitalis preparations, calcium channel blockers (verapamil or diltiazem), and beta-blockers (Table 30–3). If rapid rate control is desired, the latter two types of agents are far more effective than digitalis, which may require many hours before rate control is achieved. In addition, a common misconception is that digitalis therapy is associated with acute conversion to sinus rhythm, but carefully controlled studies have shown that conversion to sinus rhythm is no more likely with digoxin than with placebo. As emphasized later, digitalis and intravenous calcium channel blocker therapy are contraindicated in patients with Wolff-Parkinson-White syndrome and atrial fibrillation. Intravenous diltiazem has been shown to be safe and effective for patients with atrial fibrillation and heart failure.

Chronic Antiarrhythmic Therapy and Elective Cardioversion. For patients with a single, initial episode of self-limited atrial fibrillation, no specific therapy is required because recurrences may be delayed for many years. In contrast, patients who have obvious frequent recurrences may be candidates for chronic antiarrhythmic therapy (Table 30–4) with class IA (quinidine, procainamide, and disopyramide), class IC (propafenone and flecainide), or class III (sotalol, amiodarone, and dofetilide) agents, all of which are more effective than placebo in maintaining sinus rhythm.[4,5]

Unfortunately, these agents have important drawbacks. First, even with drug therapy, recurrence rates for atrial fibrillation approach 50% per year (as opposed to recurrence rates of 75% per year with placebo therapy). In addition, these agents may be associated with significant side effects. For class IA drugs, adverse effects include induction of torsades de pointes. For example, a meta-analysis compared quinidine with placebo for patients with atrial fibrillation and found that all-cause mortality was *higher* in the groups treated with quinidine. In addition, in the Stroke Prevention in Atrial Fibrillation (SPAF) trials, substantial numbers of patients were treated with antiarrhythmic agents; in patients with heart failure, those treated with class IA or IC drugs had significant excess mortality in comparison to those not treated with antiarrhythmic drugs. Great care must be exercised in the use of these agents, with the benefits balanced against the potential for adverse effects. General rules include avoidance of all

TABLE 30–3

Drugs Used for Acute Rate Control

Drug	Dose	Side Effects	Primary Metabolic Route
Digoxin	0.5 mg followed by 0.25 mg q2–6h to a total dose of 1–1.5 mg	Nausea, emesis, disturbed vision, atrial and/or ventricular arrhythmias	Renal
Diltiazem	20 mg IV as a loading dose (if necessary), followed by an infusion at 5–15 mg/hr	Hypotension, peripheral edema, headache, sinus node depression, AV block	Hepatic
Verapamil	0.15-mg/kg loading dose, 5–10 mg q30min as needed	Same as above	Hepatic
Esmolol	0.5-μg/kg/min loading dose, then infusion at 0.05–0.2 μg/kg/min	Negative inotropic effects, suppression of sinoatrial and AV nodal function, bronchospasm	Hepatic
Metoprolol	5 mg IV, up to 15 mg total	Same as above	Hepatic

IV, intravenously; AV, atrioventricular.

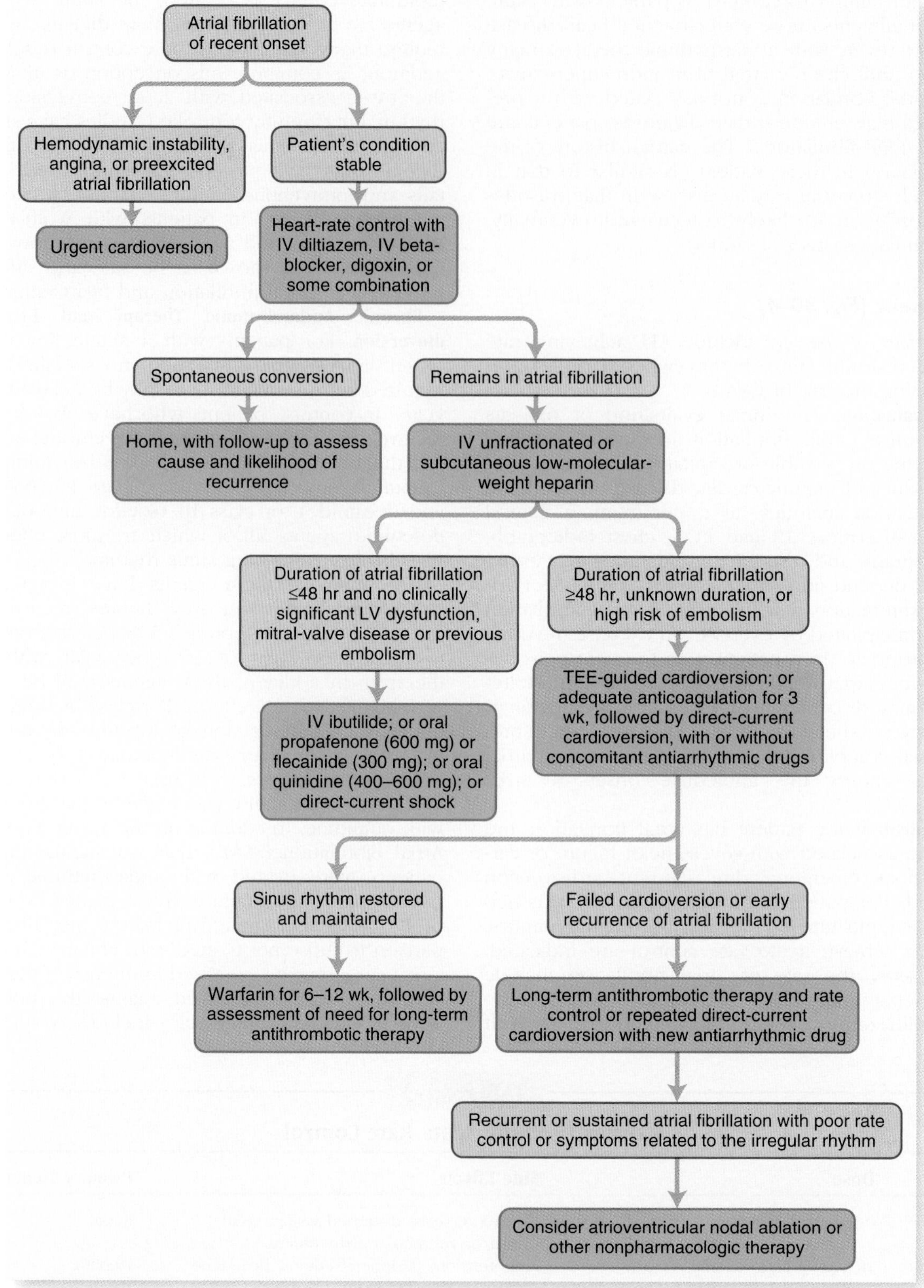

Atrial fibrillation of recent onset

Hemodynamic instability, angina, or preexcited atrial fibrillation

Urgent cardioversion

Patient's condition stable

Heart-rate control with IV diltiazem, IV beta-blocker, digoxin, or some combination

Spontaneous conversion

Home, with follow-up to assess cause and likelihood of recurrence

Remains in atrial fibrillation

IV unfractionated or subcutaneous low-molecular-weight heparin

Duration of atrial fibrillation ≤48 hr and no clinically significant LV dysfunction, mitral-valve disease or previous embolism

IV ibutilide; or oral propafenone (600 mg) or flecainide (300 mg); or oral quinidine (400–600 mg); or direct-current shock

Duration of atrial fibrillation ≥48 hr, unknown duration, or high risk of embolism

TEE-guided cardioversion; or adequate anticoagulation for 3 wk, followed by direct-current cardioversion, with or without concomitant antiarrhythmic drugs

Sinus rhythm restored and maintained

Warfarin for 6–12 wk, followed by assessment of need for long-term antithrombotic therapy

Failed cardioversion or early recurrence of atrial fibrillation

Long-term antithrombotic therapy and rate control or repeated direct-current cardioversion with new antiarrhythmic drug

Recurrent or sustained atrial fibrillation with poor rate control or symptoms related to the irregular rhythm

Consider atrioventricular nodal ablation or other nonpharmacologic therapy

FIGURE 30–4. Management of recent-onset atrial fibrillation. IV, intravenous; LV, left ventricular; TEE, transesophageal echocardiography. (Reprinted, by permission, from Falk RH: Atrial fibrillation. N Engl J Med 2001;344:1067–1078.)

TABLE 30–4

Overview of Drug Therapy for Arrhythmias

Arrhythmia	Acute Management (IV)	Chronic Therapy (Usually Oral)	Chronic Anticoagulation
Atrial fibrillation	Digoxin, verapamil, diltiazem, or metoprolol for rate control Class IC or ibutilide for cardioversion	No organic cardiac disease—classes IA or IC Heart failure—amiodarone or dofetilide Hypertension—sotalol or class IC	Yes
Atrial fibrillation with rapid rate because of Wolff-Parkinson-White syndrome	Ibutilide or procainamide; avoid IV verapamil or digoxin	Amiodarone, sotalol, or class IC	No
Atrial flutter	Digoxin, verapamil, diltiazem, or metoprolol	Amiodarone, sotalol, class IA or IC	Yes
Paroxysmal supraventricular tachycardia	Adenosine, verapamil, propranolol, or esmolol	Beta-blockers, calcium channel blockers, class IA or IC, or sotalol	No
Monomorphic ventricular tachycardia	Lidocaine, procainamide, or amiodarone	Amiodarone or sotalol	No
Polymorphous ventricular tachycardia (congenital)	Propranolol and/or cardiac pacing	ICD and beta-blockers	No
Polymorphous ventricular tachycardia (acquired)	IV magnesium; correct electrolyte abnormalities	Avoid offending drug class	No

ICD, implantable cardioverter-defibrillator; IV, intravenous.

class IA drugs in the face of torsades de pointes associated with one of these agents and avoidance of class IC agents for patients with structural heart disease. In addition, sotalol is contraindicated in patients with severe depression of left ventricular EF.

The only drugs that appear to be both effective and safe for patients with heart failure and atrial fibrillation are amiodarone and dofetilide. Amiodarone is associated with a host of both cardiac (e.g., severe sinus bradycardia or arrest or AV block) and noncardiac (e.g., thyroid abnormalities, pulmonary fibrosis) adverse effects, but low-dose amiodarone (i.e., 200 mg/day) appears to be very well tolerated. Care must be used in the treatment of patients with sinus node dysfunction. Dofetilide has a narrow therapeutic window and can cause life-threatening arrhythmias; it should be used only in patients who have highly symptomatic atrial fibrillation and are intolerant of other drugs.

Anticoagulant Therapy. The risk of CVA in patients with nonrheumatic atrial fibrillation is 4% to 7% per year.[3,5] Those at particularly high risk include patients older than 70 years or those with hypertension, a history of heart failure, increased left atrial size, or previous CVA. The risk for CVA is similar in patients with paroxysmal versus chronic atrial fibrillation. Numerous studies have documented the remarkable efficacy of warfarin in decreasing the risk of emboli by 45% to 85% in patients with nonrheumatic atrial fibrillation and a low risk of significant hemorrhage, provided that the international normalized ratio (INR) is in the range of 2.0 to 2.5.[5,6] Still controversial is the need for anticoagulant therapy in younger patients with lone atrial fibrillation because the risk of emboli is very low in this group.

The role of aspirin therapy for patients with atrial fibrillation remains controversial.[5,7] In one study, 75 mg of aspirin failed to decrease the risk of stroke in comparison to placebo (5.5% per year), and the incidence of stroke was higher with 325 mg of aspirin (4.8%) than with warfarin (3.6%). The SPAF III trials demonstrated that aspirin (325 mg/day) and fixed low-dose warfarin (1, 2, or 3 mg) were ineffective in preventing stroke.[5, 7] Therefore, the weight of current data favors warfarin with an INR of 2.0 to 3.0 as the best strategy to prevent systemic embolization.[5,6,8] Ongoing trials are assessing antithrombin agents, clopidogrel, and low-molecular-weight heparin in patients with atrial fibrillation in an attempt to find efficacious agents that will not require ongoing blood testing of the INR.

Direct-Current Cardioversion. Direct-current cardioversion is a very effective technique for restoration of sinus rhythm. Because of the benefits of sinus rhythm in terms of improved cardiac output and decreased risk of embolic phenomena in general, at least one attempt should be made to restore sinus rhythm. Several precautions are in order. The patient must be pretreated with an antiarrhythmic agent because reversion to atrial fibrillation after shock therapy is very common. In addition, unless urgent cardioversion is required because of hemodynamic decompensation or secondary ischemia, it is imperative to follow one of two options for reducing the risk of systemic embolization.

The recommended option for new-onset atrial fibrillation is to perform transesophageal echocardiography (TEE), which provides an excellent ability to detect clots in the left atrium or the left atrial appendage. Evidence from several studies indicates that detection of either a clot or spontaneous echo contrast in the left atrium is associated with a higher risk for systemic embolization.[9,10] In the absence of such findings on TEE, systemic emboli are rare, and TEE-guided therapy results in similarly low rates (<1%) of thromboembolism.[10] Therefore, patients with recent-onset atrial fibrillation and no evidence of atrial clots or spontaneous contrast by TEE may undergo direct-current cardioversion after initiation of anticoagulant therapy, but without a course of full anticoagulant treatment.[9,10] It must be appreciated that atrial function is depressed after cardioversion and that anticoagulant therapy is recommended for at least 1 month after cardioversion. For patients with clots or spontaneous echo contrast with TEE, full anticoagulant therapy at an INR of 2.0 to 2.5 is recommended for at least 2 to 3 weeks before cardioversion.

An alternative approach is for patients with new-onset atrial fibrillation to be fully anticoagulated for at least 3 consecutive weeks before attempted direct-current cardioversion and for about 4 weeks afterward to decrease the risk of an embolism after successful reversion to sinus rhythm. This approach tends to be less efficient than the TEE-guided approach for recent-onset atrial fibrillation but is an acceptable alternative for atrial fibrillation of longer duration.

Direct-current external shock is usually performed in a monitored area under the supervision of an anesthesiologist. It is wise to check arterial oxygen saturation, the serum potassium level, and digoxin or antiarrhythmic blood drug levels before cardioversion. Direct-current shocks beginning with at least 200 J are used in an attempt to achieve sinus rhythm. If the patient fails to revert after maximal external shocks (360 J), successful cardioversion can almost always be achieved by either the use of a biphasic waveform defibrillator, pretreatment with 1 mg of ibutilide, or an attempt at internal cardioversion with small-energy shocks delivered between the coronary sinus and the right atrium.

Chemical Cardioversion. Ibutilide is a short-acting class III intravenous antiarrhythmic agent that can result in prompt conversion of atrial fibrillation to sinus rhythm. The same issues of proper anticoagulation apply as with direct-current electrical cardioversion. Unlike direct-current cardioversion, ibutilide is contraindicated in patients with significant structural heart disease and is less effective at conversion to sinus rhythm. Although ibutilide obviates the need for anesthesia, close telemetry monitoring is required because of its propensity for inducing ventricular arrhythmias.

Long-Term Approach. One should be especially careful to identify patients whose atrial fibrillation might be cured. Examples include patients with hyperthyroidism, as well as those in whom other cardiac arrhythmias appear to trigger atrial fibrillation. For example, patients with atrial flutter or PSVT may experience atrial premature impulses that trigger atrial fibrillation. It is possible to apply catheter ablation in selected patients to cure the underlying arrhythmia and hence prevent the trigger for atrial fibrillation. Therefore, in the evaluation of patients with atrial fibrillation, initial testing should include obtaining a thyroid-stimulating hormone assay, an echocardiogram, and a 48-hour ambulatory ECG recording for those with paroxysmal atrial fibrillation. When analyzing these recordings, the clinician seeks evidence for triggering arrhythmias. In addition, one looks for vagal triggers of atrial fibrillation, such as sinus bradycardia associated with sleep or heavy meals, which may be initially treated with vagolytic antiarrhythmic agents such as disopyramide. Alternatively, if atrial fibrillation appears only with enhanced sympathetic tone, such as with exercise, a trial of beta-blocker therapy is appropriate.

The natural history of atrial fibrillation associated with structural cardiac disease or in patients with lone atrial fibrillation is for spontaneous recurrence of the arrhythmia. Unfortunately, no drug is universally effective, and the decision of how many drugs to try before a judgment is made to terminate antiarrhythmic drugs and focus on rate control depends on how symptomatic the patient is during atrial fibrillation. If the episodes are poorly tolerated, multiple drug trials or even various ablative procedures may be required (see later). On the other hand, if rate control can be readily achieved with drugs that block the AV node, such as digoxin, beta-blockers, or calcium antagonists, and the patient has a good symptomatic outcome, a completely acceptable alternative is to use drugs to control the rate combined with chronic anticoagulant treatment. Results from a large, randomized trial of 4060 patients showed no difference in mortality, stroke, or quality of life for the strategy of rate control and anticoagulation versus the strategy of maintaining sinus rhythm.[11] In two smaller studies[12–13] that randomized a total of about 500 patients to a rate control strategy versus a rhythm control strategy, the two groups also had generally similar outcomes. As a result, rate control is clearly an acceptable and sometimes preferred alternative to attempts to restore sinus rhythm.

Role of Catheter Ablation. Various ablative techniques have been successfully applied to the treatment of patients with symptomatic atrial fibrillation that is refractory to drug therapy. The most used technique involves the application of radiofrequency energy to the region of the AV junction to produce complete AV block (Table 30–5). In this situation, complete arrhythmia control is achieved, but chronic pacemaker therapy is required. Newer modifications of this technique involve the application of radiofrequency energy to the posterior or midseptal areas to modify, but not completely destroy, AV nodal conduction.

A number of surgical centers are currently using the maze procedure in an attempt to cure atrial fibrillation. This procedure involves placing transmural lesions over both atria in such a manner that the fibrillatory impulses cannot complete a reentrant circuit. The maze procedure involves all the risks of major open heart surgery.

In some patients with paroxysmal atrial fibrillation, a rapidly firing ectopic focus, often within the pulmonary veins, may cause atrial fibrillation. Catheter ablative procedures for attempted cure of atrial fibrillation have resulted in a long-term success rate of 50% to 60% but an unacceptably high incidence of pulmonary vein stenosis (2% to 8%).[13] More recently, newer technical approaches have yielded higher short-term success rates

TABLE 30–5

Overview of Catheter Ablation: Indications and Success Rates

Type of Arrhythmia	Site of Ablation (e.g., accessory pathway, AV node)	Indications for Ablation	Success Rate for Catheter Ablation (%)
Atrial fibrillation	AV junction	Rapid ventricular response uncontrolled with medications	100
Typical atrial flutter	Linear lesion between the inferior vena cava and tricuspid annulus	Patients who do not wish to take chronic antiarrhythmic drugs and anticoagulants or whose flutter cannot be controlled with medications	80–90
AV node reentry	Slow AV nodal pathway (see Fig. 30–7)	Symptomatic PSVT* (absolutely indicated in patients who do not want or are resistant to chronic drug therapy)	95+
Atrial tachycardia	Atrial focus	Rapid ventricular response uncontrolled with medications Patients who wish to avoid lifelong drug therapy	70–80 (right sided) 60–70 (left sided)
Wolff-Parkinson-White syndrome	Accessory pathway (see Fig. 30–9)	Episodes of PSVT* Episodes of atrial fibrillation	85–95 (right sided) 95+ (left sided)

*For PSVT, catheter ablation has matured so that it can be used as first-line therapy.
AV, atrioventricular; PSVT, paroxysmal supraventricular tachycardia.

(70% to 90%) without pulmonary vein stenosis, but longer follow-up will be needed to assess these newer methods. At the present time, pulmonary vein procedures should be reserved for highly symptomatic patients who are resistant to multiple drug trials.

Patients with persistent tachycardia may suffer from a tachycardia-induced cardiomyopathy with left ventricular failure superimposed on their native cardiac disease. Hence, in the management of patients with chronic atrial fibrillation, rate control is an important objective that must be achieved either via AV nodal blocking drugs or, failing these, with catheter ablative procedures.

When to Call a Cardiologist. At several times in the life cycle of patients with atrial fibrillation, expert consultation is strongly recommended. For clinicians who do not use antiarrhythmic agents on a regular basis, it is helpful to obtain expert consultation to sequence drug therapy, especially when agents such as propafenone, sotalol, amiodarone, ibutilide, and dofetilide are being considered. Similarly, if the clinician is not experienced in the performance of direct-current cardioversion, it is well advised to ask for expert assistance in preparing a patient for this procedure and performing it. When sinus rhythm cannot be maintained, catheter ablative procedures should be considered in patients who remain symptomatic despite attempts to control their heart rate.

Atrial Flutter

Diagnosis

Treatment of patients with atrial flutter is very similar to that of atrial fibrillation, but with several important differences. Atrial flutter has been separated into two types. *Typical* atrial flutter (90%) is usually manifested by negative flutter waves in the inferior leads and positive waves in lead V_1 (Fig. 30–5). This type has been termed *counterclockwise flutter.* Alternatively, typical flutter may show regular flutter waves that are positive in the inferior leads and negative in V_1 (*clockwise flutter*). These morphologic features are associated with a very regular flutter rate of approximately 300 complexes per minute. *Atypical* flutter (10%) shows either positive or negative flutter waves in the inferior leads, is associated with more rapid rates (350/min) that are often irregular, and may precede the onset of atrial fibrillation.

Cause, Risk Factors, and Pathophysiology of Atrial Flutter. Atrial flutter may occur in patients without cardiac disease, but it most often occurs in association with mitral or tricuspid valve disease or after repair of certain congenital abnormalities. Atrial flutter occurs commonly after cardiac surgery and is seen in approximately 5% of patients after acute myocardial infarction. In patients with atrial flutter, the rhythm may subsequently change to atrial fibrillation.

Mechanisms. Typical atrial flutter is now known to be a reentrant arrhythmia localized to the right atrium with a critical zone of conduction at the base of the right atrium between the tricuspid annulus and the eustachian ridge. With counterclockwise rotation around the flutter isthmus, a negative flutter wave is found in leads II, III, and aVF and a positive flutter wave in V_1. Clockwise flutter produces positive waves in leads II, III, and aVF and negative deflection in V_1. In contrast, in patients with atypical flutter, the precise circuit has not been defined; atrial fibrillation will often develop in these patients.

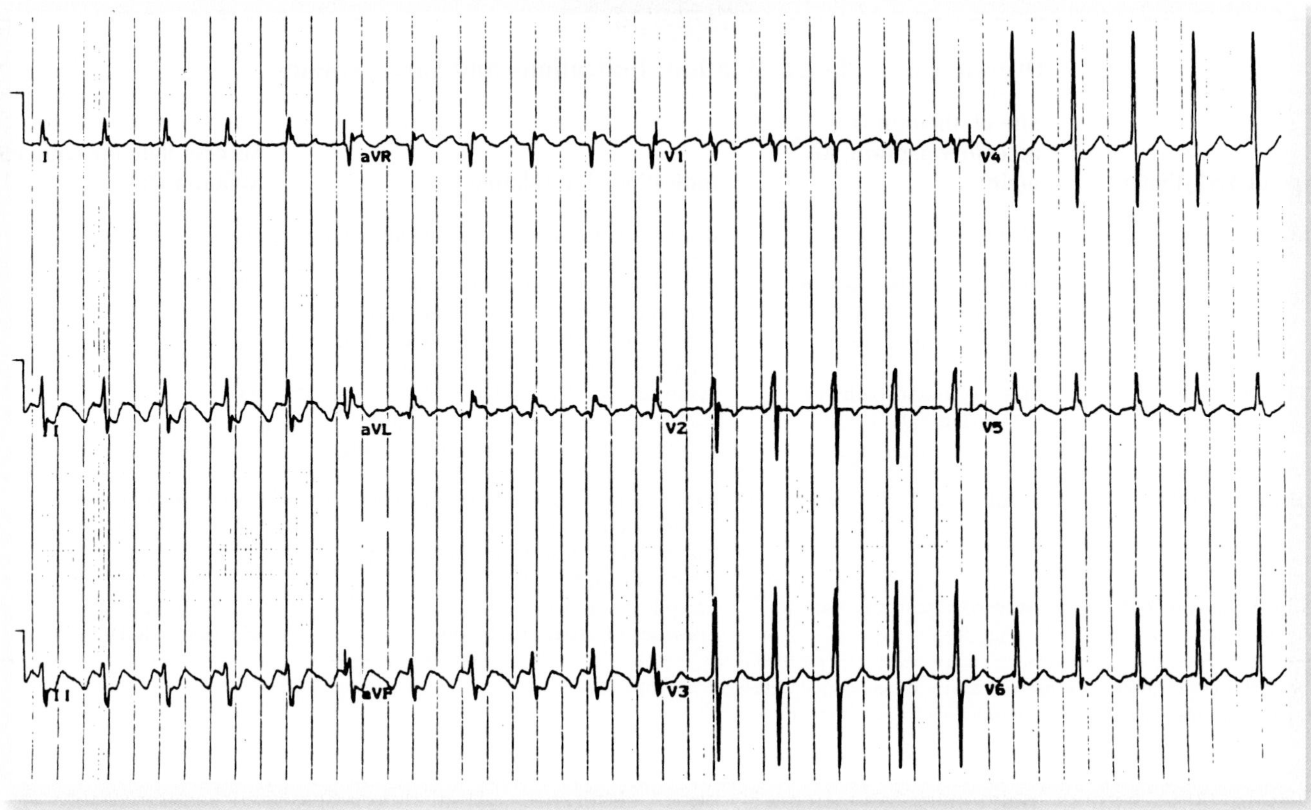

FIGURE 30–5. A 12-lead electrocardiogram shows the pattern of typical atrial flutter. Note the inverted flutter waves in the inferior leads and the positive flutter waves in V_1. Atrial flutter is accompanied by a 2:1 atrioventricular block.

Management

Initial Evaluation. Initial evaluation can proceed in an orderly fashion if the patient is hemodynamically stable despite this arrhythmia. Such evaluation includes a careful history with emphasis on the presence of cardiac disease, a 12-lead ECG, and an echocardiogram.

Treatment. Cardioversion to sinus rhythm should be considered whenever feasible. Direct-current cardioversion is very effective even at low energy, and patients with atrial flutter are often converted to sinus rhythm with 20 to 50 J of delivered energy. In patients with atrial fibrillation and hemodynamic compromise, electrical cardioversion is the indicated therapy, and it is generally recommended for all patients. Ibutilide has about a 35% to 60% acute success rate in the conversion of patients with recent-onset atrial flutter and no significant structural heart disease. A less effective alternative approach is to use AV nodal blocking drugs to slow the ventricular response (see Table 30–3), but this strategy is more difficult in patients with atrial flutter than in those with atrial fibrillation. Nevertheless, rate control is the preferred option when reversion to sinus rhythm is not possible. Patients with typical atrial flutter are generally responsive to atrial overdrive pacing; therefore, if direct-current cardioversion must be avoided or if the patient already has an atrial pacemaker lead in place, rapid overdrive pacing should be attempted to terminate this arrhythmia.

Current information suggests that patients with chronic atrial flutter have a risk of systemic embolization.[14] Anticoagulant therapy should be seriously considered in patients with chronic or recurrent atrial flutter, particularly if TEE shows spontaneous echo contrast or frank clot formation.

Long-Term Treatment. Patients with recurrent or chronic atrial flutter can be treated in a manner very similar to that outlined for patients with atrial fibrillation. This approach involves the use of antiarrhythmic drugs and AV nodal blocking agents for rate and rhythm control. However, chronic drug therapy is often ineffective in patients with atrial flutter. In contrast, catheter ablative techniques to produce a line of block between the tricuspid annulus and the inferior vena cava can interfere with the flutter circuit and have a success rate of about 85% (see Table 30–5), thus suggesting that this approach, rather than drug therapy, is the routine treatment of choice for recurrent or chronic atrial flutter. Successful ablation obviates the need not only for antiarrhythmic therapy but also for chronic anticoagulant treatment.

When to Call a Cardiologist. Because atrial flutter is often very resistant to drug therapy, the patient is best served by early referral to a cardiologist, who can aid the primary physician with cardioversion or overdrive pacing, outline drug therapy if appropriate, and recommend when to intervene with catheter ablation.

Paroxysmal Supraventricular Tachycardia

Diagnosis

The diagnosis of PSVT is suspected from a history of abrupt onset and abrupt termination of palpitations. The diagnosis is confirmed by recording a narrow-complex tachycardia during an episode of palpitations (Fig. 30–6). Evaluation of these patients should include obtaining data from an event recorder (which the patient activates) or a 24- to 48-hour ambulatory ECG recorder, depending on the frequency of symptoms. The recorded symptoms depend on the tachycardia rate, the relationship of the P-wave to the QRS complex, and associated cardiac disease. In some patients, the overriding symptom may be severe anxiety, and the episode may be misdiagnosed as a hysterical reaction or panic attack.

Most instances of PSVT (see Fig. 30–2) are due to reentrant arrhythmias involving the AV nodal region, an accessory extranodal pathway, or a circuit localized within the atrium. The most common mechanism is AV nodal reentry (AVNRT), and it is due to *dual AV nodal* pathways. These pathways are designated "fast" and "slow" conduction pathways (Fig. 30–7). The PSVT is usually triggered by a critically timed atrial premature complex that results in conduction block in the fast pathway and antegrade conduction over the slow pathway. If conduction in the slow pathway is sufficiently slow, the return impulse now finds the fast pathway excitable, and this sequence may give rise to a circus movement tachycardia involving the AV junctional area. Risk factors that may exacerbate the triggering of premature beats include stress, caffeine, and beta-receptor agonists.

A similar mechanism is known to occur in patients with *accessory AV pathways* (AVRT). In some 2 to 3 per 1000 live births in the United States each year, babies are born with an accessory pathway that is separate from the normal AV node–His axis. This pathway consists of microscopic muscular tissue that bridges the atrium to the ventricle over the AV groove. The pathway may be located almost anywhere on the right or left annulus or may occur in the septum. The accessory pathway usually has a longer refractory period than the AV node does; hence, a premature impulse will tend to block conduction in the accessory pathway and conduct over the AV node and His bundle to the ventricle. If the ventricular impulse finds the accessory pathway responsive for retrograde conduction, that impulse returns to the atrium and initiates a circus movement tachycardia (see Fig. 30–7). Because antegrade conduction usually proceeds over the AV node, the QRS complex during tachycardia will either be normal or show a pattern of aberrant supraventricular conduction.

Some 90% of patients with PSVT have one of the two mechanisms described previously (AVNRT, 50%; AVRT,

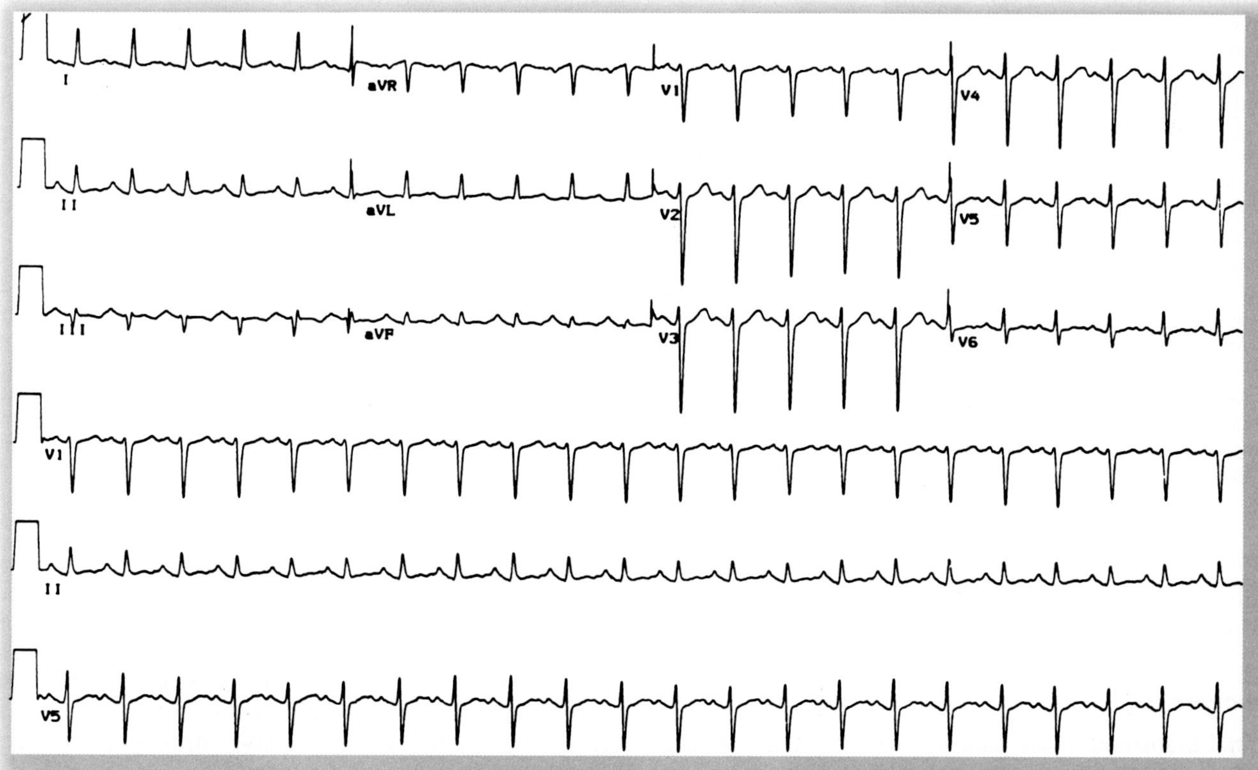

FIGURE 30–6. A 12-lead electrocardiogram of a patient with atrial tachycardia. Note that the P-wave usually just precedes the QRS in patients with atrial tachycardia.

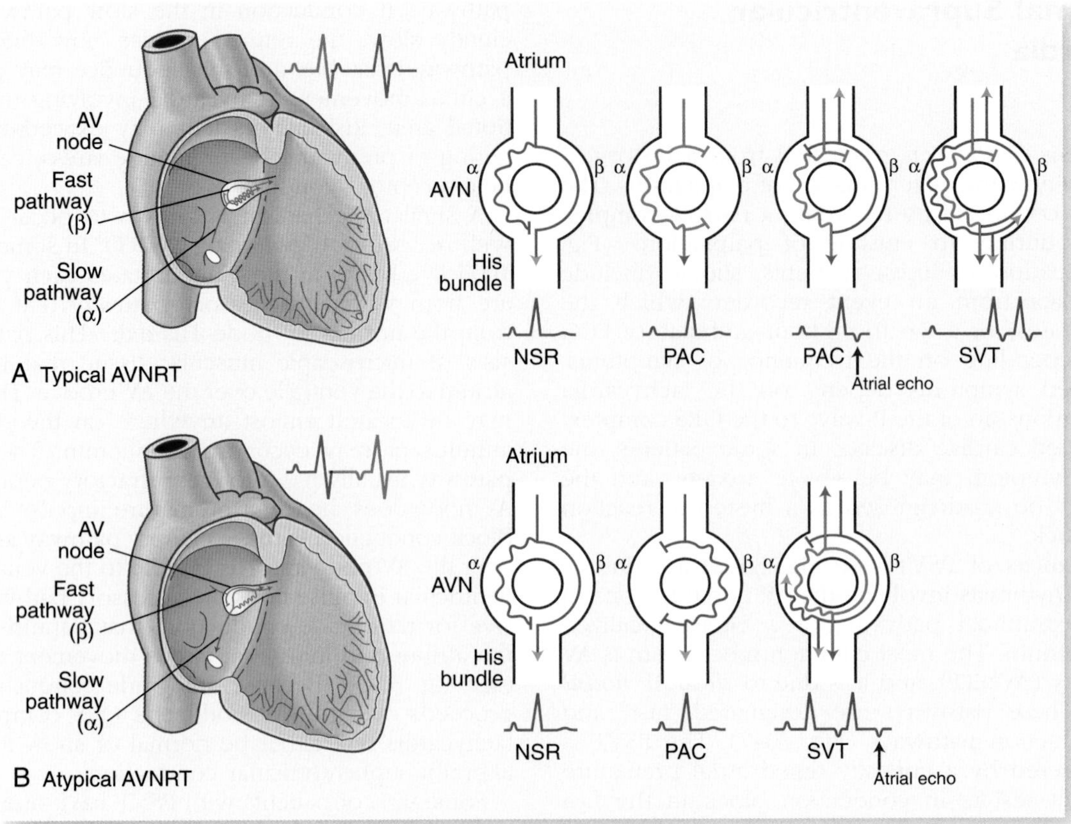

FIGURE 30–7. Schema for typical and atypical atrioventricular node reentrant tachycardia (AVNRT). *A*, Typical atrioventricular (AV) node (AVN) reentry. An impulse from the atrium enters the AV node and travels down both the slow (α) and the fast (β) pathways. It quickly travels down the fast pathway and results in activation of the ventricles with a short PR interval and in blocking of the impulse from the slow pathway when it reaches the terminal portion of the AV node because the tissue is still refractory. A premature atrial contraction (PAC) results in conduction of the impulse down the slow pathway and thus a longer PR interval. It blocks conduction in the fast pathway because that tissue has a longer refractory period. If the tissue of the fast pathway regains conduction, the impulse, after traveling down the slow pathway, can return retrogradely back to the atrium via the fast pathway and induce an atrial echo beat. A key component of the circuit is that the retrograde impulse finds the fast pathway no longer refractory. For this situation to occur, a suitable delay in antegrade conduction over the slow pathway must ensue. The QRS complex is narrow because the ventricle is being activated via the normal His-Purkinje system (HPS). Retrograde activation over the fast pathway happens quickly, and on the surface ECG the retrograde P-wave is usually "buried" or at the tail end of the QRS complex. This finding can give the appearance of a "pseudo"–right bundle branch pattern in lead V_1. This abnormality is a short RP tachycardia. *B*, When the circuit is reversed, as during atypical AV node reentry, antegrade conduction occurs over the fast pathway and retrograde conduction over the slow pathway. In atypical AV node reentry, a PAC is conducted over the fast pathway. The PR interval remains short. If retrograde activation proceeds over the slow pathway to the atrium, supraventricular tachycardia (SVT) may be initiated. The QRS complex remains narrow because activation of the ventricle is still via the normal HPS. Retrograde atrial activation over the slow pathway takes longer than conduction over the fast pathway and thereby results in a long RP interval. This abnormality is a long RP tachycardia. NSR, normal sinus rhythm. (Redrawn from Grogin HR: Supraventricular tachycardia. In Scheinman M [vol ed]: Arrhythmias: Electrophysiologic principles. In Braunwald E [series ed]: Atlas of Heart Diseases, vol 9. Philadelphia, Current Medicine, 1996, pp 5.1–5.17.)

40%). The bulk of the remainder have atrial tachycardia that may be due to reentry within the atrium or abnormal automaticity of an atrial focus.

Management

Initial Evaluation. Most patients with PSVT are young and do not have any evidence of cardiac disease; hence, except in special circumstances, extensive evaluation is not required. A number of practical points bear emphasis. The ECG during and even after an episode of rapid tachycardia will often show persistent ST depression. This finding, in and of itself, does not necessitate hospitalization and does not require coronary angiography. An echocardiogram should be obtained in selected patients with PSVT to evaluate possible occult cardiac abnormalities. For example, patients with right-sided accessory pathways may have apparent or occult Ebstein's anomaly (see Chapter 34).

Treatment. Because the predominant mechanisms of PSVT involve AV nodal conduction, initial therapy for patients with narrow-complex tachycardia involves maneuvers or drugs that block conduction at the AV node. Carotid sinus massage, for example, is a safe and often effective maneuver for termination of tachycardia. Care must be taken to exclude significant carotid stenosis (by careful auscultation over the carotids) before applying carotid massage. Children with PSVT are often treated by the application of facial cold packs, a potent vagal maneuver. These maneuvers increase vagal tone, which delays conduction and prolongs refractoriness in the AV node. If the tachycardia fails to terminate with vagal maneuvers, intravenous drug treatment is indicated.

Adenosine and verapamil are very rapidly acting, effective, and safe. Adenosine is administered in bolus infusions to adults at an initial dose of 6 mg; repeat doses of 12 and 18 mg may be attempted if the lower dose proves ineffective. The half-life of adenosine is approximately 10 seconds, so adverse effects are quickly dissipated. Adenosine is effective in approximately 95% of patients with PSVT, and the chief adverse effect is transient dyspnea and chest tightness. Intravenous verapamil is administered at a dose of 0.15 mg/kg but should not be used in patients with underlying sinus or AV node dysfunction or in those pretreated with beta-blockers. The chief advantage of adenosine is its short half-life. One advantage of verapamil is its relatively low cost, but this drug may aggravate underlying sinus or nodal disease or heart failure in patients with depressed left ventricular function. Short-acting beta-blocking agents (esmolol) or intravenous propranolol may be used, particularly if the patient fails to respond to adenosine. Medications are so effective that direct-current cardioversion is seldom required, except for conditions associated with hemodynamic collapse. Similarly, anticoagulant therapy is not required for patients with PSVT.

Special Case of the Wolff-Parkinson-White Syndrome. Patients with Wolff-Parkinson-White syndrome have an accessory pathway going from the atrium to the ventricle and bypassing the usual delay in the AV node. When the patient is in sinus rhythm, dual conduction down this pathway and through the AV node will often cause a delta wave, which is the initial slurred deflection that is seen at the beginning of the QRS complex and that results from early activation of the QRS complex by conduction over the accessory pathway (Fig. 30–8). The presence of an alternative AV pathway in patients with Wolff-Parkinson-White syndrome makes them prone to the development of PSVT, which may then cause atrial fibrillation.

Patients with Wolff-Parkinson-White syndrome or its variants, such as a short resting PR interval without a delta wave in sinus rhythm (accelerated AV nodal conduction), may initially be seen in atrial fibrillation with a rapid ventricular response. Patients with Wolff-Parkinson-White syndrome or other accessory pathways are also slightly more likely to have other congenital cardiac abnormalities that are associated with a higher risk of PSVT, atrial fibrillation, and atrial flutter.

In patients with short refractory periods of the abnormal pathway, rapid, life-threatening arrhythmias may occur (Fig. 30–9). This situation, which is recognized by an irregular wide complex (preexcited QRS) with a very rapid rate (i.e., RR intervals less than 250 msec) on the ECG, should be considered dangerous and an indication for urgent attention. Emergency direct-current countershock followed by intravenous infusion of procainamide is the treatment of choice for atrial fibrillation or atrial flutter in patients with accessory pathways and very rapid AV conduction. These patients should generally be admitted to the hospital for further evaluation by a cardiologist and should be recommended to undergo catheter ablation of the pathway. It is critical to remember *not* to use intravenous digoxin or verapamil in these patients. Lidocaine and intravenous beta-blockers are not deleterious but are not usually effective for rate control in patients with rapid atrial fibrillation via an accessory pathway, and hence their use often delays appropriate care.

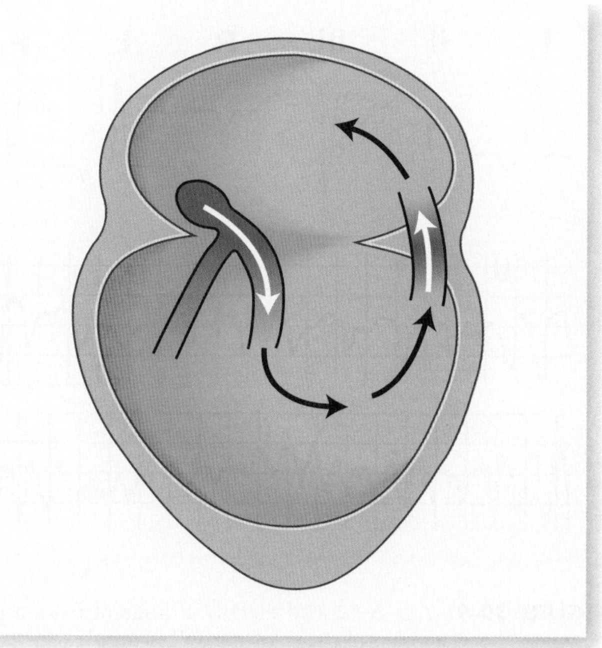

FIGURE 30–8. Schema showing a reentrant pathway in patients with accessory pathways. The tachycardia circuit usually involves antegrade conduction over the atrioventricular node and retrograde conduction over the accessory pathway.

Long-Term Treatment of Patients with Recurrent PSVT. Chronic drug therapy for patients with recurrent episodes of PSVT includes the use of agents that block conduction at the AV node (digoxin, calcium antagonists, or beta-blockers) (see Table 30–3) and agents that act primarily on fast-pathway or accessory-pathway conduction (i.e., the class IA agents quinidine, procainamide, and disopyramide or the class IC agents propafenone and flecainide) (see Table 30–4). Class III antiarrhythmic agents (amiodarone, sotalol) act on both the normal and the fast or accessory pathways. Chronic digoxin therapy is contraindicated in patients with Wolff-Parkinson-White syndrome.

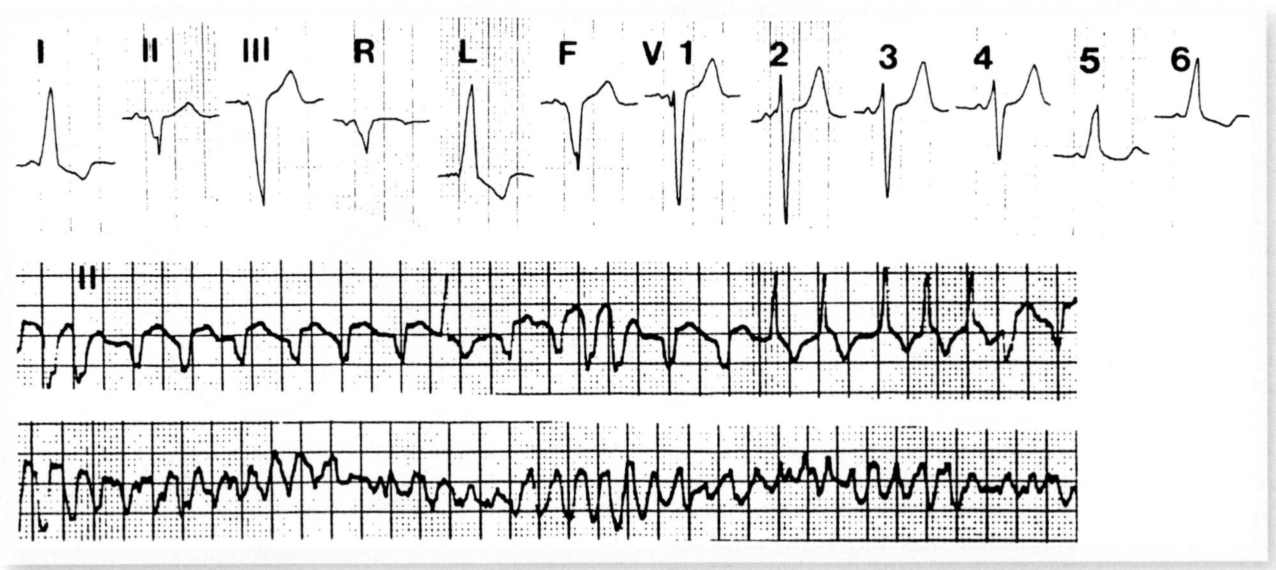

FIGURE 30–9. *Top,* A 12-lead electrocardiogram from a patient with Wolff-Parkinson-White syndrome. Note the delta wave between the P-wave and onset of the QRS complex in lead V_2. *Middle* and *bottom,* A lead II rhythm strip (not continuous) initially shows atrial fibrillation with a rapid ventricular response that quickly deteriorated into ventricular fibrillation *(bottom).* Atrial fibrillation with a rapid ventricular response is the most dangerous arrhythmia for patients with Wolff-Parkinson-White syndrome.

In patients who have recurrent SVTs of relatively short duration and who are asymptomatic except for palpitations, an alternative to catheter ablation or chronic antiarrhythmic treatment may be episodic therapy for the occasional arrhythmia. In some patients, 10 to 40 mg of propranolol or equivalent doses of other beta-blockers may be adequate to terminate a supraventricular arrhythmia; in others, a concomitant 0.25-mg dose of digoxin may provide an effective "cocktail." The use of intermittent therapy is discouraged because symptomatic prolonged pauses may develop when the arrhythmia terminates. More complex arrhythmias will commonly require chronic medications or referral to a cardiologist.

The advent of radiofrequency catheter ablative procedures has completely changed the approach to the long-term management of patients with recurrent PSVT and other SVTs[15] (see Table 30–5). These catheter techniques involve the use of invasive electrophysiologic (EP) studies to localize the abnormal pathway or pathways, which are then destroyed by the application of radiofrequency energy. The technique is effective in 90% to 98% of attempts and is associated with a very low incidence of adverse effects.

When to Refer to a Cardiologist. Referral for specialist care is indicated for all patients with possible Wolff-Parkinson-White syndrome and episodes of palpitations or syncope. Patients with Wolff-Parkinson-White syndrome carry the distinct risk of sudden cardiac death because of atrial fibrillation with a rapid rate. In addition, all patients with recurrent PSVT who either fail a course of medical therapy or are disinclined to take lifelong drug therapy are candidates for catheter ablation and should be referred to a specialist who can adequately discuss the benefits and possible adverse effects of the catheter procedure. Ablative techniques have also proved to be safe and effective in patients with atrial tachycardia.

Premature Atrial Contractions

Half or more of the adult population will have premature atrial contractions that will often be asymptomatic. Premature atrial contractions are probably the most common arrhythmic cause of palpitations (see Chapter 9) and can occasionally precipitate a sustained SVT in patients with the appropriate substrate. Frequent or recurrent premature atrial contractions may be caused by any of the stresses that precipitate sinus tachycardia, or they may be an early sign of a dilated atrium in patients with mitral or tricuspid valve disease, heart failure, or congenital heart disease.

Premature atrial contractions are preceded by a detectable P-wave that differs from the sinus P-wave by a PR interval of 0.12 second or longer. The premature contraction may or may not be associated with effective ventricular ejection and a detectable pulse, depending on whether the premature contraction is very early. For very early premature contractions, the P-wave may be difficult to find in the preceding T-wave, and some very early premature atrial contractions may be blocked because the AV node is still in its refractory period. In such situations, a blocked premature atrial contraction may be misdiagnosed as a sinus pause or sinus node dysfunction. Conducted premature atrial contractions may be associated with aberrant ventricular conduction and, hence, a wide ventricular complex. Premature atrial contractions are not commonly associated with a compensatory pause because unlike a premature ventricular contraction, they usually cause immediate resetting of the sinus node. In some patients, however, the premature atrial contraction may not be effectively conducted back into the sinus node; in these situations, a compensatory pause will occur.

Premature atrial contractions commonly require no treatment. Patients with symptomatic palpitations caused by atrial premature contractions should be reassured regarding their benign nature, and drug therapy should be discouraged. For patients in whom premature atrial contractions trigger SVTs, treatment is as described previously.

Wandering Atrial Pacemaker and Multifocal Atrial Tachycardia

When patients have more than two different P-wave morphologies, the rhythm is termed *wandering atrial pacemaker* (if the heart rate is less than 100 beats/min) or *multifocal atrial tachycardia* (if the heart rate is above 100 beats/min). Wandering atrial pacemaker is often a prelude to a sustained atrial tachycardia or, more commonly, atrial fibrillation in a patient with intrinsic heart disease. Multifocal atrial tachycardia is most commonly an arrhythmia found in patients with advanced pulmonary disease, sometimes associated with an exacerbation of the pulmonary disease itself and sometimes with the medications used to treat the pulmonary disease.

As with sinus tachycardia and premature atrial contractions, wandering atrial pacemaker and multifocal atrial tachycardia may be precipitated by a variety of noncardiac conditions whose successful treatment often results in termination of the arrhythmia. If the arrhythmia itself is causing important secondary problems, verapamil and metoprolol are the recommended medications, provided that the patient does not have severe left ventricular dysfunction.

Premature Ventricular Complexes and Nonsustained Ventricular Tachycardia

Diagnosis

Ventricular arrhythmias may be separated into various categories, including isolated *premature ventricular complexes* (PVCs) (Fig. 30–10), *nonsustained VT* (three or more successive PVCs), and *sustained monomorphic VT* (Fig. 30–11), which is defined as VT persisting for 30 seconds or requiring termination by intervention. Ventricular arrhythmias in these categories generally show a single morphology; patients with multiple types of monomorphic VT are referred to as having a *pleomorphic pattern.* A separate category of ventricular arrhythmia includes patients with *polymorphous VT,*

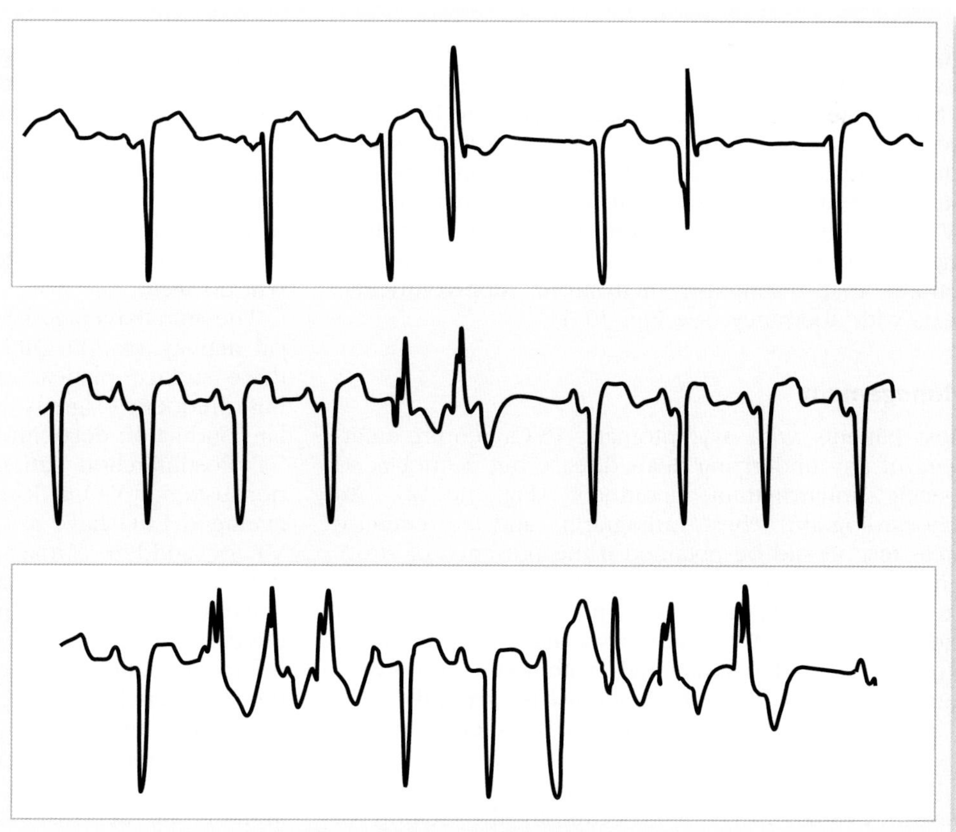

FIGURE 30–10. *Top,* Single premature ventricular complexes. *Middle* and *bottom,* Ventricular couplets and triplets, respectively.

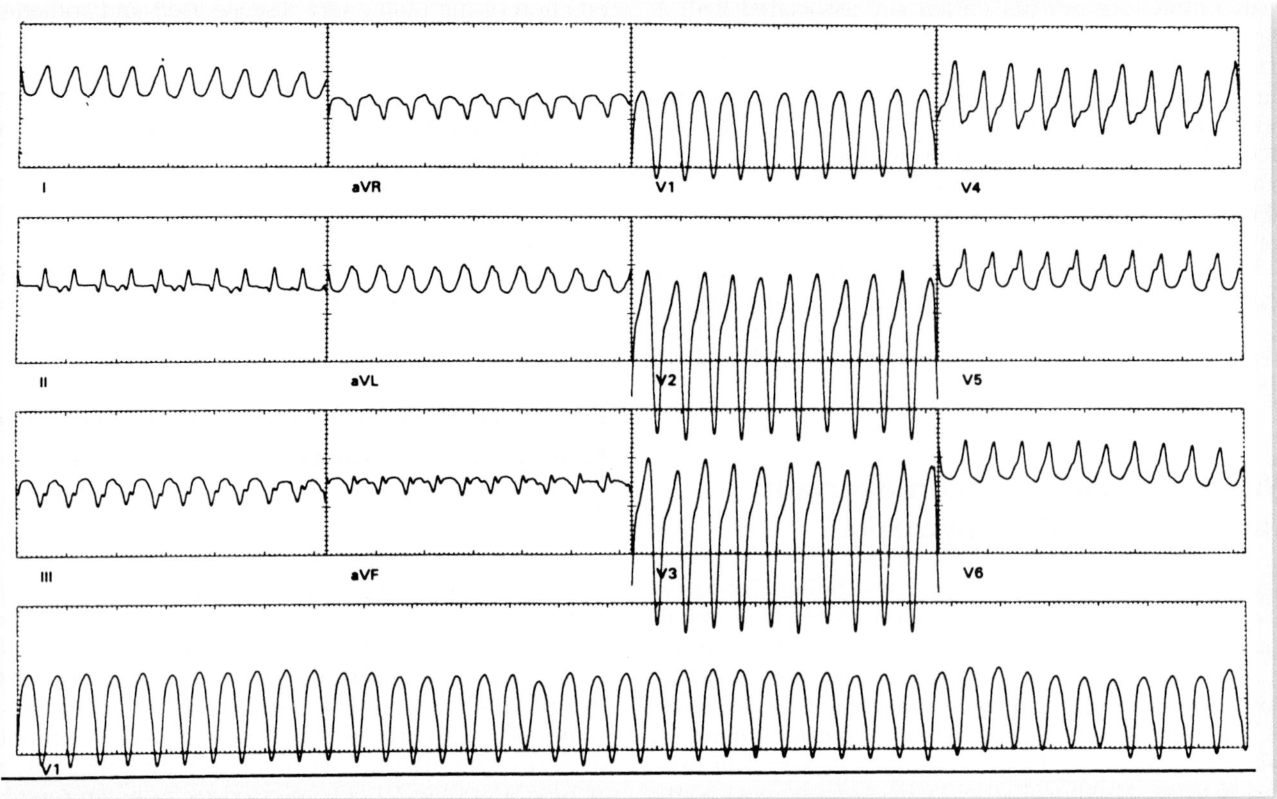

FIGURE 30–11. A 12-lead electrocardiogram shows wide-complex tachycardia. Atrioventricular dissociation is evident (best seen in lead II) and is most consistent with ventricular tachycardia.

which is defined as a rapid ventricular arrhythmia with beat-to-beat changes in the ventricular complexes.

Making the Diagnosis. Ventricular premature beats are recognized by premature wide complexes followed by compensatory pauses. The cause of the compensatory pause is related to the fact that the PVC penetrates the AV node, thereby making it refractory to the next sinus impulse. In addition, PVCs have distinct morphologic features that distinguish them from supraventricular beats with aberrancy (see Fig. 30–1).

Management

Most patients with asymptomatic PVCs require treatment of any underlying heart disease but do not need specific antiarrhythmic treatment (Fig. 30–12). An echocardiogram, chest radiograph, and an exercise stress test should be obtained if the presence of structural heart disease is uncertain or if the PVCs occur with exercise. Studies have shown that very frequent exercise-induced PVCs are associated with a worse prognosis, but that individuals with PVCs or nonsustained VT and no structural heart disease generally have a benign long-term prognosis, so no specific antiarrhythmic therapy is indicated.[16]

In patients with ventricular arrhythmias, sudden cardiac death most often occurs in the setting of ischemic cardiac disease. If the patient has just recovered from an acute myocardial infarction, the EF should be determined to assess prognosis (see Chapter 27). Patients who survive an acute myocardial infarction and who have high-density PVCs (i.e., ≥10 PVCs/hr) or complex PVCs have a higher risk of 2-year mortality. This finding is of limited value, however, because 40% of postinfarction patients will have either high-density PVCs or nonsustained VT, and most of these patients will do well.

The signal-averaged ECG, which records the electrical activity of 200 QRS complexes obtained from all three surface planes, can detect late, low-amplitude, high-frequency signals that correlate with intraventricular conduction delay and may provide the substrate for VT. Postinfarction patients with high-density PVCs (or nonsustained VT), a decreased EF, and a positive signal-averaged ECG have a 17-fold risk for either sustained VT or sudden cardiac death when compared with patients without these risk factors.

Numerous studies have documented the beneficial effects of beta-blocker therapy for post-myocardial infarction patients (see Chapter 27) and have shown that the benefits are greater in patients with poor left ventricular function. By comparison, class I agents increase morality in postinfarction patients, sotalol provides no significant reduction in mortality,[17] and amiodarone decreases arrhythmic deaths but has no significant impact on overall mortality.[18] Even when

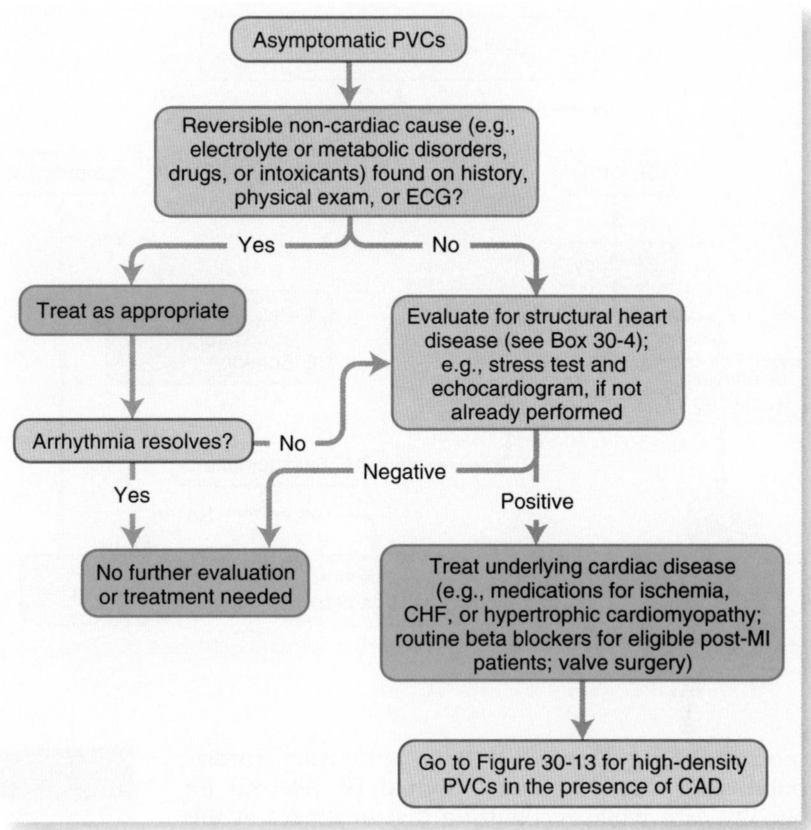

FIGURE 30–12. Management of premature ventricular complexes (PVCs). See text for details. CAD, coronary artery disease; CHF, congestive heart failure; ECG, electrocardiogram; MI, myocardial infarction.

antiarrhythmic drug therapy for nonsustained VT is guided by EP testing, it does not improve the prognosis.[19] In accordance with these data, beta-blockers should be used in all postinfarction patients who can tolerate them, but no additional specific antiarrhythmic agent can be advocated.

At the present time, noninvasive testing (including measurement of heart rate variability, the signal-averaged ECG, baroreceptor sensitivity, or T-wave alternans) has too low a positive predictive value to be of routine clinical utility. By comparison, invasive EP testing in an attempt to provoke inducible VT in patients with nonsustained VT may define the prognosis and guide therapy in high-risk patients (see later). If patients with an EF below 40% have episodes of sustained or nonsustained VT despite medications that are indicated for their heart failure (see Chapter 28), angina (Chapter 25), or postinfarction status (Chapter 27), they should be referred to a cardiologist with expertise in arrhythmias for consideration of EP testing.

High-Density Premature Ventricular Complexes and Nonsustained Ventricular Tachycardia in Patients with Structural Heart Disease

Patients with coronary artery disease and high-density PVCs or nonsustained VT and a depressed EF (<40%) should generally undergo a diagnostic EP study for further risk stratification (Fig. 30–13). Patients who do not have inducible sustained VT during invasive EP testing have a better prognosis.[20] In contrast, two randomized trials have demonstrated a significant mortality benefit of implantable cardioverter-defibrillators (ICDs) for patients who have nonsustained VT, coronary artery disease, an EF less than 40%, and inducible sustained VT on EP testing.[20,21] Another study found that ICD implantation was significantly better than amiodarone or sotalol for patients with symptomatic VT or ventricular fibrillation (VF).[22] Unfortunately, the current price for ICDs makes them more expensive than most accepted medical and surgical therapies despite their clear benefit.[23] Although current randomized trial data do not extend to postinfarction patients with high-density PVCs without sustained VT, most patients with high-density PVCs will also have nonsustained VT, as defined by three or more consecutive PVCs with a rate of 120/min or higher on continuous monitoring.

Role of the Primary Care Physician. PVCs are very frequent, and most patients with this problem do not require therapy, especially those who have no structural cardiac disease. Patients without structural heart disease do not have an increased risk of subsequent cardiac events. Even exercise-induced nonsustained VT is not associated with an increased risk of cardiac events in subjects without apparent cardiac disease. Primary care physicians should identify patients who have high-density PVCs or nonsustained VT and who also have

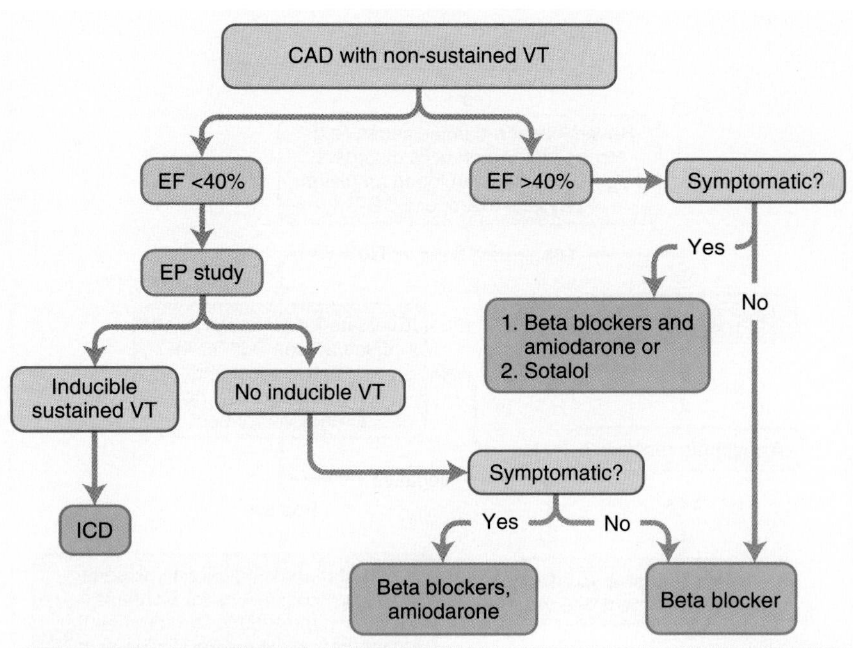

FIGURE 30–13. Coronary artery disease (CAD) with high-density (≥10/hr) premature ventricular complexes (PVCs) or nonsustained ventricular tachycardia (VT). EF, ejection fraction; EP, electrophysiologic; ICD, implantable cardioverter-defibrillator.

coronary artery disease or other underlying cardiac abnormalities. These patients should be referred for specialty care while recognizing that treatment at this time may vary among specialists.

Sustained Ventricular Tachycardia

Diagnosis

VT often occurs in the setting of high-density PVCs and should be distinguished from SVT with aberrant conduction (see Fig. 30–1). AV dissociation is the most definitive ECG finding in VT.

Patients with sustained VT deserve careful evaluation to look for specific causes (Box 30–4). Approximately 75% of patients with sustained VT have underlying coronary artery disease. For these patients, the extent of coronary disease, the presence of impaired left ventricular function, and evidence of myocardial ischemia are important prognostic factors. Sustained VT in young patients with familial hypertrophic cardiomyopathy carries a high risk of sudden cardiac death. Other causes of VT include acquired valvular heart disease, idiopathic cardiomyopathy, and congenital cardiac disease. It is now well appreciated that patients who have had successful surgery for correction of the tetralogy of Fallot or a ventricular septal defect are at risk for the late development of VT. Another recently described, but rare cause of either sustained VT or sudden cardiac death in young adults is known as *arrhythmogenic right ventricular dysplasia*, in which the right ventricular muscle is replaced by fibrofatty tissue. The diagnosis may be substantiated by an echocardiogram or by cardiac magnetic resonance imaging.

Ventricular Tachycardia without Structural Cardiac Disease. In contrast to patients with structural heart disease and VT are those in whom VT occurs in the setting of no structural disease. These patients usually have VT emanating from either the right or left ventricular outflow tract or, less commonly, from a left septal focus. Right ventricular outflow tract VTs are often induced by exercise and may respond to beta-blocker therapy. Patients with idiopathic left septal VT are characterized by an unusual form of VT that usually responds to intravenous verapamil therapy and may respond acutely to vagal maneuvers. Patients with idio-

BOX 30–4

Causes of Sustained Ventricular Tachycardia or Fibrillation

STRUCTURAL CARDIAC DISEASE	OTHER CARDIAC DISEASE
Coronary artery disease	Congenital or acquired long QT syndrome
Cardiomyopathy	Coronary artery spasm
Hypertrophic	Catecholamine-induced VT
Dilated	Right ventricular outflow VT
Restrictive	Left fascicular VT
	Brugada's syndrome

Valvular heart disease

Congenital

- Corrected congenital lesions (e.g., VSD repair, tetralogy of Fallot)
- Anomalous origin of the left coronary artery
- Right ventricular dysplasia

VSD, ventricular septal defect; VT, ventricular tachycardia.

pathic VT originating from the left or right ventricular outflow tracts, from the cusps of the aortic sinuses, or from the left septum may be candidates for permanent cure of the tachycardia by catheter ablation.

The Brugada syndrome is characterized by the development of rapid polymorphous VT or VF in patients who have a right bundle branch block pattern with ST elevation in leads V_1 and V_2 on the resting ECG.[24] In approximately 15% of these patients, a specific abnormality has been found in a sodium channel gene *(SCNA5)*. Because of the high risk of recurrent VT or VF in untreated patients, ICD therapy is recommended for this syndrome.

Management of Patients with Structural Heart Disease

Patients with VT require careful evaluation directed at diagnosing the presence, type, and severity of any underlying cardiac disease. As such, most of these patients will require echocardiography. If coronary artery disease is known or suspected, coronary arteriography is often needed to discern the extent and severity of the coronary disease. VT is commonly seen in patients with large myocardial infarctions or in areas of myocardial aneurysm formation. Invasive EP studies can guide decisions involving drug, ablative, or ICD therapy.

For patients with VT and no structural heart disease, attention is directed at obtaining a 12-lead ECG during VT to help localize the origin of this VT. In patients with exercise-induced palpitations, a treadmill test performed in the presence of experienced personnel and resuscitation equipment may be required to make the diagnosis.

Acute Management. Direct-current cardioversion should always be used in the presence of hemodynamic instability or acute cardiac ischemia. In patients who are hemodynamically stable without acute ischemia, initial therapy depends on an accurate diagnosis (see Fig. 30–1). For example, although intravenous verapamil may be highly effective in patients with SVT, this agent may be lethal in those with VT. Initial drug therapy for patients with monomorphic VT should include a bolus infusion of amiodarone or lidocaine (see Fig. 24–3), followed by a continuous drip (see Table 30–2). Intravenous therapy with procainamide may also be used if left ventricular EF is known to be preserved (EF >40%). Studies have shown that intravenous procainamide is more effective in terminating VT but that lidocaine less frequently causes hypotension. From a practical standpoint, the EF is often not known, and intravenous amiodarone is considered by many to be the drug of choice. The new Advanced Care Life Support (ACLS) guidelines also stress the use of a single antiarrhythmic agent followed by cardioversion as needed to minimize the potential proarrhythmic effects of multiple medications. Intravenous amiodarone is infused into a central venous line in a dextrose solution. An initial loading dose of 5 mg/kg is administered over a period of 30 to 45 minutes, followed by an infusion of 1 g over a 24-hour period. After stabilization, therapy is switched to oral amiodarone in doses of 200 to 400 mg/day. Intravenous amiodarone must be used with great care and should be supervised by physicians well versed in its use.

Role of the Primary Care Physician. The primary care physician should attempt to distinguish VT from SVT with aberration and should be responsible for the emergency treatment of patients with sustained VT or fibrillation (see Chapter 24). After the patient is stabilized, the evaluation is directed at establishing the cause of this arrhythmia. If a reversible cause is not found, multiple treatment options exist.

Drug Therapy. Among antiarrhythmic medications, the class III agents amiodarone and sotalol are preferable to class I drugs. In patients with sustained VT, the Antiarrhythmics vs. Implantable Defibrillators (AVID) trial showed that ICDs were significantly more effective than amiodarone in patients with ischemic heart disease and left ventricular EFs below 40%.[22] Recent substudies, however, suggest that amiodarone is as effective as ICD therapy in patients with coronary artery disease and EFs between 35% and 40%.

Device Therapy. Use of the ICD has had a dramatic impact on therapy for patients with malignant ventricular arrhythmias. These devices, placed intravenously (Fig. 30–14), detect VT or VF and then initiate either antitachycardia pacing or a rescue shock when appropriate. The current recommendations for ICDs[25] (Box 30–5) may broaden to all patients who have a low EF after acute myocardial infarction[26] (see Chapter 27) and to other patients based on the results of ongoing randomized trials. At present, ICD therapy is the preferred treatment option for patients with hemodynamically unstable sustained VT, VT poorly responsive to conventional medical therapy such as amiodarone, or VF except when in the setting of acute myocardial infarction or severe electrolyte abnormalities. Because this field is rapidly evolving, such patients should be managed in consultation with a cardiologist experienced in arrhythmias.

Catheter Ablation. Only modest success has been reported with the use of ablative techniques for patients with ischemic heart disease, in part related to the complexity of VT and the frequent occurrence of multiple reentrant circuits. Certain types of VT are, however, very effectively treated by catheter ablation. One such arrhythmia is bundle-to-bundle reentry. These patients usually have syncope or a history of aborted sudden death. The basic mechanism is reentry involving both the right and left bundle branches. Catheter ablation of the right bundle branch is curative. In selected individuals who have good left ventricular function and who need cardiac surgery for other reasons (e.g., coronary artery bypass surgery, valve surgery, or correction of congenital abnormalities), detection of a VT focus may allow surgical excision of the focus during the operation.

Ventricular Fibrillation. Evaluation of patients with VF is similar to that described for patients with VT. In the absence of obvious precipitating causes (e.g., drugs, electrolyte abnormalities, severe hypoxemia, or acidosis), these patients should be treated with an ICD. If the

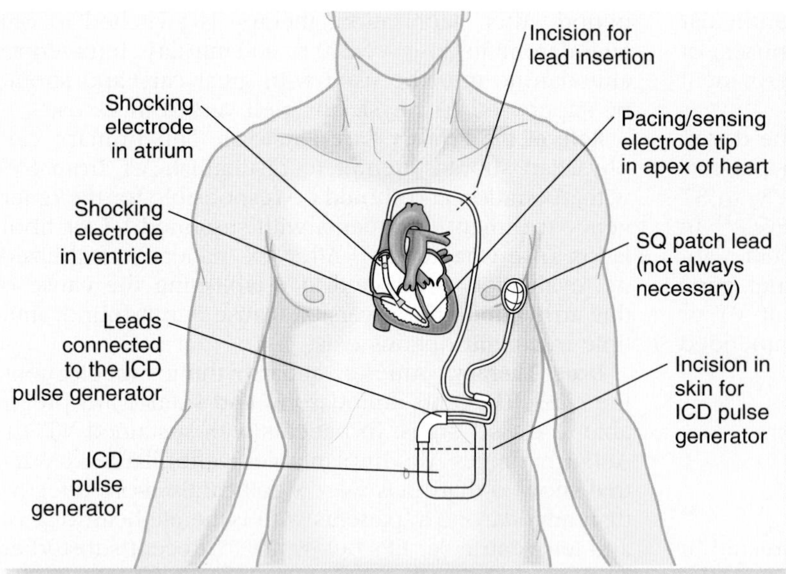

FIGURE 30–14. Nonthoracotomy lead system. Perhaps the single most significant advance in implantable defibrillator technology to date has been the development of transvenous lead systems that do not require thoracotomy for implantation. ICD, implantable cardioverter-defibrillator; SQ, subcutaneous. (Redrawn from Cockrell JL, Siu A: Implantable defibrillators for the management of cardiac rhythm disorders. In Scheinman M [vol ed]: Arrhythmias: Electrophysiologic principles. In Braunwald E [series ed]: Atlas of Heart Diseases, vol 9. Philadelphia, Current Medicine, 1996, pp 9.1–9.16; adapted from Cardiac Pacemakers, Inc., St. Paul, MN.)

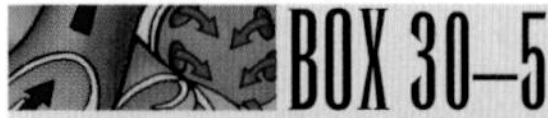
BOX 30–5

Devices for Ventricular Tachycardia: Indications for ICD

ICD INDICATED

Cardiac arrest secondary to VF or VT not due to a transient or reversible cause
Symptomatic or hemodynamically significant sustained VT
Nonsustained VT in the presence of previous MI, LV dysfunction, and inducible VT at EP study
Syncope of unknown etiology with structural heart disease and inducible VT at EP study (see Chapter 10)

ICD MAY BE INDICATED

High-risk long QT syndrome or hypertrophic cardiomyopathy
Hemodynamically stable sustained VT
Cardiac arrest presumed to be due to VF when EP testing is precluded by a medical condition
Severe symptomatic sustained VT while awaiting cardiac transplantation

ICD CONTRAINDICATED

Syncope of unexplained etiology with no inducible VT at EP study
Incessant VT or VF
VF or VT treatable by surgical or catheter ablation
VT due to a reversible cause
Terminal illness
End-stage cardiomyopathy (class IV) and not a candidate for cardiac transplantation
Psychiatric contraindications

Modified from ACC/AHA/NASPE Guideline Update for implantation of cardiac pacemakers and antiarrhythmia devices: Summary article. Circulation 2002;106:2145–2161.

EP, electrophysiologic; ICD, implantable cardioverter-defibrillator; MI, myocardial infarction; VF ventricular fibrillation; VT, ventricular tachycardia.

VF occurred as a result of acute (<48 hours) myocardial infarction, no chronic treatment may be needed. If the arrhythmia was precipitated by transient myocardial ischemia, coronary revascularization may be critical. An ICD is recommended in patients in whom the cause of the VF has not been diagnosed or in those who have a substantial risk of recurrence. As with VT, these decisions should be made in conjunction with an experienced cardiologist.

Polymorphous Ventricular Tachycardia

Diagnosis

Diagnostic Considerations. Polymorphous VT is defined as a rapid ventricular arrhythmia with beat-to-beat changes in the QRS complex. A subset of polymorphous VT is an arrhythmia denoted by the term *torsades de pointes*. This arrhythmia consists of beat-to-beat changes in QRS complex polarity so that the QRS complex appears to be rotating about the baseline. Another typical feature of torsades de pointes is its association with a long QT interval. It should be emphasized that patients with more than one form of monomorphic VT may have a pattern resembling polymorphous VT, with a change from one monomorphic configuration to another (pleomorphic VT).

The pathogenesis and treatment of polymorphous VTs are very different from that for monomorphic VT. Polymorphous VT may be divided into hereditary and acquired forms (Box 30–6).

Hereditary. Hereditary forms of polymorphic VT are known as the *idiopathic long QT syndrome*. This syndrome consists of patients at great risk for sudden cardiac death associated with prolonged QT intervals and may be inherited as an autosomal dominant trait without hearing loss (Romano-Ward syndrome) or as an autosomal recessive trait with hearing loss (Jervell and Lange-Nielsen syndrome). The syndrome should be sus-

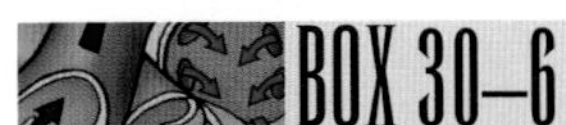

BOX 30–6

Causes of Polymorphous Ventricular Tachycardia

Congenital
- Jervell and Lange-Nielsen syndrome
- Romano-Ward syndrome (abnormalities on chromosomes 3, 4, and 7 have been described)

Acquired (drugs)
- Antiarrhythmic drugs
  - Class IA (quinidine, procainamide, disopyramide)
  - Class III (sotalol, amiodarone [rare], dofetilide)
- Psychotropic drugs
  - Tricyclic antidepressants
  - Phenothiazines
- Antibiotics
  - Erythromycin and other macrolide antibiotics, pentamidine, ampicillin, trimethoprim-sulfamethoxazole, ketoconazole
- Antihistamines
  - Terfenadine, astemizole
- Miscellaneous drugs
  - Probucol, ketanserin, cocaine, papaverine, organophosphates

Electrolyte disorders
- Hypokalemia, hypocalcemia, hypomagnesemia

Severe ischemia
- After myocardial infarction
- Coronary spasm

Normal heart, no electrolyte disorders or offending drugs
- Exercise induced
- Short coupled premature ventricular complexes

pected in children or young adults with seizures, syncope, or aborted sudden death. Untreated patients face a very high risk of sudden cardiac death as a result of polymorphous VT that degenerates into VF. A voluntary worldwide registry suggests that 75% of untreated patients will die suddenly. In contrast, those treated with beta-blockers have a much improved prognosis but still face a 6% risk of sudden cardiac death. Currently, at least six distinct genetic defects involving different cardiac ion channels have been identified as the cause of prolonged repolarization and thus a prolonged QT interval.[27] Genetic testing is currently limited to the research setting.

Acquired. The most common cause of acquired polymorphous VT is drug related (Fig. 30–15). The chief offenders appear to be class IA drugs (quinidine, procainamide, disopyramide) and sotalol, each of which prolongs the action potential duration. These agents are usually, but not always associated with QT prolongation, and the polymorphous VT is almost always provoked by a preceding pause. Other currently marketed agents incriminated in the induction of polymorphous VT include tricyclic antidepressants, phenothiazine derivatives, macrolide antibiotics, probucol, organic phosphate insecticides, and high protein liquid diets. Electrolyte abnormalities, particularly hypokalemia, hypocalcemia, and hypomagnesemia, may either cause or be associated with provoking drug-induced polymorphous VT.

Another important setting for polymorphous VT is in patients with severe ischemia. The true incidence of this arrhythmia is not known because many patients do not survive to reach the hospital. In these patients, episodes of polymorphous VT are usually preceded by sinus tachycardia and by symptoms or ECG signs of acute myocardial ischemia, but the QT interval is generally normal. Polymorphous VT may also rarely occur in patients with apparently normal hearts and no exposure to drugs or electrolyte abnormalities.

Management

A careful family and drug history, together with the baseline ECG and the ECG recorded during the arrhythmia, usually allows the clinician to differentiate acquired from congenital long QT syndrome. Patients with congenital long QT syndrome generally have a family history of syncope or sudden cardiac death at a young age. Special evaluation may be required in patients with syncope and a borderline-prolonged QT interval. Because the arrhythmia (torsades de pointes) is often precipitated by startle, attempts to provoke the arrhythmia (while the patient is under ECG monitoring) by startle are appropriate, as is the use of a stress test to assess whether the QT interval shortens appropriately with increases in heart rate. On occasion, patients with long QT syndrome will actually show lengthening of the QT interval with increases in the heart rate.

Treatment of Idiopathic Long QT Syndrome. Beta-blockers are of proven benefit and are the drug of first choice. If this therapy fails, an ICD is the next choice; even with an ICD, however, adjunctive therapy with beta-blockers and cardiac pacing may be required to decrease the frequency of ICD discharges. It should be appreciated that current ICD therapy incorporates anti-bradycardia pacing, which is also useful in these patients to prevent pauses that may trigger polymorphous VT.

Treatment of Drug-Induced Polymorphous VT. The most important aspect of treatment depends on a proper diagnosis along with prompt cessation of the offending drug (see Fig. 24–3). The diagnosis should be suspected if a patient treated with the previously mentioned drugs has syncope, seizures, or palpitations. Electrolyte abnormalities should be sought and corrected. If polymorphous VT recurs, a bolus infusion of magnesium (1 to 2 g over a 10-minute period, followed by continuous infusions) is indicated. The most effective acute therapy is insertion of a temporary transvenous cardiac pacemaker, by which the cardiac rate is adjusted to mitigate the length of the pause that appears critical for the induction of polymorphous VT. As the arrhythmia is brought under control, the paced rate is gradually reduced and the pacemaker ultimately removed.

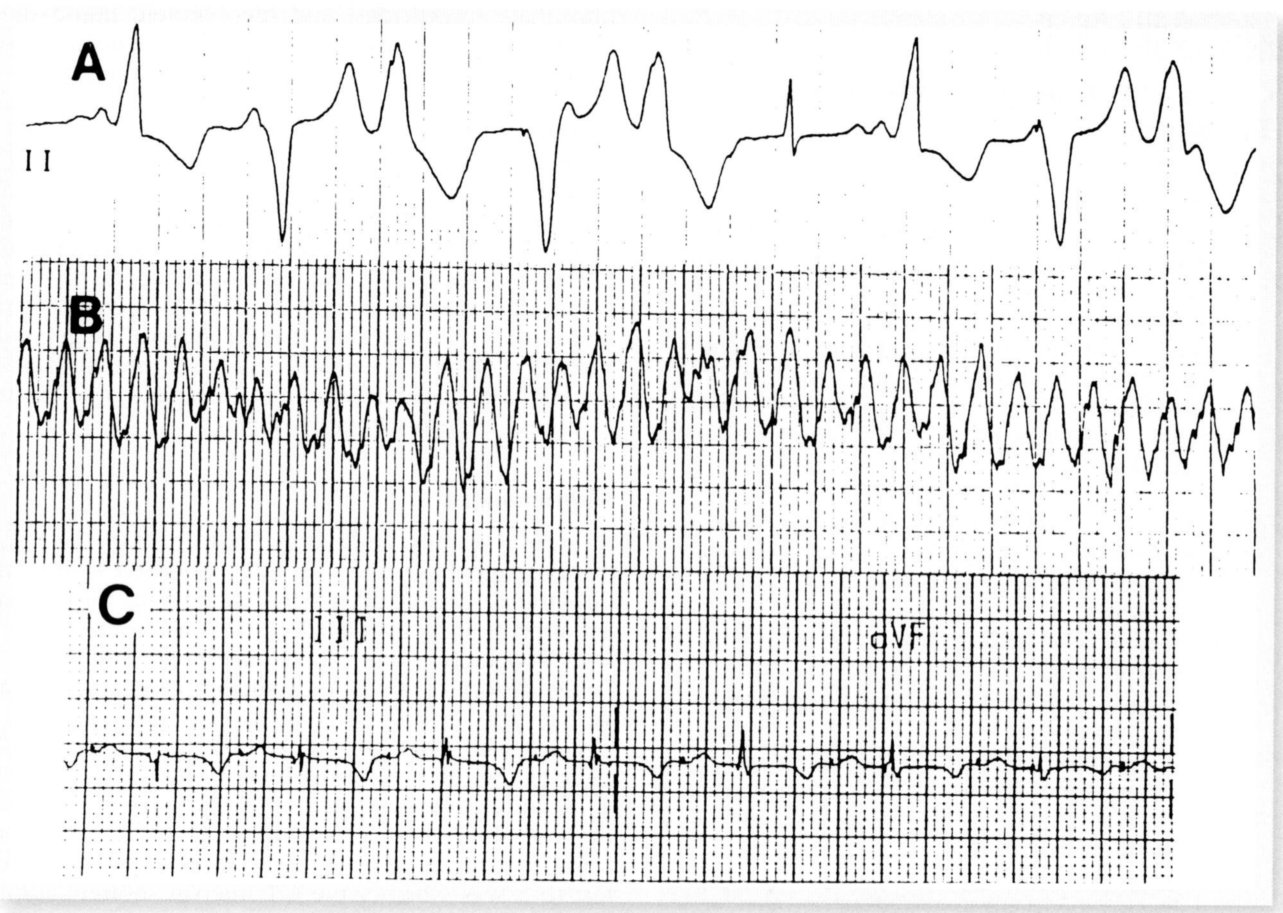

FIGURE 30–15. *A*, Strips show multiform ventricular complexes in a patient treated with quinidine. Note that the normally conducted beat (narrow QRS complex) is associated with marked prolongation of the QT interval. *B*, An episode of polymorphous ventricular tachycardia that required emergency cardioversion. *C*, The efficacy of atrial overdrive pacing.

For patients with polymorphous VT caused by unstable ischemic heart disease, treatment with beta-blockers, nitrates, or intravenous amiodarone may be effective, whereas traditional antiarrhythmic agents appear to be of limited value. When feasible, prompt revascularization is the treatment of choice.

When polymorphous VT occurs in the rare patient who has a normal heart and has not been exposed to drugs, the arrhythmia may be catecholamine (or exercise) related, may be due to coronary artery spasm, or may be of completely unknown origin. Some of these patients (especially those in the exercise-related group) may respond to beta-blockers or calcium channel blockers. Because mortality in these patients is high and drug therapy is not reliable, an ICD should be strongly considered.

The primary physician should try to distinguish between monomorphic and polymorphous VT because these arrhythmias have different mechanisms and modes of treatment. The clinician must also differentiate acquired from congenital forms of polymorphous VT. Patients with congenital long QT syndrome are rare and at very high risk for sudden cardiac death. Expert consultation is required for determining the role of drug versus ICD therapy. In addition, expert advice is often needed to resolve issues relating to genetic testing of family members, treatment of asymptomatic affected family members, and proper family counseling.

Patients Who Have Survived Sudden Cardiac Death

In patients who have survived an episode of cardiac sudden death, the precipitating arrhythmia may be a tachyarrhythmia or bradyarrhythmia.[28] In those with evidence of bradyarrhythmias, permanent pacemaker implantation is commonly indicated (see Chapter 31). If a tachyarrhythmia is known to be the cause, specific evaluation and treatment should be targeted to the known tachyarrhythmia (Fig. 30–16).

In many patients, however, the specific arrhythmic cause of sudden cardiac death cannot be determined. In those in whom the event occurred in conjunction with an obvious acute myocardial infarction, evaluation and subsequent treatment should proceed as guided by the features of the acute myocardial infarction, its com-

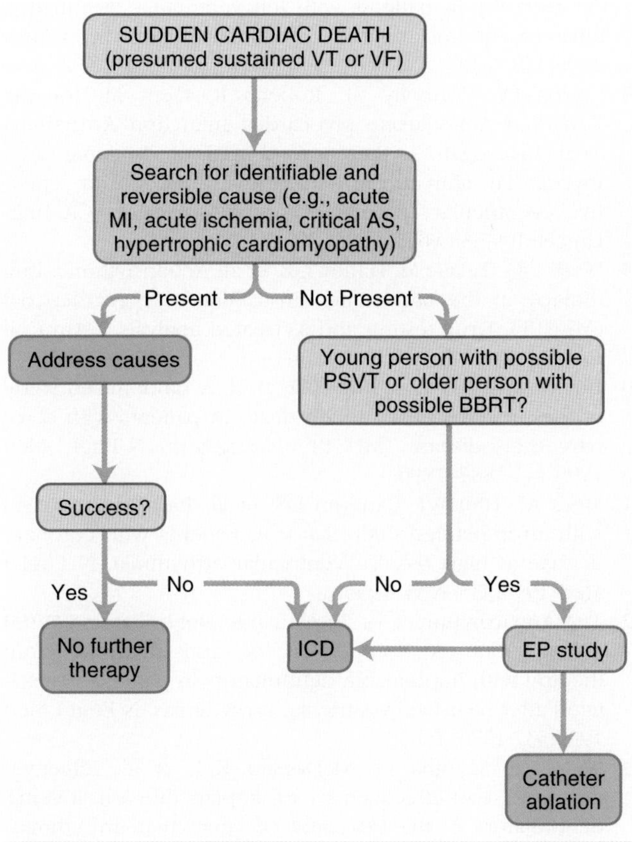

FIGURE 30–16. Management of a sudden cardiac death survivor. See text for details. AS, aortic stenosis; BBRT, bundle branch reentrant tachycardia; EP, electrophysiologic; ICD, implantable cardioverter-defibrillator; MI, myocardial infarction; PSVT, paroxysmal supraventricular tachycardia; VF, ventricular fibrillation; VT, ventricular tachycardia.

plications, and its sequelae (see Chapter 27). In other patients, the sudden cardiac death may clearly be attributed to an acute episode of myocardial ischemia, even in the absence of acute myocardial infarction. In such patients, treatment of the underlying coronary artery disease, commonly with revascularization, is paramount. Occasionally, the evaluation may reveal critical aortic valvular stenosis (Chapter 32), hypertrophic cardiomyopathy (Chapter 29), massive pulmonary embolism (Chapter 38), or other less common causes of sudden cardiac collapse, each of which has its own specific treatments.

In numerous patients, however, the episode of cardiac arrest cannot be attributed to a potentially reversible coronary or noncoronary cause. In such patients, a comprehensive clinical history and examination should be accompanied by at least an ECG, echocardiogram, and stress test to determine whether any underlying structural heart disease is present, even if it may not be directly remediable by surgical or medical means. Evaluation and treatment should proceed with standard EP testing, empiric ICD placement, or both. Treatment is then an ICD combined with medications that can prevent the need for ICD discharge in the individual patient. Evaluation and treatment of these patients should be performed in conjunction with a cardiologist experienced in arrhythmias, who would normally also participate in the follow-up care of such patients.

Evidence-Based Summary

1. Atrial fibrillation: For recent-onset atrial fibrillation, the timing of cardioversion and the duration of pre-cardioversion anticoagulation can be guided by the results of TEE. Chronic anticoagulation with warfarin (Coumadin) to maintain an INR between 2.0 and 3.0 significantly reduces the risk of stroke. Aspirin is not adequate in elderly or high-risk patients. The long-term approach of maintaining sinus rhythm has many theoretical advantages. Most authorities advocate initially attempting to maintain sinus rhythm. However, ongoing trials will provide evidence-based guidance on which patients are more likely to benefit from treatments designed to maintain sinus rhythm versus treatments that control the heart rate but leave the patient in atrial fibrillation.
2. Atrial flutter: The natural history of atrial flutter includes frequent recurrences. Studies have shown that most patients with atrial flutter can now be safely cured by catheter ablation with a high success rate.
3. Paroxysmal SVT: Patients who fail medical therapy or wish to avoid long-term medical therapy can be safely and effectively cured with catheter ablation.
4. PVCs, nonsustained VT: Patients with a normal left ventricular EF have an excellent prognosis and require no therapy. Those with nonsustained VT or with high-density PVCs (≥10/hr), a previous myocardial infarction, and an EF less than 40% require diagnostic EP testing. In the presence of inducible VT, an ICD is recommended.
5. Sustained VT: An ICD is generally recommended if the patient has a hemodynamically unstable sustained VT that is not due to a transient or reversible cause.
6. Sudden cardiac death survivor: An ICD is generally recommended if the event was not due to a transient or reversible cause.

References

1. Brugada P, Brugada J, Mont L, et al: A new approach to the differential diagnosis of a regular tachycardia with a wide QRS complex. Circulation 1991;83:1649–1659.
2. Guidelines 2000 for Cardiopulmonary Resuscitation and Emergency Cardiovascular Care. Part 6: Advanced cardiovascular life support: 7D: The tachycardia algorithms. The American Heart Association in collaboration with the

International Liaison Committee on Resuscitation. Circulation 2000;102(Suppl):I158–I165.
3. Peters NS, Schilling RJ, Kanagaratnam P, Markides V: Atrial fibrillation. Lancet 2002;359:593–603.
4. Roy D, Talajic M, Dorian P, et al: Amiodarone to prevent recurrence of atrial fibrillation. N Engl J Med 2000;342: 913–920.
5. Fuster V, Ryden LE, Asinger RW, et al: ACC/AHA/ESC guidelines for the management of patients with atrial fibrillation: Executive summary. J Am Coll Cardiol 2001; 38:1231–1265.
6. Segal JB, McNamara RL, Miller MR, et al: Anticoagulants or antiplatelet therapy for non-rheumatic atrial fibrillation and flutter. Cochrane Database Syst Rev 2001;CD001938.
7. Taylor FC, Cohen H, Ebrahim S: Systematic review of long term anticoagulation or antiplatelet treatment in patients with non-rheumatic atrial fibrillation. BMJ 2001;332:321–326.
8. Falk RH: Atrial fibrillation. N Engl J Med 2001;344: 1067–1078.
9. Klein AL, Grimm RA, Murray D, et al: Use of transesophageal echocardiography to guide cardioversion in patients with atrial fibrillation. N Engl J Med 2001;344: 1411–1420.
10. Klein AL, Murray RD, Grimm RA: Role of transesophageal echocardiography—guided cardioversion of patients with atrial fibrillation. J Am Coll Cardiol 2001;37:691–704.
11. The Atrial Fibrillation Follow-up Investigation of Rhythm Management (AFFIRM) Investigators. A comparison of rate control and rhythm control in patients with atrial fibrillation. N Engl J Med 2002;23:1825–1834.
12. Hohnloser SH, Kuck K-H, Lilienthal J: Rhythm or rate control in atrial fibrillation—Pharmacological Intervention in Atrial Fibrillation (PIAF): A randomized trial. Lancet 2000;356:1789–1794.
13. Van Gelder IC, Hagens VE, Bosker HA, et al: A comparison of rate control and rhythm control in patients with recurrent persistent atrial fibrillation. N Engl J Med 2002;347:1834–1840.
14. Elhendy A, Gentile F, Khandheria BK, et al: Thromboembolic complications after electrical cardioversion in patients with atrial flutter. Am J Med 2001;111:433–438.
15. Ganz LI, Friedman PL: Supraventricular tachycardia. N Engl J Med 1995:332;162–173.
16. Jouven X, Zureik M, Desnos M, et al: Long-term outcome in asymptomatic men with exercise-induced premature ventricular depolarizations. N Engl J Med 2000;343:826–833.
17. Waldo AL, Camm AJ, de Ruyter H, et al: Effect of D-sotalol on mortality in patients with left ventricular dysfunction after recent and remote myocardial infarction. Lancet 1996;348:7–12.
18. Cairns JA, Connolly SJ, Roberts R, Gent M, for the Canadian Amiodarone Myocardial Infarction Arrhythmia Trial Investigators: Randomised trial of outcome after myocardial infarction in patients with frequent or repetitive ventricular premature depolarisations: CAMIAT. Lancet 1997;349:675–682.
19. Wyse DG, Talajic M, Hafley GE, et al: Antiarrhythmic drug therapy in the multicenter unsustained tachycardia trial (MUSTT): Drug testing and as-treated analysis. J Am Coll Cardiol 2001;38:344–351.
20. Buxton AE, Lee LL, Fisher FD, et al: A randomized study of the prevention of sudden death in patients with coronary artery disease. (MUSTT Investigators). N Engl J Med 1999;341:1882–1890.
21. Moss AJ, Hall WJ, Cannom DS, et al: Improved survival with an implanted defibrillator in patients with coronary disease at high risk for ventricular arrhythmia. N Engl J Med 1996;335:1933–1940.
22. The Antiarrhythmics vs. Implantable Defibrillators (AVID) Investigators: A comparison of antiarrhythmic drug therapy with implantable defibrillators in patients resuscitated after near-fatal ventricular arrhythmias. N Engl J Med 1997;337:1576–1583.
23. Weiss JP, Saynina O, McDonald KM, et al: Effectiveness and cost-effectiveness of implantable cardioverter defibrillators in the treatment of ventricular arrhythmias among Medicare beneficiaries. Am J Med 2002;112:519–527.
24. Brugada J, Brugada R, Antzelevitch C, et al: Long-term follow-up of individuals with the electrocardiographic pattern of right bundle-branch block and ST-segment elevation in precordial leads V_1 to V_3. Circulation 2002;105: 73–78.
25. ACC/AHA/NASPE 2002 Guideline Update for implantation of cardiac pacemakers and antiarrhythmia devices: Summary article. Circulation 2002;106:2145–2161.
26. Moss AJ, Zareba W, Hall J, et al: Prophylactic implantation of a defibrillator in patients with myocardial infarction and reduced ejection fraction. N Engl J Med 2002;346: 877–883.
27. Khan IA: Clinical and therapeutic aspects of congenital and acquired long QT syndrome. Am J Med 2002;112: 58–66.
28. Callans DJ: Management of the patient who has been resuscitated from sudden cardiac death. Circulation 2002;105:2704–2707.

CHAPTER 31

Recognition and Management of Patients with Bradyarrhythmias

Jacob M. Mishell and Nora Goldschlager

OFFICE EVALUATION OF PATIENTS WITH BRADYARRHYTHMIAS

Patients with bradycardia are frequently encountered in the ambulatory setting. The physician may identify a slow heart rate as part of an evaluation for specific symptoms. Bradycardias can also be diagnosed incidentally on a 12-lead electrocardiogram (ECG) or physical examination. In many patients, the bradycardia can have an adverse impact on prognosis, such as when patients have syncope from low cardiac output (see Chapter 10).[1, 2] Conversely, some patients (e.g., young athletes with high vagal tone) will have slow resting heart rates that are not detrimental to their health.

In the current climate of managed heath care, primary care providers are increasingly faced with the responsibility of evaluating patients with bradyarrhythmias based on 12-lead ECGs and other outpatient tests, such as ambulatory ECG monitoring, and then correlating patients' symptoms, if any, to the particular finding. Physicians must distinguish benign conditions that can be managed conservatively from those that require referral to a cardiologist for more specialized therapies, including permanent pacemaker implantation. The goal of this chapter is to serve as a resource for the noncardiologist who encounters patients with bradyarrhythmias.

Cardiac Conduction System

In normal sinus rhythm, the heart rate is set by the sinus (sometimes called sinoatrial) node located in the high right atrium at the junction of the superior vena cava (SVC). The sinus node is a cluster of cells that have the capability of spontaneously generating an electrical impulse (automaticity). The impulse depolarizes the atria and travels via intra-atrial conduction pathways to the atrioventricular (AV) node. The three areas of the AV node or junction—atrionodal, central compact, and nodal-His portions—merge without clear separation with the His bundle. The impulse is then conducted via the bundle of His to the right and left bundle branches that terminate in the Purkinje fiber network. (Fig. 31–1).

If the cells in the sinus node fail to depolarize, or if the sinus impulse fails to exit the sinus node to depolarize the atria, other sites in the heart have the ability to serve as back-up pacemakers. Cells in the atrionodal area have a relatively fast intrinsic depolarization rate (45 to 60 beats per minute) and are responsive to autonomic nervous system input. Cells in the nodal-His region have a slower intrinsic rate (about 40 beats per minute) and, because of sparse autonomic innervation, are generally unresponsive to neural influences. Either of these sites can originate a "junctional" rhythm with a characteristic rate, responsiveness to vagal and adrenergic tone, and associated clinical symptoms. The QRS complex duration cannot be relied upon to distinguish the origin of the rhythm because rhythms originating

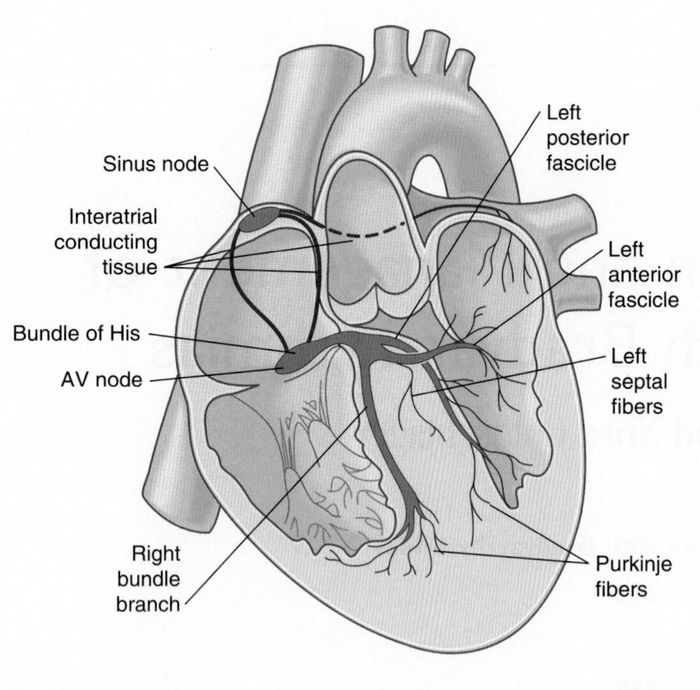

FIGURE 31–1. Schema of the AV conduction system. The sinoatrial node is located near the junction of the superior vena cava and the right atrium. Impulse formation that begins in the sinoatrial node spreads throughout the atria and to the AV node by means of interatrial conducting tissue. The atrial impulse is conducted through the AV node to the bundle of His. The major bundle branches, the left and right bundle branches, arise from the bundle of His; the left branch then divides into anterior and posterior fascicular radiations. The bundle branch fibers terminate in the Purkinje network that activates ventricular muscle.

proximal to the His bundle can have a wide QRS complex.

Symptoms and Their Underlying Pathophysiology

The clinical presentation of patients with bradycardia, due either to intrinsic abnormalities of impulse formation or to intrinsic conduction system disease, is determined by the presence of three conditions: the slow heart rate itself, the inability to increase the heart rate in response to an increase in metabolic need, and the inappropriately timed atrial and ventricular depolarization and contraction sequences (Box 31–1). Because cardiac output is the product of heart rate and stroke volume, absolute bradycardia can cause symptoms related to hypoperfusion despite normal ventricular function.

In addition to decreased cardiac output from a slow heart rate, other mechanisms may be at least as important, especially in those patients with underlying structural heart disease. For example, during periods of AV block, the atria and ventricles commonly depolarize and contract asynchronously. Right and left atrial pressures and volumes increase to variable extents, depending on the degree to which the AV valves are open or closed at the onset of ventricular systole. The resulting atrial stretch and stimulation of atrial natriuretic peptide secretion produce reflex systemic hypotension, which can cause symptoms of cerebral hypoperfusion. Additionally, the elevated left atrial pressure can lead to pulmonary vascular congestion and even frank pulmonary edema, which can be erroneously diagnosed as being due to left ventricular dysfunction. Individuals with noncompliant left ventricles, such as in the setting of left ventricular hypertrophy, may be dependent on properly-timed atrial systole.

The symptoms of bradycardia thus reflect varying degrees of cerebral hypoperfusion, low cardiac output

BOX 31–1

Clinical Presentation of Patients with Bradycardia

Symptoms due to cerebral hypoperfusion
- Presyncope and syncope
- Confusion
- Memory loss
- Bradycardia-dependent tachyarrhythmias (e.g., atrial fibrillation, polymorphic ventricular tachycardia)

Symptoms due to chronotropic incompetence
- Effort-related fatigue
- Weakness
- Dyspnea
- Hypotension

Symptoms due to AV dyssynchrony resulting from varying AV intervals or ventriculoatrial conduction
- Heart failure
- Hypotension
- AV valve regurgitation

AV, atrioventricular.

at rest or during exercise, and an impaired hemodynamic state. Syncope (see Chapter 10) is the classic symptom of cerebral hypoperfusion resulting from inadequate cardiac output due to slow heart rate. However, symptoms of presyncope such as dizziness, lightheadedness, weakness, and confusion reflect the same pathophysiology and warrant the same aggressive approach to diagnosis and management. Symptoms can be episodic or chronic and can change over time and with advancing age. Because patients often adapt their lifestyles to compensate for the impairment in heart rate, they may not volunteer significant symptoms unless they are directly questioned about their ability to perform specific activities. Patients may deny symptoms because they do not realize that they have curtailed activities to compensate for decreased stamina. Additionally, patients with cerebral hypoperfusion may not remember the details of clinical episodes and may therefore be limited in their ability to provide an accurate history. It should be noted that even seasoned clinicians have been surprised when their "asymptomatic" patients report how much better they feel after pacemaker insertion.

Chronotropic Incompetence

Some patients will complain of symptoms such as fatigue only with activity. In this circumstance, the physician must consider chronotropic incompetence, which is an impaired heart rate response to exercise. Patients with sinus node dysfunction or AV block, in which the escape focus is unresponsive to autonomic nervous system input (such as fascicular or ventricular escape foci), cannot increase their heart rates in response to increases in metabolic demand imposed by exertion. As a result, they are intolerant of effort and report symptoms of exercise-related breathlessness, weakness, and fatigue. The sometimes vague and episodic nature of the symptoms may confuse the clinician unless a high index of suspicion for this disorder is maintained. The presentation, which can be disabling, is often confused with other conditions such as ischemic heart disease, adverse medication reaction, hypothyroidism, or simply advanced age.

Bradycardia-Induced Ventricular Arrhythmias

Rarely, bradycardias can lead to a potentially lethal form of ventricular tachycardia known as pause-dependent or bradycardia-dependent ventricular tachycardia (VT). This form of VT is usually polymorphous and can be associated with a long QT interval. The precipitating event can be a nonconducted extrasystole, a postextrasystolic pause, or merely a slowing of the heart rate. Symptoms include palpitations, presyncope, or syncope. Whereas some patients can tolerate VT for a period of time, especially if the rate is less than 200 beats per minute, it is an unstable rhythm that can degenerate into ventricular fibrillation (see Chapter 30).

Approach to Patients with Bradyarrhythmias

The approach to treating patients with bradyarrhythmias is based on a careful evaluation including history taking, physical examination, and 12-lead ECG.[1] These steps form the basis for clinical decision making in terms of further testing, treatment, and referral. A detailed yet focused history and physical examination is essential to determine whether or not the patient has symptoms or signs that are attributable to the rhythm. Whereas the history and physical are the most useful tools to assess clinical impairment, the 12-lead ECG remains the most appropriate initial diagnostic test. The ECG provides useful information about the rate and rhythm, and can help establish the diagnosis. Unfortunately, since the ECG provides only a "snapshot" of the cardiac rhythm, the patient must be having the bradyarrhythmia while the test is performed for it to be diagnostic.

Further management depends on incorporating this information into a unified clinical picture. The major branch points in decision making hinge on whether or not the patient is symptomatic (Fig. 31–2). For example, patients with sinus node dysfunction will generally benefit from treatment only if symptoms are present; those without symptoms are best managed conservatively with routine follow-up. The practitioner's objective is to determine which patients may be followed clinically, which patients have symptoms that may be improved with specific treatments, and most importantly, which patients are at risk for significant morbidity and even mortality if not treated with a permanent cardiac pacing system.[1, 2]

Physical Examination

All patients with bradycardia require careful physical examination to document evidence of cardiac dysfunction as well as to identify underlying structural heart disease, if present.[1] Additionally, clues to the rhythm and presence or absence of AV synchrony may be present.

The examination includes a complete set of vital signs. In addition to the routine measurements obtained at rest, orthostatic blood pressure measurements represent a mild physiologic challenge for the cardiovascular system and can reveal more subtle degrees of impairment. For example, a patient's inability to raise his or her heart rate in response to the stress of rising from a seated position could be a subtle manifestation of chronotropic incompetence. In the setting of AV dyssynchrony, the systolic blood pressure and the intensity of the carotid upstroke may vary from beat to beat owing to changes in stroke volume. Whether the pulse is regular or irregular will also provide an important clue to the cause of the bradycardia.

The jugular venous pressure (JVP) can provide a good estimation of right atrial filling pressures. An elevated JVP may represent right-sided heart failure, which can be seen if cardiac output is low because of a bradyarrhythmia or if there is underlying structural heart

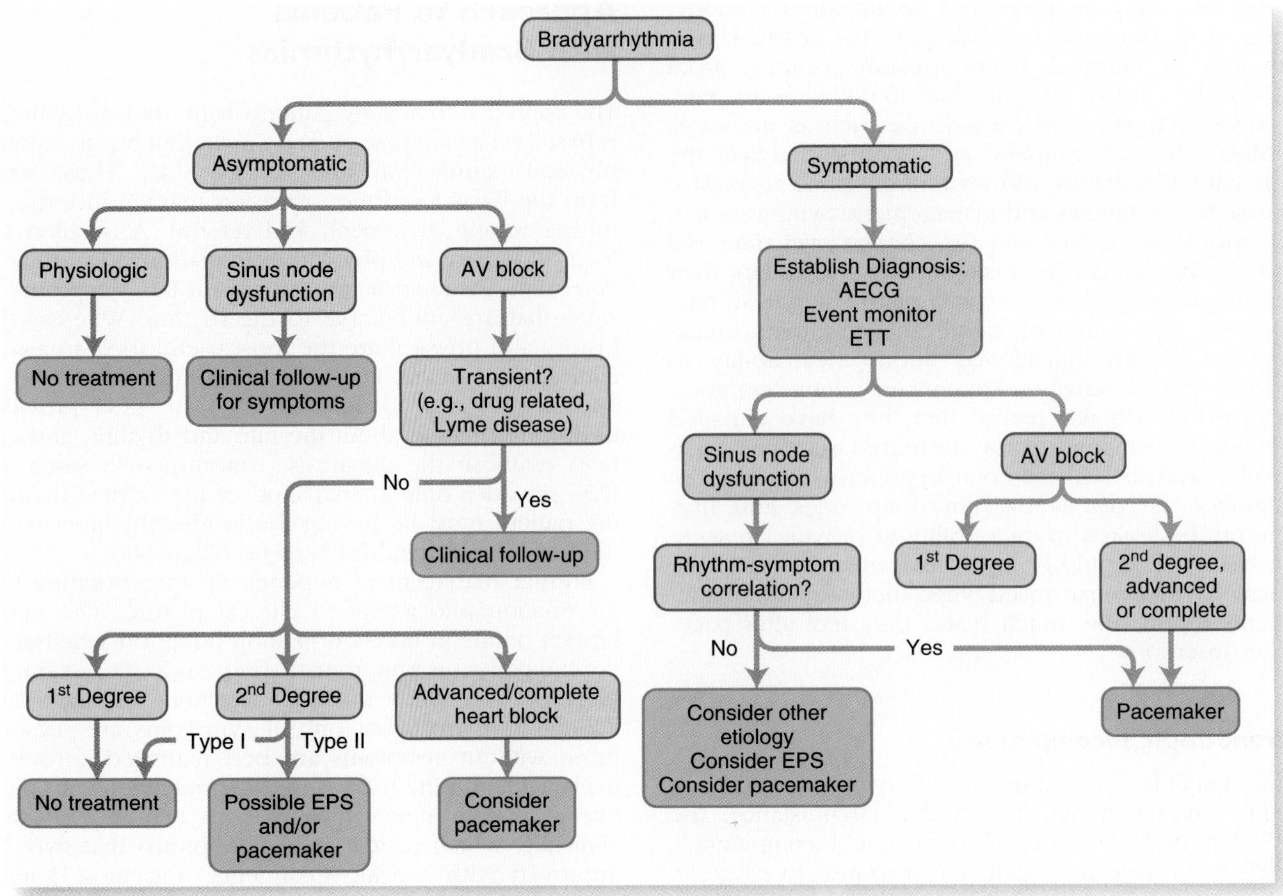

FIGURE 31–2. General approach to the patient with bradycardia. AECG, ambulatory electrocardiography; AV, atrioventricular; EPS, electrophysiologic study; ETT, exercise treadmill test.

disease, or both. Jugular venous waveform contours can provide clues to AV dyssynchrony (see Chapter 3). In patients with AV dissociation or 1:1 retrograde ventriculoatrial conduction, examination of the jugular venous pulse contour reveals cannon A-waves because of right atrial contraction against a closed tricuspid valve. Cannon A-waves should not be confused with an elevated JVP.

Examination of the precordium should focus on signs of concomitant structural heart disease. For example, the presence of an S_4 gallop and a laterally displaced point of maximal impulse raises the likelihood of left ventricular hypertrophy, diastolic dysfunction, and relative dependence on AV synchrony. Other signs of heart failure, such as rales or peripheral edema, may be present. The physical examination also serves to identify systemic disorders that may affect the cardiac conduction system; for example, hypothyroidism may be suggested by the finding of periorbital edema.

12-Lead ECG

The 12-lead ECG is a fundamental tool that can provide identification of not only the cardiac rhythm, but also clues to the existence of cardiac conditions that need to be recognized. Examples include disorders of the AV and intraventricular (IV) conduction system (such as first-degree AV block and bundle branch block), evidence of atrial abnormalities (suggesting atrial hypertrophy or intra-atrial conduction delay), and ventricular hypertrophy. Conduction system disease is often diffuse, with up to one third of patients with sinus node dysfunction having AV and IV conduction disease, and a similar percentage of patients with AV block having sinus node dysfunction. Patients with ventricular hypertrophy may be especially reliant on atrial contraction to provide optimal filling of a relatively noncompliant ventricle and to preserve an adequate stroke volume. Bradycardia can be a presenting sign of myocardial ischemia or infarction, which would require immediate transfer to an emergency department. Toxic or therapeutic effects of medications, such as beta-blockers, calcium channel blockers, or digoxin, may present as sinus node dysfunction or as AV block.

Further Testing

Ambulatory ECG Monitoring. Because the 12-lead ECG is often not sufficient to make a definitive diagnosis of episodic rhythm disturbances, ambulatory ECG (Holter) monitoring is commonly the next test to document rhythm abnormalities in patients with symptoms suggesting bradycardia. These devices employ an "alarm" button that can be activated by the patient on perception of symptoms; monitors can be programmed to retain in memory the cardiac rhythm for a specific number of seconds before and after the alarm is activated by the patient. Wristwatch monitors are less cumbersome than Holtor monitors and are preferred by many patients.

Because the patient must be able to trigger the alarm for precise correlation between the heart rhythm and symptoms, ambulatory ECG devices are best utilized in patients who have daily symptoms but who do not have frank syncope or severe presyncopal symptoms. Precise rhythm-symptom correlation is, however, difficult to obtain, in part because patients may focus on staying conscious and avoiding personal injury rather than on activating the monitor. In patients who have recurrent symptoms of cerebral hypoperfusion but do not develop symptoms during ambulatory monitoring, further diagnostic evaluation, such as event monitoring and exercise testing are indicated (see Fig. 31–2), especially if suggestive bradyarrhythmias were noted on continuous ambulatory monitoring.

Event Monitoring. In contrast to the ambulatory ECG recording device, which must be worn continuously by the patient, the event recorder is carried by the patient for weeks to months and placed on the skin and turned on only when symptoms are occurring. The device contains electrodes on its surface to record the rhythm from the skin onto a small tape. The taped rhythm can be transmitted over telephone lines to a monitoring center for immediate interpretation or can be sent in its entirety to the center for printing and interpretation. The event monitor is extremely useful in patients with inconsistent and episodic symptoms but without frank syncope or severe presyncope, because participation by the patient in the recording of the rhythm is necessary.

In both ambulatory ECG monitoring and event recording, documentation of a normal rhythm and rate during symptoms is helpful in excluding an arrhythmia as the etiology. Likewise, the correlation of symptoms with a rhythm disturbance is diagnostic. In the absence of symptoms, the physician must decide whether to proceed to additional testing.

Treadmill Testing. Formal exercise testing is necessary to evaluate the heart rate response to effort in patients suspected of having chronotropic incompetence. The importance of recognizing the condition of chronotropic incompetence has increased in recent years, in part due to the development of rate-adaptive cardiac pacemakers that, through sensor technology, can increase and decrease the pacing rate in response to activities of daily living. Special exercise protocols are often used by arrhythmia specialists to determine whether the heart rate is appropriate for various activities as well as for maximal exercise capacity.

Electrophysiologic Testing. For the majority of patients with clinically significant bradyarrhythmias, a diagnosis can be made without the use of invasive electrophysiologic (EP) testing. EP studies may be helpful in selected patients when there is a very high clinical suspicion of sinus node or AV node dysfunction that has not been documented by other means. EP studies are insensitive but highly specific for diagnosing AV node dysfunction. Situations in which EP testing can be useful include syncope in the setting of sinus bradycardia (see Chapter 10), first-degree AV block with concomitant bundle branch block, or bifascicular block. The details of the testing strategies used during EP tests for bradyarrhythmias are complex and outside the scope of this chapter, but the general principle is that the refractory times and conduction velocities are measured at specific sites of the cardiac conduction system.

Role of the Primary Care Physician

Depending upon the particular community in which a physician practices, some or all of the aforementioned noninvasive tests for bradycardia may be available; if not, referral to a specialist is warranted for expeditious evaluation of the patient. The role of the primary care physician is crucial, however, in suspecting the diagnosis of bradycardia in symptomatic patients and in planning the diagnostic approach. Similarly, the primary care physician should be able to recognize those bradycardias that are benign and without prognostic impact, thus obviating the need for expensive and unnecessary diagnostic tests.

Since most patients with symptomatic bradycardia and some with asymptomatic bradycardia require cardiac pacing, referral to a pacemaker specialist is often necessary. Pacing is also indicated when the bradycardia is due to the use of medications that must be continued to treat other medical illnesses.

SPECIFIC BRADYARRHYTHMIAS

Sinus Node

Sinus Bradycardia

Bradycardia in adults is defined by convention as a heart rate lower than 60 beats per minute; however slow heart rates are frequently found in normal individuals. Normal resting heart rates range from 46 to 93 beats per minute for men and 51 to 95 beats per minute for women. Healthy adults can have heart rates as low as 35 to 40 beats per minute, especially during sleep when vagal tone is high.

Sinus bradycardia is diagnosed when the P-waves have a normal morphology and a constant PR interval less than 200 milliseconds. Variation of the rate, or sinus arrhythmia, may be present at the same time. The mechanism is usually increased vagal or decreased sympathetic tone. Sinus bradycardia, sometimes resulting in atrial escape rhythms, is frequently observed in young healthy adults, especially athletes, and junctional escape rhythms are common (Fig. 31–3). Many conditions and medications can cause sinus bradycardia (Box 31–2); it is a common finding in the elderly.

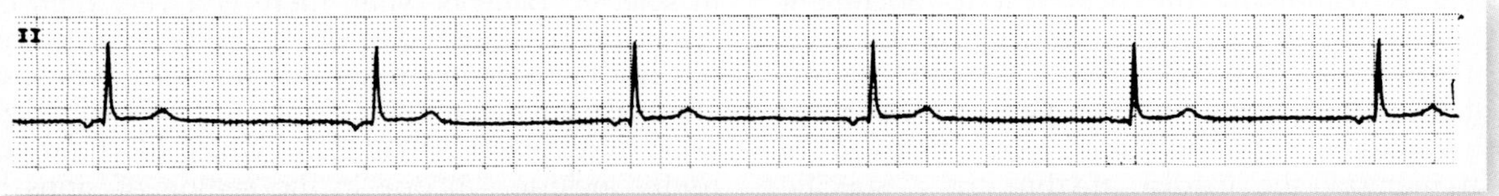

FIGURE 31–3. Lead II rhythm strip recorded in a 32-year-old, well conditioned, healthy man during a routine physical examination. The inverted P-waves in this lead indicate a junctional or low atrial focus of origin (the next to last P-wave is possibly of sinus origin). This rhythm is not in and of itself abnormal, because it may be an escape rhythm due to sinus bradycardia as is commonly seen in conditioned individuals. Neither evaluation nor treatment of the rhythm is required in cases such as this. Exercise testing, with its associated vagolysis and enhancement of sympathetic tone, would be expected to demonstrate an increase in the sinus rate.

Sinus Arrhythmia

Sinus arrhythmia refers to variability in the sinus rate. Respiratory sinus arrhythmia is a common condition in which the sinus rate increases with inspiration and decreases with expiration. It is commonly seen in young healthy adults. Non-respiratory sinus arrhythmia, in which the phasic changes in sinus rate are not due to respiration, is more commonly seen in older individuals who have underlying heart disease, but its presence in an asymptomatic individual should not prompt a cardiac evaluation. Sinus arrhythmias are almost always benign and rarely require treatment. Documentation of their existence is usually all that is required.

BOX 31–2

Causes of Bradycardia

- Idiopathic degenerative processes
- Increased intracranial pressure (e.g., meningitis, intracranial tumors)
- Hypoxia
- Hypothermia
- Hypothyroidism
- Infectious diseases
  - Chagas' disease
  - Lyme disease
  - Endocarditis
- Infiltrative processes
  - Hemochromatosis
  - Sarcoidosis
  - Amyloidosis
  - Neoplasm
- Collagen vascular diseases
- Medications
  - Beta-blockers (including ophthalmic preparations)
  - Calcium channel blockers (verapamil, diltiazem)
  - Digoxin
  - Class I antiarrhythmic agents (e.g., propafenone)
  - Class III antiarrhythmic agents (e.g., amiodarone, sotalol)
  - Clonidine
  - Lithium carbonate
- Mycardial ischemia or infarction
- Increased vagal tone (e.g., vomiting, vasovagal syncope with bradycardia)
- Iatrogentic (e.g., radiofrequency AV nodal ablation; post valve replacement, especially aortic valve)
- Electrolyte disturbances (e.g., hypokalemia, hyperkalemia)

Sinus Node Dysfunction

Sinus node dysfunction is synonymous with sick sinus syndrome (Fig. 31–4). In contrast to the benign conditions described earlier, sinus dysfunction is present when there is profound bradycardia, pauses in sinus rhythm (sinus arrest), or sinoatrial block. These rhythms can be found alone or in combination. Whereas many conditions are associated with sinus node dysfunction, it is usually due to a degenerative process involving the sinus node. The degenerative process and associated fibrosis often involve the AV node and intraventricular conduction system as well as the sinus node. As many as 25% to 30% of patients with sinus node dysfunction have evidence of AV block and bundle branch block.

When sinus node dysfunction is diagnosed, potentially reversible or treatable causes should be pursued (see Box 31–2). Sinus node dysfunction can be transient when it is medication-related and may be completely reversible when the offending agent is withdrawn. Conversely, when patients require an implicated medication, such as beta-blockers in the setting of coronary artery disease, permanent cardiac pacing is indicated so that the medication can be continued. It is important to distinguish vagally mediated sinus bradycardia from sinus node dysfunction because the former generally is a benign condition.

Sinus Pause

Sinus pause or sinus arrest is a cessation of sinus node automaticity. When there is no sinus node discharge, the atria are not depolarized and, consequently, no P-waves are seen on the ECG (Fig. 31–5). Sinus pauses are not a multiple of a basic PP interval and they vary without any discernible pattern from pause to pause. P-waves are not seen on the ECG until the sinus node regains function or until a junctional or ventricular

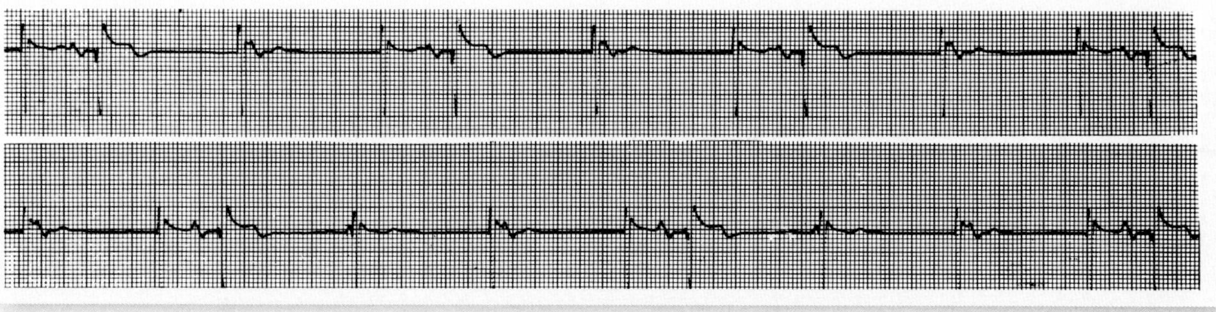

FIGURE 31–4. This rhythm strip was recorded in a 48-year-old, healthy, active man who complained of breathlessness during moderately strenuous exercise. There was no evidence of structural heart disease on physical examination, and an echocardiogram was normal. The atrial rhythm is marked sinus bradycardia at a rate of about 43 beats per minute. The narrow QRS rhythm is mostly regular at a rate of 50 beats per minute, suggesting a junctional origin. Occasionally, P-waves are associated with earlier than expected QRS complexes; these beats represent capture beats. The rhythm is thus sinus bradycardia, atrioventricular (AV) dissociation with intermittent capture, and junctional escape rhythm. The long PR interval of captured beats may not indicate AV nodal disease, because it may represent concealed retrograde conduction of the junctional impulse into the AV node, delaying transmission of the subsequent sinus depolarization. Although the sinus bradycardia was atropine-sensitive, the patient declined chronic anticholinergic therapy and opted for a dual-chamber rate-adaptive pacemaker, which allowed both appropriate rate response to physical activity and restoration of AV synchrony. The patient has remained asymptomatic.

pacemaker intervenes and depolarizes the atria as well as the ventricles. Symptoms are dependent on the rate of these "back-up" pacemakers, which are slower than the sinus node rate and may be unstable.

Treatment of sinus pauses or arrest depends both on the degree of symptoms as well as the etiology (as it does for all sinus node dysfunction). Some normal individuals without structural heart disease experience marked sinus bradycardia and pauses under conditions of high vagal tone (Fig. 31–6). In some subjects, a trigger such as vomiting can be identified. In general, vagally mediated sinus rhythm disturbances are benign. If this condition is suspected in the setting of syncope or severe presyncope, however, referral to a cardiologist is indicated (Boxes 31–3 and 31–4).

Sinoatrial Exit Block

In sinoatrial exit block, the sinus node has normal automaticity and impulse formation. However, the impulse either is delayed in its conduction to the atria or fails to depolarize the atria because it fails to exit the node. Sinoatrial block may take the form of progressive delay in transmission of the sinus-generated impulse through the sinoatrial node to the atrium, ultimately resulting in a nonconducted sinus impulse and absence of a P-wave (Wenckebach, or type I second-degree sinoatrial exit block) or abrupt failure of transmission of the sinus impulse to the atrium (type II second-degree sinoatrial exit block). In type I second-degree sinoatrial exit block, the PP intervals become progressively shorter

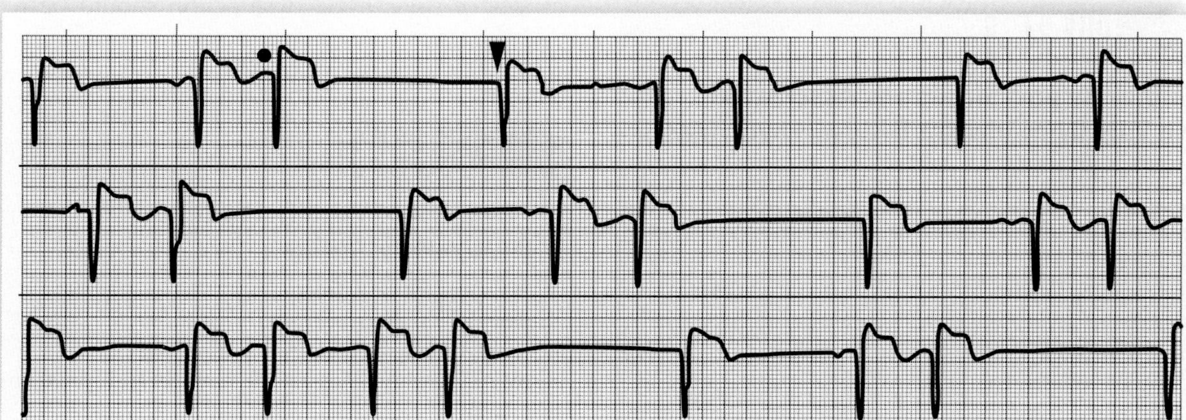

FIGURE 31–5. V_1 rhythm strip illustrating atrial bradycardia, junctional premature complexes *(closed circle),* and pauses in atrial rhythm of variable lengths in a patient with recurrent syncope. Many pauses in rhythm are terminated by junctional escape complexes *(arrow).* The P-waves are of variable morphology, and the PR intervals vary with the specific P-wave morphology. This rhythm strip illustrates sinus node dysfunction.

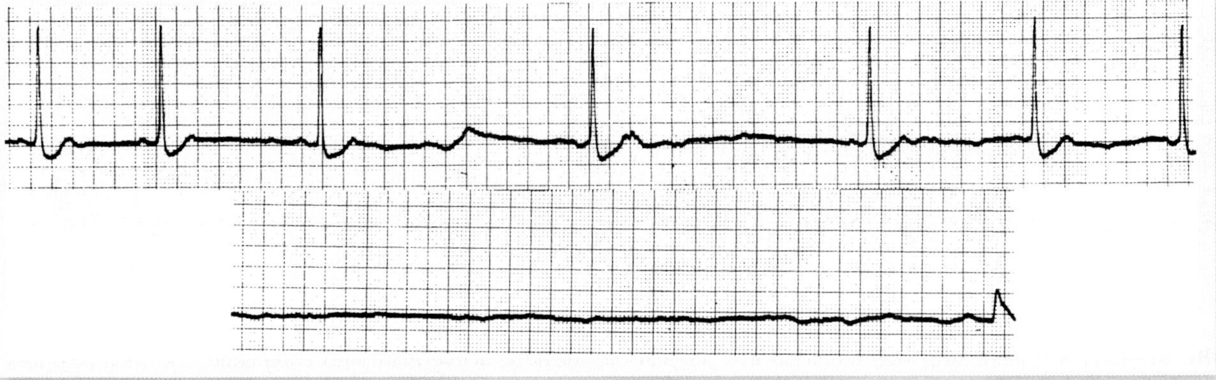

FIGURE 31–6. Vagal bradycardia and asystole in an intubated patient during suctioning. Although long pauses in rhythm as seen here are not uncommon in the hospital setting (where they require no treatment), they can occur in healthy individuals with neurocardiogenic syncopal syndromes and may be reproduced during head-up tilt-table testing.

until a P-wave fails to occur. In type II second-degree sinoatrial exit block, abrupt failure of impulse conduction to the atria can occur at 2:1, 3:1, or higher intervals. Distinguishing fixed high-grade sinoatrial exit block from sinus bradycardia on a 12-lead ECG may not be possible and is probably clinically unimportant; management will depend on the etiology and symptoms rather than on the precise electrophysiologic mechanism.

Bradycardia-Tachycardia Syndrome

Bradycardia-tachycardia syndrome is characterized by episodes of both bradycardia and supraventricular tachyarrhythmia (Fig. 31–7). Bradycardia-tachycardia syndrome is caused by diffuse disease of the cardiac conduction system but is not necessarily associated with structural heart disease. The bradycardia is due to sinus node dysfunction with associated junctional or ventricular escape rhythms. The supraventricular tachycardias may be atrial tachycardia, atrial flutter, atrial fibrillation, or AV nodal reentrant tachycardia. Importantly, individual patients may suffer from more than one type of supraventricular tachyarrhythmia. Medical therapy is difficult because drugs that may help suppress the tachyarrhythmias commonly exacerbate the bradycardia and hasten the need for a permanent pacemaker. If the tachyarrhythmia is paroxysmal atrial fibrillation, anticoagulation will be required to reduce the risk of thromboembolism (see Chapter 30), unless antiarrhythmic agents can suppress the rhythm (either without precipitating symptomatic bradycardia or with a pacemaker to protect the patient against the bradycardia).

Office Management of Sinus Node Bradycardias

The management of sinus bradycardias includes a careful evaluation for the presence or absence of symptoms as well as concomitant cardiac disease. Myocardial ischemia or infarction should always be considered if there is evidence in the history or ECG to suggest this diagnosis. The list of potentially reversible or treatable causes of sinus node dysfunction should be reviewed

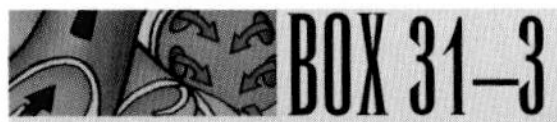

BOX 31–3

Conditions and Situations Associated with Vagally-Mediated Bradyarrhythmias

Sleep
Urination
Defecation
Swallowing
Valsalva maneuver
Vomiting
Tracheal intubation
Endoscopic procedures
Suctioning
Elevated intracranial pressure
Extreme hypertension
Isotonic exercise
Neurally-mediated syncope syndromes

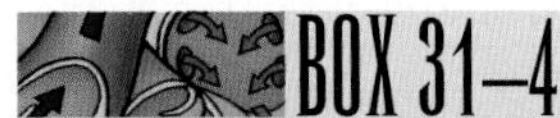

BOX 31–4

Features of Vagally-Mediated Bradyarrhythmias

Transient or situational
Slowing of sinus rate
Irregular sinus rhythm
AV block with changing PR intervals and irregular sinus rates
Atypical type I or II 2° AV block sequences, often with variable PP intervals
Variable rates of escape foci
Responds to atropine or an increase in sympathetic tone

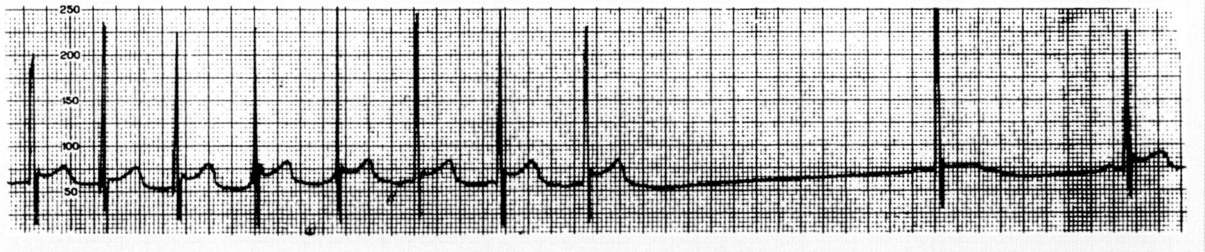

FIGURE 31–7. This rhythm strip illustrates the bradycardia-tachycardia syndrome. An accelerated junctional tachycardia at a rate of 81 beats per minute in the beginning of the strip abruptly terminates and is followed by a pause of 3.8 seconds. The subsequent rhythm is sinus bradycardia at a rate of 36 beats per minute. Patients with this syndrome frequently experience palpitations during the tachycardias and presyncopal symptoms during the bradycardias. Treatment is permanent cardiac pacing to protect against bradycardia and antiarrhythmic drugs to suppress the tachycardia.

(see Box 31–2). For example, hypothyroidism should be diagnosed and treated appropriately. Special attention should be paid to the medications the patient is receiving. Withdrawal of the offending agent can be curative. If the medications are required to treat an underlying medical condition and no other reversible cause can be identified, then cardiac pacing will be required to provide rate support.

If the history suggests that the sinus bradycardia may be vagally mediated, evaluation can be performed in the office setting if the bradycardia is present. Vagally mediated sinus bradycardias respond to intravenous atropine. The expected normal heart rate response to 2 to 3 mg of intravenous atropine is an increase in heart rate of about 15% to rates of 85 to 90 beats per minute. Walking briskly around the office or running in place also produces vagolysis and will increase the sinus rate in vagally mediated sinus bradycardias. Resolution of bradycardia with administration of atropine is suggestive but not diagnostic of a vagally mediated bradycardia; some patients with sinus node dysfunction will also demonstrate an increase in heart rate.

In general, vagally mediated bradyarrhythmias are benign and require no specific therapy. However, some patients experience highly symptomatic, vagally mediated bradycardic episodes, especially if there is also a significant vasodepressor response resulting in cerebral hypoperfusion (the neurocardiogenic syncope syndromes; see Chapter 10). These individuals often require referral to a cardiologist to confirm the diagnosis and to guide therapy.

Atrioventricular Block

Pathophysiology and Natural History

Like sinus node dysfunction, AV nodal-His block is frequently due to sclerodegenerative processes, but it can also be caused by myocardial infarction, infection, or trauma (see Box 31–2). AV block can be acquired or congenital. Patients with congenital AV block usually have escape pacemakers arising from within the AV node or His bundle. In contrast, only about 25% of patients with acquired AV block have escape pacemakers arising from within the AV node; rhythms originate within the His bundle in about 15% to 20% of patients and distal to the His bundle in about 70% of patients (Fig. 31–8).

The natural history of patients with AV block depends on the underlying cardiac condition, the site of the block, and the consequent rhythm disturbances. First-degree AV block generally has a good prognosis. Both second-degree (types I and II) and third-degree AV block can be associated with adverse outcomes, including death, unless they are vagally mediated or due to a reversible cause.

Diagnosis

His bundle electrography provides important information regarding normal and abnormal AV conduction and can diagnose the site of AV conduction delay. The technique involves positioning of a multipolar electrode catheter across the tricuspid valve in proximity to the AV node and His bundle to record electrical activity as it passes through the level of the low right atrium (A), His bundle (H), and proximal right bundle branch; ventricular activity (V) is also recorded. Normally, the conduction time through the AV node is 90 to 150 msec, and the conduction time through the His-Purkinje system is 22 to 55 msec. In patients with a prolonged PR interval on the 12-lead ECG, a long AH interval signifies conduction delay within the AV node, and a long HV time represents conduction delay within the His bundle or bundle branches.

First-Degree AV Block

First-degree AV block is defined as a PR interval greater than 0.20 seconds (Fig. 31–9). By definition, AV conduction is delayed, but, in contrast to second- and third-degree block, all atrial impulses are conducted to the ventricles. The components of the PR interval are intra-atrial conduction (10 to 50 msec), AV nodal conduction (90 to 150 msec), and intra-His and His-Purkinje conduction (25 to 55 msec). The conduction delay in first-degree AV block can thus represent prolonged

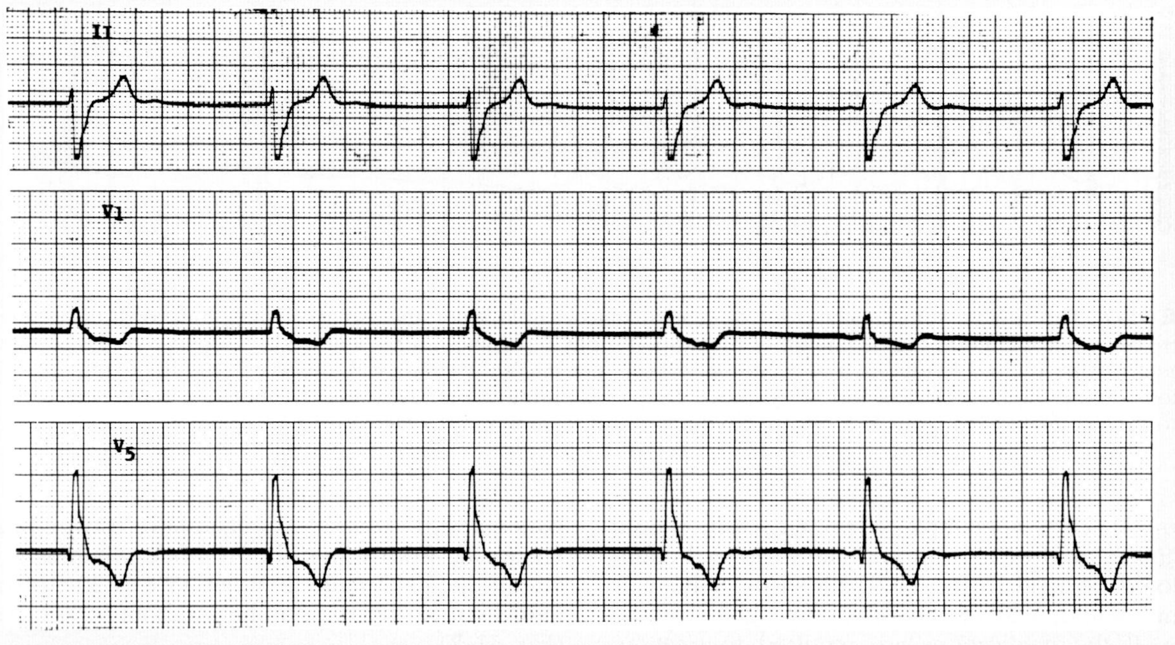

FIGURE 31–8. Simultaneously recorded leads II, V_1, and V_5 in a 42-year-old patient presenting with syncope. The QRS rhythm shows a pattern of left and superior axis deviation and right intraventricular conduction delay, suggesting a fascicular origin; the rate is about 39 beats per minute. Deformities in the early portions of the T-waves can be seen to occur at relatively constant intervals, possibly representing retrogradely (ventriculoatrial) conducted P-waves (an exception is the next to the last complex). Patients with VA conduction can have severe symptoms of cerebral hypoperfusion and exercise intolerance due both to reflex hypotension caused by the atrial stretch-mediated baroreceptor stimulation and to the inability of this cardiac pacemaker (originating in ventricular tissue) to increase its firing rate in response to metabolic need.

interatrial, intra-AV nodal, or His-Purkinje conduction. Although His bundle recordings can clarify the site of the conduction delay, such testing is rarely indicated when first-degree AV block is the only abnormality.

Second-Degree AV Block

In second-degree AV block, some, but not all of the atrial impulses, are conducted to the ventricles. Second-degree AV block is further categorized as being type I or type II.

Type I Second-Degree AV Block. Type I second-degree AV block (Wenckebach AV block) is characterized by progressive delay of conduction of the atrial impulse to the ventricles because of increasing AV nodal refractoriness. Eventually, an atrial impulse is not conducted. The AV conduction ratio in type I second-degree AV block can be 2:1, 4:3, 8:7 and so on (Fig. 31–10). Because type I second-degree AV block usually occurs within the AV node, the PR interval of the first conducted P-wave of the Wenckebach period is often prolonged. Since the conduction disturbance does not involve the bundle branches, the QRS complexes are narrow and have normal morphology, unless concomitant bundle branch disease is present (Fig. 31–11). In a classic Wenckebach period, the PR interval progressively lengthens and the RR intervals progressively shorten.

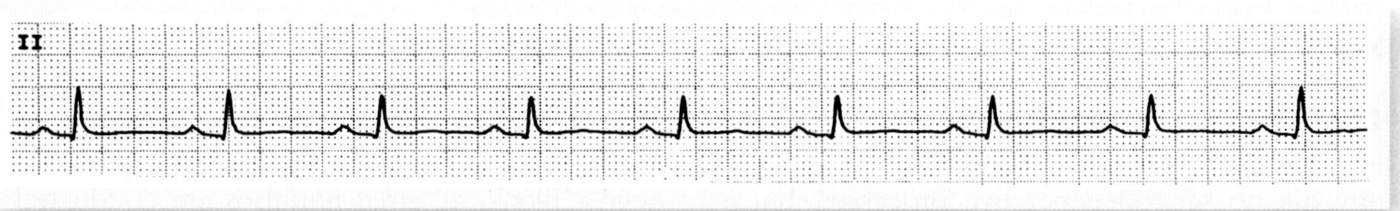

FIGURE 31–9. Lead II rhythm strip demonstrating first-degree AV block (PR interval > 0.20 sec). The PR interval is prolonged to about 0.25 seconds. The PR interval contains within it interatrial conduction, AV nodal conduction, and His-Purkinje conduction; the site of conduction delay in first-degree AV block is usually the AV node, especially if the QRS complexes are narrow and appear normal.

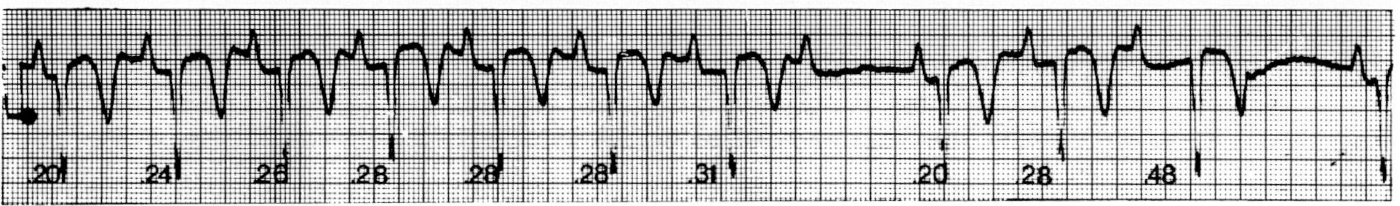

FIGURE 31–10. Type I second-degree AV block (Wenckebach) is illustrated in this rhythm strip by the increasing PR intervals (designated by the numbers) before failure of conduction of a P-wave. The sinus rate is constant at about 70 beats per minute. The first period has an 8:7 AV conduction ratio. Long AV conduction ratios are often atypical, as in this example, in which the three PR intervals before the last PR interval do not progressively increase. (Other atypical features can include failure of RR intervals to shorten before the nonconducted P-wave). The second period has a 4:3 AV conduction ratio; the nonconducted P-wave deforms the last T-wave of the period. This shorter period is typical of type I second-degree AV block. The usual site of conduction delay in type I second-degree AV block is the AV node, especially when the QRS complexes are narrow and appear normal.

Type II Second-Degree AV Block. In type II second-degree AV block, there is intermittent failure of conduction of the atrial impulse to the ventricles without prior evidence of prolongation of the AV conduction time (Fig. 31–12). In contrast to type I second-degree AV block, in which the conduction delay is in the AV node, the conduction delay in type II second-degree AV block occurs in the His bundle, or, more commonly, distal to the His bundle in the bundle branches. If the block is within the His bundle, the QRS complexes are usually narrow and appear to be normal or only mildly aberrant. If the block is distal to the His bundle, the QRS complexes will have a bundle-branch block pattern. In contrast to type I second-degree AV block, the PR interval of the conducted P-waves is essentially constant and often normal. The failure of AV conduction can be abrupt and unpredictable without a measurable increase in AV conduction delay. Special attention should be paid to patients with type II second-degree AV block because conduction can deteriorate without warning to symptomatic advanced AV block.

2:1 AV Block. A 2:1 AV conduction ratio may represent either type I or type II second-degree AV block. Because two consecutive PR intervals are not recorded, the presence or absence of progressive PR interval prolongation cannot be ascertained, and the differential

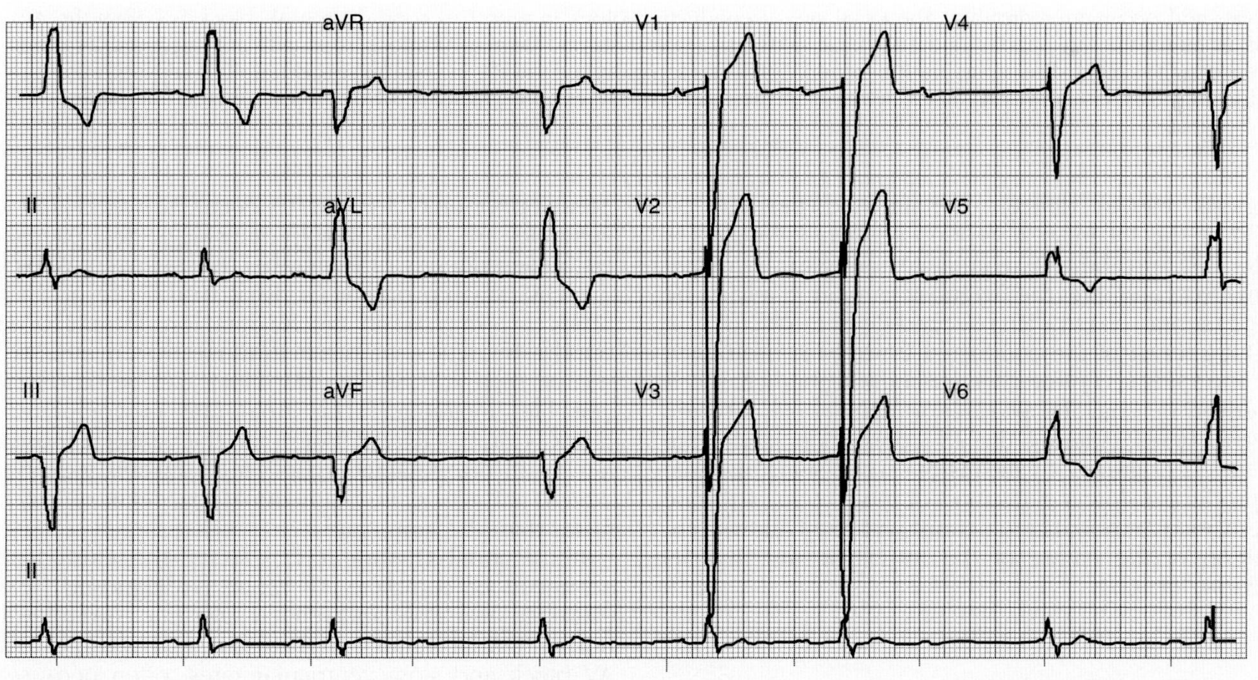

FIGURE 31–11. This 12-lead ECG was recorded in an asymptomatic patient. It illustrates sinus rhythm, a left bundle branch block pattern, and type I second-degree (Wenckebach) AV block. The Wenckebach periods are terminated by junctional escape complexes. The AV block may be occurring in either the AV node or in the right bundle branch; electrophysiologic study may be required to localize the precise site of block. Because of the possibility of trifascicular conduction system disease, permanent cardiac pacing is warranted, even in asymptomatic patients.

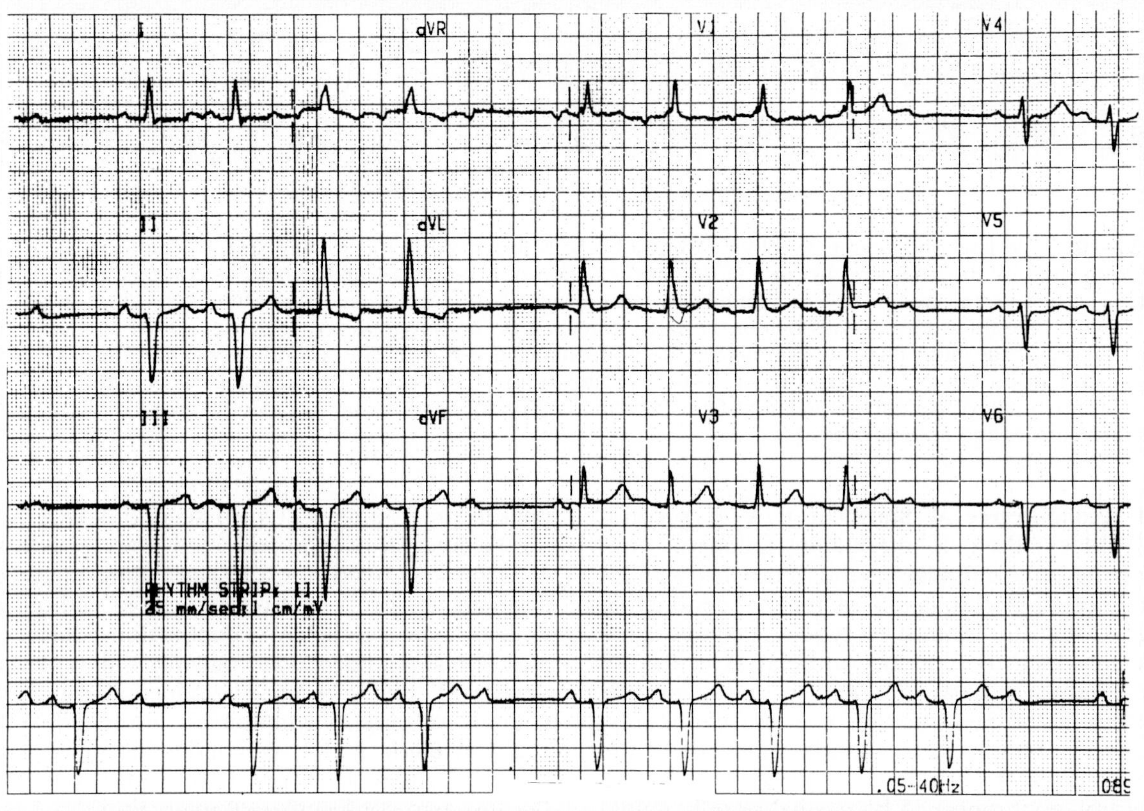

FIGURE 31–12. Type II second-degree AV block is illustrated in this 12-lead ECG and accompanying lead II rhythm strip. The sinus rate is constant at about 76 beats per minute. The PR intervals of conducted impulses are also constant. Concomitant bifascicular block is present. Nonconducted P-waves are not preceded by progressive lengthening of the PR intervals and occur unpredictably. The usual site of conduction block in type II second-degree AV block is below the AV node, in either the His bundle or the Purkinje network. Type II second-degree AV block is usually accompanied by other evidence of fascicular disease, as in this example. The prolongation of the PR interval in this example could represent conduction delay either within the AV node or in the fascicular system; the presence of AV block suggests the latter.

diagnosis may be difficult. Certain guidelines can be useful: if the PR interval of the conducted P-waves is prolonged and the QRS complexes are narrow and of normal morphology, the diagnosis is more likely to be type I (supra- or intra-His) second-degree AV block. If the PR interval of the conducted P-waves is prolonged and the QRS complexes have a bundle branch block pattern, it may not be possible to distinguish between the two types. Altering the AV conduction ratio from 2:1 to 3:2 or greater by means of carotid sinus massage (to produce a slower sinus rate) or intravenous atropine (to enhance AV nodal conduction) will often allow identification of the nature of the AV block and thus its probable location.

Advanced and Complete AV Block

In high-grade AV block, the AV conduction ratio is 3:1 or greater. Multiple levels of block may exist, causing irregularity in the PR intervals and ventricular rate (Fig. 31–13). When complete AV block occurs, no atrial impulses are conducted to the ventricles, despite temporal opportunity for this to occur; the atria and the ventricles are depolarized by their respective pacemakers, independently of each other. In advanced AV block, the QRS rhythm originates distal to the site of the AV block and may be in the AV junction, bundle of His, bundle branches, or distal Purkinje system and is an escape rhythm. Complete AV block can be paroxysmal and life-threatening. The atrial rate in complete AV block is almost always faster than the ventricular escape rate, with the notable exception of digitalis toxicity, in which an accelerated junctional pacemaker may be faster than the sinus rate.

If the atrial rhythm is not sinus, the existence of advanced or complete AV block is diagnosed by the presence of a slow and regular QRS rate. Atrial fibrillation and atrial flutter may be associated with advanced AV block and slow ventricular rates, often because of medications that are intentionally used to slow AV conduction. The rate of the ventricular rhythm, as well as the QRS morphology, will depend on the site of origin of the rhythm. In this setting, a regular ventricular rhythm will not be the result of conduction of the irregular atrial rhythm but rather will be caused by an inde-

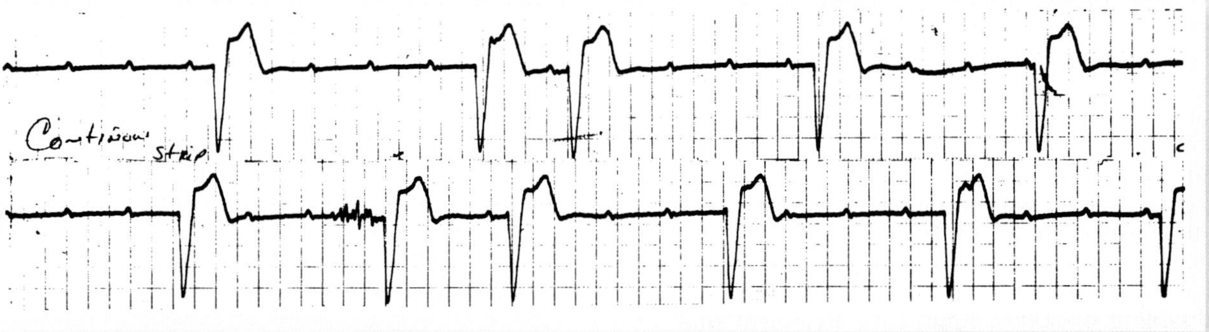

FIGURE 31–13. This continuously recorded V_1 rhythm strip was obtained in a 74-year-old man being treated with beta-blockers, calcium channel blockers, and long-acting nitrates. He presented to the emergency department with two days of dizziness and falling. The atrial rhythm is sinus, and high-degree AV block is present, with ventricular rates as low as 30 beats per minute. The QRS complexes have a left bundle branch block pattern, suggesting the possibility of advanced conduction system disease. Despite the absence of sinus bradycardia, this rhythm is assumed to be due to or exacerbated by the medications that the patient is taking, and they should be discontinued. If the AV block does not resolve after discontinuing these AV nodal blocking agents, the rhythm must be considered to be caused by intrinsic conduction system disease, which will require permanent cardiac pacing. Should the medications be necessary to treat the patient's underlying medical problems, then pacemaker implantation will be required. In this example, temporary pacing may well be required as a bridge to definitive therapy.

pendent pacemaker originating below the level of the conduction block.

Vagotonic Block. In vagotonic block, a high degree of vagal tone, such as occurs in conditioned athletes or with reduced sympathetic tone during sleep, may be associated with marked slowing of the sinus rate, pauses in rhythm, variable degrees of AV conduction delay manifested by PR interval prolongation (which is often irregular), and failure to conduct P-waves (resembling type I or type II second-degree AV block; see Box 31–4). It is crucial to recognize vagotonic block, because it usually occurs in normal individuals but can also occur in patients with inferior or right ventricular myocardial infarction or other conditions in which increased vagal tone is present (see Box 31–3). Vagally mediated bradycardia can add to the effects of certain medications, such as beta-adrenergic blocking agents, some anti-hypertensive agents, and digitalis. It can also be seen during swallowing (deglutition bradycardia), coughing (tussive bradycardia), yawning, and even assumption of an upright posture ("postural heart block"). In the critical care setting, vagally mediated bradycardia (including AV block) can occur during endotracheal suctioning or esophagogastric intubation and in patients with elevated intracranial pressure (see Fig. 31–6).

Office Management of Atrioventricular Block

Asymptomatic AV Block

Occasionally, AV block with slow ventricular rates is discovered incidentally on a routine ECG recording. As with atrial bradycardias, it is most important to obtain a thorough history, seeking evidence of symptoms of bradycardia, which can be vague, subtle, and nonspecific. If the patient is truly asymptomatic and the AV block is supra-His in location (as evidenced by narrow QRS complexes with normal morphology), frequent, careful observation may be all that is required. If the AV block is potentially infra-His (i.e., type I or II second-degree AV block in the presence of bundle branch disease), referral for EP study and possible "prophylactic" pacemaker implantation is indicated and may improve prognosis in selected patients. Many patients who have bradycardia but are unable to identify specific symptoms feel better after permanent pacemaker implantation, suggesting that they have adapted their lifestyle and expectations to match a diminished ability to raise cardiac output.

Increased Vagal Tone

High vagal tone can cause or contribute to both atrial and ventricular bradycardia even in the absence of withdrawal of sympathetic tone. Vagally mediated bradycardias are usually transient and not accompanied by symptoms of severe presyncope or syncope, and usually no specific treatment is required. If necessary, intravenous atropine can be used to facilitate AV nodal conduction and to increase the ventricular rate. However, if the atropine causes an increase in the atrial rate, paradoxical slowing of the ventricular rate can occur because of more rapid stimulation of the AV node with encroachment on the refractory period of the AV conduction system. The effects of intravenous atropine are short-lived, and its chronic use is limited by significant side effects. If the decision is made to attempt medical therapy for vagally mediated AV block, oral theophylline and transdermal scopolamine have been used with limited success.[3]

In contrast to the majority of vagally mediated bradyarrhythmias, which are asymptomatic and usually can be treated conservatively, some patients suffer from a broad category of disorders collectively known as neurocardiogenic syndromes (see Chapter 10). The pathophysiology of these syndromes is complex and includes the influence of the central nervous system on the cardiovascular system, with resulting reflex bradycardia or peripheral vasodilation, or both, which can result in profound hypotension. Patients with neurocardiogenic syndromes can suffer frequent, unpredictable, abrupt and disabling episodes. Aggressive treatment may be required, with paroxetine being of some benefit but permanent dual chamber pacing being the preferred approach if significant bradycardia occurs during these episodes (see Chapter 10).[4–6] Volume support with increased fluid intake, mineralocorticoids, and support hose may also be useful. Because left ventricular baroreceptor stimulation from vigorous systolic contraction appears to be a key pathophysiologic mechanism, drugs such as beta-blockers that have negative inotropic effects are often used to manage these conditions. Patients in whom these malignant vasovagal syndromes are suspected should be referred to a specialist.

Medications

Commonly used medications that cause or contribute to bradycardia do so by enhancing vagal tone (e.g., digitalis), reducing sympathetically mediated enhancement of AV conduction (e.g., beta-blockers), or acting directly on sinoatrial and AV conduction tissue (e.g., calcium channel blockers). Thus, a thorough review of the patient's medications is important. Withdrawal of these drugs is often associated with reversal of the AV block, and permanent cardiac pacing is not required. However, if the medications are required, then pacemaker therapy may be necessary. If the ventricular rate is slow in the absence of these agents, then intrinsic AV conduction disease is present, and referral to a cardiologist for consideration of permanent pacing is indicated.

Supraventricular Arrhythmias in Patients with AV Conduction Disease

Many patients with supraventricular arrhythmias, especially atrial fibrillation, will require treatment with agents that provide ventricular rate control by reducing the ability of the AV node to conduct impulses to the ventricles. Some of these patients have or will develop disease of the AV conduction system and will not tolerate the rate-controlling agent unless a pacemaker is implanted. Caution should be used when considering electrical cardioversion in patients with supraventricular arrhythmias and slow ventricular rates in the absence of medications that slow AV conduction. Postcardioversion bradycardia or even asystole can occur owing to the diffuse underlying conduction system disease.

Advanced and Third-Degree AV Block

Outpatients who have high-grade or complete AV block of any cause and who have symptoms (including those of myocardial ischemia or infarction) should be treated as emergencies and transferred immediately to an intensive care unit in the event that temporary or permanent transvenous pacing becomes necessary. Many patients, even the elderly, can tolerate extreme bradycardia (25 to 30 beats per minute) if they are supine and their intravascular volume is increased with intravenous fluid administration. If available, transcutaneous pacing can be used, but it is unreliable and not well tolerated for prolonged periods of time. Very rarely, cardiopulmonary resuscitative procedures are necessary.

CARDIAC PACING

Indications

Temporary or permanent cardiac pacing is indicated in any situation in which bradycardia causes symptoms of cerebral hypoperfusion or hemodynamic decompensation. The guidelines published in 1998 by the American College of Cardiology and American Heart Association,[7] which are currently being updated, classify symptomatic second-degree AV block with associated bradycardia and symptomatic third-degree or complete AV block as Class I indications for permanent cardiac pacing (Fig. 31–14). Patients with third-degree or complete AV block who are asymptomatic but who have documented periods of asystole greater than or equal to 3.0 seconds or escape rates less than 40 beats per minute while awake also are considered appropriate candidates for pacemaker implantation. Patients with asymptomatic complete AV block with ventricular rates greater than 40 while awake often have pacemakers inserted, as do patients with asymptomatic type II second-degree AV block (Class IIa ACC/AHA recommendation).[7, 8] First-degree AV block is not an indication for a pacemaker unless definite symptoms of AV dyssynchrony (the "pacemaker syndrome") are present and are alleviated by temporary pacing (Class IIa ACC/AHA recommendation). Patients with bradycardia-dependent ventricular tachycardia may require pacing to prevent pauses in rhythm, thus eliminating the tachyarrhythmia. Pacing has also been helpful in selected patients with well-documented pause-dependent atrial fibrillation. Newer indications for pacemakers include heart failure with delayed intraventricular conduction, recurrent vasovagal or unexplained syncope, and selected patients with hypertrophic cardiomyopathy.[9–12]

Temporary Pacing

Temporary cardiac pacing is best accomplished by the transvenous route in all but the most critical situations, although emergency pacing can be achieved transcutaneously. *Transcutaneous pacing,* in which electrical current is delivered to the heart via large surface electrodes, is generally reserved for standby or prophylactic use in patients at high risk for bradycardia (e.g., during acute inferior and large anterior wall myocardial

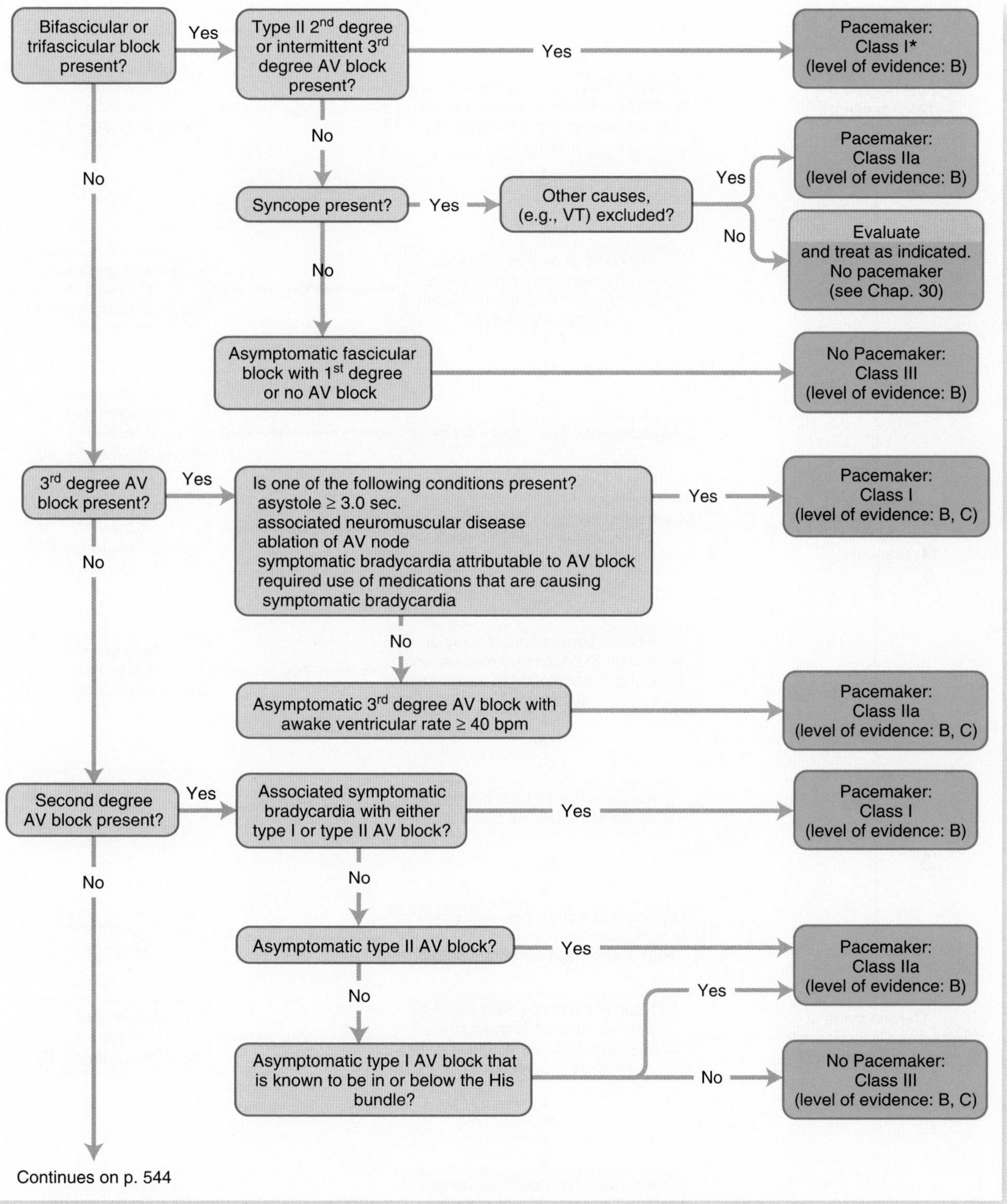

FIGURE 31–14. Diagram for selection of patients for permanent cardiac pacing based on symptoms and site of conduction system disease. *Class I, conditions for which there is either evidence or general agreement, or both, that pacemaker implantation is beneficial, useful, and effective; Class II, conditions for which there is either conflicting evidence or a divergence of opinion, or both, about the usefulness of pacemaker implantation; Class IIa, weight of evidence/opinion is in favor of usefulness/efficacy; Class IIb, usefulness/efficacy is less well established by evidence/opinion); Class III, conditions for which there is either evidence or general agreement, or both, that pacemaker implantation is not useful or effective, and in some cases may be harmful. Level of evidence A, based on data derived from multiple randomized clinical trials involving a large number of individuals; Level of evidence B, based on data derived from a limited number of trials involving a comparatively small number of patients or from well-designed data analysis of nonrandomized studies or observational data registries; Level of evidence C, based on consensus of expert opinion. AV, atrioventricular; bpm, beats per minute; HR, heart rate; LV, left ventricular; VT, ventricular tachycardia.

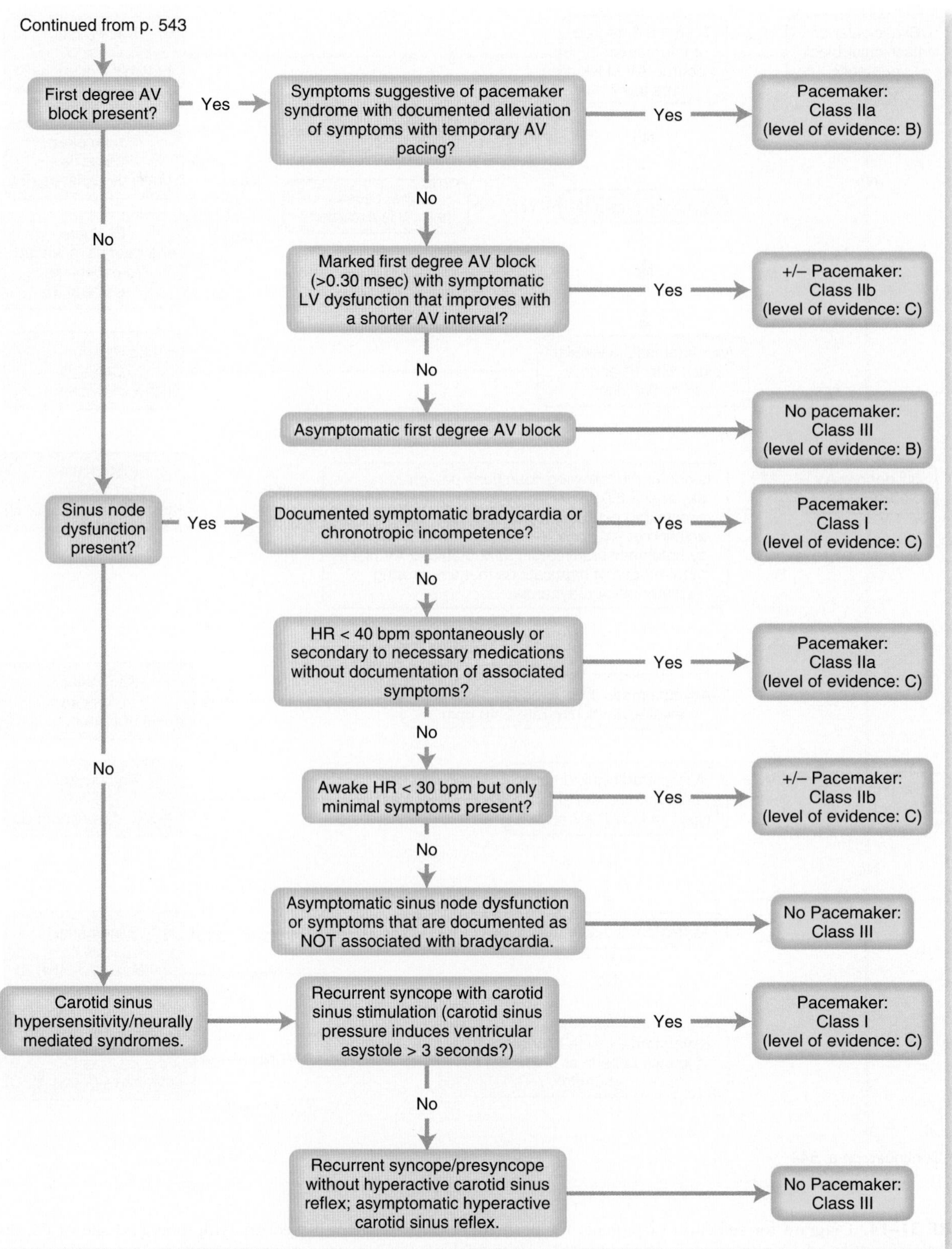

FIGURE 31–14. *Continued* (Adapted from Gregoratos G, Cheitlin MD, Conill A, et al: ACC/AHA guidelines for implantation of cardiac pacemakers and antiarrhythmia devices: A report of the American College of Cardiology/American Heart Association Task Force on Practice Guidelines [Committee on Pacemaker Implantation]. J Am Coll Cardiol 1998;31:1175–1209.)

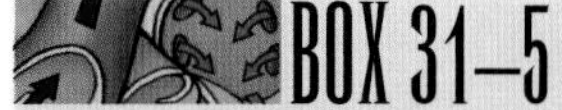

Nomenclature of Pacemaker Modes*

AAI Demand atrial pacing; output inhibited by sensed atrial signals.

AAIR Demand atrial pacing; output inhibited by sensed atrial signals. Atrial paced rates decrease and increase in response to sensor input up to the programmed sensor-based upper rate.

VVI Demand ventricular pacing; output inhibited by sensed ventricular signals.

VVIR Demand ventricular pacing; output inhibited by sensed ventricular signals. Ventricular paced rates decrease and increase in response to sensor input up to the programmed sensor-based upper rate.

VDD Paces ventricle, senses in both atrium and ventricle; synchronizes with atrial activity and paces ventricle after a preset atrioventricular interval up to the programmed upper rate.

VDDR Paces ventricle, senses in both atrium and ventricle; synchronizes with atrial activity and paces ventricle after a preset atrioventricular interval up to the programmed upper rate; ventricular paced rates decrease and increase in response to sensor input up to the programmed sensor-based upper rate.

DDD Paces and senses in both the atrium and ventricle; paces ventricle in response to sensed atrial activity up to programmed upper rate. In absence of spontaneous activity, will pace both atrium and ventricle synchronously.

DDDR Paces and senses in both the atrium and ventricle; paces ventricle in response to sensed atrial activity up to programmed upper rate. In absence of spontaneous activity, will pace both atrium and ventricle synchronously; atrial and ventricular paced rates can both increase and decrease in response to sensor input up to the programmed sensor upper limit.

*By convention, the first letter in the pacemaker-mode designation refers to the chamber(s) in which pacing occurs, the second letter to the chamber(s) in which sensing occurs, and the third letter to the response of the pacemaker to the sense signals. An R in the fourth position denotes rate-responsiveness. A, atrium; V, ventricle; D (in first or second position of mode designation), dual (both atrium and ventricle); I, inhibition; D (in third position of mode designation), inhibition and triggering (pacing in response to another event); R, rate-adaptive.

infarctions associated with bundle branch block) and in some patients who have sinus node dysfunction and who are undergoing elective cardioversion of atrial arrhythmias. Availability of transcutaneous pacemakers has heretofore been limited to hospitals and some cardiologists' offices. However, these pacemakers can be useful in cardiopulmonary resuscitation, and depending on the particular practice and community, their use should become more widespread.

The transcutaneous pacing system uses two large low-impedance surface electrodes placed on the anterior and posterior chest walls. A long pulse duration of 20 to 40 msec and programmable current output of up to 100 mA are often necessary to overcome the impedance of the chest wall and intrathoracic structures. The transcutaneous pacemaker paces the ventricle unless it senses spontaneous ventricular electrical activity, and it thus functions in VVI (demand) mode (Box 31–5). Ventricular capture (depolarization) is best seen on the pacemaker generator's oscilloscope and strip-chart recording (Fig. 31–15). Substantial distortion of the QRS complex is present on bedside rhythm monitors or ECG

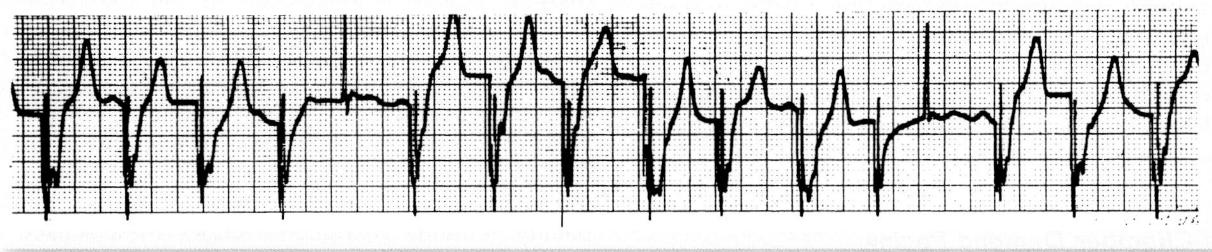

FIGURE 31–15. Rhythm strip illustrating transcutaneous cardiac pacing, recorded from the pacing device's ECG monitor. The pacing stimuli are delivered over a 40 msec interval and thus can obscure the onset of the paced QRS complexes. Transcutaneous pacing systems function in VVI mode (see text and Box 31–5) and are inhibited by spontaneous ventricular depolarizations. In this rhythm strip, the fifth and 13th QRS complexes are early and upright, are not preceded by a pacing stimulus, and are therefore native in origin; they appropriately inhibit the output of the pacing device. The pacing stimuli preceding these spontaneous QRS complexes (fourth and 12th stimuli) do not produce paced ventricular depolarizations, and therefore there are no associated T-waves (the presence of a T-wave is helpful in indicating ventricular depolarization when the QRS complexes are obscured). Thus, intermittent failure to capture is present. Paper speed changes account for the irregularity in the paced rhythm.

recordings, and paced QRS complexes cannot be identified by these means. Ventricular capture should be verified by palpating the pulse. Skeletal muscle twitching (not to be considered a sign of myocardial stimulation) occurs at a stimulus output of 30 mA, but ventricular capture does not usually occur until 35 to 80 mA. Sedation of an awake patient is usually required to mitigate the painful muscle contractions.

Transcutaneous cardiac pacing can be effective in up to 70% of patients. Most poor outcomes result from its use in advanced stages of cardiopulmonary arrest. If cardiac arrest has been present for more than 15 minutes, successful pacing is accomplished in only 33% to 45% of patients, with little effect on outcome. *Temporary transvenous and esophageal pacing,* which are performed in hospital settings and in intensive care units by specialists, are indicated when reliable emergency pacing is required (see Chapter 24).

Permanent Pacing

Permanent cardiac pacing is almost always performed through the transvenous route; in some circumstances, however, epicardial placement of electrodes via thoracotomy or a subxiphoid approach is used. When performed via the transvenous route, the lead is usually placed in or near the apex of the right ventricle. Although it has been suggested that pacing from the right ventricular outflow tract might offer some benefit over pacing from the apex in that ventricular depolarization proceeds more normally from base to apex, a randomized study comparing the two sites failed to demonstrate a difference.[13]

Pacing system design is complex, but all pacemaker generator functions are described by a standard code (Table 31–1). Current pacemakers have several functions that can be changed non-invasively by a programmer. The programmable features of a pacing system allow for optimal benefit for the patient while conserving the battery's energy. The type of pacing system, model, and serial number are indicated on an identification card supplied to the patient by the manufacturer; patients should carry this card with them at all times. It is important to note, however, that the information provided by the card does not guarantee the current status of any programmable function; pacemaker interrogation is necessary to document all programmed parameters.

Single-Chamber Demand Pacing (VVI, VVIR, AAI, AAIR)

Both sensing and pacing circuits are present in these units. When a spontaneous intracardiac signal is sensed, VVI and AAI pulse generators inhibit their output, and thus no pacemaker stimulus occurs. Electrical signals sensed by demand-pulse generators can originate not only from the heart but also from the environment (e.g., electrocautery, cellular telephones), from the patient (e.g., muscle potentials), or occasionally, from the pacing system itself. The sensed signals can inhibit output and result in pauses in paced rhythm, a phenomenon termed *oversensing,* which can cause symptoms of cerebral hypoperfusion. This problem can generally be corrected by noninvasive programming to increase the sensing threshold, thereby obviating the need for surgical revision.

TABLE 31–1

Symptoms in Patients with Pacing Systems

Symptom	Possible Pacemaker-Related Causes
Palpitations	Inappropriate rate settings or rate-adaptive parameters Pacemaker-mediated tachyarrhythmias
Weakness	Pacemaker syndrome Inappropriate rate-adaptation settings Failure to capture Oversensing leading to pauses in rhythm Battery end of life with slow rate or inadequate generator output
Breathlessness, nocturnal dyspnea, fatigue	Pacemaker syndrome Inappropriate upper rate setting Inappropriate rate-adaptation setting Battery end of life with slow rate or no output
Hiccups, cough	Diaphragmatic pacing
Muscle twitching	Lead insulation failure Unipolar stimulation
Swelling, suffusion of upper extremity	Thrombophlebitis (subclavian vein, inferior vena cava)
Dyspnea, edema	Right heart failure due to lead-related pulmonary emboli (including septic emboli)
Fever of unknown origin	Pacing system infection

P-Synchronous Pacing Systems (VDD and VDDR)

VDD(R) pacing systems are single lead systems in which electrodes are located in both the atrium and the ventricle. The lead is positioned in the right ventricular apex for ventricular sensing and pacing; the sensing atrial electrodes are located on the lead at the level of the atrium. When the atrial electrodes sense an electrical signal, a ventricular pacing stimulus is delivered after a programmable AV delay that corresponds roughly to the PR interval. If a spontaneous QRS complex occurs, the ventricular output is inhibited. Thus, the ventricular pacing stimulus is triggered either by a sensed atrial signal or inhibited by a native QRS event (Fig. 31–16).

DDD and DDDR Pacing Systems

DDD pulse generators are capable of sensing and pacing in both the atrium and the ventricle. They therefore attempt to mimic the physiology of normal AV conduction in patients who require cardiac pacing. The ability to sense retrograde atrial depolarizations can trigger ventricular pacing; if the paced ventricular

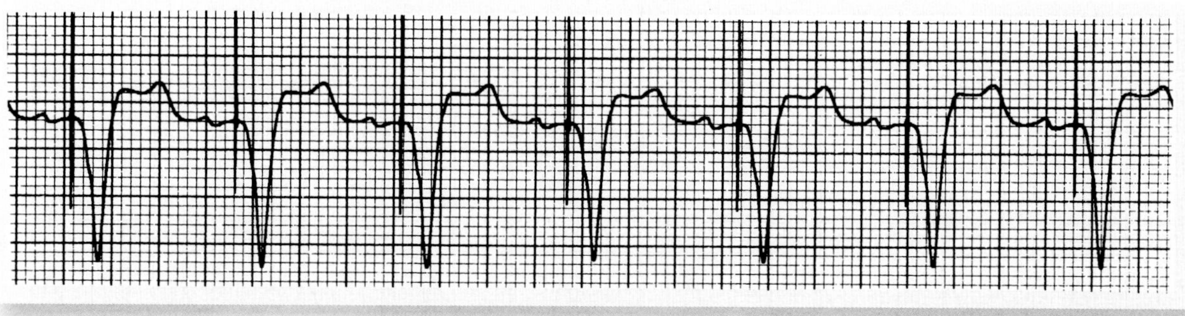

FIGURE 31–16. P-synchronous pacing in a 64-year-old woman with complete AV block. The atrial rhythm is sinus. All P-waves are sensed and followed at a constant AV interval by paced QRS complexes. Thus, "tracking" of the atrial rhythm is present. The parameters of intact pacing system function demonstrated in this illustration are atrial sensing and ventricular pacing; atrial pacing and ventricular sensing are not seen and are thus not verified. This pacing system could be either a DDD or a VDD system (see text and Box 31–5). The tracking of sinus rhythm and rate not only allows AV synchrony but also rate adaptation in response to increases in metabolic need.

depolarization conducts retrogradely to the atrium, the process can become repetitive, creating a "pacemaker-mediated tachycardia." Specific pulse-generator features are designed to terminate these tachycardias automatically.

Dual-chamber devices depend on a stable atrial rhythm for optimal function. Because rapid paced ventricular rates can occur during normal tracking function of rapid atrial rhythms, these systems should not be used in patients with atrial arrhythmias such as chronic atrial fibrillation, refractory atrial flutter, multifocal atrial tachycardia, or refractory atrial tachycardia. Instead, single-chamber VVI or VVIR devices can be used in these patients. All current devices can change their mode of function automatically from DDD(R) to single-chamber VVI(R) or dual chamber nontracking DDI(R) function if an atrial arrhythmia is sensed; such devices are appropriate for patients with paroxysmal atrial arrhythmias when there is an advantage to allowing AV synchrony during sinus or atrial-paced rhythm. Pacemakers with this "mode switching" feature are now used in virtually all patients with paroxysmal supraventricular tachyarrhythmias.

Rate Responsiveness

Rate-adaptive pacing systems (see Box 31–5) are appropriate for patients with persistent or refractory atrial arrhythmias who are not candidates for DDD(R) devices and for patients with sinus node dysfunction that prevents atrial rate acceleration in response to increases in metabolic demand. Current commonly used sensors measure muscle activity, minute ventilation or QT interval, and then adjust the paced rate. Newer pacing systems use two sensors to optimize the rate response to different types of activity and to "cross-check" the specificity of the sensor input to the pulse generator. Sensor-based pacing rates depend on the individual sensor and the programmed rate-response parameters. Patient dissatisfaction with rate-adaptive pacing almost always reflects inappropriate programmed parameters; the determination of optimal settings often requires considerable time and expertise.

ECG Patterns of Paced Complexes

The configuration of paced P-waves and QRS complexes reflects how myocardium is depolarized (Fig. 31–17). Paced atrial complexes reflect the sequence of atrial activation initiated by the pacing stimulus and thus also the site of the stimulating electrode(s). Because the atrial electrodes can be located in the atrial appendage or screwed into any portion of atrial tissue, paced P-waves will have variable contours. Atrial hypertrophy and conduction delay cannot be diagnosed if the P-waves are paced.

Pacing from the right ventricular endocardium or epicardium produces paced QRS complexes having a left bundle branch block configuration (reflecting right ventricular depolarization beginning before left ventricular depolarization). Occasionally, pacing from the interventricular septum can cause paced QRS complexes with an indeterminate conduction delay pattern; they can even be narrow and relatively normal-appearing, reflecting near-simultaneous activation of both the right and the left sides of the interventricular septum. Paced QRS complexes usually have a duration of 0.12 to 0.18 second; if they are substantially longer, intrinsic myocardial disease, rapid paced rate, hyperkalemia, or antiarrhythmic drug therapy should be suspected. Spontaneous QRS complexes occurring in patients with pacemakers often show marked T-wave inversion of unknown cause, as a result, myocardial ischemia or infarction cannot be diagnosed with certainty.

Choice of Cardiac Pacing System and Relative Costs

State-of-the-art pacing systems can be costly. The cost of single chamber, non–rate-adaptive devices, including pulse generator and lead, is about \$5500 to \$5800, and

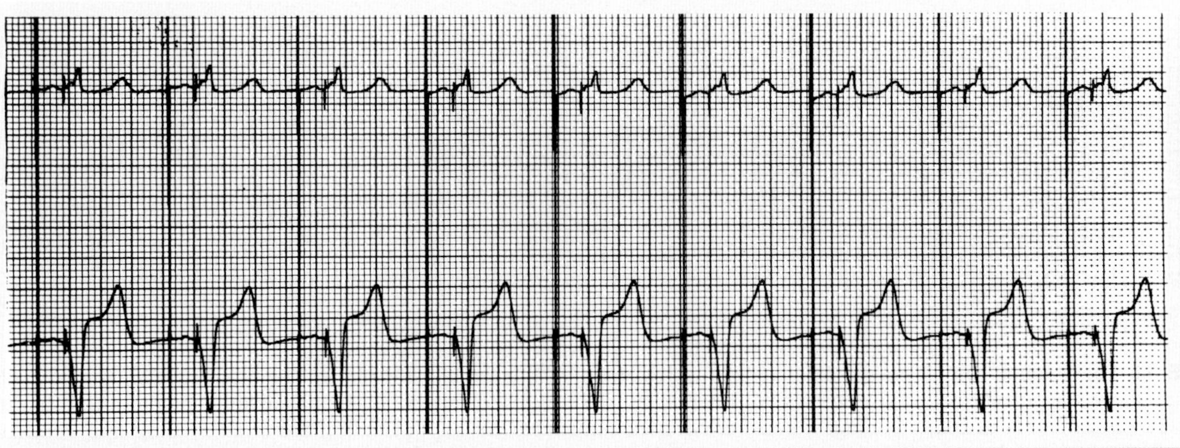

FIGURE 31–17. AV pacing is illustrated in these simultaneously recorded leads I and II. Since all P-waves and QRS complexes are paced and no native complexes are seen, sensing function cannot be evaluated. The large atrial pacing artifact is due to the unipolar configuration of the atrial lead; the smaller ventricular pacing artifact is owing to the bipolar configuration of the ventricular lead. Note the changing amplitude and polarity of the ventricular pacing stimuli, an artifact of the recording equipment. The patient's native heart rate and rhythm are not known, because all complexes are paced.

that of single-chamber, rate-adaptive devices is about $7400. Dual-chamber non–rate-adaptive (pulse generator and two leads) pacemakers can cost up to $8000, and rate-adaptive pacemakers can cost $9000 or more depending on the availability of special algorithms that recognize paroxysmal supraventricular arrhythmias and alter mode of function ("mode switching"), retain ECG data in memory, use more than one sensor, or have other sophisticated technical features.

These high up-front costs notwithstanding, studies have suggested the advantages and cost-effectiveness of appropriate device selection, including multiple programmable features. Device selection should always take advantage of the patient's spontaneous sinus rhythm to preserve AV synchrony and normal rate response provided that atrial bradycardia is not present; rate adaptation in patients with atrial bradycardia will preserve the normal sequence of depolarization and contraction and thus optimize hemodynamic function.[14] Patients with supraventricular arrhythmias should be prescribed dual-chamber devices to take advantage of normal rhythm when it is present, and potentially to reduce the frequency of paroxysmal arrhythmias. In one randomized trial, the incidence of cardiovascular death, thromboembolism, and heart failure was significantly reduced by the use of dual-chamber systems in appropriate patients after eight years of follow-up.[15] There is also evidence that dual chamber pacing reduces the incidence of atrial fibrillation and heart failure and improves quality of life.[16–19] However, randomized trials have not shown a survival benefit for dual chamber pacing compared with single chamber pacing.[18, 19]

Pacing System "Malfunctions"

Pacing system "malfunctions" fall into four general categories, the general nature of which should be recognized by the primary care physician. These include undersensing, or failure to sense; oversensing, or sensing unwanted signals; failure to capture; and failure of output (true undersensing is not present in this circumstance).

Failure to sense spontaneous complexes and to inhibit output appropriately results in the delivery of an earlier than expected pacing stimulus (Fig. 31–18). Failure to sense can occur because of lead dislodgment, fibrous reaction where the lead site meets the myocardium, or the end of battery life. Occasionally, a delay in native conduction prevents the native depolarization from reaching the lead electrode early enough to inhibit the pacing stimulus output; this phenomenon does not represent true failure to sense.

Oversensing refers to sensing of unwanted electrical signals such as T-waves, myopotentials, and environmental signals (e.g., electrocautery, cell phones).[20] Oversensing inhibits output and can produce long asystolic pauses. Programming the pulse generator to a higher sensing threshold so as to ignore lesser electrical signals will often solve the problem. When a programmer is not available or the pulse generator cannot be identified, placing a magnet over the generator will eliminate the oversensing while the patient is urgently transported for definitive care.

Failure to capture is present when pacing stimuli do not depolarize the otherwise receptive nonrefractory myocardium (Fig. 31–19). This condition may result from poor electrode position, too low a programmed output, end of battery life with resulting reduction in energy output, or an increase in myocardial stimulation threshold.

Failure to capture often can be managed by noninvasive programming to a higher energy output, but lead repositioning or replacement, or implantation of a new

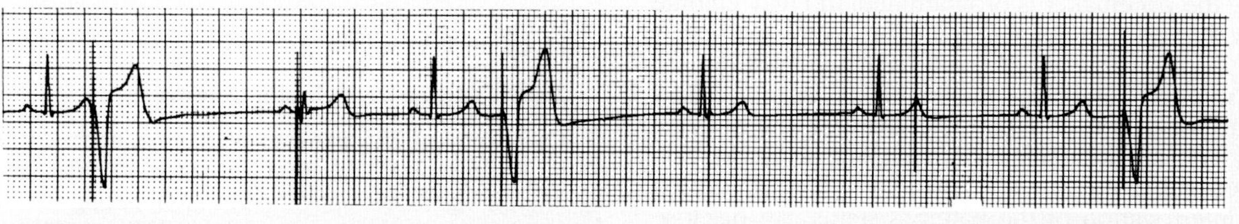

FIGURE 31–18. Failure to sense in a 37-year-old woman with a VVI pacing system (see text) implanted for "congenital complete AV block" 18 years earlier. Pacing function is intact. The pacing rate is about 39 beats per minute, and the pulse generator is at the end of its life. The failure to sense intrinsic QRS complexes results in fixed-rate asynchronous stimulus delivery. The third QRS complex is a fusion complex in which the ventricles are depolarized by both the sinus-stimulated QRS complex and the paced complex. The fourth and fifth pacing stimuli do not produce a QRS complex; however, because they fall in the refractory period of ventricular muscle, true failure to capture cannot be diagnosed.

generator, or both, may be required. Failure to pace, even if asymptomatic, requires urgent referral to a pacemaker specialist.

The difference between failure to capture in response to a delivered pacing stimulus and *absence of stimulus output* should be clearly understood. Applying a magnet will aid in determining the cause for the lack of stimulus output. If no output is present on a 12-lead ECG, the problem may be a fracture of the lead or a break in its insulation, or the pulse generator may be at the end of its life. Pacemaker interrogation is necessary to make the correct diagnosis and undertake corrective measures.

Monitoring the Patient with a Pacemaker

All patients with pacemakers should be monitored on a routine basis by a pacemaker specialist; the specialist may or may not be the implanting cardiologist but is generally not an implanting surgeon. Additional transtelephonic monitoring, set up by the pacemaker specialist, can be used routinely to reduce the number of visits to the specialist as well as to provide follow-up support for those patients who reside at considerable distances from pacemaker centers or who are physically unable to get to the center. Rhythm strips and pacemaker rate information are routinely sent to the pacemaker specialist for inclusion in the patient's pacemaker file. It is the responsibility of the specialist routinely to interrogate the pacemaker, assess battery status, perform pacing and sensing threshold(s) to optimize programmed parameters and thus prolong pulse generator life, and to assess the underlying rhythm and rate and the degree of pacemaker dependency. The pacemaker specialist also accesses rhythm and rate information stored in the pacemaker's memory to aid in arrhythmia management and optimal programming. Because it is the specialist who receives advisories of real and potential pacemaker-related problems, as well as of manufacturer—or government—initiated recalls of devices found to be actually or potentially defective, the specialist is in the best position to evaluate the patient in a timely manner in light of the potential device failures, some of which can be life-threatening.

In general, once a patient has stabilized after pacemaker implantation and the wound has been checked, routine office follow-up can be performed at 3 months, then semiannually, and finally annually until the battery nears its expected end of life, which is currently at around 5 to 7 years, but which depends substantially

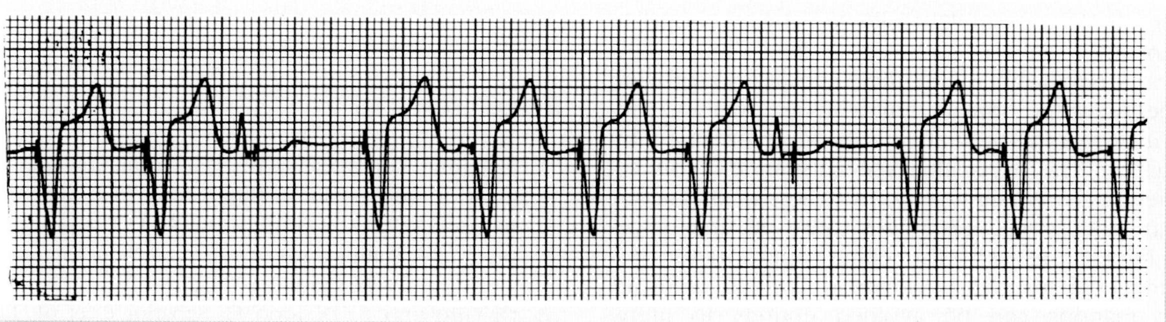

FIGURE 31–19. Asynchronous fixed-rate ventricular pacing illustrating episodic noncapture (third and eighth pacing stimuli) due to ventricular refractoriness produced by the preceding spontaneous QRS complexes. This finding should not be interpreted as failure to capture. True capture failure requires that a temporal opportunity to capture exists.

on how the pacemaker is programmed and may change with evolving technology. Depending on the particular pacing system, after about the fourth year postimplantation, monthly telephone transmissions are prescribed to ensure detection of subtle rate changes that indicate battery end of life. Telephone transmissions do not, however, substitute for office follow-up visits, during which interrogation of the battery's status can disclose information not available from rate data alone.

The primary care physician must ensure that the paced patient has formal follow-up with a cardiologist who has up-to-date, state-of-the art knowledge of cardiac pacing. Communication among the patient's physicians is necessary, so that each knows the concerns of the others. This communication is particularly important if a patient is receiving medications that can affect pacing and sensing thresholds, so that any appropriate programming changes can be made. Wound infections, upper extremity thrombophlebitis, and pacing system infections can occur months to years after implantation, and these complications must be recognized because referral to a specialist will be required.[21] Intercurrent events that can affect the pacemaker's function, such as myocardial infarction and the development of renal insufficiency, should prompt referral for additional pacemaker checks. Especially in patients with rate-adaptive pacing systems, the pacemaker specialist will want to know the perception by the primary care physician of the patient's exercise tolerance and general sense of well-being so the pacemaker can be programmed to the most appropriate rate-response settings. Patients who are undergoing surgical procedures may need antibiotic prophylaxis to prevent infection of the pacing system, but this practice varies widely among pacemaker specialists.

In patients with pacemakers, any symptoms that are new or otherwise unexplained warrant an evaluation by the pacemaker specialist (see Table 31–1) because noninvasive programming may be able to correct or ameliorate symptoms that can be identified as being related to the pacing system. In patients with unexplained fever, specialized studies such as echocardiography may be necessary to exclude infection of the pacing system, a complication that requires aggressive antibiotic therapy and, commonly, removal of the entire system. Patients who develop new pulmonary hypertension require evaluation for lead-related thromboembolism, whether septic or sterile, followed by appropriate treatment.

It is the responsibility of the specialist to provide the patient and the primary care physician with a copy of the most recent programmed settings obtained by interrogation. The pacemaker specialist should counsel the patient as to which types of activities or diagnostic or therapeutic procedures might cause adverse pacemaker interactions, so that either appropriate programming changes can be made or certain activities and occupations can be avoided entirely to allow protection of both the pacing system and the patient.[20] The primary care physician should be apprised of these conditions as well, so continued reinforcement can occur.

Evidence-Based Summary

Atrial Versus Ventricular Pacing

One study of 225 patients with sinus node dysfunction randomized to atrial versus ventricular pacing found a significant benefit from atrial pacing in reducing thromboembolic events (from 23% to 12%) at 8-year follow-up.[18] All-cause mortality was reduced by 15% (35% versus 50%), which was significant in univariate analysis but not multivariate analysis. Cardiovascular death was reduced from 34% to 17%, a significant difference even after controlling for differences in baseline characteristics ($P = .022$).

Other studies, however, have not reproduced these findings. In a study of over 400 patients 65 years of age or older with sick sinus syndrome or AV-block, no significant difference was found between patients randomized to ventricular pacing versus dual chamber pacing in death, stroke, heart failure, or quality of life at 30 months of follow-up.[18] Of note, however, 26% of patients crossed over from single to dual chamber pacing mode due to symptoms of the pacemaker syndrome. A larger study of more than 2000 patients with sinus node dysfunction, again with a crossover rate from single to dual chamber pacing of 38%, found that dual chamber pacemakers reduced the incidence of atrial fibrillation and heart failure and led, on average, to a slight but statistically significant improvement in quality of life at a median follow-up of 36 months.[19] However, there was no difference in mortality, the combined endpoint of death or stroke, or hospitalization due to heart failure. The largest trial, which randomized 2568 patients to receive physiologic (atrial or dual chamber) or ventricular pacing systems and followed them for 3 years, also failed to find a difference in the primary outcome of cardiovascular mortality or stroke, although a relative risk reduction of 18% was found in the occurrence of atrial fibrillation.[16, 17] In summary, dual chamber or physiologic pacing to preserve atrial contraction reduces the risk of atrial fibrillation and probably of heart failure, may improve quality of life in some patients, but does not appear to reduce stroke, cardiovascular mortality, or overall mortality.

References

1. Mangrum JM, DiMarco JP: The evaluation and management of bradycardia. N Engl J Med 2000;342:703–709.
2. Ashley EA, Raxwal VK, Froelicher VF: The prevalence and prognostic significance of electrocardiographic abnormalities. Curr Probl Cardiol 2000;25:1–72.
3. Di Girolamo E, Di Iorio C, Sabatini P, et al: Effects of paroxetine hydrochloride, a selective serotonin reuptake inhibitor, on refractory vasovagal syncope: A randomized, double-blind, placebo-controlled study. J Am Coll Cardiol 1999;33:1227–1230.

4. Connolly SJ, Sheldon R, Roberts RS, Gent M. The North American Vasovagal Pacemaker Study (VPS). A randomized trial of permanent cardiac pacing for the prevention of vasovagal syncope. J Am Coll Cardiol 1999;33:16–20.
5. Sutton R, Brignole M, Menozzi C, et al: Dual-chamber pacing in treatment of neurally mediated tilt-positive cardioinhibitory syncope. Pacemaker versus no therapy: A multicentre randomized study. Circulation 2000;102:294–299.
6. Ammirati F, Colivicchi F, Santini M, for the Syncope Diagnosis and Treatment Study Investigators: Permanent cardiac pacing versus medical treatment for the prevention of recurrent vasovagal syncope: A multicenter, randomized, controlled trial. Circulation 2001;104:52–57.
7. Gregoratos G, Abrams J, Epstein AE, et al: ACC/AHA/NASPE 2002 guideline update for implantation of cardiac pacemakers and antiarrhythmia devices: A report of the American College of Cardiology/American Heart Association Task Force on Practice Guidelines (ACC/AHA/NASPE Committee to Update the 1998 Pacemaker Guidelines). Circulation 2002;106:2145–2161.
8. Kusumoto FM, Goldschlager N: Device therapy for cardiac arrhythmias. JAMA 2002;287:1848–1852.
9. Bryce M, Spielman SR, Greenspan AM, Kotler MN: Evolving indications for permanent pacemakers. Ann Intern Med 2001;134:1130–1141.
10. Varma C, Camm AJ: Pacing for heart failure. Lancet 2001;357:1277–1283.
11. Cazeau S, Leclercq C, Lavergne T, et al: Effects of multisite biventricular pacing in patients with heart failure and intraventricular conduction delay. N Engl J Med 2001;344: 873–880.
12. Gold MR. Permanent pacing: New indications. Heart 2001; 86:355–360.
13. Victor F, Leclercq C, Mabo P, et al: Optimal right ventricular pacing site in chronically implanted patients: A prospective randomized crossover comparison of apical and outflow tract pacing. J Am Coll Cardiol 1999;33: 311–316.
14. Nielsen JC, Bottcher M, Nielsen TT, et al: Regional myocardial blood flow in patients with sick sinus syndrome randomized to long-term single chamber atrial or dual chamber pacing-effect of pacing mode and rate. J Am Coll Cardiol 2000;35:1453–1461.
15. Andersen HR, Nielsen JC, Thomsen PE, et al: Long-term follow-up of patients from a randomized trial of atrial versus ventricular pacing for sick-sinus syndrome. Lancet 1997;350:1210–1216.
16. Skanes AC, Krahn AD, Yee R, et al: Progression to chronic atrial fibrillation after pacing: The Canadian trial of physiologic pacing. J Am Coll Cardiol 2001;38:167–172.
17. Connolly SJ, Kerr CR, Gent M, et al: Effects of physiological pacing versus ventricular pacing on the risk of stroke and death due to cardiovascular causes. N Engl J Med 2000;342:1385–1391.
18. Lamas GA, Orav EJ, Stambler BS, et al: Quality of life and clinical outcomes in elderly patients treated with ventricular pacing as compared with dual-chamber pacing. Pacemaker Selection in the Elderly Investigators. N Engl J Med 1998;338:1097–1104.
19. Lamas GA, Lee KL, Sweeney MO, et al: Ventricular pacing or dual-chamber pacing for sinus-node dysfunction. N Engl J Med 2002;346:1854–1862.
20. Goldschlager N, Epstein A, Friedman P, et al: Environmental and drug effects on patients with pacemakers and implantable cardioverter/defibrillators: A practical guide to patient treatment. Arch Intern Med 2001;161:649–653.
21. Chamis AL, Peterson GE, Cabell CH, et al: Staphylococcus aureus bacteremia in patients with permanent pacemakers or implantable cardioverter-defibrillators. Circulation 2001;104:1029–1033.

CHAPTER 32 Recognition and Management of Patients with Valvular Heart Disease

Blase A. Carabello

Five million Americans have some form of valvular heart disease. In addition to its magnitude, further importance is added to the recognition and management of valve disease because, unlike coronary disease, which often progresses despite therapy, proper management of valvular heart disease leads to a normal life span in most instances. Misdiagnosis or improper management may result in a shortened life span or persistent congestive heart failure.

All valvular disease imparts a hemodynamic overload on either the left or the right ventricle, or both, that may be well tolerated for years. Eventually the overload can produce myocardial damage that may become irreversible. In some patients, medical therapy may forestall this damage; in others, surgical intervention is the only effective therapy. This chapter addresses the recognition of valvular heart disease and emphasizes the best modalities for evaluation and follow-up. It also focuses on when to refer patients for the specialized care leading to surgical intervention.[1]

AORTIC STENOSIS

Aortic stenosis (AS) is the most common of the primary valvular heart diseases. It is estimated that up to 1% of Americans are born with a bicuspid aortic valve, which is the most common cardiac congenital abnormality (see Chapter 34). A substantial proportion of this group eventually develops significant aortic valvular obstruction. Other patients develop stenosis of a previously normal tricuspid valve. Although once considered to be a degenerative disease, understanding of its etiology has evolved considerably over the past decade. It is now clear that the early lesion of aortic stenosis has much in common with coronary disease.[2] First, the initial valve lesion of AS is similar to that of the plaque of coronary disease. Second, there is emerging epidemiologic evidence linking AS to serum lipid abnormalities. Third, there is a strong correlation between calcium deposition in the coronary arteries (indicative of coronary disease) to calcium in the aortic valve. Fourth, HMG CoA reductase inhibitors (statins) appear able to retard the progression of both coronary disease and of AS.[3]

In industrialized societies, rheumatic heart disease rarely causes AS. In rheumatic AS, the mitral valve is almost always abnormal. Thus, the diagnosis of rheumatic AS should not be made in the face of an echocardiographically normal mitral valve.

As AS progresses, an increasingly higher left ventricular systolic pressure is required to drive blood across the obstructed valve, resulting in a pressure gradient between the left ventricle and the aorta. This extra pressure work that the left ventricle must perform results in concentric left ventricular hypertrophy. Initially, the hypertrophy is compensatory because the increased muscle mass allows the ventricle to generate the higher pressure required by the obstruction to flow. Eventually the hypertrophied myocardium takes on pathologic characteristics, resulting in the development of symptoms, morbidity, and mortality.[4]

Diagnosis

History

Most patients with AS are asymptomatic. As shown in Figure 32–1, survival is nearly normal during this asymptomatic phase. When the classic symptoms of angina, syncope, or congestive heart failure develop, there is a rapid increase in the risk of death unless aortic valve replacement is performed. Although AS is rarely the cause of angina, syncope, or congestive heart failure in the large population of patients who complain of these common symptoms, this diagnosis should never be overlooked when patients present with those symptoms, because AS is lethal if uncorrected, yet it has an excellent outcome after aortic valve surgery.

Physical Examination

AS is usually discovered because of the typical systolic ejection murmur that is heard best in the aortic area and radiates to the neck (see Chapter 11). The murmur has a harsh quality and initially may be quite loud. As the disease progresses, the murmur peaks progressively later in systole, and its intensity usually decreases as cardiac output falls. The murmur may disappear over the sternum and reappear at the apex, giving the false impression that mitral regurgitation is present (Gallivardin's phenomenon). When the severity of AS becomes hemodynamically significant, the carotid upstroke becomes reduced in volume and delayed. This may be appreciated as the physician palpates his or her own carotid pulse with one hand and simultaneously palpates the patient's carotid pulse with the other. A graphic example of this important physical finding is demonstrated in Figure 32–2. An additional finding helpful in assessing the severity of AS on physical examination is the quality of the second heart sound (S_2). As stenosis severity worsens, valve motion is reduced and the aortic component of S_2 disappears. Thus, a single soft S_2 representing the closure of the pulmonic component is a typical finding in severe AS. More rarely, S_2 may be paradoxically split.

Laboratory Studies

The electrocardiogram (ECG) in severe AS usually shows left ventricular hypertrophy. The chest x-ray may demonstrate a boot-shaped heart consistent with the development of left ventricular concentric hypertrophy. Occasionally, aortic valve calcification is seen on the lateral view. Echocardiography is the principal laboratory method by which AS is diagnosed and quantified. Two-dimensional echocardiography demonstrates thickened valve leaflets with restricted motion. It also gauges left ventricular ejection fraction and the extent of concentric left ventricular hypertrophy. Ejection fraction is the percent of the left or right ventricle's end-diastolic volume (EDV) ejected during systole (i.e., stroke volume/EDV). Precise measurement of the transvalvular gradient is afforded by Doppler interrogation of the valve (see Chapter 5) (Fig. 32–3). In general, in

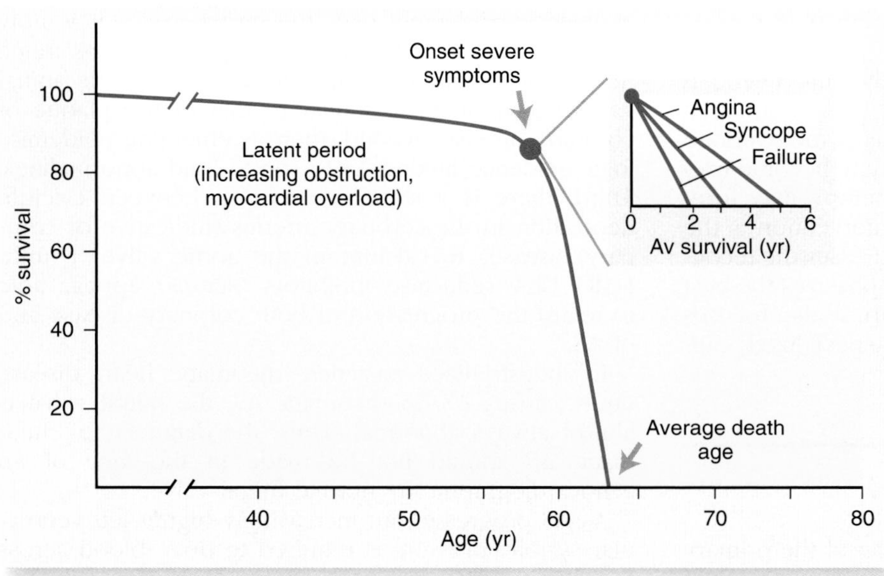

FIGURE 32–1. The natural history of aortic stenosis. There is a long latent period during which survival is about the same as that for the normal population. Once the symptoms of angina, syncope, or congestive heart failure develop, survival declines dramatically. Within 5 years, one half of the patients complaining of angina will die unless corrective surgery is performed. For patients complaining of syncope, 50% survival is only 3 years, and for patients who complain of the symptoms of congestive heart failure, 50% survival is only 2 years without aortic valve replacement. Av, average. (Redrawn from Ross J, Jr, and Braunwald E: Aortic stenosis. Circulation 38[Suppl 5]: V–61, 1968. Reproduced with permission from Circulation. Copyright 1968 American Heart Association.)

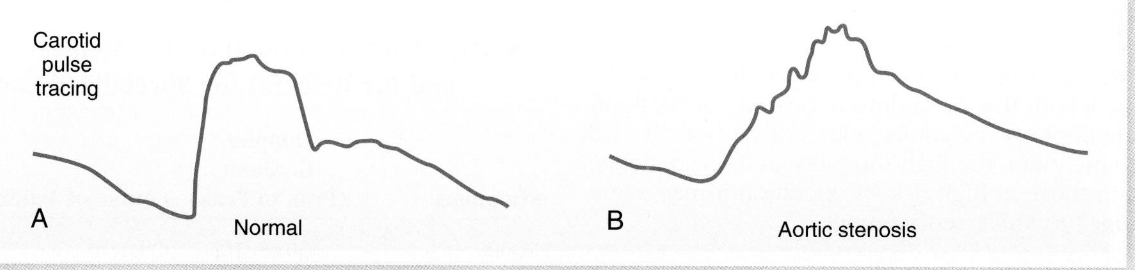

FIGURE 32–2. The carotid pulse tracing of a normal subject is demonstrated *(A)* and compared with the carotid pulse tracing of a patient with aortic stenosis *(B)*. The marked delay in upstroke that can be seen here can also be easily palpated during physical examination. (A and B, Redrawn from Boro KM, and Wynne J: External pulse recordings, systolic time intervals, apexcardiography, and phonocardiography. In Cohn PF, Wynne J [eds]: Diagnostic Methods in Clinical Cardiology. Boston, Little, Brown, 1982.)

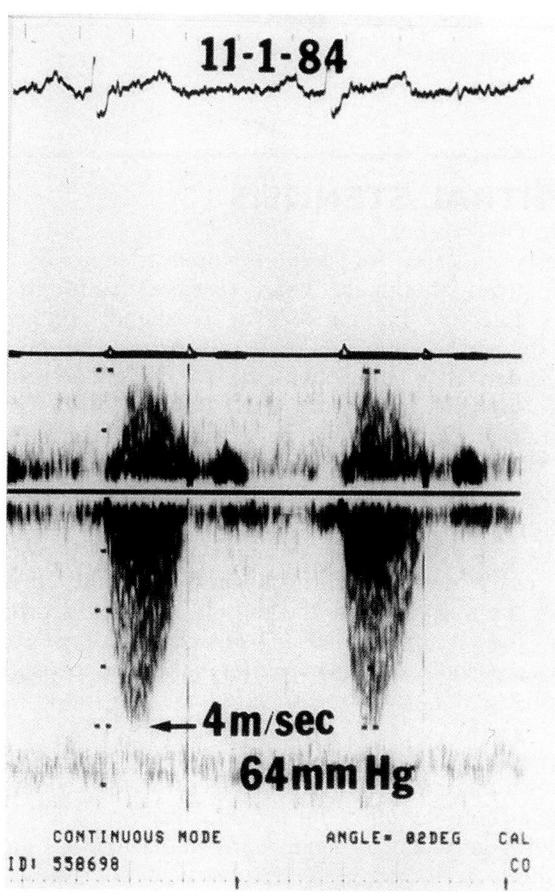

FIGURE 32–3. The Doppler interrogation of the aortic valve in a patient with aortic stenosis demonstrates high-velocity blood flow at 4 msec. Using the modified Bernoulli equation (see text), a gradient of 64 mm Hg is calculated. (From Assey ME, Usher BW, and Carabello BA: The patient with valvular heart disease. In Pepine CJ, Hill JA, Lambert CR [eds]: Diagnostic and Therapeutic Cardiac Catheterization. 2nd ed. Baltimore, Williams & Wilkins, 1994.)

resting subjects who are not in heart failure, gradients higher than 50 mm Hg indicate severe AS, although lower gradients may also signify severe stenosis when the cardiac output is reduced.

Because most patients with AS are in an age range where concomitant coronary artery disease is likely, adult patients with AS should undergo cardiac catheterization before surgery. During this procedure, coronary angiography displays the coronary anatomy and the transvalvular gradient is confirmed by direct pressure measurement.

Management

Apart from prophylaxis against infective endocarditis, there is no effective medical management for AS although statin therapy to retard progression of the valve lesion may become standard therapy in the future. If the patient is asymptomatic, no therapy is required. If the symptoms of angina, syncope, or heart failure have developed, immediate valve replacement is indicated as a lifesaving measure. Nitrates and diuretics may be employed cautiously to treat angina and heart failure, respectively, in the interim between when the diagnosis is made and when surgery is performed. Beta-blockers should be avoided in the treatment of angina because they may precipitate cardiovascular collapse. Angiotensin-converting enzyme (ACE) inhibitors and other vasodilators used prominently in the treatment of most forms of congestive heart failure may precipitate syncope and even death in AS and are relatively contraindicated. In some individuals with concomitant systemic hypertension, cautious use of vasodilators may reduce symptoms.

In severely symptomatic patients who are not candidates for aortic valve replacement (because of other life-limiting illnesses such as terminal cancer), balloon aortic valvotomy affords temporary improvement in the transvalvular gradient and may relieve symptoms in some patients. During this procedure, a large balloon catheter is advanced percutaneously from the femoral artery and over a guide wire to the aortic valve orifice. There, balloon inflation modestly increases valve cusp mobility. Unfortunately, the stenosis returns to its original severity within 6 months in approximately half of the patients in whom this procedure is carried out. Balloon aortic valvuloplasty in adults with critical, calcific AS does not ameliorate the high mortality in these patients, although in those at high risk of operation it may serve as a "bridge" to valve replacement.

Management Strategy

When AS is detected on the physical examination of an *asymptomatic* patient, an echocardiogram should be performed to quantify severity. If the peak gradient is less than approximately 50 mm Hg, the patient can be followed yearly with a history and physical examination.[5] If the peak gradient exceeds approximately 50 mm Hg, follow-up should be performed every 6 months. In patients who are physically active, repeat echocardiography is indicated if the patient reports the onset of one or more of the triad—angina, syncope, or heart failure. At that time, an echocardiogram can be repeated to determine whether there has been a change in the severity of the stenosis and whether left ventricular dysfunction has developed. At that point, the patient should be referred promptly for final workup before aortic valve replacement. In sedentary patients, more frequent echocardiograms may detect the onset of left ventricular dysfunction before the onset of symptoms. In the rare circumstance in which there has been a clear decrement in left ventricular performance in the still-asymptomatic patient, aortic valve replacement is probably advisable. Some experts have advocated aortic valve replacement in asymptomatic patients with severe AS because of a small (1%–2%) but definite risk of sudden death in such patients. This strategy exposes all patients with the disease to the risk of the operation and of harboring a prosthetic valve to benefit the small group at risk for sudden death. Exercise testing once contraindicated in patients with AS, now appears useful in helping to define a high risk group of asymptomatic patients or to demonstrate latent symptoms. In such cases, stress testing may be useful in assessing symptomatic status and its use is becoming more widespread. Exercise testing in patients with AS must be performed with extreme caution, and probably should be left in the hands of the cardiologist.

At the other end of the spectrum, even patients who present with advanced heart failure and severe left ventricular dysfunction may still benefit from aortic valve replacement, especially if the mean transvalvular gradient exceeds 30 mm Hg. In this case, surgery affords an acute reduction in left ventricular afterload, permitting immediate improvement in left ventricular performance. Thus, many such patients are still surgical candidates and should be referred for evaluation.

Table 32–1 summarizes the clinical and echocardiographic markers that guide the primary care physician's timing for referral of aortic stenosis patients for specialized care.

TABLE 32–1

Aortic Stenosis: Guidelines for Medical Therapy and for Referral for Specialized Care

Symptoms	Doppler Gradient (Peak to Peak)	Course of Action
None	<30 mm Hg	Observe
None	>30 mm Hg	Refer for exercise testing
Equivocal	>30 mm Hg	Refer for further evaluation
Angina, syncope or CHF	>30 mm Hg	Refer for further evaluation
CHF	Any level	Refer for further evaluation
Angina syncope	<30 mm Hg	Consider another cause
Symptomatic but aortic valve surgery contraindicated	>30 mm Hg	Consider balloon aortic valvotomy

CHF, congestive heart failure.

MITRAL STENOSIS

Almost all cases of acquired mitral stenosis (MS) result from rheumatic heart disease. Although the attack rate of rheumatic fever is slightly higher in men than in women, MS develops far more frequently in women than men, with a 4 : 1 female-to-male ratio. Typically, symptoms of MS develop in the fourth and fifth decades of life. In many cases, the woman with MS is asymptomatic until her first pregnancy, when increased hemodynamic demand results in cardiac decompensation. Although it has been debated for decades, it appears that in most cases of MS occurring in Western countries, the rheumatic disease spares the myocardium and muscle function is normal. Thus, the symptoms of MS usually do not accrue from contractile dysfunction but rather are caused by the obstruction to blood flow across the mitral valve itself.[6]

Opening of the normal mitral valve in early diastole creates a common chamber between the left atrium and the left ventricle, allowing for equalization of left atrial and left ventricular pressures early in diastole. As shown in Figures 32–4 and 32–5, MS obstructs blood flow and causes a persistent pressure gradient between the left atrium and the left ventricle. This obstruction to flow reduces filling of the left ventricle, raises left atrial pressure, and causes pulmonary congestion and reduced cardiac output. Thus, the classic features of left-sided congestive heart failure are manifested without overt left ventricular muscle dysfunction. Because the right ventricle has the responsibility for generating the force that drives blood across the mitral valve, the stenosis places a progressive pressure overload on the right ventricle. Secondary, reversible pulmonary vasoconstriction and pulmonary vascular thickening often develop along with the MS, further adding to the burden on the right

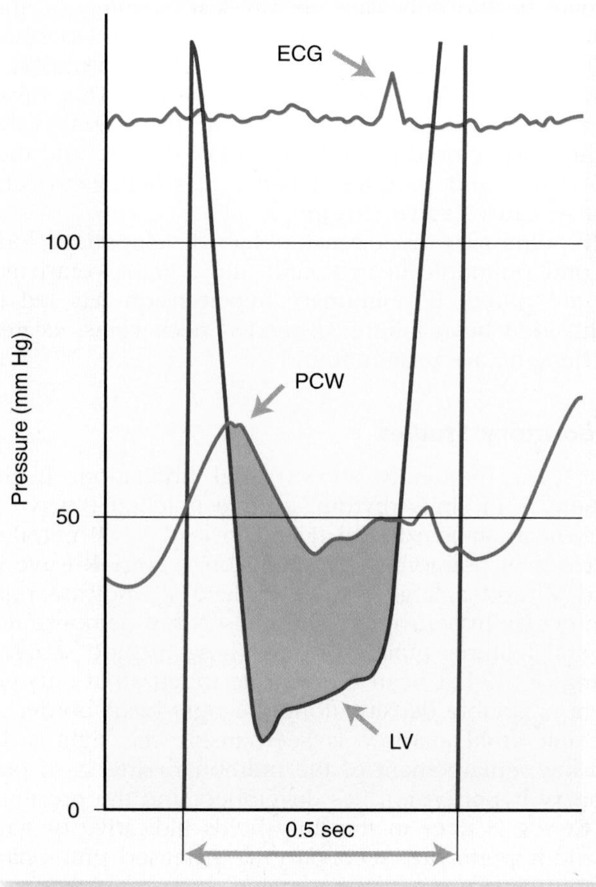

FIGURE 32–4. Pressure tracings taken from a patient with mitral stenosis demonstrate a large diastolic pressure gradient (shaded area) between the pulmonary capillary wedge pressure (PCW) representing left atrial pressure and the left ventricular pressure (LV). ECG, electrocardiogram. (Redrawn from Carabello BA, Grossman W: Calculation of stenotic valve orifice area. In Baim DS, Grossman W [eds]: Cardiac Catheterization, Angiography, and Intervention. 5th ed. Baltimore, Williams & Wilkins, 1996.)

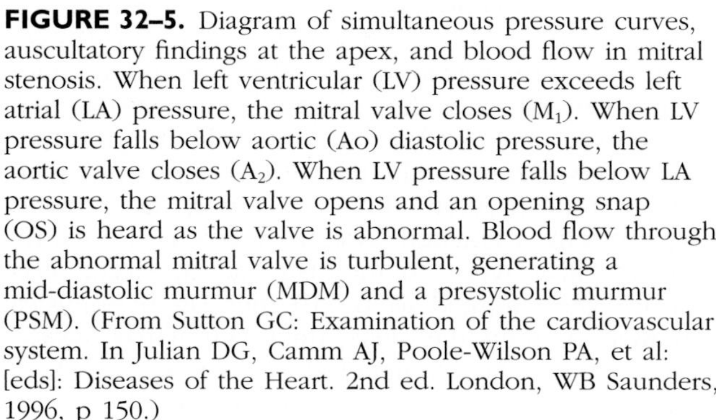

FIGURE 32–5. Diagram of simultaneous pressure curves, auscultatory findings at the apex, and blood flow in mitral stenosis. When left ventricular (LV) pressure exceeds left atrial (LA) pressure, the mitral valve closes (M_1). When LV pressure falls below aortic (Ao) diastolic pressure, the aortic valve closes (A_2). When LV pressure falls below LA pressure, the mitral valve opens and an opening snap (OS) is heard as the valve is abnormal. Blood flow through the abnormal mitral valve is turbulent, generating a mid-diastolic murmur (MDM) and a presystolic murmur (PSM). (From Sutton GC: Examination of the cardiovascular system. In Julian DG, Camm AJ, Poole-Wilson PA, et al: [eds]: Diseases of the Heart. 2nd ed. London, WB Saunders, 1996, p 150.)

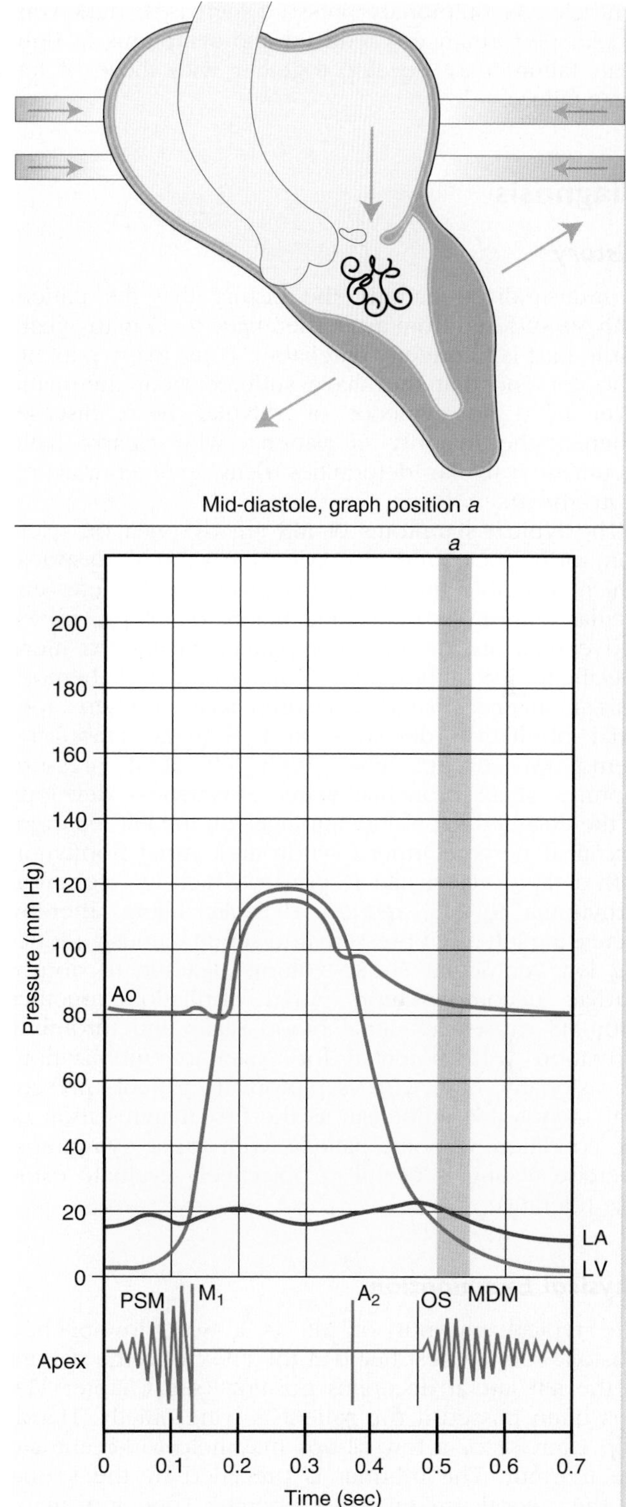

ventricle. As pulmonary pressure increases, right ventricular performance is reduced and symptoms of right heart failure may develop together with those of left heart failure.

Diagnosis

History

In industrialized nations, the history that the patient with MS suffered from acute rheumatic fever many years in the past is frequently unreliable. Thus, many patients who contend that they have suffered from rheumatic fever have no evidence of valvular heart disease, whereas the majority of patients who clearly have rheumatic valvular deformities deny ever contracting acute rheumatic fever.

The typical symptoms of MS are dyspnea on exertion, orthopnea, and paroxysmal nocturnal dyspnea, which resemble the symptoms produced by left ventricular failure. As right-sided failure develops, ascites and edema are frequent complaints. Symptoms more specific for MS (although less common) include hemoptysis, hoarseness, sudden decompensation when rapid atrial fibrillation develops, and systemic embolism. Hemoptysis occurs when high left atrial pressure ruptures small bronchial veins. Hoarseness develops as the enlarged left atrium impinges on the left recurrent laryngeal nerve (Ortner's syndrome). Atrial fibrillation with a rapid ventricular response, which is a common arrhythmia in MS, reduces diastolic filling, thereby increasing left atrial pressure and simultaneously reducing left ventricular stroke volume, leading to abrupt cardiac decompensation. Atrial fibrillation together with MS causes left atrial blood stasis and thrombus formation with potential for systemic embolization. Occasionally, otherwise asymptomatic patients present with a systemic embolism as the first manifestation of the condition. In some patients with vague symptoms, exercise testing is useful to objectively evaluate exercise tolerance.

Physical Examination

The typical murmur of MS is a soft, low-pitched diastolic rumble best heard at the apex with the patient in the left lateral decubitus position (see Chapter 11). It is often missed if the patient is lying quietly. Handgrip exercise or a few sit-ups may help to accentuate the murmur. The murmur is preceded by the sound of the stenotic mitral valve opening (opening snap) (see Fig. 32–5). High left atrial pressure in severe disease opens the mitral valve early in diastole, causing the interval between S_2 and the opening snap to be short (60 to 80 msec). In less-severe cases of MS, lower left atrial pressure delays opening of the mitral valve and the S_2-opening snap interval is longer (>100 msec).

Another important clue to the presence of MS is a loud first heart sound (S_1). In some cases where neither an opening snap nor a mitral rumble is audible, a loud S_1 may be the only clue on physical examination that MS is present. The S_1 is typically loud in MS because the transmitral gradient holds the valve open until it is closed by the force of ventricular systole. This varies from the normal condition where the mitral valve leaflets drift closed toward the end of diastole and thus move less and produce a softer S_1 when ventricular systole causes valve closure.

If pulmonary hypertension has developed, a loud second pulmonic heart sound and a right ventricular lift are noted. If pulmonary hypertension has led to right-sided heart failure, distended neck veins, ascites, and edema are usually found.

Laboratory Studies

The ECG frequently shows atrial fibrillation. If the patient is in sinus rhythm, a large notched P-wave is present in standard lead II and in lead V_1 (P mitrale). In cases of pulmonary hypertension, a large R-wave in lead V_1 and a large S-wave in lead V_6 indicate right ventricular hypertrophy. The chest x-ray demonstrates several features typical of MS. These include straightening of the left heart border due to left atrial enlargement, a double density along the right heart border as the left atrial shadow is seen inside the right atrial shadow, enlargement of the pulmonary arteries if pulmonary hypertension has developed, and the presence of Kerley B lines in the lung fields indicative of lymphatic hypertrophy secondary to increased pulmonary venous pressure.

Despite the utility of the physical examination, ECG, and chest x-ray in diagnosing MS, echocardiography is the best technique for evaluating the patient with this disorder (Fig. 32–6). Doppler interrogation (see Chapter 5) can derive the transvalvular gradient and estimate the flow rate and mitral valve orifice area. In addition, the echocardiographic appearance of the valve is an excellent guide as to whether balloon mitral valvotomy, a nonsurgical procedure for relief of the stenosis, is applicable. Those patients with relatively pliant valve leaflets, little involvement of the subvalvular apparatus, limited mitral valve calcification, and no or mild mitral regurgitation are excellent candidates for balloon mitral valvotomy. Left ventricular ejection fraction and pulmonary artery pressure can also be estimated. If even mild tricuspid regurgitation exists, Doppler interrogation of the tricuspid valve can assess the reverse gradient between the right ventricle and the right atrium during systole. This in turn can be used to calculate pulmonary artery systolic pressure. If, for instance, the echocardiographically estimated systolic gradient across the tricuspid valve were 36 mm Hg and the right atrial pressure were judged to be 10 mm Hg by physical examination, then the peak right ventricular systolic pressure would be estimated at 46 mm Hg, which, in the absence of pulmonary stenosis, would also be the pulmonary artery systolic pressure.

Cardiac catheterization is usually not necessary to define the severity of MS. Catheterization is performed in older patients to identify coronary disease or as a precursor to balloon valvotomy.

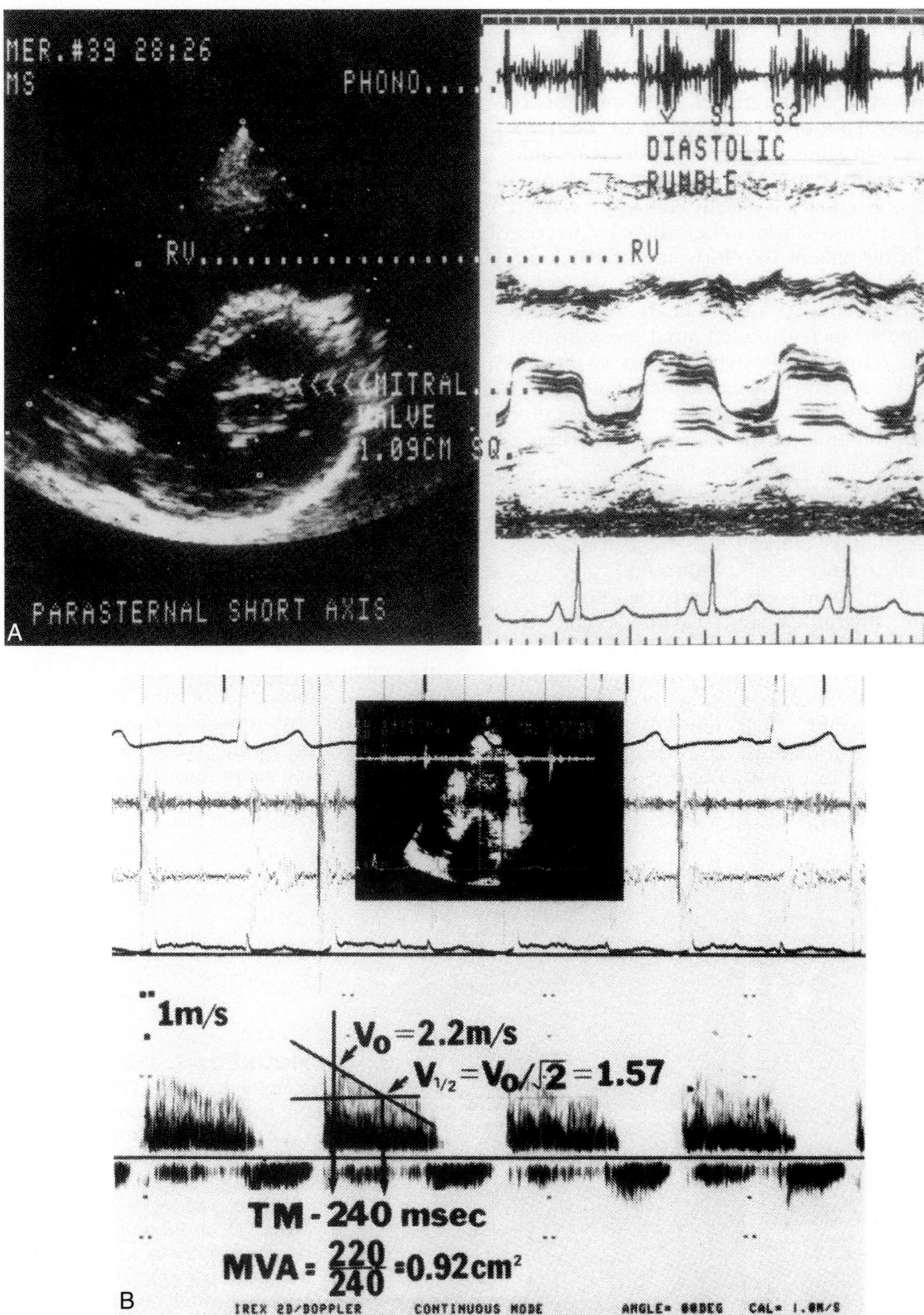

FIGURE 32–6. *A*, Cross-sectional image of the mitral valve used to planimeter its area. M-mode echocardiogram is at the right. This very stenotic valve has an orifice area of 1.09 cm^2. RV, right ventricle. *B*, The Doppler flow pattern for a patient with mitral stenosis. It demonstrates delay in decay of flow velocity that is maintained by the transmitral gradient. This principle, in turn, is used to calculate the pressure half-time that is divided into the empirical constant of 220 to calculate a mitral valve area (MVA). TM, time from T_o to $T_{1/2}$; V_o, velocity at valve opening. (A and B, From Assey ME, Usher BW, Carabello BA: The patient with valvular heart disease. In Pepine CJ, Hill JA, Lambert CR [eds]: Diagnostic and Therapeutic Cardiac Catheterization. 2nd ed. Baltimore, Williams & Wilkins, 1994.)

Management

No therapy is required in asymptomatic patients in normal sinus rhythm. Symptoms of mild pulmonary congestion usually can be controlled with diuretics alone. For patients in sinus rhythm, digitalis is of little benefit because contractile function is usually normal and the symptoms of congestive heart failure are caused primarily by valve obstruction rather than by a contractile deficit. If the patient develops atrial fibrillation, however, prompt slowing of the heart rate is necessary, because, as noted previously, a rapid heart rate reduces mitral inflow, thereby increasing left atrial pressure and reducing cardiac output. Although digoxin is usually the drug of choice for chronically maintaining control of the ventricular response, intravenous diltiazem or esmolol may be preferable in the acute setting when a more rapid reduction in heart rate is required. Once heart rate has been reduced, restoration of sinus rhythm with quinidine, procainamide, sotalol, or amiodarone is usually achieved. If this therapy fails to restore sinus rhythm, electrical cardioversion is indicated.

If atrial fibrillation cannot easily and consistently be reverted to sinus rhythm, if sinus rhythm cannot be maintained, or if symptoms increase to greater than New York Heart Association classification II, that is, if patients develop symptoms on mild or moderate exertion, or if there is evidence that pulmonary hypertension is developing, mechanical correction of MS is usually warranted because further delay worsens the prognosis. Unlike in AS, in MS, in most cases an excellent durable commissurotomy can be performed by balloon mitral valvotomy (Fig. 32–7).[7] In this procedure, transseptal catheterization is performed by advancing a sheathed catheter and needle from the right femoral vein to the right atrial side of the intra-atrial septum. The needle is advanced to puncture the septum, and the sheath is passed over the needle into the left atrium. A guide wire is passed through the sheath into the left ventricle. A balloon dilatation catheter is placed over the guide wire across the mitral orifice where it is inflated, producing a separation of the valve leaflets at the commissures. Typically, this results in doubling of the mitral valve area and reduces the transmitral valve gradient to 6 mm Hg or less, in turn improving symptomatic status. If the valve anatomy is unfavorable for balloon valvotomy, as can be determined by echocardiography (see earlier), open surgical commissurotomy or mitral valve replacement should be performed.

In patients with MS and chronic atrial fibrillation who are not candidates for operation or balloon valvotomy because of coexisting disease or refusal to undergo the procedure, anticoagulation is desirable because the combination of atrial fibrillation and MS produces an incidence of stroke of 5% to 10% per year in the absence of anticoagulation.

In summary, echocardiography should be performed when MS is suspected or first detected. Patients are then followed by repeated clinical examination and echocardiography until symptoms limit lifestyle, atrial fibrillation occurs, or pulmonary hypertension (systolic pressure ≥50 mm Hg) develops. At this time, the patient

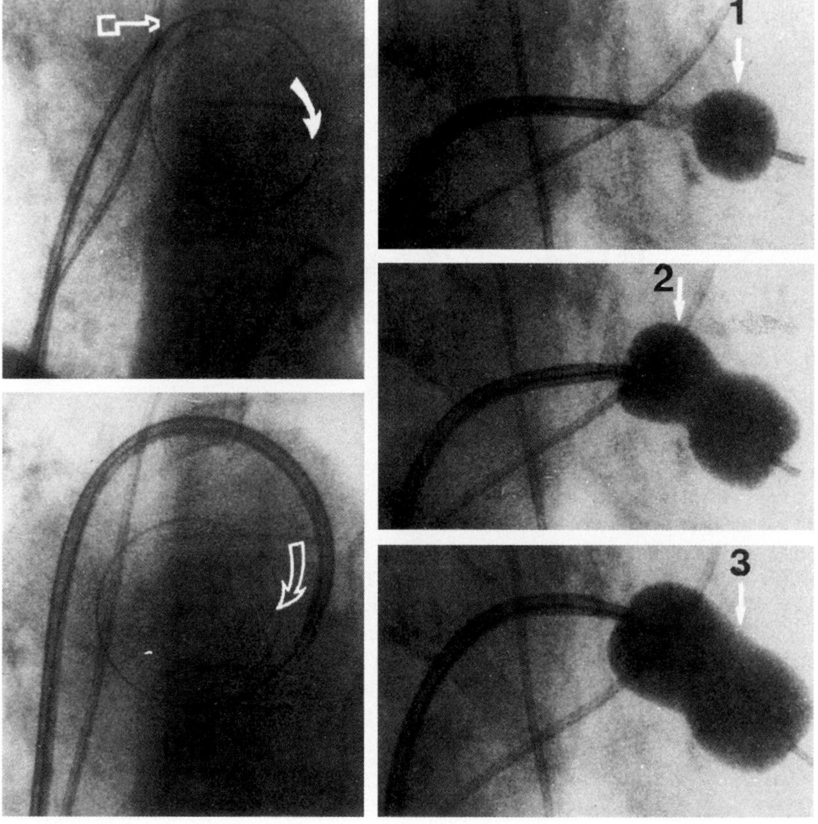

FIGURE 32–7. The steps of a balloon mitral valvotomy. *Top left,* Puncture of the interatrial septum with a guide wire *(curved arrow)* advanced across the septum through the mitral valve. *Bottom left,* A large sheath has been advanced over the guide wire *(curved arrow). Top right,* (1) An Inoue balloon catheter has been advanced across the mitral valve and the distal portion has been inflated and retracted snugly against the mitral valve. *Middle right,* (2) The proximal portion of the balloon has been partially inflated, leaving a waist at the site of the mitral valve stenosis. *Bottom right,* (3) The balloon has now been fully inflated and the waist has nearly disappeared, indicating successful separation in at least one of the commissures. (From Berman AD, McKay RG, Grossman W: Balloon valvuloplasty. In Baim DS, Grossman W [eds]: Cardiac Catheterization, Angiography, and Intervention. 5th ed. Baltimore, Williams & Wilkins, 1996.)

TABLE 32–2

Mitral Stenosis: Guidelines for Medical Therapy and for Referral for Specialized Care

Symptoms (Including Atrial Fibrillation)	Valve Area (cm^2)	Evidence of Pulmonary Hypertension (Clinical or Doppler)	Course of Action
None	>1.0	No	Observe
None	<1.0	No	Exercise to evaluate symptoms objectively; refer if exercise is severely limited
Mild	>1.0 <1.5	No	Observe
None	<1.5	Yes	Refer for further evaluation
Atrial fibrillation	<1.5	No or yes	Refer for further evaluation
Moderate	<1.5	No or yes	Refer for further evaluation

is referred for definitive mechanical correction of the stenosis.

In patients who present with far-advanced disease with severe pulmonary hypertension, surgical risk is increased. It is important to note that after successful operation, pulmonary artery pressure usually returns to or toward normal. Thus, pulmonary hypertension by itself is not a contraindication to referral for surgery or valvotomy.

Table 32–2 contains clinical and echocardiographic markers that guide the primary care physician in timing referral of mitral stenosis patients for specialized care.

MITRAL REGURGITATION

The mitral valve apparatus is composed of the mitral annulus, the mitral leaflets, the chordae tendineae, and the papillary muscles. When abnormalities of any of these four components cause mitral regurgitation (MR), the regurgitation is classified as *primary*. In disease states where ventricular dilatation and changes in ventricular geometry cause malalignment of the papillary muscles, the regurgitation is considered to be *secondary*. Common causes of primary MR include endocarditis, spontaneous rupture of chordae tendineae, rheumatic heart disease, myocardial ischemia, the mitral valve prolapse syndrome, and collagen vascular disease.

MR places a volume overload on the left ventricle. Normally, all of the blood that the left ventricle ejects enters the aorta and constitutes the effective forward cardiac output. In MR, a portion of the left ventricular end-diastolic volume is ejected into the left atrium; this regurgitation may be considered to be wasted or ineffective cardiac output.[8] Additionally, the regurgitant volume increases left atrial pressure, which is referred to the lungs where it causes pulmonary congestion. As shown in Figure 32–8, in acute MR when left ventricular hypertrophy has not yet had time to develop, there is a modest increase in end-diastolic volume as sarcomeres are stretched by the volume overload. This use of the Frank-Starling mechanism allows a modest increase in total stroke volume and also increases the work-generating capability of the ventricle. As the disease becomes more chronic, eccentric hypertrophy develops, allowing forward stroke volume to be returned toward normal. Additionally, the increased volume of both the left atrium and the left ventricle that develops with time allows the regurgitant volume to be accommodated at a lower diastolic pressure, reducing the symptoms of pulmonary congestion. This compensated stage may persist for several years but, if uncorrected, eventually leads to left ventricular muscle dysfunction.[9] A major goal of the management of MR is early recognition of left ventricular dysfunction, so that surgery can be performed to correct the MR before left ventricular dysfunction becomes permanent. It should be emphasized that the increased preload that results from the volume overload and the tendency for the regurgitant orifice to unload the ventricle during systole (reduced afterload) augment ventricular performance and cause ejection fraction to be higher than normal. In patients with MR, a fall of ejection fraction into the mid-normal range usually indicates the presence of muscle dysfunction.

Diagnosis

History

The patient with MR in the compensated phase of the disease is usually asymptomatic. Even fairly strenuous exercise is relatively well tolerated. In the acute phase before compensation has developed or later in the disease when decompensation is beginning to develop, symptoms typical of left-sided congestive heart failure (dyspnea on exertion, orthopnea, and paroxysmal nocturnal dyspnea) occur or the new onset of atrial fibrillation in the absence of other symptoms may presage the onset of left ventricular dysfunction.

Physical Examination

MR is most commonly recognized by the presence of a holosystolic murmur heard best at the apex, often radiating to the axilla (see Chapter 11). It is often accompanied by a systolic thrill. The enlarged volume-overloaded left ventricle causes a hyperactive precordium while displacing the point of maximal impulse downward and to the left. The rapid filling of the left ventricle in diastole by the large volume of blood stored in the left atrium during systole usually creates a third heart sound (S_3). As such, an S_3 in MR may simply be an indicator of the severity of the regurgitation and does

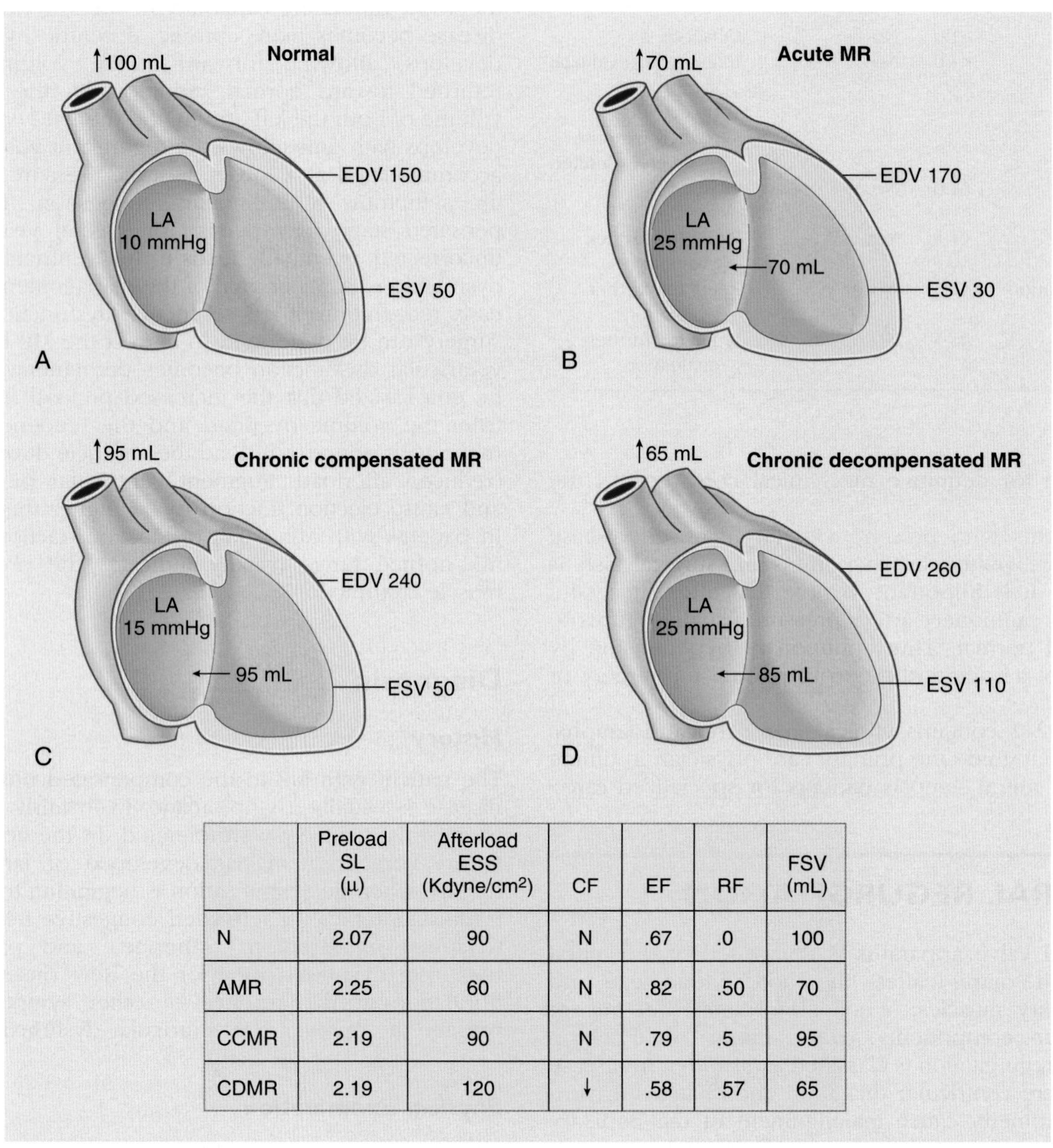

	Preload SL (μ)	Afterload ESS (Kdyne/cm²)	CF	EF	RF	FSV (mL)
N	2.07	90	N	.67	.0	100
AMR	2.25	60	N	.82	.50	70
CCMR	2.19	90	N	.79	.5	95
CDMR	2.19	120	↓	.58	.57	65

not necessarily mean that the patient is in heart failure. If secondary pulmonary hypertension has developed, findings of right-sided failure may also be present.

Laboratory Studies

The ECG often shows left atrial abnormality and left ventricular hypertrophy in severe, chronic MR. The chest x-ray shows an enlarged left ventricle and pulmonary congestion if the patient is in heart failure. The finding of a normal-sized heart on chest x-ray suggests either that the MR is relatively mild or that it is acute and eccentric hypertrophy has not yet had time to develop.

As in other valvular disorders, echocardiography is key in the assessment of mitral regurgitation (see Chapter 5) (Fig. 32–9). During echocardiography, left ventricular dimensions and performance are gauged. Color-flow Doppler provides an estimate of the severity of the MR. Often, the pathoanatomy that has produced the MR is discernible during transthoracic echocardiography. If not, transesophageal echocardiography that achieves superb imaging of the mitral valve is usually capable of diagnosing the cause of the MR.

Because the echocardiographic assessment of the severity of MR is occasionally inaccurate, cardiac catheterization usually is performed before surgery to assess hemodynamics, the ventriculographic severity of MR, and the coronary anatomy.

Management

Surgical Therapy

The only definitive treatment for MR is mitral valve surgery, which should be carried out before irreversible left ventricular dysfunction has developed. As noted earlier, the favorable loading conditions of MR augment

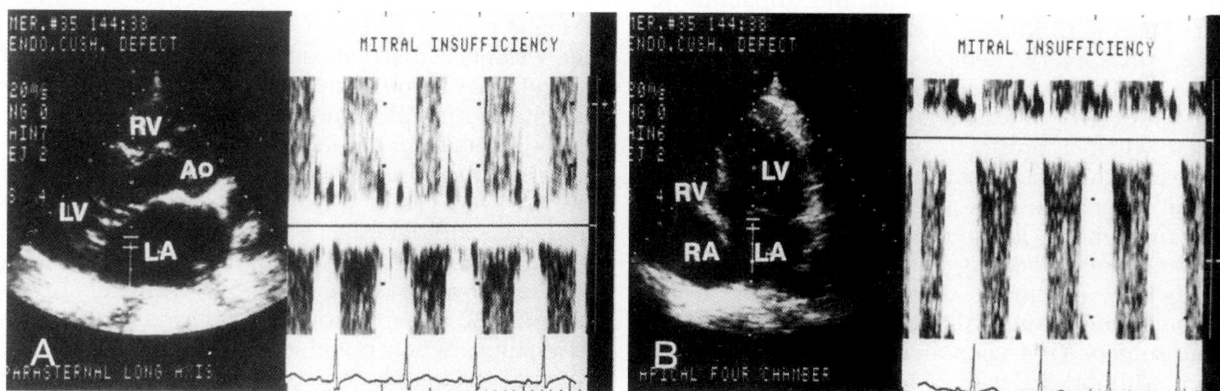

FIGURE 32–9. Parasternal long axis (*A*) and apical four-chamber (*B*) views of the heart of a patient with mitral regurgitation. Both left ventricular and left atrial enlargement are seen. Continuous-wave Doppler interrogation demonstrates mitral regurgitant flow. Ao, aorta; LA, left atrium; LV, left ventricle; RA, right atrium; RV, right ventricle. (A and B, From Assey ME, Usher BW, Carabello BA: The patient with valvular heart disease. In Pepine CJ, Hill JA, Lambert CR [eds]: Diagnostic and Therapeutic Cardiac Catheterization. 2nd ed. Baltimore, Williams & Wilkins, 1994.)

FIGURE 32–8. The pathophysiologic stages of mitral regurgitation (MR). *A* and *B*, Normal physiology (N) is contrasted with that of acute mitral regurgitation (MR). In AMR, the volume overload of MR increases sarcomere length (SL), augmenting preload. Increased SL is reflected by an increase in end-diastolic volume (EDV). The new pathologic pathway for ejection into the left atrium (LA) reduces afterload as quantified by end-systolic stress (ESS), allowing the left ventricle to eject more completely. Enhanced ejection is reflected by a fall in end-systolic volume (ESV). As a result, the total stroke volume increases to 140 mL, but because 50% is regurgitated into the LA (regurgitant fraction [RF] 0.50), forward stroke volume (FSV) falls. Ejection fraction (EF) increases, although contractile function (CF) is normal but not increased. *C*, Chronic compensated mitral regurgitation (CCMR). In this phase of MR, eccentric cardiac hypertrophy produces a further increase in EDV. This allows for a large increase in total stroke volume (190 mL) so that FSV returns to nearly normal. The now-enlarged LA can accommodate the regurgitant volume at a lower pressure, so that left atrial pressure declines. CF remains normal, and EF remains increased. *D*, Chronic decompensated mitral regurgitation (CDMR). In this phase, CF has been reduced from muscle damage caused by prolonged severe volume overload. Reduced CF reduces the effectiveness of left ventricular ejection and ESV increases. There is a further increase in diastolic volume, which is not compensatory for the increase in ESV, resulting in a fall in total and forward stroke volume. Concomitantly, increased EDV worsens the MR by annular dilatation and papillary muscle malalignment and regurgitant fraction increases. EF is reduced from the CCMR state but often remains within the normal range.

ejection performance. Thus, a supernormal ejection fraction is "normal" in MR. In order to achieve a surgical outcome that allows for a normal postoperative life span, relief of symptoms, and normal postoperative ejection performance, MR should be corrected before left ventricular ejection fraction falls below 60% or before echocardiographic end-systolic minor-axis diameter exceeds 45 mm. Further delay in operation, even in *asymptomatic* patients, may result in persistent postoperative left ventricular dysfunction or reduced life span.[10]

Currently, three types of operation are performed for the correction of MR—mitral valve replacement with removal of the mitral valve apparatus, mitral valve replacement with preservation of at least part of the mitral valve apparatus, and mitral valve repair in which a prosthetic valve is avoided and the native valve is reconstructed so that it becomes competent. Recently, the importance of the mitral valve apparatus in maintaining left ventricular function has been recognized. The mitral valve apparatus not only prevents MR but also acts as an internal skeleton integrating left ventricular contraction. Destruction of the apparatus reduces ejection performance and worsens postoperative outcome. Thus, every attempt should be made to conserve the continuity between the valve leaflet and the papillary muscle of at least a part of the mitral apparatus, even when a prosthetic valve is inserted. Mitral valve repair is the most desirable operation, because the mitral valve apparatus is conserved, retaining its function of augmenting left ventricular performance and at the same time avoiding the risks of a prosthesis, which include prosthetic valve failure, endocarditis, and thromboembolism.[11] Although controversial, some advocate surgery for asymptomatic patients with severe MR even without evidence of left ventricular dysfunction if it is nearly certain that a mitral valve repair can be effected. Arguments for this position are that operative mortality is low (<1%), no prosthesis is inserted, and that early repair "cures" the disease, obviating the need for frequent surveillance follow-up examinations. The major difficulty with this position is that an unanticipated valve replacement may be mandated because the surgeon finds the valve irreparable at the time of surgery. In this case, the patient is committed to extra years with a prosthetic valve in place increasing the risk of prosthesis-related complications.

Medical Therapy

Medical therapy in MR is reserved for acute symptomatic MR and for patients with chronic symptomatic MR deemed not to be surgical candidates. In *acute* MR, the use of vasodilators such as ACE inhibitors or nitroprusside guided by Swan-Ganz catheterization is the mainstay of therapy. By reducing afterload, vasodilators increase aortic flow preferentially, at once increasing forward flow while reducing regurgitant volume and left atrial pressure. Concomitantly, vasodilator-mediated reduction in preload helps to relieve the symptoms of pulmonary congestion and also reduces left ventricular volume, which in part restores mitral valve competence.

TABLE 32–3

Guidelines for Referral for Valve Surgery in Patients with Severe Mitral Regurgitation

Symptoms	ESD (mm)		EF	Course of Action
None	<45		>0.60	Observe
Mild	<45		>0.60	Observe
>Mild	<45		>0.60	Refer for further evaluation
None	>45	or	<0.60	Refer for further evaluation
Yes	>45	or	<0.60	Refer for further evaluation

EF, ejection fraction; ESD, end-systolic left ventricular diameter.

If acute MR has resulted in hypotension, intra-aortic balloon pumping, which reduces afterload while maintaining blood pressure, is substituted for vasodilators. In asymptomatic patients, no medical therapy is indicated.

Unlike aortic regurgitation, in which the use of vasodilators may forestall surgery in patients with asymptomatic chronic disease (see later), there is no convincing evidence that vasodilator therapy is of benefit in *chronic asymptomatic* MR. In patients with symptomatic chronic mitral regurgitation, digoxin, diuretics, and vasodilators form the mainstay of medical therapy.

In *summary*, asymptomatic patients with MR should be followed yearly with history, physical examination, and echocardiography. If symptoms develop or if ejection fraction declines to or approaches 60% or if the left ventricular end-systolic minor-axis diameter approaches 45 mm, the patient should be referred for preoperative evaluation. When possible, patients should be referred to surgeons known for excellence in mitral valve repair. In patients with far-advanced disease, referral also is indicated for assessment for surgery. These patients may still improve, provided the mitral valve apparatus can be preserved at the time of operation. If surgery is not deemed feasible, therapy with digoxin, diuretics, and an ACE inhibitor is indicated.

In severe acute MR, patients are usually unstable and require specialized therapy with intravenous vasodilators or intra-aortic balloon counterpulsation.

Table 32–3 presents markers that guide the primary care physician in the timing of referral of patients with MR for specialized care.

MITRAL VALVE PROLAPSE

Mitral valve prolapse (MVP) refers to a group of conditions in which one or both mitral valve leaflets become superior to the plane of the mitral annulus (prolapse into the left atrium) during systole.[12] The causes of MVP range from variations of normal physiology to severe anatomic deformity of the mitral valve. The former include normal subjects during the Valsalva maneuver as well as patients with atrial septal defect, in whom the left ventricle is reduced in volume; this reduces tension on the mitral apparatus, allowing the mitral valve to prolapse into the left atrium during systole. On release of the Valsalva maneuver or after repair of the atrial septal defect, left ventricular volume returns to normal and the mitral valve prolapse disappears. This variety of MVP is probably completely benign.

The most common pathologic cause of MVP is myxomatous degeneration of the valve. Other causes of pathologic prolapse include Marfan's syndrome, collagen vascular disease, and coronary artery disease. The term *mitral valve prolapse syndrome* refers to a degenerative condition of the mitral valve in which thickened and redundant leaflets are associated with atypical chest pain, autonomic dysfunction, and a modest risk of complications, including progression to severe MVP, stroke, and infective endocarditis.

Diagnosis

History

Most patients with MVP are asymptomatic. A minority complain of atypical chest pain, palpitations, fatigue, and orthostatic lightheadedness. When MR is severe, the symptoms described previously in the section on MR may be present.

Physical Examination

Another name for the MVP syndrome is the *click-murmur syndrome*, derived from the findings during physical examination of patients with the disease. Classically, MVP produces a mid-systolic click and a late-systolic murmur (see Chapter 11). The click occurs as the elongated mitral valve apparatus reaches the end of its tether in mid systole. At this point, the valve leaflets pass the point of coaptation, causing mitral valve incompetence, and the murmur of MR commences. In some patients, only the click or only the murmur is present. In others, neither physical finding is present despite MVP proved by echocardiography.

The presence of the click and murmur and their position in the systolic portion of the cardiac cycle vary with maneuvers that alter left ventricular volume (see Chapter 11). Maneuvers that decrease volume, such as assuming the upright position or the Valsalva maneuver, cause the valve to prolapse earlier, so that the click is heard earlier in systole and the murmur becomes more holosystolic in nature. Maneuvers that increase left ventricular volume, such as assuming recumbency or squatting, reduce the amount of prolapse and may cause the click and murmur to disappear entirely. With time, in some patients, degeneration of the valve worsens, so that the murmur becomes progressively more holosystolic as the severity of MR increases.

Laboratory Studies

The electrocardiogram in MVP is often normal, but it may demonstrate nonspecific ST segment and T-wave abnormalities, especially in the inferior leads.

Echocardiography (see Chapter 5) is the diagnostic modality of choice to confirm this condition. The diagnosis of MVP is based on the appearance of one or both leaflets of the mitral valve superior to the annular plane in systole. The plane of the mitral annulus is not flat but rather has the configuration of a saddle (hyperbolic paraboloid). This configuration may cause the mitral valve to appear to be prolapsing in the echocardiographic apical four-chamber view when, in fact, prolapse is absent. Thus, the diagnosis of MVP seen in the apical four-chamber view must be confirmed in the parasternal long-axis view to avoid overdiagnosis of this condition. Diagnoses of MVP made before general recognition of this principle in 1987 may, therefore, have been made in error. Perhaps more important than diagnosing the prolapse itself (which can usually be detected on physical examination), echocardiography displays the morphology of the mitral valve (Fig. 32–10). As noted earlier, it is those patients whose valves are clearly anatomically abnormal (misshapen, redundant, and thickened) who are at risk for most of the complications of the disease. Doppler interrogation of the valve also allows estimation of the degree of mitral regurgitation that might be present.

Management

The majority of patients with MVP are asymptomatic and require no therapy.[12] Those patients who have clearly abnormal valvular anatomy and who also have the murmur of MR should undergo endocarditis prophylaxis for those procedures that cause a bacteremia (see Chapter 33). In patients who complain of chest pain or palpitations, beta-blockers, diltiazem or verapamil may be effective therapy. Some patients with MVP are at risk for stroke. These appear to be those patients who have anatomically misshapen valves and the murmur of MR. It has been speculated that this combination results in valve damage or perhaps denudation of the endothelium in the left atrium, providing a nidus for clot formation, which in turn, might embolize. In patients with thickened and redundant mitral valves, daily low-dose aspirin therapy is probably indicated, although no trials have been performed to substantiate this recommendation. When MVP has led to severe MR, the regurgitation is treated using the same principles detailed previously for the treatment of mitral regurgitation from any cause.

CHRONIC AORTIC REGURGITATION

The aortic valve may become incompetent due to pathology of either the aortic valve leaflets or the aortic root. Endocarditis and rheumatic heart disease are common valvular causes of aortic regurgitation (AR). Idiopathic aortic root dilatation (annuloaortic ectasia) associated with hypertension and aging, Marfan's syn-

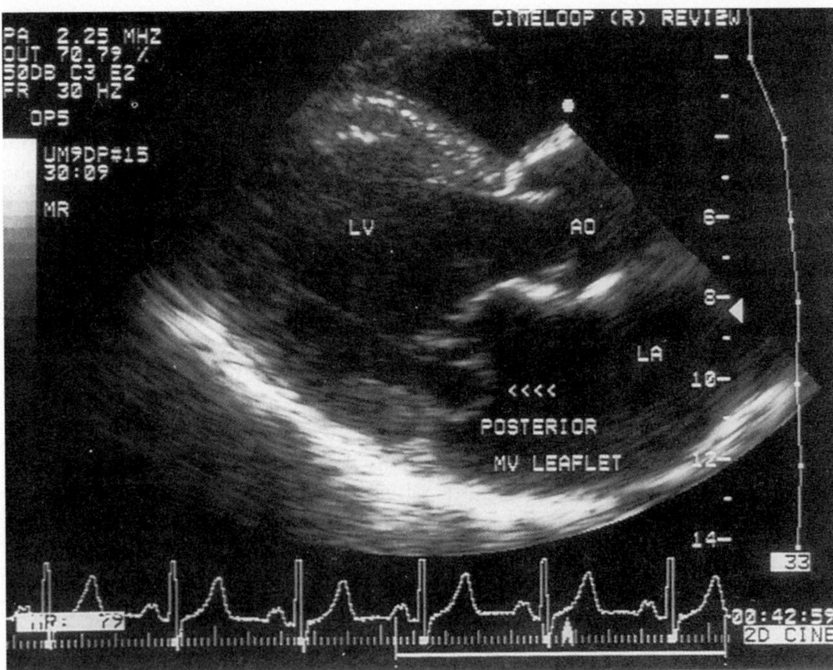

FIGURE 32–10. Two-dimensional echocardiogram shows severe prolapse of a thickened posterior mitral valve (MV) leaflet. Ao, aorta; LA, left atrium; LV, left ventricle. (From Carabello BA, Ballard WL, Gazes PC: Case #17. In Sahn SA, Heffner JE [eds]: Cardiology Pearls. Philadelphia, Hanley & Belfus, 1994.)

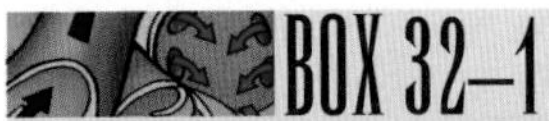

BOX 32–1

Causes of Aortic Regurgitation

AORTIC ROOT CAUSES	VALVE LEAFLET CAUSES
Aortic dissection	Infective endocarditis
Marfan's syndrome	Rheumatic heart disease
Annuloaortic ectasia	
Syphilis	
Ehlers-Danlos syndrome	
Ankylosing spondylitis	
Aortitis of any cause	
Pseudoxanthoma elasticum	
Systemic lupus erythematosus	

drome, aortic dissection, syphilis, and collagen vascular disease affect the aortic root, leading to AR. A more complete list of the causes of aortic regurgitation is provided in Box 32–1.

As in MR, AR exerts a volume overload on the left ventricle. Unlike MR, the excess stroke volume is ejected into a high-pressure chamber, the aorta, where it increases pulse pressure. Thus, systolic hypertension frequently accompanies AR, making it a combined pressure and volume overload.[8] Appropriately, the ventricular hypertrophy that occurs differs from that of MR. In AR, there are both eccentric hypertrophy to accommodate the volume overload and modest concentric hypertrophy to compensate for the pressure overload. As with severe MR, severe AR may be tolerated for a prolonged period of time. Eventually, however, left ventricular function declines. Thus, as with MR, AR should be corrected before left ventricular dysfunction becomes severe and irreversible.

Diagnosis

History

Patients with severe AR and normal left ventricular function may be remarkably asymptomatic, even during strenuous exertion. When symptoms do develop, they are usually those of left-sided congestive heart failure. Occasionally, angina occurs in patients with AR, although much less frequently than in patients with AS. Angina probably develops in part due to the relative diastolic hypotension that develops due to the valve incompetence. Because the coronary arteries fill in diastole, a lowered diastolic blood pressure reduces the driving force filling the coronary arteries and reduces coronary blood flow. When angina does occur in AR, it is frequently associated with vasodilatation and flushing. Less common complaints in patients with AR include syncope, an unpleasant awareness of the heartbeat, or carotid artery pain.

Physical Examination

The typical murmur of AR is a high-pitched, early decrescendo, blowing diastolic murmur heard best along the left sternal border when the patient is sitting upright (see Chapter 11). As the regurgitant jet impinges on the mitral valve, it may cause partial valve closure and a low-pitched rumble of physiologic MS (Austin Flint murmur). In chronic AR, the precordium is extremely active and the point of maximal impulse is displaced downward and to the left. The high total stroke volume and wide pulse pressure produce a myriad of signs (see Chapter 3). These include Corrigan's pulse (a brisk carotid upstroke with a rapid decline), de Musset's sign (bobbing of the head), Duroziez's sign (a systolic and diastolic bruit when the femoral artery is compressed by the bell of the stethoscope), Hill's sign (augmentation of the systolic femoral blood pressure of greater than 30 mm over brachial systolic pressure), and Quincke's pulse (systolic plethora and diastolic blanching of the nail bed when gentle pressure is placed on the nail).

Laboratory Studies

In severe AR, the electrocardiogram usually shows left ventricular hypertrophy. The chest x-ray demonstrates an enlarged heart, often with dilatation of the proximal aorta. The echocardiogram demonstrates an enlarged left ventricle (Fig. 32–11). The valvular or aortic root anatomy responsible for AR may be detected. Color-flow Doppler interrogation of the aortic valve demonstrates the AR and helps quantify its severity (Fig. 32–12).

When surgery is contemplated, cardiac catheterization is usually performed to confirm the echocardiographic estimate of regurgitant severity by aortography. Coronary arteriography is also performed to assess the presence of coronary artery disease.

Management

Timing of Operation

As with MR, AR must be corrected before the development of irreversible left ventricular dysfunction develops, if the symptoms of heart failure (if present) are to be relieved and the patient is to attain a normal postoperative life span. Unlike in MR, however, in most cases of AR, valve replacement instead of repair is necessary. Thus, in deciding when to operate, the risks of a prosthesis must be weighed against the risk of delaying surgery.[1] The "55 rule" has been extremely useful in making this decision. Sound studies demonstrate that a good outcome can be expected, provided that the left ventricular echocardiographic end-systolic minor-axis diameter does not exceed 55 mm and that the left ventricular ejection fraction is not lower than 55%. Thus, for asymptomatic patients, operation can be delayed until either symptoms develop or the aforementioned thresholds are approached. If end-systolic diameter is less than 40 mm, it is unlikely that ventricular dysfunction will develop within 2 years, and thus, echocardiography can safely be performed at 2-year intervals. For end-systolic diameters between 40 and 50 mm, yearly echocardiographic follow-up is recommended, and if end-systolic diameter is greater than 50 mm but less than 55 mm, echocardiographic follow-up should be performed every 6 months.[13] When symptoms of heart failure develop in a patient with severe AR, surgery should be performed regardless of the echocardiographic findings because the new onset of heart failure indicates cardiac decompensation.[14]

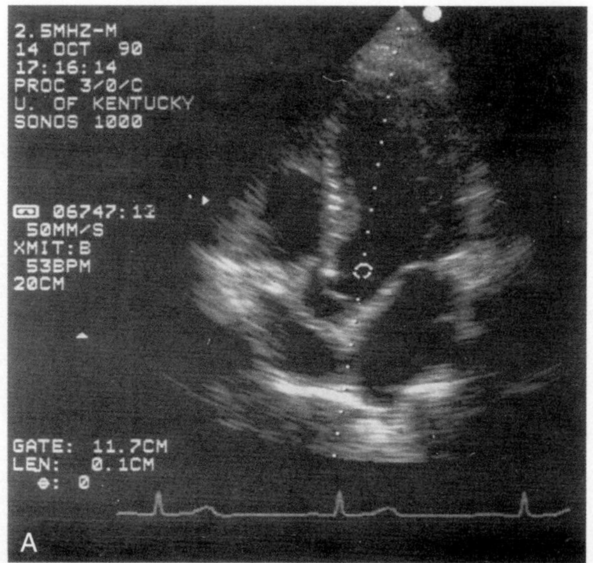

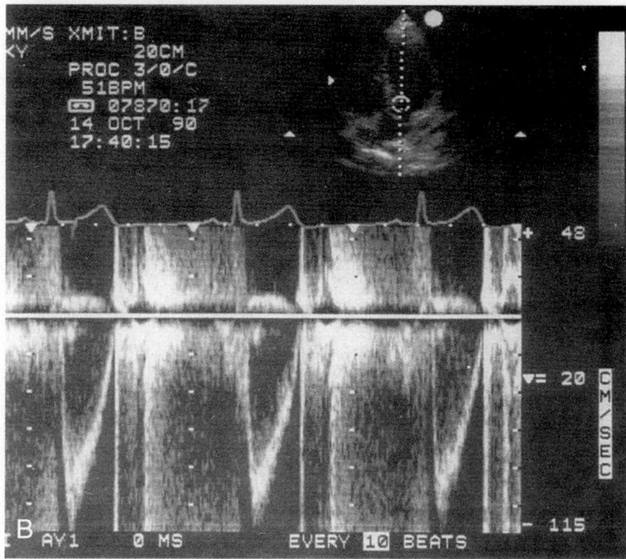

FIGURE 32–11. Pulsed-wave mapping technique for quantitating aortic regurgitation. Two-dimensional echocardiogram still frames were taken from the apical four-chamber view and show the location of the pulsed-wave sample volume (*A*) and spectral recordings from each site (*B*). Sample volume located just below the aortic valve and pulsed-wave recording demonstrate holodiastolic, high-velocity, and broad-banded signal indicative of turbulent regurgitant flow. (A and B, From Smith MD: Evaluation of valvular regurgitation by Doppler echocardiography. In Carabello BA [ed]: Valvular Heart Disease, vol 9. Philadelphia, WB Saunders, 1991.)

There is increasing evidence that vasodilator therapy in asymptomatic patients with normal left ventricular function can delay both the onset of left ventricular dysfunction and the need for surgery (Fig. 32–13).[15] The best documentation for this effect exists for nifedipine, although it is likely that other dihydropyridine calcium channel blockers and possibly ACE inhibitors may provide the same benefit.

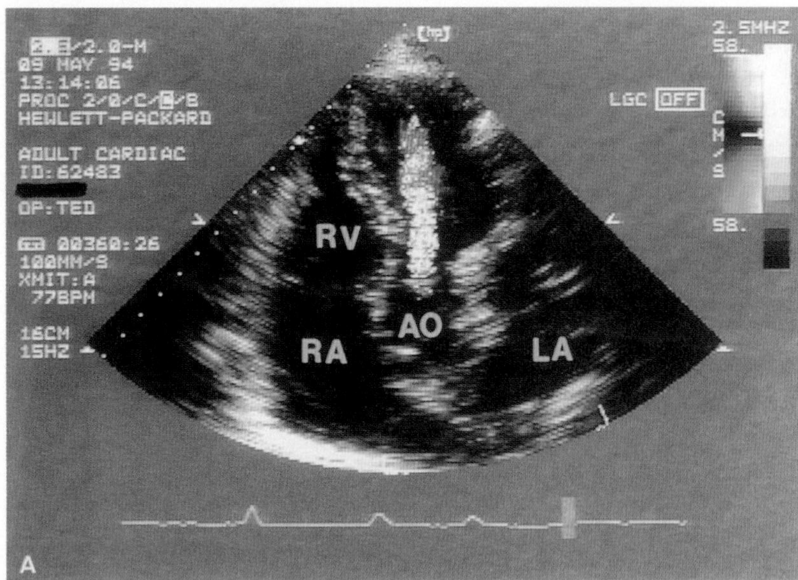

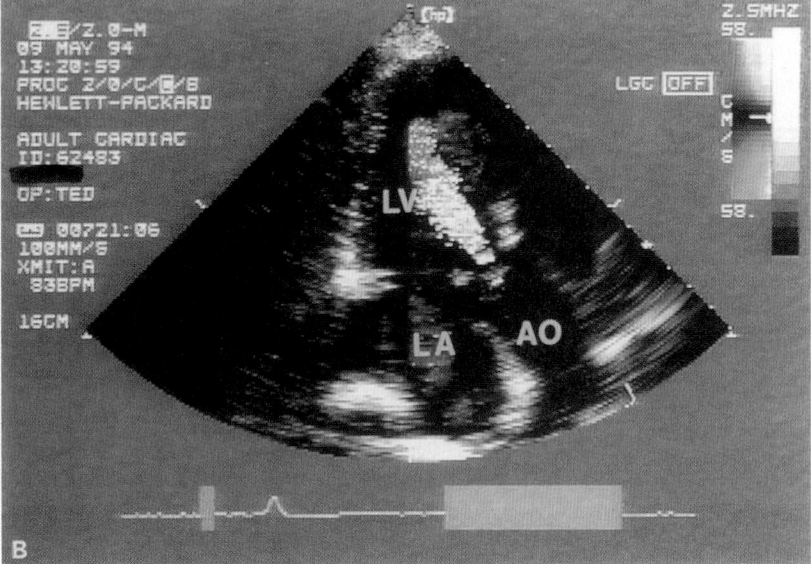

FIGURE 32–12. *A*, Apical five-chamber view of the heart with color-flow Doppler shows aortic regurgitation with a jet extending from the aortic valve leaflets almost to the apex of the left ventricle consistent with moderately severe aortic regurgitation. RV, right ventricle; RA, right atrium; LA, left atrium; AO, aorta. *B*, Apical long-axis view of the left ventricle (LV) in the same patient shows a regurgitant aortic jet extending from the aortic valve leaflets to the apex of the ventricle consistent with moderately severe aortic regurgitation. (A and B, From Young GD, St. John Sutton M: Echocardiography and Doppler ultrasound. In Julian DG, Camm AJ, Fox KM, et al [eds]: Diseases of the Heart. 2nd ed. London, WB Saunders, 1996, Plate 16.1.)

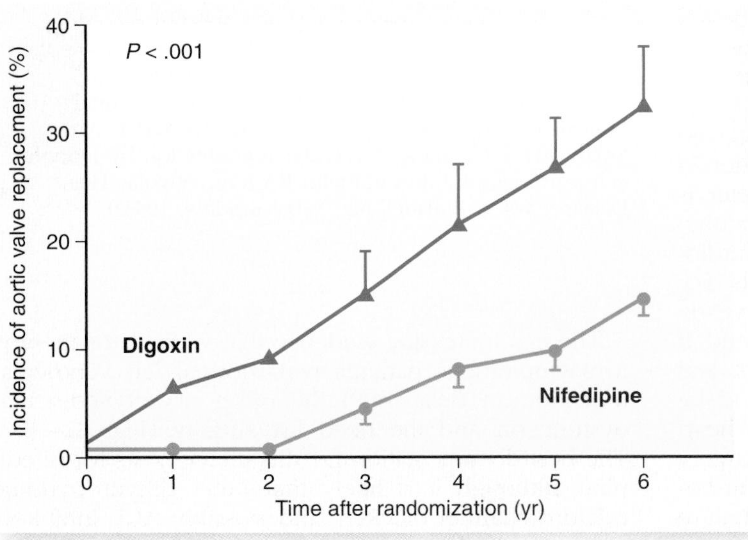

FIGURE 32–13. The need for aortic valve replacement for asymptomatic patients with aortic regurgitation is compared for a group of such patients treated with digoxin versus a group treated with nifedipine. Nifedipine delayed the onset of symptoms and reduced the need for aortic valve replacement. (Redrawn from Scognamiglio R, Rahimtoola SH, Fasoli G, et al: Nifedipine in asymptomatic patients with severe aortic regurgitation and normal left ventricular function. N Engl J Med 1994;331:689–694. Copyright 1994 Massachusetts Medical Society. All rights reserved.)

Overall Strategy

Asymptomatic patients with moderate to severe chronic AR should receive long-acting nifedipine, 30 to 60 mg per day. In the future, other vasodilators may be shown to be equally effective to nifedipine. Thus, it is probably reasonable to substitute other dihydropyridine calcium blockers such as amlodipine or an ACE inhibitor if nifedipine is poorly tolerated. Clinical and echocardiographic follow-up should be performed at intervals determined by left ventricular end-systolic dimension. When either symptoms develop or ejection fraction approaches 0.55 or end-systolic diameter approaches 55 mm, patients should be referred for preoperative workup including cardiac catheterization, aortography, and coronary arteriography. Table 32–4 provides markers that guide the primary care physician in timing of referral of the patient with AR for specialized care.

TABLE 32–4

Guidelines for Referral for Patients with Severe Chronic Aortic Regurgitation

Symptoms	ESD (mm)		EF	Course of Action
None	<55		>0.55	Begin vasodilators, observe
>Mild	<55		>0.55	Refer for further evaluation
None	≥55	or	<0.55	Refer for further evaluation
Yes	≥55	or	<0.55	Refer for further evaluation

EF, ejection fraction; ESD, left ventricular end systolic diameter.

ACUTE AORTIC REGURGITATION

Acute AR often constitutes a medical emergency, but unfortunately, this condition may be difficult to recognize. In acute AR, there is a sudden fall in cardiac output, resulting in hypotension, and a sudden rise in left ventricular diastolic pressure, both events acting in concert to reduce coronary blood flow.[16] Perhaps because of this coronary pathophysiology, the mortality of acute AR treated medically approaches 75% if even mild heart failure develops. Conversely, surgical treatment has a mortality of less than 25%. Most cases of severe acute AR are caused by infective endocarditis. Although there is a persistent fear that a prosthetic valve might become reinfected if it is implanted early in the patient's course of antibiotic therapy, reinfection is relatively rare, occurring in only 10% of prosthetic valves even when they are implanted within 48 hours of the last positive blood culture (see Chapter 33).

As noted previously, a large total stroke volume and wide pulse pressure and the resultant eccentric hypertrophy cause most of the signs of chronic AR. In acute AR, eccentric hypertrophy has not yet developed and both the wide pulse pressure and the large stroke volume are absent, as are most of the signs of AR. In fact, a short, blowing diastolic murmur may be clue of this condition on physical examination

Diagnosis

Because it is the onset of heart failure that makes the outcome of medical therapy poor, the signs of even mild heart failure should be carefully elicited on physical examination. Besides listening for the typical murmur, close attention should be directed to S_1. In severe acute AR, left ventricular filling from the aorta closes the mitral valve before ventricular systole (mitral valve preclosure), decreasing the intensity of S_1. Mitral valve preclosure suspected on physical examination and confirmed echocardiographically is an ominous sign indicating the need for urgent aortic valve replacement.

Once acute AR is suspected, prompt echocardiography is mandatory. An M-mode echocardiogram is used to search for premature mitral valve closure (Fig. 32–14), an important indicator regarding the timing of operation. In addition, aortic valve vegetations confirming the diagnosis of endocarditis and Doppler flow interrogation of the aortic valve to assess the severity of AR can be obtained.

In most cases of acute AR, cardiac catheterization is not necessary. Most cases affect younger patients in whom there is no reason to suspect coronary artery disease. Thus, the data needed to judge whether operation is necessary usually can be obtained during physical examination and echocardiography.

Management

In patients who are entirely asymptomatic, conservative management is possible. If infective endocarditis is the cause of the acute AR, appropriate antibiotic therapy is employed (see Chapter 33). Such patients should be carefully followed clinically for signs of heart failure. If these occur, referral for preoperative workup is indicated. In some cases, preoperative improvement is afforded by using hemodynamic monitoring and vasodilators. This strategy should not be used to delay surgery but rather as an attempt to improve the patient's condition preoperatively.

TRICUSPID REGURGITATION

The most important cause of primary tricuspid regurgitation (TR) is infective endocarditis (see Chapter 33). Tricuspid valve involvement occurs in only 10% of the general population who develop endocarditis but increases to 50% among users of illicit intravenous drugs who develop endocarditis. Most TR is secondary to right ventricular dilatation and failure, which in turn may be caused by left heart failure, primary lung disease, primary pulmonary hypertension, or an intracardiac

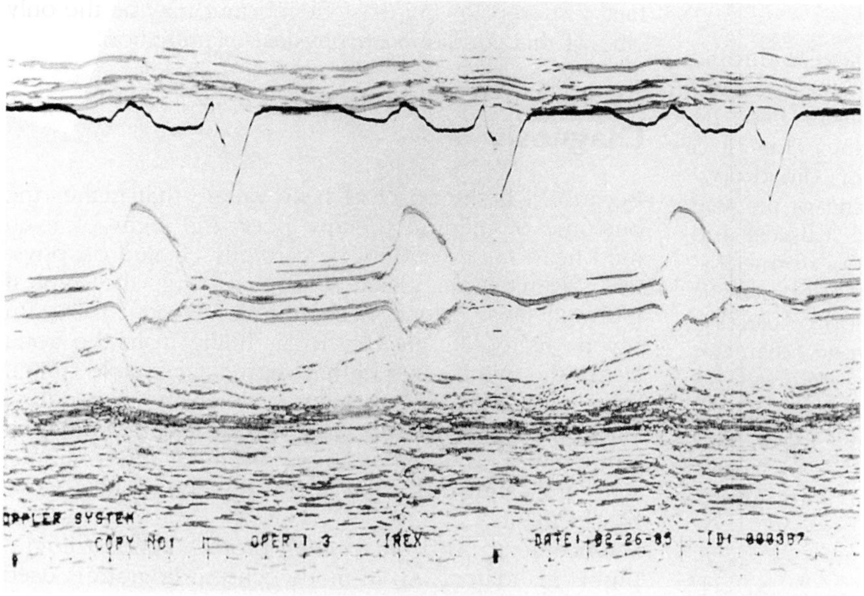

FIGURE 32–14. The M-mode echocardiogram in a patient with acute severe aortic regurgitation. The mitral valve tracings are shown just below the electrocardiogram. The mitral valve is seen to close well before the QRS (mitral valve preclosure, *arrow*), indicating very high left ventricular end-diastolic pressure and the need for urgent aortic valve replacement. (From Carabello BA, Usher BW, Gwinn NS: Cardiology. In Sahn SA, Heffner JE [eds]: Critical Care Pearls. Philadelphia, Hanley & Belfus, 1989.)

shunt. Although the volume overload imposed on the right ventricle by tricuspid regurgitation may worsen the patient's overall condition, the right ventricle tolerates TR remarkably well. Therefore, treatment is usually aimed at improving the diseases responsible for the TR rather than at surgical correction.

Diagnosis

History

There are no features in the patient's history specific for TR. Its presence worsens the symptoms of right ventricular failure, including fatigue, edema, and ascites.

Physical Examination

The murmur typical of TR is a holosystolic murmur heard along the left sternal border (see Chapter 11). The murmur increases with inspiration as negative intrathoracic pressure increases right ventricular inflow and outflow. In end-stage right ventricular failure, however, inspiration fails to augment right ventricular filling, and the inspiratory increase in the murmur does not occur. On physical examination, there are also signs of right ventricular enlargement, most commonly seen as a parasternal lift. Examination of the neck veins reveals large V-waves. This corresponds to systolic expansion of the liver, which may be palpated in the right upper quadrant. The liver may be tender if right ventricular failure has been rapid in onset.

Laboratory Studies

The ECG shows right-axis deviation and evidence of right ventricular hypertrophy. Right ventricular enlargement is seen on the chest x-ray as obliteration of the retrosternal air space.

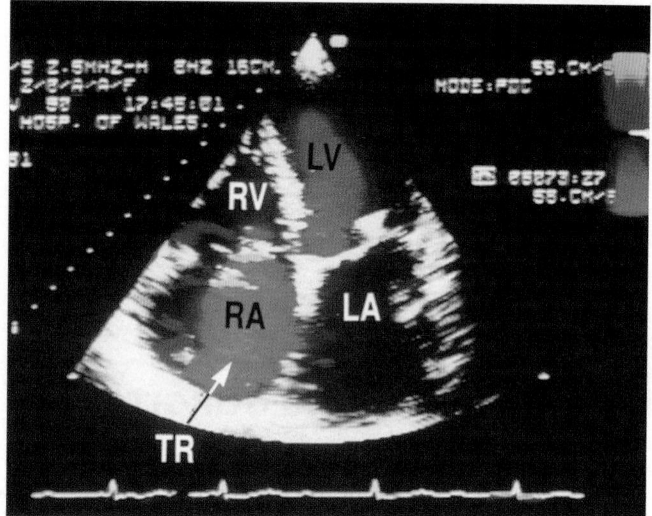

FIGURE 32–15. Apical four-chamber view with color-flow Doppler of a patient with severe tricuspid regurgitation (TR). Most of the right atrium (RA) is filled with blue, which represents the TR. RV, right ventricle; LV, left ventricle; LA, left atrium. (From Hall RJC, Nitter-Hauge S: Other valve disorders; a. tricuspid-pulmonary and mixed lesions; b. prosthetic valves. In Julian DG, Camm AJ, Fox KM, et al [eds]: Diseases of the Heart. 2nd ed. London, WB Saunders, 1996, Plate 42.1.)

The echocardiogram demonstrates both right atrial and right ventricular enlargement. Doppler interrogation of the tricuspid valve demonstrates retrograde systolic tricuspid flow (Fig. 32–15). Pulmonary artery pressure can be estimated and is used to identify pulmonary hypertension as the cause of right ventricular decompensation. If endocarditis is the primary cause of tricuspid regurgitation, vegetations are often imaged.

Cardiac catheterization is rarely indicated in the diagnosis of TR. Right ventriculography to demonstrate TR is not commonly practiced because introduction of a catheter across the tricuspid valve to perform the study can by itself cause TR, introducing the possibility of artifact into the study. If cardiac catheterization is performed, right atrial pressure tracings show large V-waves; as the TR worsens, the right atrial pressure tracing progressively resembles a right ventricular pressure tracing.

Management

The management of TR is usually aimed at treating the disease responsible for right ventricular decompensation. Thus, if left heart failure caused right heart failure, the focus is on improving left ventricular performance. In chronic secondary TR, diuretics are the mainstay of therapy in reducing right ventricular volume overload. Vasodilators, which have such an important role in the treatment of left ventricular failure, have little effect on the pulmonary vascular bed and, thus, usually do little to help reduce primary TR. Because most cases of primary TR stem from infective endocarditis secondary to illicit drug use, there is usually little enthusiasm for tricuspid valve replacement, for fear that the valve prosthesis will become infected during subsequent drug use. In some cases, however, especially those in whom infected emboli have produced pulmonary hypertension, tricuspid valve replacement may be necessary. Although there is only modest experience with tricuspid valve repair, this strategy is attractive because it avoids a prosthesis and may be appropriate therapy for some patients.

VALVE PROSTHESES

All valvular prostheses have their own inherent drawbacks.[17, 18] Although insertion of the prosthesis improves the condition for which it was inserted and, when operation is timed properly, can offer the patient a normal life span, thromboembolism, endocarditis, and primary

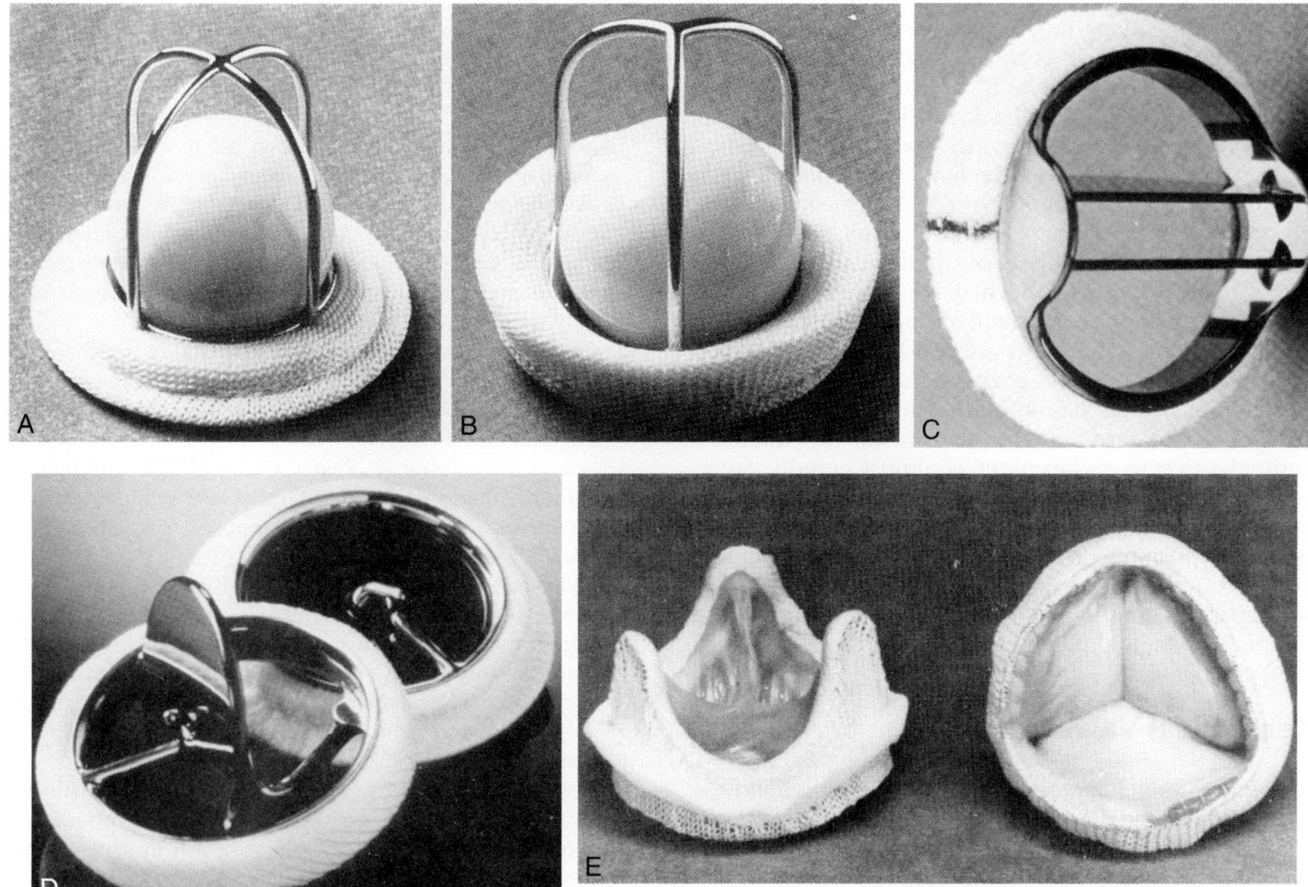

FIGURE 32–16. Several types of valve prostheses. *A*, Starr-Edwards caged-ball mitral prosthesis. *B*, Starr-Edwards caged-ball aortic prosthesis. *C*, St. Jude Medical bileaflet valve. *D*, Medtronic-Hall tilting disk valve. *E*, The Carpentier-Edwards bioprosthesis. (A–E, From Wernley JA, Crawford MH: Choosing a prosthetic heart valve. In Carabello BA [ed]: Valvular Heart Disease, vol 9. Cardiology Clinics, 1991.)

valve failure all complicate the use of prosthetic valves. Further, most prostheses are inherently stenotic compared with normal native valves. For this reason, emphasis on valve repair is increasing, and it is agreed that, whenever possible, the patient's native valve should be repaired rather than replaced with a prosthesis. Repair is now possible in most cases of nonrheumatic MR and in about 10% to 15% of cases of AR. Balloon valvotomy is successful in the long-term treatment of pulmonic stenosis and in many cases of MS, permitting correction of these conditions without the use of a prosthesis. In acquired calcific AS, however, valve degeneration is so extensive that repair is virtually impossible and a prosthesis must be inserted. Options for prosthetic valves include bioprosthetic heterografts, bioprosthetic homografts, and mechanical valves. Transplantation of the patient's pulmonary valve into the aortic position, with use of a homograft in the pulmonary position (the Ross procedure), is attractive in young patients because the pulmonary autograft can grow with the patient. Some of the commonly used prosthetic valves are demonstrated in Figure 32–16.

Bioprosthetic Heterografts

Bioprosthetic heterografts are typically made from porcine aortic valves that can be inserted in any position. Their advantage is a low incidence of thromboembolism, and therefore, anticoagulation is not required. Their major drawback is primary valve failure. The younger the patient, the sooner deterioration occurs, and the older the patient, the more delayed deterioration is. For example, in a 30-year-old patient, deterioration often occurs within 5 years of implantation, whereas in the 70-year-old patient, valvular function is likely to remain normal for at least 10 years. Thus, these valves are particularly appropriate for use in older patients. They also are used in young women who wish to become pregnant, because warfarin anticoagulation, which has a high risk for causing fetal damage, is not required. In such cases, the need for eventual valve re-replacement is almost certain. Stent-free human homograft valves are sewn into the aortic position and, occasionally, can be modified for use in the mitral position. They do not require anticoagulation and seem especially resistant to endocarditis. They appear durable, although long-term follow-up is limited.

Mechanical Valves

Mechanical valves are extremely durable, and some have an excellent hemodynamic profile with low transvalvular gradients even in small-sized valves. All require lifetime anticoagulation to avoid the high risk of thromboembolism. Mechanical valves are particularly useful in patients with a small aortic annulus and in young patients with a long life expectancy. They should be avoided in patients who are unwilling to take warfarin faithfully or who are at high risk for bleeding.

TABLE 32–5

Characteristics of Commonly Used Prosthetic Valves

Name	Type	Anticoagulant	Durability
Carpentier-Edwards	B	No, unless large LA and AF	5–15 yr
Hancock	B	Same	5–15 yr
St. Jude	M, L_2	Yes	Unlimited
Medtronic-Hall	M, TD	Yes	Unlimited
Starr-Edwards	M, CB	Yes	Unlimited

AF, atrial fibrillation; B, bioprosthesis; CB, caged ball; L_2, bileaflet; LA, left atrium; M; mechanical; TD, tilting disk.

In choosing a valve prosthesis, the need for durability, the risk of anticoagulation, the hemodynamics of the prosthesis, and patient preference must all be considered. The ultimate decision is often not made until the native valve has been examined at operation, at which time the surgeon chooses a valve that maximizes benefit and minimizes risk.

Table 32–5 lists some of the characteristics of commonly used prosthetic valves.

References

1. Bonow RO, Carabello B, deLeon AC Jr, et al: Guidelines for the management of patients with valvular heart disease: Executive summary. A report of the American College of Cardiology/American Heart Association Task Force on Practice Guidelines (Committee on Management of Patients with Valvular Heart Disease). Circulation 1998; 98:1949–1984.
2. Otto CM, Kuusisto J, Reinchenback DD, et al: Characterization of the early lesion of "degenerative" valvular aortic stenosis: Histological and immunohistochemical studies. Circulation 1994;90:844.
3. Novaro GM, Tiong IY, Pearce GL, et al: Effect of hydroxymethylglutaryl coenzyme A reductase inhibitors on the progression of calcific aortic stenosis. Circulation 2001; 104:2205–2209.
4. Pellikka PA, Nishimura RA, Bailey KR, et al: The natural history of adults with asymptomatic, hemodynamically significant aortic stenosis. J Am Coll Cardiol 1990;15:1012.
5. Otto CM, Burwash IG, Legget ME, et al. Prospective study of symptomatic valvular aortic stenosis: Clinical, echocardiographic, and exercise predictors of outcome. Circulation 1997;95:2262–2270.
6. Fawzy ME, Choi WB, Mimish L, et al: Immediate and long-term effect of mitral balloon valvotomy on left ventricular volume and systolic function in severe mitral stenosis. Am Heart J 1996;132:356–360.
7. Reyes VP, Raju BS, Wynne J, et al: Percutaneous balloon valvuloplasty compared with open surgical commissurotomy for mitral stenosis. N Engl J Med 1994;331:961.
8. Carabello BA: Progress in mitral and aortic regurgitation. Prog Cardiovasc Dis 2001;43(6):457–475.

9. Carabello BA: The pathophysiology of mitral regurgitation. J Heart Valve Dis 2000;9(5):600–608.
10. Enriquez-Sarano M, Tajik AJ, Schaff HV, et al: Echocardiographic prediction of survival after surgical correction of organic mitral regurgitation. Circulation 1994;90:830.
11. Mohty D, Orszulak TA, Schaff HV, et al: Very long-term survival and durability of mitral valve repair for mitral valve prolapse. Circulation 2001;104(12 Suppl 1):I1–17.
12. Freed LA, Levy D, Levine RA, et al: Prevalence and clinical outcome of mitral-valve prolapse. N Engl J Med 1999;341:1–7.
13. Bonow RO, Lakatos E, Maron BJ, et al: Serial long-term assessment of the natural history of asymptomatic patients with chronic aortic regurgitation and normal left ventricular systolic function. Circulation 1991;84:1625.
14. Klodas E, Enriquez-Sarano M, Tajik AJ, et al: Optimizing timing of surgical correction in patients with severe aortic regurgitation: Role of symptoms. J Am Coll Cardiol 1997;30:746–752.
15. Scognamiglio R, Rahimtoola SH, Fasoli G, et al: Nifedipine in asymptomatic patients with severe aortic regurgitation and normal left ventricular function. N Engl J Med 1994;331:689.
16. Mann T, McLaurin L, Grossman W, et al: Assessing the hemodynamic severity of acute aortic regurgitation due to infective endocarditis. N Engl J Med 1975;293:108.
17. Lindblom D, Lindblom U, Qvist J, et al: Long-term relative survival rates after heart valve replacement. J Am Coll Cardiol 1990;15:566.
18. Hammermeister K, Sethi GK, Henderson WG, et al: Outcomes 15 years after valve replacement with a mechanical versus a bioprosthetic valve: Final report of the Veterans Affairs randomized trial. J Am Coll Cardiol 2000;36:1152–1158.

CHAPTER 33

Recognition and Management of Patients with Infective Endocarditis

Adolf W. Karchmer

The morbidity and mortality associated with infective endocarditis (IE) can be significantly reduced by early diagnosis and initiation of effective therapy. Because symptoms associated with IE are often nonspecific and prosaic, patients with this infection are likely to seek initial medical care from their primary care physicians. Accordingly, understanding the clinical presentations of IE, an efficient approach to diagnosis, effective therapy for various forms of IE, and the appropriate role of subspecialty physicians in the management of these patients is essential to achieve an optimal outcome.[1–4]

EPIDEMIOLOGY

Microbial infection of the endothelial surface of the heart results in the syndrome of infective endocarditis. This infection most commonly involves heart valves but occasionally occurs on the low-pressure side of a septal defect, on a chordae tendineae, or on a patch of mural endocardium that has been injured by an aberrant stream of blood. The actual lesion produced, called a *vegetation,* is an amorphous mass of platelets and fibrin in which is enmeshed the proliferating causative microorganism. In developed countries, IE is a relatively infrequent disease. Its occurrence ranges from 1.7 to 6.2 cases per 100,000 overall population but increases progressively after 30 years of age, so that rates exceed 15 cases per 100,000 population greater than 50 years of age. Among all cases of IE in developed countries, 10% to 20% of infections occur on prosthetic valves (prosthetic valve endocarditis [PVE]). Actuarial estimates suggest that 1.4% to 3.1% of valve recipients develop IE within the initial year after valve surgery and by 5 years 3.2% to 5.7% have developed PVE. Intravenous drug abuse entails an even greater risk for IE than that associated with prosthetic valves or rheumatic heart disease. The rate of IE in this group is 2% to 5% per patient-year. The risk of IE among patients with mitral valve prolapse is small to moderate; nevertheless, because of the high frequency of this valvular pathology in the population, mitral valve prolapse is a common predisposition for IE. Among persons with mitral valve prolapse, those with mitral regurgitation or thickened valve leaflets are at increased risk for IE.

CLINICAL FEATURES

The clinical presentation of IE ranges from marked systemic toxicity and rapid development of intracardiac and extracardiac complications (acute endocarditis) to an indolent prolonged illness with modest fever and toxicity and, in some instances, scant evidence of infection or cardiac disease on examination (subacute endocarditis). Although the clinical features of IE are primarily non-specific (Table 33–1), their occurrence in a patient with an underlying cardiac condition or behavior pattern (intravenous drug abuse) known to predispose to endocarditis, particularly in the absence of an overt focal infection, should elicit consideration of IE. Additional important clues to the presence of IE include bacteremia with organisms that commonly cause IE or an embolic event (pulmonary or systemic) that is not attributable to an apparent underlying illness or that occurs in the context of a non-specific febrile illness. Similarly, new or rapidly progressive cardiac valvular dysfunction in a patient with unexplained fever may be indicative of IE. Occasionally, patients with indolent IE present with renal dysfunction that is the consequence of immune complex-mediated glomerulonephritis. Some findings on the physical examination are suggestive of IE: *splinter hemorrhages* (i.e., subungual dark red streaks) (Fig. 33–1), *Osler nodes* (i.e., small, tender nodules on the finger or toe pads) (Fig. 33–2), and *Janeway lesions* (i.e., small hemorrhages on the palms and soles), are characteristic, although not pathognomonic, of IE. Systemic emboli, which are often a presenting or early complication of IE, occur in 20% to 40% of pateints with IE and commonly involve the central nervous system. Fortunately, the frequency of embolic events decreases rapidly with effective therapy, from 13 per 1,000 patient days at onset of therapy to 1.2 per 1,000 patient days after 2 weeks of antibiotic therapy. Mycotic cerebral aneurysms occur in 1% to 5% of patients with IE (see Extracardiac Complications).

A high index of suspicion is required in order to avoid overlooking the diagnosis of IE. This is particularly true when IE occurs in patients without a previously known predisposition to valvular infection or when the cardinal symptom of fever is blunted or absent (the very elderly or those with azotemia, severe debility, or congestive heart failure).

The clinical features of IE among drug abusers and patients with prosthetic heart valves merit special mention. Left-sided IE among intravenous drug abusers is clinically similar to IE among nonaddicts. However, 65% to 75% of IE in this group involves the right heart

TABLE 33–1

Frequency of Signs and Symptoms in Patients with IE

Symptoms	%	Signs	%
Fever	80–85	Fever	80–90
Chills	40–75	Heart murmur	80–85
Sweats	25	Changing or new murmur	10–40
Anorexia	25–55		
Weight loss	25–35	Systemic embon	20–40
Malaise	25–40	Splenomegaly	15–50
Cough	25	Clubbing	10–20
Stroke	15–20	Osler's nodes	7–10
Headache	15–40	Splinter hemorrhage	5–15
Myalgia/arthralgia	15–30	Janeway lesions	6–10
Back pain	7–10	Retinal lesions (Roth's spots)	4–10
Confusion	10–20		

Adapted from Karchmer AW: Infective endocarditis. *In* Braunwald E, Zipes DP, Libby P (eds). Heart Disease. 6th ed, Philadelphia, WB Saunders, 2001, p. 1730.

IE, infective endocarditis.

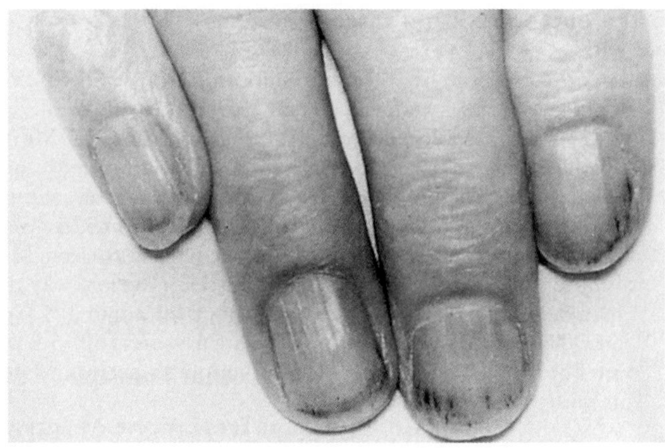

FIGURE 33–1. Splinter hemorrhages in a patient with infective endocarditis. (From Freeman R, Hall RJC: Infective endocarditis. In Julian DG, Camm AJ, Fox KM, et al [eds]: Diseases of the Heart, 2nd ed. London: WB Saunders, 1996, p 896.)

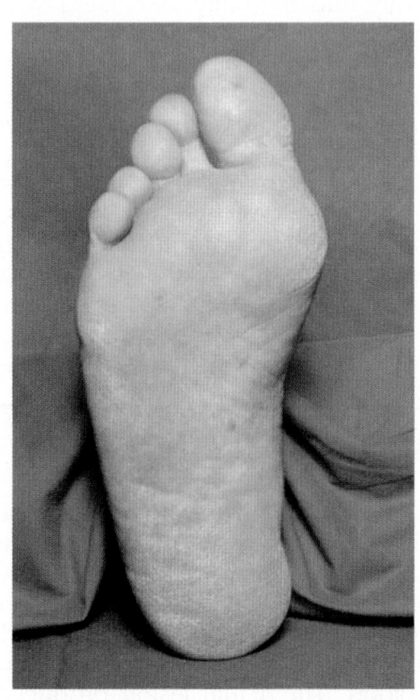

FIGURE 33–2. Osler's node on the great toe. (From Mir MA: Atlas of Clinical Diagnosis. London, WB Saunders, 1995, p 243.)

valves, particularly the tricuspid valve. Patients with right-sided IE, which is often caused by *Staphylococcus aureus,* present abruptly with cough, dyspnea, hemoptysis, or pleuritic chest pain, in addition to the usual features of IE. Chest radiographs in these patients commonly reveal nodular infiltrates due to septic pulmonary infarcts. These infiltrates may subsequently become necrotic, cavitate, and result in a pyopneumothorax. Patients with PVE developing within 60 days of cardiac surgery may have postoperative complications that mask the usual prosaic symptoms of IE. In these patients, as well as in those with later onset of PVE, valve dysfunction with new regurgitant murmurs and findings of congestive heart failure are encountered commonly. Perivalvular infection with dehiscence of the valve from the annulus and paravalvular leakage or with abscess formation complicates approximately 45% of patients with PVE involving mechanical or bioprosthetic valves and is particularly prevalent when PVE occurs within 1 year after cardiac surgery or involves an aortic valve prosthesis.

DIAGNOSIS

The clinical, laboratory, and echocardiographic features of IE have been codified into a scheme, the so-called Duke criteria, that provide a sensitive and specific approach to the clinical diagnosis of IE (Box 33–1).[6] Finding two major criteria, one major and three minor criteria, or five minor criteria allows a definite diagnosis of IE. Occasional patients fall just short of the diagnosis of definite IE and yet have no alternative diagnosis to explain their febrile illness. If one major and one minor criteria or three minor criteria are present, these patients are classified as possible IE and treated for it. To use as a criterion a positive blood culture for organisms that often contaminate these cultures—that is, coagulase-negative staphylococci or diphtheroids—or that rarely cause IE, such as gram-negative bacilli, requires additional rigor. To do so, blood cultures must be persistently positive or multiple cultures must be positive with a single clone. Alternative sites of infection must be ruled out. If the possibility of IE is considered early in the workup of a febrile patient and the evaluation is conducted with care, it is unlikely that the diagnosis of IE will be rejected erroneously when using these guidelines. Alternatively, the diagnosis of culture-negative IE may be accepted erroneously in patients when nonbacterial thrombotic vegetations are detected echocardiographically (e.g., marantic endocarditis, cryptic collagen-vascular disease, and antiphospholipid antibody syndrome).

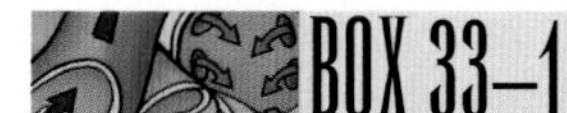

BOX 33–1

Criteria Used in the Diagnosis of IE

MAJOR CRITERIA

1. Positive blood culture
   A. Two separate blood cultures yielding organisms typically causing IE: Viridans streptococci, *Streptococcus bovis,* HACEK; community-acquired *Staphylococcus aureus,* or community-acquired enterococci, in the absence of a primary focus of infection
   B. Microorganisms consistent with IE from persistently positive blood cultures: At least two positive cultures of blood drawn >12 hr apart, or all three of three, or a majority of four or more separate blood cultures (first and last cultures drawn at least 1 hr apart)
   C. Single positive blood culture for *Coxiella burnetii* or antiphase I IgG antibody titer >1:800
2. Evidence of endocardial involvement
   A. Positive echocardiogram of IE
      (1) Oscillating intracardiac mass on a valve or supporting structures, in the path of regurgitant jets, or on implanted material in the absence of an alternative anatomic explanation
      (2) Abscess
      or
      (3) New partial dehiscence of a prosthetic valve
   B. New valvular regurgitation (worsening or changing of preexisting murmur not adequate)

MINOR CRITERIA

1. Predisposing heart condition or intravenous drug use
2. Fever: temperature ≥38.0°C
3. Vascular phenomena: major arterial emboli, septic pulmonary infarcts, mycotic aneurysm, intracranial hemorrhage, conjunctival hemorrhages, and Janeway lesions
4. Immunologic phenomena: glomerulonephritis, Osler's nodes, Roth's spots, and rheumatoid factor
5. Microbiologic evidence: Positive blood culture but less than a major criterion (see earlier)* or serologic evidence of active infection with an organism consistent with IE

*Excludes a single positive blood culture for coagulase-negative staphylococci or organisms that do not cause IE.

IE, infective endocarditis; HACEK, *Haemophilus* species, *Actinobacillus actinomycetemcomitans, Cardiobacterium hominis, Eikenella* species, *Kingella kingae.*

Adapted from Li JS, Sexton DJ, Mick N, et al: Proposed modification of the Duke criteria for the diagnosis of infective endocarditis. Clin Infect Dis 2000;30:633–638.

Blood Cultures

The diagnostic scheme appropriately emphasizes blood cultures and echocardiographic findings. Among patients with IE caused by organisms other than those that are highly fastidious, more than 95% of all blood cultures obtained will be positive. Accordingly, three separate sets of blood cultures, obtained over 24 hours from separate venipunctures, should be sufficient both to identify the causative organism and to demonstrate that the bacteremia is continuous, a finding characteristic of this infection and few others. In spite of technologic advances in microbiology laboratories that enhance the yield of organisms from blood cultures, 5% to 15% of patients with clinically diagnosed IE have negative blood cultures. Of those IE patients with negative blood cultures, approximately 50% have received antibiotics before the cultures were obtained, a factor that likely accounts for the negative cultures. Given the importance of isolating the causative organism in establishing optimal therapy, as well as the diagnosis of IE, treatment should be delayed for several days when evaluating hemodynamically stable patients with subacute presentations who have received antibiotics within the previous 2 weeks. This delay is not likely to allow otherwise preventable complications to occur but will allow repeat blood cultures to be obtained without further confounding by antimicrobial therapy.

Echocardiography (See Also Chapter 5)

Although echocardiographic findings are not required to diagnose definite IE clinically, identification of vegetations or perivalvular complications consistent with IE markedly enhances one's ability to make this diagnosis. The sensitivity of a single transesophageal echocardiographic examination (TEE) to identify vegetations in patients with clinically diagnosed native valve IE ranges from 90% to 94%; the sensitivity of the transthoracic echocardiographic (TTE) approach is significantly lower (45% to 75%).

Because of obesity, pulmonary disease, and chest wall deformity, visualization of valves by TTE is inadequate in up to 20% of adults. TTE is significantly less adequate than TEE in detecting infection on prosthetic valves, perivalvular abscesses, leaflet perforations, or intracardiac fistulae. The sensitivity and specificity of TEE for detecting perivalvular infection are 75% to 100% and 94%, respectively, and for imaging vegetations on prosthetic valves they are 86% to 94%, and 88% to 100%, respectively. The diagnostic accuracy of TEE is increased by multiplanar (>2 planes) imaging. Nevertheless, false-negative rates for imaging vegetations with TEE may approach 10%. Although experts differ on the echocardiographic strategy for evaluating a patient with suspected IE, most agree that a technically adequate, negative TTE in a patient with a less than 4% prior probability of IE is sufficient to exclude the diagnosis. If the prior probability is 5% to 55% (this includes patients with vascular catheter-associated *S. aureus* bacteremia), initial evaluation by TEE is more cost effective than a strategy of TTE which, if negative, is followed by a TEE. In patients with a high prior probability of IE (>55%) treatment for IE is usually indicated regardless of the echocardiographic evaluation.

Echocardiography is not sufficiently sensitive to rule out IE in a patient in whom the clinical suspicion is high; and hence, negative findings should not dissuade one from treatment. Among patients where there is an intermediate level of suspicion, a negative TEE does not rule out the diagnosis; on the contrary, further evaluation, including another TEE, is required in this situation. Figure 33–3 depicts a strategy for echocardiographic evaluation of patients with suspected IE.

Other Diagnostic Tests

In most patients, efforts to diagnose IE are not significantly enhanced by tests other than blood cultures, echocardiography, and rheumatoid factor. Serologic tests are helpful when blood cultures are negative. Some of the studies typically obtained, although not diagnostically helpful, are important in the management of patients: complete blood counts, serum creatinine, selected liver function tests, and urinalysis. Other tests that have been obtained often in the past, including circulating immune complex titer, quantitative immunoglobulins, cryoglobulins, C-reactive protein, and sedimentation rate, although often abnormal, rarely aid in the diagnosis of IE or the assessment of response to treatment, and generally can be omitted. Among patients with apparent culture-negative IE that is not attributable to prior antibiotic therapy, serologic tests to identify infection caused by *Brucella* species, *Legionella* species, *Coxiella burnetii* (the causative agent of Q fever), *Chlamydia* species, and *Bartonella* species may aid in diagnosing IE. Peripheral arterial emboli or resected valves and vegetations extracted surgically can be cultured as well as examined histologically and by polymerase chain reaction for genetic material from microorganisms to establish a causative diagnosis. The sequential evaluation of patients with suspected IE and selected symptoms is outlined in Table 33–2.

MICROBIOLOGY

A relatively small number of bacterial species cause the majority of cases of IE. This observation is embodied in the major criteria of the Duke diagnostic scheme and enhances the specificity of the scheme. The frequency with which these organisms cause IE varies somewhat among the various clinical subtypes of IE (Table 33–3). Although virtually any bacterial or fungal species can cause IE, understanding the common causes is essential when designing empirical antibiotic therapy for IE or when evaluating the possibility of IE among bacteremic patients. Among patients with community-acquired native valve IE that is unassociated with narcotic addiction, *S. aureus* is the predominant cause of the acute endocarditis syndrome. Streptococci, enterococci, coagulase-negative staphylococci, and the HACEK group of organisms (*Haemophilus* species, *Actinobacillus actinomycetemcomitans, Cardiobacterium hominis, Eikenella* species, and *Kingella kingae*) are the major causes of IE presenting in a subacute fashion. Nosocomial IE is primarily caused by *S. aureus*, coagulase negative staphylococci, and enterococci and is an infrequent complication of intravascular device-related bacteremia or bacteremia associated with genitourinary tract manipulations. *S. aureus* strains causing IE among intravenous drug abusers are frequently methicillin-resistant (also resistant to oxacillin, nafcillin, imipenem, and the cephalosporins). The coagulase-negative staphylococci that cause PVE during the initial year after valve placement are predominantly *Staphylo-*

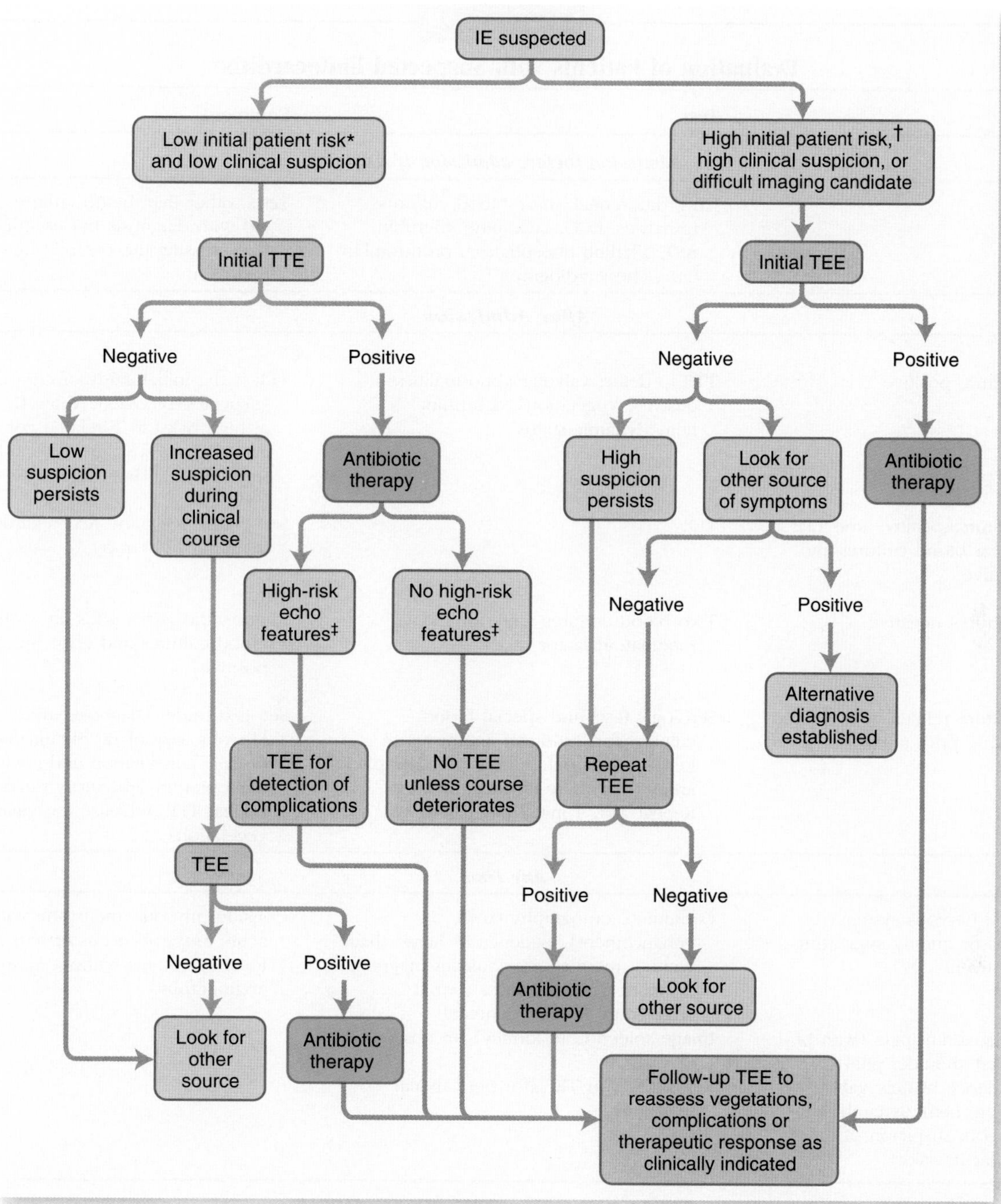

FIGURE 33–3. An approach to the diagnostic use of echocardiography in suspected infective endocarditis (IE). *A patient with low initial risk might have fever and a previously known heart murmur, and no other stigmata of IE, for example. †High initial patient risks include prosthetic heart valves, many congenital heart diseases, previous endocarditis, new murmur, heart failure, and other stigmata of endocarditis. ‡High-risk echocardiographic features include large or mobile vegetations, or both, valvular regurgitation, suggestion of perivalvular extension, or secondary ventricular dysfunction (see text).TEE, transesophageal echocardiogram; TTE, transthoracic echocardiogram. (From Bayer AS, Bolger AF, Taubert KA, et al: (Ad Hoc Writing Group for the American Heart Association): Diagnosis and management of infective endocarditis and its complications. Circulation 1998;98:2936–2948.)

coccus epidermidis, and 85% of these strains are resistant to methicillin and other beta-lactam antibiotics. Of the coagulase-negative staphylococcal strains causing PVE 1 year or more after cardiac surgery, 50% are species other than *S. epidermidis* and only 30% are resistant to methicillin.

When, in the absence of confounding prior administration of antibiotics, blood cultures from patients with

TABLE 33–2

Evaluation of Patients with Suspected Endocarditis*

Timing	Test	Comment
	Admission (before admission if stable)	
	CBC, differential, three blood cultures, urinalysis, ECG, creatinine, bilirubin, AST, alkaline phosphatase, prothrombin time, chest radiograph	Tests, other than blood cultures, do not aid with diagnosis but establish baseline for assessing the complications of IE or treatment
	After Admission	
24–48 hr Blood culture positive	TTE to detect valvular abnormalities, describe vegetations, determine hemodynamic status	TEE is the initial study of choice with suspected prosthetic valve IE, patients at high risk for IE-related complications, and patients who are difficult to manage by TTE
48–72 hr Blood cultures positive and TTE negative, or blood cultures and TTE negative	TEE	See Figure 33–4 and text regarding initiation of therapy
72–96 hr Blood cultures negative	Two blood cultures daily for 2 days, rheumatoid factor	Rheumatoid factor adds little value if blood cultures and echocardiogram are positive
Days 7–10 Blood culture remain negative (no confounding prior antibiotics given)	Serologic tests and special blood cultures for fastidious organisms Retrieve material embolic to a peripheral artery for culture and examination Repeat TEE if initially negative	See text under Diagnosis and Microbiology of IE; obtain infectious disease consultation and advice of microbiology laboratory director Repeat TEE; increase the yield for vegetations
	Any Time	
Focal central nervous system symptoms or finding suggesting localized event	Computed tomography (with enhancement); evidence of hemorrhage without mass effect, consider magnetic resonance angiogram or formal angiogram, lumbar puncture	Consider mycotic aneurysm; with acute *Staphylococcus aureus* IE or new focal symptoms without infarct, consider angiography
Left upper quadrant pain (with or without left shoulder pain)	Image spleen (and kidney) for abscess	
Clinical evidence of new valve dysfunction, hemodynamic deterioration, suspicion of perivalvular invasion	Repeat TTE or TEE (for perivalvular invasion)	

*For patients who are hemodynamically stable and have a subacute presentation.

AST, aspartate transaminase; CBC, complete blood count; ECG, electrocardiogram; IE, infective endocarditis; TEE, transesophageal echocardiography; TTE, transthoracic echocardiography.

convincing clinical evidence of IE remain negative after 7 to 10 days of incubation, the causes of culture-negative IE must be evaluated. In addition to the fastidious variants of the common bacterial causes of IE, for example, HACEK group organisms and L-cysteine- or pyridoxal-requiring streptococci (nutritionally deficient streptococci now speciated as *Abiotrophia)* infection caused by fungi, *Brucella* species, *Legionella* species, *Bartonella* species, *Chlamydia* species, Tropheryma whipplei, and *Coxiella burnetii* must be considered. Clinical and epidemiologic circumstances may suggest one of these unusual organisms as the cause of blood culture-negative IE. Special blood culture handling should be requested to isolate these organisms. Additionally, noninfectious causes of fever with associated heart murmur or systemic emboli that mimic IE—including acute rheumatic fever, marantic endocarditis, Libman-Sacks endocarditis, antiphospholipid antibody syndrome, atrial myxoma, carcinoid syndrome, and renal cell cancer—must be considered. The possibility that the heart murmur, which has raised the question of IE, is in fact coincidental and that the presenting syndrome is a "fever of unknown origin" must be considered.

TABLE 33–3

Microbiology of IE in Specific Clinical Situations: Number of Cases (%)

	Native Valve Endocarditis*		Prosthetic Valve Endocarditis† Time of Onset after Valve Surgery			Endocarditis in Drug Addicts†	
Organism	***Community Acquired (n = 603)***	***Nosocomial (n = 82)***	***<2 mo (n = 144)***	***2–12 mo (n = 31)***	***>12 mo (n = 194)***	***Right-Sided (n = 346)***	***Left-Sided (n = 204)***
Streptococci‡	186 (31)	6 (7)	2 (1)	3 (9)	61 (31)	17 (5)	31 (15)
Pneumococci	8 (1)	—	—	—	—	—	—
Enterococci	53 (9)	13 (16)	12 (8)	4 (12)	22 (11)	6 (2)	49 (24)
Staphylococcus aureus	217 (36)	45 (55)	32 (22)	4 (12)	34 (18)	267 (77)	47 (23)
Coagulase-negative staphylococci	28 (5)	8 (10)	47 (33)	11 (32)	22 (11)	—	—
Fastidious gram-negative coccobacilli (HACEK group)	18 (3)	—	—	—	11 (6)	—	—
Gram-negative bacilli	21 (3)	4 (5)	9 (13)	1 (3)	11 (6)	17 (5)	26 (13)
Fungi, *Candida* species	5 (1)	3 (4)	12 (8)	4 (12)	3 (1)	—	25 (12)
Polymicrobial/ miscellaneous	36 (6)	1 (1)	4 (3)	2 (6)	9 (5)	28 (8)	20 (10)
Diphtheroids	—	—	9 (6)	—	5 (3)	—	—
Culture	31 (5)	2 (2)	7 (5)	2 (6)	16 (8)	10 (3)	6 (3)

*Data from Karchmer AW: Prevention and treatment of infective endocarditis. *In* Antman EM (ed): Cardiovascular Therapeutics. Philadelphia, WB Saunders, 2002, pp 1082, 1083.

†Data from Karchmer AW: Infective endocarditis. *In* Braunwald E, Zipes DP, Libby P (eds): Heart Disease: A Textbook of Cardiovascular Disease, 6th ed. Philadelphia, WB Saunders, 2001, p 1725.

‡Includes *Viridans* streptococci, *Streptococcus bovis*, other non-group A, groupable streptococci.

HACEK, *Haemophilus* species, *Actinobacillus actinomycetemcomitans*, *Cardiobacterium hominis*, *Eikenella* species, and *Kingella kingae*.

ANTIMICROBIAL THERAPY

Optimal antimicrobial therapy requires the use of an agent or combination of agents that is bactericidal for the organism causing IE.[7] The regimens recommended for therapy are based on the precise susceptibility of the causative organism and prior clinical experience in the treatment of IE caused by the organism. Selection of treatment must also consider individual patient limitations, including allergies, renal or hepatic dysfunction, potential interactions with other required therapy, and the risk of adverse events. The regimens generally recommended for the treatment of the common bacterial causes of IE are similar for patients with infection of native and prosthetic valves (Table 33–4). Treatment of PVE is, however, usually several weeks longer than that used for native valve IE, and staphylococcal PVE is treated with a combination regimen that includes rifampin.[5]

Initiating Therapy

The evaluation and treatment of a patient with suspected IE begins with a careful history and physical examination, with particular attention to the clinical manifestations and possible complications of IE (see Table 33–2, Fig. 33–4). Baseline laboratory tests should include complete blood counts, platelet count, serum creatinine, liver function tests, chest radiograph, electrocardiogram, and three separately drawn blood cultures. An echocardiogram should also be obtained (see Fig. 33–3). If focal extracardiac complications are suspected, the area in question should be studied with appropriate imaging techniques.

Pressures to contain medical cost often cause physicians to begin empirical antimicrobial therapy for suspected IE immediately after blood cultures have been obtained. This practice is appropriate when patients present with highly toxic, acute endocarditis, which may rapidly destroy cardiac valves, or with severe hemodynamic decompensation for which emergency valve surgery will be required (see Fig. 33–4). Prompt treatment of these patients may forestall valve damage or may quench infection and reduce the risk of reinfection after emergency valve replacement. Among hemodynamically stable patients with suspected subacute endocarditis, precipitous initiation of therapy before blood cultures have yielded an isolate may be counterproductive. When initial blood cultures are negative because the patient has taken antibiotics, this precipitous therapy compromises the opportunity to obtain additional cultures that are not confounded by antibiotic therapy (see Diagnosis). It is prudent to delay therapy for several days in the hemodynamically stable patient while awaiting the results of the initial blood cultures. It is unlikely that empirical therapy initiated a few days earlier will prevent complications.

TABLE 33–4

Recommended Antibiotic Therapy for IE

Infecting Organism	Antibiotic	Dose and Route*	Duration (wk)[†]	Comments
1. Penicillin-susceptible viridans streptococci, *Streptococcus bovis*, and other streptococci, penicillin MIC ≤ 0.1 μg/mL	A. Penicillin G	12–18 million units IV daily in divided doses q 4 hr	4	
	B. Penicillin G plus gentamicin[‡]	12–18 million units IV daily in divided doses q 4 hr 1 mg/kg IM or IV q 8 hr	4 2	Avoid aminoglycoside-containing regimens when potential for nephrotoxicity or ototoxicity is increased.[‡]
	C. Penicillin G plus gentamicin[‡]	Same doses as noted previously	2	See text
	D. Ceftriaxone	2 gm IV or IM daily as single dose	4	Can be used in patients with nonimmediate penicillin allergy. IM administration of ceftriaxone is painful.
	E. Vancomycin[§]	30 mg/kg IV daily in divided doses q 12 hr	4	Use for patients with immediate or severe penicillin or cephalosporin allergy. Infuse doses over 1 hr to avoid histamine release (red man syndrome).
2. Relatively penicillin-resistant streptococci Penicillin MIC 0.2–0.5 μg/mL	A. Penicillin G plus gentamicin[‡]	18–24 million units IV daily in divided doses q 4 hr 1 mg/kg IM or IV q 8 hr	4 2	
Penicillin MIC > 0.5 μm/mL	B. Penicillin G plus gentamicin[‡]	See regimens recommended for enterococcal endocarditis	4	Preferred for nutritionally variant (pyridoxal- or cysteine-requiring) streptococci.
3. Enterococci (in vitro evaluation for MIC to penicillin and vancomycin, beta-lactamase production, and high-level resistance to gentamicin and streptomycin required)	A. Penicillin G plus gentamicin[‡]	18–30 million units IV daily in divided doses q 4 hr 1 mg/kg IM or IV q 8 hr	4–6	See text for use of streptomycin instead of gentamicin in these regimens. Four wk of therapy recommended for patients with shorter history of illness (<3 mo) who respond promptly to treatment.
	B. Ampicillin plus gentamicin[‡]	12 gm IV daily in divided doses q 4 hr Same dose as noted previously	4–6 4–6	
	C. Vancomycin[§] plus gentamicin[‡]	30 mg/kg IV daily in divided doses q 12 hr Same dose as noted previously	4–6 4–6	Use for patients with penicillin allergy. Do not use cephalosporins.

4. Staphylococci infecting native valves (assume penicillin resistance), methicillin-susceptible	A. Nafcillin or oxacillin plus optional addition of	12 gm IV daily in divided doses q 4 hr	4–6	Penicillin—18–24 million units daily in divided doses q 4 hr can be used instead of nafcillin, oxacillin, or cefazolin if strains do not produce beta-lactamase.
	gentamicin[‡]	1 mg/kg IM or IV q 8 hr	3–5 days	
	B. Cefazolin plus optional addition of	2 gm IV q 8 hr	6	Cephalothin or other first-generation cephalosporin in equivalent doses can be used.
	gentamicin[‡]	Same dose as previously	3–5 days	
	C. Vancomycin[§]	30 mg/kg IV in divided doses q 12 hr	6	Use for patients with immediate penicillin allergy.
5. Staphylococci infecting native valves, methicillin-resistant	A. Vancomycin[§]	30 mg/kg IV in divided doses q 12 hr	6	
6. Staphylococci infecting prosthetic valves, methicillin-susceptible (assume penicillin resistance)	A. Nafcillin or oxacillin	12 gm IV daily in divided doses q 4 hr	6	First-generation cephalosporin or vancomycin could be used in penicillin-allergic patients. Use gentamicin during initial 2 wk. See text for alternatives to gentamicin. For patients with immediate penicillin allergy, use regimen 7.
	plus gentamicin[‡]	1 mg/kg IV or IM q 8 hr	2	
	plus rifampin[§]	300 mg orally q 8 hr	6	
7. Staphylococci infecting prosthetic valves, methicillin-resistant	A. Vancomycin[§]	30 mg/kg IV in divided doses q 12 hr	6	Use gentamicin during the initial 2 wk of therapy. See text for alternatives to gentamicin. Do not substitute a cephalosporin or imipenem for vancomycin.
	plus gentamicin[‡]	1 mg/kg IV or IM q 8 hr	2	
	plus rifampin[‖]	300 mg orally q 8 hr	6	
8. HACEK organisms[¶]	A. Ceftriaxone	2 gm IV or IM daily as a single dose	4	Cefotaxime or other third-generation cephalosporin in comparable doses may be used.
	B. Ampicillin	12 gm IV daily in divided doses q 4 hr	4	Test organism for beta-lactamase production. Do not use this regimen if beta-lactamase is produced.
	plus gentamicin[‡]	1 mg/kg IV or IM q 8 hr	4	

*Recommended doses are for adults with normal renal and hepatic function. Doses of gentamicin, streptomycin, and vancomycin must be adjusted in patients with renal dysfunction. Use ideal body weight to calculate doses (men = 50 kg + 2.3 kg per inch over 5 ft; women = 45.5 kg + 2.3 kg per inch over 5 ft).

[†]All durations in weeks except where specifically noted (4.A and B with gentamicin).

[‡]Aminoglycosides should not be administered as a single daily dose in patients with normal renal function.

[§]Peak levels obtained 1 hr after completion of the infusion should be 30–45 µg/mL.

[‖]Rifampin increases the dose of warfarin or dicumarol required for effective anticoagulation.

[¶]HACEK organisms include *Haemophilus species, Actinobacillus actinomycetemcomitans. Cardiobacterium hominis, Eikenella corrodens,* and *Kingella kingae.*

IE, infective endocarditis; IM, intramuscular; IV, intravenous; MIC, minimal inhibitory concentration.

From Karchmer AW: Treatment of infective endocarditis. *In* Antman EM (ed): Cardiovascular Therapeutics, 2nd ed. Philadelphia, WB Saunders, 2002, pp 1082–1099.

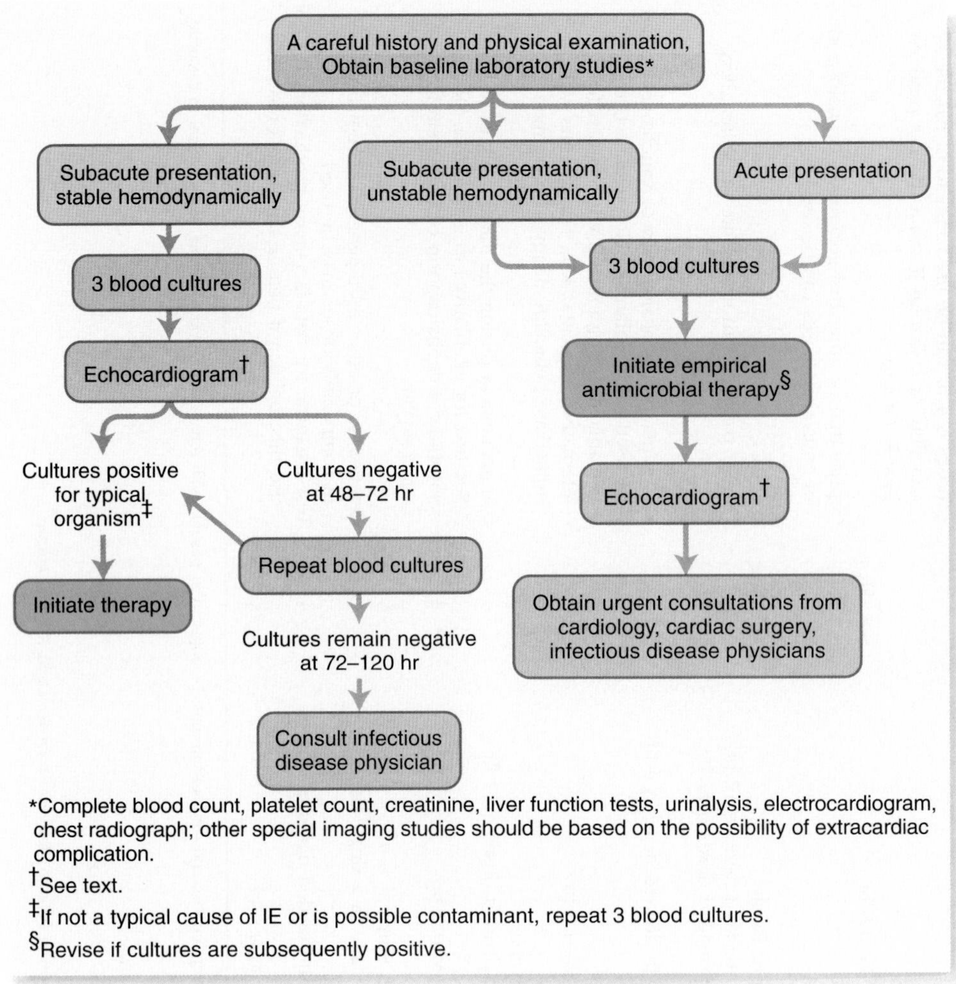

FIGURE 33–4. Diagnostic evaluation and the initiation of therapy in patients with suspected endocarditis. IE, infective endocarditis.

Selecting Therapy

Consensus regimens have been developed by an ad hoc writing group for the American Heart Association for treatment of patients with commonly encountered forms of IE (see Table 33–4). It is prudent to administer the regimen as it is specified. Compromises in the agent selected, dose, route of administration, and duration of therapy, in general, should be avoided, however, and if necessary, they should be approached with the assistance of an infectious disease consultant.

Outpatient Therapy

Home health care systems with well-trained staff combined with technical advances in infusion therapy enable physicians to safely administer antibiotic therapy for IE in an outpatient setting. Even multiple daily dose regimens, including regimens using two antibiotics, can be administered to outpatients using portable, programmable computer-driven pumps. Physicians must exercise clinical judgment in identifying appropriate patients for outpatient antibiotic therapy. The patient must be reliable and compliant regarding treatment. Underlying conditions must not impair management outside of the hospital setting. The home setting, including the family and professional support services, must be capable of managing the complexities of parenteral therapy, that include suitable storage of antibiotic solutions and infusion materials, sterile initiation and discontinuation of intravenous infusions, and maintenance of intravenous access. The symptoms of IE and the risk of complications should have abated before embarking on outpatient treatment. In particular, the patient should have been afebrile for 3 to 4 days and free of clinical evidence suggesting impending complications: unstable hemodynamics, poorly controlled heart failure, new conduction abnormalities, and new or unstable neurologic signs and symptoms. To this end, echocardiographic assessment of the site of infection and cardiac function should be obtained before discharge, and blood cultures should have become negative.

Guidelines for the transition of patients to outpatient therapy are not clearly established. The initial 2 weeks of treatment encompass the period of greatest risk for complications which in turn require prompt diagnosis and treatment to achieve optimal results. Thus, only patients with uncomplicated IE or at low risk for complications should be treated as outpatients during this period and even these patients may merit daily physician or treatment team assessment. After two weeks of treatment, patients with uncomplicated IE who are stable can be considered for outpatient treatment. Patients at high risk for complications, that is, those with prosthetic valve endocarditis, acute IE, infection with a highly virulent organism (*S. aureus*, pneumococci) are poor candidates for outpatient treatment during the initial 2 weeks of treatment or possibly for a longer period contingent upon their clinical course.

Careful physician and laboratory monitoring for complications of IE or therapy are necessary during outpatient therapy. Patients should be examined daily or every 3 to 7 days depending on the duration of prior therapy and the patient's clinical stability. Laboratory tests are monitored to detect early antibiotic toxicities and thus vary with the regimen used (see Monitoring during Antimicrobial Therapy). The availability of convenient outpatient infusion centers or the ability of the home health care system to assist with monitoring, including the maintenance of intravenous access and obtaining periodic laboratory tests, is an important variable in the decision to administer outpatient antimicrobial therapy.

Before being discharged to outpatient treatment, patients should be advised that unpredictable complications may occur and should be instructed to report untoward events promptly. Outpatient therapy must not result in compromised suboptimal antimicrobial therapy.

Specific Treatment Regimens

Streptococcal IE (Fig. 33–5)

The vast majority of the streptococci that cause IE are highly susceptible to penicillin (minimal inhibitory concentration [MIC] ≤ 0.1 μg/mL) and can be effectively treated with any of the recommended regimens (see Table 33–4, 1.A–E).[7] The 2-week regimen (see Table 33–4, 1.C), although effective for uncomplicated streptococcal IE, should not be used to treat IE caused by pyridoxal- or L-cysteine-requiring strains (Abiotrophia spp.) streptococcal PVE, or IE complicated by myocardial abscess, mycotic aneurysm, or focal extracardiac infection. The ceftriaxone regimen (see Table 33–4, 1.D) is easily administered in an outpatient setting and can usually be given to patients with a history of penicillin allergy that does not suggest an immediate allergic reaction (urticaria, angioedema, or symptoms suggestive of anaphylaxis). Vancomycin (see Table 33–4, 1.E) is recommended for patients with a history of an immediate allergic reaction to a penicillin or a cephalosporin. Patients with PVE caused by penicillin-susceptible streptococci should be treated for 6 weeks with penicillin or ceftriaxone (see Table 33–4, 1.A or D); gentamicin 1 mg/kg every 8 hours (adjusted for decreased renal function) should be given intravenously during the initial 2 weeks.

Relative resistance to penicillin (MIC ≥ 0.2 μg/mL) is detected in 15% of streptococci that cause IE. IE caused by these organisms, as well as that caused by Abiotrophia spp, and the potentially more virulent Lancefield group B streptococci (*S. agalactiae*), is optimally treated with a regimen that includes gentamicin (see Table 33–4, 2.A and B).

Enterococcal IE

Enterococcus faecalis and *Enterococcus faecium* cause 85% and 10% of the episodes of enterococcal IE, respectively. Enterococci are inhibited rather than killed by penicillin, ampicillin, and vancomycin and are not susceptible to cephalosporins or the antistaphylococcal penicillinase-resistant penicillins (nafcillin and oxacillin). The bactericidal antibiotic effect needed for optimal treatment of enterococcal IE requires the synergistic interaction of a cell wall-active antibiotic (penicillin, ampicillin, or vancomycin) that inhibits the organism at concentrations achievable clinically and an aminoglycoside (primarily gentamicin or streptomycin) that, in the presence of the cell wall-active agent, is able to exert a lethal effect.

The standard regimens recommended for the treatment of enterococcal IE (see Table 33–4, 3.A–C) provide synergistic bactericidal therapy if, as noted previously, the organism is inhibited by clinically achievable concentrations of the cell wall-active agent and does not exhibit high-level resistance to the aminoglycoside.[9] Treatment of enterococcal IE with a nonbactericidal cell wall-active agent alone, that is, ampicillin, penicillin, or vancomycin, is successful in only 30% to 40% of patients. In contrast, the bacteriologic cure rate for therapy with a synergistic bactericidal combination of antibiotics is 85%. Streptomycin, 7.5 mg/kg (not to exceed 500 mg/dose) given intramuscularly or intravenously every 12 hours to achieve peak serum concentrations of approximately 20 μg/mL, can be used instead of gentamicin if the causative strain does not possess high-level resistance to streptomycin. Patients who are allergic to penicillins must be treated with either the vancomycin regimen (see Table 33–4, 3.C) or with a penicillin or ampicillin regimen (see Table 33–4, 3.A and B) after being cautiously desensitized to penicillin.

Antimicrobial resistance among enterococci is increasingly common and complex. Thus, enterococci causing IE must always be tested in vitro for susceptibility to ampicillin and vancomycin, for beta-lactamase production, and for high-level resistance to streptomycin and gentamicin. The complexity of the regimens for treatment of enterococcal IE, their potential toxicity, and evolving antibiotic resistance among enterococci suggest that patients with enterococcal IE should be seen by an infectious disease consultant to aid in the selection of optimal therapy.

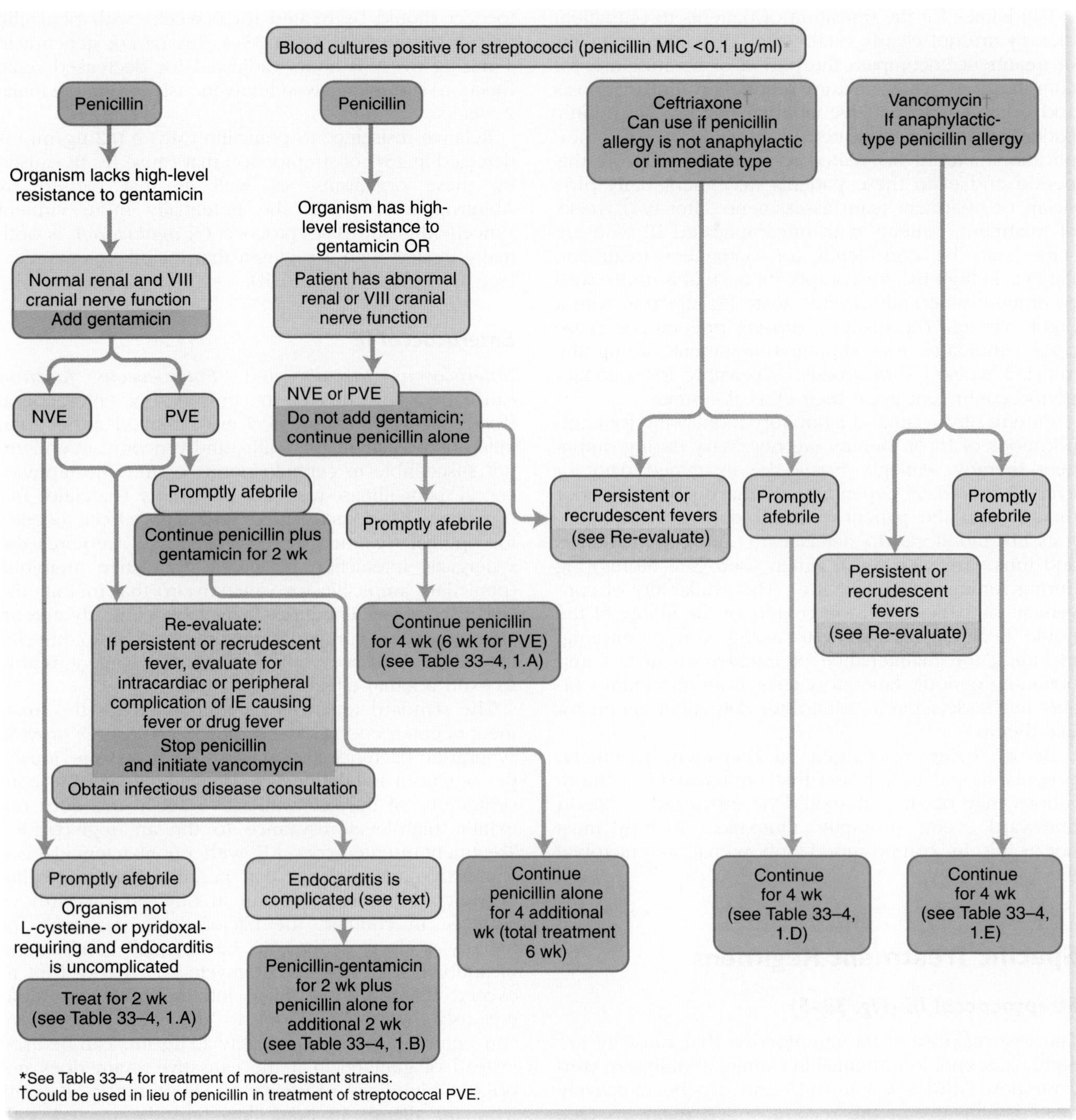

FIGURE 33–5. Treatment of streptococcal endocarditis. IE, infective endocarditis; MIC, minimal inhibitory concentration; NVE, native valve endocarditis; PVE, prosthetic valve endocarditis.

Staphylococcal IE (Fig. 33–6)

The overwhelming majority of coagulase-negative staphylococci and *S. aureus* produce penicillinase and are resistant to penicillin and ampicillin. Many coagulase-negative staphylococci and some *S. aureus*, particularly those causing nosocomially acquired IE, are resistant to methicillin and to all other currently available beta-lactam antibiotics. Fortunately, the vast majority of methicillin-resistant strains remain susceptible to vancomycin.

Nafcillin, oxacillin, and cefazolin are the primary agents recommended for the treatment of native valve IE caused by methicillin-susceptible staphylococci. Although not proven to enhance survival, gentamicin is often given concurrently during the initial 3 to 5 days of therapy in an attempt to accelerate control of the infection through the synergistic interaction of

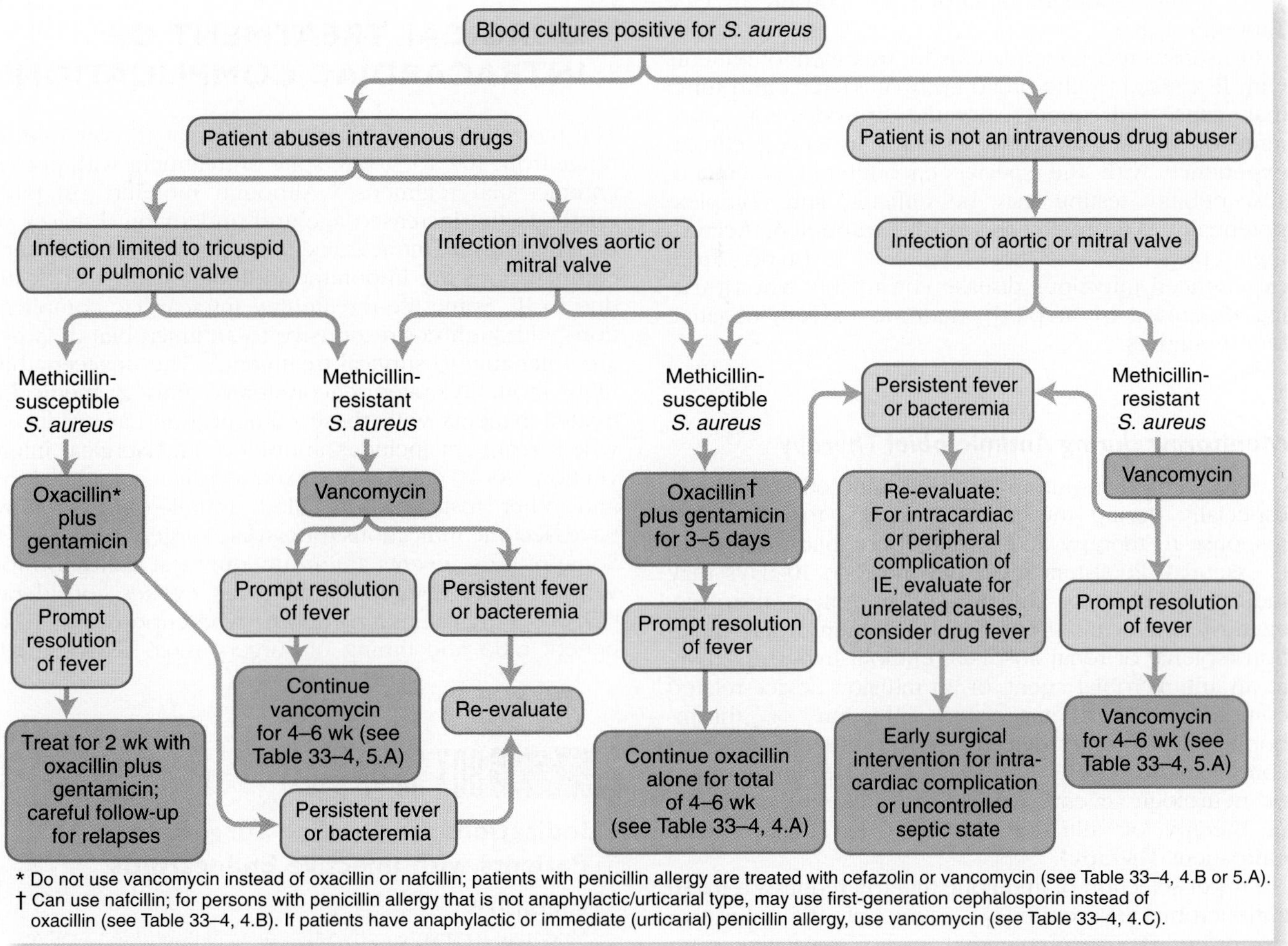

FIGURE 33–6. Treatment of native valve endocarditis caused by *Staphylococcus aureus*. IE, infective endocarditis.

the beta-lactam antibiotic and gentamicin (see Table 33–4, 4.A and B). Longer courses of gentamicin are not advocated because of potential nephrotoxicity. If beta-lactams cannot be used because of hypersensitivity, treatment with vancomycin is recommended (see Table 33–4, 4.C). An aminoglycoside is not routinely combined with vancomycin because of the potential enhanced nephrotoxicity of this combination. Vancomycin is not as bactericidal for methicillin-susceptible staphylococci as are beta-lactam agents and should not be used to treat staphylococcal IE for reasons of convenience only. Optimal treatment of native valve IE caused by methicillin-resistant staphylococci requires vancomycin (see Table 33–4, 5.A). Rifampin is not routinely used in the treatment of staphylococcal native valve IE.

If IE caused by methicillin-susceptible *S. aureus* among intravenous drug addicts is limited to the right-sided valves, 2 weeks of therapy using a semisynthetic penicillinase-resistant penicillin plus gentamicin (1 mg/kg every 8 hours) is highly effective among those patients who promptly become afebrile and do not have focal extracardiac infection. Vancomycin is not an effective alternative to the beta-lactam agent in this abbreviated regimen.

Staphylococcal infection involving prosthetic valves or other intracardiac foreign material is optimally treated with a multidrug regimen for a minimum of 6 and often 8 weeks (see Table 33–4, 6.A and 7.A). In this setting, rifampin plays a pivotal role in the killing of staphylococci that are adherent to foreign material. Because resistance to rifampin emerges easily in this setting, an additional agent that is known to be effective against the staphylococcus should be added to the beta-lactam antibiotic or vancomycin that serves as primary treatment. Gentamicin is the preferred agent; however, some strains will be resistant to gentamicin. In that case, an effective alternative aminoglycoside or fluoroquinolone should be used. Treatment with rifampin ideally should be delayed until the two agents have been used for a few days.

IE Caused by HACEK and Other Organisms

Some HACEK organisms produce beta-lactamase and are resistant to ampicillin. Accordingly, ceftriaxone has become the treatment of choice for HACEK IE (see Table 33–4, 8.A).

Consensus recommendations for treatment of patients with IE caused by the broad array of bacteria and fungi that cause infrequent sporadic episodes of valve infection are not available. In many instances, clinical experience with the species encountered is limited, susceptibility testing may be difficult, and complex, potentially toxic regimens may be warranted. Accordingly, physicians are urged to seek assistance from experienced infectious disease consultants when treating IE caused by atypical organisms or with negative blood cultures.

Monitoring during Antimicrobial Therapy

Careful clinical monitoring during antibiotic treatment, especially during the initial 2 weeks, to assess the response to therapy and to detect complications of IE is essential. Persistent fever beyond 7 to 10 days may indicate a failure of antimicrobial treatment, the presence of a myocardial abscess, focal extracardiac infection (splenic or renal abscess), emboli, hypersensitivity to an antimicrobial agent, or an infusion device-related complication (catheter-related infection or thrombophlebitis). Prompt detection of these events or other complications of IE (hemodynamic decompensation or neurologic event) may allow lifesaving revisions of therapy or initiation of adjunctive therapy (see Outpatient Therapy).

Proper selection of antibiotic therapy requires reliable antimicrobial susceptibility testing of the causative organism. The recommended organism-specific consensus regimens (see Table 33–4) result in predictably high bactericidal antimicrobial activity in the patient's serum from dose to dose. As a result, measurement of the serum bactericidal titer, the highest dilution of the patient's blood at a given time that kills 99.9% of a standard inoculum of the infecting organism, is no longer recommended. It is, however, appropriate to monitor serum concentrations of vancomycin and aminoglycosides when they are used. This allows dose adjustments, which ensures optimal therapy and reduces adverse events. Serum creatinine must be monitored when treatment employs vancomycin or an aminoglycoside. Complete blood counts should be checked weekly in patients receiving a beta-lactam antibiotic or vancomycin, and liver function tests should be monitored every 7 to 10 days in those receiving oxacillin or nafcillin.

Routine blood cultures in patients on therapy who no longer have fever are not indicated. Persistence or recrudescence of fever during therapy should be evaluated with blood cultures. Doing so may detect breakthrough bacteremia or new infections. Several blood cultures to document cure of IE are often obtained 2 to 8 weeks after completion of treatment. Recurrence of fever during this period after treatment demands blood cultures to assess the possibility of relapsed IE.

SURGICAL TREATMENT OF INTRACARDIAC COMPLICATIONS

The mortality rates for various forms of IE continue to range from 10% to 50% in spite of treatment with potent antimicrobial regimens.[10] Although mortality, in part, relates to the increased age and underlying diseases of patients with IE, intracardiac and central nervous system complications are important additional causes of death due to IE. Some life-threatening intracardiac complications, although not responsive to antimicrobial therapy, are amenable to surgical treatment.[11] The unacceptably high mortality rates encountered among medically treated patients with these complications are reduced when treatment includes antibiotics and surgical intervention. As a result, these intracardiac complications and other instances of failed antimicrobial therapy have become indications for cardiac surgery (Box 33–2). Some of these events are an unequivocal indication for surgery. More commonly, an event evokes consideration of surgical intervention, whereupon the risk-benefit ratio and timing of surgery must be weighed.

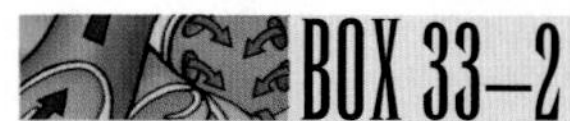

BOX 33–2

Indications for Cardiac Surgery in Patients with Infective Endocarditis

INDICATIONS*

Moderate to severe congestive heart failure due to valve dysfunction
Partially dehisced unstable prosthetic valve
Persistent bacteremia in the face of optimal antimicrobial therapy
Absence of effective, bactericidal therapy
Fungal endocarditis
Relapse of PVE after optimal antimicrobial therapy
Persistent unexplained fever (≥10 days) in culture-negative PVE
Staphylococcus aureus PVE

RELATIVE INDICATIONS†

Perivalvular extension of infection (myocardial, septal, or annulus abscess, intracardiac fistula)
Poorly responsive *Staphylococcus aureus* endocarditis involving the aortic or mitral valve
Relapse of native valve IE after optimal antimicrobial therapy
Large (>10 mm diameter) hypermobile vegetations
Persistent unexplained fever (≥10 days) in culture-negative native valve IE
Endocarditis due to highly antibiotic-resistant enterococci or gram-negative bacilli

*Cardiac surgery required for optimal outcome.
†Surgery, although not always required, must be carefully considered.
IE, infective endocarditis; PVE, prosthetic valve endocarditis.

When these circumstances arise, patients should be hospitalized in a setting where urgent cardiac surgery is available, if needed. At this juncture, multiple specialists—including cardiologists, cardiac surgeons, and infectious disease physicians—should be involved in the care of the patient. In patients with active IE (still receiving antimicrobial therapy) treated surgically for these indications, 30-day postoperative mortality rate is 7% to 10% and recurrent endocarditis occurs overall in about 7% (3% in natural valve IE and 10% to 17% in prosthetic valve IE).

Specific Indications

Valvular Dysfunction and Heart Failure

Patients with moderate to severe heart failure (New York Heart Association class III or IV) resulting from IE-induced valve dysfunction who are treated medically experience a mortality rate of 50% to 90% during hospitalization and over the ensuing 6 months. Among patients with comparable hemodynamic disability who undergo valve surgery, survival rates of 60% to 80% and 45% to 65% are achieved for native valve IE and PVE, respectively. Patients with aortic valve regurgitation deteriorate more rapidly than those with mitral valve regurgitation and require earlier surgical intervention. Occasionally, large vegetations significantly obstruct the orifice of the valve, particularly prosthetic mitral valves, necessitating surgery to relieve valve stenosis.[12]

Perivalvular Extension of Infection

Extension of infection beyond the valve into adjacent tissues, often with abcess formation, complicates 10% to 15% of patients with native valve IE and 45% to 60% of cases of PVE. This complication, which occurs more frequently with aortic versus mitral IE and is often associated with severe heart failure, is suggested by persistent unexplained (by an extracardiac source) fever in spite of appropriate antibiotic therapy. Pericarditis in patients with infection at the aortic valve site suggests extension through the annulus into the pericardial space. New onset and persistent electrocardiographic conduction abnormalities (otherwise unexplained), especially with aortic valve IE, although not sensitive, are a highly specific indicator of paravalvular infection. TEE with Doppler and color-flow Doppler evaluation is far more sensitive than TTE for the detection of perivalvular infection, abscess, and fistula. Persistent unexplained fever in spite of 10 days or more of appropriate antibiotic therapy for PVE and relapse of PVE after appropriate therapy are usually indicative of invasive infection and the need for surgical intervention. Although occasional patients with invasive infection will be cured with antibiotics alone, most appear to require surgical intervention to débride abscesses and repair structural damage. Overall operative mortality is less than 10% with increased rates for more extensive abscesses.[13]

Uncontrolled Infection

Persistent unexplained fever or continued positive blood cultures suggests uncontrolled infection. This may be the result of anatomic situations (undébrided abscess), antibiotic-resistant infecting organisms (highly resistant enterococci, *Pseudomonas aeruginosa,* gram-negative facultative bacilli, fungi). Before ascribing persistent fever to antibiotic failure, the susceptibility of the infecting organism to current therapy must be reassessed, extracardiac foci of infection must be excluded, and noninfectious causes of fever, including drug fever, must be evaluated. Scattered reports of medical cure of *Candida* species IE with prolonged antifungal therapy have been published. Although it may be possible to chronically suppress *Candida* IE with prolonged (over years) fluconazole treatment, medical cure of this entity remains unlikely.

S. aureus *IE*

A patient with *S. aureus* infection of the mitral or aortic valve whose course suggests invasive infection or who remains septic during the initial week of therapy, with or without bacteremia, is more likely to survive with surgical intervention than with continued antibiotics alone. The likelihood of curing patients with *S. aureus* PVE is markedly improved if these patients, especially those with intracardiac complications, are treated surgically. In contrast, intravenous drug addicts with *S. aureus* IE restricted to the right heart valves can usually be cured with continued antibiotic therapy, even in the face of several weeks of fever. It is likely that these patients will return to drug abuse and be at risk for recurrent IE; hence, it is prudent to avoid valve replacement, when possible.

Culture-Negative IE

Persistence of fever during empirical antimicrobial therapy in patients with echocardiographically confirmed, blood culture-negative IE suggests that either antibiotic therapy is inadequate or invasive infection is present. Accordingly, after excluding extracardiac infection and noninfectious causes of fever, including marantic endocarditis, these patients should be considered for surgery.

Large, Hypermobile Vegetations

The risk of arterial embolization appears greater among patients with large vegetations (>10 mm), particularly when these are pedunculated or hypermobile, than among patients with smaller or no echocardiographically demonstrable vegetations. Central nervous system emboli remain an important source of morbidity and mortality in patients with IE. Nevertheless, large vegetations in and of themselves are not an established indication for cardiac surgery to prevent emboli. Importantly, most emboli occur before diagnosis or in the initial days of treatment. Furthermore, the risk of embolism decreases significantly after 2 weeks of effective antimicrobial therapy. Thus, timing is an important variable. The role of surgery in the management of patients with large vegetations remains controversial. Occasionally exceptionally large vegetations may serve as an indication for surgery. More often, however, vegetation characteristics should be one of multiple clinical and echocardiographic observations weighed when considering surgery.

Timing of Cardiac Surgery

If the potential for cardiac surgical intervention to reduce mortality and morbidity in patients with IE is to be realized, primary care physicians must not only recognize the indications for surgery but also understand the optimal timing of surgery for each indication. Delayed surgery may result in preventable morbidity or mortality. Surgery to correct valve dysfunction that has caused congestive heart failure must be performed before intractable hemodynamic deterioration occurs, regardless of the duration of prior antibiotic therapy. It is clear that survival after surgery is inversely proportional to the severity of the preoperative hemodynamic disability. Uncontrolled infection also requires early surgical intervention. Delaying surgery in order to administer additional antibiotic therapy to patients who are failing antibiotic therapy does not improve outcome. In contrast, if the hemodynamic status is stable and infection is controlled, other considerations should determine the timing of surgery. For example, in a patient with valve dysfunction that requires surgery but who is hemodynamically compensated and in whom infection is controlled, surgery can be delayed until nearing the completion of the planned antibiotic regimen. In a patient who will ultimately require surgery because of valve dysfunction, detection of a very large vegetation may prompt surgery earlier than originally planned in an effort to reduce emboli. The high likelihood of severe neurologic deterioration postoperatively is offered as a contraindication to cardiac surgery in patients with central nervous system embolic infarcts or hemorrhage. In fact, the risk of neurologic deterioration decreases to 15% and 10% 2 and 3 weeks after an infarct, respectively. Thus, if cardiac surgery is considered lifesaving, it can be performed with acceptable neurologic risk at this time. Worsening of preexisting cerebral hemorrhage during cardiac surgery, however, remains a risk for at least 1 month after the original hemorrhage and makes surgical intervention hazardous throughout the period of active IE.

EXTRACARDIAC COMPLICATIONS

Focal extracardiac septic complications occasionally require treatment that differs significantly from that given for IE. Unique treatment may entail a longer duration of antibiotic therapy or drainage of a localized abscess. Splenic abscess, which complicates 3% to 5% of cases of IE, can be identified by ultrasound or computed tomography. Successful therapy almost always requires drainage percutaneously or splenectomy. Effective therapy for vertebral osteomyelitis may require a longer course of therapy than that for IE itself.

Mycotic aneurysms complicate 2% to 10% of cases of IE, and half of these aneurysms are located intracranially. Focal neurologic symptoms, persistent headache, or embolic events may be a harbinger of an aneurysm. Intracranial mycotic lesions that hemorrhage should be resected, if possible, to avoid further bleeding. Unruptured aneurysms may resolve with antibiotic therapy. Thus, these are followed angiographically. Failure to resolve or progressive enlargement during therapy is an indication for resection if technically feasible.

CONSULTATIVE SERVICES

The high cure rates for uncomplicated, subacute, viridans streptococcal and enterococcal IE suggest to the inexperienced physician that patients with IE are easily managed. In fact, IE is a treacherous disease, in part because the site of infection cannot be examined directly to assess progress. In addition, life-threatening complications—for example, arterial emboli, rupture of a mycotic aneurysm, valve destruction, and congestive heart failure—may occur without warning. As a result, it is prudent to seek infectious disease and other subspecialty consultative assistance when treating any patient with IE except those with uncomplicated viridans streptococci infection (Box 33–3). Because of the high mortality rates and the high frequency of invasive infection, patients with left-sided *S. aureus* IE and all

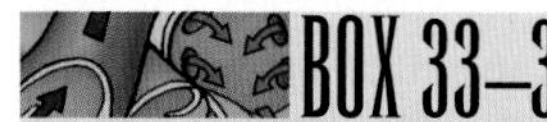

BOX 33–3

Situations Warranting Subspecialty Consultation in the Treatment of Infective Endocarditis

- Uncertain diagnosis
- Apparent culture-negative endocarditis
- Patient allergic to or intolerant of recommended therapy
- Endocarditis caused by an unusual organism or an unusually resistant organism
- Enterococcal endocarditis
- *Staphylococcus aureus* left-sided endocarditis
- Prosthetic valve endocarditis
- Relapse after appropriate therapy
- Persistent bacteremia or fever during therapy
- An indication or relative indication for cardiac surgical intervention (see Table 16–6)
- Neurologic complication
- Arterial embolic event
- Cerebral or peripheral mycotic aneurysm

patients with PVE should be seen in consultation by an infectious disease specialist. If these patients have been admitted to a hospital where cardiac surgery cannot be performed, provisional arrangements for urgent transfer to such a facility should be made at the time of diagnosis. Additionally, interpretation of enterococcal susceptibility tests and design of optimal therapy may require subspecialty consultation.

PREVENTION

The rationale and regimens for prophylaxis of IE are based on the recognition of the lesions that predispose to IE, the bacteria that cause IE, and the procedures that generate a moderately high frequency of transient bacteremia with these organisms.[14] Although experimental models of the pathogenesis and prophylaxis of IE support the concept of antibiotic prophylaxis to prevent IE, no randomized, controlled human trial has established the efficacy of chemoprophylaxis. Furthermore, most episodes of IE arise in patients unrelated to events for which prophylaxis is indicated. Although it is likely that optimal prophylaxis prevents only a small fraction of IE episodes, efforts to provide prophylaxis remain the standard of care. An American Heart Association expert committee has identified the patients likely to benefit from prophylaxis and the procedures warranting prophylaxis (Boxes 33–4 through 33–6) and has suggested regimens for use to prevent IE (Tables 33–5 and 33–6). By recognizing the cardiac lesions at risk for IE,

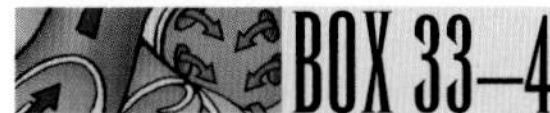
BOX 33–4

Risk of Infective Endocarditis Associated with Cardiac Abnormalities

HIGH RISK

Prosthetic heart valves
Prior bacterial endocarditis
Complex cyanotic congenital heart disease
Surgically constructed systemic-pulmonary shunts

MODERATE RISK

Congenital cardiac malformations (other than high- or low-risk lesions)
Acquired valvular dysfunction
Hypertrophic cardiomyopathy
Mitral valve prolapse with valvular regurgitation or thickened leaflets

LOW OR NEGLIGIBLE RISK

Isolated ostium secundum atrial septal defect
Surgically repaired atrial or ventricular septal defect or patent ductus arteriosus
Prior coronary artery bypass surgery
Mitral valve prolapse without valvular regurgitation
Physiologic, functional, or innocent heart murmurs
Prior Kawasaki's disease or rheumatic fever without valvular dysfunction
Cardiac pacemakers and implanted defibrillators

Adapted from Dajani AS, Taubert KA, Wilson W, et al: Prevention of bacterial endocarditis: Recommendations by the American Heart Association, from the Committee on Rheumatic Fever, Endocarditis, and Kawasaki Disease, Council on Cardiovascular Diseases in the Young. JAMA 1997;277:1794–1801.

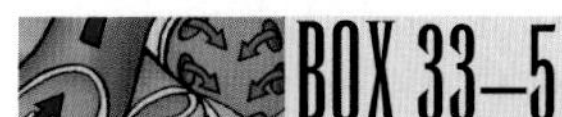
BOX 33–5

Dental Procedures for Which Infective Endocarditis Prophylaxis Is Considered

PROPHYLAXIS RECOMMENDED

Dental extractions
Periodontal procedures (surgery, scaling, root planing, probing)
Dental implant placement, reimplantation of avulsed teeth
Endodontic instrumentation (root canal) or surgery beyond the apex
Subgingival placement of antibiotic fibers or strips
Initial placement of orthodontic bands (not brackets)
Intraligamentary local anesthetic injections
Prophylactic cleaning of teeth or implants when bleeding is anticipated

PROPHYLAXIS NOT RECOMMENDED

Restorative dentistry (operative and prosthodontic) with or without retraction cord
Local anesthetic injection (not intraligamentary)
Intracanal endodontic treatment (postplacement and buildup)
Placement of rubber dams
Suture removal
Placement of removable prosthodontic or orthodontic appliances
Taking oral impressions or radiographs
Orthodontic appliance adjustment
Shedding primary teeth

Adapted from Dajani AS, Taubert KA, Wilson W, et al: Prevention of bacterial endocarditis: Recommendations by the American Heart Association, from the Committee on Rheumatic Fever, Endocarditis, and Kawasaki Disease, Council on Cardiovascular Diseases in the Young. JAMA 1997;277:1794–1801.

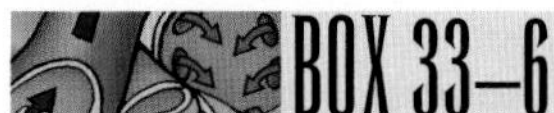
BOX 33–6

Procedures for Which Infective Endocarditis Prophylaxis Is Considered

PROPHYLAXIS RECOMMENDED	PROPHYLAXIS NOT RECOMMENDED
Respiratory Tract	
Surgical operation involving mucosa	Endotracheal intubation
Bronchoscopy with rigid bronchoscope	Bronchoscopy with flexible bronchoscope with or without biopsy*
	Tympanostomy tube insertion
Gastrointestinal Tract[†]	
Sclerotherapy for esophageal varices	Transesophageal echocardiography
Dilatation of esophageal stricture	Endoscopy with or without biopsy*
Endoscopic retrograde cholangiography with biliary obstruction	
Biliary tract surgery	
Surgery involving intestinal mucosa	
Genitourinary Tract	
Prostate surgery	Vaginal hysterectomy*
Cystoscopy	Vaginal delivery*
Urethral dilatation	Cesarean section
	In the absence of infection: Urethral catheterization, uterine dilatation and curettage, therapeutic abortion, sterilization, insertion/removal of intrauterine device
Other	Cardiac catheterization, coronary angioplasty
	Implantation of pacemakers, defibrillators, coronary stents
	Clean surgery
	Circumcision

*Prophylaxis is optional for high-risk patients.

[†]Recommended for high-risk patients; optional for moderate-risk group.

Adapted from Dajani AS, Taubert KA, Wilson W, et al: Prevention of bacterial endocarditis: Recommendations by the American Heart Association, from the Committee on Rheumatic Fever, Endocarditis, and Kawasaki Disease, Council on Cardiovascular Diseases in the Young. JAMA 1997;277:1794–1801.

repetitively reminding patients that they are at risk, and prescribing appropriate antibiotic prophylaxis, the primary care physician is ideally positioned to prevent IE. In addition to prevention of IE by antibiotic prophylaxis, the primary care physician can reduce the risk of IE by encouraging patients to maintain good oral hygiene through regular dental care.

Patients with cardiac abnormalities can be divided into those at high, moderate, and low or negligible risk for developing IE (see Box 33–4). Prophylaxis is not recommended for those at low or negligible risk. By 6 months after repair without residue, the moderate risk for IE associated with patent ductus arteriosus, ventricular septal defect, ostium primum atrial septal defect, and coarctation of the aorta is eliminated. The role of prophylaxis in patients with mitral valve prolapse (MVP), a common occurrence in the population, is controversial. The risk for IE in patients with MVP appears to be 5 to 10 times higher than in the general population but 100 times lower than that in patients with rheumatic valvular disease. In MVP, the risk for IE relates to regurgitant blood flow across the mitral valve and thickened valve leaflets, or both. Prophylaxis is recommended for patients with clinical evidence of MVP (systolic click) and a murmur of mitral regurgitation and patients over 45 years of age who on prior echocardiography have evidence of MVP and thickened leaflets, even in the absence of regurgitation at rest. Routine echocardiographic screening for MVP to identify candidates for prophylaxis is not recommended, however.

Prophylaxis is advised for procedures likely to induce bacteremia with IE-prone bacteria (see Boxes 33–5 and 33–6). When multiple dental procedures are required in close sequence, it may be desirable to separate them by 1 to 3 weeks to lessen the potential for selecting antibiotic-resistant oral flora. When surgery is to be performed on the genitourinary tract, cultures should be obtained preoperatively and infection eradicated before proceeding with surgery.

The regimens recommended for use as prophylaxis are targeted to the IE-prone bacteria likely to be encountered in the manipulated areas (see Tables 33–5 and 33–6). Antibiotic regimens to prevent recurrence of acute rheumatic fever are not adequate for prophylaxis of IE. Because patients receiving these regimens may have oral cavity flora that are resistant to penicillins, clindamycin or clarithromycin should be used for prophylaxis of IE. Surgical procedures on infected tissues, including incision and drainage, may induce bacteremia; consequently, prophylaxis should be

TABLE 33–5

Regimens for IE Prophylaxis in Adults: Oral, Respiratory Tract, or Esophageal Procedures

Setting	Antibiotic	Regimen*
Standard	Amoxicillin	2.0 gm PO 1 hr before procedure
Unable to take oral medication	Ampicillin	2.0 gm IM or IV within 30 min of procedure
Penicillin-allergic patients	Clindamycin	600 mg PO 1 hr before procedure or IV 30 min before procedure
	Cephalexin[†]	2.0 gm PO 1 hr before procedure
	Cefazolin[†]	1.0 gm IV or IM 30 min before procedure
	Cefadroxil[†]	2.0 gm PO 1 hr before procedure
	Clarithromycin	500 mg PO 1 hr before procedure

*For patients in the high-risk group, administer one half the dose 6 hr after the initial dose; dosing for children: amoxicillin, ampicillin, cephalexin, or cefadroxil use 50 mg/kg PO; cefazolin IV 25 mg/kg; clindamycin 20 mg/kg PO, 25 mg/kg IV; clarithromycin 15 mg/kg PO.

†Do not use cephalosporins in patients with immediate hypersensitivity (urticaria, angioedema, anaphylaxis) to penicillin.

IE, infective endocarditis; PO, by mouth; IM, intramuscular; IV, intravenous.

Adapted from Dajani AS, Taubert KA, Wilson W, et al: Prevention of bacterial endocarditis: Recommendations by the American Heart Association, from the Committee on Rheumatic Fever, Endocarditis, and Kawasaki Disease, Council on Cardiovascular Diseases in the Young. JAMA 1997;227:1794–1801.

TABLE 33–6

Regimens for IE Prophylaxis in Adults: Genitourinary and Gastrointestinal* Tract Procedures

Setting	Antibiotic	Regimen[†]
High-risk patients	Ampicillin plus gentamicin	Ampicillin 2.0 gm IV/IM plus gentamicin 1.5 mg/kg within 30 min of procedure, repeat ampicillin 1.0 gm IV/IM or amoxicillin 1.0 gm PO 6 hr later
High-risk, penicillin-allergic patients	Vancomycin plus gentamicin	Vancomycin 1.0 gm IV over 1–2 hr plus gentamicin 1.5 mg/kg IM/IV infused or injected 30 min before procedure; no second dose recommended
Moderate-risk patients	Amoxicillin or ampicillin	Amoxicillin 2.0 gm PO 1 hr before procedure or ampicillin 2.0 gm IM/IV 30 min before procedure
Moderate-risk, penicillin-allergic patients	Vancomycin	Vancomycin 1.0 gm IV infused over 1–2 hr and completed within 30 min of procedure

*Excludes esophageal procedures (see Table 33–5).

†Dosing for children: Ampicillin 50 mg/kg IV/IM, vancomycin 20 mg/kg IV, gentamicin 1.5 mg/kg IV/IM (children's doses should not exceed adults doses).

IE, infective endocarditis; IV, intravenous; IM, intramuscular; PO, by mouth.

Adapted from Dajani AS, Taubert KA, Wilson W, et al: Prevention of bacterial endocarditis: Recommendations by the American Heart Association, from the Committee on Rheumatic Fever, Endocarditis, and Kawasaki Disease, Council on Cardiovascular Diseases in the Young. JAMA 1997;277:1794–1801.

considered when IE-prone patients undergo these procedures. When *S. aureus* is the likely infecting organism, prophylaxis regimens should use an antistaphylococcal penicillin, a first-generation cephalosporin, or if methicillin-resistant *S. aureus* is anticipated, vancomycin.

References

1. Bayer AS, Scheld WM: Endocarditis and intravascular infections. In Mandell GL, Bennett JE, Dolin R (eds): Principles and Practice of Infectious Diseases, 5th ed. New York, Churchill Livingstone, 2000, pp 857–902.
2. Karchmer AW: Infective endocarditis. In Braunwald E, Zipes DP, Libby P (eds): Heart Disease: A Textbook of Cardiovascular Medicine, 6th ed. Philadelphia, WB Saunders, 2001, Philadelphia, pp 1723–1748.
3. Karchmer AW: Prevention and treatment of infective endocarditis. In Antman EM (ed): Cardiovascular Therapeutics: A Companion to Braunwald's Heart Disease. Philadelphia, WB Saunders, 2002, pp 1082–1099.
4. Mylonakis E, Calderwood SB: Infective endocarditis in adults. N Engl J Med 2001;345:1318–1330.
5. Karchmer AW: Infections of prosthetic valves and intravascular devices. In Mandell GL, Bennett JE, Dolin R (eds): Principles and Practice of Infectious Diseases, 5th ed. Philadelphia, Churchill Livingstone, 2000, pp 903–917.
6. Li JS, Sexton DJ, Mick N, et al: Proposed modifications to the Duke criteria for the diagnosis of infective endocarditis. Clin Infect Dis 2000;30:633–638.
7. Wilson WR, Karchmer AW, et al: Antibiotic treatment of adults with infective endocarditis due to viridans streptococci, enterococci, other streptococci, staphylococci, and HACEK microorganisms. JAMA 1995;274:1706–1713.
8. Andrews MM, von Reyn CF: Patient selection criteria and management guidelines for outpatient parenteral antibiotic therapy for native valve infective endocarditis. Clin Infect Dis 2001;33:203–209.
9. Bayer AS, Bolger AF, Taubert KA, et al: Diagnosis and management of infective endocarditis and its complications. Circulation 1998;98:2936–2948.
10. Bishara J, Leibovici L, Gartman-Israel D, et al: Long-term outcome of infective endocarditis: The impact of early surgical intervention. Clin Infect Dis 2001;33:1636–1643.
11. Alexiou C, Langley SM, Stafford H, et al: Surgery for active culture-positive endocarditis: Determinants of early and late outcome. Ann Thorac Surg 2000;69:1448–1454.

12. Gillinov AM, Shah RV, Curtis WE, et al: Valve replacement in patients with endocarditis and acute neurologic deficit. Ann Thorac Surg 1996;61:1125–1130.
13. d'Udekem Y, David TE, Feindel CM, et al: Long-term results of operation for paravalvular abscess. Ann ThoracSurg 1996;62:48–53.
14. Dajani AS, Taubert KA, Wilson W, et al: Prevention of bacterial endocarditis: Recommendations by the American Heart Association, from the Committee on Rheumatic Fever, Endocarditis, and Kawasaki Disease, Council on Cardiovascular Diseases in the Young. JAMA 1997;277: 1794–1801.

CHAPTER 34

Recognition and Management of Adults with Congenital Heart Disease

Elyse Foster and Melvin D. Cheitlin

Congenital heart disease occurs in 1% of all live births,[1] and most patients are recognized in infancy or childhood and appropriately treated. Since cardiopulmonary bypass capabilities were developed in the early 1950s, amazing advances in the surgical treatment of infants and children with major congenital heart lesions have permitted survival into adulthood.[2] Most patients who have major congenital heart disease and who have been surgically corrected or palliated will reach adulthood and childbearing age. Even lesions such as transposition of the great arteries, which was invariably fatal in the first year of life, are now surgically ameliorated. Thus, it is estimated that the number of patients with congenital heart disease reaching adulthood is approximately 20,000 per year in the United States alone.[1] Because such patients have an increased risk of bearing offspring with congenital heart disease, the prevalence of this disease in newborns may also be rising.

The embryology of the formation of the heart and cardiovascular system is complex, and abnormalities can occur at many stages and lead to a wide variety of congenital heart defects.[3,4] All congenital heart lesions fall into one or more of the following anatomic-pathophysiologic categories (Table 34–1): (1) predominant left-to-right shunts, (2) predominant right-to-left shunts, (3) stenotic or atretic valves and hypoplastic ventricles, (4) abnormalities of the great vessel, (5) positional abnormalities, and (6) other congenital syndromes. The relative incidences of these defects vary widely (Table 34–2).

Therefore, the aims of this chapter are as follows:

1. Describe the clinical features, recommended diagnostic evaluation, and indications for surgery for the most common unoperated congenital lesions encountered in adult patients (Tables 34–3 and 34–4).
2. Describe the most common complications that arise after palliative surgery for congenital heart disease.
3. Describe the interaction between congenital heart disease and systemic illnesses.

Prospective clinical trials comparing treatment of the various types of congenital heart disease have not been performed. Recommendations for treatment are based on experience and the well-documented natural history of the disease.[5] It is not reasonable to expect a primary care physician to manage patients with complicated congenital heart disease without the aid of a cardiologist experienced in the care of these patients.

TABLE 34–1

Anatomic-Pathophysiologic Classification of Congenital Heart Disease

Abnormality	Definition	Level	Example
I. Left-right shunt	Pulmonary venous return shunted to the right heart (PBF > SBF)	Venous	Pulmonary vein draining into the superior vena cava or right atrium
		Atrial	Atrial septal defect
		Ventricular	Intraventricular septal defect
		Arterial	Patent ductus arteriosus
II. Right-left shunt	Systemic venous return shunted to the left heart (SBF > PBF) "Cyanotic heart disease"	Venous	Superior vena cava into the left atrium
		Atrial	Tricuspid atresia
		Ventricular	Tetralogy of Fallot
		Arterial	Transposition of the great vessels
			Truncus arteriosus
III. Stenotic and hypoplastic valves or ventricles			Congenital aortic stenosis
			Congenital pulmonic stenosis
			Pulmonary atresia
			Left heart hypoplasia
IV. Great vessel abnormalities		Arterial	Coarctation of the aorta
		Venous	Total anomalous pulmonary venous drainage
V. Positional abnormalities			Corrected transposition (*L*-transposition)
			Dextrocardia and dextroposition
			Transposition of the great vessels
VI. Other congenital syndromes with aortic involvement			Marfan's syndrome
			Muscular dystrophy

PBF, pulmonary blood flow; SBF, systemic blood flow.

TABLE 34–2

Incidence of Specific Congenital Lesions According to Age at Diagnosis

Lesion	Incidence at Birth (per 1000 Births)	Incidence in Adults (per 1000)	Specific Chromosomal Abnormalities	Associated Syndromes/Other
Atrial septal defect	0.9	0.6		Holt-Oram syndrome
Ventricular septal defect	3	0.3		
Patent ductus arteriosus	0.6	0.5		
Pulmonary stenosis	0.6	0.5		Congenital rubella, Noonan's syndrome
Aortic stenosis	0.3	0.25		
Coarctation	0.7	0.6		
Tetralogy of Fallot	0.3	0.2	Chromosome 22 deletions (11%)	
Atrioventricular septal defect	0.25	0.15	Trisomy 21	Down's syndrome
Transposition of the great vessels	0.2	0.1		

Nevertheless, with a greater number of individuals surviving to adulthood with complex disease, these patients will come to primary care physicians for routine health care and for treatment of complications or subsequent acquired disease.[6] Therefore, it is important that the primary care physician establish a relationship with a cardiologist who is knowledgeable about congenital heart disease and who can serve as a consultant in the care of these patients. Many of these patients will require at least periodic ongoing follow-up in a specialized center for adults with congenital heart disease.[7]

The primary care physician will see adult patients with congenital heart disease in the following ways:

1. *Minor congenital abnormalities*. Examples include single anomalous pulmonary vein, bicuspid aortic valve, and mild coarctation of the aorta. In these conditions, the challenge for the primary care physician is to first recognize the abnormality and,

TABLE 34–3

Findings in Selected Uncomplicated Congenital Cardiac Defects*

Type	Physical Findings	ECG	Chest Radiograph
Atrial septal defect	Ejection murmur across pulmonic valve Widely and fixed split S_2 Diastolic flow murmur across tricuspid valve Parasternal (RV) impulse	rSr′ or rSr′s′; left axis with ostium primum defect	Large pulmonary artery and increased pulmonary vascular markings (pulmonary plethora)
Ventricular septal defect	Holosystolic left parasternal murmur ± thrill Normal or moderately split S_2 Diastolic flow murmur and S_3 Apical impulse prominent and displaced laterally; also parasternal impulse	Biventricular or left ventricular hypertrophy	Cardiomegaly Prominent pulmonary artery and pulmonary plethora
Patent ductus arteriosus	Widened arterial pulse pressure Hyperdynamic apical impulse Continuous "machinery" murmur	LV hypertrophy	Prominent pulmonary artery and pulmonary plethora; enlarged LA, LV; occasionally calcified ductus
Congenital valvular aortic stenosis	Decreased pulse pressure and carotid upstroke Sustained apical impulse S_4; systolic ejection murmur ± thrill Single or paradoxical splitting of S_2 Concomitant aortic regurgitation common	LV hypertrophy	Poststenotic aortic dilatation Prominent LV
Valvular pulmonic stenosis	Large jugular A-wave RV parasternal impulse Pulmonic ejection sound Systolic ejection murmur ± thrill at second left intercostal space Widely split S_2 with soft (or inaudible) P_2 Right ventricular S_4	RV hypertrophy RA abnormality	Pulmonary blood flow normal or reduced Poststenotic dilatation of main or left pulmonary artery RA and RV enlargement
Coarctation of aorta	Reduced lower extremity blood pressure; delayed, diminished femoral pulses Mid-systolic coarctation murmur at left sternal border or posterior left intrascapular area Continuous murmur from collaterals Sustained apical impulse; S_4 Evidence of associated bicuspid aortic valve common	LV hypertrophy	Prominent ascending aorta; LV enlargement Poststenotic aortic dilatation Notching of inferior rib surfaces from collateral flow in intercostal arteries
Ebstein's anomaly	Acyanotic or cyanotic (right-to-left shunt from increased RA pressure) Increased jugular pressure and regurgitant wave Systolic murmur of tricuspid regurgitation increased with inspiration Wide splitting of S_2; S_4 and S_3	RA abnormality Right bundle branch block PR prolongation Ventricular preexcitation	Enlarged RA Pulmonary vascularity normal or decreased
Tetralogy of Fallot	Usually cyanotic Clubbing may be present Prominent ejection murmur at left sternal border Soft or absent P_2	RV hypertrophy RA abnormality	"Boot"-shaped heart from RV hypertrophy, small pulmonary artery, and small LV Pulmonary vascularity normal or reduced

*Findings vary depending on the severity of lesions and associated abnormalities (see text).

ECG, electrocardiogram; LA, left atrium; LV, left ventricle; RA, right atrium; RV, right ventricle; S_2, second heart sound; P_2, second pulmonic heart sound.

From Andreoli TE, Bennett JC, Carpenter CCJ, Plum F: Congenital heart disease. *In* Cecil Essentials of Medicine, 4th ed. Philadelphia, WB Saunders, 1997, p 41.

TABLE 34–4

Indications for Primary Surgery, Common Postoperative Complications, and Indications for Reoperation in Congenital Heart Disease

Lesion	Indication for Primary Repair	Post-Repair Complications	Indication for Reoperation
Atrial septal defect	Qp : Qs ≥ 1.8 : 1 and/or dilated right ventricle Paradoxical embolism	Atrial fibrillation, CVA* Patch leak	Secundum: large residual shunt Primum: MR
Ventricular septal defect	Qp : Qs ≥ 1.8 : 1 and/or dilated left ventricle	Patch leak Endocarditis† Progressive PHTN	Patch leak when Qp : Qs ≥ 1.5 : 1
Patent ductus arteriosus	Audible shunt (i.e., murmur)	Persistent shunt Endoarteritis† Progressive PHTN	Persistent shunt
Atrioventricular septal defect	Qp : Qs > 1.5 : 1 Hemodynamically significant MR	Patch leak Endocarditis Progressive MR Atrial fibrillation Atrioventricular block	MR Patch leak
Anomalous pulmonary venous drainage	Qp : Qs > 1.5 : 1	Obstruction of the pulmonary veins	N/A
Tetralogy of Fallot	No previous repair	Patch leak Pulmonary insufficiency Residual PS Heart block Ventricular and atrial arrhythmias Sudden death Endocarditis	Hemodynamically significant PI or PS
Transposition of great vessel	N/A	**Post-atrial switch** RV failure Tricuspid regurgitation Baffle leak Baffle obstruction Atrial arrhythmias Heart block Endocarditis **Post-arterial switch** Supravalvar aortic stenosis Coronary artery stenosis	**Post-atrial switch** Significant baffle obstruction Progressive RV failure TR **Post-arterial switch** Significant supravalvar stenosis Coronary stenosis with ischemia
Ebstein's anomaly	Severe TR RV failure	Atrial arrhythmias Progressive TR	Severe TR
Tricuspid atresia	N/A	**Post-Fontan** Atrial arrhythmias Protein-losing enteropathy Ascites	Conduit obstruction
Aortic stenosis	AVA < 0.8 cm^2 and symptoms	**Post-valvotomy** Progressive AI or restenosis Ventricular arrhythmias Sudden death Endocarditis	Severe AS or AI and symptoms or LV dysfunction
Subaortic stenosis	Gradient >30 mm Hg or the development of AI at a lower gradient	Progressive AI Restenosis Endocarditis	Severe AI or recurrent stenosis and symptoms
Pulmonary stenosis	Transpulmonary gradient >50 mm Hg Transpulmonary gradient <50 mm Hg with RV hypertrophy or symptoms	Restenosis PI Endocarditis rare	Severe PS or PI and symptoms
Coarctation of aorta	Upper extremity HTN Transcoarctation gradient >25 mm Hg	Residual HTN Saccular aneurysm Dissecting aneurysm Circle of Willis aneurysm—CVA Premature CAD AS/AI Endocarditis or endarteritis	Recurrent coarctation AS/AI CAD Saccular or dissecting aneurysm

*These complications are most common when repaired in adults older than 40 years.

†Endocarditis and endarteritis are likely only in the presence of a persistent shunt.

AI, aortic insufficiency; AS, aortic stenosis; AVA, aortic valve area; CAD, coronary artery disease; CVA, cerebrovascular accident; MR, mitral regurgitation; PHTN, pulmonary hypertension; PI, pulmonic valve insufficiency; PS, pulmonic valve stenosis; Qp : Qs, pulmonary-to-systemic flow ratio; RV, right ventricle; TR, tricuspid regurgitation.

TABLE 34–5

Primer of Palliative Surgery

	Anatomy	**Comment**
	Systemic Arterial–Pulmonary Arterial	
Classic Blalock-Taussig	Subclavian artery directly to PA	Absent ipsilateral radial pulse; continuous murmur
Modified Blalock-Taussig	Subclavian to PA conduit	Preserved pulse; continuous murmur
Central shunt	Aorta to pulmonary artery conduit	Continuous murmur
Waterston	Ascending aorta to RPA	Continuous murmur*
Potts	Descending aorta to LPA	Continuous murmur*
	Systemic Venous to PA	
Glenn	Superior vena cava to PA	No murmur secondary to shunt; arrhythmias uncommon
Fontan	Total cavopulmonary shunt	No murmur; atrial arrhythmias common
	Other	
Mustard and Senning	Atrial baffle for TGV	No murmur Obstruction and atrial arrhythmias common
Jatene	Arterial switch for TGV	Possible murmur from aortic insufficiency or supravalvar stenosis
Rastelli	Right ventricle–pulmonary artery	Valve degeneration may lead to pulmonary insufficiency murmur

*A continuous murmur may disappear in the presence of pulmonary hypertension.

LPA, left pulmonary artery; PA, pulmonary artery; RPA, right pulmonary artery; TGV, transposition of the great vessels.

Adapted from Foster E, Cheitlin M: Hemodynamically unstable presentations of congenital heart disease. In Brown DL (ed): Adults in Cardiac Intensive Care. Philadelphia, WB Saunders, 1997.

second, understand the natural history of these lesions. For instance, a patient with a bicuspid aortic valve may do well until 40 or 50 years of age, when progressive valve calcification leads to severe aortic stenosis.

2. *Major untreated congenital heart disease.* At times, significant congenital heart disease can be overlooked during childhood. The most common lesion is an atrial septal defect, but a ventricular septal defect or even a patent ductus arteriosus is occasionally missed. A second type of patient has untreated congenital heart disease because no adequate palliative surgical procedure was available previously or at present. Patients with pulmonary vascular disease and pulmonary hypertension can be very difficult to treat; usually, their only option is lung transplantation with or without heart transplantation or intracardiac repair. Lesions that markedly restrict pulmonary blood flow because of small pulmonary arteries could neither be grafted nor shunted successfully in the past; innovative surgery available in specialized centers may palliate selected patients with these lesions and relieve their cyanosis. Rarely, previously untreated patients will have "single-ventricle" lesions, usually associated with pulmonary stenosis in those surviving to adulthood.
3. *Significantly palliated lesions.* This category includes the most frequently seen patients with significant congenital heart disease. The palliation can be partial; for instance, patients with a Blalock-Taussig or Potts shunt for the tetralogy of Fallot have persistent cyanosis. However, late post-repair complications also occur in patients who have had total correction of the tetralogy of Fallot or who have had an atrial switch procedure to provide physiologic correction of transposition of the great arteries. None can be considered completely cured (see Tables 34–4, 34–5).
4. *Patients who have been "cured."* These patients are the least common ones with congenital heart disease and consist of some patients with closure of an atrial or ventricular septal defect and ligation and division of a patent ductus arteriosus.

The primary care physician will usually see only the most common of the congenital heart lesions: atrial septal defect, ventricular septal defect, patent ductus arteriosus, tetralogy of Fallot, coarctation of the aorta, and congenital aortic stenosis. The differential diagnosis of congenital heart disease in adults requires a thorough history and physical examination, a chest radiograph, and an electrocardiogram (ECG). A definitive diagnosis, together with an extensive amount of information concerning pathophysiology, can often be obtained with a complete echocardiographic examination. Additional information can be obtained by magnetic resonance imaging (MRI); for example, the size of the pulmonary arterial branches may be better seen with this noninvasive technique. Cardiac catheterization and angiography are indicated after a noninvasive evaluation when pulmonary vascular resistance must be measured or the pulmonary and coronary arteries must be examined.

LESIONS CHARACTERIZED BY A LEFT-TO-RIGHT SHUNT

Interatrial Septal Defect

Pathophysiology

In this group of lesions, a defect in the interatrial septum allows pulmonary venous return to pass from the left to the right atrium. Because this left-to-right shunt increases venous return to the right ventricle, right ventricular stroke volume and pulmonary blood flow are increased in comparison to systemic blood flow (Fig. 34–1).

The three types of atrial septal defects are (1) ostium secundum defects in the center of the atrial septum, (2) ostium primum defects in the lower part of the septum and frequently associated with abnormalities of the mitral or tricuspid valves with resultant valvular regurgitation, and (3) sinus venosus defects, which are usually superior and posterior in relation to the superior vena cava and are frequently associated with anomalous drainage of one or more pulmonary veins into the right atrium or superior vena cava. In addition, up to 15% of the normal population may have a patent foramen ovale with the potential for right-to-left shunting, which can cause embolic stroke or put the individual at higher risk for decompression illness or high-altitude sickness.[8]

Recognition and Diagnosis

History and Physical Examination. Young patients with atrial septal defects are frequently asymptomatic and identified only because of a murmur, an abnormal chest radiograph, or an abnormal ECG. With increased diastolic filling of the right ventricle and increased right ventricular stroke volume, the patient often has a right ventricular precordial lift. The most significant abnormality on physical examination is the wide and fixed split second heart sound (S_2), which is caused by a consistent increase in right ventricular diastolic filling unaltered by the respiratory cycle. A grade II or III/VI, rarely grade IV/VI systolic ejection murmur is heard in the second interspace to the left of the sternum because of the increased pulmonary flow across a normal pulmonic outflow tract and valve. A rumbling mid-diastolic murmur may also be heard along the left sternal border as a result of increased diastolic flow across a normal

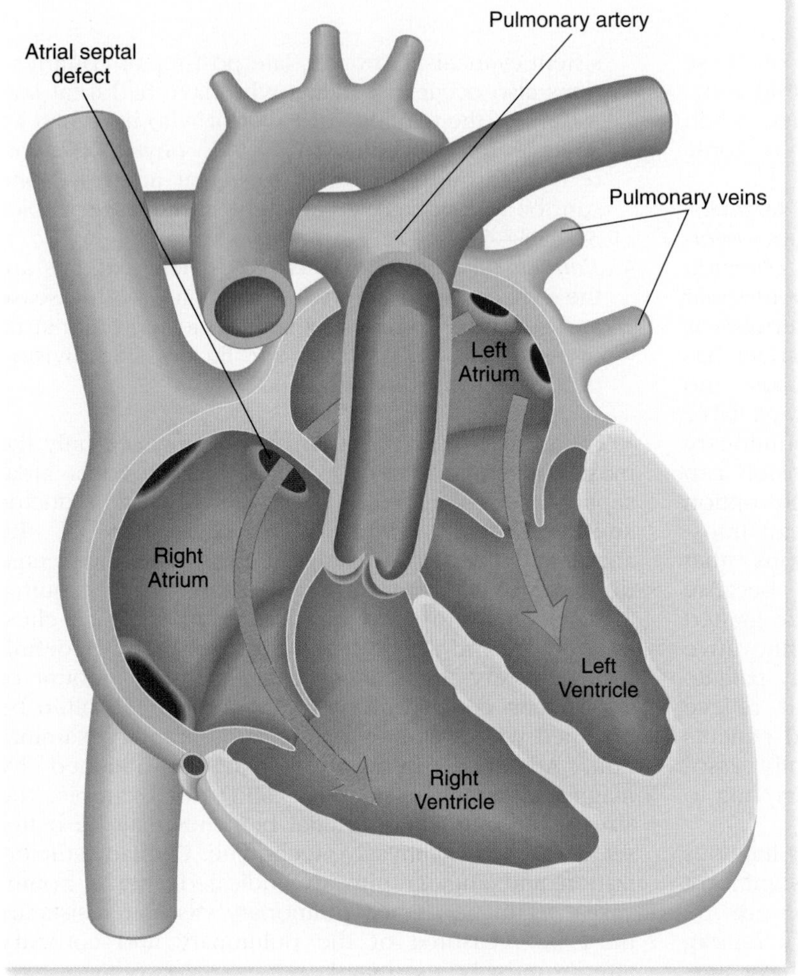

FIGURE 34–1. This diagram shows the typical location of an ostium secundum atrial septal defect. *Arrows* depict the direction of blood flow in the absence of pulmonary vascular disease. (Reprinted, by permission, from Brickner ME, Hillis LD, Lange RL: Congenital heart disease [first of two parts]. N Engl J Med 2000;342:256–263.)

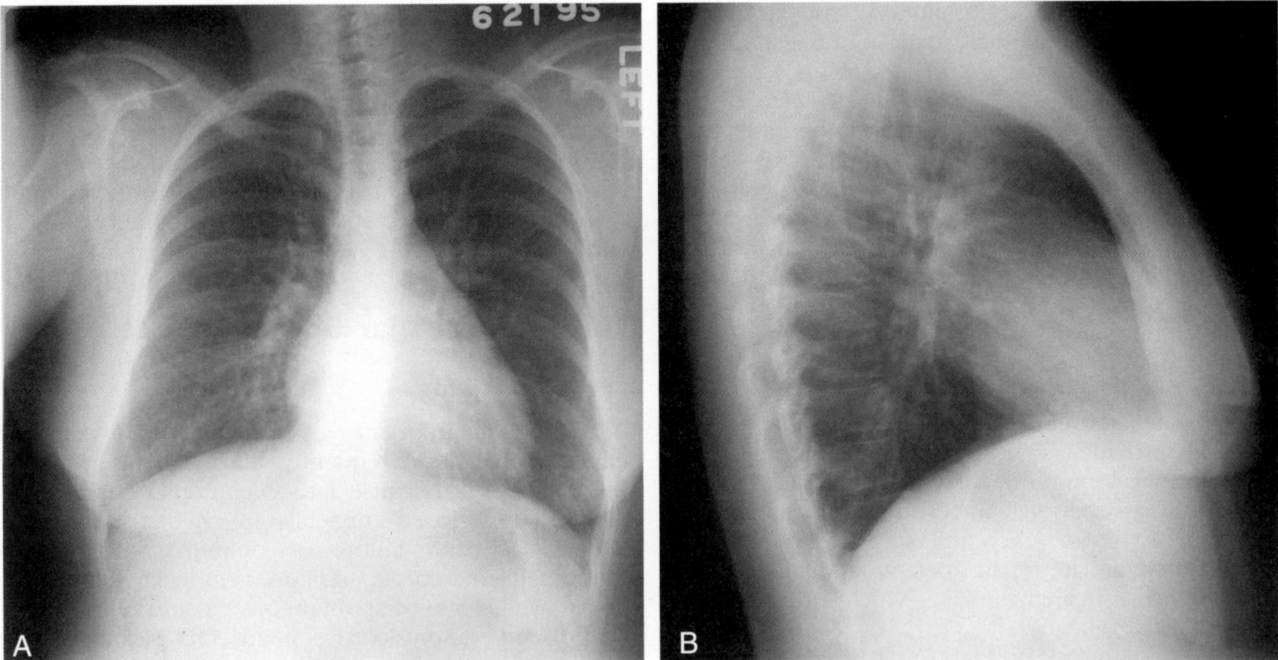

FIGURE 34–2. *A,* Chest radiograph, posteroanterior view, of a 32-year-old woman with an ostium secundum atrial septal defect. Note the prominent pulmonary vascular markings and increased cardiothoracic ratio. *B,* Chest radiograph, lateral view. Note the right ventricular enlargement.

tricuspid valve. With an ostium primum defect, the associated cleft mitral valve may cause an apical pansystolic murmur of mitral regurgitation. The murmur may be well heard along the left sternal border because the jet may be directed into the right atrium through the low atrial septal defect.

Laboratory

Chest Radiograph. With a significant left-to-right shunt, the cardiac silhouette is enlarged mainly because of the right ventricular dilatation. Pulmonary vascular markings are increased (Fig. 34–2).

ECG. The ECG shows signs of right ventricular enlargement with an rsR′ pattern in V_1. Patients with an ostium primum atrial septal defect have characteristic severe left axis deviation because of the abnormal course of the conduction system, in addition to the rsR′ in V_1.

Other Diagnostic Procedures and Referral for Cardiology Consultation. Transthoracic echocardiography (TTE) with a contrast study should be the initial investigation in patients with a suspected atrial septal defect. Although the defect is rarely visualized directly in adults, indirect evidence of an atrial septal defect includes right-sided chamber enlargement and the appearance of saline contrast in the left heart chambers. Doppler echocardiography can demonstrate flow across the atrial septum. The next step in the evaluation would be referral to a cardiologist for transesophageal echocardiography (TEE) (Fig. 34–3) or catheterization and for coronary angiography in patients older than 40 years to detect possible coronary artery disease. These studies should determine the need for referral for closure of the defect.

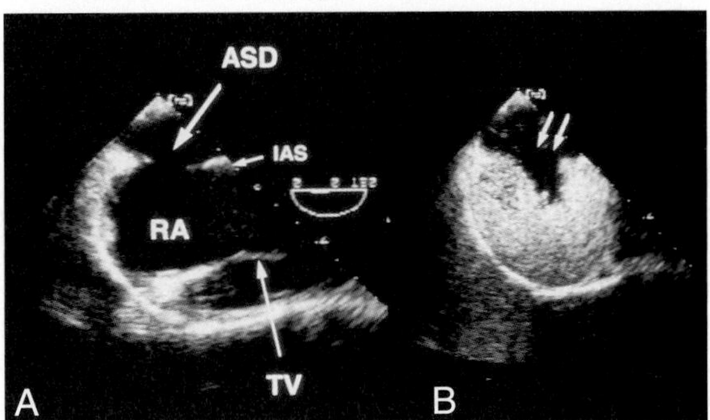

FIGURE 34–3. Transesophageal echocardiogram of a 24-year-old man with an ostium secundum atrial septal defect (ASD). *A,* The defect is located in the midportion of the interatrial septum (IAS). RA, right atrium; TV, tricuspid valve. *B,* Negative contrast effect of intravenously injected saline solution when unopacified left atrial blood enters the right atrium *(double arrow).*

Course and Complications

Most patients are asymptomatic or minimally symptomatic into early adulthood. Young women tolerate pregnancy well if significant pulmonary hypertension has not developed. However, if the left-to-right shunt is large, most patients will eventually have symptoms of heart failure and, frequently, atrial fibrillation. In older patients without pulmonary vascular disease, the magnitude of the left-to-right shunt can increase as left ventricular compliance falls because of diastolic dysfunction. Whereas aging alone may reduce diastolic compliance, hypertension and coronary artery disease may make it even worse. Pulmonary vascular disease with pulmonary hypertension, reversal of the shunt, and the development of cyanosis occurs in approximately 10% to 15% of patients. Even in the absence of pulmonary hypertension, patients with an unoperated atrial septal defect do not have a normal life expectancy. Early natural history studies demonstrated only about a 50% survival rate beyond age 40 years.[3] If atrioventricular (AV) valvular regurgitation is present in a patient with an ostium primum defect, heart failure may occur at an earlier age. Because of the abnormal interatrial communication, paradoxical embolization may occasionally result in systemic embolization, even in the absence of pulmonary hypertension.

Primary or patch closure of an atrial septal defect in childhood provides excellent operative results and nearly normal long-term survival in adults. Surgical closure is also superior to medical therapy in persons older than 40 years when the shunt ratio is 1.7 or higher.[9] However, late repair does not appear to reduce the incidence of arrhythmias, which are generally related to atrial dilatation.[10]

Treatment

Operative patch closure is generally recommended if the shunt is large with a pulmonary blood flow–to–systemic blood flow ratio of 1.8:1 or higher and right ventricular enlargement. Percutaneous closure with a variety of devices is increasingly becoming available and can be considered in adults. Several of these devices have been approved by regulatory agencies. In the presence of atrial arrhythmias or a history of cerebral ischemia, a period of post-procedure anticoagulation should be considered. Patients with smaller shunts caused by true atrial septal defects or by a patent foramen ovale have a lower incidence of heart failure, pulmonary hypertension, and arrhythmias. The risk for paradoxical embolization is also lower with smaller defects, but a defect of any size can be associated with paradoxical embolization, which is usually considered an indication for closure regardless of the size of the shunt. Even in elderly patients with large shunts, operative and now percutaneous closure can be performed at low risk and with good results in reducing symptoms. If the patient has severe pulmonary vascular disease and a reversed (right-to-left) shunt with arterial oxygen saturation at rest below 90% and little or no residual left-to-right shunt, closure is contraindicated.

In patients with ostium primum defects, surgical valve repair with or without annuloplasty may reduce the severity of the mitral and tricuspid regurgitation. If severe mitral regurgitation persists, valve re-repair or replacement is necessary. In sinus venosus defects, it is frequently necessary to patch the atrial septal defect in such a way as to ensure that the anomalous pulmonary venous drainage is diverted into the left atrium.

Management of Postoperative Patients. If an atrial septal defect was closed during childhood, patients can lead a completely normal life without any need to impose exercise restrictions unless the patient has persistent or progressive pulmonary hypertension. Likewise, in the absence of pulmonary hypertension, pregnancy is safe. Atrial fibrillation is common, so anticoagulation is indicated in postoperative patients with this arrhythmia because of the high risk of stroke. However, the risk of endocarditis is extremely low, and prophylactic antibiotics are recommended for only the first 6 months after surgery or successful percutaneous closure, unless other lesions such as mitral regurgitation are also present.

Interventricular Septal Defect

Pathophysiology

Patients with unoperated ventricular septal defects are encountered less frequently than patients with atrial septal defects because large ventricular septal defects are usually closed surgically in childhood when evidence of heart failure or pulmonary hypertension becomes apparent; in addition, ventricular septal defects have a high rate of spontaneous closure in infancy and childhood. A ventricular septal defect permits a left-to-right shunt to occur at the ventricular level (Fig. 34–4). When the increased pulmonary blood flow returns to the left ventricle, left ventricular diastolic volume and stroke volume increase.

Ventricular septal defects can be classified by anatomic location: perimembranous ventricular septal defects, AV canal ventricular septal defects, multiple muscular ventricular septal defects, and the so-called supracristal ventricular septal defect.

Recognition and Diagnosis

History and Physical Examination. A murmur is frequently detected shortly after birth. A young adult with an uncorrected ventricular septal defect and normal pulmonary artery pressure is usually asymptomatic but may have suffered an episode of endocarditis. When the shunt ratio exceeds 2:1 to 3:1, exertional dyspnea may develop after the age of 30 years; symptoms are rare in patients with smaller shunts. The most disabled group, those with pulmonary hypertension and cyanosis (i.e., Eisenmenger's physiology), is discussed separately.

If the ventricular septal defect is small (restrictive), a large pressure difference can be noted between the left and the right ventricles in systole. The resulting high-velocity jet across the defect causes the loud, frequently grade IV/VI, pansystolic murmur that is characteristic of this lesion and heard along the left sternal border in the third or fourth intercostal space.

If the ventricular septal defect is large (nonrestrictive), no pressure difference occurs between the left and the right ventricles; in this case, the magnitude of the shunt depends on the ratio of pulmonary to systemic vascular resistance. If pulmonary vascular resistance is lower than systemic vascular resistance, the left-to-right shunt can be large, and the pansystolic murmur may be loud. As pulmonary vascular resistance approaches systemic vascular resistance, the left-to-right shunt diminishes, and the systolic murmur becomes softer and finally disappears.

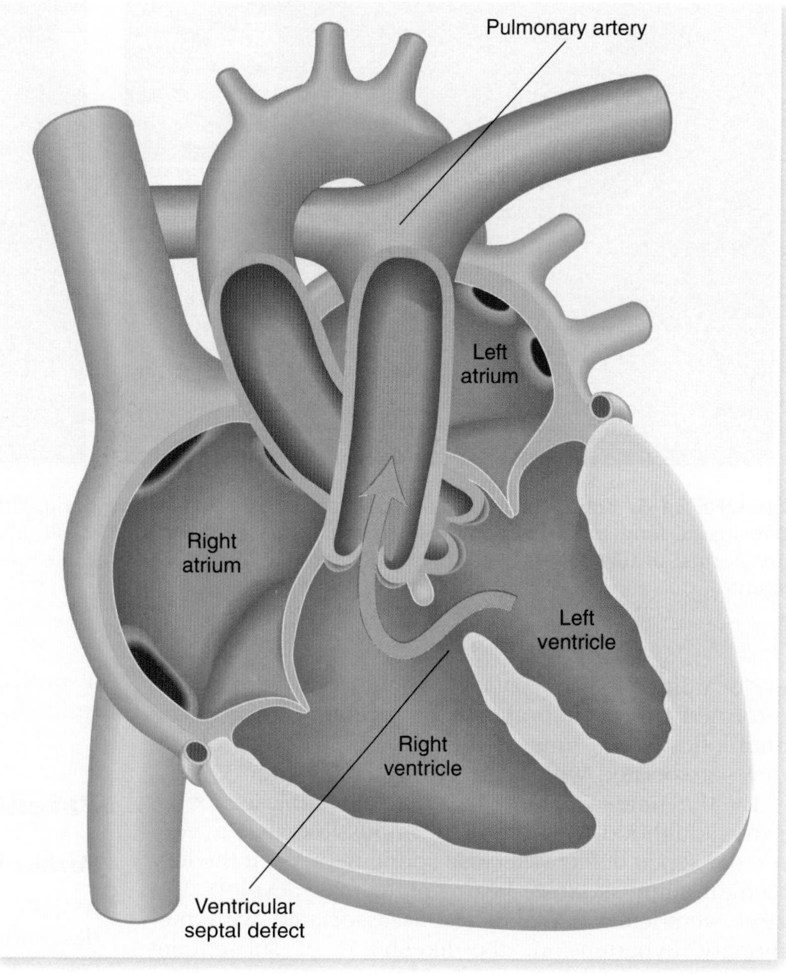

FIGURE 34–4. Diagram showing the typical location of a perimembranous ventricular septal defect, with the *green arrow* depicting the direction of blood flow in the absence of pulmonary hypertension. (Reprinted, by permission, from Brickner ME, Hillis LD, Lange RL: Congenital heart disease [first of two parts]. N Engl J Med 2000;342:256–263.)

With large left-to-right shunts, the left ventricle dilates and becomes hypertrophied, and a hyperdynamic, displaced left ventricular apex results. A diastolic rumbling murmur may be heard at the apex because of increased blood flow in diastole across the mitral valve. If pulmonary pressure is high, the pulmonic component of S_2 becomes loud, and a right ventricular lift may develop.

A diastolic blowing murmur of aortic regurgitation may occur in patients with a supracristal ventricular septal defect because of prolapse of the right coronary cusp. A pansystolic murmur followed immediately by a blowing diastolic murmur may simulate a continuous murmur.

Laboratory

Chest Radiograph. With a small left-to-right shunt, the chest radiograph may be normal. With a large left-to-right shunt, cardiomegaly may be caused by left ventricular dilatation, left atrial dilatation, and possibly right ventricular dilatation. The main pulmonary artery is prominent, and pulmonary vascular markings are increased. When pulmonary vascular resistance is increased, the chest radiograph will show evidence of right ventricular prominence, dilatation of the main pulmonary artery, and peripheral "pruning" of the pulmonary vessels. With severe, long-standing pulmonary hypertension, calcification of the proximal pulmonary arteries may be seen.

ECG. The ECG may be within normal limits, or it may show left ventricular or biventricular hypertrophy, depending on the size of the shunt and pulmonary artery pressure.

Other Diagnostic Procedures and Referral for Cardiology Consultation. TTE with color-flow Doppler imaging usually defines the location and size of a ventricular septal defect (Fig. 34–5). If the left-to-right shunt is large, the left atrium and left ventricle are dilated. Right ventricular dimensions are normal unless pulmonary hypertension is present. Pulmonary artery systolic pressure can usually be estimated by Doppler. The presence of associated defects (e.g., pulmonary valve stenosis) or expected complications (e.g., aortic insufficiency with a supracristal ventricular septal defect) can be confirmed.

Once a clinically significant ventricular septal defect is diagnosed, referral to a cardiologist is recommended to assist in deciding whether cardiac catheterization or surgical closure is indicated.

Course and Complications

With a small perimembranous or muscular ventricular septal defect, the only danger is that of infective

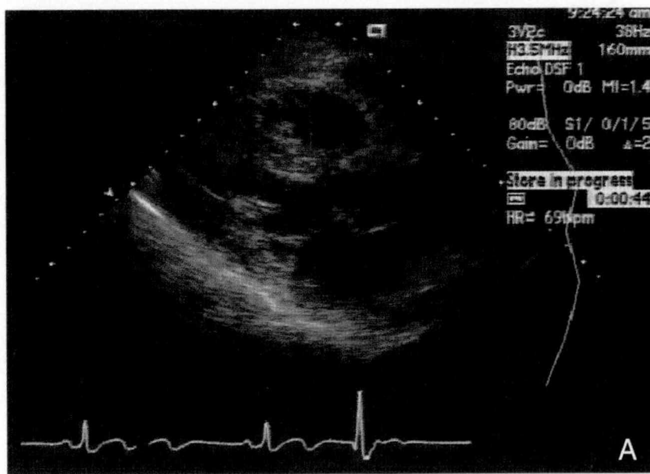

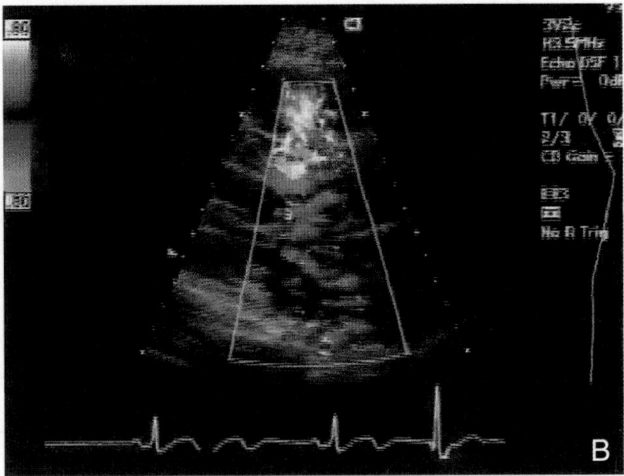

FIGURE 34–5. Transthoracic echocardiogram of an adult with a perimembranous ventricular septal defect (VSD). *A,* A parasternal long-axis view demonstrates the defect *(arrow).* The left atrium (LA), left ventricle (LV), and right ventricle (RV) are normal in this patient with a small shunt. *B,* A high-velocity color-flow Doppler jet is visible and due to a left-to-right shunt.

endocarditis.[11] The patient should repeatedly be informed of the importance of receiving appropriate antibiotics at the time of dental work or other procedures associated with bacteremia (see Chapter 33).

By the time a patient has reached adolescence or early adulthood, it is virtually impossible that a ventricular septal defect will close spontaneously. If the left-to-right shunt is large, heart failure may develop. If a large ventricular septal defect is associated with pulmonary hypertension, the likelihood of subsequent pulmonary vascular disease is high. In adults in whom a ventricular septal defect has been diagnosed, the overall 10-year survival rate after diagnosis is approximately 75%. A functional class worse than 1 (see Chapter 4), cardiomegaly, and elevated pulmonary artery pressure (>50 mm Hg) are clinical predictors of an adverse prognosis.

Treatment

With a small ventricular septal defect, prophylaxis against infective endocarditis should be recommended. With a large ventricular septal defect in an adolescent or adult, closure of the defect should be performed if a dominant left-to-right shunt is present. Once pulmonary vascular resistance exceeds 60% to 70% of systemic vascular resistance and the left-to-right shunt diminishes, closure of a ventricular septal defect is no longer indicated. If aortic regurgitation develops in a patient with a supracristal ventricular septal defect, closure of the ventricular septal defect will help prevent progression of the aortic regurgitation and is therefore indicated.

Management of Postoperative Patients. A patient whose ventricular septal defect was closed in childhood usually leads a normal life, without any need to impose restrictions on exercise or pregnancy unless progressive pulmonary hypertension is present. Prophylactic antibiotics are indicated only for the first 6 postoperative months, except in patients with a residual defect.

Patent Ductus Arteriosus

Pathophysiology

A patent ductus arteriosus connects the proximal descending aorta with the pulmonary artery at its bifurcation (Fig. 34–6). The magnitude of the left-to-right shunt depends on the size of the patent ductus and the ratio of pulmonary to systemic vascular resistance, in a manner similar to that of a ventricular septal defect. In the absence of pulmonary vascular disease, aortic pressure exceeds pulmonary artery pressure throughout the cardiac cycle, thereby resulting in continuous left-to-right shunting of blood and a "continuous murmur" or "machinery murmur."

When a patent ductus arteriosus is large and pulmonary vascular resistance is low in comparison to systemic vascular resistance, a large left-to-right shunt causes a loud, continuous, so-called machinery murmur. The marked increase in pulmonary blood flow results in left-sided volume overload with an increase in the size of the left atrium, left ventricle, ascending aorta, and aortic arch. The left ventricular volume overload can result in heart failure. As with a large ventricular septal defect, the high-pressure, high-flow state of a patent ductus arteriosus can cause severe pulmonary hypertension as a result of pulmonary vascular disease.

Recognition and Diagnosis

History and Physical Examination. If the patent ductus arteriosus is small, the heart will be normal and the only finding will be the continuous murmur, usually loudest under the left clavicle or in the second interspace along the left sternal border. With a large patent ductus

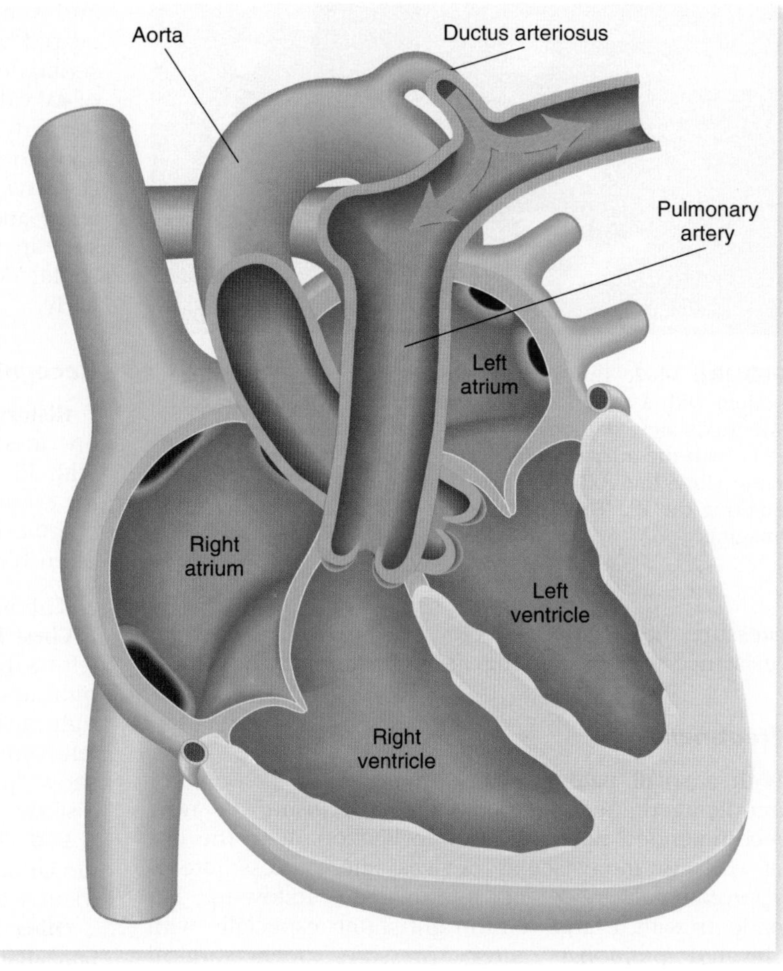

FIGURE 34–6. Diagram showing the location of a patent ductus arteriosus, with the *arrow* depicting the direction of flow in the absence of pulmonary hypertension. (Reprinted, by permission, from Brickner ME, Hillis LD, Lange RL: Congenital heart disease [first of two parts]. N Engl J Med 2000;342:256–263.)

arteriosus and relatively low pulmonary vascular resistance, the continuous murmur will be louder, the left ventricular apex will be displaced and hyperactive, and a low-pitched diastolic murmur may be heard at the apex because of increased diastolic flow across a normal mitral valve.

With a large patent ductus arteriosus and high pulmonary vascular resistance, the murmur is no longer continuous; it may be heard only in systole or may even be absent. The pulmonic component of S_2 is increased, and the only audible murmur might be the high-pitched, decrescendo murmur of pulmonary valve regurgitation along the left sternal border—a murmur that may be indistinguishable from the murmur of aortic regurgitation. In patients with a patent ductus arteriosus and pulmonary vascular disease with reversed shunting, the key to diagnosis is the presence of "differential cyanosis and clubbing" in the lower extremities (i.e., toes) and the absence of these findings in the fingers (see "Former Left-to-Right Shunts with Pulmonary Vascular Disease [Eisenmenger's Physiology]").

Laboratory

Chest Radiograph. With a small patent ductus arteriosus, the chest radiograph may be normal. With a large patent ductus arteriosus and a large left-to-right shunt, the left ventricle and left atrium may be enlarged. The main pulmonary artery and major branches of the pulmonary artery are increased, as are the pulmonary vascular markings. The pulmonary arteries are pruned in the presence of pulmonary hypertension.

ECG. With a large patent ductus arteriosus, left ventricular hypertrophy and left atrial enlargement may be seen on the ECG. With increased pulmonary vascular resistance, right ventricular hypertrophy often occurs.

Other Diagnostic Procedures and Referral for Cardiology Consultation. On two-dimensional echocardiography, the ductus itself is rarely seen, but abnormal, continuous, high-velocity "aliased" flow is seen within the main pulmonary artery near the left branch on color-flow Doppler imaging (Fig. 34–7). If a patent ductus arteriosus is suspected, referral to a cardiologist is indicated to assist in the definitive diagnosis and in the decision about whether closure is needed.

Course and Complications

With a small patent ductus arteriosus, the only danger is that of infective endocarditis; prophylactic antibiotics should be given at the time of dental work or other procedures that may cause bacteremia. With a large left-to-right shunt, especially with high pulmonary artery

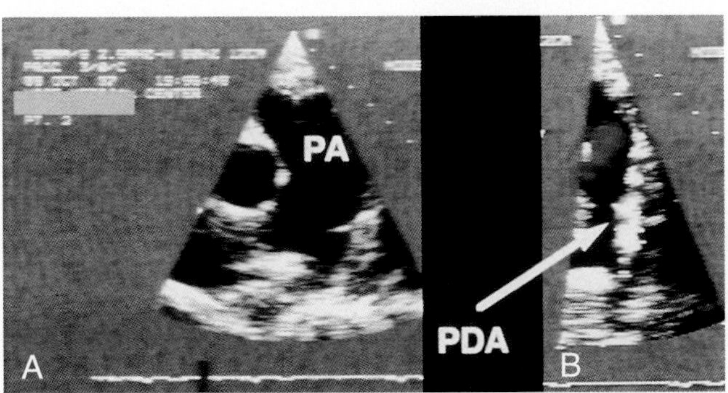

FIGURE 34–7. Transthoracic echocardiogram of an adult patient with a patent ductus arteriosus (PDA). *A,* A basal short-axis view demonstrates the dilated pulmonary artery (PA) with the adjacent circular ascending aorta. *B,* In the same view, the color-flow jet through the PDA is seen entering the PA. The flow was continuous on real-time imaging.

pressure, heart failure or elevated pulmonary vascular resistance with Eisenmenger's syndrome may develop.

Treatment

With a small patent ductus arteriosus in a young or middle-aged person, percutaneous closure is now recommended rather than open ligation. With the use of coils or intravascular devices, the success rate is approximately 95% at intermediate follow-up. In patients with a large left-to-right shunt, especially with elevated pulmonary artery pressure, open surgical ligation of the patent ductus arteriosus, preferably with division, is indicated at any age.

In a patient older than 60 to 65 years with a small patent ductus arteriosus, the risk of infective endarteritis must be balanced against the potential complications of surgery or percutaneous intervention. In an older, asymptomatic patient, antibiotic prophylaxis is indicated, but correction is not generally recommended. Occasionally, a small "silent" patent ductus arteriosus is detected serendipitously on Doppler echocardiography performed for another indication. Closure is not usually recommended in patients with inaudible shunts, but antibiotic prophylaxis is prudent.

Management of Postoperative Patients. After closure of a patent ductus arteriosus early in childhood before the development of pulmonary hypertension, the patient usually leads a normal life.[4] Prophylactic antibiotics are recommended only when a murmur persists postoperatively, and their use is controversial when the shunt is detected only by color-flow Doppler imaging.

Complete AV Septal Defect (AV Canal Defect)

Pathophysiology

This lesion is characterized by failure of the endocardial cushions to complete their task of closing the atrial and ventricular septa and forming the mitral and tricuspid valves. As a result, patients have a ventricular septal defect, an atrial septal defect, and varying degrees of AV valve regurgitation. *Atrioventricular* septal defects, formerly known as endocardial cushion defects, are commonly encountered in children with trisomy 21 (Down's syndrome). With large left-to-right shunts at the atrial and ventricular levels and high (systemic) pressure in the right ventricle because of the ventricular septal defect, pulmonary vascular disease occurs very early.

Recognition and Diagnosis

History and Physical Examination. Most adults with uncorrected complete AV septal defects are cyanotic with Eisenmenger's syndrome and are not candidates for correction. When the repair has been performed in childhood, residual mitral or tricuspid regurgitation often remains.

Laboratory

Chest Radiograph. Depending on the severity of the left-to-right shunt and the AV valve regurgitation, the right and left ventricles are dilated, as are the left and right atria. Pulmonary vascularity is increased when a left-to-right shunt persists; the pulmonary arteries show "pruning" in the presence of pulmonary vascular disease.

ECG. The characteristic ECG shows severe left axis deviation suggestive of a left anterior hemiblock. Biventricular hypertrophy can also be seen.

Other Diagnostic Procedures and Referral for Cardiology Consultation. The echocardiogram demonstrates complete absence of the crux of the heart, with both low atrial and high ventricular septal defects. In adults, color-flow imaging and Doppler studies show regurgitation through both AV valves and evidence of pulmonary artery hypertension.

Adults with this lesion should be referred to a cardiologist experienced in congenital heart disease to determine their suitability for primary repair or to evaluate and treat residual disease.

Course, Complications, and Treatment

Because most untreated patients with complete AV septal defects will not survive the first year, these children are usually corrected in infancy. Surgery consists of patch closure of the atrial and ventricular septal defects and repair of the AV valves. An unoperated adult with a complete AV septal defect is rarely a candidate for complete repair because of the frequent and early development of pulmonary vascular disease, but this person may be a candidate for heart-lung transplantation or lung transplantation with intracardiac repair.

Management of Postoperative Patients. For patients who have been corrected in infancy, the most common postoperative sequela is progressive mitral valve regurgitation as a result of inadequate repair. Tolerance for pregnancy depends on the presence of pulmonary hypertension and the severity of valvular dysfunction.

Mitral valve regurgitation places the patient at continued risk for endocarditis, and prophylactic antibiotics are indicated. Complete heart block is relatively common after surgical repair, may appear late in the postoperative course, and requires a pacemaker.

Anomalous Pulmonary Venous Drainage

Pathophysiology

One, more than one, or all the pulmonary veins can drain anomalously into the right heart and create a left-to-right shunt, which increases venous return to the right ventricle and increases right ventricular stroke volume as in an atrial septal defect. When all the pulmonary veins drain anomalously into the systemic venous system, an atrial septal defect must be present to return oxygenated blood to the left side of the heart.

Recognition and Diagnosis

History and Physical Examination. Patients with a single anomalous vein but no concomitant atrial septal defect are usually asymptomatic and have a normal physical examination. With multiple anomalously draining pulmonary veins, right ventricular overload is usually present, and a systolic ejection murmur is heard at the left base, findings similar to those of an atrial septal defect. Similarly, if even a single anomalous pulmonary vein is associated with a sinus venosus atrial septal defect, the patient will have findings of the atrial septal defect.

Laboratory

Chest Radiograph. Anomalous veins may be visible on the radiograph. With multiple anomalous pulmonary veins, the pulmonary vascular markings will be increased, and the right ventricle will be enlarged.

ECG. The ECG may be normal unless the left-to-right shunt is large, in which case an rsR′ pattern or right ventricular hypertrophy will be present.

Other Diagnostic Procedures and Referral for Cardiology Consultation. Color-flow Doppler imaging may reveal a flow disturbance when the vein drains into the inferior vena cava. TEE can be used to identify the entrance of the pulmonary veins. MRI and computed tomography (CT) are excellent imaging techniques for identifying anomalous pulmonary veins. Referral to a cardiologist experienced in congenital heart disease is indicated to determine the need for surgery.

Course, Complications, and Treatment

The benign course of patients with a single anomalous pulmonary vein supports the recommendation that surgical correction is not indicated in the absence of an associated sinus venosus atrial septal defect. If multiple veins are draining anomalously, the course and complications are similar to those of an interatrial septal defect. When pulmonary blood flow is increased to 1.8 to 2 times systemic blood flow, surgical repair with redirection of the pulmonary veins into the left atrium should be performed. The rare adult seen de novo with total anomalous pulmonary venous drainage usually remains a surgical candidate.

PREDOMINANT RIGHT-TO-LEFT SHUNTS (CYANOTIC HEART DISEASE)

Cyanosis in an adult patient with congenital heart disease is almost always associated with reduced pulmonary blood flow and a right-to-left shunt. The approach to diagnosis in a cyanotic patient is outlined in Figure 34–8.

Former Left-to-Right Shunts with Pulmonary Vascular Disease (Eisenmenger's Physiology)

Pathophysiology

In an adult with cyanotic congenital heart disease, Eisenmenger's physiology is the most common cause. In patients with an interatrial septal defect, interventricular septal defect, or patent ductus arteriosus, pulmonary vascular disease develops only in those with a large left-to-right shunt. With a large ventricular septal defect or patent ductus arteriosus, pulmonary hypertension may be present from birth. The excessive pulmonary blood flow and high pulmonary artery pressure inevitably result in intimal hyperplasia, medial arterial smooth muscle hypertrophy, and a relative paucity of small pulmonary arteries as the lung grows (Fig. 34–9). Once pulmonary vascular resistance reaches 60% to 70% of systemic vascular resistance, the process is irreversible and may progress even if the shunt is closed. In patients with atrial septal defects, pulmonary vascular resistance and pressure fall after birth. The development of pulmonary hypertension is more insidious but is usually established by adolescence or early adulthood if it is going to occur.

Because of the development of pulmonary vascular disease, pulmonary vascular resistance is markedly increased. The left-to-right shunt is decreased in magnitude or even absent. The severe pulmonary hypertension, which presents an afterload burden to the right ventricle, causes right ventricular hypertrophy and, finally, right heart failure. The shunt then becomes balanced or predominantly right to left.

Recognition and Diagnosis

History and Physical Examination. Patients are symptomatic with limitations in physical activity because of dyspnea and fatigue. Other symptoms include syncope, chest pain, and hemoptysis. A history of endocarditis or septic embolization may be elicited. Headaches and fatigability may be due to secondary erythrocytosis.

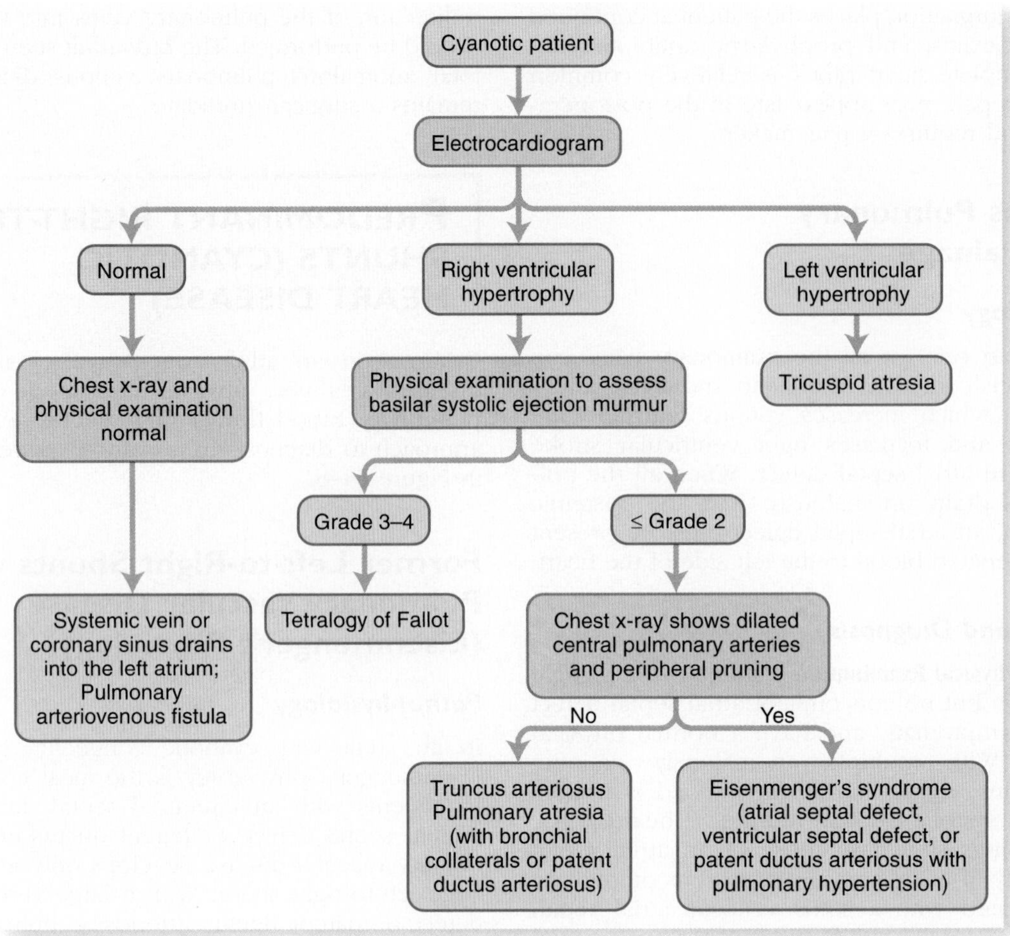

FIGURE 34–8. Diagnostic approach to a cyanotic patient with suspected congenital heart disease.

Physical examination reveals cyanosis of the lips, fingers, and toes and clubbing of the fingers and toes[12] (Box 34–1). The murmurs of the respective shunt lesions are no longer typical and may be entirely absent. The physical findings may confirm right heart failure with increased central venous pressure, tricuspid regurgitation, pulmonic regurgitation, and right-sided third and fourth heart sounds.

All three anatomic lesions have a similar clinical manifestation when pulmonary vascular disease is present, and they may be difficult to distinguish from one another. However, with a patent ductus arteriosus, the desaturated blood passes through the ductus and down the aorta, thereby causing the toes to be cyanotic while the fingers of the right hand or both hands are pink, depending on whether the desaturated blood goes into the left subclavian artery.

Laboratory. Oxygen saturation is low, with evidence of secondary erythrocytosis and an increased hematocrit. The bleeding time may be prolonged because of an associated bleeding diathesis. Uric acid levels may be elevated.

Chest Radiograph. The chest radiograph shows evidence of right ventricular enlargement, prominent proximal pulmonary arteries and even calcification, and "pruning" (Fig. 34–10) of the peripheral pulmonary vessels.

ECG. The ECG shows evidence of right atrial enlargement and right ventricular hypertrophy, usually with a rightward axis. A superior axis suggests an ostium primum atrial septal defect or an AV septal defect as the underlying cause (Fig. 34–11).

Other Diagnostic Procedures and Referral for Cardiology Consultation. TTE demonstrates right atrial enlargement and severe right ventricular hypertrophy with varying degrees of right ventricular dilatation and dysfunction. If the shunt is intracardiac, it can usually be detected by echocardiography in conjunction with color-flow Doppler and injection of agitated saline contrast. A patent ductus arteriosus may be difficult to diagnose by echocardiography in an adult with Eisenmenger's physiology. Pulmonary artery systolic pressure can be estimated from the peak velocity of the tricuspid regurgitant jet.

Referral to a cardiologist is indicated to confirm the diagnosis and to determine whether the pulmonary vascular disease is reversible or not. The latter determination may require cardiac catheterization.

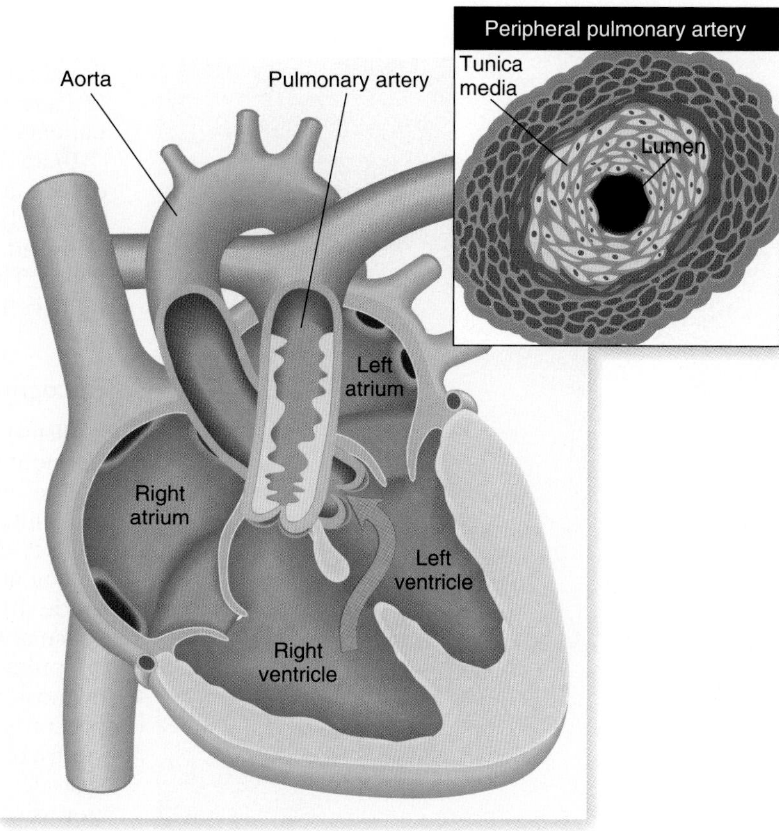

FIGURE 34–9. Eisenmenger's physiology caused by a large ventricular septal defect. The *inset* illustrates the pathologic changes seen in the pulmonary arteries on biopsy: intimal hyperplasia, medial hypertrophy, and secondary luminal thrombosis. (Reprinted, by permission, from Brickner ME, Hillis LD, Lange RL: Congenital heart disease [second of two parts]. N Engl J Med 2000;342:334–342.)

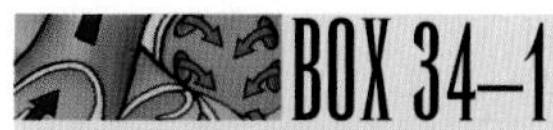
BOX 34–1

Findings of Eisenmenger's Physiology*

Signs of pulmonary arterial hypertension
- Prominent jugular A-wave (decreased ventricular compliance as a result of RV hypertrophy)
- Jugular regurgitant wave (if functional tricuspid regurgitation is present)
- Left parasternal (right ventricular) lift
- Palpable pulmonary artery pulsation (second left intercostal space)
- Pulmonic ejection murmur
- Loud P_2
- Diastolic decrescendo murmur of pulmonic insufficiency (Graham Steell's murmur)
- Holosystolic murmur of tricuspid regurgitation

Cyanosis
Clubbing of fingers and toes (left hand and toes in PDA)
Erythrocytosis

*Not all findings are present in each case.
RV, right ventricular; P_2, second pulmonic heart sound; PDA, patent ductus arteriosus.
From Andreoli TE, Bennett JC, Carpenter CCJ, Plum F: Congenital heart disease. *In* Cecil Essentials of Medicine, 4th ed. Philadelphia, WB. Saunders, 1977, p 42.

Course and Complications

Death occurs from the middle of the third decade to as late as the sixth decade of life.[13] Although life expectancy is shortened in patients with Eisenmenger's physiology, careful medical management may reduce mortality. The most common causes of death include pulmonary infarction and hemoptysis, arrhythmias with sudden death, progressive right ventricular failure, and brain abscess. Pregnancy carries an extremely high fetal and maternal mortality (in excess of 50%) and should be avoided.[5] A sudden drop in blood volume or systemic vascular resistance can markedly reduce pulmonary blood flow, increase arterial desaturation, and ultimately result in cardiogenic shock and death.

Treatment

When pulmonary vascular resistance is high enough to cause a predominant right-to-left shunt, surgical closure of the defect is contraindicated. Patients with Eisenmenger's physiology should be monitored in specialized centers for adults with congenital heart disease. When the patient is sufficiently symptomatic, right ventricular failure has occurred, or ventricular arrhythmias causing syncope have developed, heart and lung transplantation or lung transplantation with intracardiac repair should be considered.

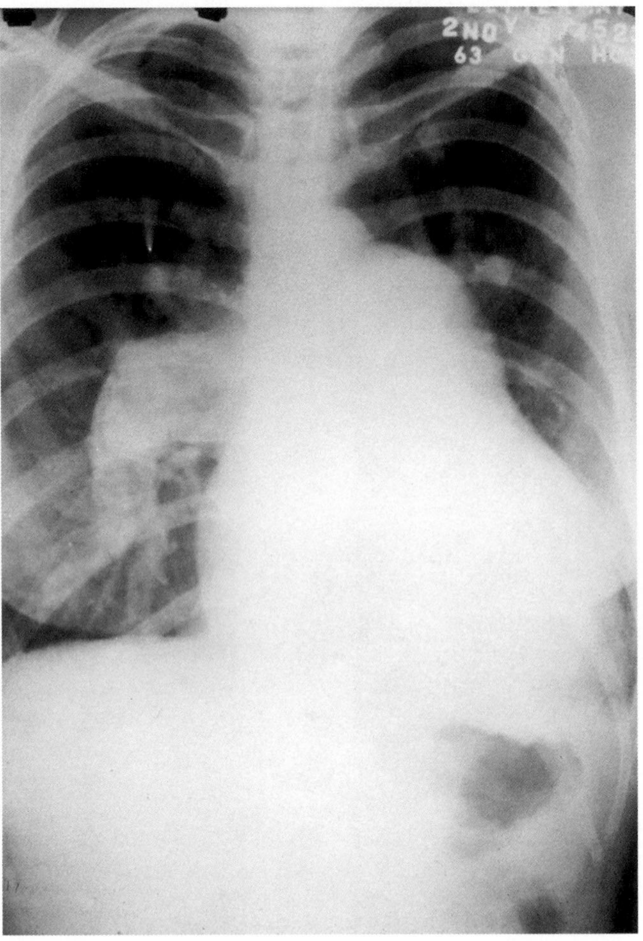

FIGURE 34–10. Chest radiograph, posteroanterior view. The patient is a 40-year-old woman with Eisenmenger's syndrome caused by a ventricular septal defect. Note the enlarged heart and monstrous enlargement of the pulmonary artery and proximal branches of the right pulmonary artery. An atherosclerotic calcification is present in the right pulmonary artery. Note the clear lateral lung fields ("pruning").

Tetralogy of Fallot

Pathophysiology

Tetralogy of Fallot refers to a combination of lesions consisting of an interventricular septal defect, infundibular stenosis with or without valvular pulmonic stenosis, and an aorta overriding the ventricular septal defect. The fourth lesion inferred by the word *tetralogy* is right ventricular hypertrophy, which is a compensatory response to the other lesions (Fig. 34–12). The right ventricular obstruction and large ventricular septal defect result in high right ventricular pressure that is similar to left ventricular pressure. When the resistance from right ventricular outflow obstruction is greater than systemic vascular resistance, a right-to-left shunt, arterial desaturation, and if severe, cyanosis can develop. If the right ventricular outflow obstruction is not severe, little or no right-to-left shunt may occur. The shunt may even be left to right, and the pulmonary valve and arteries may be normal or large. This lesion is sometimes referred to as the "pink" or "acyanotic" tetralogy of Fallot. The aortic arch is right sided in about 10% of patients.

In an adult with a perimembranous ventricular septal defect, acquired hypertrophy of the right ventricular muscle bundles can result in dynamic outflow obstruction and a pathophysiology similar to the tetralogy of Fallot. This entity has been termed "double-chambered right ventricle."

Recognition and Diagnosis

History and Physical Examination. Tetralogy of Fallot is frequently diagnosed in infancy when cyanosis appears at the usual time of ductal closure. The rare adult encountered with untreated tetralogy of Fallot usually has severe exercise intolerance.

Patients have a systolic ejection murmur, usually grade III or IV/VI, in the second to third intercostal space at the left sternal border caused by the infundibular pulmonic stenosis. S_2 is single. Later, clubbing and cyanosis of the upper and lower extremities develop. A precordial lift may be present as a result of right ventricular hypertrophy. After primary total repair, a systolic murmur of residual infundibular pulmonic stenosis and a short murmur of pulmonary insufficiency can usually be heard. If the patient has had a palliative systemic-to-pulmonary shunt (see later), a continuous murmur is audible.

Laboratory

Chest Radiograph. The size of the heart is normal, and the apex is rounded and lifted off the left hemidiaphragm. These findings give the appearance of a boot-shaped heart (Fig. 34–13). The pulmonary arteries are normal or small, and the lung fields are clear. A right-sided aortic arch may be present.

ECG. Right ventricular hypertrophy is always present. After primary repair, a right bundle branch block is frequently noted, and varying degrees of AV block may be present.

Other Diagnostic Procedures and Referral for Cardiology Consultation. In patients with unrepaired tetralogy of Fallot, TTE demonstrates severe hypertrophy of the right ventricle, including the infundibulum, usually with a thickened, malformed pulmonary valve. A large ventricular septal defect is seen in the vicinity of the membranous septum (i.e., perimembranous), with evidence of right-to-left shunting and a dilated overriding aorta. The gradient across the right ventricular outflow tract can be measured by Doppler. In patients who have undergone total primary repair, some degree of residual stenosis is usually present, and pulmonic valve insufficiency is almost always observed. Referral to a cardiologist is indicated to determine eligibility for surgery in unrepaired patients and to determine the severity of residual lesions in repaired patients.

When TTE is nondiagnostic, biplane or multiplane TEE may be helpful. In patients being considered for surgery, catheterization is indicated to measure pul-

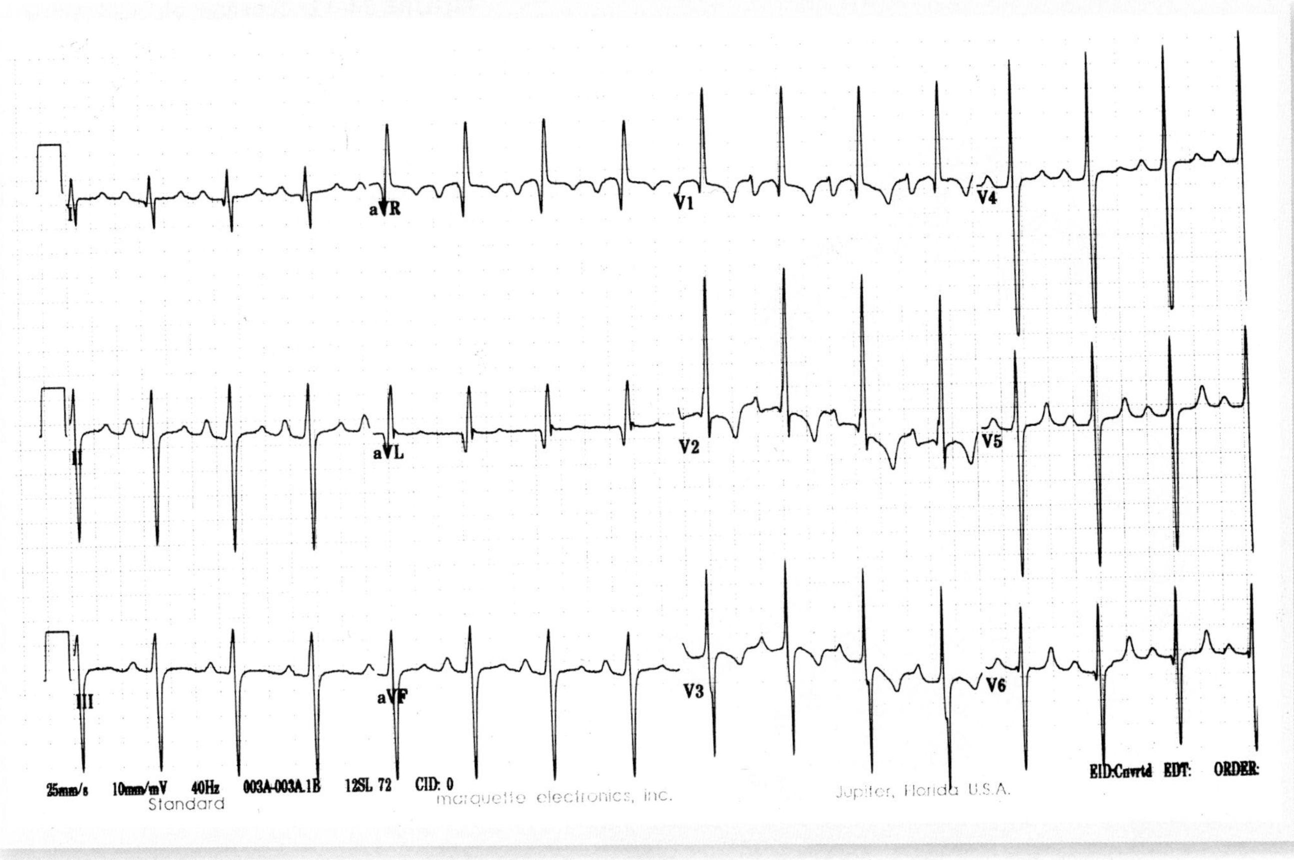

FIGURE 34–11. Electrocardiogram from a 36-year-old patient with Eisenmenger's syndrome caused by an atrioventricular septal (canal) defect. Note the evidence of right ventricular and biatrial enlargement with a superior and leftward QRS axis.

monary vascular resistance, especially in those with preexisting palliative shunts, and to define the anomalous origin of the coronary arteries and the size of the pulmonary arteries.

Course and Complications

Most patients with tetralogy of Fallot have had palliative operations or corrective surgery by the time that they are teenagers. Occasionally, a patient reaches the third decade of life without surgery. Sometimes, patients are initially seen with only palliative systemic-to-pulmonary artery shunts such as a Blalock-Taussig shunt (subclavian to the pulmonary artery), a Potts shunt (descending aorta to the left pulmonary artery), or a Waterston shunt (ascending aorta to the right pulmonary artery). Before surgical correction was possible, most patients died in the second decade of life.

Although it is an extremely successful operation, total intracardiac repair (see later) for tetralogy of Fallot can leave several significant postoperative residua, including right ventricular outflow tract obstruction, pulmonary valve regurgitation, and arrhythmias. In the early and intermediate follow-up period, important residual right ventricular outflow tract obstruction appears to be the major source of morbidity and mortality. However, in the late follow-up period, pulmonary valve insufficiency with eventual right ventricular failure as a result of volume overload and ventricular arrhythmias may lead to disability and even death. The survival rate at about 30 years after surgery for the tetralogy of Fallot is about 90%.[14] Sudden death accounts for approximately 50% of the late deaths.[15]

Treatment

All patients who have not had surgery should be evaluated for surgical correction. The feasibility of surgical correction depends on the anatomy of the pulmonary arteries. Patients with only palliative shunts should have these shunts taken down and surgical repair performed unless pulmonary vascular resistance has become severely elevated. The operation consists of patching the ventricular septal defect and relieving the right ventricular outflow tract obstruction.

Management of Postoperative Patients. After palliative procedures or total intracardiac repair, patients are at risk for endocarditis and should receive antibiotic prophylaxis during procedures associated with bacteremia. Patients are at risk for tachyarrhythmias (atrial and

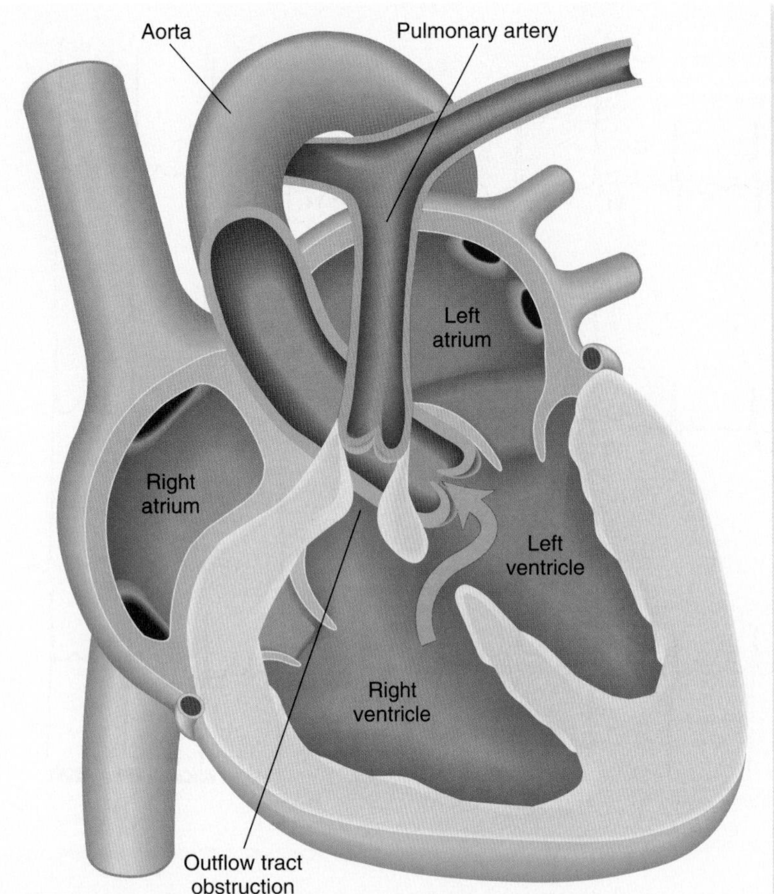

FIGURE 34–12. Tetralogy of Fallot with a ventricular septal defect, overriding aorta, outflow tract obstruction from infundibular hypertrophy and a hypoplastic pulmonary artery, and severe right ventricular hypertrophy. The *arrow* depicts the right-to-left direction of flow across the ventricular septal defect. (Reprinted, by permission, from Brickner ME, Hillis LD, Lange RL: Congenital heart disease [second of two parts]. N Engl J Med 2000;342:334–342.)

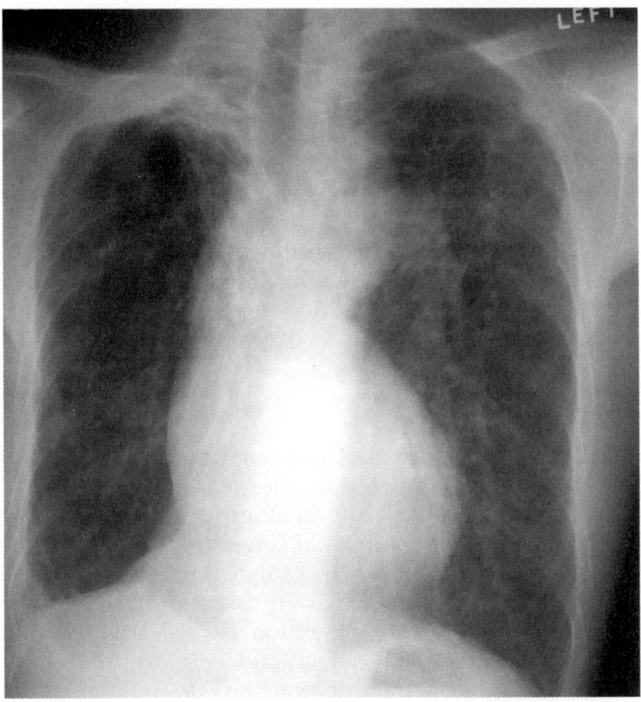

FIGURE 34–13. Chest radiograph, posteroanterior view. The patient is a 52-year-old man with the tetralogy of Fallot and a left-sided aortic arch. Note the "elevated" left ventricular apex. Interstitial lung markings are increased in this patient because of chronic pulmonary disease.

ventricular) and complete heart block after intracardiac repair. A QRS duration greater than 180 msec is predictive of sudden death.[15] Premature ventricular contractions, which are extremely common, do not have prognostic significance and should not be treated empirically. Patients with a markedly prolonged QRS interval, nonsustained ventricular tachycardia, or syncope should be referred to an electrophysiologist with experience in congenital heart disease.

Hemodynamic residua after total intracardiac repair may include right ventricular outflow tract obstruction, pulmonary valve insufficiency, peripheral pulmonary artery stenosis of one or both pulmonary arteries, and ventricular septal patch leaks. The presence and severity of residual lesions can usually be determined noninvasively, and patients should be monitored by an experienced cardiologist to decide whether and when repeat surgery is indicated. Pregnancy is generally well tolerated if the residual right ventricular outflow obstruction is not severe. Unless right ventricular failure is present, pulmonic valvular insufficiency is not a contraindication to pregnancy.

Transposition of the Great Arteries

These infants are born with the great arteries originating from the wrong ventricle. The aortic valve arises anteriorly from the right ventricle and the pulmonic valve posteriorly from the left ventricle. Without cross-connections, such as a patent foramen ovale, atrial septal defect, ventricular septal defect, or patent ductus arteriosus, this lesion is incompatible with life.

Infants with this condition rarely survive without intervention; thus, with only rare exceptions, adults have had a palliative atrial switch procedure (such as the Mustard or Senning procedures), after which the right ventricle usually continues to serve the systemic circulation. More recently, an arterial switch operation, the Jatene procedure, was developed to reconnect the great arteries to their proper ventricle, reconnect the coronary arteries to the new aortic location, and restore a "normal" circulation.

Patients with an atrial switch procedure are at risk for failure of the systemic "right" ventricle, obstruction of the systemic or pulmonary veins by the intra-atrial baffle, intra-atrial baffle leaks with paradoxical embolization, and especially atrial tachyarrhythmias. Patients with the arterial switch operation (Jatene procedure) can have coronary artery obstruction, aortic valvular regurgitation, and supravalvular obstruction at the site of the aortic and pulmonary artery anastomoses. Postoperative patients should be monitored by a cardiologist experienced in congenital heart disease. Medical therapy to treat failure of the systemic right ventricle includes afterload reduction with vasodilators, digoxin, and diuretics. Noninvasive and invasive studies may demonstrate a need for further surgical palliative procedures.

Ebstein's Anomaly

Pathophysiology and Natural History

In Ebstein's anomaly, the septal and posterior leaflets of the tricuspid valve are dysplastic and displaced from the tricuspid annulus apically into the body of the right ventricle. Thus, a portion of the right ventricle is above the tricuspid valve (the atrialized right ventricle) and enlarges the true right atrium. The valve may be regurgitant, and if the patient has a patent foramen ovale or an atrial septal defect, a large right-to-left shunt may be present. These patients are cyanotic, are likely to be recognized initially in infancy, and may have undergone palliative procedures with closure of the atrial septal defect. Symptoms in adolescents or adults are more likely related to progressive tricuspid regurgitation with heart failure or arrhythmias than to cyanosis. Nevertheless, some patients with severe displacement of the tricuspid valve can live normal lives with minimal symptoms.

Recognition and Diagnosis

History and Physical Examination. A history of dyspnea and intermittent cyanosis leading to exercise intolerance, atypical chest pain, and palpitations or syncope may be present. On physical examination, these patients frequently have a widely split S_1 and S_2. After one or more loud systolic clicks from prolapse of the redundant leaflets, a systolic murmur of tricuspid regurgitation with accentuation on inspiration may be heard. Because the regurgitant jet may be eccentric as a result of the displaced leaflet, it is not unusual to hear the tricuspid regurgitation murmur best at the apex, similar to the murmur of mitral regurgitation.

Laboratory

Chest Radiograph. Classically, the chest radiograph shows a globular heart with a long sweep of right atrium. The lung fields are usually normal but may have diminished pulmonary blood flow. The normal prominent bulge of the main pulmonary artery segment may be absent.

ECG. The classic ECG reveals a low-voltage right bundle branch block, often a first-degree AV block, and right atrial abnormality. Wolff-Parkinson-White syndrome may be present, and the patient may have runs of paroxysmal atrial tachycardia.

Other Diagnostic Procedures and Referral for Cardiology Consultation. The echocardiogram is diagnostic and demonstrates the morphology of the abnormal tricuspid valve as well as a tricuspid regurgitant jet arising apically within the right ventricle. Referral to a cardiologist is indicated for evaluation of symptomatic patients. Catheterization is rarely needed but may be indicated preoperatively when surgical treatment is necessary. Electrophysiology studies should be performed in a center where radiofrequency ablation is available to treat bypass tract–related arrhythmias.

Course and Complications

Once the patient has survived childhood, the prognosis is favorable, even with severe displacement of the tricuspid valve. If the tricuspid regurgitation is severe, the ability to increase cardiac output may be diminished, and the patient may have progressive limitation in activity with fatigability.

Treatment and Management Issues

If an unoperated patient is symptomatic, closure of an atrial septal defect and reconstruction of the tricuspid valve by annuloplasty or even replacement have been performed with success. If atrial tachycardia is present with an anomalous muscle connection, radiofrequency ablation of the AV pathway can successfully treat the paroxysmal atrial tachycardia. Patients with persistent tricuspid regurgitation after valve repair and those who have had tricuspid valve replacement require antibiotic prophylaxis.

Other Cyanotic Lesions

Tricuspid atresia, single ventricle, and truncus arteriosus are uncommon lesions that are almost uniformly fatal in childhood without palliative surgical procedures. Whenever possible, these patients should be managed in conjunction with a service specializing in adult congenital heart disease.

STENOTIC AND ATRETIC VALVES AND HYPOPLASTIC VENTRICLES

Congenital Aortic Stenosis

Pathophysiology

The pathophysiology of congenital aortic stenosis is similar to that of acquired aortic stenosis (see Chapter 32). However, in congenital left ventricular outflow tract obstruction, the anatomic level of obstruction can be valvular, supravalvular, or subvalvular, whereas in acquired aortic stenosis, it is almost always valvular. Valvular aortic stenosis is due to a malformed valve that is usually functionally bicuspid. Patients with the most severely malformed and stenotic valves may require intervention in childhood. Even with a less restricted orifice, the disturbed flow through the valve causes progressive thickening and calcification and may eventually result in severe stenosis and varying degrees of valvular insufficiency that develop later in life. Intervening endocarditis may hasten valve destruction and cause predominant valvular insufficiency.

In supravalvular aortic stenosis, the narrowing is usually above the level of the sinuses of Valsalva. Therefore, the coronary arteries arise from the aorta proximal to the obstruction and are subject to an elevated systolic pressure equal to that of the left ventricle. The high pressure causes coronary artery dilatation and may accelerate atherosclerosis.

In the most common form of subaortic stenosis, a discrete membrane immediately below the aortic valve causes a systolic jet that traumatizes the valve leaflets and results in aortic regurgitation. Patients also often have associated left ventricular outflow tract obstruction with coarctation of the aorta and mitral valve abnormalities. Obstructive hypertrophic cardiomyopathy is discussed in Chapter 29.

Recognition and Diagnosis

History and Physical Examination. Congenital valvular aortic stenosis has findings similar to those of acquired disease and is covered in Chapter 32. In congenital aortic stenosis, an ejection click is usually heard as long as the leaflets remain flexible. This click disappears as calcification and immobility of the valve progress. Other aspects of the physical examination are similar to that of acquired disease.

With supravalvular aortic stenosis, the obstruction is above the aortic valve, and thus no ejection click or aortic regurgitation is present. The systolic jet arises in the ascending aorta, and the percussion wave is directed into the innominate artery. This mechanism raises systolic blood pressure in the right arm by 10 to 20 mm Hg in comparison to that in the left arm.

In patients with discrete membranous subaortic stenosis, no ejection click occurs. Eighty percent of patients have a murmur of aortic regurgitation.

Laboratory

Chest Radiograph. The chest radiograph is similar to that in patients with acquired aortic stenosis and may show poststenotic dilatation of the aorta and calcification of the valve. The findings in supravalvular aortic stenosis are similar, with one important distinction—no poststenotic dilatation of the ascending aorta. Calcification can be seen in the atherosclerotic dilated coronary arteries of some patients. Similarly, in patients with discrete membranous subvalvular aortic stenosis, the chest radiograph shows no poststenotic dilatation.

ECG. In young patients with severe aortic stenosis, the ECG may be normal, and thus the absence of left ventricular hypertrophy on the ECG does not exclude the diagnosis in this population.

Other Diagnostic Procedures and Referral for Cardiology Consultation. TTE is diagnostic in valvular aortic stenosis, with direct visualization of the valve leaflets by two-dimensional imaging and measurement of the pressure gradient across the left ventricular outflow tract by Doppler interrogation. The valve area can be accurately calculated. However, surface imaging is limited in its ability to visualize a subaortic membrane or supravalvar stenosis; in these cases, TEE may be indicated.

Referral to a cardiologist is recommended for symptomatic patients or patients with moderate or severe asymptomatic stenosis or to clarify the severity of the stenosis when a discrepancy exists between the clinical findings and the noninvasive data.

Course and Complications

Complications of congenital aortic stenosis in adults are similar to those of acquired aortic stenosis. As soon as symptoms begin, a rapid increase in mortality is noted, with one quarter to one third of deaths occurring suddenly. With discrete membranous subvalvular aortic stenosis, progressive aortic regurgitation can develop.

After aortic valvotomy for severe stenosis during childhood, approximately one fourth of patients will need repeat surgery for recurrent stenosis or progressive aortic insufficiency in the next 25 years.[16] With medical treatment, approximately one third of children with systolic gradients below 50 mm Hg and about 80% of those with gradients of 50 to 79 mm Hg will need surgery within 25 years.[16]

Treatment

With symptomatic, hemodynamically significant valvular aortic stenosis (i.e., an aortic valve area less than $0.8\,cm^2$) and a flexible noncalcified valve, balloon valvotomy may have therapeutic success similar to that of operative valvotomy, even in adults. However, when calcification or associated aortic insufficiency is noted, valve replacement is required. The Ross procedure, which places a homograft in the pulmonary valve position and uses the patient's own pulmonary valve in the aortic position, has had promising early to intermediate results when performed by experienced surgeons. One advantage of this innovative, though technically challenging approach is that it obviates the need for anticoagulation and does not entail the use of a bioprosthetic valve, which may degenerate over time.

Indications for repair of supravalvular aortic stenosis are a significant gradient, coronary artery dilatation, or both. In patients with discrete membranous subvalvular aortic stenosis and any associated aortic regurgitation, operative repair with adequate resection of the membrane and underlying myocardium should be performed in an attempt to prevent progressive aortic regurgitation or regrowth of the membrane.

Management of Postoperative Patients. Patients treated surgically for valvular, supravalvular, and subvalvular aortic stenosis in childhood are at risk for endocarditis, regardless of the type of surgery performed. Those who underwent surgical valvotomy, as well as those with previous resection of a subaortic membrane, must be monitored for progressive aortic insufficiency.

Pulmonic Valvular Stenosis

Pathophysiology

Although pulmonic valve stenosis may be progressive, it is congenital in origin. The obstruction to outflow puts an afterload burden on the right ventricle and results in concentric right ventricular hypertrophy. Severe right ventricular hypertrophy with increased systolic compression may compromise intramural coronary flow. Because of the increased right ventricular myocardial oxygen demand, this situation can lead to subendocardial ischemia.

Recognition and Diagnosis

History and Physical Examination. Symptoms vary with the severity of obstruction. In patients with severe obstruction (peak right ventricular–pulmonary artery pressure gradient >80 mm Hg), dyspnea, fatigue, symptoms of right ventricular failure, and syncope may be present. In adults, symptoms may first appear during pregnancy when the higher cardiac output leads to an increasing gradient. On physical examination, the sound of pulmonary closure is inaudible or soft. A fourth heart sound and prominent A-waves in the jugular venous pulse are often present. Typical findings include a right ventricular heave, a right parasternal systolic thrill, and a systolic ejection sound that characteristically decreases with inspiration, followed by a loud (≥III/VI) systolic ejection murmur at the upper left sternal border.

Laboratory

Chest Radiograph. The chest radiograph usually shows normal overall heart size but with right ventricular prominence, normal pulmonary vascularity, and poststenotic dilatation of the main and left pulmonary arteries.

ECG. The ECG typically shows right axis deviation and exhibits right ventricular hypertrophy and right atrial enlargement.

Echocardiography. Two-dimensional echocardiography shows the stenotic, doming pulmonary valve and thickening of the free wall of the right ventricle. Accurate measurement of the pressure gradient across the right ventricular outflow tract is possible with Doppler interrogation. Referral to a cardiologist is indicated for catheterization and pulmonary arteriography when needed and to assist in the decision to intervene.

Course and Complications

It is unusual to see an adult with severe valvular pulmonary stenosis. Adult patients with valvular pulmonary stenosis generally do well; eventually, however, right ventricular failure can occur. In children treated medically for pulmonary stenosis without surgical intervention, the likelihood of symptomatic stenosis requiring surgery depends on the initial gradient: less than 25 mm Hg, 5%; 25 to 49 mm Hg, 20%; and 50 to 79 mm Hg, 76%. Symptoms may occur during pregnancy in patients with moderately severe or severe pulmonary stenosis.

Surgical valvotomy has been an extremely successful operation for long-term relief of pulmonary valve obstruction. A recent natural history study of surgically treated severe (gradient ≥80 mm Hg) pulmonic stenosis demonstrated an excellent 25-year survival rate of 95%, equivalent to that of the normal population. Approximately 50% of patients had residual mild to moderate regurgitation, but reoperation was rarely necessary (5%) at 25 years.[17]

Treatment

In an adult, severe pulmonary valve stenosis requiring intervention is defined as a peak systolic gradient in excess of 60 mm Hg. The decision to treat moderate stenosis (gradient between 40 and 60 mm Hg) is based on the presence of symptoms, the age of the patient, and the degree of right ventricular hypertrophy.

In patients with severe valvular pulmonary stenosis, percutaneous balloon valvuloplasty is the current treatment of choice and has replaced surgical valvotomy in those with flexible valves (see Chapter 32). In patients with mild to moderate pulmonary stenosis, especially if right ventricular hypertrophy is not present, observation plus a recommendation for prophylactic antibiotics to prevent infective endocarditis is indicated without surgical or nonsurgical intervention.

Management of Postoperative Patients. Recurrent valvular pulmonary stenosis is uncommon, and routine serial echocardiography is not indicated, although a baseline study is recommended when an adult patient is first encountered. Thereafter, additional studies should be performed only when a change in clinical status is suggested by the development of symptoms or after a change in the physical examination. Patients treated either surgically or by balloon valvuloplasty for valvular pulmonary stenosis in childhood have a low risk for endocarditis. Thus, antibiotic prophylaxis is recommended only in those with a murmur of residual stenosis or insufficiency.

GREAT VESSEL AND CORONARY ARTERY ABNORMALITIES

Coarctation of the Aorta

Pathophysiology

The most common form of aortic coarctation is characterized by narrowing at the level of the ligamentum arteriosum (Fig. 34–14). The constriction may take the form of a localized hourglass narrowing or a hypoplastic segment of the distal arch proximal to the ligamentum. On occasion, the aorta can be completely interrupted at that level.

Proximal to the aortic obstruction, arterial hypertension is usually present. Because of lower pressure in the aorta distal to the obstruction, the brachiocephalic vessels form collateral arterial channels with the intercostal arteries and the superior and inferior recurrent epigastric arteries, which carry blood around the coarctation to the distal aorta. The key physical findings are femoral pulses that are either absent or delayed and diminished in comparison to the right brachial pulse. The blood pressure differential between the upper and the lower extremities reflects the pressure drop across the coarctation.

As many as 80% of patients with coarctation of the aorta have an associated bicuspid aortic valve. Aortic aneurysms can occur around the area of the coarctation or elsewhere in the aorta and branches of the circle of Willis (so-called berry aneurysms).

Recognition and Diagnosis

History and Physical Examination. An adult with uncorrected coarctation is usually asymptomatic. Nonspecific symptoms may develop, including exertional dyspnea, headache, epistaxis, and leg fatigue, as well as symptoms of heart failure. Unfortunately, the initial manifestation of untreated coarctation, most commonly seen between the ages of 15 and 40 years, may be catastrophic as a result of aortic rupture or dissection, infective endocarditis or endarteritis, or cerebral hemorrhage.

Hypertension is present in the right arm or both arms. Usually, hypertension is not severe in an adult with coarctation and is predominantly systolic. On palpation, the femoral pulses are diminished and delayed in comparison to the brachial pulses and may even be absent.

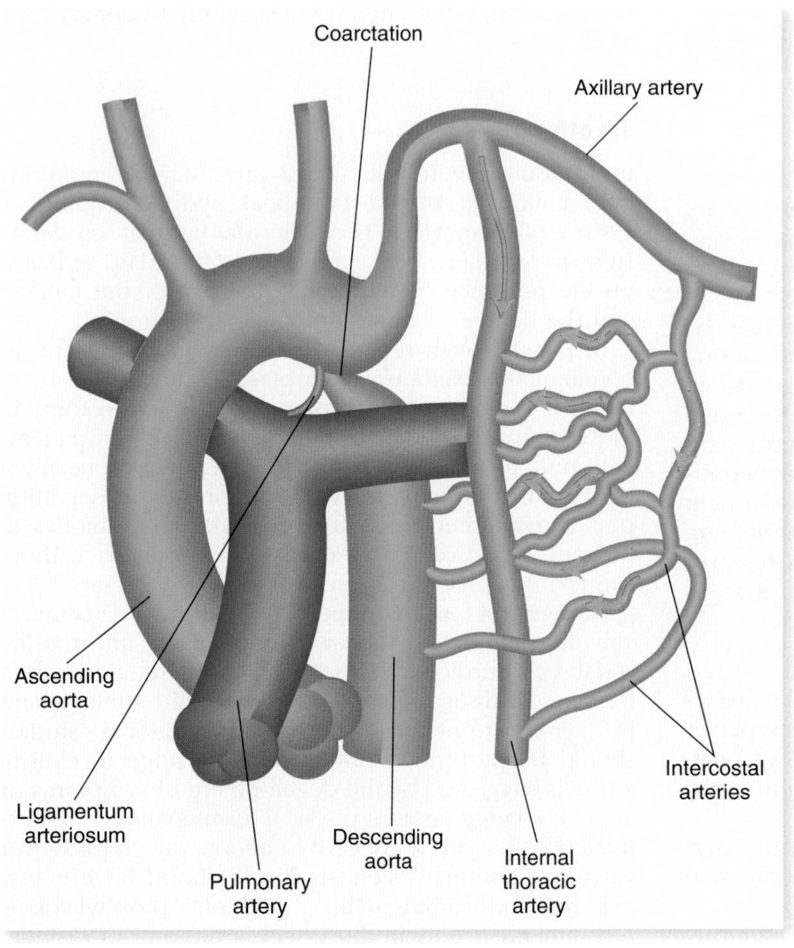

FIGURE 34–14. Arterial circulation in the presence of aortic coarctation. The internal thoracic artery and the intercostal arteries are dilated and providing collateral flow to the lower part of the body. (Reprinted, by permission, from Brickner ME, Hillis LD, Lange RL: Congenital heart disease [first of two parts]. N Engl J Med 2000;342:256–263.)

Normally, systolic blood pressure is 10 to 20 mm Hg higher in the legs; in coarctation, blood pressure in the thighs is lower than in the arms, especially after exercise. With the patient leaning forward, arterial pulsation may be felt posteriorly in the intercostal spaces because of the pulsations of the enlarged collateral periscapular and intercostal vessels.

Coarctation of the thoracic aorta causes a late systolic ejection murmur that is usually audible in the second and third interspaces at the left sternal border, but also posteriorly to the left of the spine in the interscapular area. At times, the murmur is best heard in the back. Patients with a bicuspid aortic valve may also have a basilar systolic ejection murmur, a faint aortic regurgitation murmur, and a systolic ejection click.

Laboratory

Chest Radiograph. The aortic knob may be enlarged because of lateral displacement of the left subclavian artery. On barium swallow, the esophagus can be seen to have a double indentation, the so-called reversed-3 sign, as a result of the aortic knob superiorly and a second indentation caused by poststenotic dilatation of the descending aorta distal to the coarctation. Frequently, notching of the inferior surfaces of the ribs posteriorly may occur in an adult owing to erosion of the ribs by the collateral arteries (Fig. 34–15).

ECG. The ECG is frequently normal or shows left ventricular hypertrophy.

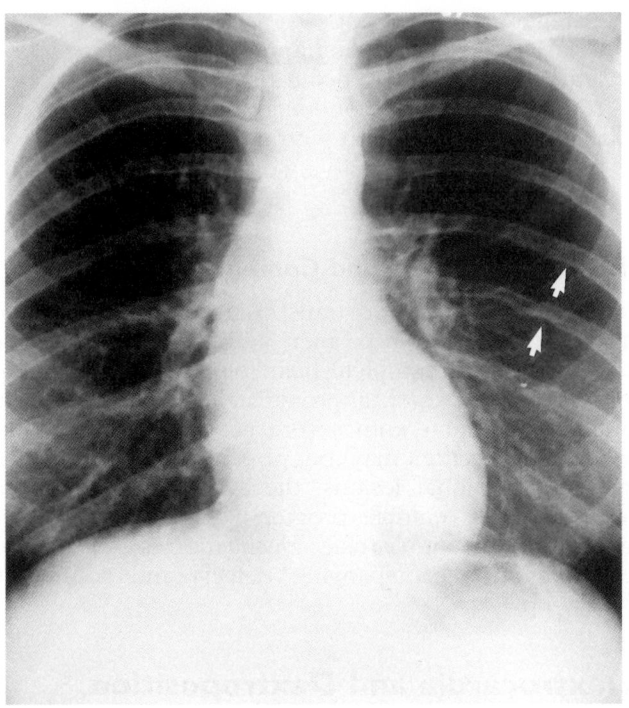

FIGURE 34–15. Chest radiograph, posteroanterior view, of a 25-year-old patient with coarctation of the aorta and a bicuspid aortic valve. Note the prominence of the ascending aorta as a result of poststenotic dilatation secondary to the bicuspid aortic valve and rib notching, especially in the left posterior ribs *(arrows)*.

Other Diagnostic Procedures and Referral for Cardiology Consultation. It is difficult to visualize the actual site of the coarctation in an adult patient with two-dimensional TTE. However, Doppler studies of the descending aorta in the suprasternal notch view may identify and measure the degree of obstruction, even when images are suboptimal. An associated bicuspid aortic valve can also be identified by surface two-dimensional imaging. Angiography or MRI is usually needed to define the site and extent of narrowing.

Referral to a cardiologist is advised to assist with the often-difficult decision of when to operate on patients, especially those with milder degrees of coarctation. Coronary angiography should be performed preoperatively in most adults older than 30 years because of the high incidence of premature coronary artery disease.

Course and Complications

The patient may be asymptomatic. However, coarctation and hypertension can lead to the complications of hypertension—stroke, heart failure, and premature coronary artery disease and its complications. In the pre-repair era, 50% of patients died by about age 30 years and 90% by age 60 years. Before the age of 30 years, proximal aortic rupture, aortic dissection, and cerebral hemorrhage from rupture of a berry aneurysm are the major complications. After the age of 40 years, the incidence of heart failure increases. Infective endarteritis (at the site of coarctation) and endocarditis (on a bicuspid aortic valve) are a danger at all ages.

Treatment

If the coarctation is severe enough to cause proximal hypertension with a gradient greater than 25 to 30 mm Hg across the coarctation, repair should be undertaken. Most of these patients will have multiple collateral vessels seen on aortography, as well as atheromatous changes at the site of the coarctation; each of these problems makes surgery more challenging. If the gradient is less than 20 mm Hg and no collaterals are present, repair is not indicated. In some patients, primary balloon dilatation with stenting may be successful.

Management and Treatment of Postoperative Patients. Patients with repaired coarctation require continued close clinical follow-up. Hypertension requiring medical therapy is likely to persist in patients repaired after the first 10 years of life. Postoperative patients require antibiotic prophylaxis because of the persistent danger of endocarditis on the bicuspid aortic valve and endarteritis at the site of repair. A preexisting aneurysm of the circle of Willis may cause a cerebrovascular accident even after repair of the coarctation.

MRI should be performed as a baseline examination in all postoperative adults after coarctation repair for detection of potential complications, including recoarctation, focal saccular aneurysms, and dissecting aneurysms. The incidence of recurrent coarctation requiring surgery at 20-year follow-up is about 3%.

Focal saccular aortic aneurysms may develop at the site of the repair. Rupture of these aneurysms, more likely in women and during pregnancy, is heralded by the occurrence of paraspinal pain and hemoptysis. Thus, a woman with an aneurysm who is contemplating pregnancy should probably undergo prophylactic reoperation before conception. In addition, patients have an ongoing risk of aortic dissection even without an aneurysm.

Mortality at 20-year follow-up after successful repair is approximately 5%, mostly secondary to cardiovascular disease and cerebrovascular accidents. Approximately 10% of patients require subsequent cardiovascular surgery, most commonly for aortic valve replacement of the coexisting bicuspid aortic valve.

Coronary Artery Anomalies

Although coronary artery anomalies are rare, they should be considered a potential cause in young patients (usually in the second or third decade of life) with symptoms suggestive of ischemia, including exertional syncope or chest pain.[18] Suspicion of a coronary anomaly should be highest when the patient does not have any risk factors for premature atherosclerotic disease or evidence of valvular heart disease or cardiomyopathy. The most common coronary anomalies seen in adults are anomalous origin of the left circumflex coronary artery from the right sinus of Valsalva, coronary-to-pulmonary artery fistulas, coronary cameral fistulas (fistulous connections between the coronary artery and the coronary chamber, usually the right atrium or right ventricle), and abnormal origin of the left coronary artery from the anterior sinus of Valsalva or the right coronary artery from the left posterior sinus of Valsalva. Hypoplasia of the coronary arteries with small underdeveloped distal epicardial vessels is a rare condition.

As with other forms of ischemia, the ECG may be normal at rest, and exercise testing may be required to detect an abnormality. However, in patients with anomalous origin of a coronary artery, ischemia may not be precipitated by stress, even in those who have had a previous serious ischemic episode. TTE is rarely diagnostic, although on rare occasion an anomalous coronary artery may be detected serendipitously when an echocardiogram is obtained for another purpose.

Referral to a cardiologist is indicated for diagnosis and treatment. In some cases, TEE, MRI, or CT can accurately identify an anomalous origin of the proximal coronary arteries. However, coronary angiography is mandatory in patients requiring surgery and is usually the next study after an exercise test. When ischemia is definitively demonstrated or the patient has had a syncopal episode during exertion, surgical intervention is the only treatment. Management of asymptomatic anomalies is less certain and depends on the anticipated potential for ischemic complications. With coronary arteriovenous fistulas or coronary cameral fistulas, surgical closure is indicated when the left-to-right shunt exceeds 1.5:1.

POSITIONAL ABNORMALITIES

Physiologically "Corrected" Transposition (*l*-Transposition)

Pathophysiology

This lesion is characterized by malposition of the great vessels and ventricular inversion, with the left ventricle connected to the right atrium and pulmonary artery and the right ventricle connected to the left atrium and aorta. Blood flow is physiologically correct, but an anatomic right ventricle serves as the systemic ventricle. Most adults in whom this lesion was previously undiagnosed have no other abnormalities.

Recognition and Diagnosis

History and Physical Examination. Corrected transposition is frequently discovered as a result of the physical findings from accompanying congenital defects such as a ventricular septal defect or subpulmonic valve stenosis. When no other abnormalities are present, this lesion may remain undetected until the patient has syncope as a result of complete heart block. Because the aortic valve is leftward and anterior, in the position of the normal pulmonic valve, S_2 may be very loud and similar to the S_2 in a patient with pulmonary hypertension.

Laboratory

Chest Radiograph. Radiographic findings depend on whether accompanying defects are present.

ECG. Reversal of the conduction system causes abnormal septal depolarization with no R-wave in V_1 and no Q-waves in V_5 and V_6. Varying degrees of AV block may be present.

Treatment, Course, and Complications

Patients with corrected transposition may live to old age if they have no other additional lesions. The development of complete heart block is common and occurs at a rate of approximately 5% per year in adults. In patients with severe accompanying lesions, surgical correction may be possible. However, even without additional lesions, the systemic ventricle, an anatomic right ventricle, progressively fails and requires medical treatment. Cardiac consultation is indicated to evaluate any accompanying defects and coordinate follow-up.

Dextrocardia and Dextroposition

Pathophysiology

With dextrocardia and situs inversus, the vena cava, atria, ventricles, and great vessels are all reversed and thus connected appropriately. Frequently, associated congenital heart lesions are present, and the right lung may be hypoplastic.

Recognition and Diagnosis

History and Physical Examination. Patients are asymptomatic in the absence of other lesions. The abnormality is suspected by palpating the cardiac activity over the right side of the chest instead of the left. The position of the left ventricular point of maximal impulse can be extremely helpful in making a diagnosis, with it being either in the right mid-clavicular line (dextrocardia) or at the right sternal border or epigastrium (dextroposition).

Laboratory

Chest Radiograph. A definitive diagnosis is made by the radiographic appearance of dextrocardia. The cardiac mass and the stomach bubble are on the right. With dextroposition, the stomach bubble is on the left, as it is normally.

ECG. With dextrocardia, the frontal leads are characteristically changed, and the right and left arm leads appear to be reversed, but with the R-wave diminishing from V_1 to V_6. Cardiac consultation is indicated to evaluate whether any associated cardiopulmonary defects are present.

CONGENITAL SYNDROMES ASSOCIATED WITH CARDIAC ANOMALIES

Marfan's Syndrome

Marfan's syndrome, a genetic disorder of connective tissue, is by far the most common syndrome likely to be encountered in adult patients. It is transmitted as an autosomal dominant trait but has a 30% rate of spontaneous mutation. The most important cardiac manifestations are aortic root dilatation and mitral valve prolapse with mitral regurgitation. The aortic root dilatation is progressive and may be complicated by aortic valve insufficiency, aortic dissection, and rupture without dissection. These patients should be monitored by serial echocardiography, and prophylactic aortic root repair is generally advised when the aortic diameter exceeds 5.0 cm (see Chapter 36). Aortic dissection may occur even before the aorta enlarges to such a degree, and pregnant women are at particularly high risk. Prophylactic therapy with beta-blockers significantly reduces the rate of aortic dilatation and probably the incidence of aortic insufficiency and dissection.[19] In addition to the aortic complications, progressive mitral regurgitation may occur, especially in patients with endocarditis and chordal rupture.

A related connective tissue disorder is Ehlers-Danlos syndrome, which is associated with similar cardiac features.

Muscular Dystrophies

Many forms of muscular dystrophy have associated involvement of the myocardium or cardiac conduction system, and these cardiac abnormalities may also be present in some heterozygotic carriers who may not have obvious abnormalities in skeletal muscle function. A baseline ECG and chest radiograph should be obtained, and patients with cardiac symptoms or abnormalities on these screening tests should be referred for cardiac consultation.

SYSTEMIC MANIFESTATIONS OF CONGENITAL HEART DISEASE AND OTHER LIFE ISSUES

Hematology

Secondary erythrocytosis develops in patients with significant cyanosis from congenital heart disease. When these patients are in the "compensated" state, they are asymptomatic with a stable hematocrit (usually <65%) and no evidence of iron deficiency. The absolute value of the hematocrit does not determine the clinical state, and occasional patients may tolerate even a hematocrit of 70%. "Decompensated" patients have increasing hematocrit values (>65%) and symptoms of hyperviscosity (headache, fatigability, and coagulation abnormalities). Phlebotomy should be performed, preferably at an experienced center, for headache, fatigability, and a hematocrit greater than 65% in patients with symptoms. Isovolumetric saline replacement is indicated unless heart failure is present. Additionally, iron deficiency should be excluded as a cause of the symptoms and treated if present. A mild bleeding diathesis is also associated with cyanotic heart disease and necessitates preoperative phlebotomy to a hematocrit just below 65% before elective surgery.

Hyperuricemia

The mechanism of hyperuricemia in cyanotic congenital heart disease is poorly understood but does not seem to be based on red cell turnover alone and is probably related to decreased urate clearance by the kidneys. Gout is fairly common and can be treated with conventional therapy; nephrolithiasis is uncommon.[13]

Pulmonary Disease

Hemoptysis most commonly occurs in patients with cyanotic heart disease secondary to Eisenmenger's syndrome. It has multiple causes, including pulmonary edema, pulmonary infection, pulmonary infarction, and pulmonary arteriolar rupture. Moreover, multiple thoracic surgeries, hypoplastic lungs, and a predisposition to frequent pulmonary infections may lead to chronic lung disease. It is important to consider the confounding role of pulmonary disease in patients with symptomatic dyspnea. In patients with obstructive lung disease, bronchodilator therapy must be used with caution to avoid exacerbating any underlying arrhythmias. Conversely, in patients requiring treatment of arrhythmias with amiodarone, it is important to monitor

TABLE 34–6

Risk of Endocarditis in Congenital Heart Disease According to Defect

Defect	Associated Defects	Risk of Endocarditis	Prophylaxis Indicated
		Acyanotic	
Bicuspid AV	Coarctation	High	Yes
Valvar PS	VSD (see TOF), Noonan's syndrome	Low (mild PS)	Yes
		Intermediate (severe PS)	Yes
ASD secundum	Mitral valve prolapse	Low	No*†
ASD primum, AV canal	Bridging AV leaflets, trisomy 21	Intermediate (with MR)	Yes
VSD	PS (see TOF), AI	Intermediate-high (unoperated or w/AI)	Yes
		Low (operated w/o AI)	No*
PDA	Coexists with many complex syndromes	Low (ligated)	No
		Intermediate (patent)	Yes
Coarctation	Bicuspid AV	Low (operated‡)	Yes
		Intermediate (untreated)	Yes
C-TGV	VSD, infundibular PS	Low (isolated C-TGV)	No†
Ebstein's anomaly	ASD PFO	Low-intermediate	Yes
		Cyanotic	
TOF	RAA, ASD	Intermediate	Yes
Eisenmenger's syndrome	VSD, ASD, PDA	Intermediate	Yes
Tricuspid atresia	Pul Atr, ASD, VSD	?	Yes
Pul Atr/intact septum		?	Yes
D-TGV	ASD, PFO, PDA, VSD, PS	Intermediate	Yes
		Postoperative	
Blalock-Taussig		High	Yes
Prosthetic valve		High	Yes
Right ventricle–pulmonary artery conduit		High	Yes

*Indicated for first 3 months postoperatively.

†Indicated in the presence of other lesions.

‡Unless an associated bicuspid AV is present.

AI, aortic insufficiency; ASD, atrial septal defect; AV, aortic valve; C-TGV, congenitally corrected transposition of the great vessels; D-TGV, transposition of the great vessels; MR, mitral regurgitation; PDA, patent ductus arteriosus; PFO, patent foramen ovale; PS, pulmonic stenosis; Pul Atr, pulmonary atresia; RAA, right-sided aortic arch; TOF, tetralogy of Fallot; VSD, ventricular septal defect.

Adapted from Foster E: Congenital heart disease in adults. In Crawford M (ed): Clinical Cardiology. Norwalk, CT, Appleton & Lange, 1994. Based on American Heart Association recommendations, 1997.

their pulmonary status with serial pulmonary function tests.

Infectious Disease and Endocarditis Prophylaxis

The major risk of infection in patients with congenital heart disease is endocarditis and endarteritis[20] (see Chapter 33). Indications for prophylactic antibiotics according to the American Heart Association consensus document are summarized in Table 34–6.[21] Endocarditis is much less frequent with right-sided, low-pressure tricuspid and pulmonic valve lesions. Persistent fever in any patient with congenital heart disease warrants a careful examination for the stigmata of endocarditis. Blood cultures should be obtained if endocarditis is at all suspected, but the decision to treat while awaiting results depends on the clinical status of the patient. Careful attention to dental hygiene, skin infections, and other potential sources of bacteremia (e.g., genitourinary tract, especially in sexually active women) is an important adjunctive part of the preventive medical regimen.

Reproductive Issues

As patients with congenital heart disease reach reproductive age, birth control and pregnancy must be specifically addressed. The method of contraception should be individualized and chosen after consideration of a number of important issues, including (1) the risk of pregnancy and childbirth for the patient (surgical sterilization might be considered for those at highest risk, i.e., patients with Eisenmenger's and Marfan's syndromes); (2) the social situation, including the number of partners and the frequency of sexual intercourse; (3) the risk of thrombotic disorders; and (4) the presence of hypertension (e.g., in a patient with unrepaired coarctation). For example, barrier methods (e.g., diaphragm, condom, vaginal sponge) may be used when sexual intercourse is infrequent and the risk of pregnancy is minimal or low. Current hormonal methods—including low-dose estrogen pills, progesterone-only pills, and implanted progesterone—appear to be associated with a low risk of thromboembolic disease and hypertension. Intrauterine devices are relatively contraindicated because of the risk of salpingitis, especially in patients with multiple partners and patients at highest risk for endocarditis. The relative advantages and disadvantages of each of these methods should be addressed in conjunction with an experienced gynecologist to help the patient make the most suitable choice.

In a patient who wishes to become pregnant, advance planning is desirable. The patient will then be able to weigh the risks of pregnancy, as determined by her functional class and specific lesion, against her desire to conceive and proceed with pregnancy. Because of the risk of transmission of congenital heart disease (approximately 5% for the mother and somewhat lower for the father), fetal echocardiography is strongly recommended.[22] Some data suggest that folate supplementation in women of childbearing age may reduce the risk of congenital heart disease. Nevertheless, with careful management, more and more women with congenital anomalies are able to have successful pregnancies. Both maternal mortality and fetal mortality depend on the maternal functional class.[5] In Eisenmenger's syndrome, maternal mortality is extremely high (in excess of 50%), but it is much lower with other cyanotic lesions. However, these patients should be aware that the rate of fetal demise may be as high as 50%; intrauterine growth retardation and prematurity are common.

Regardless of the nature of their congenital heart disease, patients who are in functional class III or IV, as well as those with pulmonary vascular disease and Marfan's syndrome, should be strongly advised against pregnancy. For all but the lowest risk patients (functional class I), prenatal care should generally include a high-risk obstetrics service in association with a specialized adult congenital heart service. Other issues to consider for maternal and fetal welfare include the presence of ventricular dysfunction and arrhythmias (and their therapy) and the need for antibiotic prophylaxis and anticoagulation. The safest management of anticoagulation during pregnancy for patients with prosthetic valves is an unresolved issue and should therefore be planned on an individual basis in consultation with a high-risk obstetrics service and a cardiologist.

Genetic Counseling

Although knowledge of the genetic basis of congenital heart disease has grown recently, few specific recommendations can be made with regard to counseling (see Table 34–2). Marfan's, Holt-Oram (heart-hand syndrome associated with atrial septal defect), and Noonan's (associated with pulmonic valve stenosis) syndromes are autosomal dominant traits with a 50% likelihood of transmission to offspring. In the DiGeorge syndrome, a chromosome 22 deletion is associated with conotruncal cardiac abnormalities, including ventricular septal defects, pulmonary atresia, coarctation of the aorta, and hypoplastic left heart syndrome; approximately 10% of patients with the tetralogy of Fallot have this genetic disorder. A reasonable recommendation is that prospective parents with congenital heart disease or a child with congenital heart disease be referred for genetic counseling if pregnancy is contemplated.

Exercise Guidelines

Adult patients with congenital heart disease frequently request guidelines for physical exercise and participation in sports (Table 34–7). However, exercise prescriptions must be individualized with an emphasis on the severity of the lesion and the patient's clinical status.[23] Clinical features that seriously limit exercise tolerance and increase the risk of exercise include cyanosis, pulmonary hypertension, ventricular dysfunction, and arrhythmias. Specific lesions considered to place the patient at highest risk during exercise are severe aortic stenosis, anomalous origin of the left coronary artery, Marfan's syndrome, and severe mitral valve prolapse. Exercise testing to detect ischemia, arrhythmias, and hemodynamic instability may be helpful in evaluating the safety of exercise in an individual patient. Because isometric (i.e., static) exercise raises blood pressure to high levels in a short time, patients with lesions potentially exacerbated by increased afterload (e.g., those with aortic insufficiency or a systemically functioning right ventricle) should avoid weightlifting and similar activities.

Occasionally, physicians are consulted regarding the safety of scuba diving in cardiac patients. During decompression, gas bubbles are found in the venous circulation. In the presence of an abnormal intracardiac communication, such as an uncorrected ventricular septal defect or atrial septal defect, paradoxical embolization of these gas bubbles may occur. Patients with uncorrected atrial or ventricular septal defects should therefore refrain from recreational or professional diving. Divers who suffer decompression sickness also appear to have a greater than normal prevalence of a patent foramen ovale, so a percutaneous device or surgical closure can be considered for a patent foramen ovale in individuals who refuse to refrain from this activity.

Work, Travel, and Insurance

Many people with congenital heart disease have been successful in school and are gainfully employed. The work must be tailored to any physical limitations (see earlier). The ability to maintain employment is critical to the patient's overall well-being, and effort should be made to help the patient continue working.[5]

The fall in arterial oxygen saturation during airplane travel in cyanotic patients is similar to that in normal patients and is generally well tolerated.[24] Thus, if the

TABLE 34–7

Exercise Guidelines for Patients with Congenital Heart Disease

Unrestricted	Low-Intensity Sports*	No Competitive Sports
ASD, VSD—operated† or small	ASD, VSD—moderate	ASD, VSD with CHF or Eisenmenger's syndrome
PDA—operated† or small	PDA—moderate	PDA with CHF or Eisenmenger's syndrome
PV stenosis (<50 mm Hg)	PV stenosis (>50 mm Hg)	Severe PV stenosis with symptoms
AV stenosis (<25 mm Hg‡)	AV stenosis (25–49 mm Hg‡)	AV stenosis (>50 mm Hg‡)
Coarctation—treated§	Coarctation (<20 mm Hg differences)	Coarctation (>20 mm Hg differences)
	Unoperated or palliated cyanotic heart disease	
Repaired TOF w/o residua	Repaired TOF with mild RV pressure or volume overload	Repaired TOF with severe residua
TGS s/p arterial switch	TGA s/p atrial switch	
	Anomalous left coronary artery	
	Marfan's syndrome‖	

*Low-intensity sports include those with low static and dynamic activity: billiards, bowling, cricket, curling, golf, and riflery.

†Operated, without residual pulmonary hypertension.

‡Peak gradient.

§Treated without residual blood pressure difference and without significant hypertension.

‖No body contact sports.

ASD, atrial septal defect; AV, aortic valve; CHF, congestive heart failure; PDA, patent ductus arteriosus; PV, pulmonic valve; RV, right ventricular; s/p, status post; TGA, transposition of the great arteries; TOF, tetralogy of Fallot; VSD, ventricular septal defect.

Adapted from Graham TP, Bricker JT, James FW, Strong WB: 26th Bethesda Conference: Recommendations for determining eligibility for competition in athletes with cardiovascular abnormalities. Task force 1: Congenital heart disease. Circulation 1994;93:272–276. Adapted with permission from ACCSAP, 1995.

risk of travel is not excessive because of other medical considerations (e.g., heart failure or arrhythmias), air travel is probably safe without any need for supplemental oxygen.

Medical insurance and life insurance are frequently unavailable to many patients with congenital heart disease. Thus, in the current medical environment, the high-cost medical care that these patients require may be difficult to deliver, thereby posing important ethical and economic issues.

Evidence-Based Summary

Several consensus guidelines apply broadly to adult patients with congenital heart disease. However, like all the recommendations in this chapter, they are based on expert consensus and not on data from randomized trials.

- Primary care physicians should identify a regional center to which their patients with congenital heart disease can be referred. Reliance on the patient's pediatric cardiologist for continuing care is discouraged, and the primary care physician should assist the patient in making the transition to appropriate facilities. It is desirable for every patient with congenital heart disease to be evaluated in a regional center at least once.[1]
- Records should date back to the time of the original diagnosis and should include reports of operations, cardiac catheterizations, and other diagnostic tests. The primary care physician should encourage patients to keep their own copies of these documents in the form of a "health passport."[6,25]
- Education about healthy behavior, including dental hygiene, antibiotic prophylaxis, and contraception, is critically important. Risk factor intervention for acquired heart disease should not be overlooked.
- The primary care physician should ensure that diagnostic procedures, including echocardiography, MRI, and cardiac catheterization, are performed in laboratories experienced in congenital heart disease.
- In patients with complex congenital heart disease, empiric treatment of arrhythmias is discouraged. Referral to an electrophysiologist experienced in congenital heart disease is advised for curative ablation, antiarrhythmic management, and intracardiac defibrillators.
- Surgery for congenital heart disease should generally be performed in regional centers by cardiac surgeons trained in such surgery. Exceptions may include closure of an ostium secundum atrial septal defect or ligation of a patent ductus arteriosus.
- When a patient with congenital heart disease requires noncardiac surgery, risk stratification is based on the patient's functional class and ventricular function, as well as the presence of pulmonary hypertension and cyanosis. In patients with adverse risk factors, noncardiac surgery should be performed at a regional center.

- Pregnancy is contraindicated in women with pulmonary hypertension. Women who have other adverse risk factors, including heart failure, poor ventricular function, and cyanotic heart disease, should be managed by an interdisciplinary team within an adult congenital heart disease center. Genetic counseling is advisable.
- Guidelines for exercise have been published (Table 34–7). Competitive athletics is contraindicated in most patients with complex lesions or severe or symptomatic simple lesions.
- Patients should be encouraged to work at jobs commensurate with their level of medical disability. Continuous health insurance coverage is essential in these patients, and referral to appropriate resources is encouraged. Patients should be screened for depression.[6]

References

1. Warnes CA, Liberthson R, Danielson GK Jr, et al: 32nd Bethesda Conference: Care of the adult with congenital heart disease. Task Force 1: The changing profile of congenital heart disease in adult life. J Am Coll Cardiol 2001;37:1170–1175.
2. Perloff JK, Warnes CA: Challenges posed by adults with repaired congenital heart disease. Circulation 2001;103: 2637–2643.
3. Brickner ME, Hillis LD, Lange RL: Congenital heart disease in adults (first of two parts). N Engl J Med 2000;342: 256–263.
4. Brickner ME, Hillis LD, Lange RL: Congenital heart disease in adults (second of two parts). N Engl J Med 2000;342: 334–342.
5. Morris C, Menashe V: 25-year mortality after surgical repair of congenital heart defect in childhood. A population-based cohort study. JAMA 1991;266:3447–3452.
6. Foster E, Graham TP Jr, Driscoll DJ, et al: 32nd Bethesda Conference: Care of the adult with congenital heart disease. Task Force 2: Special health care needs of adults with congenital heart disease. J Am Coll Cardiol 2001;37: 1176–1183.
7. Warnes CA, Liberthson R, Danielson G: Task Force 1: The changing profile of congenital heart disease in adult life. J Am Coll Cardiol 2001;37:1161–1198.
8. Kerut EK, Norfleet WT, Plotnick GD, Giles TD: Patent foramen ovale: A review of associated conditions and the impact of physiological size. J Am Coll Cardiol 2001;38: 613–623.
9. Attie F, Rosas M, Granados N, et al: Surgical treatment for secundum atrial septal defects in patients >40 years old. J Am Coll Cardiol 2001;38:2035–2042.
10. Gatzoulis MA, Freeman MA, Siu SC, et al: Atrial arrhythmia after surgical closure of atrial septal defects in adults. N Engl J Med 1999;340:839–846.
11. Gabriel H, Heger M, Innerfofer P, et al: Long-term outcome of patients with ventricular septal defect considered not to require surgical closing during childhood. J Am Coll Cardiol 2002;39:1066–1071.
12. Myers KA, Farquhar DR: Does this patient have clubbing? JAMA 2001;286:341–347.
13. Cantor WJ, Harrison DA, Moussadji JS, et al: Determinants of survival and length of survival in adults with Eisenmenger syndrome. Am J Cardiol 1999;84:677–681.
14. Nollert G, Fischlein T, Bouterwek S, et al: Long-term survival in patients with repair of tetralogy of Fallot: 36 year follow-up of 490 survivors of the first year after surgical repair. J Am Coll Cardiol 1997;30:1374–1383.
15. Gatzoulis MA, Balaji S, Webber SA, et al: Risk factors for arrhythmia and sudden cardiac death late after repair of tetralogy of Fallot: A multicentre study. Lancet 2000;356: 975–981.
16. Keane JF, Driscoll DJ, Gersony WM, et al: Second natural history study of congenital heart defects. Results of treatment of patients with aortic valvar stenosis. Circulation 1993;87(2 Suppl):I16–I27.
17. Hayes CJ, Gersony WM, Driscoll DJ, et al: Second natural history study of congenital heart defects. Results of treatment of patients with pulmonary valvar stenosis. Circulation 1993;87(2 Suppl):I28–I37.
18. Angelini P, Velasco JA, Flamm S: Coronary anomalies: Incidence, pathophysiology, and clinical relevance. Circulation 2002;105:2449–2454.
19. Shores J, Berger KR, Murphy EA, Pyeritz RE: Progression of aortic dilatation and the benefit of long-term beta-adrenergic blockade in Marfan's syndrome. N Engl J Med 1994;330:1335–1341.
20. Morris CD, Reller MD, Menashe VD: Thirty year incidence of infective endocarditis after surgery for congenital heart disease. JAMA 1998;279:599–603.
21. Dajani AS, Taubert KA, Wilson W, et al: Prevention of bacterial endocarditis. Recommendations by the American Heart Association. Circulation 1997;96:358–366.
22. Whittemore R, Wells JA, Castellsague X: A second-generation study of 427 probands with congenital heart defects and their 837 children. J Am Coll Cardiol 1994;23: 1459–1467.
23. Graham TP, Bricker JT, James FW, Strong WB: 26th Bethesda Conference: Recommendations for determining eligibility for competition in athletes with cardiovascular abnormalities. Task Force 1: Congenital heart disease. J Am Coll Cardiol 1994;24:867–873.
24. Harnick E, Hutter PA, Hoorntje TM, et al: Air travel and adults with cyanotic congenital heart disease. Circulation 1996;93:272–276.
25. Webb CL, Jenkins KJ, Karpawich PP, et al: Collaborative care for adults with congenital heart disease. Circulation 2002;105:2318–2323.

CHAPTER 35 Recognition and Management of Patients with Pericardial Disease

Rick A. Nishimura and Kenneth R. Kidd

Diseases of the pericardium are relatively uncommon in routine clinical practice but are important to recognize because a delayed or incorrect diagnosis or therapy may be life threatening. Acute pericarditis can mimic other disease entities that require their own specific urgent attention, such as myocardial infarction or aortic dissection. Pericardial tamponade is a medical emergency for which immediate pericardiocentesis is required, whereas constrictive pericarditis causes a syndrome of progressive heart failure that can be completely cured by pericardiectomy.

The pericardial lining around the heart consists of an inner visceral pericardium and a tough outer parietal pericardium. The pericardium completely encircles the outer cardiac structures and extends superiorly to wrap around the base of the great vessels. Normally, less than 50 mL of fluid in the pericardial space (between the visceral and parietal pericardium) is thought to "lubricate" the surfaces of the pericardium. In reality, the true function of the pericardium remains unknown. It has been speculated that the pericardium stabilizes the cardiac structures or prevents the spread of infection, but patients without a pericardium (because of either congenital absence or surgical removal) have normal cardiac function.

The pericardium is a "silent" structure that normally causes no sound on auscultation and no findings on inspection or palpation. Because it is less than 2 mm in thickness, it cannot be visualized on echocardiography. On higher resolution imaging modalities such as computed tomography (CT) or magnetic resonance imaging (MRI), the normal pericardium may be seen as a thin layer around the heart, particularly if it is separated by a fatty layer. The pericardium may become inflamed, effusive, or constrictive. In diseases of the pericardium, symptoms are caused by either the pain of pericardial or pleural irritation or the hemodynamic consequences when proper filling of the cardiac chambers is prohibited by pericardial restraint.

ACUTE PERICARDITIS

The diagnosis of acute uncomplicated pericarditis can usually be made on the basis of the history, physical examination, and electrocardiogram (ECG). An accompanying pericardial effusion, with or without tamponade, can be assessed by the physical examination, chest radiograph, and echocardiogram. It must be remembered, however, that acute pericarditis does not always cause pericardial effusion, that very small pericardial effusions may be seen in normal individuals, and that a pathologic pericardial effusion may be a sign of a pericardial diagnosis other than acute viral or idiopathic pericarditis.

The most common cause of acute pericarditis in a young, previously healthy individual is spontaneous idiopathic pericarditis or viral pericarditis (Box 35–1).

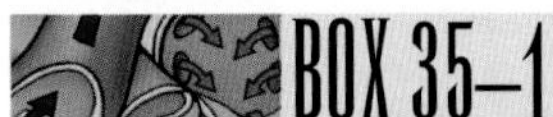

BOX 35–1

Causes of Pericarditis

Idiopathic (nonspecific)
Viral infections: Coxsackie A virus, Coxsackie B virus, echovirus, adenovirus, mumps virus, infectious mononucleosis, varicella, hepatitis B, acquired immunodeficiency syndrome
Tuberculosis
Acute bacterial infections: pneumococci, staphylococci, streptococci, gram-negative septicemia, *Neisseria meningitidis, Neisseria gonorrhoeae*
Fungal infections: histoplasmosis, coccidioidomycosis, *Candida*, blastomycosis
Other infections: toxoplasmosis, amebiasis, *Mycoplasma, Nocardia*, actinomycosis, echinococcosis, Lyme disease
Acute myocardial infarction
Uremia: untreated uremia; in association with hemodialysis
Neoplastic disease: lung cancer, breast cancer, leukemia, Hodgkin's disease, lymphoma
Radiation: cardiac injury
Autoimmune disorders: systemic lupus erythematosus, rheumatoid arthritis, scleroderma, mixed connective tissue disease, Wegener's granulomatosis, polyarteritis nodosa, acute rheumatic fever
Other inflammatory disorders: sarcoidosis, amyloidosis, inflammatory bowel disease, Whipple's disease, temporal arteritis, Behçet's disease
Drugs: hydralazine, procainamide, phenytoin, isoniazid, phenylbutazone, dantrolene, doxorubicin, methysergide, penicillin (with hypereosinophilia)
Trauma: including chest trauma; hemopericardium after thoracic surgery for pacemaker insertion or cardiac diagnostic procedures; esophageal rupture; pancreatic-pericardial fistula
Delayed myocardial-pericardial injury syndromes: post–myocardial infarction (Dressler's) syndrome; post-pericardiotomy syndrome
Dissecting aortic aneurysm
Myxedema
Chylopericardium

In some patients, pericarditis develops as part of an infectious process (e.g., acute bacterial pericarditis, tuberculosis), a known systemic disease (e.g., a disseminated malignancy, a polyserositis associated with a collagen vascular disease, or uremia), or a specific cardiac insult (e.g., acute myocardial infarction, trauma, cardiac surgery, or irradiation). In patients without an obvious cause at the time of initial evaluation, viral or idiopathic pericarditis accounts for the overwhelming majority of cases, but tumors, tuberculosis, other infections, and collagen vascular diseases each account for an important minority of cases[1, 2] (Table 35–1).

TABLE 35–1

Final Diagnosis of the Causes of Acute Pericarditis in 331 Patients without an Obvious Etiology at the Time of Initial Evaluation

Idiopathic/viral	277 (84%)
Neoplastic	20 (6%)
Tuberculous	13 (4%)
Other infections	9 (3%)
Collagen vascular disease	5 (1.5%)
Other	7 (2%)

Pooled data from Permanyer-Miralda G, Sagristà-Sauleda J, Soler-Soler J: Primary acute pericardial disease: A prospective series of 231 consecutive patients. Am J Cardiol 1985;56:623–629; and Zayar R, Anguita M, Torres F, et al: Incidence of specific etiology and role of methods for specific etiologic diagnosis of primary acute pericarditis. Am J Cardiol 1995;75:378–382.

Clinical Features

Patients with symptoms of acute pericarditis may seek care at an outpatient office or an emergency department, and the major initial symptom is usually chest pain, which can be quite intense or relatively mild. The pain is generally described as "sharp and stabbing," although it can also be a dull ache. It is typically located in the substernal area and may radiate to the neck, jaw, arms, back, and shoulders. A characteristic of pericardial pain is that it commonly has a pleuritic component that is exacerbated by deep inspiration or changes in position. Leaning over usually lessens the pain, whereas the supine position may intensify the pain, perhaps because the inflamed pericardium comes into closer contact with the diaphragm. The pain generally increases gradually over hours and persists for many hours or days; it waxes and wanes but never completely disappears.

Other common symptoms are low-grade fever and palpitations from sinus tachycardia or, less commonly, atrial tachyarrhythmias. Symptoms of infectious diseases or systemic processes may be important clues to the presence of malignancy, uremia, collagen vascular diseases, or infections other than self-limited viral diseases. Dyspnea may be caused by a large pericardial effusion (see later), or the patient may feel short of breath because the pain inhibits full inspiration.

Acute pericarditis must be differentiated from acute myocardial ischemia (Table 35–2), as well as other cardiac and noncardiac causes of chest pain (Table 35–3 and Tables 6–2 and 6–3). It is important to remember that primary causes of chest pain, such as acute myocardial infarction (see Chapter 27), aortic dissection (see Chapter 36), lung cancer, and bacterial pneumonia, can also secondarily involve the pericardium.

Physical Examination

A patient with acute pericarditis often looks uncomfortable and does not want to change position for fear

TABLE 35–2

Chest Pain in Acute Pericarditis versus Acute Myocardial Ischemia

	Acute Pericarditis	Acute Ischemia
Onset	More often sudden	Usually gradual, crescendo
Main location	Substernal or left precordial	Same or confined to zones of radiation
Radiation	May be the same as ischemic, also trapezius ridge(s)	Shoulders, arms, neck, jaw, back; not trapezius ridge(s)
Quality	Usually sharp, stabbing; "background" ache or dull and oppressive	Usually "heavy" (pressure sensation) or burning
Inspiration	Worse	No effect unless with infarction pericarditis
Duration	Persistent; may wax and wane	Usually intermittent; < 30 min each recurrence, longer for unstable angina
Body movements	Increased	Usually no effect
Posture	Worse on recumbency; improved on sitting, leaning forward	No effect or improvement on sitting
Nitroglycerin	No effect	Usually relief

From Spodick DH: The Pericardium: A Comprehensive Textbook. New York, Marcel Dekker, 1997.

of exacerbating the pain. Shallow breaths are taken to avoid the inspiratory exacerbation of pain. The most common rhythm abnormality in a patient with acute pericarditis is sinus tachycardia, which is also the most sensitive sign of impending hemodynamic compromise, even when systemic blood pressure remains normal. Sinus bradycardia or other rhythms such as atrial fibrillation should suggest the presence of other diseases.

Blood pressure is usually normal unless the pericarditis is associated with a large pericardial effusion. Similarly, jugular venous pulsations (see Chapter 3) can usually be seen in the supine position and disappear below the clavicle with the patient sitting at 45 degrees if hemodynamic compromise has not occurred. Hypotension, a narrow pulse pressure, pulsus paradoxus, and elevated venous pressure, especially in the absence of an inspiratory decrease, all suggest pericardial tamponade, a medical emergency (see later).

The sine qua non of acute pericarditis is a pericardial rub heard on auscultation. This rub typically has three components, each corresponding to a time when the cardiac chambers expand within the pericardial sac: one during ventricular systole, a second during rapid ventricular filling in early diastole, and a third in late diastole at the time of atrial contraction. In less severe cases, the rub may have only two or even just one component. A pericardial rub, which is differentiated from a murmur by its scratchy quality, is sometimes localized to a small area on the chest wall and may come and go spontaneously or with changes in position. To hear a rub, it may be necessary to auscultate the heart with the patient in multiple positions, especially sitting up

TABLE 35–3

Differential Diagnosis of Pericarditis from Other Cardiovascular Causes of Acute Chest Pain

Condition	Symptoms	Examination	Electrocardiogram	Chest Radiograph	Echocardiogram
Acute pericarditis	Gradual onset of pleuritic chest pain ± dull ache	Pericardial friction rub ± pleural rub; ± elevated JVP	Diffuse concave upward ST elevation; PR depression in leads II, III, aVF; PR elevation in aVR	Normal or globular cardiac silhouette	Normal or effusion
Myocardial infarction/unstable angina	Acute or stuttering chest pain; coronary risk factors	S_4, MR murmur, no rub	Localized ST elevation or depression	Normal or pulmonary congestion	Wall motion abnormality
Pulmonary embolism	Pleuritic chest pain, dyspnea	Pleural rub; increased P_2	T inversion in V_1–V_3; S_1, Q_3 pattern	Normal or infiltrate	Dilated RV
Aortic dissection	Acute onset of severe chest pain	Pulse deficit, AR murmur, hypertension		Dilated aorta	Dilated aorta

AR, aortic regurgitation; JVP, jugular venous pressure; MR, mitral regurgitation; RV, right ventricle.

and leaning forward while holding a full expiration. Despite these maneuvers, a rub is sometimes not audible or may be evanescent. In a patient with a large pericardial effusion, the heart sounds are often soft and hard to hear.

Diagnostic Tests

Laboratory Tests. In most patients with acute pericarditis, acute inflammation results in an elevated erythrocyte sedimentation rate, C-reactive protein level, and white blood cell count. The presence of atypical lymphocytes on a peripheral smear suggests a viral cause of the pericarditis.

All patients should have a tuberculin skin test and test of renal function (Box 35–2). The MB band of creatine kinase (CK-MB) or troponin levels (or both) should be measured. Even without any evidence by history or physical examination, patients may have had a myocardial infarction with secondary pericardial inflammation, or they may have a myocarditis caused by inflammation from the adjacent pericarditis. Other blood tests are useful in selected situations.

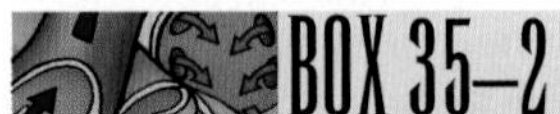

BOX 35–2

Selected Diagnostic Tests in Acute Pericarditis

IN ALL PATIENTS

Tuberculin skin test (and control skin test to exclude anergy)
BUN and creatinine to exclude uremia
Erythrocyte sedimentation rate
Electrocardiogram
Chest radiograph

IN SELECTED PATIENTS

Echocardiogram
ANA and rheumatoid factor to exclude systemic lupus erythematosus or rheumatoid arthritis in patients with acute arthritis or pleural effusion
TSH and T_4 to exclude hypothyroidism in patients with clinical findings suggestive of hypothyroidism and in asymptomatic patients with unexplained pericardial effusion
HIV test to exclude the possibility of AIDS in patients with risk factors for HIV disease or a compatible clinical syndrome
Blood cultures in febrile patients to exclude associated possible infective endocarditis and bacteremia
Fungal serologic tests in patients from endemic areas or in immunocompromised patients
ASO titer in children or teenagers with suspected rheumatic fever
Heterophil antibody test to exclude mononucleosis in young or middle-aged patients with a compatible clinical syndrome or acute fever, weakness, and lymphadenopathy

AIDS, acquired immunodeficiency syndrome; ANA, antinuclear antibody; ASO, antistreptolysin O; BUN, blood urea nitrogen; HIV, human immunodeficiency virus; T_4, thyroxine; TSH, thyroid-stimulating hormone.

Electrocardiogram. Sinus tachycardia may be present, but other rhythm abnormalities are rare in uncomplicated acute pericarditis. Ventricular arrhythmias suggest myocardial ischemia or a myocarditis complicating the pericarditis. In patients with a large pericardial effusion, low voltage is commonly found. Classic ST and PR segment abnormalities occur on the 12-lead ECG in the acute phase of pericarditis (Fig. 35–1). Typically, ST segment elevation occurs diffusely in the precordial and limb leads, unlike the pattern of myocardial infarction, in which ST elevation in one region is accompanied by reciprocal ST depression in other regions (Fig. 35–2). In pericarditis, the contour of the ST elevation is usually concave upward (up-sloping like a smile), a pattern not seen with the ST elevation of myocardial infarction.

Another diagnostic feature of the ECG of acute pericarditis is PR segment depression, which is best seen in the inferior leads (see Fig. 35–1), with reciprocal PR segment elevation in lead aVR. These PR segment changes are not seen in patients with myocardial infarction.[3]

Three subsequent, less specific ECG stages may follow the diffuse concave upward ST changes (stage 1) that are initially seen in patients with acute pericarditis. Other than the finding of PR segment elevation/depression, these phases cannot be reliably distinguished from a variety of other conditions.

Chest Radiograph. The chest radiograph is usually normal in patients with uncomplicated acute pericarditis. Small pleural effusions may develop because the pleura is frequently inflamed, and a unilateral left pleural effusion is sometimes present. If cardiomegaly with a globular silhouette is seen (Fig. 35–3), an associated pericardial effusion should be suspected.

Echocardiography. Echocardiography is not required in patients with uncomplicated acute pericarditis, but two-dimensional transthoracic echocardiography is indicated in patients in whom hemodynamic compromise (as assessed by elevated jugular venous pressure, hypotension, or pulsus paradoxus) is suspected or cardiomegaly is present. Echocardiography is also indicated in patients who have other concomitant illnesses such as renal failure or collagen vascular disease, previous radiation therapy, or malignancies because the natural history of pericarditis caused by these conditions may not be as benign as the natural history of viral or idiopathic pericarditis.

The presence and size of a pericardial effusion, which is seen as an echo-free space around the heart (Fig. 35–4), can be readily assessed by echocardiography (see Chapter 5). In acute pericarditis, however, an effusion may not be seen on echocardiography (sometimes called "dry" pericarditis). In addition, normal individuals frequently have a tiny pericardial effusion detected by echocardiography. If an effusion is present, Doppler echocardiography can aid in determining its hemodynamic significance (see "Pericardial Tamponade")

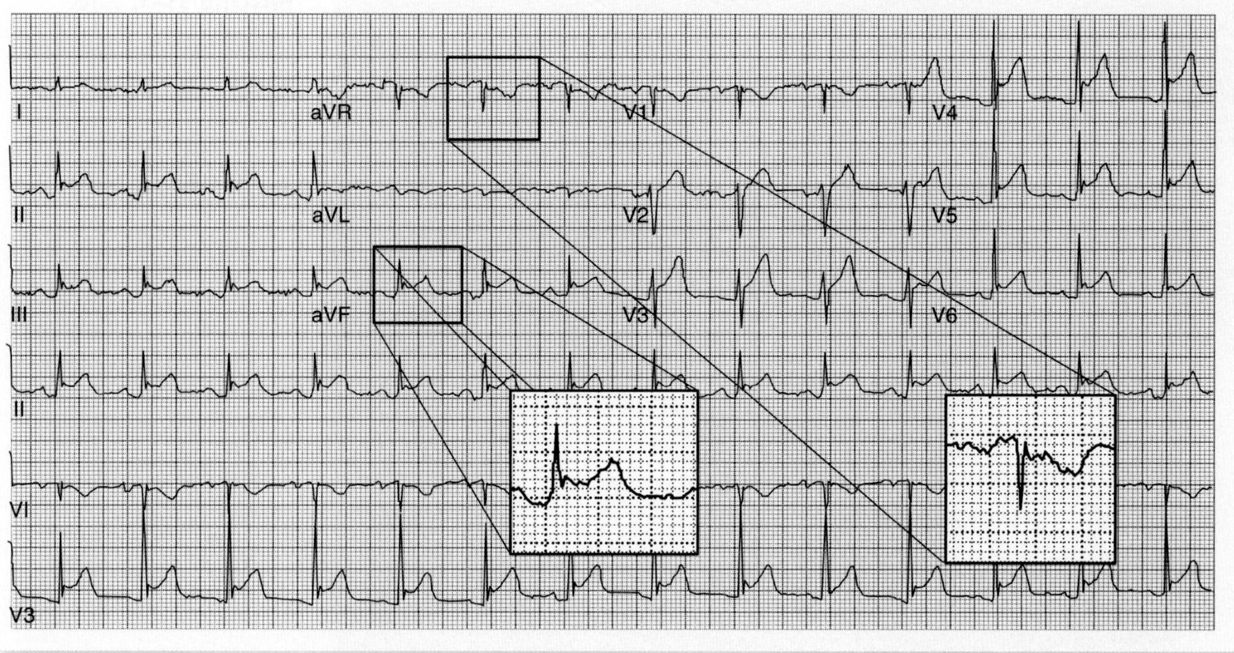

FIGURE 35–1. A classic 12-lead electrocardiogram from a patient with acute pericarditis. Concave upward ST elevation is present in all leads (*left box insert*). In addition, PR elevation (*arrow*) is noted in lead aVL (*right box insert*).

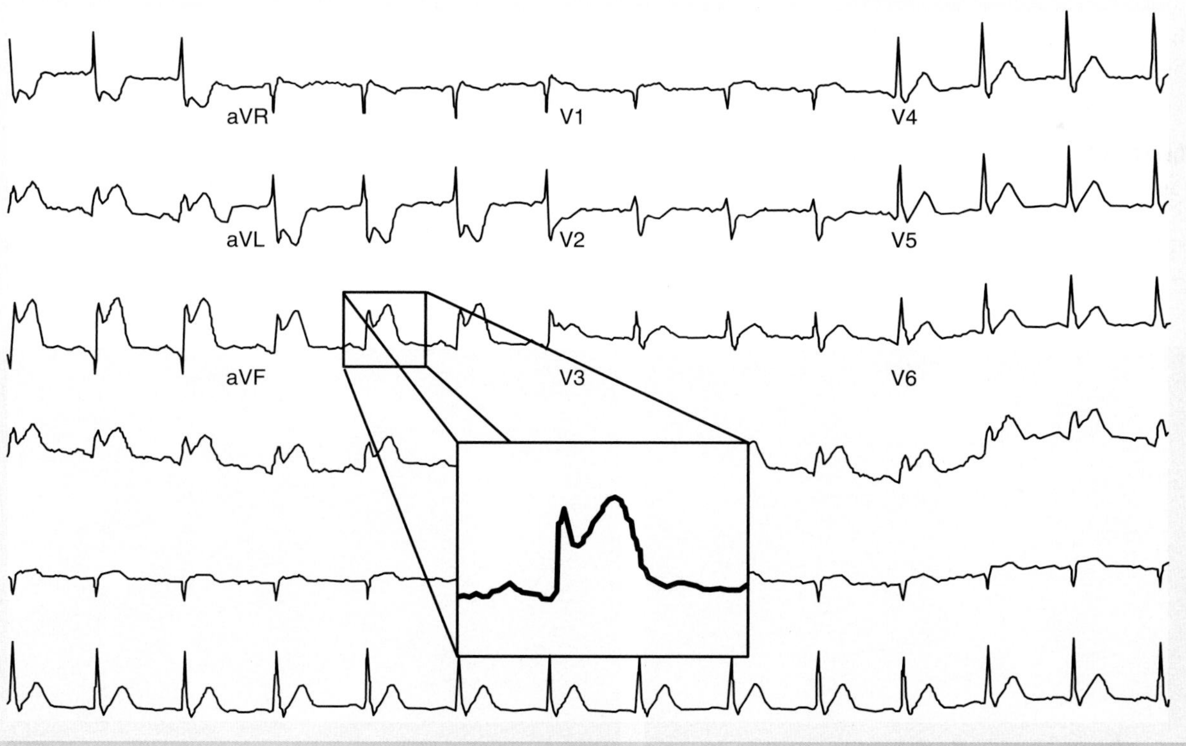

FIGURE 35–2. A 12-lead electrocardiogram from a patient with an acute myocardial infarction. The ST segment morphology is different from what is seen in a patient with pericarditis in that the ST segments are not concave upward (*box insert*). Reciprocal ST depressions are also seen in the high lateral leads.

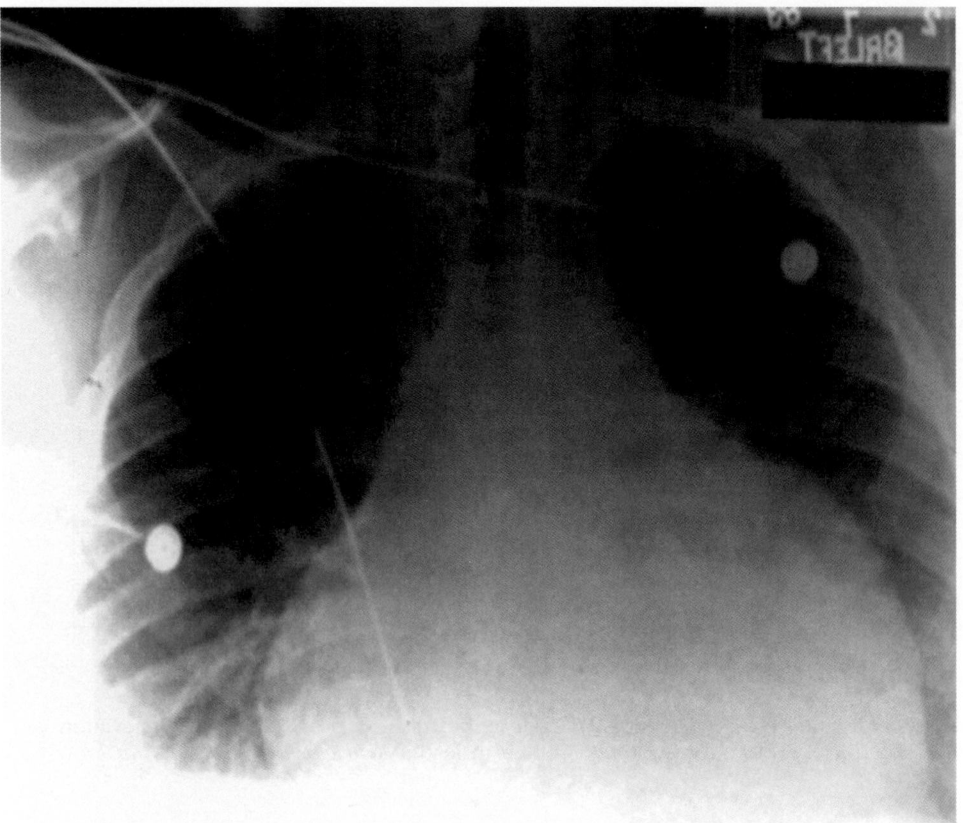

FIGURE 35–3. Large "globular" cardiac silhouette seen on a chest radiograph in a patient with a pericardial effusion.

and whether emergency pericardiocentesis is required (Fig. 35–5).

Treatment

Patients who appear acutely ill with a high fever should be hospitalized. Hospitalization is also warranted for patients with any signs of impending hemodynamic compromise or a pericardial effusion in the setting of any cause of acute pericarditis other than viral or idiopathic because patients with these other causes may have an effusion that accumulates rapidly and causes subsequent tamponade. If no effusion is present, patients can usually be monitored in an outpatient setting. In patients with an equivocal history or suspicious ECG changes, or both, treatment for a possible acute coronary syndrome (see Chapters 26 and 27) must

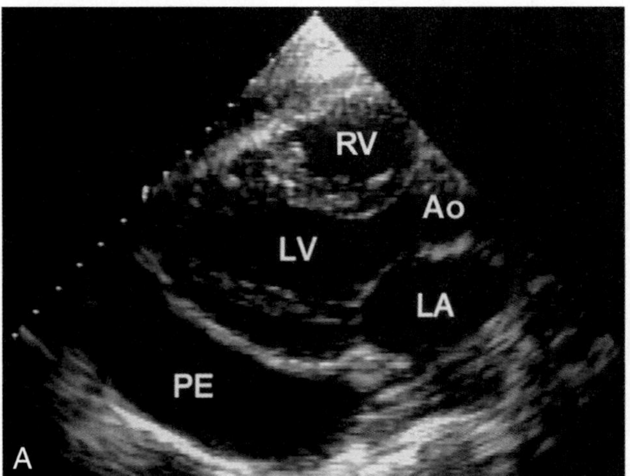

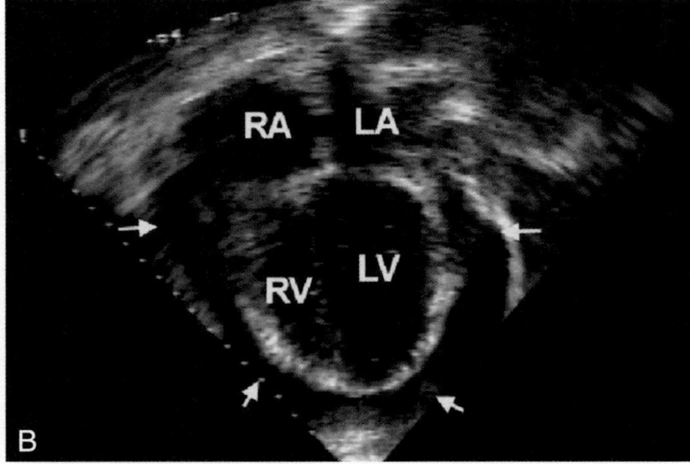

FIGURE 35–4. Two-dimensional echocardiograms from two patients with large pericardial effusions (PE), which are seen as an echo-dense space around the heart. *A*, Parasternal long-axis view with the pericardial effusion located mainly posterior to the heart. *B*, Apical four-chamber view with a circumferential pericardial effusion (*arrows*). Ao, aorta; LA, left atrium; LV, left ventricle; RA, right atrium; RV, right ventricle.

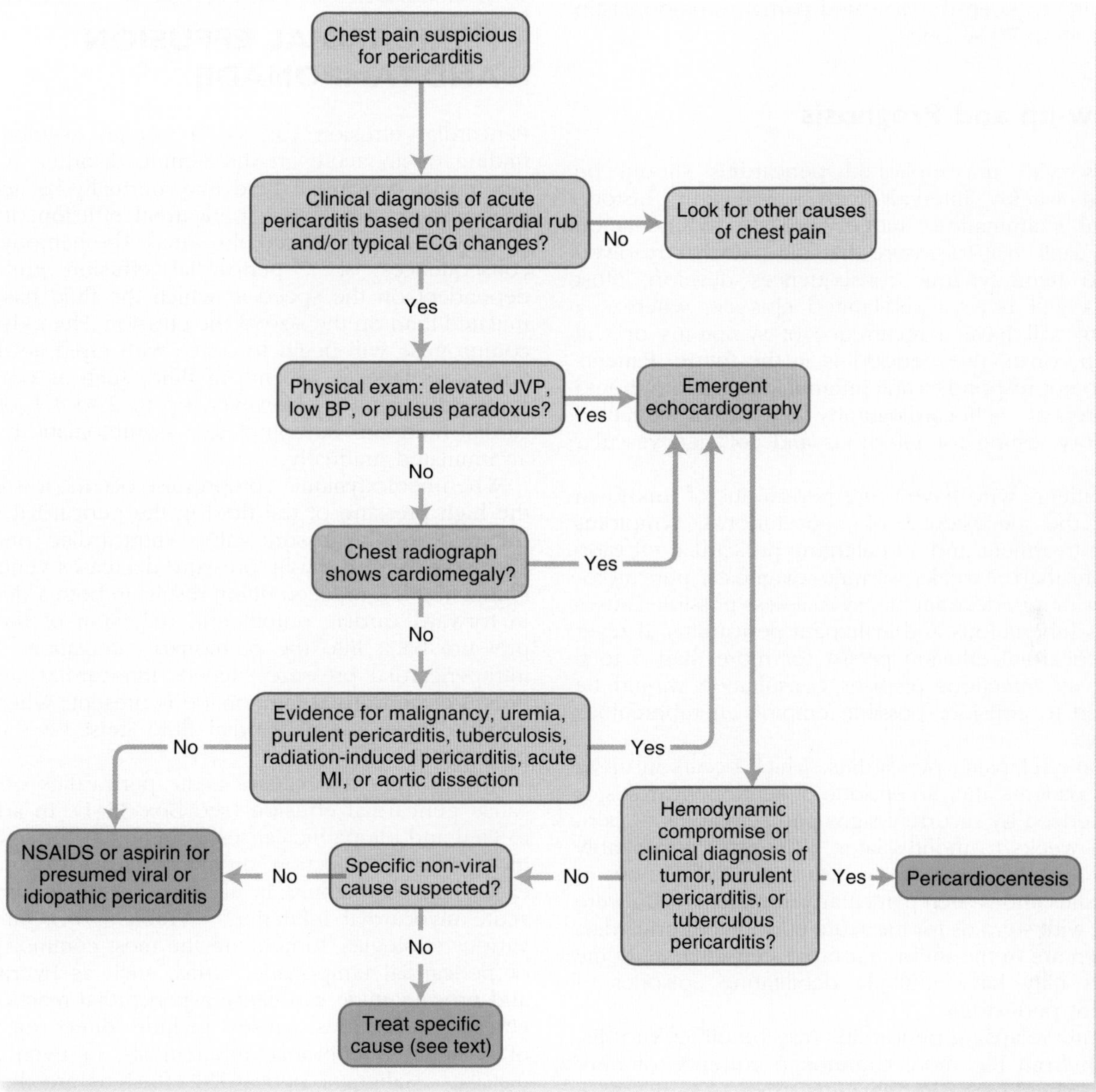

FIGURE 35–5. Evaluation of a patient with suspected acute pericarditis.

be considered. Echocardiography may be especially helpful in these equivocal situations because regional wall motion abnormalities suggest ischemia and the absence of pericardial effusion means that anticoagulation or antithrombotic therapy is probably safe.

Treatment of most cases of acute pericarditis is the institution of oral high-dose salicylates or other nonsteroidal anti-inflammatory drugs (NSAIDs). Corticosteroids provide relief of the inflammatory process but should not be used in patients with acute idiopathic pericarditis because recurrent episodes of pericarditis may develop when the steroids are tapered. Salicylates should be given as three to four 325-mg tablets every 4 hours while awake. For other NSAIDs, the dose should be the equivalent of 50 mg of indomethacin three times a day; parenteral ketorolac can be used in severe cases. NSAIDs or salicylates should be given for 1 month and then tapered over a 2-week period. Symptoms and the erythrocyte sedimentation rate can be monitored to ensure that the taper is not too rapid.

Pericardiocentesis is not indicated in acute pericarditis unless purulent or tuberculous pericarditis is clinically suspected or the patient fails to respond to 2 to 3 weeks of NSAID therapy. In patients taking warfarin, it should generally be continued under careful monitoring unless the patient has a pericardial effusion. For patients who have an effusion but may absolutely require anticoagulation (e.g., patients with prosthetic heart valves), consultation with a cardiologist and a hematologist is recommended; options include continuing the warfarin or switching to a continuous infusion of intravenous unfractionated heparin, which has a short half-life and can be rapidly reversed with protamine to keep the activated partial thromboplastin time at 55 to 70 seconds.

Follow-up and Prognosis

Patients with uncomplicated pericarditis should be seen at weekly intervals with a follow-up history, physical examination, and erythrocyte sedimentation rate at each visit to ensure that the pain has resolved and no hemodynamic consequences develop. Most patients will have a self-limited episode, whereas a minority will have a recurrence of symptoms or will develop constrictive pericarditis in the future. Patients who do not respond to anti-inflammatory agents should have repeat echocardiography and more detailed laboratory testing for infectious and collagen vascular diseases.

In patients who have acute pericarditis of unknown cause, the persistence of constitutional symptoms despite treatment and an enlarging pericardial effusion for more than 3 weeks warrants diagnostic pericardiocentesis or a pericardial biopsy to assess possible causes such as tuberculous and malignant pericarditis. If fever and pericardial effusion persist for more than 5 to 6 weeks, an infectious diseases consultation should be obtained to consider possible empiric antituberculous therapy.

Chronic relapsing pericarditis, which occurs in up to 20% of patients after an episode of acute pericarditis, is characterized by recurrent signs and symptoms of pericarditis weeks to months later. This entity is probably due to an autoimmune response to the initial bout of pericarditis and is seen particularly in patients who were treated with steroids for the acute episode of pericarditis and then are in the midst of a rapid steroid taper. Some patients may have multiple debilitating episodes of recurrent pericarditis.

Chronic relapsing pericarditis may be difficult to distinguish from the more common occurrence of nonspecific chest pain after an initial bout of pericarditis. In a patient with recurrent vague chest pain but neither a pericardial rub nor an elevated erythrocyte sedimentation rate, the diagnosis of chronic relapsing pericarditis should be questioned.

When pericarditis relapses in a patient who is rapidly weaned from steroid therapy, the treatment of choice is high-dose NSAIDs or salicylates during a slow steroid taper. Steroids should be tapered over a period of 1 month to a dose equivalent to approximately 15 to 20 mg of prednisone per day while high-dose NSAIDs or salicylates are being given. The taper should then occur very slowly, with the steroid dose decreased by approximately 1 mg/wk. If the pericarditis recurs during this taper, the steroids should then be increased back to 20 mg of prednisone per day, with a slower taper of 1 mg every other week. A trial of colchicine at 1 to 2 mg/day has been suggested for patients with relapsing pericarditis,[4] but the effectiveness of this therapy is controversial. If the patient cannot be weaned off steroids, surgery to remove the pericardium may be effective in preventing recurrent pericarditis.

PERICARDIAL EFFUSION AND TAMPONADE

Pericardial effusion can be a benign asymptomatic finding or an acute life-threatening disorder. A small amount of pericardial fluid may normally be seen on echocardiography, but a pericardial effusion of more than 50 mL is considered abnormal. The hemodynamic consequences of a pericardial effusion are more dependent on the speed at which the fluid has accumulated than on the size of the effusion. Hemodynamic compromise will begin to occur with rapid accumulation of as little as 150 mL of fluid, such as occurs in myocardial rupture. However, up to 2 to 3 L of pericardial fluid can be completely asymptomatic if it has accumulated gradually.

When hemodynamic compromise occurs, it is due to the high pressure of the fluid in the pericardial space. Intrapericardial pressure raises intracardiac pressure. The increase in diastolic pressure decreases ventricular filling, and the reduced filling results in both a decrease in forward cardiac output and reflection of the high pressure back into the pulmonary circulation.[5] When intrapericardial pressure exceeds intracardiac diastolic pressure, pericardial tamponade is present. When tamponade develops, pericardial fluid must be removed emergently.

Any process that causes acute pericarditis can also cause pericardial effusion (see Box 35–1). In addition to viral and idiopathic causes, common systemic causes include tumor, infection, uremia, collagen vascular diseases, and heart failure; local causes include trauma and acute myocardial infarction[6, 7] (Table 35–4). Of these various etiologies, tumors are the most common cause of pericardial tamponade. Drugs such as hydralazine and procainamide can cause a pericardial reaction and effusion. Infectious causes include direct extension of bacterial pneumonia, tuberculosis, or even fungal diseases. Malignant pericardial effusions are the most common cause of effusion with tamponade, usually

TABLE 35–4

Causes of Moderate to Large Asymptomatic Pericardial Effusions in 464 Patients in Two Recent Studies[6, 7]

Cause	Patients
Idiopathic/viral	172 (37%)
Neoplastic	86 (19%)
Iatrogenic/trauma	60 (13%)
Tuberculous or purulent	26 (6%)
Acute myocardial infarction	26 (6%)
Collagen vascular disease	20 (4%)
Heart failure	20 (4%)
Uremia	20 (4%)
Radiation induced	10 (2%)
Aortic dissection	10 (2%)
Hypothyroidism	5 (1%)
Other	9 (2%)

from a breast, lung, or hematologic source; sometimes the pericardial fluid has malignant cells, whereas other cases are related to "paraneoplastic" pericardial irritation from an adjacent tumor. Other more acute processes causing severe hemodynamic compromise include myocardial rupture (from trauma or myocardial infarction), aortic dissection, and bleeding after open heart surgery.

History and Physical Examination

A detailed history should be taken to determine whether any past history or current symptoms indicate the possible presence of malignancy, uremia, pneumonia, other infections, collagen vascular disease, heart failure, or any drugs (hydralazine, procainamide) that might cause a pericardial effusion.

Asymptomatic Pericardial Effusion. Patients with an isolated pericardial effusion that has accumulated slowly are often completely asymptomatic because the slow accumulation allows the pericardium to expand with little elevation in intrapericardial pressure. Findings on physical examination may be normal, although the heart sounds may be muffled. The diagnosis is usually made by a chest radiograph showing cardiomegaly with a globular heart. In other patients, the diagnosis may be made serendipitously when an echocardiogram, CT scan, or MRI is performed for another indication and demonstrates a pericardial effusion. Other patients who have disease entities that are known to cause pericardial effusion, such as hypothyroidism, uremia, or collagen vascular disease, may have an asymptomatic pericardial effusion discovered during their evaluation.

Pericardial Tamponade. Patients with pericardial tamponade who are not in cardiogenic shock have the predominant symptoms of fatigue and shortness of breath. Patients with tamponade nearly always have tachycardia, usually a sinus tachycardia, as a result of reflex sympathetic stimulation from low cardiac output. Blood pressure is usually low with a narrow pulse pressure, but systemic pressure can sometimes initially be normal because of arterial vasoconstriction.

Pulsus paradoxus occurs with pericardial tamponade and is due to a marked drop in filling of the left ventricle with inspiration, which results in lower cardiac output manifested as a greater than normal reduction in blood pressure during inspiration (Fig. 35–6). Detection of pulsus paradoxus can be accomplished rapidly at the bedside. The blood pressure cuff should be inflated to the level at which systolic pressure is first heard. The inflation should be kept at the systolic blood pressure level, and the Korotkoff sounds should be auscultated during spontaneous inspiration and expiration. If the sound disappears with inspiration, the cuff should be deflated another 5 mm Hg and the sounds auscultated again during inspiration and expiration. These steps should be repeated until the Korotkoff sounds are heard during both inspiration and expiration. The difference in systolic pressure during inspiration and expiration is the degree of pulsus paradox. Normally, this difference is less than 10 mm Hg. If the pulsus paradoxus is greater than 10 mm Hg, pericardial tamponade should be suspected. Pulsus paradoxus can also be seen in situations in which negative intrathoracic pressure is accentuated during inspiration, such as during an acute exacerbation of asthma, pulmonary embolism, tension pneumothorax, or circulatory shock. Jugular venous pressure is universally elevated in tamponade.

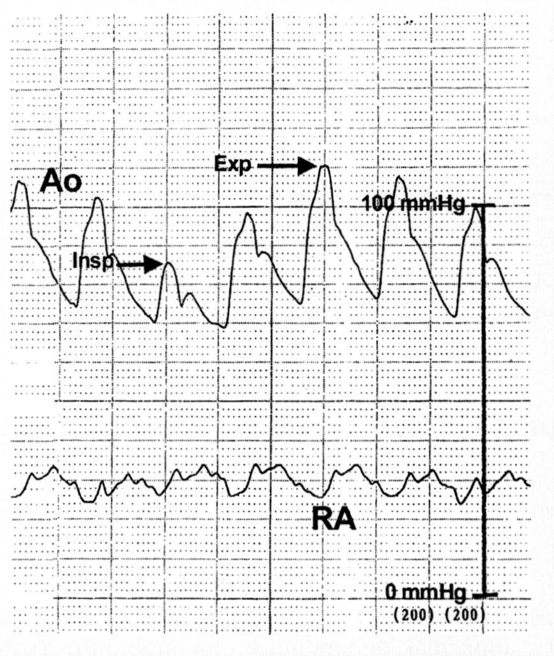

FIGURE 35–6. Pressure curves from the ascending aorta (Ao) and right atrium (RA) in a patient with pericardial tamponade. During inspiration (Insp), systolic pressure decreases 25 mm Hg, in addition to a decrease in pulse pressure. Right atrial pressure is severely elevated to 30 mm Hg with an X descent but no Y descent. Exp, expiration.

Pericardial Tamponade and Cardiogenic Shock. Cardiogenic shock can accompany pericardial tamponade if pericardial fluid accumulates very rapidly because of conditions such as myocardial rupture (from trauma or a myocardial infarction), aortic dissection, or bleeding after open heart surgery. These patients will be seen in extremis with a rapid thready pulse and peripheral vasoconstriction. Blood pressure may completely disappear during inspiration as a result of the large pulsus paradoxus.

Diagnostic Testing

Blood Tests. The laboratory evaluation of pericardial effusion should be similar to the approach for acute pericarditis (see Box 35–2). Specific causes of pericardial effusion, including hypothyroidism, uremia, and collagen vascular diseases, can be diagnosed by obtaining thyroid function studies, blood urea nitrogen and creatinine levels, and serologic studies for rheumatoid arthritis and systemic lupus erythematosus (SLE).

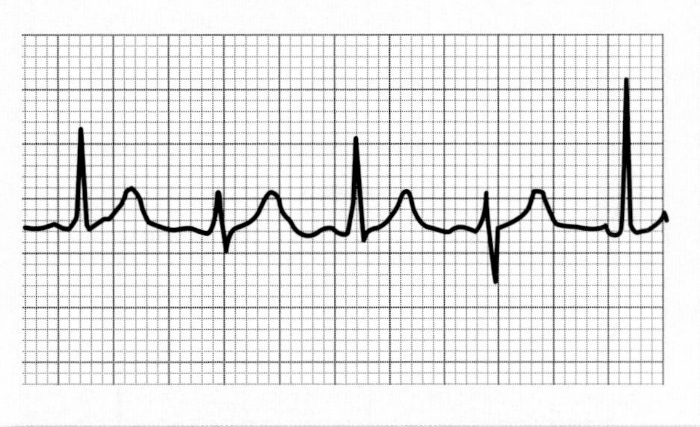

FIGURE 35–7. An electrocardiographic strip from a patient with pericardial effusion and pericardial tamponade. Electrical alternans, with a shift in axis every other beat, is present.

Chest Radiograph. The chest radiograph may or may not be abnormal, depending on the amount of pericardial fluid. When a large amount of fluid is present, the cardiac silhouette is enlarged with a globular configuration (see Fig. 35–3).

Electrocardiogram. In patients with a sizable pericardial effusion, the ECG usually has low voltage. If active inflammation is present, the classic signs of acute pericarditis may be seen (see Fig. 35–1). In extreme circumstances, patients may have electrical alternans, in which an axis shift occurs every other beat because of the increased mobility of the heart within the pericardial fluid (Fig. 35–7).

Echocardiography. The diagnosis of pericardial effusion is made by two-dimensional echocardiography (see Fig. 35–4), which is the diagnostic modality of choice in visualizing fluid around the pericardium. All patients in whom pericardial effusion is suspected should undergo echocardiography, including (1) patients with acute pericarditis who have elevated venous pressure or pulsus paradoxus, (2) patients who have cardiomegaly on a chest radiograph and have known or suspected pericarditis or conditions associated with pericarditis, and (3) patients with acute pericarditis and concomitant medical problems that may lead to a rapidly accumulating effusion (malignancies, uremia, irradiation). The echocardiographer can frequently estimate the amount of pericardial fluid, which is seen as a dark echo-free space surrounding the entire heart.

Other Imaging Modalities. Although echocardiography is the procedure of choice for the diagnosis of pericardial effusion, other noninvasive imaging modalities such as CT and MRI can diagnose pericardial effusion. However, CT cannot differentiate between pericardial fluid and pericardial thickening.

Once the diagnosis of pericardial effusion is made, it is important to document whether the patient has hemodynamic compromise and pericardial tamponade.[5, 8] In most instances, this distinction can be made by the patient's clinical findings and physical examination. When the results of the physical examination are equivocal, echocardiographic findings of right atrial and ventricular collapse or typical Doppler velocity patterns can be used to diagnose pericardial tamponade noninvasively[9] (Fig. 35–8). In unusual cases in which the diagnosis of pericardial tamponade remains equivocal after echocardiography, many experts recommend diagnostic pericardiocentesis, whereas others prefer first to perform cardiac catheterization to assess whether diastolic pressures are elevated and equalized in all four cardiac chambers (Fig. 35–9).

Treatment

The urgency and type of treatment of pericardial effusion are dependent on whether hemodynamic compromise is present.

Asymptomatic Pericardial Effusion. In a patient who is completely asymptomatic and has no hemodynamic compromise, treatment of the pericardial effusion is not urgent.[10, 11] A detailed history should be taken to deter-

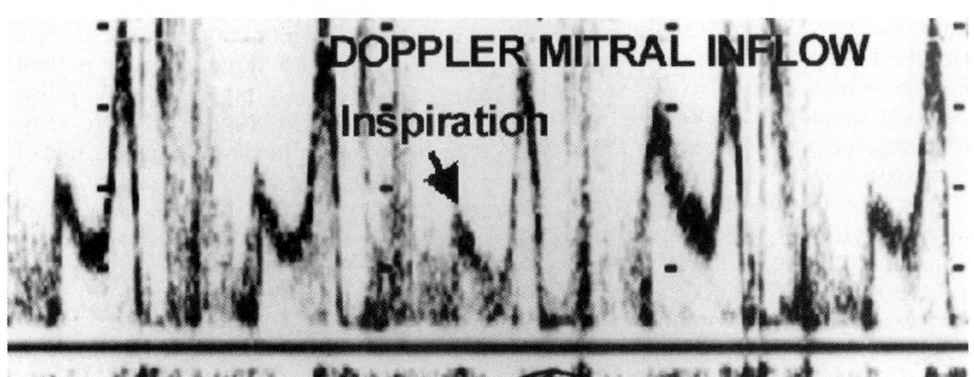

FIGURE 35–8. Doppler echocardiogram from a patient with pericardial tamponade. Patients with cardiac tamponade have an increase in the size of the right ventricle during inspiration as a result of increased venous return to the right side of the heart. Because of pericardial restraint from the high-pressure intrapericardial fluid, ventricular interaction between the right and left ventricles is enhanced. Therefore, as the right ventricle expands during inspiration, flow into the left ventricle decreases as demonstrated by the decrease in the initial velocity during inspiration on the mitral flow velocity curve (*arrow*).

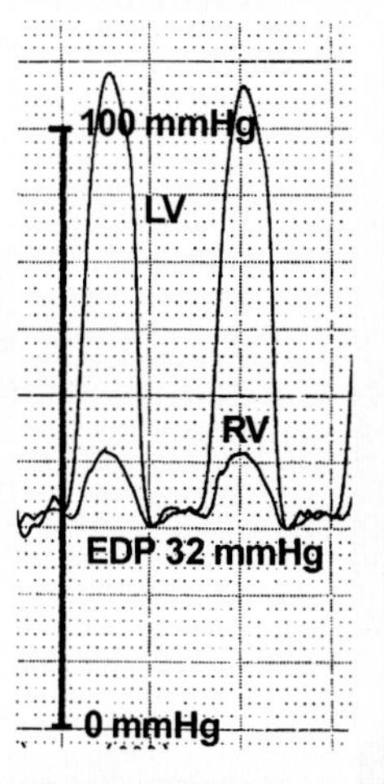

FIGURE 35–9. Cardiac catheterization recording of pressure from the left ventricle (LV) and right ventricle (RV) in a patient with pericardial tamponade. Diastolic pressure is severely elevated and equalized in these two chambers, with an end-diastolic pressure (EDP) of 32 mm Hg. An early rapid filling wave is not seen.

mine whether any past history of malignancy, pneumonitis, or other infections (e.g., acquired immunodeficiency syndrome or tuberculosis) or any drugs (e.g., hydralazine, procainamide) might be causing the pericardial effusion. In a patient with a high suspicion of malignancy, diagnostic pericardiocentesis with cytologic examination of the fluid is recommended to determine whether metastatic disease is causing the effusion.[12, 13] However, in most instances, careful follow-up without either diagnostic aspiration or therapeutic drainage is adequate for a patient with an asymptomatic pericardial effusion and no clear underlying cause or evidence of hemodynamic compromise. If evidence of acute inflammation is noted, such as an accompanying pericardial rub or an elevated erythrocyte sedimentation rate, treatment should be instituted with salicylates or NSAIDs as for acute pericarditis.

Pericardial Tamponade. In a patient with hemodynamic compromise, treatment is removal of the pericardial fluid. In rare cases, the aspiration should be performed on an emergency basis at the bedside. More commonly, an expeditious pericardiocentesis can be performed by a cardiologist under echocardiographic guidance.[7, 8]

To help stabilize the patient until pericardiocentesis can be performed, the patient should be administered intravenous fluid to increase preload. An afterload-reducing agent such as nitroprusside should also be given to treat the arteriolar vasoconstriction. The combination of fluids and nitroprusside may stabilize the patient until pericardiocentesis can be performed.

In patients undergoing pericardiocentesis, as much fluid as possible should be drained at the time of the procedure. Malignant, idiopathic, and even viral pericardial effusions are often bloody; chemistry panels and cell counts of the pericardial fluid are rarely helpful except when a very low glucose level points to an infectious cause. In patients with tamponade, fluid should always be sent for cytologic analysis. Because pericardial effusions may rapidly reaccumulate, especially if caused by tumor invading the pericardium, a catheter should be left in the pericardial space for 2 to 3 days for continued drainage. If the drainage does not stop, consultation with a surgeon is recommended. Because patients with continued pericardial drainage have a high rate of recurrent tamponade, removal of the pericardium or obliteration of the pericardial space should be considered.

Follow-up and Prognosis

Asymptomatic Pericardial Effusion. Asymptomatic, small to moderate pericardial effusions rarely result in pericardial tamponade and usually resolve spontaneously.[11] Careful clinical follow-up with a repeat echocardiogram is recommended at 1 month and monthly thereafter until the effusion resolves (Fig. 35–10). If the effusion remains stable for 6 months, echocardiography can be repeated at longer intervals, such as every 6 months or 1 year, if the patient remains clinically stable.

In patients with large idiopathic effusions persisting for 6 months or longer, tamponade can unpredictably develop in as many as 30% over long-term follow-up; diagnostic pericardiocentesis will occasionally detect a neoplastic or tuberculous cause. Therapeutic pericardiocentesis, with prolonged drainage if necessary, will resolve many chronic large pericardial effusions. Pericardiectomy may be indicated for recurrences of the effusion.[10] The long-term prognosis in patients with chronic effusions is primarily dependent on the cause of the effusion.

Pericardial Tamponade. In patients with pericardial tamponade, the in-hospital mortality rate is now less than 10%, in part because of the safety and efficacy of echocardiography-guided pericardiocentesis.[12–14] Over the subsequent year, the mortality rate in hospital survivors with a malignant effusion is about 75%, whereas patients with other causes of tamponade have only about a 3% to 5% subsequent annual mortality.

CONSTRICTIVE PERICARDITIS

Constrictive pericarditis occurs when a thickened and fibrotic pericardium restricts the inflow of blood into the right and left ventricles.[15, 16] Constrictive pericarditis can result in severe signs and symptoms of heart failure that mimic advanced myocardial or valvular disease. The diagnosis of constrictive pericarditis can be difficult to make and requires a high index of clinical suspicion to pursue proper diagnostic testing. Complete pericardiectomy can resolve the symptoms of constrictive pericarditis and result in normal longevity.[15]

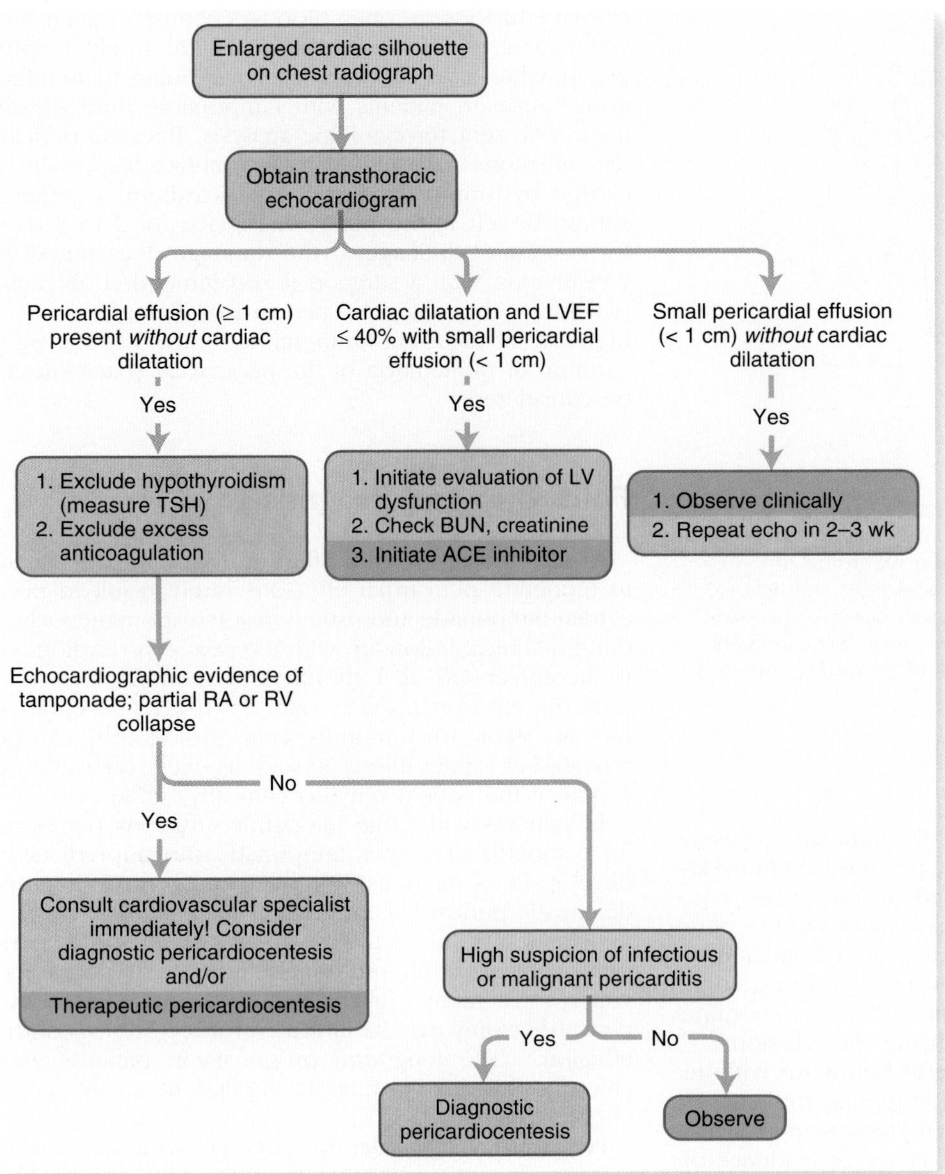

FIGURE 35–10. Management of asymptomatic pericardial effusion in patients with a normal physical examination. ACE, angiotensin-converting enzyme; BUN, blood urea nitrogen; EF, ejection fraction; LV, left ventricular; RA, right atrial; RV, right ventricular; TSH, thyroid-stimulating hormone.

History and Clinical Features

Patients with constrictive pericarditis predominantly have right-sided heart failure that is out of proportion to the left-sided failure; substantial pulmonary congestion is rare. Fatigue, hepatomegaly, ascites, and lower extremity edema are typically found. Many patients are first thought to have cirrhosis when they truly have congestive hepatomegaly secondary to constrictive pericarditis.

Over half of patients with constrictive pericarditis do not have a known underlying etiology.[15] In these patients, the pericardial process is probably due to a fibrotic reaction to a previous viral pericarditis. In modern series, tuberculosis is confirmed in only a small minority of cases, even when the excised pericardium is evaluated.[16] However, an increasing number of patients are now being seen with constrictive pericarditis caused by either previous mantle radiation therapy for a malignancy or a pericardial reaction after previous open heart surgery. Therefore, patients with right-sided failure and a history of mantle radiation or open heart surgery should be suspected of having constrictive pericarditis.

Physical Examination

Patients with severe constrictive pericarditis may have cardiac cachexia with wasting of the upper body muscles, ascites, and edema. Blood pressure is frequently low, and sinus tachycardia or atrial fibrillation may be present. Severe elevation of venous pressure is consistently found unless the patient is dehydrated. The contour of the venous pressure is also abnormal, with rapid "X" and "Y" descents (see Chapter 3). These rapid descents occur as blood from the right atrium flows rapidly into the right ventricle during diastole and then

TABLE 35–5

Differentiation of Constrictive Pericarditis from Restrictive Cardiomyopathy

Type of Evaluation	Constrictive Pericarditis	Restrictive Cardiomyopathy
Physical examination	Regurgitant murmurs uncommon	Regurgitant murmurs common
Chest radiography	Pericardial calcification may be present	Pericardial calcification absent
Echocardiography	Normal wall thickness Prominent early diastolic filling with abrupt displacement of the interventricular septum	Increased wall thickness, thickened cardiac valves, and granular sparkling texture (amyloid). Enlarged atria and low ejection fraction favor restrictive cardiomyopathy
Doppler studies	Early mitral flow is reduced with the onset of inspiration and a reciprocal effect on tricuspid flow Expiratory increase in hepatic vein diastolic flow reversal	No respiratory variation in diastolic flow Inspiratory increase in hepatic vein diastolic flow reversal Mitral and tricuspid regurgitation common
Cardiac catheterization	RVEDP and LVEDP usually equal RV systolic pressure < 50 mm Hg RVEDP greater than one third of RV systolic pressure	LVEDP often > 5 mm Hg more than RVEDP, but may be identical
Endomyocardial biopsy	May be normal or show nonspecific myocyte hypertrophy or myocardial fibrosis	May reveal specific cause of restrictive cardiomyopathy
CT/MRI	Pericardium may be thickened ≥ 3 mm	Pericardium usually normal

CT, computed tomography; LV, left ventricular; LVEDP, left ventricular end-diastolic pressure; MRI, magnetic resonance imaging; RV, right ventricular; RVEDP, right ventricular end-diastolic pressure.

From Mayosi BM, Volmink JA, Commerford PJ: Pericardial disease: An evidence-based approach to diagnosis and treatment. In Yusuf S, Cairns JA, Camm AJ, et al (eds): Evidence Based Cardiology. London, BMJ Books, 1998, pp 765–784.

pressure rises abruptly from the abnormal pericardial restraint, which further restricts blood flow. The heart sounds are commonly without murmurs, but an early diastolic pericardial knock may be audible in severe cases.

Hepatomegaly is common, and palpation of the liver may reveal a pulsatile sensation that reflects the rapid descents seen on jugular venous pressure. Ascites and lower extremity edema may be present.

Diagnosis

Constrictive pericarditis should be suspected in any patient with severe signs and symptoms of heart failure in the absence of other etiologies. An echocardiogram may reveal other causes of heart failure such as left ventricular systolic dysfunction, valvular heart disease, or pulmonary hypertension. If the patient has nearly normal left ventricular systolic function in the absence of significant valvular disease or pulmonary hypertension, constrictive pericarditis should be considered.

In patients with severe right heart failure and no other known cause, the differential diagnosis is constrictive pericarditis versus a restrictive cardiomyopathy (Table 35–5). In constrictive pericarditis, pericardial restraint prevents normal filling of the ventricles, thereby resulting in elevated intracardiac pressures and heart failure. In restrictive cardiomyopathy, the heart muscle itself is stiff and noncompliant, so the ventricles cannot fill properly.[17] Both constrictive pericarditis and restrictive cardiomyopathy will cause elevated diastolic pressure in all four cardiac chambers. It is important to differentiate between constrictive pericarditis and restrictive cardiomyopathy because pericardiectomy will cure constrictive pericarditis whereas there is no generally successful treatment for restrictive cardiomyopathy (see Chapter 29).

Constrictive pericarditis can be very difficult to confirm. In about 25% of cases, it results in calcification of the pericardium, best seen on a lateral chest radiograph[15, 16] (Fig. 35–11); pleural effusions are present in about 60% of cases. When no calcification is seen on the chest radiograph, assessment of the pericardium by either CT or MRI can show thickening of the pericardium (Fig. 35–12).

The diagnosis can also be established by cardiac catheterization, in which the classic findings are elevation and equalization of diastolic pressures in all four cardiac chambers, with a "dip and plateau" contour seen in the ventricular diastolic pressure (Fig. 35–13). The stiff, noncompliant heart muscle in a patient with restrictive cardiomyopathy may produce similar findings. In some patients, especially those with previous radiation therapy or open heart surgery, mixed pericardial and myocardial disease may be present. Although newer diagnostic approaches involving Doppler echocardiography and catheterization may help distinguish between these two entities,[18] a definitive diagnosis of constrictive pericarditis may require exploratory thoracotomy.

Treatment

The only treatment of constrictive pericarditis is surgical pericardiectomy.[15] The operative risk, which depends on the severity of the illness and co-morbid

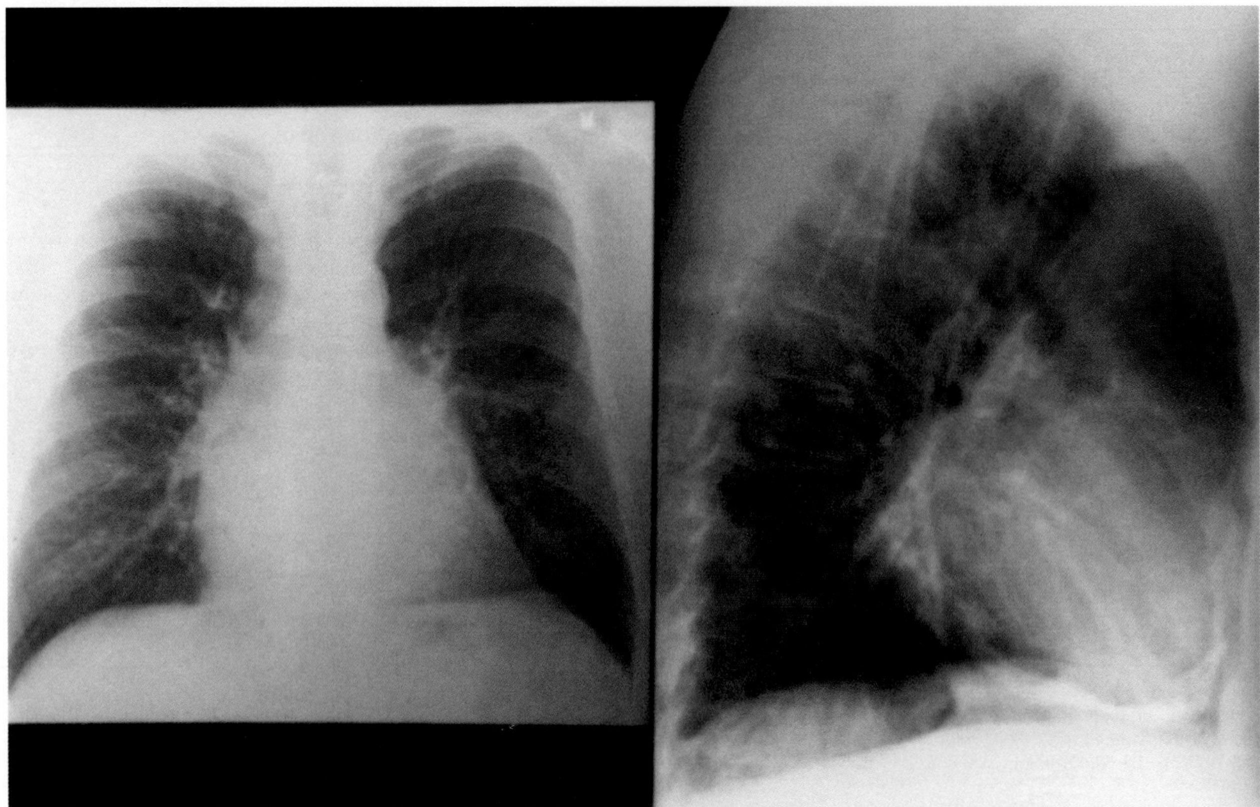

FIGURE 35–11. Posteroanterior and lateral chest radiographs in a patient with constrictive pericarditis. Severe calcification is present around the heart and is specifically seen in the lateral view.

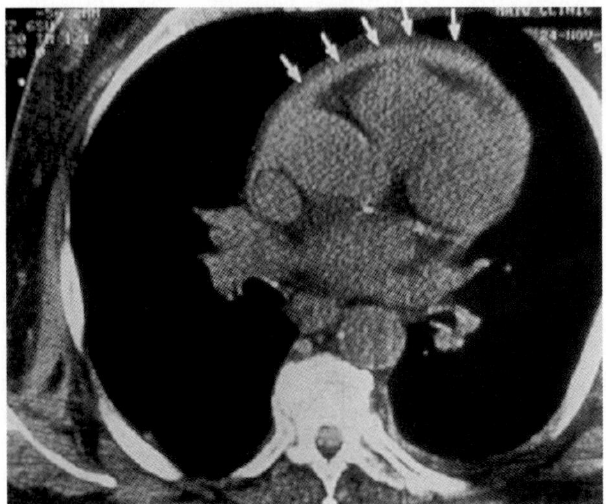

FIGURE 35–12. Computed tomographic scan from a patient with constrictive pericarditis. Increased pericardial thickness (*arrows*) is evident.

factors, ranges from 5% to 25%. After successful pericardiectomy, most patients can return to a normal lifestyle with apparently normal longevity. Patients with radiation-induced constriction do poorly because many have combined myocardial and pericardial disease. It is necessary to perform a complete pericardiectomy from phrenic nerve to phrenic nerve because incomplete resections may not achieve optimal hemodynamic benefit.

SPECIFIC FORMS OF PERICARDIAL DISEASE

Effusive-Constrictive Pericarditis

Effusive-constrictive pericarditis occurs when pericardial tamponade is combined with pericardial constriction. Patients initially have findings of tamponade, but even after pericardiocentesis they continue to have elevated intracardiac pressure because of an underlying constrictive pericarditis. If symptoms persist, the treatment is pericardiectomy.

Postcardiotomy Syndrome

The postcardiotomy syndrome is an acute pericarditis that occurs weeks to months after open heart surgery.[19] Patients have typical symptoms of acute pericarditis manifested as fever, pleuritic chest pain, tachycardia, a pericardial rub, and an elevated erythrocyte sedimentation rate. This syndrome is characterized by the presence of antimyocardial antibodies and is thought to be

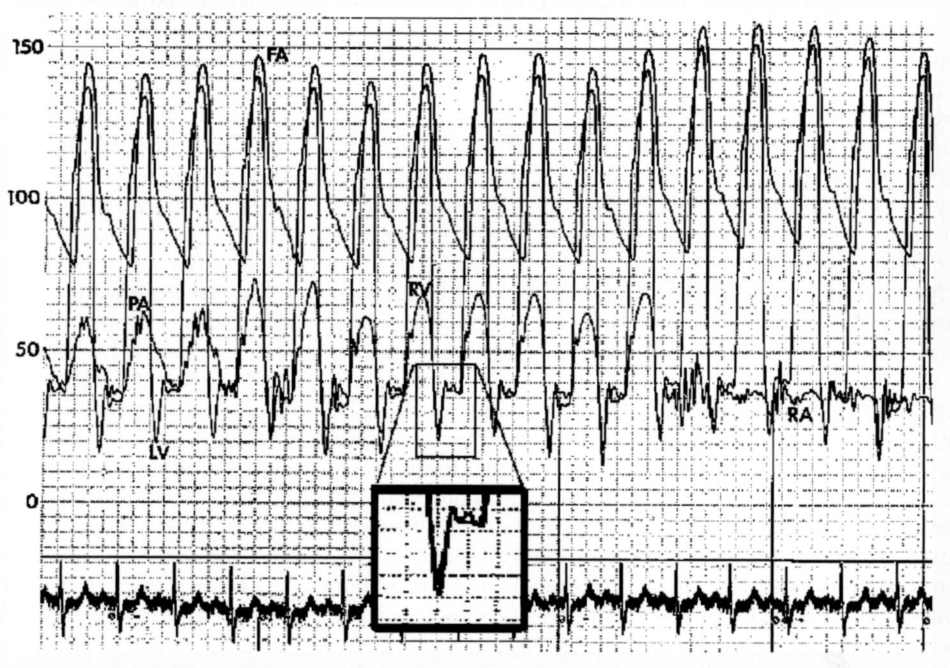

FIGURE 35–13. Cardiac catheterization pressures in a patient with constrictive pericarditis. Femoral artery (FA) and left ventricular (LV) pressures are shown with "pull-back" from the pulmonary artery (PA) to the right ventricle (RV) to the right atrium (RA). The pressures in all cardiac chambers are elevated and equalized. In addition, a typical "dip and plateau" pattern can be seen in the left ventricular and right ventricular diastolic pressures from early rapid filling and then sudden pericardial restraint (*box insert*).

due to an autoimmune reaction. A similar clinical picture is seen with the postperfusion syndrome caused by cytomegalovirus (CMV) infection in patients who were previously uninfected but were exposed to CMV-positive blood during cardiopulmonary bypass or transfusions. In CMV infection, atypical lymphocytes are usually seen and are often accompanied by elevated liver enzymes.

Treatment of postcardiotomy syndrome is similar to treatment of acute pericarditis. NSAIDs or salicylates should be given for 1 month and then tapered slowly over a period of 2 weeks. In patients taking anticoagulation agents, the pericardial effusion can be bloody and lead to pericardial tamponade. In patients who require anticoagulation, it should be stopped only if evidence of hemodynamic compromise exists. In some patients who have had open heart surgery, late pericardial constriction develops without preceding acute pericarditis. The constrictive physiology may be caused by bleeding in and around the open pericardium, with subsequent inflammatory reaction, scarring, and fibrosis. If active inflammation is present, as documented by an elevated sedimentation rate, a trial of anti-inflammatory agents may be instituted. However, surgical removal of the blood and clot is usually indicated, oftentimes accompanied by more extensive pericardiectomy.

Post–Myocardial Infarction Pericarditis, including Dressler's syndrome

Acute pericarditis can develop several days after an acute myocardial infarction, usually because of transmural extension of the infarction to the pericardial surface. This syndrome is now less common in the reperfusion era (see Chapter 27) as the size of acute infarctions has diminished. Anticoagulation should be temporarily withheld to avoid the evolution of a bloody effusion into pericardial tamponade.

A late autoimmune pericarditis, termed Dressler's syndrome, may also develop weeks to months after a myocardial infarction. Diagnosis and treatment are similar to that for acute pericarditis.

Uremic Pericarditis

Pericardial effusion may develop in patients with severe renal failure, especially those undergoing dialysis. In these patients, treatment of the renal failure with aggressive dialysis may decrease the pericardial effusion.

Infectious Pericarditis

Purulent Bacterial Pericarditis. Purulent bacterial pericarditis may occur from direct extension of bacterial pneumonia, from direct extension of pleural empyema, or rarely from peritonitis or a subphrenic abscess. Most patients have an acute illness with systemic sepsis, and acute tamponade develops in the majority of these patients. The most common organisms are gram positive, especially streptococci, pneumococci, and staphylococci. Pericardiocentesis usually shows leukocytosis and occasionally frank pus, and the fluid glucose level is usually markedly depressed.

In as many as 50% of patients, the diagnosis is made only at autopsy. In patients in whom pericarditis is diagnosed antemortem, pericardiocentesis (often with an indwelling catheter or repeated taps to drain recurrent fluid) combined with antimicrobial therapy leads to a high survival rate, although late constrictive pericarditis requiring pericardiectomy will develop in 30% to 40% of patients.[20] Instillation of antibiotics into the pericardial space is not generally recommended. The key to both short- and long-term survival is high clinical suspicion with urgent diagnostic and therapeutic pericardiocentesis.

Tuberculous Pericarditis. Tuberculous pericarditis remains common in developing countries but now accounts for less than 5% of cases of acute pericarditis in developed countries, where it is seen most commonly in those who are immunosuppressed, especially patients positive for human immunodeficiency virus. Tuberculous pericarditis commonly has insidious manifestations with nonspecific symptoms; acute painful pericarditis is rare. Most patients have an effusive-constrictive physiology or pericardial constriction, and tamponade is rare. The chest radiograph suggests active pulmonary tuberculosis in about 30% of cases, and a pleural effusion is present in 40% to 60% of cases. The echocardiogram typically shows fibrinous strands in the pericardial effusion with multiple echo densities adherent to the pericardial surface.

Pericardiocentesis is recommended whenever tuberculous pericarditis is suspected. With modern culture techniques, about 75% of patients will have a positive culture for the tubercle bacillus, which is rarely seen on a stained smear of pericardial fluid. Measurement of the adenosine deaminase level in pericardial fluid may be helpful. In one series, an adenosine deaminase level of 40 U/L or greater had a positive predictive value of 96% for tuberculous pericarditis; however, only about 75% of patients with ultimately confirmed tuberculous effusions had adenosine deaminase levels this high.[21] In some centers, sensitive and specific polymerase chain reaction testing has been used successfully to diagnose tuberculosis from body fluids. Pericardial biopsy may be positive in situations in which the pericardial fluid does not show tuberculosis, and biopsy is recommended when tuberculous pericarditis is strongly suspected. Tuberculin skin testing is not usually helpful because many patients are anergic.

All patients with confirmed tuberculous pericarditis should be treated, and empiric treatment will oftentimes be strongly considered in patients with a consistent clinical picture. A combination of rifampicin, isoniazid, and pyrazinamide for 2 months followed by isoniazid and rifampicin for an additional 4 months yields a cure rate of about 85% to 90%. Adjuvant prednisolone may lead to better outcomes, but current data are not sufficient to recommend routine adjuvant steroid therapy.

Even when tuberculous pericarditis is promptly diagnosed and treated, constrictive pericarditis will develop in 30% to 60% of patients. When late constrictive pericarditis develops after antituberculous therapy, surgical pericardiectomy is the treatment of choice, with 95% or more of patients doing well after pericardiectomy.

When patients have tuberculous constrictive pericarditis in the absence of previous therapy, the constrictive physiology may resolve with appropriate medical treatment in up to 75% of patients. Adjuvant steroids have been associated with a better outcome, although the results in the largest randomized trial did not reach conventional statistical significance. In general, pericardiectomy is recommended if the constrictive physiology does not improve after 4 to 6 weeks of therapy or if calcification is present.

Fungal Pericarditis. Fungal pericarditis is uncommon. The most common fungal syndrome is histoplasmosis pericarditis, which usually resolves in several weeks and can be treated successfully with NSAIDs. In some patients, however, acute tamponade may rapidly develop, so it is generally recommended that patients with confirmed histoplasmosis pericarditis be hospitalized initially. Specific antifungal therapy is recommended only in patients with disseminated histoplasmosis.

Other types of fungal pericarditis usually occur in patients who have disseminated fungal infection, commonly because they are immunosuppressed, have received broad-spectrum antibiotics, or are recovering from cardiac surgery. Prolonged intravenous amphotericin therapy is generally required, along with surgical drainage of the pericardial space.

Pericardial Disease and Cancer

Malignant Pericarditis. Tumors account for approximately 6% of cases of acute pericarditis that is initially without an obvious cause (see Table 35–1) and close to 20% of cases of moderate to large pericardial effusions (see Table 35–4). In patients with pericardial tamponade, the percentage is even higher. About 80% of cases of malignant pericarditis are due to breast cancer, leukemia, and lymphoma. Melanoma is a relatively uncommon cause of malignant pericarditis, but a large proportion of patients with melanoma have pericardial involvement.

Most patients have direct tumor involvement of the pericardium, commonly from extension of an adjacent malignant lesion or from hematogenous or lymphatic spread. "Paraneoplastic" pericardial effusions may develop in patients with mediastinal lymphoma as a result of pericardial irritation or compromised lymphatic drainage. Up to 50% of women with metastatic breast cancer have pericardial effusions, which often are small and asymptomatic.

Pericardiocentesis is critical for both diagnosis and management. Fluid cytology is positive in about 85% of patients; optically guided percutaneous pericardioscopy is a useful supplemental diagnostic procedure. Complete drainage with an indwelling catheter for 2 or 3 days is the treatment of choice. If the drainage does not stop, pericardial surgery is recommended.[12]

The prognosis depends on the success of treatment of the underlying malignancy. Patients with lymphous or breast cancer have a better outcome than do patients whose malignant pericarditis and tamponade is due to lung cancer or other metastatic carcinomas.[22] Overall, the 1-year mortality rate can be 80% or more, depending on the tumor and its response to therapy.

Postradiation Pericarditis. In patients who receive mantle radiation for Hodgkin's disease, postradiation pericarditis develops in about 2%. After irradiation for breast cancer, the incidence of radiation-induced pericarditis is between 0.4% and 5%. The radiation-induced pericardial injury may appear acutely during the course of treatment, but more commonly it takes months or even a decade before clinical appearance. The initial pericarditis and effusion may resolve spontaneously; however, constrictive pericarditis develops in some patients, oftentimes with adjacent myocarditis and even coronary artery damage. Differentiation of radiation pericarditis from malignant pericarditis is a critical diagnostic challenge.

Pericardiocentesis may be indicated early in the course to perform cytologic studies or biopsy when malignant pericardial disease is suspected. Concomitant radiation-induced hypothyroidism is common and can contribute to or even cause the effusion. Pericardiectomy is the treatment of choice for recurrent pericarditis and for large recurrent pericardial effusions.

Autoimmune Pericarditis

Systemic Lupus Erythematosus and Rheumatoid Arthritis. Up to 50% of patients with SLE have pericarditis, usually during an acute flare of the disease[23] when polyserositis, rheumatic symptoms, and other manifestations of the disease are seen. The initial symptoms of autoimmune pericarditis are usually acute pericarditis or an asymptomatic effusion. Pericardial tamponade is uncommon, and progressive restrictive pericarditis is highly unusual. Unless purulent pericarditis is suspected, pericardiocentesis is not usually required either diagnostically or therapeutically. The underlying SLE should be treated aggressively. Steroids, which are not generally recommended for acute pericarditis because of the risk of recurrence, are a mainstay of therapy for SLE.

Acute pericarditis or asymptomatic pericardial effusions can develop in patients with advanced rheumatoid arthritis. The process is usually self-limited or responds to aggressive treatment of the underlying rheumatoid arthritis. Pericardial tamponade, though unusual, can develop.

Pericarditis is an occasional complication of scleroderma and mixed connective tissue disease. It is rare in sarcoidosis, in which it must be distinguished from tuberculous or fungal pericarditis.

Drug-Related Pericarditis. Among the medications that cause pericarditis, the most common are procainamide, hydralazine, isoniazid, and phenytoin. Hypersensitivity pericarditis has also been reported with amiodarone, sulfa drugs, and penicillins. Hemopericardium can develop in patients treated with anticoagulants or thrombolytic agents, especially in those with preexisting pericardial inflammation or insult.[5]

Myopericarditis

Myocarditis may develop in patients with pericarditis, especially when it is due to an underlying collagen vascular disease, drugs, or viral or bacterial infection. Patients with myocarditis will be more likely to have ECG conduction delays and ventricular arrhythmias. Elevated levels of CK-MB or troponin (or both) are common, and myocardial scintigraphy may be positive. Patients with underlying myocarditis may also be susceptible to heart failure and pulmonary edema, which are uncommon in pericardial disease alone. In some situations, the mechanism for the underlying myocarditis appears to be direct extension of the inflammatory process, whereas in others it appears to be an immune mechanism. No specific treatment is available.

Acute or progressive heart failure develops in some patients after pericardiectomy for constrictive pericarditis or even after drainage of a large pericardial effusion. This syndrome, which is thought to be precipitated acutely by ventricular dilatation, may also be a manifestation of underlying myocarditis.[5]

Evidence-Based Summary

- Although no controlled trials have been conducted, NSAIDs have been effective in the treatment of acute pericarditis. Steroids are also effective but are probably associated with a higher risk of relapse, so NSAIDs are preferred.[24]
- Purulent pericarditis requires emergent complete drainage combined with aggressive systemic antibiotics.
- Case series indicate that most asymptomatic pericardial effusions can be managed conservatively as outlined in Figure 35–11.
- For neoplastic pericardial disease and pericardial disease secondary to collagen vascular disorders, aggressive treatment of the underlying systemic disease is critical.
- Constrictive pericarditis should be treated with pericardiectomy, which markedly improves symptoms and can oftentimes result in normal longevity.
- Antituberculous medications dramatically improve outcomes in tuberculous pericarditis. Adjuvant prednisolone trials have led to marginal improvement in the outcomes of tuberculous pericardial effusions and tuberculous constrictive pericarditis.

References

1. Permanyer-Miralda G, Sagristà-Sauleda J, Angel J, Soler-Soler J: Primary acute pericardial disease: A prospective series of 231 consecutive patients. Am J Cardiol 1985;56: 623–629.
2. Zayar R, Anguita M, Torres F, et al: Incidence of specific etiology and role of methods for specific etiologic

diagnosis of primary acute pericarditis. Am J Cardiol 1995;75:378–382.

3. Baljepally R, Spodick DH: PR-segment deviation as the initial electrocardiographic response in acute pericarditis. Am J Cardiol 1998;81:1505–1506.
4. Adler Y, Finkelstein Y, Guindo J, et al: Colchicine treatment for recurrent pericarditis. A decade of experience. Circulation 1998;97:2183–2185.
5. Spodick DH: Pericardial diseases. In Braunwald E, Zipes DP, Libby P (eds): Heart Disease: A Textbook of Cardiovascular Medicine. Philadelphia, WB Saunders, 2001, pp 1823–1876.
6. Sagristà-Sauleda J, Mercé J, Permanyer-Miralda G, et al: Clinical clues to the causes of large pericardial effusions. Am J Med 2000;109:95–100.
7. Nugue O, Millaire A, Porte H, et al: Pericardioscopy in the etiologic diagnosis of pericardial effusion in 141 consecutive patients. Circulation 1996;94:1635–1641.
8. Spodick DH: Bedside diagnosis of cardiac tamponade. Tex Heart Inst J 1996;23:239.
9. Nishimura RA, Tajik AJ: Evaluation of diastolic filling of left ventricle in health and disease: Doppler echocardiography is the clinician's Rosetta Stone. J Am Coll Cardiol 1997;30:8–18.
10. Sagristà-Sauleda J, Angel J, Permanyer-Miralda G, Soler-Soler J: Long-term follow-up of idiopathic chronic pericardial effusion. N Engl J Med 1999;341:2054–2059.
11. Mercé J, Sagristà-Sauleda J, Permanyer-Miralda G, Soler-Soler J: Should pericardial drainage be performed routinely in patients who have a large pericardial effusion without tamponade? Am J Med 1998;105:106–109.
12. Tsang TS, Seward JB, Barnes ME, et al: Outcomes of primary and secondary treatment of pericardial effusion in patients with malignancy. Mayo Clin Proc 2000;75:248–253.
13. Tsang TS, Enriquez-Sarano M, Freeman WK, et al: Consectutive 1127 therapeutic echocardiographically guided pericardiocenteses. Mayo Clin Proc 2002;77:429–436.
14. Tsang TSM, Oh JK, Seward JB: Diagnosis and management of cardiac tamponade in the era of echocardiography. Clin Cardiol 1999;22:446–452.
15. Ling LH, Oh JK, Schaff HV, et al: Constrictive pericarditis in the modern era: Evolving clinical spectrum and impact on outcome after pericardiectomy. Circulation 1999;100:1380–1386.
16. Ling LH, Oh JK, Breen JF, et al: Calcific constrictive pericarditis: Is it still with us? Ann Intern Med 2000;132:444–450.
17. Ammash NM, Seward JB, Bailey KR, et al: Clinical profile and outcome of idiopathic restrictive cardiomyopathy. Circulation 2000;101:2490–2496.
18. Hurrell DG, Nishimura RA, Higano ST, et al: Value of dynamic respiratory changes in left and right ventricular pressures for the diagnosis of constrictive pericarditis. Circulation 1996;93:2007–2013.
19. Tsang TS, Barnes ME, Hayes SN, et al: Clinical and echocardiographic characteristics of significant pericardial effusions following cardiothoracic surgery and outcomes of echo-guided pericardiocentesis for management: Mayo Clinic experience, 1979–1998. Chest 1999;116:275–276.
20. Goodman LJ: Purulent pericarditis. Curr Treat Options Cardiovasc Med 2000;2:343–350.
21. Mayosi BM, Volmink JA, Commerford PJ: Pericardial disease: An evidence-based approach to diagnosis and treatment. In Yusuf S, Cairns JA, Camm AJ, et al (eds): Evidence Based Cardiology. London, BMJ Books, 1998, pp 765–784.
22. Levine MJ, Lorell BH, Diver DJ, Come PC: Implications of echocardiographically-assisted diagnosis of pericardial tamponade in contemporary medical patients: Detection prior to hemodynamic embarrassment. J Am Coll Cardiol 1991;17:59–65.
23. Moder KG, Miller TD, Tazelaar HD: Cardiac involvement in systemic lupus erythematosus. Mayo Clin Proc 1999;74:275–284.
24. Hoit BD: Management of effusive and constrictive pericardial heart disease. Circulation 2002;105:2939–2942.

CHAPTER 36

Recognition and Management of Patients with Diseases of the Aorta: Aneurysms and Dissection

Patrick T. O'Gara

The Normal Aorta

The aorta is the primary conduit through which the cardiac output is delivered to the systemic arterial bed. It is divided at the level of the diaphragm into thoracic and abdominal segments. The thoracic aorta can be further subdivided into the ascending, arch, and descending portions. The ascending aorta arises from the base of the left ventricle and courses superiorly and rightward. The aortic arch gives rise to the brachiocephalic vessels. The descending thoracic aorta is a posterior mediastinal structure with attachments to the thoracic cage and constitutes the segment between the left subclavian artery and the diaphragm. The abdominal aorta extends from the diaphragmatic hiatus to its bifurcation into the common iliac arteries and is divided into suprarenal and infrarenal segments.

The wall of the aorta, like that of other arteries, is composed of three layers: intima, media, and adventitia. Its tensile strength derives primarily from the elastic lamellar units of the media and secondarily from smooth muscle cells, collagen, and ground substances. With age, the elastic fibers of the media degenerate, a process accelerated by hypertension or inflammatory conditions that predispose the aorta to aneurysmal enlargement or dissection. The terms *aneurysm* and *dissection* are not synonymous. The former implies pathologic enlargement or expansion, whereas the latter refers to the process by which a cleavage plane is created between the inner and the outer portions of the wall by the surging column of blood as it is propelled forward during each cardiac contraction. An aortic dissection can occur in a previously aneurysmal segment. Alternatively, the dissection process may lead to aneurysm formation if the false lumen continues to expand.

AORTIC ANEURYSM

Classification

Ectasia and *aneurysm* are descriptive terms indicative of vessel enlargement. The former refers to mild dilatation and usually some degree of uncoiling or tortuosity, whereas the latter implies luminal expansion beyond 1.5 to 2.0 times the normal aortic diameter. Aneurysms are generally of three types: fusiform (diffuse) (Fig. 36–1), saccular (asymmetric and protruding), and false. Fusiform and saccular aneurysms are "true" aneurysms in that their walls are composed of all three aortic layers. "False" aneurysms are contained ruptures whose outer walls are composed of periadventitial hematoma (Box 36–1).

Thoracic Aortic Aneurysm

Ascending Aortic Aneurysms

Aneurysms of the ascending aorta are asymptomatic in the majority of patients and are usually first detected on a chest radiograph obtained for other indications (Fig. 36–2). In some patients, enlargement of the aortic root,

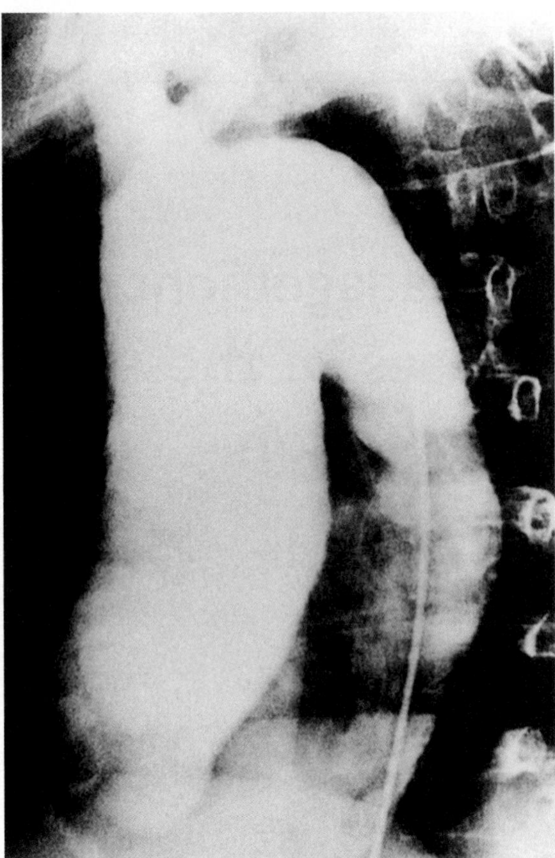

FIGURE 36–1. Contrast aortogram in the left posterior oblique projection demonstrates diffuse aneurysmal enlargement of the entire ascending and arch portions of the thoracic aorta. (From Creager MA, Halperin JL, Whittemore AD: Aneurysmal disease of the aorta and its branches. In Loscalzo J, Creager MA, Dzau VJ [eds]: Vascular Medicine: A Textbook of Vascular Biology and Diseases. Boston, Little, Brown, 1992, pp 903–930.)

BOX 36–1

Classification of Aortic Aneurysms

TYPE
Fusiform
Saccular
False (pseudo-)

LOCATION
Thoracic
- Ascending
- Arch
- Descending

Thoracoabdominal
Abdominal
- Suprarenal
- Infrarenal

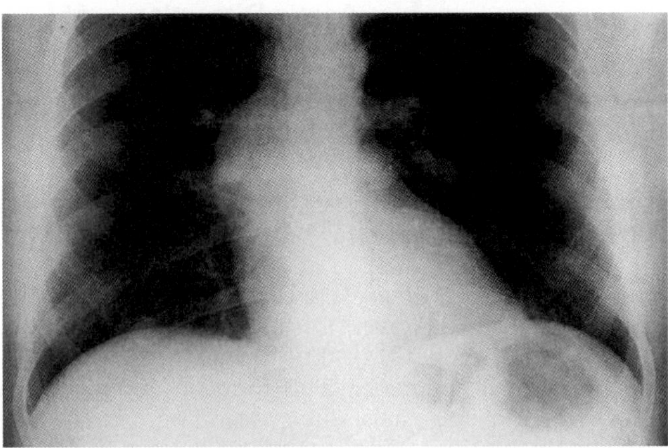

FIGURE 36–2. Chest x-ray of a 43-year-old man with an asymptomatic ascending aortic aneurysm. (From Creager MA, Halperin JL: Aortic and arterial aneurysms. In Creager MA [vol ed]: Vascular Disease. Braunwald E [ser ed]: Atlas of Heart Diseases. Philadelphia, Current Medicine, 1996, pp 1.1–1.19.)

especially when it exceeds 5 cm in diameter, is accompanied by a murmur of aortic regurgitation due to malcoaptation of the leaflets. Radiation of the murmur predominantly to the right, rather than to the left, of the sternum suggests that the regurgitation is secondary to disease of the aortic root rather than of primary valvular origin. Rarely, a right superior parasternal pulsation can be appreciated.

Cause. The majority of ascending aortic aneurysms are fusiform. The most common cause is cystic medial necrosis, a noninflammatory degenerative process of the aortic media with fragmentation of elastic fibers, drop-out of smooth muscle cells, and pooling of mucoid-like ground substances. This process weakens the wall of the aortic root and predisposes to aneurysm formation or dissection, or both. Specific diseases associated with cystic medial necrosis include Marfan's syndrome and, less commonly, other inherited disorders of connective tissue, such as Ehlers-Danlos syndrome, osteogenesis imperfecta, and the mucopolysaccharidoses (Hunter's and Hurler's syndromes).

Marfan's syndrome is caused by a mutation in the gene for *fibrillin*, a protein that is critical to the structural integrity of the aortic media. Common clinical manifestations of the syndrome include an abnormally long arm span, arachnodactyly, ectopia lentis, high-arched palate, scoliosis, pectus excavatum, and aortic and mitral regurgitation. Ehlers-Danlos type IV is associated with a defect in the gene for type III procollagen. A novel familial aortic aneurysm gene has been localized on chromosome 11.[1] Not all patients with cystic medial necrosis on pathologic examination of an aortic aneurysm specimen have a recognizable connective tissue disorder, but certain clinical clues are commonly present, such as a history of spontaneous pneumothoraces or inguinal hernias. The term *annuloaortic ectasia* is a clinical and pathoanatomic descriptor that is applied to the condition affecting a subset of patients with aneurysms involving the aortic root, associated with aortic regurgitation, but not accompanied by other evidence of connective tissue abnormalities.[2]

Atherosclerosis is a distinctly *uncommon* cause of ascending aortic aneurysm. When atherosclerotic changes are present in this portion of the aorta, evidence of the disease in other segments of the aorta and systemic vascular beds is usually quite obvious. In contrast to aneurysms that result from cystic medial necrosis, which are confined to the ascending aorta, atherosclerotic changes extend into and, often, beyond the arch.

There has been an increasing appreciation for the importance of inflammatory conditions that affect the aorta and predispose to its aneurysmal enlargement.[3] These include *giant cell arteritis,* which predominantly affects the large and medium-sized muscular arteries, often including the temporal arteries, and occurs most commonly in older women. Associated symptoms such as low-grade fever, fatigue, headache, and proximal girdle stiffness (polymyalgia rheumatica) are common. The involvement of the aorta typically occurs in the ascending portion but spares the root and annulus. Both the arch and the descending thoracic aorta can be involved as well. Aortic dissection has also been described.

Takayasu's arteritis affects a younger population (mean age at diagnosis is 29 years), 90% of whom are women.[4] Although traditionally described as "pulseless disease" due to proximal obliteration of the major arch vessels, there are both aneurysmal and stenotic variants, even in the same patient. The granulomatous inflammation within the adventitial and medial layers can cause systemic inflammation, with fever and weight loss, pain and tenderness over affected arteries, hypertension, and symptoms of vascular insufficiency of the upper extremities.

A *congenital sinus of Valsalva aneurysm* is a pathologic enlargement of the aorta confined to one of the three sinuses. This condition does not usually become clinically evident until the aneurysm ruptures spontaneously, typically into a right heart chamber, causing chest pain, dyspnea, and a loud, continuous, or to-and-fro murmur. Men are affected more commonly than are women and usually during young adulthood.

Aortic Arch Aneurysms

Isolated aneurysms of the aortic arch are uncommon. Pathologic conditions affecting this portion of the aorta typically involve either or both the ascending and descending segments. Cystic medial necrosis, inflammation, and atherosclerosis are the most common causes. Since the major vessels originate from the arch, the surgical approach to this portion of the aorta is complex.

Descending Thoracic Aortic Aneurysms

Atherosclerosis is by far the most common cause of descending thoracic aortic aneurysm. Aneurysms of the descending thoracic aorta are usually asymptomatic and are most often detected on chest x-rays performed for the evaluation of other problems. When symptoms do occur, they range from a nondescript, dull ache in the left posterior chest to dysphagia secondary to extrinsic compression of the esophagus, to hoarseness because of impingement of the left recurrent laryngeal nerve, or to dyspnea, cough, wheezing, or stridor due to compression of the left main stem bronchus or its major branches. When aneurysms of the descending aorta cross the diaphragm, they are termed *thoracoabdominal aneurysms,* which may present with symptoms or signs related chiefly to the abdominal component, such as a prominent epigastric pulsation.[5]

Trauma due to a rapid deceleration injury, such as a motor vehicle accident, may result in transection of the descending thoracic aorta and subsequent false aneurysm formation. Because of the threat of rupture, prompt surgical repair of posttraumatic aneurysms is mandated.

Approach to the Patient (Fig. 36–3)

The history should include special reference to those symptoms that imply aortic expansion or threatened rupture—that is, pain or features such as dysphagia or hoarseness that suggest encroachment on adjacent structures. In the presence of aortic valve involvement by an aneurysm leading to aortic regurgitation, left ventricular failure may be a warning sign of aneurysmal expansion. Questions should also be posed regarding familial involvement (suggesting Marfan's syndrome, or other inheritable disorders of connective tissue), associated problems that suggest a connective tissue or inflammatory condition, prior trauma, infections, and a history of the risk factors for atherosclerotic vascular disease, such as hypercholesterolemia, hypertension, cigarette smoking, or diabetes.

Physical Examination

The physical examination should note body size and habitus. The blood pressure should be measured in all four extremities, and careful notation should be made of all major arterial pulses. The presence of a bruit over the carotid, subclavian, and femoral arteries, as well as the abdominal aorta, should be sought. The cardiac examination should ascertain heart size and the presence of heart murmurs, especially aortic regurgitation. The skin, eyes, skeletal system, and joints should be examined for any clues as to the presence of an underlying connective tissue or systemic inflammatory condition.

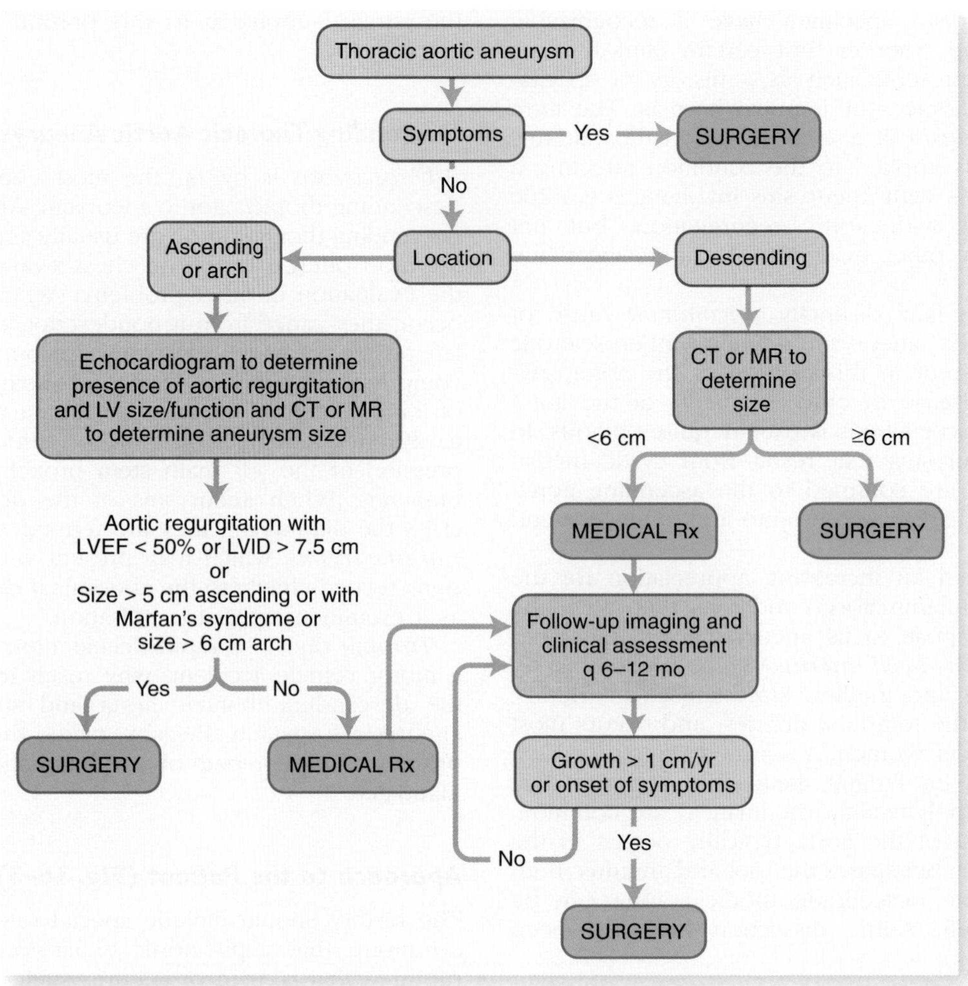

FIGURE 36–3. Approach to the patient with a thoracic aortic aneurysm. The first branch point is to ascertain whether symptoms suggestive of growth (pain, compression of adjacent structures) are present. If so, prompt surgical referral should be made. The location, extent, and size of the aneurysm should otherwise be documented. For any patient with Marfan's syndrome, referral to a cardiovascular specialist should be made. An additional concern in the patient with an ascending aortic aneurysm is the possible coexistence of aortic valve regurgitation, the presence of which may pose another set of criteria for surgical repair independent of the aneurysm's size. Isolated arch aneurysms are rare and are usually addressed in concert with either the ascending or the descending aortic component. A schedule of clinical and radiographic surveillance must be established to ensure continued aggressive medical therapy (e.g., against hypertension) and to measure the size and rate of growth of the aneurysm. AR, aortic regurgitation; CT, contrast chest computed tomography scan; ECHO, transthoracic echocardiogram; F/U, follow-up; LVEF, left ventricular ejection fraction; LVID, left ventricular internal diastolic dimension; MED Rx, medical therapy; MR, magnetic resonance scan; q, every; SURG, surgery.

Diagnostic Tests

The location, extent, size, shape, and, when possible, the rate of growth of the aneurysm should then be defined. A chest radiograph is a very useful starting point, and every effort should be made to obtain previous chest films for comparison. Simple visual comparison of radiographs often allows an appreciation of the rate of growth of the aneurysm.

Every patient with an aneurysm of the ascending aorta and an aortic diastolic murmur should have transthoracic echocardiography (TTE) to define the severity of the regurgitation, to measure left ventricular chamber size, and to assess left ventricular systolic function. Because the ascending aorta is an anterior structure within the mediastinum, TTE can also provide clear images for several centimeters above the level of the aortic valve in most patients. TTE, however, is much *less* useful for the evaluation of aneurysms of the aortic arch and descending thoracic aorta. Transesophageal echocardiography (TEE) is more valuable for the latter, but noninvasive cross-sectional imaging, as can be accomplished with contrast computed tomography (CT) (Fig. 36–4) or magnetic resonance imaging (MRI) (Fig. 36–5), is more appropriate for an elective examination. Both of the latter modalities offer a relatively wider field of view and greater resolution. In the assessment of the patient with an ascending aortic aneurysm with or without aortic regurgitation, if the TTE windows prove technically inadequate or if concern is raised that the

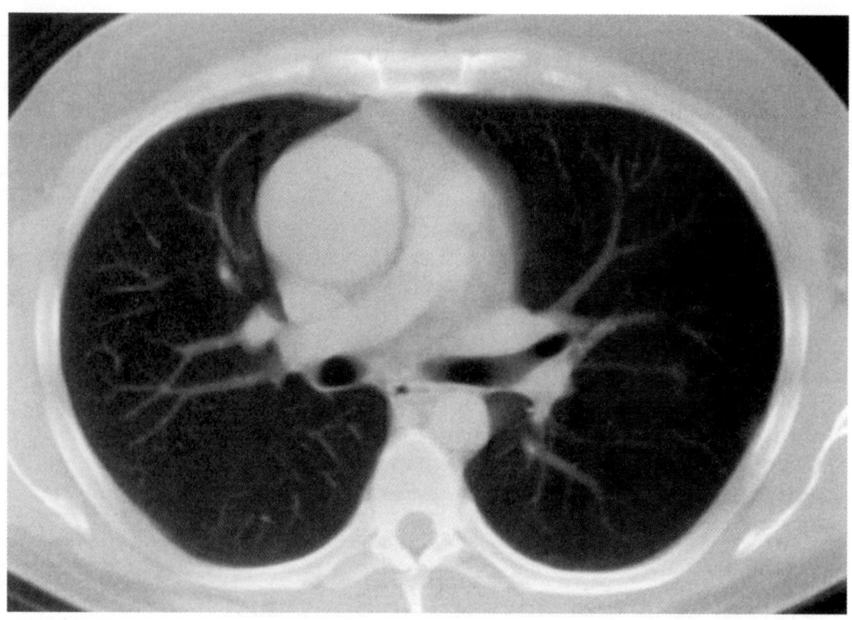

FIGURE 36–4. Contrast chest computed tomography (CT) scan of the same patient as in Figure 36–2. This image is obtained at the level of the right ventricular outflow tract and confirms the presence of an ascending aortic aneurysm. (From Creager MA, Halperin JL: Aortic and arterial aneurysms. In Creager MA [vol ed]: Vascular Disease. Braunwald E [series ed]: Atlas of Heart Diseases. Philadelphia, Current Medicine, 1996, pp 1.1–1.19.)

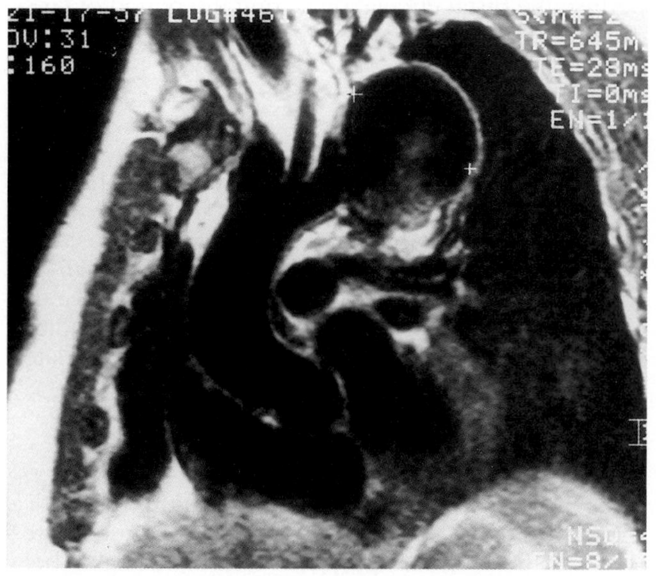

FIGURE 36–5. Magnetic resonance imaging (MRI) scan through the long axis of the aorta of a 28-year-old man with a large saccular aneurysm. This man had undergone repair of an aortic coarctation 10 years earlier and developed a false aneurysm at the proximal suture line that incorporated the origin of the left subclavian artery.

aneurysm extends beyond the field of view, then either a contrast CT scan or MRI should be obtained to provide better clarification and definition. The choice of which modality to pursue depends primarily on local expertise. Invasive contrast aortography is usually not necessary for screening, diagnosis, or assessment of the growth of the aneurysm, but it may be useful in planning surgical repair.

Patients with suspected Marfan's syndrome should undergo TTE even in the absence of findings that suggest the presence of aortic root involvement, since this portion of the aorta may be hidden within the cardiomediastinal silhouette on chest radiographs. Because the prognosis in these patients is dependent on the size of the aortic root, it is important to measure this dimension accurately and to follow it closely on serial measurements. The echocardiogram is also a useful means for assessing the mitral valve apparatus that can often be involved in patients with Marfan's syndrome. The need for and type of laboratory testing depend on the suspected cause and associated complications. There is no specific laboratory testing that is routine. A rapid plasma reagin test for syphilis should be obtained in appropriate patients with a calcified aneurysm of the ascending aorta. An erythrocyte sedimentation rate or C-reactive protein level may be a helpful guide to immunosuppressive therapy in patients with an inflammatory aortitis (giant cell, Takayasu's). Blood cultures should be obtained in patients with suspected infection of an aortic aneurysm. Genotyping among patients with suspected familial aneurysm disease (Marfan's and others) is not routinely available.

Management

The natural history of thoracic aortic aneurysms is variable and depends on the underlying cause, size, and associated features that promote continued expansion. Aneurysmal size and rates of enlargement are the strongest predictors for rupture. Aneurysms greater than 5 cm in maximal diameter or that grow rapidly (a diameter increase greater than 0.5 cm/yr) are at high risk for rupture, as are those associated with pain, which also suggests expansion.[6] The incidence of rupture does *not* seem to be related to the anatomic segment of the thoracic aorta involved. Surveillance imaging should be done on an annual basis, or every 6 months should there be concern about rapid growth. Such imaging may be accomplished with simple posteroanterior and lateral chest films for some patients with a descending thoracic aortic aneurysm, but it usually must involve contrast CT scanning or MRI studies in patients with ascending or arch involvement.

As extrapolated from the experience with the medical management of patients with acute aortic dissection, as well as from a randomized controlled trial in patients with Marfan's syndrome,[7] treatment with a beta-blocker to control blood pressure and its rate of rise appears to be useful in slowing expansion and decreasing the associated risk of rupture. Additional antihypertensive therapy may be necessary. The corrective surgery for a thoracic aortic aneurysm is difficult, usually requires circulatory bypass, and should be undertaken only in centers with a skilled and experienced surgical team. Because aneurysms in patients with Marfan's syndrome have a higher risk of rupture than atherosclerotic aneurysms, these patients must be managed more aggressively.[8]

TABLE 36–1

Indications for Surgery of Aortic Aneurysms

Ascending Thoracic	Descending Thoracic	Thoracoabdominal	Abdominal Aorta
Pain	Pain	As for descending thoracic or abdominal aorta	Pain, tenderness
Severe AR	Compression of adjacent structures		Atheroemboli
Size ≥6 cm Marfan's ≥5 cm	Size ≥6 cm		Size ≥5 cm
Growth ≥1 cm/yr	Growth ≥1 cm/yr		Growth ≥2 cm/yr

Adapted from Creager MA, Halperin JL: Aortic and arterial aneurysms. In Creager MA (vol ed): Vascular Disease. Braunwald E (ser ed): Atlas of Heart Diseases. Philadelphia, Current Medicine, 1996, pp 1.1–1.19.

Referral to a Cardiovascular Specialist

Patients with an aneurysm of the thoracic aorta should be referred to a cardiovascular specialist with the presence of any of the following:

1. Symptoms, especially pain
2. Marfan's syndrome
3. Maximal aortic diameter greater than 5.0 cm
4. Associated aortic regurgitation
5. Rate of growth greater than 0.5 cm/yr
6. Hypertension that is difficult to control
7. Suspected false aneurysm, regardless of size
8. Associated coronary or peripheral vascular disease that would potentially complicate surgical management
9. Suspected inflammatory disease of the aorta (Takayasu's giant cell aortitis)

The optimal timing of surgery for thoracic aortic aneurysms remains a subject of controversy, given the variable natural history as a function of cause, the high prevalence of associated cardiovascular disorders that independently affect long-term outcome, and the inherent risks of such technically demanding surgery. Surgical repair is recommended as shown in Table 36–1.[9,10] These size recommendations are subject to change as surgical techniques and outcomes continue to improve.

Aneurysms that involve the root of the aorta and that are accompanied by severe aortic regurgitation usually require combined replacement of the ascending aorta and aortic valve, which adds to the risk of operation. Aneurysms that extend from the ascending aorta into the arch are also more difficult to repair, and such surgery entails a higher risk of cerebrovascular complications, with stroke or neuropsychiatric changes occurring in as many as 10% to 15% of patients.[13] The most feared complication of surgery on the descending aorta is postoperative paraplegia from ischemic spinal cord damage, which occurs in approximately 5% of patients despite the adoption of a variety of techniques to perfuse the distal circulation during the period of cross-clamping.[10]

Endovascular Stenting

Endovascular stent grafting of descending thoracic aortic aneurysms of several different etiologies has been the subject of intense interest and of increasing clinical success.[11] Several anatomic and radiographic criteria apply, but the technique, first utilized as a "bail-out" strategy in patients not thought to be candidates for thoracotomy because of significant medical co-morbidities, may supplant conventional surgery for appropriately selected patients in the near future.

Postoperative Management

After the patient's recovery from operation, it is critical for the primary care physician to (1) continue aggressive efforts at blood pressure control, using a beta-blocker whenever possible; (2) modify aggressively other cardiovascular risk factors; (3) establish a schedule of periodic imaging studies to screen for complications related to the operation (such as late false aneurysm formation) and to ensure that aneurysmal disease does not appear or progress in other segments of the aorta, especially in susceptible persons, such as those with Marfan's syndrome or those previously identified as having involvement of multiple aortic segments; and (4) supervise appropriate anticoagulation and antibiotic prophylaxis in patients with mechanical prosthetic valves.

Thoracoabdominal Aortic Aneurysms

Classification

Thoracoabdominal aneurysms are classified into four anatomic groups: Type I involves most of the descending thoracic and suprarenal abdominal aorta; type II extends from just beyond the origin of the left subclavian artery to the aortic bifurcation with involvement of visceral and renal arteries; type III begins in the mid- to distal portion of the descending thoracic aorta and extends to the bifurcation of the abdominal aorta; type IV begins at or just superior to the diaphragmatic hiatus and extends beyond the origin of the renal arteries, usually to the bifurcation.[5] Type IV aneurysms are essentially synonymous with abdominal aortic aneurysms, which are discussed later. Atherosclerosis is by far the most common cause of thoracoabdominal aneurysms, which occur more commonly in men than in women.

Imaging

Attention is usually drawn to the presence of a thoracoabdominal aneurysm when the thoracic component is identified on a routine chest radiograph or when an abdominal aortic aneurysm is first appreciated by physical examination. The extent of thoracoabdominal aortic involvement and the degree of luminal enlargement can be assessed with either contrast CT scanning or MRI. Adjunctive abdominal ultrasound examinations to assess the size or rate of growth of the abdominal aortic component should not be necessary, provided that the CT or MRI studies are obtained with the appropriate windows that should extend to the pelvis. Surgical planning may require contrast aortography for precise delineation of the relationship between the aneurysm and the major aortic branch vessels, although three-dimensional (3-D) contrast computed tomographic angiography (CTA) is rapidly becoming the procedure of choice for this assessment.

Management

Medical management of patients with thoracoabdominal aortic aneurysm should follow the general principles outlined previously for the thoracic aneurysms. Namely, the blood pressure must be strictly controlled, using a beta-blocker whenever possible, and efforts at smoking cessation and lipid management should be intensified. Concomitant renal disease should be identified, since this may be an indicator of the presence of renal artery stenosis, which may also need to be addressed at the time of surgical repair. The indications for surgery, as for thoracic aneurysms, can be reduced to the following three: (1) symptoms of expansion, especially pain; (2) thoracic diameter greater than 6 cm or abdominal diameter greater than 5 cm; and (3) rate of growth (>1 cm/yr). Involvement of visceral vessels is a contraindication to endovascular stent grafting.

The major postoperative complications include paraplegia (in thoracic aneurysm), renal failure (which occurs in as many as 5% to 10% of patients), and myocardial infarction. Longer-term, postoperative medical management is similar to that for patients with thoracic aortic aneurysms.

Abdominal Aortic Aneurysms

Aneurysms of the abdominal aorta, which are most commonly caused by atherosclerosis, are subdivided into two major classes: suprarenal (or pararenal) and infrarenal. Nearly 90% are in the latter category. Genetic factors may play a causative role, because there is a distinct familial incidence of abdominal aortic aneurysm in families with decreased type III collagen and elastin or increased collagenase or metalloproteinase activity within the aortic wall. As many as 25% of patients with an abdominal aortic aneurysm have an affected first-degree relative.[12] There is also a 10% to 15% incidence of coexistent popliteal artery aneurysms. Infrarenal abdominal aortic aneurysms occur in men two to five times as frequently as in women. Their prevalence increases with age and is higher among active smokers and patients with evidence of coexistent atherosclerotic peripheral vascular disease.

Rupture

Spontaneous rupture is the most feared complication of abdominal aortic aneurysm. Risk factors for rupture include large size, rapid rate of enlargement, and pain. In an autopsy review of 591 cases of abdominal aortic aneurysm, 118 of which had ruptured, Darling and colleagues reported that rupture occurred in 10% of aneurysms smaller than 4.0 cm in maximal diameter, 25% of those 4.0 to 7.0 cm, 45% of those 7.0 to 10.0 cm, and 60% of aneurysms greater than 10.0 cm.[13] Several other previously reported large series support the contention that the risk of rupture becomes unacceptably high once the aneurysm reaches a maximal diameter of 5.0 cm. Two prospective trials,[13a,13b] however, suggested that surgery can be deferred in some patients until the aneurysm reaches 5.5 cm in size. These are patients who remain asymptomatic and who can undergo either CT or ultrasound examination every 6 months.[13a,13b] Rapid expansion, defined as an increase in diameter of more than 1.0 cm over the course of 1 year, is also an indicator of high risk. Likewise, pain in the flank, low back, or abdomen or tenderness localized to the epigastric pulsation may herald rupture. Aneurysmal rupture is an extremely hazardous condition; approximately 60% of patients die before reaching the operating room, and of those operated on, the mortality is 50%.

Approach to the Patient (Fig. 36–6)

In asymptomatic persons, the examiner should be able to detect an abdominal aortic aneurysm 4.0 cm or larger in diameter on palpation, except perhaps in obese individuals or in those with an unusual body habitus. Suspicion of the presence of an aneurysm should be raised if the common femoral or popliteal arteries feel unusually large. It is not uncommon for the diagnosis to be established only after an abdominal or lumbar spine imaging study obtained for other clinical reasons.

Abdominal ultrasonography can detect aortic aneurysms with nearly 100% sensitivity and provide an

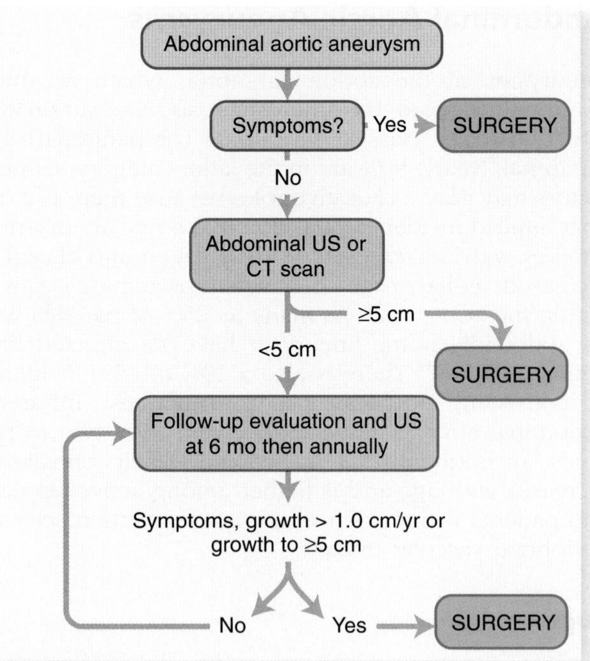

FIGURE 36–6. Approach to the patient with an abdominal aortic aneurysm. Symptoms referable to the aneurysm (pain) are an indication for surgical repair. In the vast majority of patients, the aneurysm can be sized accurately with abdominal ultrasonography. A maximal diameter greater than 5.0–5.5 cm, a growth rate in excess of 1.0 cm per year, or the development of symptoms during follow-up should also prompt surgical referral. The presence of significant comorbid conditions, however, may argue against this recommendation. Alternatively, consideration may be given to endoluminal stenting, if available. Medical therapy should focus on the control of hypertension and on the reduction of associated risk factors for atherosclerotic disease, particularly smoking cessation. CT, contrast computed tomography; SURG, surgery; US, ultrasound.

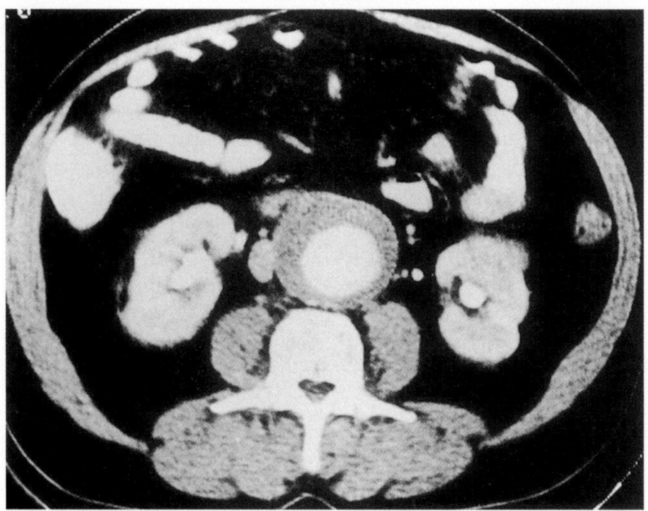

FIGURE 36–7. Contrast abdominal CT scan demonstrates an abdominal aortic aneurysm just anterior to the vertebral body. Extensive mural thrombus is present within the aneurysm. (From Creager MA, Halperin JL, Whittemore AD: Aneurysmal disease of the aorta and its branches. In Loscalzo J, Creager MA, Dzau VJ [eds]: Vascular Medicine, 2nd ed. Boston, Little, Brown, 1996, pp 901–926.)

assessment of size in the transverse and anteroposterior dimensions to within 3 mm.[10] This technique defines the longitudinal extent of the aneurysm less well, but it is otherwise extremely useful for screening and follow-up. It is safe, reproducible, noninvasive, and does not entail exposure to contrast media or ionizing radiation. Ultrasonography can also provide an assessment of mural thrombus in aneurysms. This technique, however, does not suffice for surgical planning, because it does not allow for an appreciation of the relationship between the aneurysm and branch vessels.

Both contrast CT scanning (Fig. 36–7) and MRI offer wider fields of view and better resolution than does ultrasonography in the accurate depiction of the size, shape, and extent of abdominal aortic aneurysms.[10] Newer, three-dimensional computer-generated reconstruction techniques can define the relationship between the major visceral vessels and the aneurysm. In obese patients or those with an unusual body habitus, these cross-sectional techniques are more accurate than is ultrasonography in assessing the rate of growth. In many surgical centers, operative planning can proceed on the basis of these noninvasive imaging modalities, although contrast aortography is still preferred by some surgeons. The presence on clinical examination of important, coexistent peripheral arterial occlusive disease, especially when it affects the iliofemoral systems, should trigger angiography.

Surveillance Imaging. Given the known propensity for aneurysms to enlarge (usually by 0.2 to 0.4 cm/yr), a schedule of surveillance imaging studies must be established on the initial detection of an asymptomatic abdominal aortic aneurysm (luminal diameter >3.0 cm). Much variability in the rate of enlargement exists, however. Annual ultrasonographic examinations should suffice for asymptomatic individuals whose maximal aortic diameter is less than 4.0 cm. Once aneurysm size reaches 4.0 cm, however, repeat examinations every 6 months are advised. More frequent follow-up examinations are also recommended in patients whose aneurysm's diameter has increased more than 0.5 cm within the past 12 months.

The majority of patients with abdominal aortic aneurysms have concomitant coronary artery disease. Since perioperative myocardial ischemia or infarction is the most frequent complication of such surgery, patients with risk factors for or symptoms to suggest coronary artery disease should undergo careful clinical evaluation before surgery (see Chapter 14).[14,15] Clinical markers of increased perioperative risk include previous myocardial infarction, ongoing poorly controlled angina pectoris, heart failure, diabetes, and advanced age. A "high-risk" stress test with exercise-induced ischemia at a low workload or involving multiple myocardial segments on myocardial perfusion scintigraphy (see

Chapter 4) is an additional and independent predictor of increased risk.

Management

Aggressive efforts at blood pressure control, risk factor modification, and lifestyle changes are appropriate. Because the risk of rupture appears to increase substantially once the aneurysm reaches a diameter of 5.0 cm, it is this size that should prompt referral for surgical repair. Patients with *symptomatic* aneurysms of smaller dimensions should also be referred. The risks of operation, however, are substantial, and the perioperative mortality rates are still in the range of 2% to 4%. Surgical referral of the asymptomatic patient with a 5-cm aneurysm and significant comorbid conditions that would independently pose a significant risk of mortality or major morbidity over the course of the next 2 years may not be appropriate. One- and 5-year survival rates after elective abdominal aortic aneurysm repair are in the range of 95% and 65%, respectively.[10]

Referral to a cardiologist is appropriate whenever doubt persists regarding the relative safety of proceeding with surgery on the aneurysm.

Endovascular Stenting. Early reports of the use of endovascular stenting for the treatment of abdominal (and thoracic) aortic aneurysms were quite promising. Stenting has been widely applied in the treatment of coronary, renal, and distal peripheral arterial occlusive disease. With this technique, arterial access is gained via a direct cutdown on the femoral artery and the stent is delivered to the site of the aneurysm over a balloon catheter. Using a combination of angiographic and fluoroscopic techniques, the operator deploys the stent so that its edges protrude just beyond the margins of the aneurysm itself (Fig. 36–8). This technique essentially "excludes" the aneurysm from the circulation. Blood flow is maintained through the stent, and the circumferential arterial lumen gradually thromboses. Stenting may become the procedure of choice in patients who are considered to be at high surgical risk. It is anticipated that the technique will continue to improve and that extension to a lower-risk population may become appropriate. Several endovascular stents have been investigated for the management of abdominal aortic aneurysms and results among them may vary. Concerns about the incidence of early- to short-term endoleaks (micro-leakage of contrast material in or around the stent on angiography or computed tomography), of the need for conversion to open surgical repair, and of late rupture are actively debated.[16–17a]

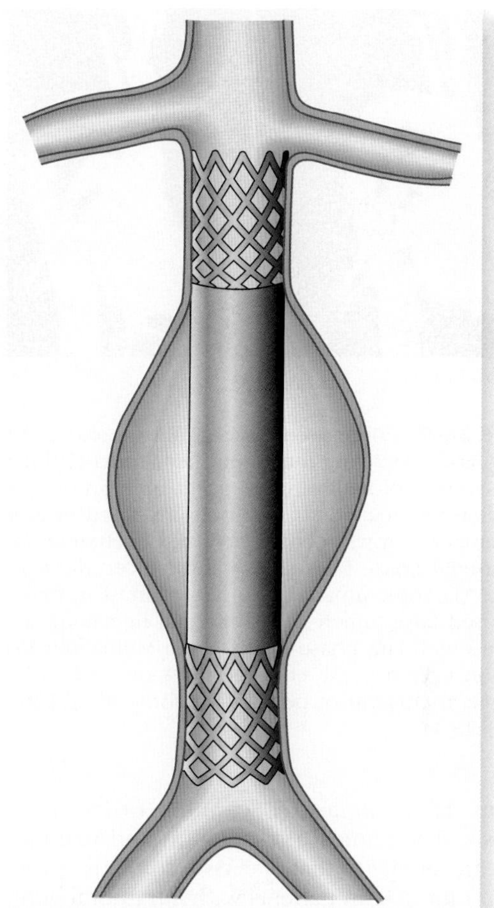

FIGURE 36–8. Diagram showing an intraluminal stent graft within an infrarenal abdominal aortic aneurysm. (From Parodi C, Palmaz JC, Barone HD: Transformed intraluminal graft implantation for abdominal aortic aneurysms. Ann Vasc Surg 1991;5:491.)

AORTIC DISSECTION

Acute dissection of the aorta is an uncommon clinical event, yet one that is fraught with catastrophic consequences. There is an annual U.S. incidence of approximately 2000 cases, which accounts for 3% to 4% of all sudden cardiovascular deaths. Untreated, mortality during the first day occurs at a rate of 1%/hr, is 75% at 2 weeks, and exceeds 90% by 1 year.

Pathogenesis

Most commonly, a tear or rent in the intima allows luminal blood to gain access to the aortic media and, driven by the force of the systolic pressure, to separate the inner two-thirds from the outer one-third of the aortic wall. The dissection propagates in an anterograde direction for a variable length and then typically reenters at a more distal location. Less commonly, propagation proceeds in a retrograde fashion or even bidirectionally. In a large majority of patients with dissection who undergo postmortem examination, an intimal tear can be identified with one or more reentry sites.

The use of cross-sectional imaging techniques has spawned a greater appreciation for two other mechanisms by which medial hematoma formation can occur in the wall of the aorta.[18] Spontaneous intramural hemorrhage (IMH) represents a continued leakage of blood into the aortic media from ruptured branches of the vasa

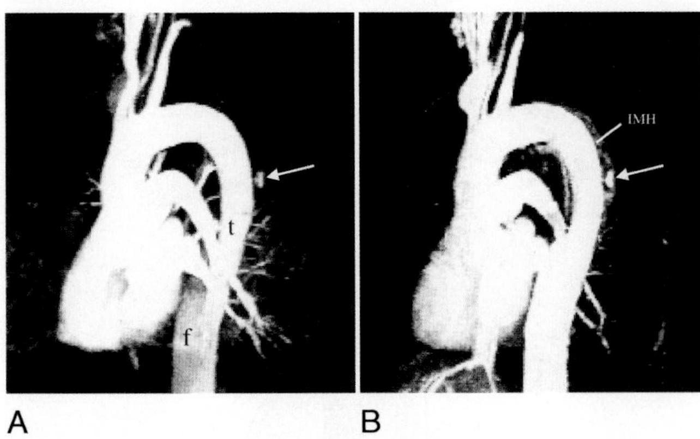

FIGURE 36–9. Contrast-enhanced MRA (a, arterial phase; b, late phase) depicting intramural hematoma (IMH) in outer curvature of wall of distal aortic arch and in proximal descending thoracic aorta, with button-shaped focal signal enhancement (arrows) consistent with penetrating aortic ulcer. Arterial phase MRA shows aortic ulcer and true (t) and false (f) aortic lumina, with less contrast in partially thrombosed false lumen and intramural hematoma when compared with late phase MRA. (From Mohiaddin RH, McCrohon J, Francis JM, et al: Contrast-enhanced magnetic resonance angiogram of penetrating aortic ulcer. Circulation 2001;103:18.)

vasorum. TEE, contrast CT scanning, or MRI is useful in diagnosis. The clinical presentation and natural history of IMH are similar to that of classic aortic dissection, with a higher mortality in patients with intramural hematomas of the ascending than of the descending aorta.

In patients with advanced atherosclerotic involvement of the aorta, luminal blood may burrow under a deep atherosclerotic plaque and erode through the internal elastic lamina and gain access to the medial layer. This may result in formation of a localized ulcer—that is, a penetrating aortic ulcer (Fig. 36–9),[19] false aneurysm, or frank rupture. Penetrating aortic ulcers are found almost exclusively in the mid- to distal portion of the descending thoracic aorta in older patients with hypertension and a heavy atherosclerotic burden. Current cross-sectional imaging techniques are useful for detecting false aneurysms resulting from penetrating atherosclerotic ulcers. Because of the risk of rupture, such false aneurysms constitute an indication for operation.

Any process that leads to the weakening and degeneration of the components of the aortic media (elastic fibers, smooth muscle) can predispose to aortic dissection. Aging is accompanied by medial degeneration, a process that is further accelerated by hypertension. Aortic dissection is most common among patients in the sixth and seventh decades of life, 80% of whom are hypertensive. It is seen earlier in patients with the inheritable disorders of connective tissue such as Marfan's and Ehlers-Danlos syndromes. Cystic medial necrosis is the pathologic expression of these syndromes and has been described as well in patients with bicuspid aortic valve disease or aortic coarctation, disorders that have also been associated with a higher than expected incidence of aortic dissection. A long list of other diseases has been associated with aortic dissection, including Turner's syndrome, Noonan's syndrome, polycystic kidney disease, and the inflammatory aortitides. About half of the reported aortic dissections in young women occur during the third trimester of pregnancy or in the early postpartum period. Many of these women may have previously unrecognized disorders of connective tissue. Because of the very high risk of spontaneous dissection or rupture, recognition of an aneurysm of the ascending aorta in a pregnant woman with Marfan's syndrome should be an indication for consideration of the termination of the pregnancy and urgent aortic repair.

Traumatic dissection can occur as a complication of catheterization or cannulation of the aorta, during the performance of cardiovascular procedures requiring aortic cross-clamping, after incision of the aorta for aortic valve replacement, or even with the excision of small buttons of aorta for the construction of proximal vein graft anastomoses. The presence of an aortic transection with the formation of a false aneurysm must be excluded in any motor vehicle accident victim with widening of the mediastinum on chest x-ray. This can be accomplished by any of the imaging techniques useful in assessing the thoracic aorta—TEE, noninvasive cross-sectional imaging (CT or MRI), or contrast aortography.

Classification

Aortic dissections are classified both temporally and anatomically. A dissection is considered to be *acute* if the patient is seen within 2 weeks of its inception. Chronic dissections are of greater than 2 weeks' duration. The most widely used anatomic schema is the Stanford classification, which divides aortic dissections simply into two types (Fig. 36–10). Type A dissections involve the ascending aorta (regardless of the site of entry or origin), whereas type B dissections do not involve the ascending aorta. The importance of this distinction lies in the recognition of the natural history. Type A dissections are associated with a relatively higher incidence of early fatal complications (rupture with tamponade, severe aortic regurgitation, and stroke) compared with Type B dissections. This simple distinction also underlies the treatment strategies that have evolved since the mid-1960s.

Nearly two thirds of aortic dissections arise within the ascending aorta, just a few centimeters above the level of the aortic valve, where the hydrodynamic and torsional forces are greatest. About one fifth occur just beyond the origin of the left subclavian artery where the relatively mobile arch becomes fixed to the posterior thoracic cage. A minority of dissections arise either in the arch itself or in the abdominal aorta.

Clinical Examination

History

Chest pain is the most common presenting feature of aortic dissection. Adjectives such as "ripping" and

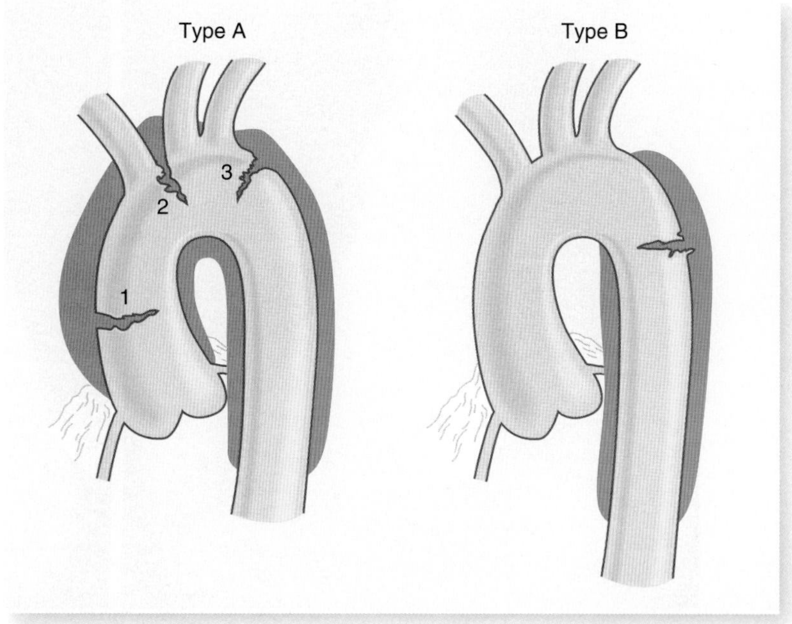

FIGURE 36–10. The Stanford classification system for aortic dissection. Type A refers to any dissection that involves the ascending aorta, regardless of its site of origin. In the example shown, entry site 1 is in the proximal ascending aorta, site 2 is in the arch after the take-off of the innominate artery, and site 3 is in the proximal descending thoracic aorta just beyond the origin of the left subclavian artery. Type B dissections are those that do not involve the ascending aorta. (Redrawn from Miller DC, Stinson EB, Oyer PE, et al: Operative treatment of aortic dissections: Experience with 125 patients over a 16-year period. J Thorac Cardiovasc Surg 1979;78:365.)

"tearing" have often been used to describe the pain of dissection but these attributes are less common than previously thought.[20] The pain usually begins abruptly and is often very severe. Patients can often recall the exact time at which the pain arose. Type A dissections usually are accompanied by anterior chest pain, but a posterior component may also occur. Patients with type B dissections typically describe pain in the interscapular or midback region almost exclusively.

Physical Examination

Helpful findings on physical examination include asymmetry of pulse or blood pressure, a new murmur of aortic regurgitation, evidence of pericardial involvement, stroke, or signs of limb ischemia. Most patients lack such features and are usually tachycardic and hypertensive.[20] Pericardial involvement is suggested by the presence of a friction rub, jugular venous distention, or pulsus paradoxus (see Chapter 35), and it implies contained rupture of a type A dissection into the pericardial space. The left pleural space is the second most common site of rupture and may be associated with both type A and type B dissections.

Diagnostic Tests

The absence of acute ischemic electrocardiographic changes is notable and helps to distinguish the severe pain of dissection from that associated with acute myocardial infarction. The chest radiograph is abnormal in about 85%–90% of patients with aortic dissection (Fig. 36–11).[20] When possible, the film on presentation should be compared with a previous study. The most common finding is mediastinal widening due to aortic expansion. On occasion, an asymmetric bulge along the edge of the aorta that corresponds to the site of origin of the dissection can be identified. The "calcium sign" refers to a 1 cm or greater displacement of intimal calcium from the soft tissue border of the aorta, typically noted in the region of the aortic knob. This finding is uncommon. Cardiac enlargement may signify the presence of a pericardial effusion. A left pleural effusion of variable magnitude may also be present. Effusions do not indicate rupture per se but rather are usually the expression of a sympathetic reaction to the intense aortic mural inflammation caused by the dissecting hematoma.

The diagnosis of aortic dissection can be made after careful integration of the information obtained from the history, physical examination, and chest radiograph in only about 60% of patients. Assessment of three clinical variables (aortic pain, mediastinal widening, pulse differential) should permit correct identification of more than 90% of patients and allow stratification into high-, intermediate-, and low-probability groupings of disease.[21] Because time is of the essence, definitive diagnostic testing should proceed promptly and efficiently.

Imaging

Four diagnostic imaging modalities for the detection and characterization of aortic dissection can be pursued, each with its own relative advantages and disadvantages.[12] The choice of technique should be based largely on imaging availability and local expertise. Collaboration among the primary care physician, cardiovascular specialist, radiologist, and surgeon is of paramount importance to deal successfully with this cardiovascular emergency.

In most institutions, TEE or contrast CT scanning is the procedure of choice (Fig. 36–12). TEE can be performed within 15 to 20 minutes by an expert operator

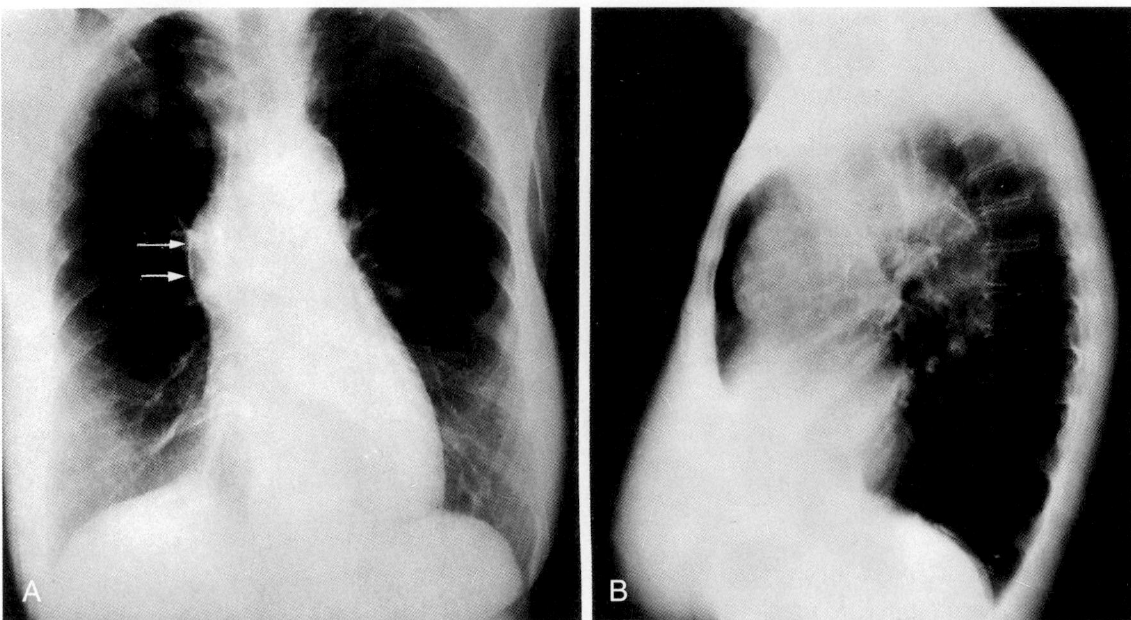

FIGURE 36–11. Posteroanterior *(A)* and lateral *(B)* chest x-rays of a 42-year-old woman with Marfan's syndrome and an acute type A dissection. There is an obvious bulge in the ascending aorta, which can be appreciated on both radiographic projections. The dissection originated at this point and extended into the descending thoracic aorta. (From O'Gara PT, DeSanctis RW: Aortic dissection. In Loscalzo J, Creager MA, Dzau VJ [eds]: Vascular Medicine, 2nd ed. Boston, Little, Brown, 1996, p 901.)

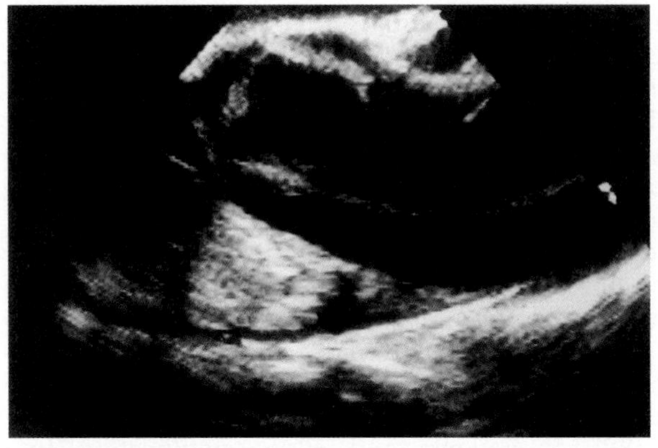

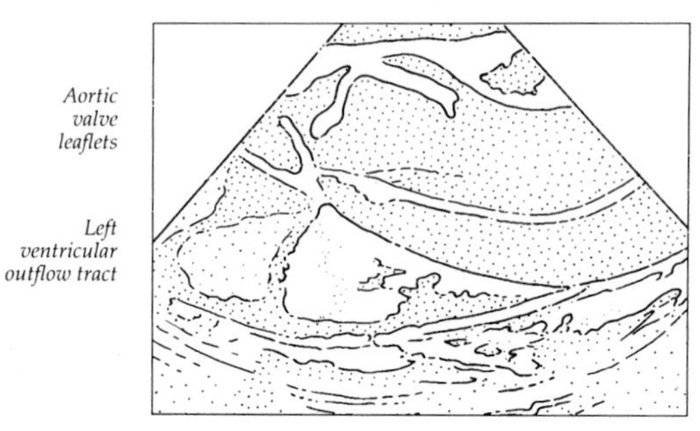

FIGURE 36–12. Transesophageal echocardiogram in a long-axis projection demonstrates a type A dissection with an intimal flap within the root and proximal ascending aorta. (From Cigarroa JE, Isselbacher EM, DeSanctis RW, Eagle KA: Diagnostic imaging in the evaluation of suspected aortic dissection: Old standards and new directions. N Engl J Med 1993;328:35. Copyright 1993, Massachusetts Medical Society. All rights reserved.)

with adjunctive sedation and the usual precautions necessary for the prevention of aspiration. The blood pressure must be monitored carefully during the performance of the procedure and the passage of the probe. Information regarding the presence or absence of involvement of the ascending aorta, concomitant aortic valve regurgitation, the status of left ventricular function, and the pericardial space can be quickly and accurately ascertained. On occasion, a TTE study might suffice, but precious minutes should not be wasted before moving promptly to a TEE investigation. The sensitivity of TEE for the detection of aortic dissection exceeds 95%. The early experience in which the specificity of this technique was less than optimal (75%) has been rectified by the introduction of multiplane probes that allow image acquisition across a 180-degree spectrum. In addition to providing information regarding cardiac structure and function, TEE may allow visualization of the coronary ostia to determine their possible involvement by the dissection. This information has obviated the need for selective coronary angiography, a procedure that was performed far more frequently in the past. One of the possible disadvantages of TEE is that it cannot provide information regarding the extent of the dissection into the abdomen and beyond. Such information is infrequently necessary for the planning

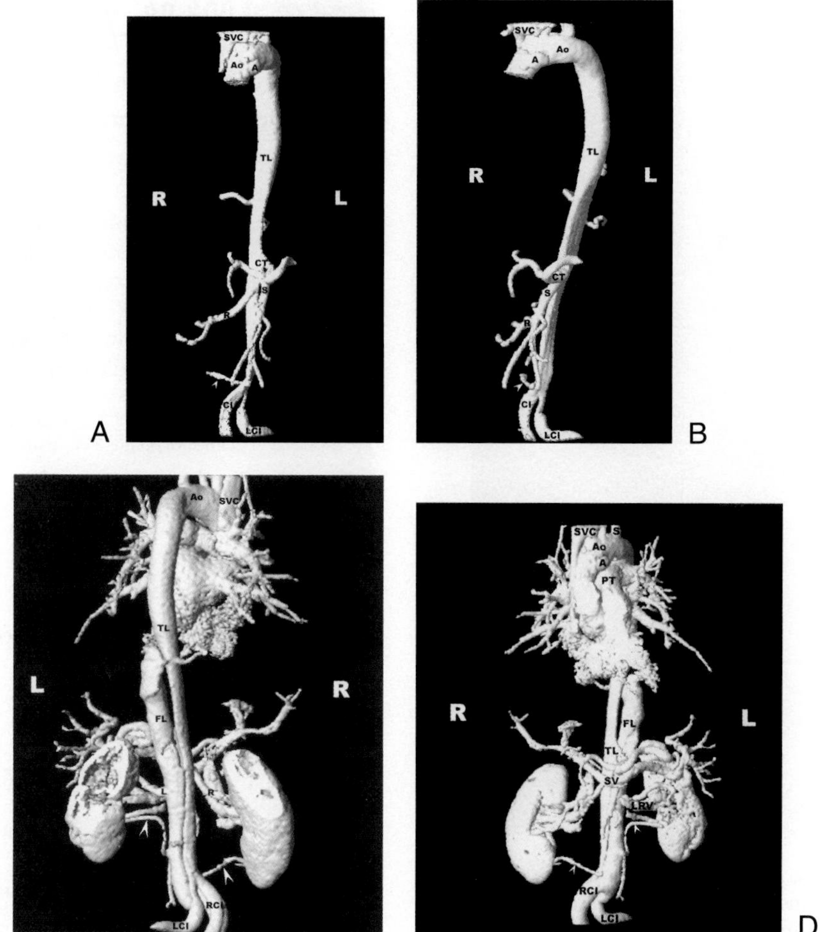

FIGURE 36–13. *A.* Coronal projection of first scan (breath-hold contrast-enhanced MRA) of patient with dissection in ascending and descending aorta. Heart and pulmonary vasculatures were removed from data set. Right renal artery and an accessory right renal artery (*arrowhead)* branch off true lumen. Note that no left renal artery is visible and no filling as yet of false lumen. A, aneurysm; Ao, aorta; CI, right common iliac artery; CT, celiac trunk; large L, left side of patient; LCI, left common iliac artery; large R, right side of patient; R, right renal artery; S, superior mesenteric artery; SVC, superior vena cava; TL, true lumen. *B.* Left anterior oblique view of same data set as in A. This image better shows relation of aneurysm to ascending aorta. In descending aorta, tapering of lumen and absence of left renal and left lumbar arteries can be appreciated. *C.* Coronal projection of second scan, which was acquired directly after the first, shows emergence of false lumen that is excluded from descending aorta. Left renal artery and accessory renal artery branch off this false lumen. *Arrowheads* point to accessory renal arteries. FL, false lumen; LRV, left renal vein; PT, pulmonary trunk; RCI, right common iliac artery; S, left subclavian artery; SV, splenic vein. *D.* Dorsal projection of second scan. This image shows connection between true and false lumina at origin of iliac arteries. False lumen fills retrogradely through this connection. Note that dissection continues into right common iliac artery. Small L indicates left renal artery; small R, right renal artery. (From Leiner T, Elenbaas T, Kaandorp D, et al: Magnetic resonance angiography of an aortic dissection. Circulation 2001;103:76.)

and performance of emergency surgery, however, and it can be obtained later via other imaging modalities.

Worldwide, CT scanning is the most frequently performed initial test for suspected aortic dissection.[20] With current generation software, sensitivity and specificity exceed 95%. CT scanning can be performed quickly, efficiently, and noninvasively, but it involves exposure to contrast media and ionizing radiation. Three-dimensional reconstruction of CT angiographic images can provide detailed information on branch vessel involvement but not on the presence or absence of aortic valve regurgitation.

The sensitivity and specificity of MRI for the detection of aortic dissection both exceed 95% (Fig. 36–13; see also Fig. 36–9). Use of this modality is constrained at many institutions by issues of limited access, cost, and the problems inherent in studying acutely ill patients on intravenous medications within a magnet that is usually housed at a distance from the emergency room or operating theater. Nevertheless, there is increasing enthusiasm for the use of MRI at many centers with an interest in diseases of the aorta.

Contrast aortography was the standard for the diagnostic evaluation of patients with suspected aortic dissection for many years (Fig. 36–14). Studies have suggested, however, that its sensitivity (88%) is actually lower than that demonstrated with TEE, contrast CT scanning, and MRI.[10] Contrast aortography may require

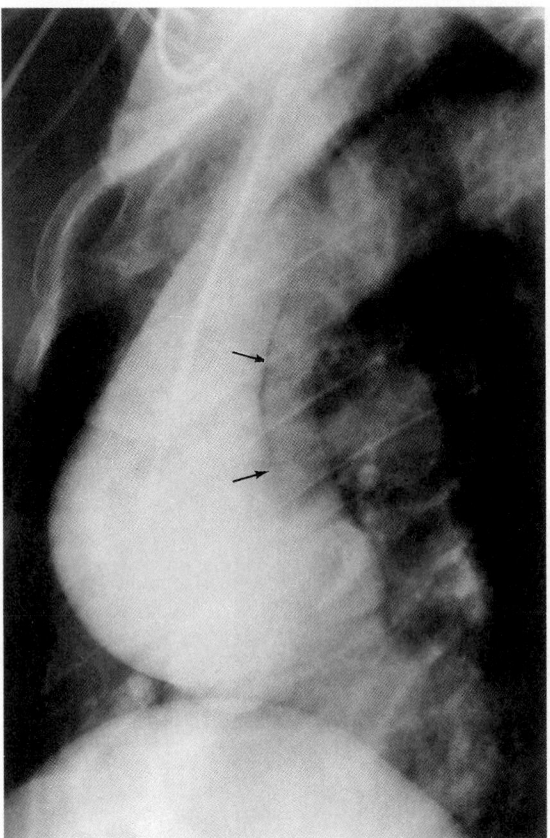

FIGURE 36–14. Contrast aortogram in the left posterior oblique projection demonstrates a type A dissection complicating a fusiform aneurysm of the ascending aorta. The intimal flap *(arrows)* separates the true and the false lumina.

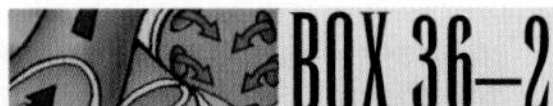

Approach to the Patient with Acute Aortic Dissection

Perform directed history and physical examination
Obtain chest x-ray
Obtain ECG to exclude myocardial ischemia
Contrast chest CT scan or TEE
  Contrast chest CT scan if TEE unavailable
Institute intravenous drug therapy (beta blockade, nitroprusside) to lower blood pressure and heart rate
Obtain surgical consultation

ECG, electrocardiogram; CT, computed tomography; TEE, transesophageal echocardiogram; TTE, transthoracic echocardiogram.

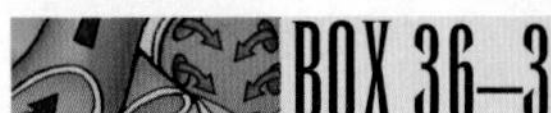

Indications for Surgery of Aortic Dissection

Acute type A dissection
Chronic type A dissection with severe aortic regurgitation, localized aneurysm, or symptoms related to compression
Acute type B dissection with rupture, rapid expansion, refractory pain, extension, or vital organ ischemia
Chronic type B dissection with aneurysmal enlargement (>6 cm)
Marfan's syndrome

more than 30 to 60 minutes to accomplish and exposes the patient to contrast media and ionizing radiation. In addition, contrast aortography may actually be least sensitive for the detection of spontaneous intramural hemorrhage, as the absence of an intimal flap may create the false impression that the aorta is not pathologically involved. Its potential advantages include its familiarity to generations of clinicians, its ability to demonstrate involvement of the aortic valve and major aortic branches, and the provision of information relative to the proximal portions of the coronary arteries. In current practice, contrast aortography has been supplanted by the cross-sectional techniques reviewed previously.

Management

Patients with suspected acute aortic dissection should be referred to the emergency department for prompt evaluation by a physician team including medical and surgical cardiovascular specialists (Box 36–2). Emergency medical measures to control the blood pressure and its rate of rise should be instituted without delay, even as the diagnostic workup is proceeding. Intravenous beta blockade (metoprolol 5 mg intravenously every 5 min for three doses) should be started unless specific contraindications (see Chapter 25) exist. A continuous intravenous infusion of sodium nitroprusside is the antihypertensive agent of choice (0.25 to 10 μg/kg per min) should the blood pressure remain elevated after institution of beta blockade. Monitoring of the heart rate and blood pressure is essential, especially during transport and the performance of diagnostic testing.

Surgical Treatment

Recognition of involvement of the ascending aorta mandates emergency surgical repair unless substantial comorbidities exist, such as a dense, severe stroke, oligoanuric renal failure, and advanced age (Box 36–3). The ascending aorta should be approached primarily even if the entry tear is in a more distal segment of the aorta and the dissection has propagated in retrograde fashion. Such surgery is performed through a median sternotomy, and cardiopulmonary bypass is instituted via the femoral vessels. When concomitant aortic valve replacement surgery is necessary, a valve-graft conduit is constructed and the coronary arteries are reimplanted into the conduit. Perioperative surgical mortality for type A dissections remains in the range of 25%, even in experienced centers.[20]

Medical Management

Medical therapy is initially preferred for the management of type B dissections. This preference is based on the observation that patients with acute type B dissections are at relatively lower risk for early death compared with patients with type A dissections. Patients with type B dissections also tend to be older and have a higher prevalence of associated cardiovascular morbidity, which increases their perioperative risk. For patients with initially uncomplicated type B dissections, outcomes with medical therapy are generally better (10% mortality) than those with surgical therapy,[20] in large measure related to the morbidity of the surgical procedure.[22] There are specific situations, however, in which acute surgical intervention is advised, including rupture, rapid expansion with or without formation of a localized saccular aneurysm, uncontrolled pain, and ischemia of a vital organ. In addition, acute surgical intervention is strongly recommended for all patients with type B dissections and Marfan's syndrome.

Medical therapy is also advised for the management of *chronic* dissection of either the type A or the type B variety. Patients who present 2 or more weeks after the acute event are a "self-selected" group of survivors for whom surgical therapy has not been shown to offer any benefit over that which can be achieved with tight medical management alone. Surgery may be necessary for complications of the dissection, such as aneurysm formation or the development of significant aortic regurgitation with heart failure.

Endovascular Stent Grafting

There are several reports of the use of endovascular stent grafts for the management of acute and chronic type B aortic dissections. The results in carefully selected patients are very encouraging and suggest that this technique may compare favorably with medical therapy as initial treatment for patients with Type B dissection.[22,23] Many investigators hope that application of this technique may prevent complications, such as expansion and rupture, that would force emergency surgery with its attendant high risks.

The management of patients with a spontaneous intramural hemorrhage in whom no intimal flap can be identified mirrors that for patients with classic dissection. Patients with penetrating aortic ulcers are usually managed similarly to those with type B dissections. Given the propensity for rupture, the re-emergence of pain after a period of quiescence should prompt surgery.

Five-year survival for the entire cohort of hospital survivors of acute aortic dissection is in the range of 80% and does not appear to differ significantly according to the type of dissection (A vs. B or acute vs. chronic) or the definitive therapy rendered (surgical vs. medical).[17] The important long-term complications include the development of aortic regurgitation, recurrent dissection, or aneurysm formation (true or false).

Long-Term Care

The primary care physician should coordinate a program of strict antihypertensive control and surveillance noninvasive imaging with the cardiovascular specialist for all patients with aortic dissection, that is, those treated surgically and those treated medically. A chest radiograph should be obtained every 3 months for the first year, and either a contrast CT scan or an MRI study should be performed every 6 months for the first year and annually thereafter. A beta-blocker[24] or, when that is contraindicated, a rate-slowing calcium channel antagonist with negative inotropic properties (verapamil or diltiazem) should form the mainstay of antihypertensive therapy. Additional agents may be necessary to control blood pressure.

Late complications occur not infrequently in survivors of surgical treatment. The incidence of subsequent aneurysm formation at sites remote from the initial surgical repair is approximately 20% over a mean follow-up of 18 months. Aneurysm formation is attributable to continued expansion of the false lumen, the walls of which are thin and inherently weak. Approximately one third of late deaths after successful surgery can be attributed to rupture of the false lumen.

References

1. Vaughan CJ, Casey M, He J, et al: Identification of a chromosome 11q23.2-q24 locus for familial aortic aneurysm disease, a genetically heterogeneous disorder. Circulation 2001;103:2469–2475.
2. Lemon DK, White CW: Annuloaortic ectasia with aortic valve insufficiency. Am J Cardiol 1978;41:482.
3. Evans JM, O'Fallon WM, Hunder GG: Increased incidence of aortic aneurysm and dissection of giant cell (temporal) arteritis. A population-based study. Ann Intern Med 1995;122:502.
4. Kerr GS, Hallahan CW, Giordano J, et al: Takayasu's arteritis. Ann Intern Med 1994;120:919.
5. Creager MA, Halperin JL, Whittemore AD: Aneurysmal disease of the aorta and its variants. In Loscalzo J, Creager MA, Dzau VJ (eds): Vascular Medicine, 2nd ed. Boston, Little, Brown, 1996, p 901.
6. Dapunt OE, Galla JD, Sadeghi AM, et al: The natural history of thoracic aortic aneurysms. J Thorac Cardiovasc Surg 1994;107:1323–1332.
7. Shores J, Berger KR, Murphy EA, Pyeritz RE: Progression of aortic dilatation and the benefit of long-term beta-adrenergic blockade in Marfan's syndrome. N Engl J Med 1994;330:1335.
8. Gott VL, Greene PS, Alejo DE, et al: Replacement of the aortic root in patients with Marfan's syndrome. N Engl J Med 1999;340:1307–1313.
9. Dzau VJ, Creager MA: Diseases of the aorta. In Braunwald E, Fauci AS, Kasper DL, et al (eds): Harrison's Principles of Internal Medicine, 15th ed. New York, McGraw-Hill, 2001, pp 1430–1434.

10. Isselbacher EM: Diseases of the aorta. In Braunwald E (ed): Heart Disease, 6th ed. Philadelphia, WB Saunders, 2001, pp 1422–1456.
11. Bortone AS, Schena S, Mannatrizio G: Endovascular stent-graft treatment for diseases of the descending thoracic aorta. Eur J Cardiothorac Surg 2001;20:514–519.
12. Webster MW, Ferrell RE, St. Jean PL, et al: Ultrasound screening of first-degree relatives of patients with an abdominal aortic aneurysm. J Vasc Surg 1991;13:9.
13. Darling RC, Messina CR, Brewster DC, Ottinger LW: Autopsy study of unoperative abdominal aortic aneurysms: The case for early resection. Circulation 1977;56(Suppl II):161–164.
13a. Lederle FA, Wilson SE, Johnson GR, et al: Immediate repair compared with surveillance of small abdominal aortic aneurysms. N Engl J Med 2002;346:1437–1444.
13b. The UK Small Aneurysm Trial Participants: Long-term outcomes of immediate repair compared with surveillance of small abdominal aortic aneurysms. N Engl J Med 2002;346:1445–1452.
14. Hallett JW, Bower TC, Cherry KJ, et al: Selection and preparation of high-risk patients for repair of abdominal aortic aneurysms. Mayo Clin Proc 1994;69:763.
15. Eagle KA, Berger PB, Calkins H, et al: ACC/AHA Guideline update for perioperative cardiovascular evaluation for non-cardiac surgery: Executive summary. Report of the American College of Cardiology/American Heart Association Task Force on Practice Guidelines. Committee on Perioperative Cardiovascular Evaluation for Non-Cardiac Surgery. J Am Coll Cardiol 2002;39:542–553.
16. Howell MH, Strickman N, Mortazavi A, et al: Preliminary results of endovascular abdominal aortic aneurysm exclusion with the AneuRx stent-graft. J Am Coll Cardiol 2001;38:1040–1046.
17. Chuter TAM: Endovascular aneurysm repair with the AneuRx stent graft is safe, but is it effective? J Am Coll Cardiol 2001;38:1047–1048.
17a. Teufelsbauer H, Prusa A, Wolff K, et al: Endovascular stent grafting versus open surgical operation in patients with infrarenal aortic aneurysms. Circulation 2002;106: 782–787.
18. Nienaber CA, Von Kodolitsch Y, Petersen B, et al: Intramural hemorrhage of the thoracic aorta. Circulation 1995;92:1465.
19. Stanson AW, Kazmier FJ, Hollier LH, et al: Penetrating atherosclerotic ulcers of the thoracic aorta: Natural history and clinical pathological correlations. Ann Vasc Surg 1986;1:15.
20. Hagan PG, Nienaber CA, Isselbacher EM, et al: The International Registry of Acute Aortic Dissection (IRAD): New insights into an old disease. JAMA 2000;283:897–903.
21. von Kodolitsch Y, Schwartz AG, Nienaber CA: Clinical prediction of acute aortic dissection. Arch Int Med 2000; 19:2977–2982.
22. Nienaber CA, Fattori R, Lund G, et al: Nonsurgical reconstruction of thoracic aortic dissection by stent-graft placement. N Engl J Med 1999;340:1539–1545.
23. Karmy-Jones R, Aldea G, Boyle EM Jr: The continuing evolution in the management of thoracic aortic dissection. Chest 2000;117:1221–1223.
24. Genoni M, Paul M, Jenni R, et al: Chronic B-blocker therapy improves outcome and reduces treatment costs in chronic type B aortic dissection. Eur J Cardiothorac Surg 2001;19;5:606–610.

CHAPTER 37 Recognition and Management of Peripheral Arterial Disease

Alan T. Hirsch

Peripheral arterial disease (PAD), a common manifestation of systemic atherosclerosis, is defined by progressive stenosis or occlusion of the arteries of the lower extremities. It is estimated that between 8 and 12 million Americans are affected by this disease in the United States, with an equal or greater number suffering from PAD in Europe.[1–4] PAD shares with coronary artery disease (CAD) similar, albeit nonidentical atherosclerosis risk factors.[1] PAD increases in prevalence and progresses to more severe clinical stages in the presence of modifiable (diabetes, smoking, hypertension, and hypercholesterolemia) and nonmodifiable (e.g., age, gender, family history) risk factors. Treatment of these risk factors in primary care practice can modify the natural history of PAD and decrease ischemic event rates.

The clinical features of PAD are dependent on the severity and chronicity of the decrease in leg arterial blood flow, and clinicians should recognize the full spectrum of PAD stages. As many as half of all patients with PAD may not suffer any recognizable limb ischemic symptoms and yet remain at very high risk for systemic ischemic cardiovascular events. Between 25% and 50% of individuals with PAD may experience claudication, which has a profound impact on quality of life. A minority of individuals with PAD (5% to 8%) will have symptoms of severe limb ischemia during their lifetime, and these patients are subject to ischemic pain at rest, nonhealing wounds, gangrene, amputation, and profoundly decreased survival.

HIGH PREVALENCE OF PERIPHERAL ARTERIAL DISEASE

PAD is a common syndrome that affects a large proportion of most adult populations worldwide.[5–8] The age-specific annual incidence of intermittent claudication defined from the Framingham cohort for ages 30 to 44 was 6 per 10,000 men and 3 per 10,000 women, and this incidence increased to 61 per 10,000 men and 54 per 10,000 women within the ages of 65 to 74.[6] The Framingham Heart Study reported a twofold increased risk for intermittent claudication in men versus women. Overall, however, the broader epidemiologic database suggests that the risk for PAD is equal in men and women, although the incidence of PAD does not rise as rapidly in women; it follows the typical 10-year delay in clinical manifestations until after menopause, as occurs for CAD.

Criqui and colleagues evaluated the prevalence of PAD in an older defined population of 613 men and women in southern California with a battery of four noninvasive tests (Rose questionnaire, pulse examination, ankle-brachial index [ABI], and pulse wave velocity) to assess the prevalence of PAD[7] (Fig. 37–1). Use of the Rose questionnaire severely underestimated the prevalence of PAD, thus demonstrating the insensitivity of this tool to assess true population rates for PAD. Basing the diagnosis solely on the history and physical examination also resulted in low sensitivity for detecting PAD. PAD detection increased two to seven times over the detection rate of the Rose questionnaire when the ABI and pulse wave velocity techniques were applied. On the other hand, an abnormal limb pulse examination overestimated the prevalence by twofold. With the objective noninvasive ABI and pulse wave velocity techniques, the prevalence of PAD in this population was 2.5% in individuals younger than 60 years, 8.3% in those between 60 and 69 years of age, and 18.8% in those older than 70 years.

The relevance of these epidemiologic data to current office-based practice has been documented in the PAD Awareness, Risk and Treatment: New Resources for Survival (PARTNERS) program.[9] This large national survey assessed the prevalence of PAD in American primary care practices by performing the ABI during the course of routine office practice in 350 large primary care practices in 25 American cities. In this study, a targeted cohort of 6979 patients were evaluated on the basis of the risk factors of age older than 70 years or age of 50 to 69 years along with a history of cigarette smoking, diabetes, or both. The PAD diagnosis was established by either a previous chart diagnosis or demonstration of an ABI of 0.90 or less during the study screening. With this technique, PAD was detected in 29% of the population; 13% had PAD only and 16% had both PAD and another form of atherosclerotic cardiovascular disease (e.g., CAD, cerebrovascular disease, or aortic aneurysmal disease). Although PAD was obviously prevalent in this targeted population, the diagnosis was newly established in 55% of patients with "PAD only" and in 35% of patients who had both PAD and other cardiovascular disease. PARTNERS also demonstrated "undertreatment" of atherosclerosis risk factors in patients with PAD whose diagnosis was not previously established in comparison to those with other cardiovascular diseases. Thus, PAD is highly prevalent, but often not promptly diagnosed in American office practice. The linkage between underdiagnosis and undertreatment offers tremendous opportunities to improve care and prevent ischemic events.

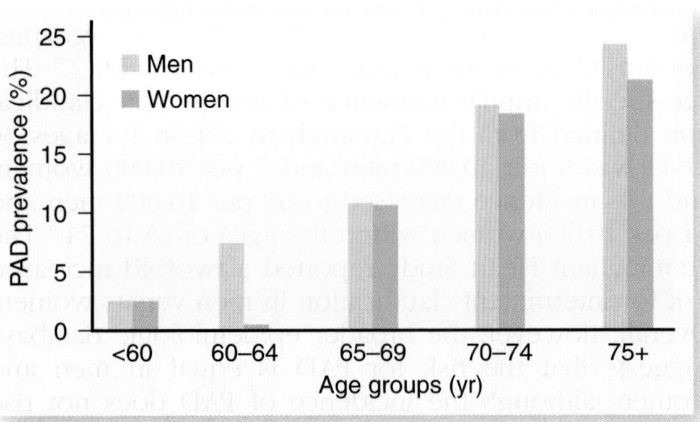

FIGURE 37–1. Bar chart illustrating the increased prevalence of peripheral arterial disease in men and women with advancing age. (Modified from Criqui MH, Fronek A, Barrett-Connor E, et al: The prevalence of peripheral arterial disease in a defined population. Circulation 1985; 71:510–515.)

ATHEROSCLEROSIS RISK FACTORS FOR THE DEVELOPMENT OF PERIPHERAL ARTERIAL DISEASE

The development of peripheral arterial, coronary arterial, and cerebrovascular disease is predicated on exposure of individuals to traditional risk factors, which include smoking, diabetes, family history, hypertension, and hyperlipidemia.[10] The relative risk (RR) for the development of PAD is most closely associated with diabetes (RR = 4.05), current smoking (RR = 2.55), increasing age (in 5-year increments (RR = 1.54), hypertension (RR = 1.51), hyperhomocystinemia (RR = 1.44), and elevated total cholesterol (RR = 1.10 per 10-mg/dL increment). When compared with the impact of these risk factors on CAD prevalence rates, the impact of smoking and diabetes is particularly prominent in the development of PAD.

Smoking is one of the primary risk factors for PAD, especially in young individuals[11] (see Chapter 21). Smoking causes damage to the vascular endothelium, promotes coagulation, and accelerates the progression of atherosclerosis. In the Cardiovascular Health Study, the RR for PAD was 2.5 for current smokers.[12] Another study found that the RR for PAD was increased as much as 7-fold in ex-smokers and as much as 16-fold in current smokers when compared with those who had never smoked. Just as the prevalence of PAD is known to be directly related to population-based smoking rates, so too has the prevalence of PAD been shown to decrease with a decline in current smoking rates. The Reykjavik Study prospectively observed Icelandic males for 18 years and identified smoking and serum cholesterol level as the only significant risk factors, other than age, that predicted the incidence of intermittent claudication in this defined population.[13] Smoking increased the risk for intermittent claudication 8- to 10-fold, and this rate fell sharply after 1970 as exposure of the population to modifiable atherosclerotic risk factors decreased. The impact of continued tobacco use on PAD progression has also been demonstrated by the work of Jonason and coworkers,[13a] who demonstrated that as many as 18% of patients with PAD who continue to smoke face a markedly increased risk for critical limb ischemia (CLI). Continued tobacco use markedly increases the 5-year mortality of individuals with PAD to approximately 40% to 50%, primarily because of myocardial infarction or stroke. Patients with PAD who continue to smoke after vascular bypass procedures have lower patency rates and higher amputation rates than those who quit.

Diabetes mellitus promotes the atherosclerotic process in all arterial circulations via complex pathophysiologic mechanisms that include both the direct biochemical effects of hyperglycemia and the increased frequency of hypertension and hyperlipidemia in patients with glucose intolerance. Populations with PAD more frequently include individuals with the "metabolic syndrome," which is defined by insulin resistance, increased triglycerides, decreased high-density lipoprotein (HDL), and small dense low-density lipoprotein (LDL) particles. In a number of studies, the relative risk for the development of PAD was increased over fourfold in those with diabetes. Individuals with PAD and diabetes more often suffer multisegmental, distal arterial stenoses. More severe and disseminated stenoses, associated neuropathy, a propensity for infection, and impaired wound healing may contribute synergistically to the higher incidence of amputation in individuals with PAD and diabetes.

Hyperlipidemia promotes atherosclerosis in the lower extremity arteries via a complex process that includes promotion of endothelial dysfunction, inhibition of nitric oxide production, and subsequent vascular inflammation, monocyte inspissation, and platelet adhesion to arterial walls. An elevation in LDL cholesterol levels is associated with an increased risk for both CAD and PAD. In the Framingham study, individuals with cholesterol levels over 270 mg/dL had twice the incidence of intermittent claudication.[14]

Twenty-four percent of the U.S. population has *hypertension*, and thus the impact of this risk factor on PAD prevalence rates is high. Hypertension also leads to endothelial dysfunction, medial hypertrophy, and decreased vascular compliance. In addition, hypertension is now recognized as a major risk factor for PAD.

Interest is increasing in the association between the development of PAD and selected newer risk factors such as hyperhomocystinemia. Elevated homocysteine levels have also been shown to be an independent risk factor for the development of PAD and other manifestations of atherosclerosis.[15] A genetic mutation in the enzyme involved in homocysteine metabolism, or a deficiency in essential B vitamins, leads to elevated homocysteine levels. Homocysteine is a highly reactive amino acid that is known to cause endothelial cell dysfunction and injury; it results in platelet activation, thrombosis, and increased vascular smooth muscle proliferation, thereby leading to more aggressive atherogenesis. It is not yet known whether treatment to lower plasma homocysteine levels improves outcomes in patients with PAD. Recent studies have also shown that markers of vascular inflammation, such as an elevated C-reactive protein (CRP) value, may predict a future risk for PAD.[16] In the Physicians' Health Study, the Women's Health Study, and the MONICA (Monitoring Trends and Determinants in Cardiovascular Disease) trials, individuals with the highest CRP levels at baseline showed a twofold to sevenfold higher risk for stroke, threefold to sevenfold higher risk for myocardial infarction, and fourfold to fivefold higher risk for severe PAD or vascular events in comparison to the control group.[17]

Peripheral Arterial Disease: A Marker of Systemic Atherosclerosis

The presence of PAD should be considered a marker for systemic atherosclerosis, and individuals with PAD have a higher coprevalence of CAD and cerebrovascular disease. Patients found to have lower extremity arterial occlusive disease should undergo a focused physical examination to ascertain the presence of symptoms or signs suggestive of concomitant coronary artery, carotid artery, or aortic aneurysmal disease. Ness and Aronow evaluated elderly patients (older than 62 years) in a long-term care facility and demonstrated that 25% of these individuals had at least two other clinical manifestations of atherosclerosis.[18] Of the patients with PAD, 58% had clinical CAD and 34% had suffered an ischemic stroke. A comparable overlap of PAD with other evidence of systemic atherosclerosis was defined in the recent community-based Minnesota Regional Peripheral Arterial Disease Screening Program.[19] This population, recruited for evaluation from both urban and rural communities by age (mean age, 73 years) and the presence of exertional limb pain, assessed cardiovascular health in those with PAD and those without PAD. Of the subjects with PAD, a history of cerebrovascular disease was present in 14% and a history of CAD was present in 56.5%. Non-PAD subjects had much less disease burden; despite advanced age, only 2% had clinical cerebrovascular disease, in addition to less than half the burden (26%) of those with CAD. Identification of individuals with PAD in practice permits one to provide care to a population with a high atherosclerotic disease burden, a group in whom preventive efforts are likely to be particularly effective.

PAD as a Marker of Increased Risk for Cardiovascular Ischemic Events. Patients with PAD have an increased risk for angina, fatal and nonfatal myocardial infarction, fatal and nonfatal stroke, congestive heart failure, and death in comparison to those without PAD. Patients with PAD have a 20% to 40% increased risk for nonfatal myocardial infarction, 60% risk of congestive heart failure, and a twofold to sevenfold increased risk for death (Fig. 37–2). The 5-year longitudinal Edinburgh Artery Study demonstrated an equivalent increased risk for coronary ischemic events and death in both symptomatic and asymptomatic patients with PAD. The ABI was shown to be a powerful predictor of cardiovascular events in patients with PAD in the Edinburgh Artery Study, as well as an independent risk factor in the Cardiovascular Health Study.[12] The lower the ABI, the greater the rate of occurrence of a fatal or nonfatal myocardial infarction. The 5-year mortality is approximately 30% and 50% in patients with an ABI of 0.70 and 0.40, respectively, and even minimal decrements in ABI portend a heightened mortality.[20]

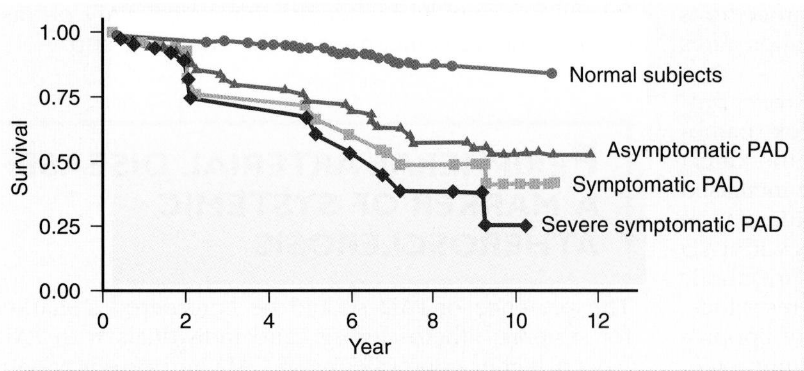

FIGURE 37–2. All-cause mortality in patients with peripheral arterial disease (PAD). The mortality of patients with PAD is high and better predicted by the presence of PAD itself than by the severity of the initial ischemic symptoms. (Modified from Criqui MH, Langer RD, Fronek A, et al: Mortality over a period of 10 years in patients with peripheral arterial disease. N Engl J Med 1992;326:381–386.)

PAD Progression to Critical Limb Ischemia. The lack of recognition of early manifestations of PAD in clinical practice may contribute not only to high rates of cardiovascular ischemic events but also to unremitting progression to the most severe manifestations of lower extremity ischemia. CLI occurs when PAD progresses to such severe impairment in limb blood flow that basic metabolic functions of the limb at rest cannot be adequately maintained. Patients have pain at rest that worsens with either recumbency or leg elevation and improves in the sitting or standing position, thus frustrating efforts to sleep. Minor wounds in limbs with CLI are prone to severe infection and can rapidly progress to frank gangrene or amputation—a great cost to the patient, family, and society. Although this most severe manifestation of PAD is easily recognized in primary care practice, it occurs relatively infrequently. Most patients with intermittent claudication (75%) experience stable exertional symptoms, CLI will develop in less than 15% to 20%, and less than 5% to 10% may undergo amputation.[21] Although no prospective clinical trials to decrease the progression of claudication to CLI have ever been performed, physicians have an intrinsic mandate to provide appropriate atherosclerotic risk interventions in all patients with PAD, and such interventions should presumably improve disease progression in all arterial beds at risk.

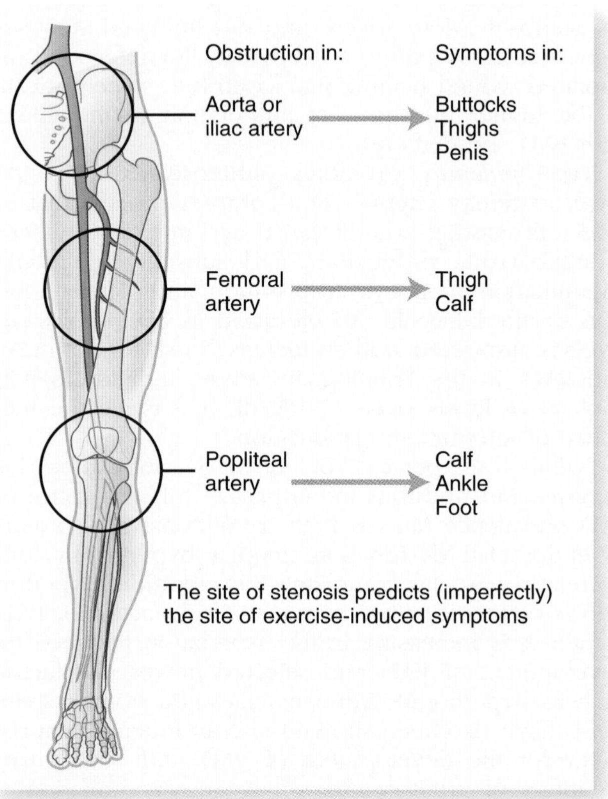

FIGURE 37–3. The relationship between peripheral arterial disease anatomy and occurrence of claudication symptoms. In contrast to coronary artery or cerebrovascular disease, peripheral arterial disease offers an opportunity to clinicians to relate the anatomic site of lower extremity arterial stenoses (from the physical examination) to patient symptoms.

OFFICE-BASED DIAGNOSIS OF PERIPHERAL ARTERIAL DISEASE

History and Physical Examination

The diagnosis of PAD can often be established from the history and physical examination alone. Classic intermittent claudication is typically described as a reproducible aching, fatigue, discomfort, or frank pain that occurs in the muscles of the legs on walking and promptly resolves with rest. A history of claudication can provide an important clue to the anatomic site of PAD, and this clue can then guide subsequent noninvasive evaluation or the therapeutic approach (Fig. 37–3). Claudication of the buttock or thigh is often associated with stenosis in the aortoiliac arterial segments, and physical examination may reveal a diminished femoral pulse or femoral bruit, or both. Stenosis of the superficial femoral artery or popliteal artery, the most common anatomic sites of PAD, is often manifested as calf claudication. Though significantly less common, severe distal PAD (as in diabetic patients) involving the infrapopliteal vessels may cause distal calf or foot claudication.

Primary care physicians should not assume that patients with PAD and claudication will spontaneously have a classic exertional history of leg pain, just as patients with angina only rarely have a classic history of central chest pressure accompanied by a positive Levine sign. The description of claudication is often atypical and may include exertional muscle symptoms, as well as symptoms from concomitant disease that can mask "classic" claudication. In the PARTNERS study database, less than 11% of patients with PAD as their sole atherosclerotic syndrome complained of "typical" claudication symptoms, whereas over half of these patients had atypical limb symptoms (including some leg discomfort at rest or discomfort that persisted after exercise). In addition, "typical" lower extremity ischemic symptoms may have such an indolent onset that patients attribute their exercise intolerance to the deconditioning of aging. Thus, many patients will not offer such a history of exertional leg pain as a "chief complaint" to their primary care clinician. Self-imposed exercise restrictions may be noted first by a spouse or other close family member rather than the patient. Because of these limitations in obtaining a claudication "chief complaint," a history of walking impairment should be considered part of a standard "review of systems" for adult patients to reveal both PAD and other important lifestyle-limiting conditions.

The physical examination also provides important clues to the diagnosis of PAD. The femoral, popliteal, and both ankle pulses can usually be readily assessed by palpation and should be recorded in the medical record. The abdomen should be examined for signs of an abdominal aneurysm and the feet carefully inspected for signs of ischemia such as discoloration, cool skin, chronic trophic skin changes, and skin breakdown (Fig. 37–4). However, although the clinical examination can provide important signs of PAD, primary care clinicians should be aware that peripheral pulse examination has significant limitations and may not be adequately sensitive to accurately diagnose PAD in many patients. In a study by Criqui and colleagues,[7] the sensitivity of any abnormal pulse was 77%, the specificity was 86%, the positive predictive value was 40%, and the negative predictive value was 97%. A study by Hiatt and associates[3,4] revealed that the sensitivity of an absent pulse for PAD was only 5% and thus the positive predictive value of an abnormal pulse was as low as 20%. This limitation of the pulse examination by even experienced examiners serves to highlight the importance of co-reliance on the ABI and the noninvasive vascular laboratory to diagnose PAD, in a manner analogous to use of the 12-lead electrocardiogram and the noninvasive cardiac laboratory to provide better diagnostic sensitivity for CAD in those at risk.

The Noninvasive Vascular Laboratory

The noninvasive vascular laboratory provides a powerful set of tools that should be applied to objectively assess the status of PAD and thereby accelerate the creation of a therapeutic plan. The provision of both physiologic data (blood pressure and Doppler blood flow velocity) and anatomic imaging studies (duplex ultrasound) can provide information that may be central to

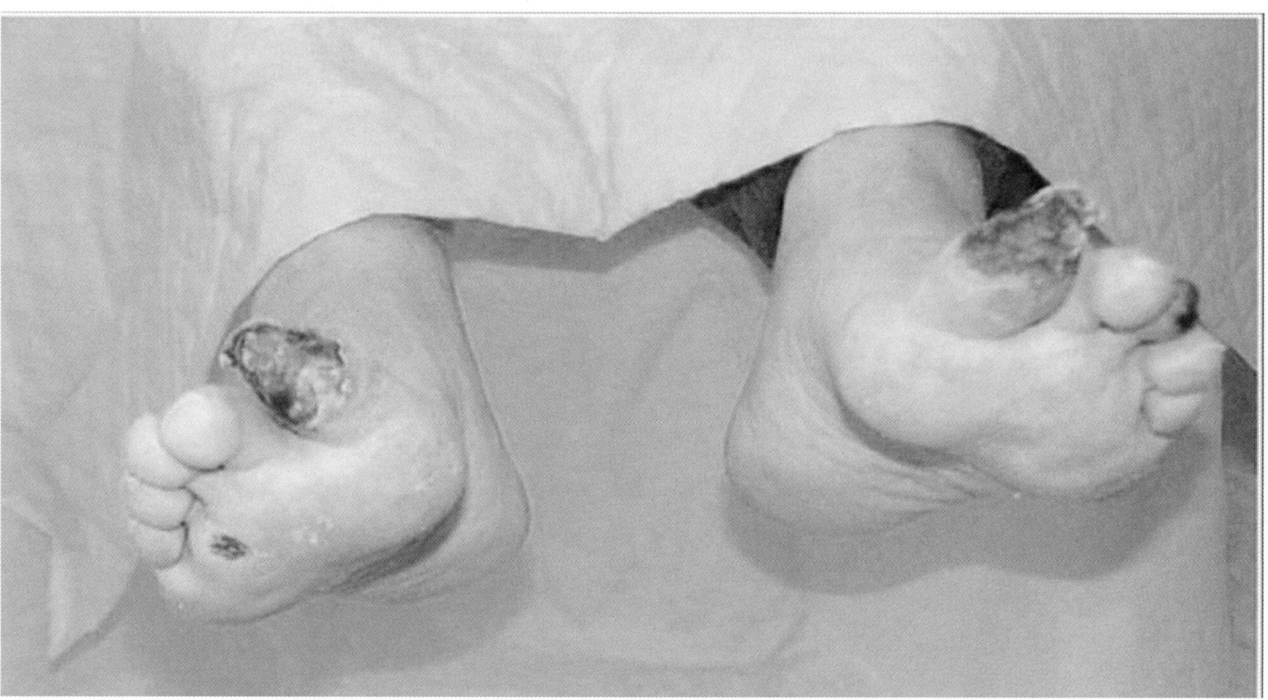

FIGURE 37–4. Ischemic foot ulceration.

the choice of therapeutic pathways. When these studies are appropriately chosen, they are cost-effective, are performed with negligible risk, and provide prognostic information. Noninvasive vascular laboratory examination of the arterial circulation of the lower extremity should be performed (1) to objectively establish the diagnosis of PAD, (2) to quantitatively assess the severity of PAD, (3) to localize specific arterial stenoses if revascularization is considered, and (4) to determine the patency of revascularized segments after revascularization (e.g., impending bypass graft failure). Potential indications for specific noninvasive vascular tests are summarized in Box 37–1 and are reviewed in the following sections.

Ankle-Brachial Index. For most patients with asymptomatic PAD or mild to moderate claudication, measurement of the ABI provides objective data that confirm the diagnosis of PAD and predict the individual's risk for CLI and amputation, the propensity for wound healing, and patient survival (Fig. 37–5). The ABI can

BOX 37–1

Role of the Noninvasive Vascular Laboratory in Patients with Peripheral Arterial Disease

CLINICAL FINDINGS	NONINVASIVE VASCULAR TEST
Asymptomatic PAD	ABI
Claudication	ABI, PVR, segmental pressures, duplex US, exercise Doppler stress test
Possible pseudoclaudication	Exercise Doppler stress test
Functional assessment of claudication	
Postoperative vein graft follow-up	ABI, Duplex US
Femoral pseudoaneurysm	Duplex US
Thoracic outlet syndrome	Arm arterial and venous duplex US with abduction maneuvers
Suspected aortic aneurysm	Abdominal US, CT, or MRA
Serial AAA follow-up	

AAA, abdominal aortic aneurysm; ABI, ankle-brachial index; CT, computed tomography; MRA, magnetic resonance angiography; PAD, peripheral arterial disease; PVR, pulse volume recording; US, ultrasound.

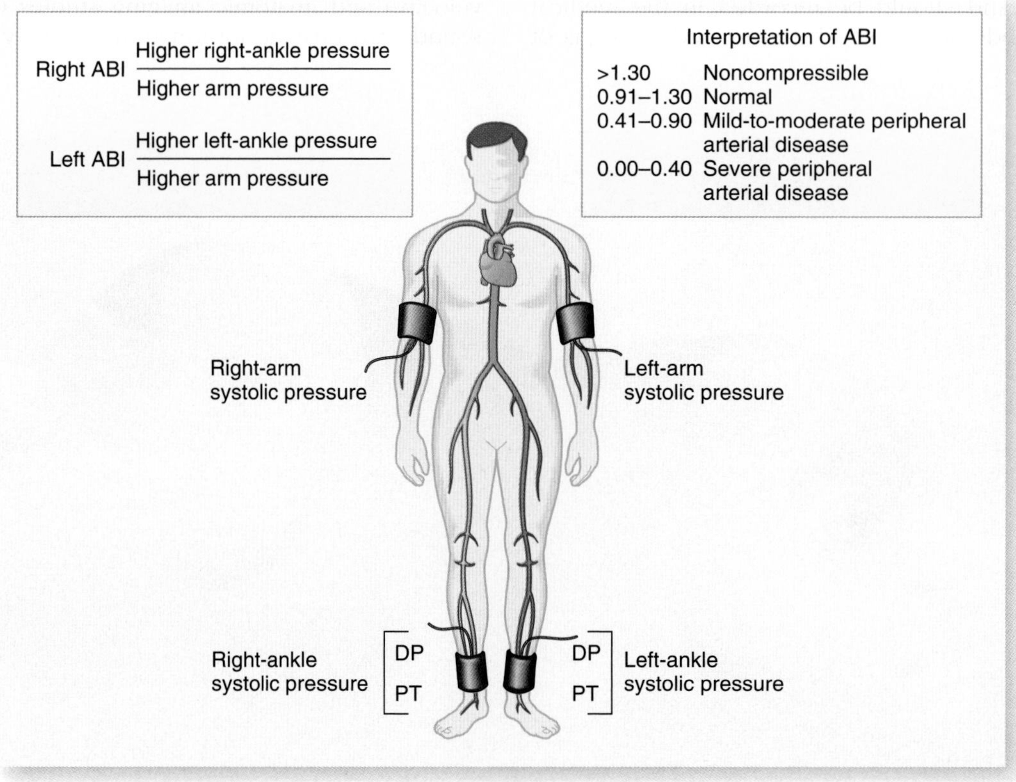

FIGURE 37–5. The ankle-brachial index (ABI) measurement. (From Hiatt WR: Medical treatment of peripheral arterial disease and claudication. N Engl J Med 2001:344:1608–1621.)

be used either as a screening tool for PAD or to monitor the efficacy of therapeutic interventions.

The ABI test requires only the use of standard office blood pressure cuffs placed on the upper part of the arm and above each ankle, and systolic pressure is recorded with a hand-held 5- or 10-MHz Doppler instrument. Normal individuals should have a minimal (<12 mm Hg) inter-arm systolic pressure gradient during a routine examination. Both arm pressures must be recorded because atherosclerotic subclavian and axillary arterial stenoses occur with relative frequency in this population. If an inter-arm blood pressure gradient is noted, the higher brachial blood pressure should be used for subsequent blood pressure ratio calculations. In healthy individuals without PAD, ankle systolic pressure is 10 to 15 mm Hg higher than brachial systolic pressure, and thus the normal ankle-arm systolic blood pressure ratio is greater than 1.0. Abnormal ABI values represent a continuous variable that is less than 0.90. ABI values are often considered to be mildly to moderately diminished when they are between 0.41 and 0.90 and moderately diminished when less than 0.40. These relative categories have prognostic value because the lower the ABI, the greater the risk of progression to CLI.

The ABI may not be accurate in individuals in whom ankle systolic blood pressure cannot be abolished by inflation of the blood pressure cuff to abnormally high values. The incidence of noncompressible, calcified conduit arteries is highest in diabetics and elderly patients. Despite the artifactually high ABI in such patients, PAD may nevertheless be quite severe. It is also possible for the ABI to be normal in patients with severe and chronic aortoiliac PAD if sufficient arterial collaterals are present. If a patient has symptoms that strongly suggest claudication, a normal ABI value should not be considered adequate to rule out PAD, and a confirmatory diagnostic vascular test (e.g., Doppler waveform analysis or duplex ultrasound) should be performed.

The ABI can be measured in any primary care office, usually in less than 15 minutes, and it provides immediate diagnostic results that can alter care. The following individuals should have ABI testing:

1. Those with exertional lower extremity discomfort
2. Those with nonhealing wounds
3. Those older than 70 years
4. Those older than 50 with a history of smoking or diabetes (or both)

Establishment of the diagnosis in a primary care setting (in lieu of a vascular laboratory) has several potential advantages: it permits immediate education of the patient regarding the cause of the symptoms, permits immediate initiation of atherosclerosis risk reduction strategies, and is less costly. Establishment of the diagnosis of PAD changes atherosclerosis risk factor treatment targets to the most stringent goals (equivalent to the targets used for patients with established CAD).

Segmental Pressure Measurements. Although the ABI provides a facile PAD diagnosis, it does not permit localization of the site of arterial stenosis. Leg arterial pressure can be measured sequentially along the limb with plethysmographic cuffs to localize significant pressure gradients (Fig. 37–6). Segmental blood pressure cuffs are usually placed at the upper thigh, lower thigh, upper calf, and lower calf areas. In most laboratories, any gradient greater than 15 to 20 mm Hg between adjacent sites may represent a physiologically important focal stenosis. Segmental leg systolic blood pressure can also be indexed relative to the brachial artery pressure in a manner analogous to the ABI. A primary care provider can easily interpret this segmental pressure analysis to determine the location of individual arterial stenoses. For example, a systolic pressure gradient between the brachial artery and the upper part of the thigh usually signifies the presence of an aortoiliac stenosis. A pressure gradient between the upper and lower thigh cuffs indicates a probable superficial femoral artery stenosis. Gradients between the lower thigh and upper calf cuffs identify a distal superficial femoral or popliteal arterial stenosis, and gradients between the upper and lower calf cuffs identify infrapopliteal disease.

Exercise Doppler Stress Tests. Patients with PAD and claudication should be considered for exercise testing to objectively assess their functional capacity. Traditionally, patients with PAD have been thought to be poor candidates for cardiovascular treadmill testing because many standard exercise testing protocols may be inordinately arduous for many patients with claudication. Subjects with PAD and claudication will less frequently reach workloads that provide optimal sensitivity to evaluate coronary ischemic symptoms. Nevertheless, treadmill testing may be extremely useful in objectively documenting the magnitude of limb symptom limitations, and it can provide correlative data regarding coronary ischemia at such "real-world" workloads as might occur either during activities of daily living or during a program of supervised exercise. Common treadmill tests for patients with claudication use less intense progressive workloads (e.g., the Gardner-Skinner, Hiatt, or Naughton protocols) and should record the time of onset of specific leg symptoms (pain-free walking time), the presence of associated coronary ischemic symptoms, and the maximal walking time.

When exercise testing is performed in association with pre-exercise and postexercise ABI measurements, the data may be helpful in differentiating vascular from nonvascular etiologies of exercise-induced leg pain (e.g., pseudoclaudication). In normal individuals, brachial and ankle blood pressure values rise together, and the ABI remains normal before and after exercise. In contrast, in patients with PAD, exercise induces the usual rise in systemic (brachial) blood pressure, but ankle blood pressure falls as a result of maximal exercise-induced ischemic vasodilatation in the claudicating limb. Thus, in an individual with true vasculogenic claudication, the postexercise ABI will demonstrate a classic fall from its baseline value. In contrast, a patient with pseudoclaudication from spinal stenosis will have a normal postexercise ABI despite exercise-limiting symptoms suggestive of PAD.

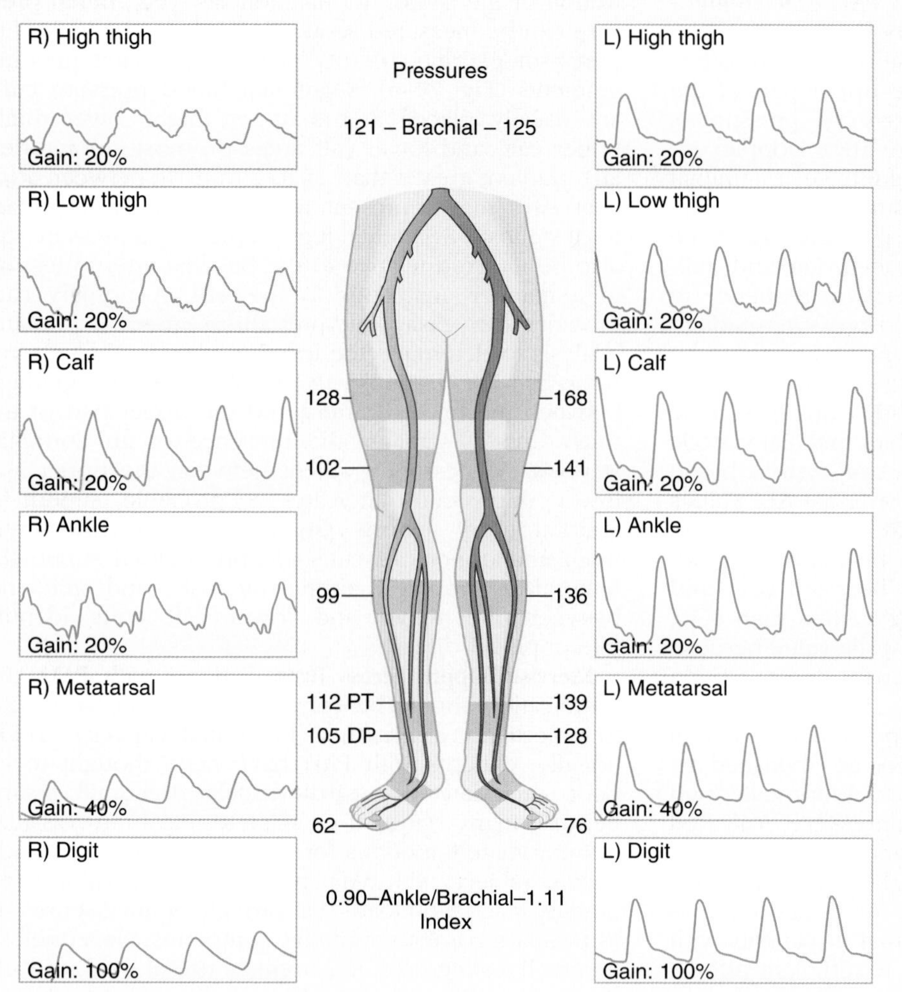

FIGURE 37–6. Pulse volume recordings and segmental pressure measurements. (Adapted from Primary Care Series, Volume 6, Society for Vascular Medicine and Biology, 1999.)

Pulse Volume Recordings. Many diagnostic vascular tests can be provided in an office setting in addition to ABI and exercise tests. The diagnosis of PAD can also be established via the use of simple plethysmographic techniques that measure the pulsatility of arterial flow in the lower extremity. Pulse volume recordings provide a method to evaluate the effect of arterial pulse pressure on limb volume via the use of either a pneumoplethysmograph or a mercury-in-Silastic strain gauge. These devices are usually applied in a segmental manner from the thigh to the ankle to measure pulse volume from normal to more distal arterial segments. A normal pulse volume recording is characterized by a rapid arterial upstroke and preserved pulse amplitude, both of which are blunted distal to significant arterial stenosis (see Fig. 37–6).

Duplex Scanning. Duplex ultrasound techniques use both two-dimensional imaging and Doppler waveform analysis and provide highly reliable diagnostic information to assess the anatomic site and functional significance of PAD. This technique assesses sequential blood flow velocity along imaged arterial segments and can thus localize specific stenoses or sites of arterial occlusion. Duplex studies can assess plaque morphology and surgical graft or stent patency and can establish the presence of aneurysms or arteriovenous fistulas. Although the duplex ultrasound technique has become a standard in most vascular laboratories, this test requires a proficient and experienced vascular technologist, may require extensive time for a complete examination, and is significantly more expensive than the physiologic testing techniques described earlier. Duplex ultrasound is not appropriate for use as a screening tool and should generally be reserved for patients in whom more precise anatomic information is needed. For example, duplex techniques may be helpful in assessing proximal aortoiliac stenoses that may be amenable to angioplasty or stent placement, in demonstrating the continued patency of arterial bypass grafts or arterial stents, and in patients with incompressible vessels, in whom ABI and segmental pressure examinations are not likely to be accurate.

Transcutaneous Oximetry. In many practice settings, the most pressing clinical problem is assessment of the probability of healing of an ischemic wound. Although routine physiologic testing (such as demonstration of an

ABI <0.40 or a markedly blunted pulse volume waveform) can provide some prognostic data, more precise vascular laboratory measurements can be useful in determining whether tissue perfusion is adequate to prevent ulceration from progressing to frank gangrene. Measurements of transcutaneous oxygen tension ($TcPO_2$) offer data regarding the net adequacy of both large arterial and arteriolar perfusion to the threatened limb. Transcutaneous oximetry is performed with oxygen-sensing electrodes attached to the skin in a normal region (e.g., a reference electrode placed on the chest) and at calf or foot sites. Normal $TcPO_2$ values are usually greater than 50 to 60 mm Hg; in contrast, $TcPO_2$ values less than 20 to 30 mm Hg suggest severe local ischemia and bode poorly for future wound healing. In summary, $TcPO_2$ studies provide an excellent method for the assessment of patients with concomitant large-vessel and microvascular disease, such as diabetic patients and patients with severe atheroembolic lesions.

Contrast Angiography. Angiography is almost never needed to establish the diagnosis of PAD and should not generally be used if limb revascularization is not imminent. The diagnostic noninvasive vascular laboratory techniques noted earlier are adequate to establish the diagnosis of PAD and to plan most therapeutic interventions. In many medical centers, angiography is now performed only in patients in whom endovascular or surgical revascularization is mandated because of CLI or in whom severe claudication persists despite a program of maximal medical management (exercise and pharmacotherapy).

MEDICAL TREATMENT OF PERIPHERAL ARTERIAL DISEASE IN PRIMARY CARE PRACTICE

Risk Factor Normalization

The natural history of PAD can be improved with aggressive medical management and normalization of atherosclerosis risk factors (see Chapter 18). Such risk factor interventions lead to reductions in cardiovascular ischemic event rates (myocardial infarction, stroke, and death). Hypertension and diabetes should be aggressively treated in all patients with PAD, but no prospective trials to date have demonstrated a PAD-specific endpoint that is altered by aggressive normalization of blood pressure or by glycemic control.

Smoking cessation is the single most important intervention that can improve the well-being of patients with PAD.[11,13] Successful abstinence from tobacco use is associated with a dramatic improvement in survival. In addition, PAD patients who successfully quit smoking achieve a slowed rate of progression of PAD to pain at rest or to CLI. Individuals with PAD who quit smoking enjoy improved limb bypass graft and endovascular procedure patency rates and decreased amputation rates.

Several randomized trials have shown that patients with PAD have better outcomes with lipid lowering. The Cholesterol Lowering Atherosclerosis Study (CLAS) and the St. Thomas trial demonstrated a beneficial effect of lipid normalization: aggressive LDL lowering was associated with both plaque stabilization (less progression) and frank regression of femoral atherosclerosis.[22] In patients with CAD who are treated aggressively to normalize LDL cholesterol, the progression of femoral arterial atherosclerosis is blunted, and the development of symptomatic claudication is decreased.[23] Current lipid-lowering guidelines from the National Cholesterol Education Program suggest that individuals with PAD should achieve an LDL cholesterol concentration of less than 100 mg/dL and receive therapy for elevated serum triglyceride levels.[24]

Antiplatelet therapy has also been demonstrated to alter the natural history of PAD by diminishing cardiovascular ischemic event rates and perhaps by blunting the progression of atherosclerosis. The potential beneficial effects of aspirin and an aspirin-dipyridamole combination on rates of progression of femoral arterial atherosclerosis were reported by Hess and colleagues in a small cohort of patients monitored over a 2-year time span.[25] Over this short period of observation, progression of femoral atherosclerosis was diminished by dual antiplatelet therapies. The effects of long-term administration of aspirin on the natural history of atherosclerotic arterial disease have also been reported from the Physicians Health Study.[26] This randomized, double-blind, placebo-controlled trial evaluated the effects of low-dose aspirin in 22,071 male physicians over an average of 60 months of treatment. Individuals who used aspirin required only half as many surgical limb revascularization procedures as those in the placebo cohort. These data suggest that aspirin decreases the frequency of thrombotic events that convert stable claudication to CLI.

The relative benefits of aspirin and clopidogrel on rates of myocardial infarction, stroke, and death were reported from the prospective Clopidogrel vs. Aspirin in Patients at Risk of Ischemic Events (CAPRIE) investigation.[27] Patients entered the CAPRIE study with clinical signs of systemic atherosclerosis; qualifying conditions included a history of recent myocardial infarction, ischemic stroke, or established PAD. Inasmuch as CAPRIE included 6452 individuals with PAD, the study is the largest prospective randomized trial ever performed to evaluate any medical therapy for PAD. Clopidogrel treatment was more effective than aspirin in preventing the combined endpoint of ischemic stroke, myocardial infarction, or vascular death in the total study population (an 8.7% relative risk reduction). Additionally, post hoc analysis demonstrated a more impressive 23.8% relative risk reduction in favor of clopidogrel versus aspirin treatment alone for the combined ischemic event endpoint in patients with PAD. Overall, patients with PAD should receive antiplatelet therapy to prevent ischemic events unless otherwise contraindicated.

Medical Treatment of Claudication (Box 37–2)

Intermittent claudication is present in 30% to 50% of patients with PAD, and it is presumed that approximately 1 to 4 million Americans suffer this functional limitation.[5] Patients with intermittent claudication have cramping, aching, fatigue, or discomfort in the muscles of the calves, thighs, or buttocks that is reproducibly elicited by walking and consistently relieved by rest (see Fig. 37–3). Because claudication represents an exercise-induced mismatch between the metabolic demand of the working muscles of the lower extremities and inadequate blood supply during volitional exercise, most patients with claudication compensate by decreasing their ambulatory pace (to less than 1 to 2 mph) and the distance exercised (to less than two to four street blocks) to avoid this discomfort. This decrease in functional capacity is associated with a major diminution in quality of life that decreases the individual's ability to participate in both work-related and leisure activities. In past decades, this detrimental impact on patient quality of life was treated less aggressively than were ischemic symptoms in other vital circulations (e.g., angina or transient ischemic attacks).

Exercise Therapy. A program of supervised exercise should be considered a primary treatment modality for improving claudication symptoms in primary care practice. It should be noted that the casual prescription of exercise in a home or "unsupervised" setting has been demonstrated to be ineffective in treating claudication. It is rare for such a "home exercise" prescription to be associated with adequate compliance to the minimal exercise frequency, duration, and workload known to improve pain-free walking. In contrast, prescription of a program of supervised walking exercise can be expected to result in an increase in the speed, distance, and duration walked, with improvements first observed within 4 to 8 weeks and increasing over 12 or more weeks. This program of "PAD rehabilitation" requires the performance of treadmill or track-based exercise for 45 to 60 minutes three or more times a week for a minimum of 12 weeks. Such exercise is supervised by a physical therapist, nurse, or exercise physiologist so that safety and compliance are maximized.

Treadmill exercise has been shown to be more effective than other exercise modalities (e.g., weight training, bicycling), presumably because treadmill walking conditions the muscle groups that are required for claudication-free walking in the community setting. The initial treadmill workload should be set to a speed and grade that elicit claudication symptoms within 3 to 5 minutes. Patients are asked to continue to walk at this workload until they achieve claudication of moderate severity, followed by a brief period of rest to permit the symptoms to resolve. The exercise-rest-exercise cycle is repeated several times during the hour of supervision. Such a program requires that patients be reassessed as they continue the program so that the workload, modified by treadmill grade or speed (or both), can be increased to allow patients to achieve increased pain-free and maximal walking distances until completion of the program. Typical benefits of such a program include a more than doubling in peak exercise performance, significant improvements in walking speed and distance, and improvements in physical function and vitality.

Despite the documented efficacy of structured exercise programs for claudication, few have historically been available because of limited reimbursement by health care payers. Publication of the 2001 American

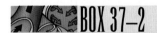

Proposed Claudication Detection and Treatment Algorithm

First Visit

- Suspected peripheral arterial disease
  - *Individual risk factors (diabetes, hypercholesterolemia, hypertension, smoking)*
  - *Age older than 70 yr or age older than 50 yr with a history of smoking or diabetes*
  - *History of exertional leg pain (suspected claudication)*
  - *Nonhealing wound*
- Document the diagnosis of peripheral arterial disease
  - *Perform an ankle-brachial index, segmental pressures, or other vascular laboratory tests*
- Document the impact of claudication (chart note, exercise tolerance test)
  - *What degree of functional improvement is needed?*
  - *What are the specific risks of each therapeutic strategy to the patient?*
- Normalize all risk factors; begin antiplatelet therapy
- Consider the role of supervised exercise and medications (cilostazol [Pletal])
- Consider the role of revascularization
  - *Refer to a vascular specialist—obtain a duplex arterial ultrasonogram (especially with suspicion of aortoiliac or proximal femoral stenosis)*
- Return for an office visit in 3–4 mo

Follow-up Visit

- *Re-evaluate functional improvement in 3–4 mo*
- *Re-evaluate success of atherosclerosis risk factor normalization*

Medical Association Current Procedural Terminology Manual and associated code (93668) for PAD rehabilitation is expected to accelerate the availability of such programs in the near future.

Pharmacotherapy. Numerous medications have historically been proposed for the treatment of claudication; however, the current range of clinically relevant medications remains limited.

Pentoxifylline. Patients with PAD have been shown to have hemorheologic defects, including nondeformable red cells, elevated fibrinogen levels, and increased platelet aggregation leading to increased blood viscosity. Pentoxifylline is an agent that improves red cell deformability, lowers fibrinogen levels, decreases platelet aggregation, and elicits small increases in walking distance in patients with PAD.[28] Pentoxifylline produced a 22% improvement over placebo in walking distance before the onset of claudication and a 12% improvement in maximal walking distance in initial investigations. Pentoxifylline has not been demonstrated to improve quality of life in patients with PAD and claudication. Moreover, the quite modest improvements in pain-fee or maximal walking distance that are achieved with pentoxifylline have led to less reliance on this medication as alternative claudication treatment strategies become available.

Cilostazol. Cilostazol is a phosphodiesterase III inhibitor that is known to promote arteriolar vasodilatation via increases in cyclic adenosine monophosphate (AMP) in vascular smooth muscle cells. Increases in cyclic AMP in platelets also cause mild inhibition of antiplatelet activation. In addition, cilostazol has antiproliferative properties that inhibit vascular smooth muscle cell proliferation in vitro. In several randomized, controlled clinical trials, cilostazol has been demonstrated to increase pain-free walking time by 30% to 50% and maximal walking time by 50% to 80% in patients with claudication.[29] This improvement in pain-free and maximal walking ability is usually established after a 2- to 3-month treatment period, but patient education is required so that compliance is maintained long enough to judge clinical efficacy. Cilostazol is generally well tolerated but can elicit adverse effects that include headache, palpitations, nausea, or loose stool. Cilostazol use has been shown to be associated with significant improvements in functional status and quality of life. In a single prospective trial, cilostazol was also more effective than pentoxifylline in improving claudication symptoms.[30] Cilostazol is the only claudication medication that, like exercise training, can elicit small improvements in the patient's lipid profile; the usually prescribed 100 mg twice daily causes increases in HDL cholesterol and decreases in fasting triglyceride levels. Thus, cilostazol appears to be an effective medication to ameliorate symptoms in patients with claudication.

Cilostazol is contraindicated in patients with any clinical history of heart failure. This "black box warning" is due to concern regarding the potential long-term adverse effects of phosphodiesterase III inhibitors, as a class, in increasing mortality in patients with severe heart failure (specifically, left ventricular systolic dysfunction, usually defined as an ejection fraction less than 40%). Suspicion of underlying heart failure in a patient with PAD and claudication should lead to noninvasive measurement of left ventricular function, such as with an echocardiogram or radionuclide ventriculogram. If left ventricular function is proved to be normal, cilostazol therapy may be considered.

Revascularization Options

Although supervised exercise and pharmacologic therapy are effective for most patients with PAD and claudication, revascularization may be beneficial for selected patient groups, including those for whom (1) exercise is ineffective because the patient is not adequately motivated to comply with the exercise prescription, the patient lacks access to a supervised PAD rehabilitation program, or compliance with such a program has not resulted in adequate improvement; (2) cilostazol or pentoxifylline is contraindicated, adverse effects, cost, or noncompliance has resulted in limited efficacy of these medications, or the therapeutic response has not been adequate; and (3) the arterial anatomy of the limb is favorable for revascularization and the risks of the revascularization procedure are low. The prescription of supervised exercise, pharmacologic therapy, or both in a primary care practice before potential revascularization is no longer considered "conservative therapy" but may be "medically appropriate therapy." Selection of a revascularization strategy must be customized to the individual patient's presumed risk-benefit ratio (e.g., associated cardiovascular risk, potential nephrotoxicity, risk of limb jeopardy), and the probable durability of the chosen revascularization strategy must also be taken into account.

Revascularization may be performed by either percutaneous transluminal angioplasty (PTA), with or without stenting, or surgical bypass, depending on the site and severity of the patient's lesions. Focal lesions less than 10 cm long have classically been amenable to these endovascular procedures. On completion of all revascularization procedures, patients have a continued, lifelong need for lifestyle and pharmacologic interventions to decrease rates of progressive atherosclerosis, myocardial infarction, stroke, and death. Thus, patients always require a continuation of exercise and medical therapy after successful revascularization strategies.

Percutaneous Transluminal Angioplasty and Stents. Patients with high-grade localized lesions in the iliac or common femoral arterial sites may be ideal candidates for endovascular procedures inasmuch as long-term (5-year) patency has been demonstrated at these "proximal" sites (Fig. 37–7). The long-term durability of PTA, with or without stents, is diminished with stenoses in the distal superficial femoral, popliteal, or infrapopliteal arteries. Angioplasty alone may provide adequate initial and long-term results in patients with short, proximal stenoses in large-caliber arteries, but patency rates may be incrementally improved by primary deployment of stents. Eccentric or long-segment stenoses may also be best treated by PTA with stent placement, and stents

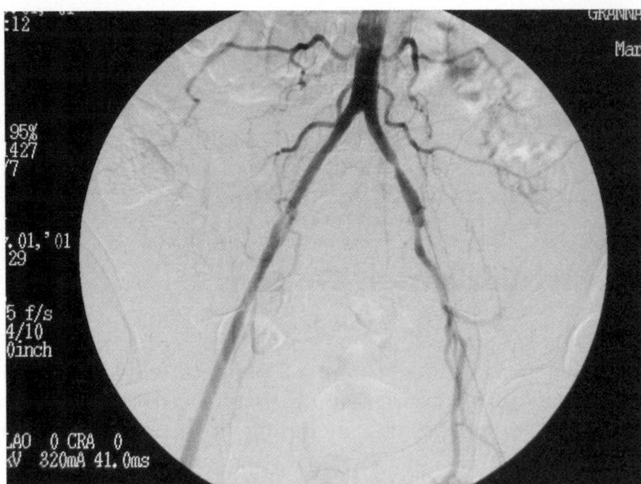
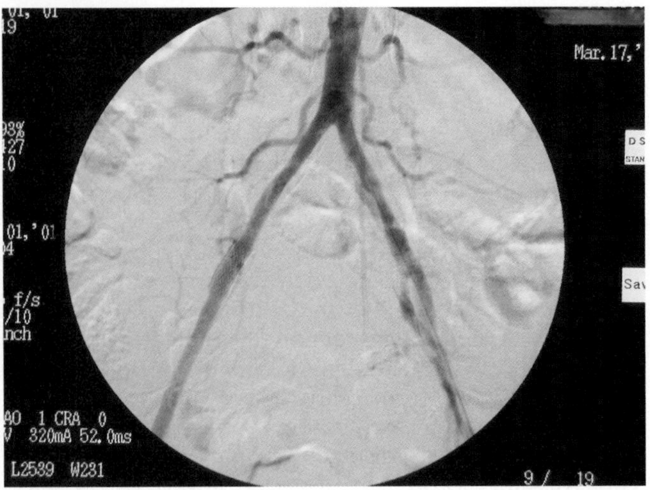

FIGURE 37–7. Iliac arterial angioplasty. *A,* Diagnostic angiogram of high-grade bilateral common iliac artery stenoses in a patient with bilateral buttock and calf claudication. *B,* Angiogram demonstrating successful angioplasty and stent deployment in the common iliac arteries in a patient with bilateral buttock and calf claudication.

may be required for arterial dissection or failure of PTA because of elastic recoil.

Surgical Revascularization. Limb arterial bypass surgery, alone or in combination with endovascular procedures, is indicated for patients who have critical, limb-threatening ischemia. Vascular surgical bypass can also be useful in selected patients in whom exercise, pharmacotherapy, and endovascular interventions are not effective. Surgical bypass is not usually considered a first-line treatment modality for patients with intermittent claudication, both because less invasive options are available and because patients with PAD have a relatively high perioperative risk for cardiovascular ischemia. Whereas distal aortic and proximal femoral lesions provide extremely favorable targets for vascular surgical bypass, this arterial anatomy is not common in patients with claudication. Although more distal femoral-popliteal or femoral-distal bypass can be achieved in many patients with claudication, long-term patency greater than 5 years requires continued graft surveillance. Prompt referral for vascular bypass (with or without PTA and stenting) is essential for all patients with CLI if amputation is to be avoided.

Factors that predict improved outcomes after surgical bypass include proximal arterial disease (above the common femoral artery), preserved infrapopliteal arterial supply to the ankle (at least one vessel runoff), and a low perioperative risk for cardiovascular ischemia. In summary, the ideal patient for surgical bypass is one with disabling claudication or critical limb ischemia, relatively few co-morbid conditions, and good rehabilitative potential.

Indications for Hospitalization

Hospitalization is indicated for patients who require surgical revascularization or treatment of CLI. It is rarely required for most patients with PAD or for those with claudication in whom outpatient treatment will usually suffice. The development of CLI (manifested by pain at rest, a nonhealing ischemic wound, or gangrene) should prompt immediate referral to vascular specialty care. Such care may include the use of intravenous antibiotics, analgesics, and wound débridement and, for many patients, will lead to angiographic imaging and a revascularization procedure.

References

1. Management of peripheral arterial disease (PAD). Trans-Atlantic Inter-Society Consensus (TASC). Eur J Vasc Endovasc Surg 2000;19(Suppl A):i–xxviii, 1–250.
2. Criqui MH, Langer RD, Fronek A, et al: Mortality over a period of 10 years in patients with peripheral arterial disease. N Engl J Med 1992;326:381–386.
3. Hiatt WR, Hoag S, Hamman RF: Effect of diagnostic criteria on the prevalence of peripheral arterial disease: The San Luis Valley Diabetes Study. Circulation 1995;91: 1472–1479.
4. Hiatt WR, Marshall JA, Baxter J, et al: Diagnostic methods for peripheral arterial disease in the San Luis Valley diabetes study. J Clin Epidemiol 1990;43:597–606.
5. Hiatt WR: Medical treatment of peripheral arterial disease and claudication. N Engl J Med 2001;344:1608–1621.
6. Kannel WB: The demographics of claudication and the aging of the American population. Vasc Med 1996;1:60–64.
7. Criqui MH, Fronek A, Barrett-Connor E, et al: The prevalence of peripheral arterial disease in a defined population. Circulation 1985;71:510–515.
8. Leng GC, Lee AJ, Fowkes FGR, et al: Incidence, natural history and cardiovascular events in symptomatic and asymptomatic peripheral arterial disease in the general population. Int J Epidemiol 1996;25:1172–1181.
9. Hirsch AT, Criqui MH, Treat-Jacobson D, et al: Peripheral arterial disease, detection, awareness, and treatment in primary care. JAMA 2001;286:1317–1324.

10. Murabito JM, D'Agostino RB, Silbershatz H, Wilson PW: Intermittent claudication: A risk profile from the Framingham heart study. Circulation 1997;96:44–49.
11. Hirsch AT, Treat-Jacobson D, Lando HA, Hatsukami DK: The role of tobacco cessation, antiplatelet and lipid-lowering therapies in the treatment of peripheral arterial disease. Vasc Med 1997;2:243–251.
12. Newman AB, Shemanski L, Manolio TA, et al: Ankle-arm index as a predictor of cardiovascular disease and mortality in the Cardiovascular Health Study. Arterioscler Thromb Vasc Biol 1999;19:539–545.
13. Ingolfsson IÖ, Sigurdsson G, Sigvaldason H, et al: A marked decline in the prevalence and incidence of intermittent claudication in Icelandic men 1968–1986: A strong relationship to smoking and serum cholesterol—the Reykjavik Study. J Clin Epidemiol 1994;47:1237–1243.

13a. Jonason T, Bergstrom R: Cessation of smoking in patients with intermittent claudication. Acta Med Scand 1987; 21:253–260.

14. Kannel WB, Skinner JJ, Schwartz MJ, Shurtleff D: Intermittent claudication: Incidence in the Framingham study. Circulation 1970;41:875–883.
15. Molgaard J, Malinow MR, Lassvik C, et al: Hyperhomocyst(e)inemia: An independent risk factor for intermittent claudication. J Intern Med 1992;231:273–279.
16. Ridker PM, Cushman M, Stampfer MJ, et al: Plasma concentrations of C-reactive protein and risk of developing peripheral vascular disease. Circulation 1998;97:425–428.
17. Koenig W, Sund M, Frohlich M, et al: C-reactive protein, a sensitive marker of inflammation, predicts future risk of coronary heart disease in initially healthy middle-aged men: Results from the Monica (Monitoring Trends and Determinants in Cardiovascular Disease) Augsburg Cohort Study, 1984 to 1992. Circulation 1999;99:237–242.
18. Ness J, Aronow WS: Prevalence of coexistence of coronary artery disease, ischemic stroke, and peripheral arterial disease in older persons, mean age 80 years, in an academic hospital–based geriatrics practice. J Am Geriatr Soc 1999;47:1255–1256.
19. Hirsch AT, Halverson S, Treat-Jacobson D, et al: The Minnesota Regional Peripheral Arterial Disease Screening Program: Toward a definition of community standards of care. Vasc Med 2001;6:87–96.
20. Vogt MT, Cauley JA, Newman AB, et al: Decreased ankle/arm blood pressure index and mortality in elderly women. JAMA 1993;270:465–469.
21. Weitz JI, Byrne J, Clagett P, et al: Diagnosis and treatment of chronic arterial insufficiency of the lower extremities: A critical review. Circulation 1996;94:3026–3049.
22. Blankenhorn DH, Azen SP, Crawford DW, et al: Effects of colestipol-niacin therapy on human femoral atherosclerosis. Circulation 1991;83:438–447.
23. Pedersen TR, Kjekshus J, Pyorala K, et al: Effect of simvastatin on ischemic signs and symptoms in the Scandinavian Simvastatin Survival Study (4S). Am J Cardiol 1998;81:333–335.
24. Executive Summary of the Third Report of the National Cholesterol Education Program (NCEP) Expert Panel on Detection, Evaluation, and Treatment of High Blood Cholesterol in Adults (Adult Treatment Panel III). JAMA 2001;285:2486–2497.
25. Hess H, Miewtaschk A, Deichel G: Drug-induced inhibition of platelet function delays progression of peripheral occlusive arterial disease: A prospective, double-blind arteriographically controlled trial. Lancet 1985;1:415–419.
26. Goldhaber SZ, Manson JE, Stampfer MJ, et al: Low-dose aspirin and subsequent peripheral arterial surgery in the Physicians Health Study. Lancet 1992;340:143–145.
27. CAPRIE Steering Committee: A randomised, blinded, trial of clopidogrel versus aspirin in patients at risk of ischaemic events (CAPRIE). Lancet 1996;348:1329–1339.
28. Girolami B, Bernardi E, Prins MH, et al: Treatment of intermittent claudication with physical training, smoking cessation, pentoxifylline, or nafronyl: A meta-analysis. Arch Intern Med 1999;159:337–345.
29. Beebe HG, Dawson DL, Cutler BS, et al: A new pharmacological treatment for intermittent claudication: Results of a randomized, multicenter trial. Arch Intern Med 1999;159:2041–2050.
30. Dawson DL, Cutler BS, Hiatt WR, et al: A comparison of cilostazol and pentoxifylline for treating intermittent claudication. Am J Med 2000;109:523–530.

CHAPTER 38

Pulmonary Embolism, Deep Venous Thrombosis, and Cor Pulmonale

Samuel Z. Goldhaber

Pulmonary embolism (PE), deep venous thrombosis (DVT), and cor pulmonale are common disorders that occasionally cause death but more often confer disability and impair quality of life. Patients afflicted with this illness often have serious underlying medical problems. Optimal management requires familiarity with risk factors, the differential diagnosis, treatment options, and preventive strategies. The Food and Drug Administration (FDA) has approved treatment of acute DVT on an outpatient basis, thus highlighting the role of the primary care provider. Mastering the management of this disorder is an important component in the repertoire of the generalist.

EPIDEMIOLOGY AND RISK FACTORS

The etiology of PE and DVT is often not clear. Many patients with PE have an inherited hypercoagulable state that remains clinically silent until exacerbated by an acquired cause of venous thrombosis (Box 38–1). The most common inherited hypercoagulable disorder is the factor V Leiden genetic mutation, which causes resistance to activated protein C because of a single amino acid missense mutation in factor V.

The most common acquired hypercoagulable states are surgery, trauma, and immobilization. Patients frequently ask their primary care providers for advice about the risk of PE during air travel. The risk of venous thromboembolism (VTE) increases with the distance traveled. The risk of PE during a flight that exceeds a distance of 10,000 km is about 50-fold higher than the risk of PE during a flight that is less than 5000 km.[1]

In one cohort study, the incidence of VTE was 1.8 per 1000 per year.[2] In those older than 75 years, the incidence was 1 per 100 per year. In this community-based observational study, VTE occurred at home (rather than in patients already hospitalized) in 63% of the affected population, 16% of whom had been hospitalized within the previous 3 months.

The International Cooperative Pulmonary Embolism Registry enrolled 2454 consecutive PE patients from 52 participating hospitals in seven countries.[3] After exclusion of patients in whom PE was first discovered at autopsy, the 3-month mortality rate was 15.3%. Age older than 70 years increased the likelihood of death by 60%. Six other risk factors independently increased the likelihood of mortality by a factor of twofold to threefold: cancer, clinical congestive heart failure, chronic obstructive pulmonary disease, systemic arterial hypotension with a systolic blood pressure less than

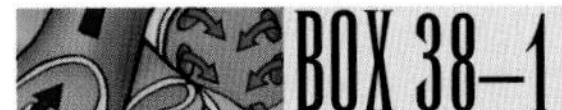

Acquired and Inherited Causes of Venous Thrombosis

INHERITED

Common
- G1691A mutation in the factor V gene (factor V Leiden)
- G20210A mutation in the prothrombin (factor II) gene
- Homozygous c677T mutation in the methylenetetrahydrofolate reductase gene

Rare
- Antithrombin deficiency
- Protein C deficiency
- Protein S deficiency

Very rare
- Dysfibrinogenemia
- Homozygous homocystinuria

Probably inherited
- Increased levels of factor VIII, factor IX, factor XI, or fibrinogen*

ACQUIRED
- Surgery and trauma
- Prolonged immobilization
- Older age
- Cancer
- Myeloproliferative disorders
- Previous thrombosis
- Pregnancy and the puerperium
- Use of contraceptives or hormone replacement therapy
- Resistance to activated protein C that is not due to alterations in the factor V gene
- Antiphospholipid antibodies
- Mild to moderate hyperhomocysteinemia

*Levels of factor VIII and fibrinogen may also increase as part of the acute phase response.

Adapted from Seligsohn U, Lubetsky A: Genetic susceptibility to venous thrombosis. N Engl J Med 2001;344:1222–1231.

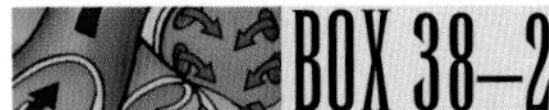

Major Clinical Manifestations of Deep Venous Thrombosis

SYMPTOMS AND SIGNS
- Pulling and aching sensation in lower part of calf (common)
- Warmth, swelling, tenderness (common)
- Palpable cord (occasional)
- Superficial venous collateral vessels (occasional)
- Fever (rare)

DIFFERENTIAL DIAGNOSIS
- Venous insufficiency (acute or chronic)
- Cellulitis or septic phlebitis
- Hematoma
- Muscle sprain
- Ruptured Baker's cyst

90 mm Hg, tachypnea, and right ventricular hypokinesis on echocardiography.

When PE is not fatal, it can cause chronic thromboembolic pulmonary hypertension with disabling fatigue and breathlessness. It can also exert a psychological toll because of the high risk of recurrence after anticoagulation is discontinued. Within 10 years of follow-up, as many as 30% of VTE patients may suffer recurrence.[4]

DIAGNOSIS

Clinical Manifestations

Acute DVT. DVT occurs two to three times more frequently than PE. Most patients in whom DVT or PE is ultimately diagnosed initially seek care from a primary care physician. The first manifestation of *DVT* is often an annoying "pulling sensation" at the insertion of the lower calf muscle into the posterior portion of the lower part of the leg. This feeling may become more pronounced over a period of several days as leg warmth, swelling, and erythema develop. Tenderness may be present along the course of the involved veins, and a cord may be palpable. Additional signs may include increased tissue turgor, distention of superficial veins, and the appearance of prominent venous collaterals. *Homans' sign,* defined as increased resistance or pain during dorsiflexion of the foot, is unreliable and nonspecific. The differential diagnosis includes muscle sprain, minor occult trauma, venous insufficiency without thrombosis, cellulitis, hematoma, and ruptured Baker's cyst (Box 38–2).

Acute PE. Despite modern diagnostic algorithms, a correct antemortem diagnosis of *PE* is made in less than half the patients who ultimately die of this disease.[5] Dyspnea is the most frequent symptom, and tachypnea is the most frequent sign of PE. Whereas dyspnea, syncope, or cyanosis usually indicates massive PE, the presence of pleuritic pain, cough, or hemoptysis often suggests a small embolism located distally near the pleura.

On physical examination, young and previously healthy individuals with a large acute PE may simply appear anxious but otherwise seem deceptively well. They need not have "classic" signs such as tachycardia or low-grade fever. In older patients who complain of vague chest discomfort, the diagnosis of PE may not be apparent unless signs of right heart failure are present, including neck vein distention, an accentuated pulmonic component of the second heart sound, and a murmur of tricuspid regurgitation. This murmur is loudest at the left lower sternal border and increases in prominence during inspiration. Because acute coronary ischemic syndromes are so common, one may overlook the possibility of life-threatening PE and

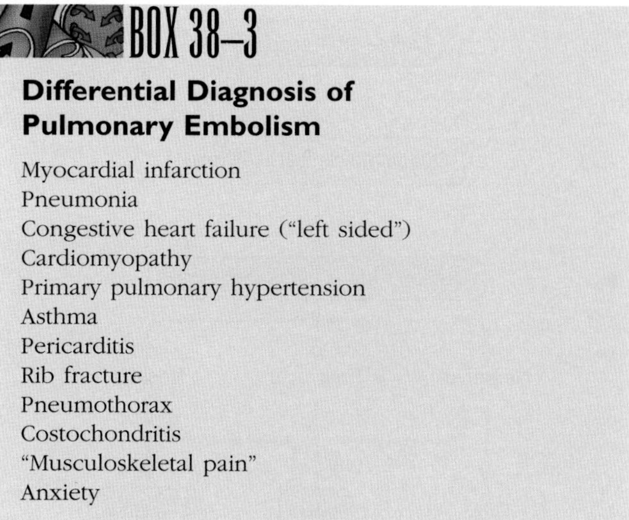

BOX 38–3

Differential Diagnosis of Pulmonary Embolism

Myocardial infarction
Pneumonia
Congestive heart failure ("left sided")
Cardiomyopathy
Primary pulmonary hypertension
Asthma
Pericarditis
Rib fracture
Pneumothorax
Costochondritis
"Musculoskeletal pain"
Anxiety

inadvertently discharge these patients from the hospital after the exclusion of myocardial infarction with serial markers of cardiac injury and serial electrocardiograms (ECGs).

The differential diagnosis of PE is broad (Box 38–3). Although PE has been called "the great masquerader," quite often another illness will simulate PE. For example, occasionally the proposed diagnosis of PE is supposedly confirmed with a combination of dyspnea, chest pain, and an abnormal lung scan. Perhaps 12 hours later, the correct diagnosis of pneumonia might become apparent when an infiltrate blossoms on the chest radiograph, productive purulent sputum is first produced, and high fever and shaking chills develop.

Some patients have PE and a coexisting illness such as pneumonia or heart failure. In such circumstances, a clue to the possible coexistence of PE is the lack of clinical improvement despite standard medical treatment of the concomitant illness.

DVT: Imaging Tests

Duplex Venous Ultrasonography. When DVT is suspected, duplex venous ultrasonography should ordinarily be the first test ordered (Fig. 38–1). This test combines (1) pulsed wave Doppler interrogation (with or without color), spectrum analysis, and measurement of blood flow velocity and (2) direct visualization of thrombus and assessment of vein compressibility by B-mode imaging. Normally, in patients without DVT, the manual pressure of the transducer applied to the surface of the skin will cause the vein walls to collapse. The cardinal criterion for diagnosing venous thrombosis by ultrasonography is loss of venous compressibility with the ultrasound transducer held transverse to the artery and vein. This imaging test is usually excellent for diagnosing or excluding an initial episode of DVT in symptomatic patients. However, for reasons that are not clear, duplex venous ultrasonography does not consistently detect asymptomatic DVT.

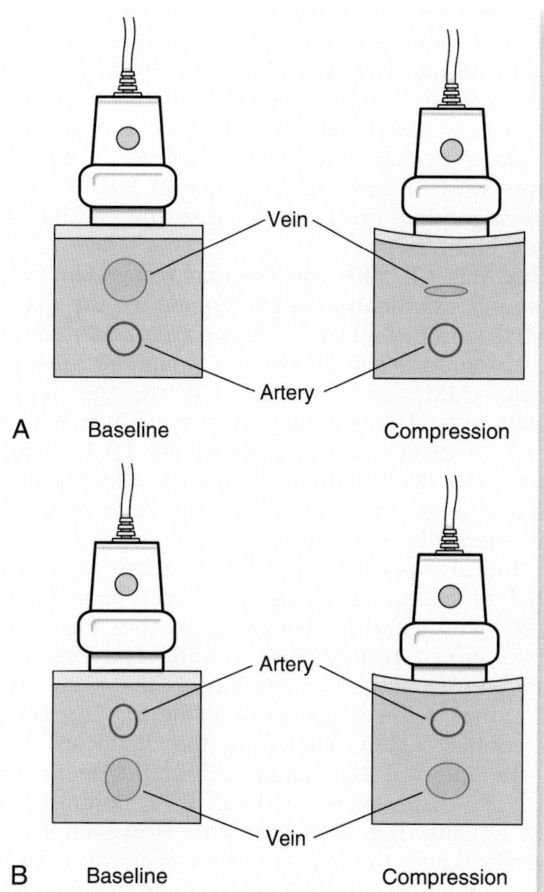

FIGURE 38–1. Compression venous ultrasonography. *A,* The compression maneuver is performed with the transducer held transverse to the vein. Pressure is applied to the surface of the skin through the transducer and then transmitted to the deeper structures, where it causes the vein walls to collapse. Normally, as in this panel, the vein collapses easily. *B,* An abnormal compression ultrasound is defined as failure to appose the walls of the deep vein while pressure is applied to the skin through the transducer. Sufficient pressure is applied to deform the arterial wall slightly. An ancillary finding is distention of the vein. Finding echogenic material in the vein lumen reinforces the diagnosis of DVT. (From Polak JF: Peripheral Vascular Sonography. A Practical Guide. Baltimore, Williams & Wilkins, 1992, pp 176–177.)

Doppler flow is evaluated in longitudinal axis images as an adjunct to the gray-scale compression technique. Color Doppler may improve the detection of venous thrombosis by (1) differentiating arteries from veins, (2) diagnosing nonocclusive thrombus when flow is detected around a nonechoic mass within the veins, and (3) helping locate deep calf veins. These small veins are often difficult to distinguish from other structures when examined solely by the gray-scale ultrasound compression technique. Whether isolated calf vein thrombosis is accurately detected on ultrasound examination depends on the skill of the sonographers at individual institutions.

Most emboli are caused by leg or pelvic DVT that embolizes. Venous ultrasonography is used at times instead of lung or chest computed tomography (CT) as a less expensive, more readily available surrogate for investigating suspected PE. However, the absence of DVT does not exclude the diagnosis of PE. Many patients with PE have no evidence of DVT by venous ultrasonography, probably because the thrombus has already embolized.

Pelvic Vein CT, MRI, and Contrast Venography. Venous ultrasound examination is inadequate for the diagnosis of pelvic vein thrombosis. When ovarian or other pelvic vein thrombosis is suspected, magnetic resonance imaging (MRI) and contrast CT are the preferred imaging tests. Ultrasonography may suffice for detection of an extensive upper extremity DVT. However, because the clavicle may hinder the identification of small and medium thromboses, MRI or contrast venography should be considered.

If clinical suspicion of DVT remains high despite normal ultrasound findings, this discrepancy may be further investigated by obtaining another imaging test, either *contrast venography* or MRI. The biggest disadvantage of contrast venography is that with massive DVT, none of the deep veins of the leg can be filled with contrast agent. Therefore, the diagnosis of DVT must be inferred by failure to fill the deep venous system. To diagnose isolated calf DVT, contrast venography remains the gold standard. However, for DVT above the knee, the results from a properly performed MRI examination are at least as definitive as contrast venography. MRI can also help determine whether a visualized thrombus is acute, subacute, or chronic. Unlike venography, MRI is noninvasive and therefore has greater patient and physician acceptability. No contrast agent is needed, so the risk of anaphylaxis and renal failure is averted.

The diagnoses of *recurrent DVT* and *acute venous insufficiency* can mimic one another, yet their management differs markedly. Recurrent DVT requires immediate and intensive anticoagulation, whereas venous insufficiency can be managed by prescribing vascular compression stockings, without hospitalization. Therefore, distinguishing between these two conditions is crucial. Duplex scanning can most reliably identify new DVT when detected in a different location from previous DVT. If ultrasound examination is inadequate to differentiate between acute and chronic DVT, MRI or contrast venography may resolve this diagnostic dilemma.

DVT: Integrated Diagnostic Approach

In most clinical circumstances, patients suspected of having DVT will quickly undergo Duplex venous ultrasonography even if the likelihood of DVT is low. Contrast venography is rarely required to establish or exclude the diagnosis of DVT because duplex venous ultrasonography almost always suffices. The most important role for contrast venography is before planned intervention such as catheter-directed thrombolysis, suction thrombectomy, or angioplasty and stenting (Fig. 38–2).

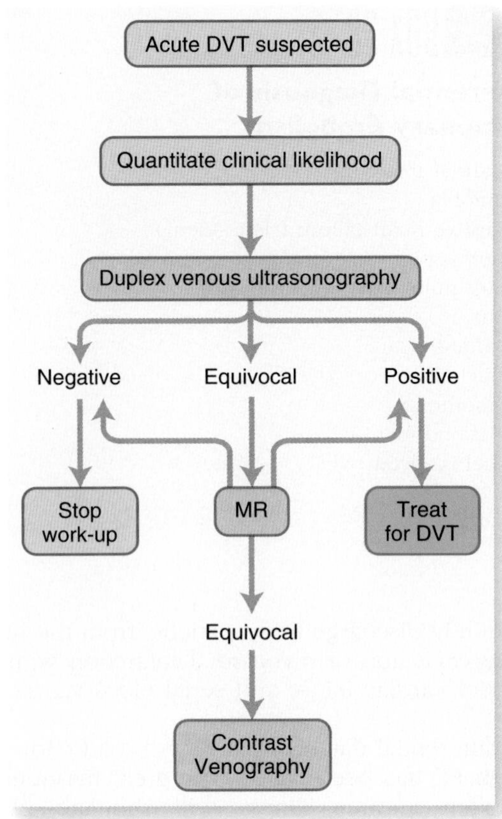

FIGURE 38–2. Algorithm for the workup of suspected acute deep venous thrombosis (DVT). MR, magnetic resonance imaging.

PE: Nonimaging Tests

Arterial Blood Gases. Arterial blood gases, used for a generation for the diagnostic evaluation and triage of patients with suspected PE, are in fact quite often misleading. An abnormally low PaO_2 on room air does not differentiate between patients who have PE at angiography and those who are suspected of having PE but have normal pulmonary angiograms. Likewise, a normal alveolar-arterial O_2 gradient does not exclude PE. Therefore, the routine use of arterial blood gases no longer has a role in the workup of PE.

D-Dimer. The quantitative plasma D-dimer enzyme-linked immunosorbent assay (ELISA) is elevated (>500 ng/mL) in at least 90% of patients with PE because of breakdown of fibrin by plasmin and endogenous (though clinically ineffective) thrombolysis.[6] Although ELISA measurements of D-dimer were cumbersome, slow, and costly in the past, automated testing with rapid turnaround is now available. The strategy of screening patients by D-dimer testing for suspected PE is useful in the absence of co-morbid conditions that elevate D-dimer such as myocardial infarction, pneumonia, cancer, sepsis, or the postoperative state. Normal

D-dimer ELISA levels have a high negative predictive value and almost always reliably exclude the diagnosis of acute PE.

Unfortunately, most hospital laboratories do not have assay kits for the plasma D-dimer ELISA and are able to perform only the less sensitive latex agglutination D-dimer test. Recently, a more sensitive latex D-dimer assay has been tested and appears to reliably exclude patients who do not have VTE.[7] Another approach is the use of a whole blood assay for D-dimer that can be performed and interpreted at the bedside within 5 minutes. The combination of low clinical suspicion and a normal D-dimer value makes PE exceedingly unlikely.[8]

Electrocardiography. The ECG is most useful for helping exclude acute myocardial infarction. Some patients with PE, especially massive PE, have right ventricular strain with a new right bundle branch block, right axis deviation, an S-wave in lead I, a Q-wave in lead III, and T-wave inversion in lead III or new T-wave inversions in leads V_1 to V_4. PE can cause inferior myocardial ischemia, probably from extrinsic compression of the right coronary artery because of right ventricular dilatation.

PE: Imaging Tests

Chest Radiography. A normal or nearly normal chest radiograph in a dyspneic patient suggests PE. Classically described but rarely observed abnormalities include focal oligemia (Westermark's sign), a peripheral wedged-shaped density above the diaphragm (Hampton's hump), or an enlarged right descending pulmonary artery. About one quarter of all chest radiographs in PE patients are completely normal. The most common abnormality is cardiomegaly, but it is neither sensitive nor specific. Importantly, the chest radiograph is being used with increasing frequency as a rapid, inexpensive substitute for ventilation lung scanning. In most patients with clinically suspected PE, the combination of a chest radiograph and perfusion lung scintigraphy reliably replaces ventilation-perfusion lung scanning.[9]

Lung Scanning. A perfusion scan defect indicates absent or decreased blood flow, possibly because of PE. Small particulate aggregates of albumin or microspheres labeled with a gamma-emitting radionuclide are intravenously injected and become trapped in the pulmonary capillary bed. Ventilation scans, obtained with radiolabeled inhaled gases such as xenon or krypton, improve the specificity of the perfusion scan. Abnormal ventilation scans indicate abnormal nonventilated lung, thereby providing possible explanations for perfusion defects other than acute PE.

Lung scanning is particularly useful if the results are normal, nearly normal (Fig. 38–3*A*), or high probability (Fig. 38–3*B*) for PE. A high-probability scan for PE is defined as having two or more segmental perfusion defects in the presence of normal ventilation. The diagnosis of PE is very unlikely in patients with normal and near-normal scans and, in contrast, is about 90% certain in patients with high-probability scans. Interpretation of moderate- or indeterminate-probability scans is especially difficult.

The lung scan was for many years the principal imaging test in the diagnostic workup of PE. However, this technique is rapidly losing popularity and has ceded its position as the premier imaging test to chest CT scanning. Many problems are associated with lung scanning. First, the Prospective Investigation of Pulmonary Embolism Diagnosis[10] study found that high-probability lung scans identify less than half of hospitalized patients with PE. Second, most lung scans are nondiagnostic, which means that the clinician is not provided with a definitive diagnosis or exclusion of acute PE. A "nondiagnostic" test is time consuming, costly, and frustrating for the physician and patient alike. Finally, the criteria for diagnosing PE are complicated and cumbersome, with large interobserver variability. The revised probability criteria for PE are extraordinarily complicated, as shown in Box 38–4.

Chest CT. This technique is rapidly becoming the principal imaging test for suspected acute PE. CT has two major advantages over lung scanning: (1) direct visualization of thrombi and (2) establishment of alternative diagnoses on lung parenchymal images that are not evident on chest radiographs. CT scans are performed during a single breath-hold, thereby reducing respiratory motion. While patients advance through the scanner, the x-ray source and detector array rotate around them. Because scans are performed in less than 30 seconds, excellent vascular opacification of the pulmonary arteries with contrast agent can usually be achieved. The major limitation of conventional chest CT has been failure to detect emboli beyond third-order pulmonary arterial branches.

With the use of newer multirow detector CT scans, four slices can be acquired simultaneously during each rotation of the x-ray source. The gantry rotates around the patient in less than 1 second, and the total examination time is eight times faster than with conventional single-row detector systems. Fewer motion artifacts occur, resolution increases from 5 to 1.25 mm, and subsegmental vessels can generally be well visualized. The combination of shorter scan times, narrow collimation, and narrow reconstruction intervals greatly enhances accuracy (Fig. 38–4). When compared with conventional spiral CT, the sensitivity of multirow detector scanners increases from about 70% to more than 90% for the diagnosis of acute PE.[11]

Echocardiography. This technique should not be used routinely in clinically stable patients to diagnose suspected PE because about half of patients with PE have normal echocardiograms.[12] Nevertheless, finding the combination of a normal left ventricle and a dilated, hypokinetic right ventricle in a breathless patient should raise the possibility of PE (Fig. 38–5) and lead to further imaging, usually chest CT. On rare occasion, thrombus can be visualized directly in the right or left main pulmonary artery. Transesophageal echocardiography may be particularly useful for direct detection of PE. In general, however, we rely on indirect signs of PE when using echocardiographic imaging (Box 38–5). Echocar-

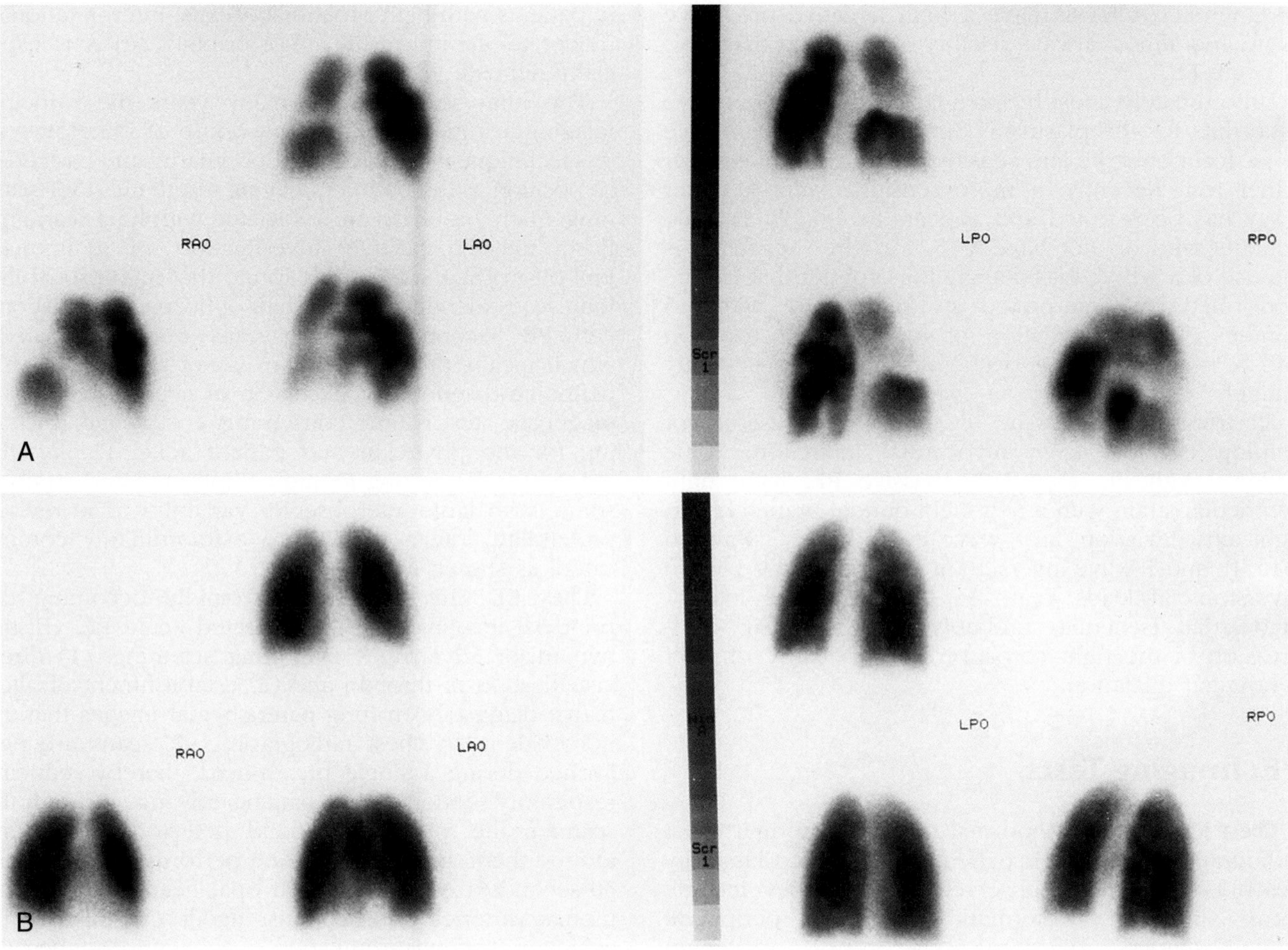

FIGURE 38–3. Lung scans. *A,* Nearly normal lung scan (after thrombolysis) from a 68-year-old woman who presented with acute PE. *B,* High-probability perfusion lung scan of the same patient, before thrombolysis. Her scan is notable for multiple bilateral segmental perfusion defects. The ventilation scan (not shown) and chest radiograph (not shown) were nearly normal. The discrepancy between near-normal ventilation and very abnormal perfusion is called "$\{\dot{V}\}/\{\dot{Q}\}$ mismatch."

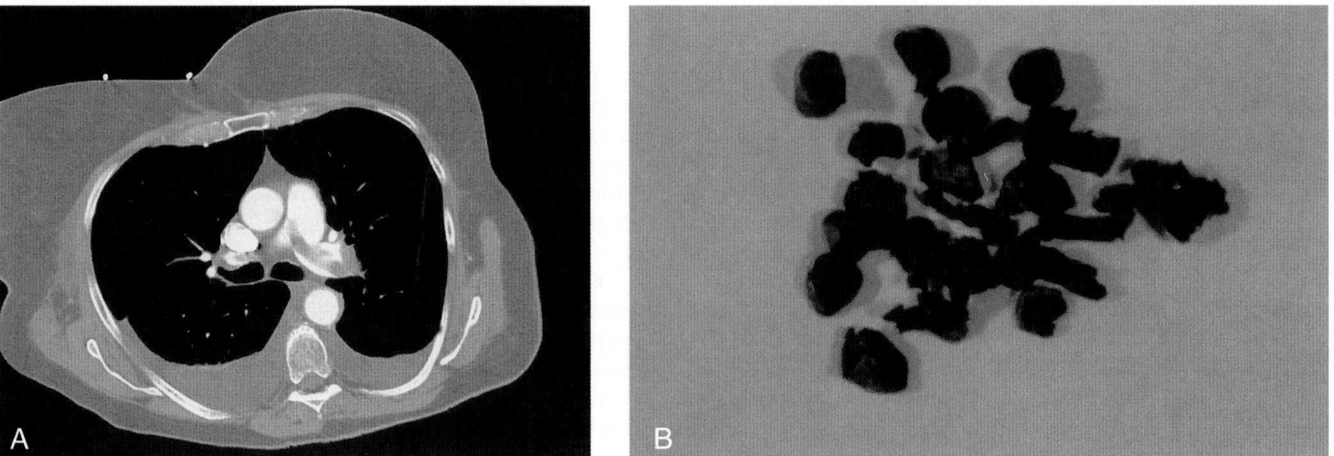

FIGURE 38–4. *A,* This 72-year-old woman suffered an acute idiopathic pulmonary embolism (PE). Multidetector chest computed tomographic scanning revealed a massive saddle embolism. *B,* Because of moderately severe right ventricular dysfunction, she underwent surgical pulmonary embolectomy. Massive PE was confirmed at surgery, and the central thromboembolism was removed. She recovered uneventfully.

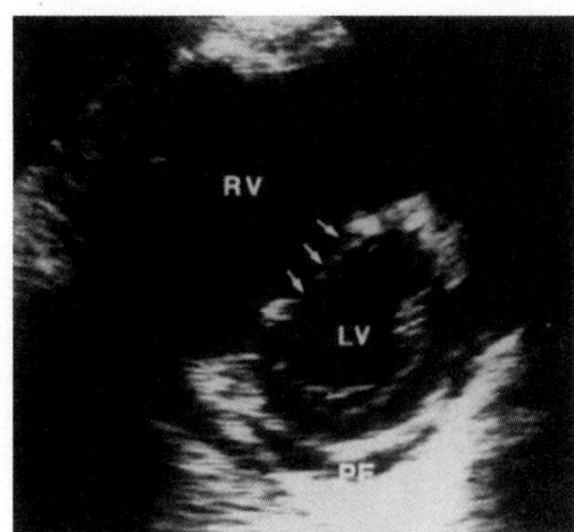

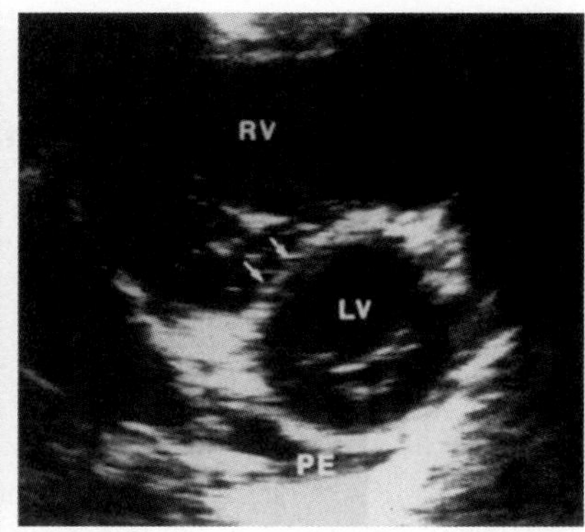

FIGURE 38–5. Parasternal short-axis views of the right ventricle (RV) and left ventricle (LV) in diastole (*left*) and systole (*right*). The diastolic and systolic bowing of the interventricular septum (*arrows*) into the left ventricle is compatible with left ventricular volume and pressure overload, respectively. The right ventricle is appreciably dilated and markedly hypokinetic, with little change in apparent right ventricular area from diastole to systole. PE, small pericardial effusion. (From Come PC: Echocardiographic evaluation of pulmonary embolism and its response to therapeutic interventions. Chest 1992;101(4 Suppl):151–162.)

BOX 38–4

Revised PIOPED Lung Scan Interpretation Criteria

HIGH PROBABILITY

- 2 large (>75% of a segment) segmental perfusion defects without corresponding ventilation or CXR abnormalities
- 1 large segmental perfusion defect and ≥2 moderate (25%–75% of a segment) segmental perfusion defects without corresponding ventilation or CXR abnormalities
- 4 moderate segmental perfusion defects without corresponding ventilation or CXR abnormalities

INTERMEDIATE PROBABILITY

- 1 moderate to <2 large segmental perfusion defects without corresponding ventilation or CXR abnormalities
- Corresponding $\dot{V}/\dot{Q}$ defects and CXR parenchymal opacity in the lower lung zone
- Corresponding $\dot{V}/\dot{Q}$ defects and small pleural effusion
- Single moderate matched $\dot{V}/\dot{Q}$ defects with normal CXR findings
- Difficult to categorize as low or high probability

LOW PROBABILITY

- Multiple matched $\dot{V}/\dot{Q}$ defects, regardless of size, with normal CXR findings
- Corresponding $\dot{V}/\dot{Q}$ defects and CXR parenchymal opacity in the upper/middle lung zone
- Corresponding $\dot{V}/\dot{Q}$ defects and large pleural effusion
- Any perfusion defects and large pleural effusion
- Any perfusion defects with a substantially larger CXR abnormality
- Defects surrounded by normally perfused lung (stripe sign)
- Single or multiple small (<25% of a segment) segmental perfusion defects with a normal CXR
- Nonsegmental perfusion defects (cardiomegaly, aortic impression, enlarged hila)

NORMAL

- No perfusion defects and perfusion outlines the shape of the lung seen on CXR

CXR, chest x-ray; PIOPED, Prospective Investigation of Pulmonary Embolism Diagnosis. Adapted from Gottschalk A, Sostman HD, Coleman RE, et al: Ventilation-perfusion scintigraphy in the PIOPED study. Part II. Evaluation of the scintigraphic criteria and interpretations. J Nucl Med 1993;34:1119–1126.

diography is an especially valuable diagnostic tool in hemodynamically unstable patients in whom the differential diagnosis includes pericardial tamponade, right ventricular infarction, and dissection of the aorta, as well as PE.

In patients with established PE, echocardiography can assist in the rapid triage of acutely ill patients. Detection of right ventricular dysfunction secondary to PE helps in stratifying risk and planning optimal management.

Integrated Diagnostic Approach. The optimal diagnostic strategy for PE necessitates an approach that integrates clinical findings, nonimaging tests (such as an ECG, chest radiograph, D-dimer, or a combination of these tests), and imaging tests (such as chest CT, lung scans, and ultrasonography of leg veins). In most circumstances, the diagnostic workup can stop after a normal D-dimer value or, if it is elevated, a normal chest CT scan (Fig. 38–6).

Workup for Hypercoagulability

Once PE or DVT is diagnosed, the primary care provider must decide whether to investigate specific causes of hypercoagulability. Many cases of PE and DVT occur when an underlying genetic predisposition is exacerbated by a specific stress such as immobilization or

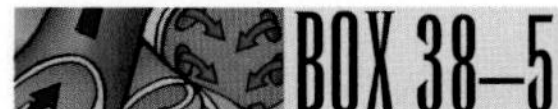

BOX 38–5

Echocardiographic Signs of Pulmonary Embolism

ABNORMAL FINDING	DESCRIPTION
Right ventricular dilatation and hypokinesis	Associated with leftward septal shift; the ratio of RVEDA to LVEDA exceeds the upper limit of normal (0.6). Associated with right atrial enlargement and tricuspid regurgitation
Septal flattening and paradoxical septal motion	Right ventricular contraction continues even after the left ventricle starts relaxing at end systole; therefore, the interventricular septum bulges toward the left ventricle
Diastolic left ventricular impairment with a small difference in left ventricular area during diastole and systole, a finding indicative of low cardiac output	Caused by septal displacement and reduced left ventricular distensibility during diastole; consequently, Doppler mitral flow exhibits a prominent A-wave, much higher than the E-wave, with an increased contribution of atrial contraction to left ventricular filling
Direct visualization of pulmonary embolus	Only if the pulmonary embolus is large and centrally located; much more easily visualized on transesophageal than transthoracic echocardiography
Pulmonary arterial hypertension detected by Doppler flow velocity in the right ventricular outflow tract	Shortened acceleration time, with peak velocity occurring close to the onset of ejection. Biphasic ejection curve, with a mid-systolic reduction in velocity
Right ventricular hypertrophy	Mildly increased right ventricular thickness (often about 6 mm, with 4 mm as the upper limit of normal); clear visualization of right ventricular muscle trabeculations
Patent foramen ovale	When right atrial pressure exceeds left atrial pressure, the foramen ovale may open and cause worsening hypoxemia or stroke

LVEDA, left ventricular end-diastolic area; RVEDA, right ventricular end-diastolic area.

pregnancy. In the Nurses' Health Study, the most important predisposing risk factors for PE were obesity, heavy cigarette smoking, and hypertension.[13] Marked obesity conferred a threefold increased risk of PE. These risk factors can be modified by the collaborative effort of the patient and primary care provider.

My workup for hypercoagulability in VTE patients includes factor V Leiden, prothrombin gene mutation, plasma homocysteine, and anticardiolipin antibodies to identify the antiphospholipid antibody syndrome. Hyperhomocysteinemia can usually be treated successfully with folic acid. The antiphospholipid antibody syndrome places patients at risk for recurrent thrombosis, especially if anticoagulant therapy is discontinued.

The classically described coagulation protein deficiencies such as antithrombin III, protein C, and protein S can be found in about 5% of patients with venous thrombosis. In most circumstances, determining whether they are present will be low yield and not cost-effective.

In patients with newly diagnosed VTE, the cancer rate is more than three times the expected rate over the ensuing year. For the next 5 years, the cancer rate remains excessively high. Cancer occurs 50% more often when VTE is "idiopathic" and unrelated to surgery or trauma.

Continued controversy surrounds the issue of defining the optimal cost-effective workup for occult malignancy in patients with newly diagnosed DVT. The available evidence indicates that a comprehensive medical history, physical examination with an emphasis on testicular and pelvic assessment, and routine laboratory tests such as a chest radiograph, urine analysis, complete blood count, chemistry panels, and stool for occult blood should suffice, along with mammography. Ordinarily, chest, abdominal, and pelvic CT or MRI does not appear to be justified. If cancer is identified with the whole-body imaging approach, it is usually advanced and widespread adenocarcinoma that is virtually refractory to treatment.

MANAGEMENT

Heparin

Heparin anticoagulation is the foundation for immediate management of acute PE or DVT. Heparin helps prevent new thrombus from forming and "buys time" for endogenous fibrinolytic mechanisms to lyse clots. If acute VTE is strongly suspected, heparin should be initiated immediately, even before chest CT, lung scanning, or venous ultrasonography is undertaken.

Unfractionated Heparin. Consensus guidelines for the use of unfractionated heparin (UFH) are listed in Box 38–6. For patients with PE or DVT, the traditional order for 5000 U UFH followed by infusion at 1000 U/hr often results in inadequate anticoagulation. An average-sized patient who is otherwise in good health should probably receive an initial bolus of 5000 to 10,000 U heparin, followed by an infusion of approximately 1250 U/hr.

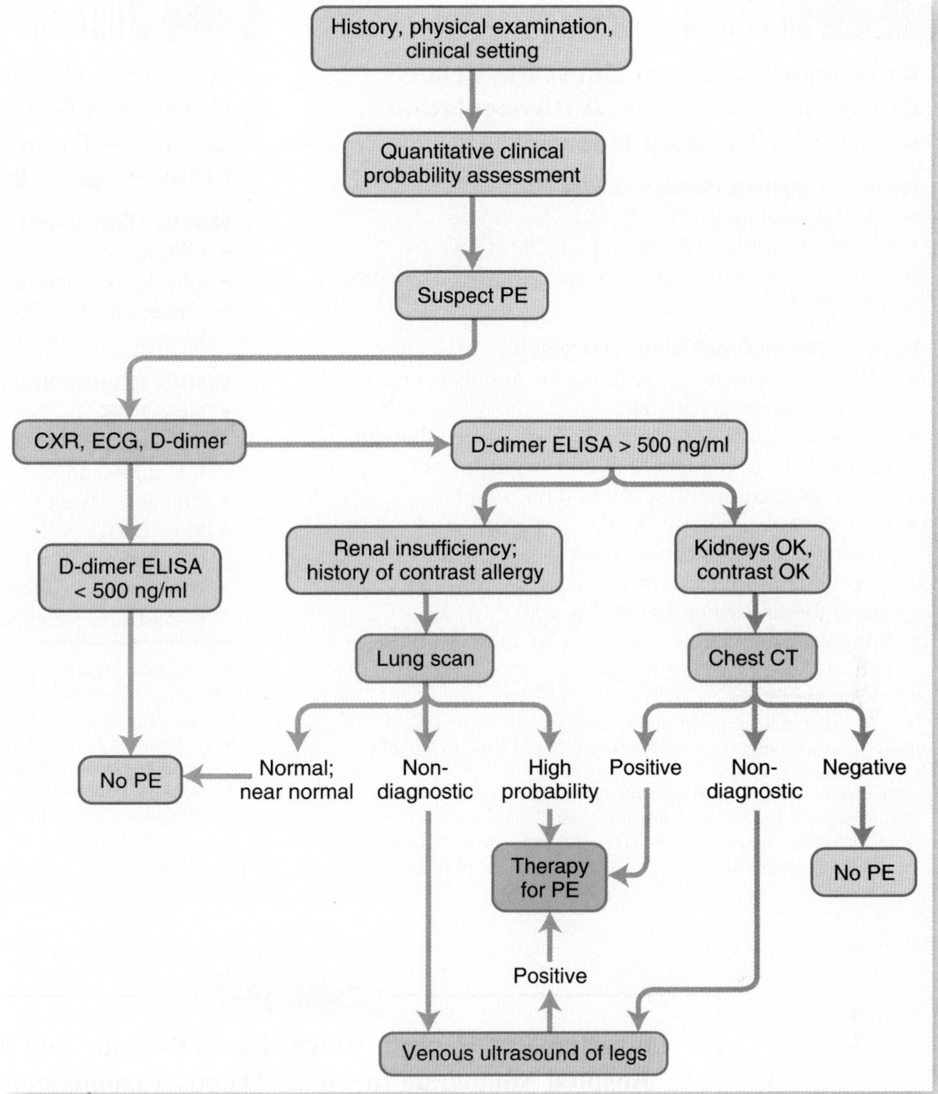

FIGURE 38–6. Integrated diagnostic approach for suspected pulmonary embolism (PE). CT, computed tomography; CXR, chest x-ray; ECG, electrocardiogram, ELISA, enzyme-linked immunosorbent assay

The Brigham and Women's Hospital nomogram, which is useful in achieving effective and safe levels of anticoagulation, is shown in Table 38–1.

Low-Molecular-Weight Heparin. Low-molecular-weight heparin (LMWH) inhibits activated coagulation factor Xa—via conformational change of the antithrombin III molecule—more efficiently than it inhibits thrombin. Because factor Xa acts earlier in the coagulation cascade than thrombin does, LMWH is often a more effective anticoagulant than UFH (Table 38–2). LMWH also reacts less with platelets than UFH does and therefore causes fewer episodes of heparin-induced thrombocytopenia.[14]

For the primary care provider, the most important advantages of LMWH are improved bioavailability and a prolonged half-life. The development of weight-adjusted dosing regimens for DVT treatment avoids cumbersome and costly laboratory monitoring (Box 38–7). In contrast to UFH, which is mainly cleared by the liver, elimination of LMWH occurs mostly via the kidneys.

A meta-analysis of more than 3000 patients who participated in acute DVT trials showed that those receiving LMWH had a lower mortality rate, lower recurrence rate, and lower rate of heparin-induced thrombocytopenia than those receiving UFH did.[15] LMWH was also much more cost-effective than UFH. The FDA-approved regimen for outpatient LMWH is enoxaparin, 1 mg/kg twice daily. Ordinarily, no blood testing is required for LMWH dosing. However, patients with massive obesity or renal insufficiency require special dosing protocols, as well as blood testing to monitor anti-Xa levels (Table 38–3).

Adverse Effects of Heparin. Heparin can cause bleeding, thrombocytopenia, and with chronic use, osteopenia. Before initiating heparin, patients should be screened for clinical evidence of active bleeding (Box 38–8). If anticoagulation is urgent, the baseline laboratory evaluation—which should include a complete blood count, platelets, partial thromboplastin time, prothrombin time, and urine dipstick for hematuria—can be completed after heparin has been started. It appears

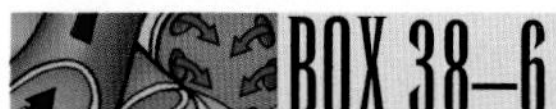

BOX 38–6

American College of Chest Physicians Consensus Guidelines: Anticoagulation with Unfractionated Heparin*

VENOUS THROMBOEMBOLISM SUSPECTED

- Obtain baseline aPTT, PT, and CBC
- Check for contraindications to heparin therapy
- Order imaging study; consider giving heparin, 5000 IU IV

VENOUS THROMBOEMBOLISM CONFIRMED

- Rebolus with heparin, 80 IU/kg IV, and start maintenance infusion at 18 U/kg
- Check aPTT at 6 hr to keep aPTT in a range that corresponds to a therapeutic blood heparin level
- Check platelet count between days 3 and 5
- Start warfarin therapy on day 1 at 5 mg and adjust subsequent daily dose according to the INR
- Stop heparin therapy after at least 4–5 days of combined therapy when the INR is >2.0
- Anticoagulate with warfarin for at least 3 mo at an INR of 2.5; range, 2.0 to 3.0

*For subcutaneous treatment with unfractionated heparin, give 250 IU/kg subcutaneously every 12 hours to obtain a therapeutic aPTT at 6 to 8 hours.

aPTT, activated partial thromboplastin time; CBC, complete blood count; INR, international normalized ratio; PT, prothrombin time.

From Hyers TM, Agnelli G, Hull RD, et al: Antithrombotic therapy for venous thromboembolic disease. Chest 2001;119(1 Suppl):176–193.

BOX 38–7

American College of Chest Physicians Consensus Guidelines: Anticoagulation for Acute Deep Venous Thrombosis with LMWH* as a "Bridge" to Warfarin

VENOUS THROMBOEMBOLISM SUSPECTED

- Obtain baseline aPTT, PT, and CBC
- Check for contraindication to heparin therapy
- Order imaging study; consider giving unfractionated heparin, 5000 U IV, or LMWH

VENOUS THROMBOEMBOLISM CONFIRMED

- Give LMWH
- Start warfarin therapy on day 1 at 5 mg and adjust the subsequent daily dose according to the INR
- Check a platelet count between days 3 and 5
- Stop LMWH therapy after at least 4–5 days of combined therapy when the INR is >2.0
- Anticoagulate with warfarin for at least 3 mo at an INR of 2.5; range, 2.0–3.0

*Enoxaparin sodium, 1 mg/kg every 12 hours subcutaneously or 1.5 mg/kg/day subcutaneously. A single daily dose should not exceed 180 mg (approved in both the United States and Canada).

aPTT, activated partial thromboplastin time; CBC, complete blood count; INR, international normalized ratio; LMWH, low-molecular-weight heparin; PT, prothrombin time.

Adapted from Hyers TM, Agnelli G, Hull RD, et al: Antithrombotic therapy for venous thromboembolic disease. Chest 2001;119 (1 Suppl):176–193.

TABLE 38–1

Unfractionated Heparin Weight-Based Brigham and Women's Hospital Nomogram for Acute Venous Thromboembolism

PTT	Repeat Bolus	Stop Infusion	Rate Change	Repeat PTT
<35	70 U/kg*	0 min	Increase 3 U/kg/hr	6 hr
35–59	35 U/kg†	0 min	Increase 2 U/kg/hr	6 hr
60–80—target	0	0 min	No change	6 hr
81–100	0	0 min	Decrease 2 U/kg/hr	6 hr
>100	0	60 min	Decrease 3 U/kg/hr	6 hr

*Maximal bolus, 10,000 U.

†Maximal bolus, 5000 U.

PTT, partial thromboplastin time.

that in most circumstances, the use of LMWH rather than an intravenous continuous infusion of UFH can minimize the potential adverse effects of heparin.

The effort expended in prompt diagnosis and expeditious initial treatment of VTE will be negated unless a reliable system is established to maintain effective and safe levels of outpatient anticoagulation. Although outpatient management of oral anticoagulation may be monotonous, repetitive, and time intensive, fastidious outpatient monitoring and follow-up are obligatory.

Warfarin

Warfarin is a vitamin K antagonist that prevents gamma-carboxylation activation of coagulation factors II, VII, IX, and X. The full anticoagulant effect of warfarin may not be apparent for 5 days, even if the prothrombin time, which is used to monitor warfarin's effect, becomes elevated more rapidly. The major adverse effect of warfarin is bleeding. Rare complications include alopecia (which develops slowly over months, particularly in light-haired women), rash, and skin necrosis.

TABLE 38–2

Comparison of Unfractionated Heparin with Low-Molecular-Weight Heparin

Characteristic	UFH	LMWH
Molecular weight (average in daltons)	15,000	5000
Ratio of anti-Xa to anti-IIa (thrombin) activity	1	>1
Metabolism	Hepatic	Renal
Bioavailability	Fair	Excellent
Frequency of subcutaneous administration	2–3×/day	Once daily
Frequency of heparin-induced thrombocytopenia	1%–2%	0.1%–0.2%
Osteoporosis after prolonged exposure	Rare	Very rare
Laboratory assay of anticoagulant effect	Activated partial thromboplastin time	Anti-Xa level
Reversal of anticoagulant effect	Protamine	Protamine
Spinal/epidural anesthesia	OK	Heed the FDA warning

Adapted from Goldhaber SZ: Prophylaxis of venous thrombosis. Curr Treat Options Cardiovasc Med 2001;3:225–235.

TABLE 38–3

Low-Molecular-Weight Heparin Weight-Based Brigham and Women's Hospital Nomogram for Enoxaparin in the Presence of Renal Insufficiency or Marked Obesity

	Enoxaparin Dose	Anti-Xa Monitoring (Heparin Level)
Renal Insufficiency		
Creatine clearance (mL/min)		
>70	1 mg/kg q12h	None
35–69	0.75 mg/kg q12h	3–6 hr after the 3rd injection
<35	1 mg/kg q24h	3–6 hr after the 3rd injection
Obese Weight (kg)		
<100 kg	1 mg/kg q12h	None
100–130 kg	1 mg/kg q12h	3–6 hr after the 1st injection
>130 kg	130 mg q12h	3–6 hr after the 1st injection

The prothrombin time, used to adjust the dose of warfarin, is reported as the International Normalized Ratio (INR), which is essentially a "corrected" prothrombin time that standardizes the results from the several dozen assays used in North American and European laboratories. The risk of bleeding increases as the INR increases. The risk of thromboembolism increases when the INR falls below the lower limit of the target range.

BOX 38–8

American College of Chest Physicians Consensus Guidelines: Initial Anticoagulation Regimen for Acute DVT or PE—Low-Molecular-Weight Heparin versus Unfractionated Heparin

1. We recommend that patients with DVT or PE be treated acutely with LMWH unfractionated IV heparin, or adjusted-dose subcutaneous heparin.
2. When unfractionated heparin is used, we recommend that the dose be sufficient to prolong the aPTT to a range that corresponds to a plasma heparin level of 0.2–0.4 IU/ml by protamine sulfate or 0.3–0.6 IU/mL by an amidolytic anti-Xa assay.
3. When compared with unfractionated heparin, LMWH offers the major benefits of convenient dosing and facilitation of outpatient treatment. LWMH treatment may result in slightly less recurrent venous thromboembolism and may offer a survival benefit in patients with cancer. We recommend that clinicians use LMWH over unfractionated heparin.

INITIAL ANTICOAGULATION WITH HEPARIN

1. We recommend that treatment with heparin or LMWH be continued for at least 5 days and that oral anticoagulation be overlapped with heparin or LMWH for at least 4–5 days. For most patients, treatment with warfarin can be started together with heparin or LMWH. The heparin product can be discontinued on day 5 or day 6 if the INR has been therapeutic for 2 consecutive days.
2. For massive PE or severe thrombosis, we recommend a longer period of heparin therapy of approximately 10 days.

aPTT, activated partial thromboplastin time; DVT, deep venous thrombosis; INR, international normalized ratio; LMWH, low-molecular-weight heparin; PE, pulmonary embolism.
From Hyers TM, Agnelli G, Hull RD, et al: Antithrombotic therapy for venous thromboembolic disease. Chest 2001;119(1 Suppl):176–193.

We initiate warfarin at a dose of 5 mg daily for an ordinary sized adult rather than initiating higher "loading doses." Subsequently, we favor gentle dose adjustments, usually no more than 20% of the warfarin dose. This gentle approach helps avoid wide swings in warfarin dosing, which I term *the yo-yo effect.* Because 2% to 3% of patients have a genetic mutation that results in slow metabolism of warfarin,[15] we test the INR after several doses of warfarin rather than waiting for 5 days after initiation of therapy. Finally, for patients who require lifelong anticoagulation, we consider prescribing point-of-care INR testing machines, which they use at home by obtaining a drop of their own blood by finger puncture. We then train them to self-adjust their warfarin doses based on the results of the INR.[16]

When the INR exceeds 5.0 in the absence of clinical bleeding, we withhold further warfarin doses and administer oral vitamin K, usually in a dose of 2.5 mg.

We prefer to administer vitamin K orally, but we give vitamin K subcutaneously to patients whose gastrointestinal absorption is uncertain. This strategy replaces the previous classic teaching in which patients were prescribed 10 mg of subcutaneous vitamin K, often for 3 consecutive days. This latter approach, now abandoned, effectively reversed warfarin's effect but created resistance to resumption of anticoagulation for at least the ensuing week.

Occasionally, patients require immediate reversal of excessive anticoagulation, which can be accomplished by the emergency administration of fresh frozen plasma, usually 2 U. However, to ensure continued reversal, vitamin K should be administered concomitantly.

Outpatient Treatment. Most patients with acute, uncomplicated DVT can be managed as outpatients with LMWH used as a "bridge" to warfarin (Box 38–9). Candidates for outpatient treatment must be reliable and have excellent family or community support services to ensure the success of this strategy. Often, the primary care provider will be the most knowledgeable individual about the feasibility of outpatient treatment or an abbreviated hospital stay.

Optimal Duration of Anticoagulation. Determining the optimal duration of anticoagulation for patients with acute DVT or PE is the most controversial issue in VTE management. Schulman and coworkers found that 6 months of oral anticoagulation halved the recurrence rate over the ensuing 2 years when compared with a strategy of 6 weeks of anticoagulation.[17] Consequently, 6 months of anticoagulation is the usual duration of therapy for proximal DVT or PE (Box 38–10).

Special Management Issues

Isolated Calf Vein Thrombosis. More than one fourth of cases of isolated calf DVT propagate proximally to the knee or thigh if left untreated and may cause paradoxical embolism and even fatal PE. Therefore, patients with isolated calf DVT should ordinarily receive 3 months of anticoagulation.

Cancer Patients. Cancer patients with DVT or PE may be resistant to the usual doses of warfarin and may require more intensive anticoagulation than usual. Patients in whom thrombosis occurs in more than one extremity (in particular, superficial thrombosis in one limb and DVT in a different extremity) have "Trousseau's syndrome" and may require lifelong LMWH to avoid recurrent thrombosis.

Antiphospholipid Antibody Syndrome. The risk of recurrent thrombosis is high in this patient population.[18] Therefore, whenever possible, patients with DVT or PE who also have the antiphospholipid antibody syndrome should be maintained, often indefinitely, at a target INR of at least 3.0.

Overall DVT Management Plan

Anticoagulation is the foundation of DVT treatment (Fig. 38–7). Ordinarily, effective, safe, and appropriately dosed therapy can be initiated with the FDA-approved regimen of enoxaparin, 1 mg/kg injected twice daily. Patients with marked leg discomfort, iliofemoral DVT, contraindications to anticoagulation, or concomitant major medical problems require hospitalization. Those with psychosocial problems that preclude home injections and home adjustments in warfarin dosing also require initial hospitalization until appropriate follow-up can be arranged. I find that psychosocial problems are far more often a barrier to home treatment than extenuating medical problems.

Patients with newly diagnosed DVT and active major bleeding should undergo placement of an inferior vena cava filter if they have pelvic or proximal leg DVT (Box 38–11). The filter usually prevents fatal PE from arising from the pelvic or deep leg veins. Ironically, filters predispose patients to an increased long-term risk of DVT.[19] Therefore, anticoagulation should be initiated if the bleeding problem is correctable or subsides.

BOX 38–9

American College of Chest Physicians Consensus Guidelines: Minimal Elements for Early Discharge or Outpatient Therapy for Acute Deep Venous Thrombosis

Responsible physician must ensure the following:

- Patient in stable condition with normal vital signs
- Low bleeding risk
- Absence of severe renal insufficiency
- Practical system for administration of low-molecular-weight heparin and warfarin with appropriate monitoring.
- Practical system for surveillance and treatment of recurrent venous thromboembolism and bleeding complications

From Hyers TM, Agnelli G, Hull RD, et al: Antithrombotic therapy for venous thromboembolic disease. Chest 2001;119(1 Suppl):176–193.

BOX 38–10

American College of Chest Physicians Consensus Guidelines: Optimal Duration of Anticoagulation

RISK FACTORS	DURATION
Reversible (transient)	≥3 mo
Idiopathic first episode	≥6 mo
Recurrent idiopathic	≥12 mo
Continuing risk factor	≥12 mo

From Hyers TM, Agnelli G, Hull RD, et al: Antithrombotic therapy for venous thromboembolic disease. Chest 2001;119(1 Suppl):176–193.

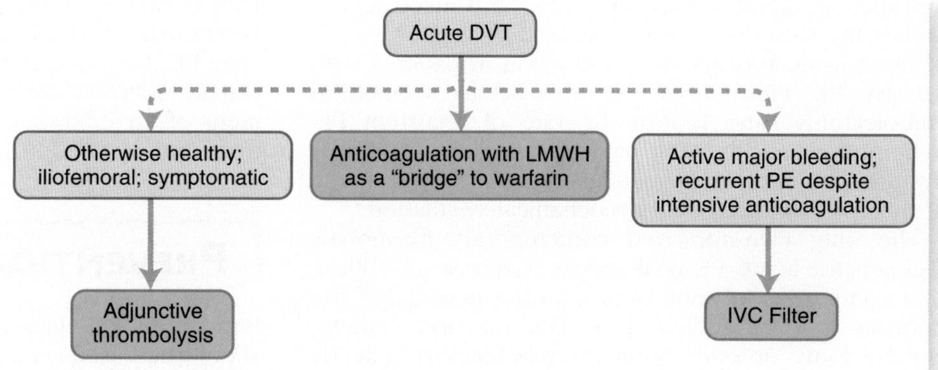

FIGURE 38–7. Deep venous thrombosis (DVT) treatment plan. IVC, inferior vena cava; LMWH, low-molecular-weight heparin; PE, pulmonary embolism.

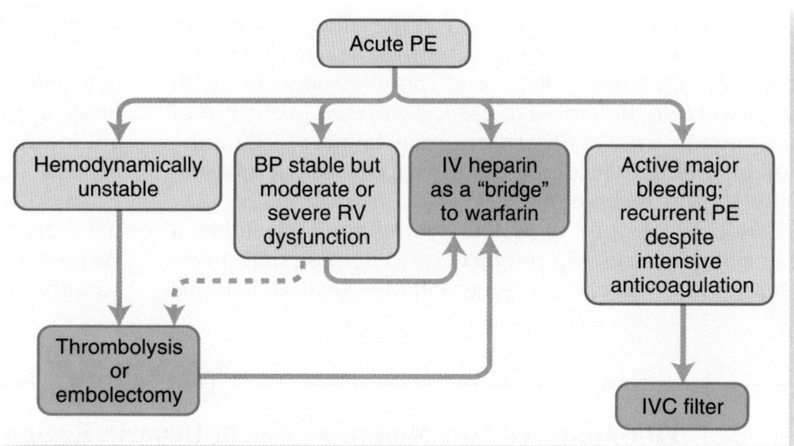

FIGURE 38–8. Pulmonary embolism (PE) treatment plan. BP, blood pressure; IV, intravenous; IVC, inferior vena cava; RV, right ventricular.

BOX 38–11

American College of Chest Physicians Consensus Guidelines: Inferior Vena Cava Filters

"We recommend placement of an inferior vena caval filter when there is a contraindication or complication of anticoagulant therapy in an individual with or at high risk for proximal vein thrombosis or PE. We also recommend placement of an inferior vena caval filter for recurrent thromboembolism that occurs despite adequate anticoagulation, for chronic recurrent embolism with pulmonary hypertension, and with the concurrent performance of surgical pulmonary embolectomy or pulmonary thromboendarterectomy."

From Hyers TM, Agnelli G, Hull RD, et al: Antithrombotic therapy for venous thromboembolic disease. Chest 2001;119(1 Suppl):176–193.

The rare patient with massive iliofemoral or upper extremity venous thrombosis should be considered for thrombolytic therapy if no contraindications are present. The ideal candidate is young and has no other medical problems. In my practice, such patients account for only about 1% of those who have DVT.

Secondary Prevention versus Primary Therapy for PE

Anticoagulation, the cornerstone of PE management, is called "*treatment*" but also represents *secondary prevention* of recurrent PE. Emboli differ markedly in size and physiologic effect. Therefore, *risk stratification* is crucial to determine which patients will do well with anticoagulation alone and which patients should be considered candidates for primary treatment with fibrinolysis or embolectomy or for secondary prevention with filter placement (Fig. 38–8). Rarely, patients with well-documented recurrent PE have absolute contraindications to anticoagulation or will have failed intensive anticoagulation. Such individuals warrant placement of an inferior vena cava filter (see Box 38–11).

Fibrinolysis. PE fibrinolysis remains a debatable indication because large clinical trials using survival as an endpoint have not been carried out.[20] Nevertheless, successful thrombolysis reverses right heart failure rapidly and safely, thereby preventing the usual cause of death from PE. Fibrinolysis may also prevent chronic pulmonary hypertension in the long term and thus improve exercise tolerance and quality of life. Thrombolysis should be considered only for patients at high risk for an adverse clinical outcome with anticoagulation alone, such as those with right ventricular dilatation or dysfunction, elevated troponin levels,[21] advanced age, or underlying cardiopulmonary disease.

Fibrinolysis appears to be lifesaving in patients with massive PE. Fibrinolysis may also act as a "medical embolectomy" and reduce the rate of recurrent PE. In hemodynamically stable patients with right ventricular dysfunction, thrombosis reduces the need for escalation of therapy with pressors or mechanical ventilation.[21a]

The only FDA-approved contemporary fibrinolytic regimen for acute PE is alteplase at a dose of 100 mg as a continuous infusion over a 2-hour period.[22] If fibrinolysis is contraindicated or fails, suction catheter embolectomy or open surgical embolectomy may be considered for hemodynamically unstable patients. Proceeding with these interventions as quickly as possible can maximize the likelihood of success with fibrinolysis or embolectomy. Waiting for the development of pressor-dependent cardiogenic shock leads to an unfavorable metabolic state and poor prognosis, with increased catecholamine release, decreased perfusion of vital organs, and multisystem organ failure. Ordinarily, patients being considered for thrombolysis or embolectomy should receive subspecialty consultation.

Echocardiography in patients with large emboli has a major role in assessing prognosis and helping determine whether anticoagulation alone will be effective. Patients with normal systemic arterial pressure and normal right ventricular function generally have a good prognosis after PE. For such individuals, secondary prevention is usually adequate with anticoagulation alone or placement of an inferior vena cava filter if major bleeding from anticoagulation is ongoing.

PREVENTION

Prevention strategies are of paramount importance and should be based on a patient's level of risk. Virtually all hospitalized patients whose anticipated length of stay exceeds 1 to 2 days should receive mechanical, pharmacologic, or combined mechanical and pharmacologic prophylaxis against VTE.

Mechanical (nonpharmacologic) measures include graduated compression stockings, intermittent pneumatic compression of the legs or feet, or placement of an inferior vena cava filter. *Pharmacologic measures* include minidose UFH, LMWH, and warfarin.

Two LMWH formulations, enoxaparin and dalteparin, have been approved for prophylaxis against VTE in various dosing regimens for orthopedic and general surgery (Table 38–4). This information should be espe-

TABLE 38–4

FDA-Approved Low-Molecular-Weight Heparin Regimens for Orthopedic and General Surgical Prophylaxis

Indication	Drug and Dose	Duration	Timing of Initial Dose
Hip replacement with enoxaparin	Enoxaparin, 30 mg q12h	≤14 days	12–24 hr postoperatively, provided that hemostasis has been achieved
Hip replacement ("European style") with enoxaparin	Enoxaparin, 40 mg q24h	≤14 days	12 ± 3 hr preoperatively
Hip replacement with dalteparin (option 1)	Dalteparin, 2500 U preoperatively and first dose postoperatively, followed by 5000 U q24h	≤14 days	First dose within 2 hr preoperatively; second dose at least 6 hr after first dose, usually on evening of the day of surgery; omit second dose on day of surgery if surgery is done in the evening
Hip replacement with dalteparin (option 2)	Dalteparin, 5000 U q24h	≤14 days	First dose on preoperative evening; second dose on evening of the day of surgery (unless surgery is performed in the evening)
Extended hip prophylaxis	Enoxaparin, 40 mg q24h	An additional 3 wk after initial hip replacement prophylaxis	After initial hip replacement prophylaxis regimen has been completed
General surgery with enoxaparin	Enoxaparin, 40 mg q24h	≤12 days	2 hr preoperatively
General surgery with dalteparin (moderate risk for venous thromboembolism)	Dalteparin, 2500 U q24h	5–10 days	1–2 hr preoperatively
General surgery with dalteparin (high risk for venous thromboembolism: option 1)	Dalteparin, 5000 U q24h	5–10 days	Preoperative evening
General surgery with dalteparin (high risk for venous thromboembolism: option 2)	Dalteparin, 2500 U preoperatively and first dose postoperatively, followed by 5000 U q24h	5–10 days	First dose 1–2 hr preoperatively; second dose 12 hr later

BOX 38–13

Diagnostic Classification of Pulmonary Hypertension

Pulmonary hypertension associated with disorders of the respiratory system and/or hypoxemia
- Parenchymal lung disease (chronic obstructive pulmonary disease, interstital pulmonary fibrosis, and cystic fibrosis)
- Chronic alveolar hypoxemia (exposure to long-term low oxygen tension such as at high altitudes)

Pulmonary venous hypertension
- Mitral valve disease
- Chronic left ventricular dysfunction
- Pulmonary veno-occlusion disease

Pulmonary hypertension from chronic thrombotic and/or embolic disease
- Thromboembolic obstruction of proximal pulmonary arteries
- Obstruction of distal pulmonary arteries

Pulmonary arterial hypertension
- Primary pulmonary hypertension (sporadic, familial)
- Pulmonary arterial hypertension related to collagen vascular disease (scleroderma, lupus, rheumatoid arthritis) congenital systemic-to-pulmonary shunts (Eisenmenger's syndrome), portoprimary hypertension, human immunodeficiency virus infection, and drugs and toxins

Pulmonary hypertension from disorders directly affecting the pulmonary vasculature
- Inflammatory
- Pulmonary capillary hemangiomatosis

From Gaine S: Pulmonary hypertension. JAMA 2000;284:3160–3168.

BOX 38–12

Clinical Manifestations of Cor Pulmonale

SYMPTOMS

Dyspnea on exertion
Weight gain (from fluid retention)
Abdominal distention
Syncope

GENERAL PHYSICAL EXAMINATION

Peripheral cyanosis and acrocyanosis
Digital clubbing
Distended neck veins
Abdominal ascites and peripheral edema
Hepatic congestion with right upper quadrant tenderness
Hepatojugular reflux

CARDIAC EXAMINATION

Right ventricular lift
Palpable P_2; widely split S_2 with increased P_2 intensity
Right-sided S_3
Murmurs of tricuspid regurgitation and pulmonic insufficiency

cially useful to primary care physicians who are evaluating patients for clearance before potential surgery. The FDA has also approved enoxaparin for VTE prophylaxis in medically ill patients.

Despite the available strategies for prevention of venous thrombosis, several groups of patients remain at high risk. DVT commonly develops in critically ill patients at rates that vary from about 20% to 80%, depending on patient characteristics.[23] In approximately 60% of trauma patients, DVT develops within the first 2 weeks of admission. Minidose heparin, defined as 5000 U of subcutaneous UFH administered two or three times daily, appears to decrease the incidence by 20%, and LMWH decreases the incidence by an additional 30% or so. DVT develops in about one quarter to one third of neurosurgical patients not receiving prophylaxis. Finally, without prophylaxis, the incidence of DVT in acute spinal cord injury patients probably exceeds 50%. One challenge in prevention of VTE is ensuring that known prophylactic measures are used and not ignored. A computerized reminder system can increase the use of preventive care for hospitalized patients. With respect to VTE prophylaxis, computerized reminders almost doubled the rate of ordering prophylactic heparin.[24]

COR PULMONALE

Cor pulmonale is usually manifested as right heart failure associated with pulmonary hypertension (Box 38–12) and can be caused by a wide spectrum of respiratory and pulmonary vascular diseases[25] (Box 38–13). Undoubtedly, chronic obstructive pulmonary disease is the most common cause of cor pulmonale. Restrictive lung diseases resulting from intrinsic pathology (e.g., interstitial fibrosis) or extrinsic causes (e.g., obesity or kyphoscoliosis) can also precipitate pulmonary hypertension from alveolar hypoxia.

PE is the most common pulmonary vascular cause of cor pulmonale. Patients with acute PE and cor pulmonale should be considered for primary therapy with thrombolysis or embolectomy.

Patients with chronic PE and cor pulmonale warrant lifelong anticoagulation and, in addition, may be candidates for lifelong continuous oxygen therapy.[26] However, pulmonary thromboendarterectomy is necessary if one wishes to correct the underlying problem. After the institution of cardiopulmonary bypass and deep hypothermia, incisions are made in both pulmonary arteries and continued into the lower lobe branches to remove organized thrombi. When successful, pulmonary hypertension will abate over the first few postoperative months, and quality of life will improve.

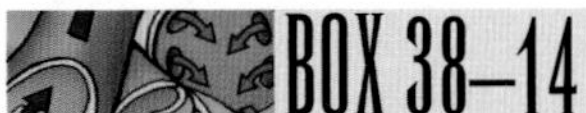

BOX 38–14

Indications for Subspecialty Referral

DIAGNOSTIC DILEMMAS

Discordance between venous ultrasound or chest CT and clinical suspicion
MRI not readily available or results indeterminate
Suspected recurrent DVT with equivocal ultrasound
Allergy to contrast agent or renal insufficiency

THERAPEUTIC DILEMMAS

Pregnancy
Iliofemoral venous thrombosis (massive DVT)
Massive PE
PE with normal systemic arterial pressure but right ventricular dysfunction on echocardiogram
Consideration of thrombolysis

COMPLICATIONS OF THERAPY

Hemorrhage
Heparin-induced thrombocytopenia

MECHANICAL INTERVENTION

Angioplasty
Stenting
Suction thrombectomy or embolectomy
Surgery

DIFFICULT MANAGEMENT ISSUES

Duration of anticoagulation
Genetic counseling and future pregnancies
Recurrent PE or DVT
Cor pulmonale from pulmonary vascular disease

CT, computed tomography; DVT, deep venous thrombosis; MRI, magnetic resonance imaging; PE, pulmonary embolism.

In properly selected patients at experienced centers, the mortality rate for thromboendarterectomy is between 5% and 10%. Balloon pulmonary angioplasty may be a treatment option for patients who are not surgical candidates.

SUBSPECIALTY REFERRAL

Despite the variety of algorithms available to help diagnose and manage PE and DVT, these conditions often pose difficult dilemmas for the primary care provider. Many patients have problems outside the realm of standard critical pathways. In such circumstances, subspecialty referral is appropriate (Box 38–14). Management of cor pulmonale secondary to pulmonary vascular disease almost always requires subspecialty consultation. Many patients need warfarin anticoagulation, which the primary care physician can regulate. The primary care provider is key in helping maintain cessation of cigarette smoking and in encouraging patients to comply with therapy.

Evidence-Based Summary

Epidemiology and Risk Factors

The incidence of VTE in adults is approximately 1.8 per 1000 per year, with about twice as many thrombi as emboli.[2] In the largest prospective PE registry, the 3-month mortality rate was 15%, and more than half the deaths were probably attributable to PE. Risk factors for death include age older than 70 years, cancer, congestive heart failure, chronic obstructive pulmonary disease, systemic arterial hypotension, tachypnea, and right ventricular hypokinesis on echocardiography.[2]

Diagnosis

The diagnosis of DVT is usually confirmed by duplex venous ultrasonography, but many PE patients do not have evidence of DVT on venous ultrasonography, probably because the thrombus has already embolized. For outpatients with suspected acute PE, a normal D-dimer ELISA has a high (approximately 95%) negative predictive value and may suffice to "rule out" PE.[27] CT scanning is rapidly replacing lung scanning as the principal imaging test for suspected PE. Multirow detector CT scanners increase the sensitivity of CT from about 70% to over 90% for the diagnosis of acute PE.[11]

Management

Anticoagulation is the foundation of therapy for VTE. For DVT management, early discharge or completely outpatient treatment may be feasible because LMWH (specifically, the FDA-approved regimen of enoxaparin, 1 mg/kg twice daily), in the absence of renal insufficiency or massive obesity, has replaced continuous infusion of intravenous UFH. A meta-analysis of more than 3000 patients who participated in acute DVT trials showed that those receiving LMWH have a lower mortality rate, lower recurrence rate, and lower rate of heparin-induced thrombocytopenia than do those receiving UFH.[28] LMWH should be administered as a "bridge" to oral anticoagulation with warfarin at a target INR of 2.0 to 3.0. For PE management, fewer studies support the use of LMWH or early hospital discharge.

The duration of anticoagulation remains controversial, but most proximal DVT and PE patients should receive at least 6 months of therapy. This recommendation is based on a Swedish randomized trial in which individuals receiving 6 months of anticoagulation had half the recurrence rate of those receiving 6 weeks of therapy.[17]

Prevention

Virtually all hospitalized patients whose anticipated length of stay exceeds 1 to 2 days should receive mechanical, pharmacologic, or combined mechanical and pharmacologic prophylaxis against VTE.[29] This strategy will decrease the DVT rate by about one third.

Cor Pulmonale

Cor pulmonale is far more often due to secondary pulmonary hypertension than to primary pulmonary hypertension. Chronic thromboembolic pulmonary hypertension causing cor pulmonale can often be successfully managed surgically with pulmonary thromboendarterectomy.[26] Patients with primary pulmonary hypertension benefit from lifelong anticoagulation and high-dose calcium channel blocking agents, continuous infusion of prostacyclin, or newer agents that are being introduced into clinical practice.[25]

References

1. Lapostolle F, Surget V, Borron SW, et al: Severe pulmonary embolism associated with air travel. N Engl J Med 2001;345:779–783.
2. Oger E: Incidence of venous thromboembolism: A community-based study in Western France. EPI-GETBP Study Group. Groupe d'Etude de la Thrombose de Bretagne Occidentale. Thromb Haemost 2000;83:657–660.
3. Goldhaber SZ, Visani L, DeRosa M: Acute pulmonary embolism: Clinical outcomes in the International Cooperative Pulmonary Embolism Registry (ICOPER). Lancet 1999;353:1386–1389.
4. Heit JA, Mohr DN, Silverstein MD, et al: Predictors of recurrence after deep vein thrombosis and pulmonary embolism: A population-based cohort study. Arch Intern Med 2000;160:761–768.
5. Pineda LA, Hathwar VS, Grant BJ: Clinical suspicion of fatal pulmonary embolism. Chest 2001;120:791–795.
6. Sijens PE, van Ingen HE, van Beek EJ, et al: Rapid ELISA assay for plasma D-dimer in the diagnosis of segmental and subsegmental pulmonary embolism: A comparison with pulmonary angiography. Thromb Haemost 2000;84:156–159.
7. Bates SM, Grand'Maison A, Johnston M, et al: A latex D-dimer reliably excludes venous thromboembolism. Arch Intern Med 2001;161:447–453.
8. Ginsberg JS, Wells PS, Kearon C, et al: Sensitivity and specificity of a rapid whole-blood assay for D-dimer in the diagnosis of pulmonary embolism. Ann Intern Med 1998;129:1006–1011.
9. de Groot MR, Turkstra F, van Marwijk KM, et al: Value of chest X-ray combined with perfusion scan versus ventilation/perfusion scan in acute pulmonary embolism. Thromb Haemost 2000;83:412–415.
10. The PIOPED Investigators: Value of the ventilation/perfusion scan in acute pulmonary embolism: Results of the Prospective Investigation of Pulmonary Embolism Diagnosis (PIOPED). JAMA 1990;263:2753–2759.
11. Qanadli SD, Hajjam ME, Mesurolle B, et al: Pulmonary embolism detection: Prospective evaluation of dual-section helical CT versus selective pulmonary arteriography in 157 patients. Radiology 2000;217:447–455.
12. Miniati M, Monti S, Pratali L, et al: Value of transthoracic echocardiography in the diagnosis of pulmonary embolism: Results of a prospective study in unselected patients. Am J Med 2001;110:528–535.
13. Goldhaber SZ, Grodstein F, Stampfer MJ, et al: A prospective study of risk factors for pulmonary embolism in women. JAMA 1997;277:642–645.
14. Weitz JI: Low-molecular-weight heparins. N Engl J Med 1997;337:688–698.
15. Aithal GP, Day CP, Kesteven PJ, Daly AK: Association of polymorphisms in the cytochrome P450 CYP2C9 with warfarin dose requirement and risk of bleeding complications. Lancet 1999;353:717–719.
16. Sawicki PT: A structured teaching and self-management program for patients receiving oral anticoagulation: A randomized controlled trial. Working Group for the Study of Patient Self-Management of Oral Anticoagulation. JAMA 1999;281:145–150.
17. Schulman S, Rhedin AS, Lindmarker P, et al: A comparison of six weeks with six months of oral anticoagulant therapy after a first episode of venous thromboembolism. Duration of Anticoagulation Trial Study Group. N Engl J Med 1995;332:1661–1665.
18. Greaves M: Antiphospholipid antibodies and thrombosis. Lancet 1999;353:1348–1353.
19. White RH, Zhou H, Kim J, Romano PS: A population-based study of the effectiveness of inferior vena cava filter use among patients with venous thromboembolism. Arch Intern Med 2000;160:2033–2041.
20. Goldhaber SZ: Thrombolysis in pulmonary embolism: A debatable indication. Thromb Haemost 2001;86:444–451.
21. Giannitsis E, Muller-Bardorff M, Kurowski V, et al: Independent prognostic value of cardiac troponin T in patients with confirmed pulmonary embolism. Circulation 2000;102:211–217.

21a. Konstantinides S, Geibel A, Heusel G, et al: Heparin plus alteplase compared with heparin alone in patients with submassive pulmonary embolism. N Engl J Med 2002; 347:1143.

22. Goldhaber SZ, Haire WD, Feldstein ML, et al: Alteplase versus heparin in acute pulmonary embolism: Randomised trial assessing right ventricular function and pulmonary perfusion. Lancet 1993;341:507–511.
23. Attia J, Ray JG, Cook DJ, et al: Deep vein thrombosis and its prevention in critically ill adults. Arch Intern Med 2001;161:1268–1279.
24. Dexter PR, Perkins S, Overhage JM, et al: A computerized reminder system to increase the use of preventive care for hospitalized patients. N Engl J Med 2001;345:965–970.
25. Gaine S: Pulmonary hypertension. JAMA 2000;284:3160–3168.
26. Fedullo PF, Auger WR, Kerr KM, Rubin LJ: Chronic thromboembolic pulmonary hypertension. N Engl J Med 2001;345:1465–1472.
27. de Moerloose P, Desmarais S, Bounameaux H, et al: Contribution of a new, rapid, individual and quantitative automated D-dimer ELISA to exclude pulmonary embolism. Thromb Haemost 1996;75:11–13.
28. Gould MK, Dembitzer AD, Doyle RL, et al: Low-molecular-weight heparins compared with unfractionated heparin for treatment of acute deep venous thrombosis: A meta-analysis of randomized, controlled trials. Ann Intern Med 1999;130:800–809.
29. Goldhaber SZ: Prophylaxis of venous thrombosis. Curr Treat Options Cardiovasc Med 2001;3:225–235.

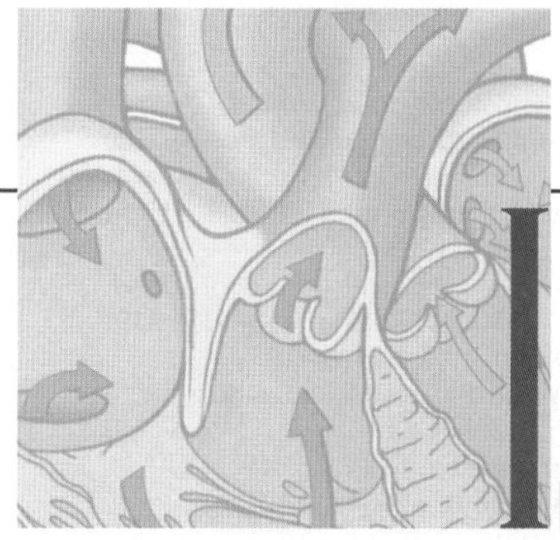

Index

Note: Page numbers followed by the letter b refer to boxed material; those followed by the letter f refer to figures and t to tables.

Q